ISOLATION AND IDENTIFICATION OF DRUGS

Edited by

E. G. C. CLARKE

AMENDMENTS

August 1971

page 14

Paracetamol and Phenacetin:

delete lines 2 and 3 ['Although. . . *p*-aminophenol'] and *substitute* 'Both drugs are excreted mostly as conjugates of *p*-acetamidophenol (paracetamol) which gives *p*-aminophenol on acid hydrolysis.'

lines 5–6: *delete* 'To 1 ml of urine is added 2 to 3 drops of 10% hydrochloric acid and the solution cooled;' and *substitute* 'To 1 ml of urine is added an equal volume of 5N hydrochloric acid and the solution is boiled and cooled;'

page 52

SYSTEM T10:

LOCATION: *delete* detail and *substitute*: '(1) *Mercurous nitrate spray*, which produces black spots, except with bromoureides. (2) *Potassium permanganate spray*, which produces yellow-brown spots on a purple background in the presence of compounds with an unsaturated side-chain. (3) *Zwikker's reagent spray*, which produces pink spots in the presence of 5,5-disubstituted barbiturates (except bromobarbiturates) and green spots in the presence of thiobarbiturates; faint pink spots are produced in the presence of bromobarbiturates and of certain 1,5,5-substituted barbiturates; the test is not particularly sensitive. (4) *Fluorescein spray*, which produces pink spots in the presence of bromobarbiturates and bromoureides; the plates are sprayed with sodium hydroxide solution (10% w/v) and heated at 100° for five minutes before applying the fluorescein spray.'

pages 52–54

SYSTEMS T10 to T13:

NOTE. The *mercurous nitrate spray* gives dark spots, fading slowly, with concentrated solutions. With more dilute solutions the spots fade rapidly. With very dilute solutions white spots on a grey background are seen; but similar spots are given by water only.

page 177, column 1

Ajmaline: Colour Tests, lines 1–2: *delete* 'sulphuric acid–formaldehyde test—purple (*sensitivity*: 1·0 μg);' [in the presence of traces of nitric acid vapour a purple colour is produced with sulphuric acid–formaldehyde]

page 219, column 1

Bephenium Hydroxynaphthoate: Quantitative Estimation, line 1: *for* 'Rogers (1958)' *read* 'Rogers (1958b)' page 260, column 1

Chlorthalidone: Ultraviolet Absorption Spectrum, line 3: *for* '600' *read* '60'; line 4: *for* '450' *read* '45'

page 284, column 2

Dequalinium Chloride: Toxicity, line 2: *for* 'between 1 and 3 mg' *read* 'between 1 and 3 g'

page 285, column 2

Desipramine: Ultraviolet Absorption Spectrum, line 3: *for* '363' *read* '307'; lines 3–4: *delete* '(E1%, 1 cm 294)'

page 294, column 2

Diazepam: Metabolism, paragraph 3, lines 2–3: *for* '0·2 mg%' *read* '0·02 mg%'

page 319, column 2

Distigmine Bromide: Ultraviolet Absorption Spectrum, line 3: *for* '111' *read* '160'

page 377, column 2

Hyoscine Butylbromide: *delete* detail *after* the graphic formula up to the beginning of the paragraph on Metabolism and *substitute* the following:

'A white crystalline powder. M.p. 139° to 141°.

Solubility. Soluble 3 in 1 of water, 1 in 50 of ethanol, 1 in 5 of chloroform, and 1 in 2500 of ether.

Extraction. Hyoscine butylbromide is a quaternary ammonium compound (see p. 29).

Chromatography. PAPER: system P1—Rf 0·52 (location reagent: *iodoplatinate spray*, strong reaction).

THIN-LAYER: system T1—Rf 0·08 (location reagent *acidified iodoplatinate spray*, positive reaction).

Colour Test. MICRO: Vitali's test— –/–/purple (*sensitivity*: 0·1µg).

Crystal Test. MICRO: *potassium bismuth iodide solution*—oily plates and needles, best viewed under polarised light (*sensitivity*: 1 in 1000).

Ultraviolet Absorption Spectrum. Hyoscine butylbromide in 0·1N sulphuric acid, maxima at 251 mµ (E1%, 1 cm 4), 257 mµ (E1%, 1 cm 5), and 263 mµ (E1%, 1 cm 3·8).'

page 379, column 2

Imipramine: Ultraviolet Absorption Spectrum, line 3: *for* '238' *read* '298'; line 4: *delete* '(E1%, 1 cm 189)'

page 430, column 1

Metyrapone: Ultraviolet Absorption Spectrum, line 3: *for* '597' *read* '470'; line 4: *delete* '(E1%, 1 cm 553)'

page 431, column 2

Morphine: Ultraviolet Absorption Spectrum, line 5: *for* '255' *read* '192' and *for* '116' *read* '87'

page 440, column 2

Nicotinamide: *delete* paragraph on Infra-red Absorption Spectrum

page 461, column 2

Oxypertine: *Proprietary Names*: Forit and Integrin are proprietary preparations of oxypertine and *not* of oxypertine hydrochloride

page 462, column 2

Oxyphenbutazone: Ultraviolet Absorption Spectrum, line 5: *for* '1500' *read* '750'

page 465, column 2

Paracetamol: Metabolism, lines 5–6: *delete* 'Deacetylation occurs to yield *p*-aminophenol.'

page 473, column 2

Pentazocine: Ultraviolet Absorption Spectrum, line 2: *for* '298 mμ' *read* '278 mμ'; line 4: *for* '278 mμ' *read* '298 mμ'

page 482, column 1

Phenelzine: Infra-red Absorption Spectrum, lines 1–2: *for* 'phenelzine (base)' *read* 'phenelzine sulphate'

page 493, column 1

Phenylbutazone: Quantitative Estimation, lines 7–8: *for* 'Tompsett (1967a)' *read* 'Tompsett (1967b)'

page 503, column 2

Piperazine: Quantitative Estimation, lines 3–4: *for* 'Rogers, 1958' *read* 'Rogers, 1958a'

page 532, column 1

Quinidine: Toxicity, CASE EXAMPLES, lines 9–11: *for* '17 mg%', '146 mg%', '58 mg%', and '1144 mg%' *substitute*, respectively, '1·7 mg%', '14·6 mg%', '5·8 mg%', and '114·4 mg%'

page 570, column 1

THIAMINE HYDROCHLORIDE, lines 4–5: *delete* 'M.p. about 207°' and detail

page 605, column 2

after '139 Thiethylperazine . . .' *insert* '139–141 Hyoscine Butylbromide, p. 377'
delete '143–144 Hyoscine Butylbromide, p. 377'

page 609, column 1

delete '207d Thiamine Hydrochloride, p. 570'

page 619

under '0·52' *after* 'Ethoheptazine. . .' *insert*
'Hyoscine Butylbromide, p. 377 — *iodoplatinate spray*'

page 627

under '0·93' *delete* 'Hyoscine Butylbromide' and detail

page 638

after '0·07' and detail *insert*
'0·08 Hyoscine Butylbromide, p. 377 . . . *acidified iodoplatinate spray*'

page 650

under '0·79' *delete* 'Hyoscine Butylbromide' and detail

page 663

Purple/Violet, column 1: *delete* 'Ajmaline, p. 177'

page 674

under '257' *after* 'Etafedrine. . .' *insert*
'Hyoscine Butylbromide, p. 377. . . 251, 263'

page 678

under '276' *delete* 'Hyoscine Butylbromide, p. 377'
under '278' *after* 'Levomethorphan . . .' *insert* 'Pentazocine, p. 473'

page 680

delete '298 Pentazocine, p. 473'

page 682

delete '278 Pentazocine, p. 473'

page 683

under '298' *add* 'Pentazocine, p. 473'

page 691

after '744' *delete* 'Nicotinamide (B), p. 440 . . . 748'

page 704

under '1300' *delete* 'Nicotinamide (A), p. 440 . . . 748'

page 705

under '1324' *delete* 'Nicotinamide (A), p. 440 . . . 748'

page 748, column 2

delete infra-red spectrum for Nicotinamide

page 753, column 1, second spectrum

for 'Phenelzine' *read* 'Phenelzine Sulphate'

page 820, column 2

before 'Rogers, E. W. (1958)' *insert* 'Rogers, E. W. (1958a) *Br. med. J.* **1** 136'
for 'Rogers, E. W. (1958)' *read* 'Rogers, E. W. (1958b)'

ISOLATION AND IDENTIFICATION OF DRUGS

AN EXTRA PHARMACOPOEIA COMPANION VOLUME
General Editor: R. G. TODD, F.P.S.

ISOLATION AND IDENTIFICATION OF DRUGS

in pharmaceuticals, body fluids
and post-mortem material

Edited by

E. G. C. CLARKE

M.A., Ph.D., D.Sc., F.R.I.C.

Professor of Chemical Toxicology in the University of London
at the Royal Veterinary College

Assisted by

Judith Berle, M.Sc.

Produced in the Department of Pharmaceutical Sciences
THE PHARMACEUTICAL SOCIETY OF GREAT BRITAIN

London

THE PHARMACEUTICAL PRESS

17 Bloomsbury Square WC1

First published 1969
Reprinted 1971

ISBN 0 85369 061 8

Made and printed in Great Britain by
William Clowes & Sons, Limited, London, Beccles and Colchester

Contents

Preface

During the period which has elapsed since the end of the second World War, the identification of drugs and other potentially poisonous substances has become increasingly urgent and increasingly difficult.

The urgency of the problem can be seen from the figures for the number of deaths due to accidental and suicidal poisoning in England and Wales during the decade 1956 to 1965:

Year	*1956*	*1957*	*1958*	*1959*	*1960*	*1961*	*1962*	*1963*	*1964*	*1965*
Suicide	860	835	877	899	943	1131	1441	1833	1928	1916
Accident	356	353	349	372	448	464	573	672	732	719
Total	1216	1188	1226	1271	1391	1595	2014	2505	2660	2635

Disquieting as these figures are, it must be realised that they take no account of the much larger number of cases of non-fatal poisoning which occur every year nor do they give any idea of the extensive loss of life among domestic animals and wild creatures due to the widespread use of chemicals on the land.

The increasing difficulty of the task is mainly due to the vast increase in the numbers of compounds—drugs, pesticides, solvents, and so on—which have come into everyday use during this period. Apart from the problem arising from the sheer number of the substances for which tests must now be made, a further difficulty stems from the fact that many of these compounds come on the market before any technique for isolating and identifying them has been described. Furthermore, this multiplicity means that many of the classical tests, long regarded as specific for certain substances, are now given by a dozen or more compounds, thus necessitating the carrying out of additional confirmatory reactions.

It is for these reasons that this book has been produced.

We have attempted to make it of value to as wide a readership as possible and have thus included rapid screening techniques for the hospital biochemist working in circumstances where speed may make the difference between life and death, precise methods for the forensic scientist whose findings must stand up to cross examination in a court of law, simple techniques for the chemist working under primitive conditions in the field, and sophisticated procedures for the research worker with full instrumentation at his disposal.

It would not have been possible to produce this book without the unstinting help given me from many sources, and my most grateful thanks are due to Judith Berle for her unfailing help and enthusiasm during the last four years, to my collaborators, D. I. Chapman, A. S. Curry, C. Daglish, R. H. Fox, G. Higgins, J. V. Jackson, H. Leach, M. S. Moss, R. L. Smith, and H. M. Stevens, not only for writing the chapters in Part 1 of this book but also for giving so generously of their time in trying out techniques and checking figures in their own laboratories, to H. V. Street for investigating the behaviour of several hundred compounds by reversed phase paper chromatography, to W. J. Wilson for providing physical constants, to S. C. Jolly for checking the structural formulae, to Linda Dawe for secretarial assistance, to Sandra Roper and Betty Forman for technical help, to the various individuals and firms mentioned on p. *xxii* whose generous gifts of drugs made possible the experimental work undertaken to produce many of the tests given in this book, and finally to R. G. Todd and the staff of the Extra Pharmacopoeia, especially Edith J. Condon, Maureen A. Dempsey, and B. J. D. Morgan, for their skilled and able assistance in turning an Idea into a Book.

London
January 1969 E. G. C. C.

Introduction

The book is divided into four parts.

Part 1 contains ten chapters which include practical details for carrying out the procedures referred to in the subsequent parts of the book. Seven of these chapters deal with particular analytical techniques—paper, thin-layer, and gas chromatography, ultraviolet and infra-red spectrophotometry, colour tests, and crystal tests. The remaining three chapters are devoted to rapid screening methods, extraction techniques, and the metabolism of drugs.

Part 2 consists of a series of monographs on over 1000 drugs and related compounds, arranged in alphabetical order of their main titles. Each monograph gives the name of the compound with synonyms and proprietary names, its chemical name, structural formula, molecular weight, and physical properties, followed by the relevant analytical data and notes on its metabolism and toxicity.

Part 3 is an arrangement of the more important analytical data of Part 2 in sequential order and tabular form.

Part 4 comprises three appendixes. Appendix 1 describes the reagents and Appendix 2 the tests employed in the analytical procedures referred to in Parts 1 and 2. Appendix 3 is a bibliography of the 900 references cited in the text.

In using the data in Part 2, the following notes may be helpful.

Nomenclature

The main titles of the monographs in Part 2 are usually British Approved Names but for those substances for which such names have not been adopted, preference has been given to International Non-Proprietary Names or United States Adopted Names, where these exist; for pesticides, the British Standard Recommended Common Names have been used. The main title is generally that of the free acid or base as this is the form in which the compound will usually be isolated in an analysis; details of the commonly available salts are included in subsidiary paragraphs within the monographs.

Chemical names are in accord with the current practice in Great Britain and generally follow the recommendations of the Chemical Society. The names used for complex radicals or groups are those recommended by the British Pharmacopoeia Commission, namely:

Recommended Name	*Chemical Name*
acetonide	isopropylidene ether of a dihydric alcohol
amsonate	4,4′-diaminostilbene-2,2′-disulphonate
camsylate	camphorsulphonate
closylate	*p*-chlorobenzenesulphonate

Recommended Name	*Chemical Name*
cypionate	β-cyclopentylpropionate
edisylate	ethane-1,2-disulphonate
eglumine	*N*-ethylglucamine
embonate	4,4′-methylenedi-(3-hydroxy-2-naphthoate)
enanthate	heptanoate
esylate	ethanesulphonate
gluceptate	glucoheptonate
isethionate	2-hydroxyethanesulphonate
meglumine	*N*-methylglucamine
mesylate	methanesulphonate
napadisylate	naphthalene-1,5-disulphonate
napsylate	naphthalene-2-sulphonate
pivalate	trimethylacetate
theoclate	8-chlorotheophyllinate
tosylate	toluene-*p*-sulphonate

Classification
At the head of each monograph an indication is given of the classification of the compound according to its therapeutic or commercial use or its pharmacological action.

Physical Properties
Only those physical properties likely to be useful to the analyst have been given. The melting-points recorded in the individual monographs are listed in sequential order on pages 603 to 611. Unless otherwise specified in the text, the stated solubilities are within the temperature range 15° to 25°.
Temperatures are expressed throughout the text in degrees Celsius (centigrade).

Screening Tests
These tests are intended primarily for the use of hospital biochemists and others who need to obtain results in the minimum of time without carrying out detailed analyses—see pages 3 to 15.

Extraction
This entry in the monographs in Part 2 indicates briefly the fraction in which the compound is likely to be encountered; it should be used in conjunction with the extraction scheme outlined on page 26.

Paper Chromatography
Details of the various systems used will be found on pages 34 to 42. The main system for screening for basic drugs is system P1, page 34. Iodoplatinate spray and bromocresol green spray are the best location reagents for this system but, should they fail to react, any of the other reagents listed on page 34 may be used. A list of Rf values for system P1, in sequential order, is given on pages 612 to 627. System P2, page 34, may be used for screening for barbiturates and systems P6 and P7, page 37, for neutral drugs. Other systems are included which deal with particular groups, such as salicylates, corticosteroids, and thiazide diuretics.

Reversed phase chromatography, systems RP1a and RP1b, pages 41 and 42, is useful in that it may be employed for acidic, basic, or neutral drugs. Rf values, in sequential order, for system RP1a will be found on pages 630 to 633 and for RP1b on pages 633 to 636.

Thin-layer Chromatography

Details of the various systems used are given on pages 46 to 58. The main system for screening for basic drugs is system T1. The best location reagents are acidified iodoplatinate spray and potassium permanganate spray. A list of Rf values for this system, in sequential order, is given on pages 637 to 650. System T10, page 52, may be used for barbiturates. Other systems are included which deal with particular groups, such as corticosteroids, cardiac glycosides, and sulphonamides.

Gas Chromatography

Details of the various systems used are given on pages 82 and 83 and lists of the relative retention times, in sequential order, on pages 656 to 662. The choice of method depends to some extent on the equipment available. System G2/225 is useful for general screening and system G5 for barbiturates.

Ultraviolet Spectrophotometry

See pages 84 to 102. It would, of course, have been desirable to have reproduced the actual curve for each compound but the cost would have been prohibitive. Instead, the wavelengths of the principal peak, of any subsidiary peaks, and of any significant inflexions or shoulders are recorded for the individual compounds in their respective monographs in Part 2.

A list of the principal peaks for compounds in acid solution is given in Table A on pages 670 to 680. Table B on pages 680 to 683 lists the principal peaks for compounds in alkaline solution when values for these compounds in acid solution are not recorded in Part 2 or when the values in alkaline solution differ significantly from those in acid solution, and Table C on pages 683 to 687 lists the principal peaks in neutral solution for compounds for which values in acid or alkaline solution are not recorded in Part 2.

Infra-red Spectrophotometry

See pages 103 to 122. Wherever possible, absorption spectra obtained with potassium bromide disks have been chosen. An index of principal peaks in ascending order of wavenumber will be found on pages 689 to 723 and reproductions of the absorption spectra on pages 727 to 793. Instructions on how to use the former are given on page 688.

Colour Tests

See pages 123 to 134. Where the entries under this heading in the monographs in Part 2 are preceded by the word MICRO, this means that they are carried out by the microtechnique described on page 133. The sensitivity given is that of the smallest quantity that may be expected to give a satisfactory result.

The colours produced by the various compounds in response to the sulphuric acid–formaldehyde test—the Marquis test—are listed on pages 663 to 669.

Crystal Tests

Where the entries under this heading in the monographs in Part 2 are preceded by the word MICRO, this indicates that the tests are carried out by the micro-technique described on page 136. The sensitivity given is that of the most dilute solution from which crystals may be expected to form.

Metabolism

Under this heading in the monographs in Part 2 a brief statement is made on the metabolic fate of each drug where this is known.

Dose

The dose recorded under this heading in the monographs in Part 2 usually indicates the maximum daily adult dose that may be given by mouth for therapeutic purposes. It is intended solely as a guide in deciding whether the amount taken by an individual falls within the therapeutic range.

Toxicity

Lethal doses in animals are given in milligrams per kilogram body-weight (mg/kg), the route of administration being indicated. Lethal doses in man are, of course, rough approximations. Where possible, examples of actual cases recorded in the literature have been cited; in choosing suitable examples, preference has been given to case reports in which the levels of the drug in body fluids and tissues have been recorded.

Use of Italic Type

In the text of Part 2, the names of those reagents that are defined in Appendix 1, page 797, are printed in *italic* type. Italic type is also used for botanical names and names of micro-organisms.

How to use the book

In cases of emergency

Turn to the chapter on rapid screening starting on page 3. This gives simple methods for identifying the common drugs that are responsible for about 90% of the cases of poisoning requiring hospital treatment.

When there is strong presumptive evidence of the identity of the drug under investigation

Turn to Part 2 and consult the monograph on the compound in question, apply the suggested method of extraction, details of which will be found in the chapter starting on page 16, and then submit the isolated material to any of the methods of identification given in the monograph. The choice of method will depend on the nature of the compound, the expertise of the analyst, the equipment available, and the urgency of the problem.

When there is no clue to the identity of the drug

Apply one of the general extraction methods outlined on pages 21 to 28, submit the residues from the various fractions to suitable chromatographic screening procedures, make a provisional identification by means of the analytical indexes in Part 3, and confirm the identification by carrying out the tests suggested in the appropriate monograph in Part 2.

Thus, for example, a residue in the acid ether fraction might be submitted to paper chromatography by system P2, page 34, or thin-layer chromatography by system T10, page 52. An Rf value of 1·40 in the former case or 0·44 in the latter would, by reference to the analytical indexes in Part 3, suggest quinalbarbitone, page 530. This could then be confirmed by gas chromatography (system G5, page 83—retention time relative to barbitone, 3·02) or by infra-red spectrophotometry (principal peaks at 1559, 1648, and 1690 cm^{-1}—see page 761).

Similarly, a residue in the alkaline chloroform fraction submitted to chromatography by the paper system P1, page 34, might give an absorbing spot, positive with iodoplatinate, at Rf 0·31, and by the thin-layer system T1, page 46, a spot at Rf 0·23, also positive with iodoplatinate. If reference is now made to the tables of Rf values for the P1 and T1 systems, pages 612 and 637, and lists are made of all the spots fulfilling the above conditions between 0·29 and 0·33 on the former system and 0·21 and 0·25 on the latter, it will be found that strychnine, page 545, is the only compound common to both lists. Should no instrumentation be available, confirmation may be made (1) by rerunning the test material on paper and thin-layer chromatograms against a known sample of strychnine, (2) by evaporating a microdrop (see page 133) of a solution of the test material in dilute acetic acid with a microdrop of a 0·5 per cent solution of ammonium vanadate, moistening the residue with a microdrop of concentrated sulphuric acid, and observing the colour change—blue → purple → red, and (3) by mixing a microdrop of a similar solution of the unknown with a microdrop of a 5 per cent solution of platinic chloride by the hanging drop technique described on page 136 and observing the shape of the crystals formed.

Comment se servir de ce livre

Dans les cas d'urgence
Consulter le chapitre sur les méthodes de dépistage rapides commençant à la page 3. Ce chapitre décrit des méthodes simples permettant d'identifier les produits toxiques communs qui sont la cause d'environ 90% des cas d'empoisonnement nécessitant un traitement hospitalier.

Lorsque des preuves suffisamment évidentes permettent de soupçonner l'identité du produit toxique que l'on recherche
Consulter, dans la Deuxième Partie, la monographie du composé en question et appliquer les méthodes d'extraction suggérées dont les détails sont donnés dans le chapitre commençant à la page 16. Soumettre ensuite le produit isolé à n'importe laquelle des méthodes d'identification indiquées dans la monographie. Le choix de la méthode dépendra de la nature du produit, de l'expérience de l'analyste, des appareils disponibles et du degré d'urgence du problème.

Lorsqu'il n'existe aucune indication quant à l'identité du produit toxique
Appliquer une des méthodes générales d'extraction décrites de la page 21 à la page 28 et soumettre les résidus des diverses fractions à des tests appropriés d'identification chromatographique. Faire une identification préliminaire en consultant les tableaux analytiques de la Troisième Partie et confirmer l'identification en procédant aux tests suggérés dans la monographie appropriée de la Deuxième Partie.

Ainsi, par exemple, un résidu dans la fraction éther acide peut être soumis à la chromatographie sur papier suivant le système P2, page 34, ou à la chromatographie en couche mince suivant le système T10, page 52. Une valeur Rf de 1,40 dans le premier cas et de 0,44 dans le second, confrontées aux tableaux analytiques de la Troisième Partie, laisseraient supposer qu'il s'agit de sécobarbital (quinalbarbitone), page 530. Ceci peut ensuite être confirmé par chromatographie gazeuse (système G5, page 83—temps de rétention relatif au barbital, 3,02) ou par spectrophotométrie aux rayons infrarouges (valeurs maximales principales à 1559, 1648 et 1690 cm^{-1}—voir page 761).

De même, un résidu dans la fraction chloroforme alcalin soumis à la chromatographie sur papier selon le système P1, page 34, peut donner un point d'absorption positif avec le platiiodure à Rf 0,31, et selon le système T1 en couche mince, page 46, un point à Rf 0,23, positif également avec le platiiodure. Si l'on consulte alors les tableaux des valeurs Rf relatives aux systèmes P1 et T1, pages 612 et 637, et si l'on dresse les listes de tous les points remplissant les conditions ci-dessus, entre 0,29 et 0,33 pour le premier système, et 0,21 et 0,25 pour le second, on verra que la strychnine, page 545, est le seul produit commun aux deux listes. Si l'on ne dispose d'aucun appareil, il est possible d'obtenir confirmation, (1) en comparant les chromatogrammes sur papier et en couche mince du produit testé avec ceux d'un échantillon que l'on sait être de la strychnine; (2) en faisant évaporer une microgoutte (voir page 133) d'une solution du produit testé dans de l'acide acétique dilué, avec une microgoutte d'une solution de vanadate d'ammoniaque à 0,5%, en humidifiant ensuite le résidu avec une microgoutte d'acide sulfurique concentré, et en observant le virage—bleu → pourpre → rouge; et (3) en mélangeant une microgoutte d'une solution semblable du produit inconnu avec une microgoutte d'une solution de chlorure de platine à 5%, suivant la technique de la goutte en suspension décrite à la page 136, et en observant la forme des cristaux qui se forment.

Anleitung zum Gebrauch des Buches

Im Notfall
Schlagen Sie das auf Seite 3 beginnende Kapitel auf, das schnelle Prüfungsmethoden beschreibt. Hier finden Sie einfache Verfahren zum Nachweis der gebräuchlichen Arzneimittel, die für ungefähr 90% aller Spitalbehandlung benötigenden Vergiftungen verantwortlich sind.

Wenn deutliche Anzeichen die Identität des Arzneimittels, die untersucht wird, vermuten lassen
Schlagen Sie Teil 2 auf und suchen Sie in der Einzelabhandlung über die in Frage stehende Verbindung Rat, wenden Sie das vorgeschlagene Verfahren zur Absonderung, über welches Sie näheres in dem auf Seite 16 beginnendem Kapitel finden, an und unterziehen Sie dann den abgetrennten Stoff irgendeiner der in der Abhandlung genannten Methoden der Identifizierung. Die Wahl der Methode hängt von der Beschaffenheit der Verbindung, der Erfahrung des Untersuchers, der verfügbaren Apparatur und der Dringlichkeit der Aufgabe ab.

Wenn keine Hinweise auf die Identität des Arzneimittels bestehen
Wenden Sie eines der auf Seite 21–28 kurz beschriebenen allgemeinen Absonderungsverfahren an, unterziehen Sie die Rückstände der verschiedenen Fraktionen den geeigneten chromatographischen Untersuchungen, und unternehmen Sie eine vorläufige Identifizierung mit Hilfe der analytischen Tabellen im Teil 3. Bestätigen Sie den Befund durch die Prüfungen, die in den entsprechenden Abhandlungen in Teil 2 vorgeschlagen werden.

So zum Beispiel kann ein Rückstand im sauren Ätheranteil nach System P2, Seite 34 der Papierchromatographie unterzogen werden, oder der Dünnschichtchromatographie nach System T10, Seite 52. Ein Rf-Wert von 1,40 im ersten Falle oder 0,44 im zweiten weist, wenn man in den analytischen Tabellen im Teil 3 nachsieht, auf Quinalbarbiton, Seite 530. Dieser Befund kann durch Gaschromatographie bestätigt werden (System G5, Seite 83—Retentionszeit bezüglich auf Barbiton, 3,02), oder durch Infrarotspektroskopie (Hauptbanden bei 1559, 1648, und 1690 cm^{-1}—siehe Seite 761).

In ähnlicher Weise kann ein Rückstand des alkalischen Chloroformanteils, wenn er einer chromatographischen Untersuchung nach dem Papiersystem P1, Seite 34 unterzogen wird, einen Absorptionsflecken geben, der bei Rf 0,31 mit Jodoplatinat positiv reagiert. Nach dem Dünnschichtsystem T1, Seite 46, kann er einen Flecken bei Rf 0,23 geben, der gleichfalls mit Jodoplatinat positiv ist. Wenn man sich jetzt auf die Tabellen der Rf-Werte für die P1 und T1 Systeme, Seite 612 und 637, bezieht, und Listen aller Flecken anlegt, die den obigen Bedingungen zwischen 0,29 und 0,33 im ersten System und zwischen 0,21 und 0,25 im zweiten System genügen, dann findet man, dass Strychnin, Seite 545, die einzige Verbindung ist, die beiden Listen gemeinsam ist. Falls keine Instrumente zur Verfügung stehen, kann eine Bestätigung gefunden werden durch (1) vergleichende Papier- und Dünnschichtchromatogramme des zu untersuchenden Stoffes und einer sicheren Strychninprobe, (2) durch Verdampfen eines Mikrotropfens (siehe Seite 133) einer Lösung des zu untersuchenden Stoffes in verdünnter Essigsäure mit einem Mikrotropfen einer 0,5 prozentigen Lösung von Ammoniumvanadat, Befeuchten des Rückstandes mit einem Mikrotropfen konzentrierter Schwefelsäure und Beobachten des Farbumschlages—blau → purpur → rot, und (3) indem man einen Mikrotropfen einer ähnlichen Lösung des unbekannten Stoffes mit einem Mikrotropfen einer 5 prozentigen Lösung von Platintetrachlorid im Verfahren der hängenden Tropfen mischt (das Verfahren wird auf Seite 136 beschrieben) und die Gestalt der sich bildenden Kristalle beobachtet.

Cómo usar el libro

En las urgencias médicas
Consultar el capítulo sobre cribado rápido que comienza en la página 3. En él se describen métodos sencillos para la identificación de drogas comunes, que son las responsables de un 90% de los casos de envenenamiento que precisan hospitalización.

Cuando existan pruebas bien fundadas acerca de la identidad de la droga que se está investigando
Pásese a la Parte 2 y consúltese la monografía correspondiente al compuesto investigado, aplicando el método de extracción que se sugiera, según los datos que se encontrarán en el capítulo que comienza en la página 16; someter entonces la substancia aislada a cualquiera de los métodos de identificación indicados en la monografía. El método a utilizar dependerá de la naturaleza del compuesto, la pericia del analista, del equipo de que se disponga, y de la urgencia del caso.

Cuando no haya pista alguna identificadora de la droga
Aplíquese uno de los métodos generales de extracción indicados en las páginas 21 a 28, sometiendo los resíduos de las diversas fracciones a procedimientos adecuados de cribado cromatográfico, haciendo una identificación provisional utilizando los índices analíticos de la Parte 3, y confirmando la identificación mediante las pruebas sugeridas en la correspondiente monografía de la Parte 2.

Así, por ejemplo, un resíduo en la fracción ácida de éter podría someterse a cromatografía sobre papel siguiendo el sistema P2, página 34, o a cromatografía de capa delgada según el sistema T10, de la página 52. Un valor Rf = 1,40, en el primer caso, o de 0,44 en el segundo, al hacer comparación con los índices analíticos de la Parte 3, sugeriría la presencia de secobarbital (quinalbarbitone), página 530. Esto podría confirmarse entonces mediante cromatografía en fase gaseosa (sistema G5, página 83—tiempo de retención relativo al barbital, 3,02) o mediante espectrofotometría infrarroja (máximas principales a 1559, 1648, y 1690 cm^{-1}—véase página 761).

De igual modo, un resíduo en la fracción alcalina de cloroformo sometido a cromatografía sobre papel siguiendo el sistema P1, página 34, pudiera dar una mancha de absorción, positiva empleando yodoplatinato, a Rf = 0,31, y mediante el sistema T1 de capa delgada, página 46, una mancha a Rf = 0,23, igualmente positiva con yodoplatinato. Si ahora consultamos las tablas de valores Rf correspondientes a los sistemas P1 y T1, páginas 612 y 637, y se preparan listas a base de todas las manchas que cumplen las anteriores condiciones comprendidas entre 0,29 y 0,33 para el primer sistema, y entre 0,21 y 0,25 para el segundo, encontraremos que la estricnina, página 545, es el único compuesto común a ambas listas. De no disponerse de los instrumentos necesarios, la confirmación puede verificarse (1) volviendo a hacer avanzar a la substancia problema sobre cromatogramas obtenidos mediante papel y capa delgada de una muestra conocida de estricnina, (2) evaporando una microgota (véase la página 133) de una solución problema en ácido acético diluído, con una microgota de una solución al 0,5 por ciento de vanadato amónico, humedeciendo el resíduo con una microgota de ácido sulfúrico concentrado, y observando el cambio de color—azul → púrpura → rojo, y (3) mediante la mezcla de una microgota de una solución semejante del problema, con una microgota de una solución al 5 por ciento de cloruro platínico, siguiendo la técnica de la gota suspendida, según se describe en la página 136, y estudiando la forma de los cristales que se hayan formado.

Abbreviations

A—ampere(s)
Å—ångström(s)
AMA—American Medical Association
ASTM—American Society for Testing Materials
B.P.—British Pharmacopoeia
b.p.—boiling-point
B.P.C.—British Pharmaceutical Codex
cal—calorie(s)
cm—centimetre(s)
cm^3—cubic centimetre(s)
cm^{-1}—reciprocal centimetre(s)
ed.—editor; edited by
Edn—edition
e.g.—*exempli gratia*, 'for example'
et al.—et alii, 'and others'
eV—electronvolt(s)
FAO/WHO—Food and Agricultural Organisation (and the) World Health Organisation
f.p.—freezing point
g—gramme(s)
gal—gallon(s)
g/kg—gramme(s) per kilogram
GLC—gas-liquid chromatography
GSC—gas-solid chromatography
i.e.—*id est*, 'that is'
in—inch
I.R.—infra-red
kg—kilogram(s)
l—litre(s)
lb—pound(s)
LD50—a dose lethal to 50% of the specified animals
λ—wavelength
M—molar
m—metre(s)
m^2—square metre(s)
max—maximum
mEq—milliequivalent(s)
mg—milligram(s)
mg/kg—milligram(s) per kilogram
mg/l—milligram(s) per litre
mg/ml—milligram(s) per millilitre
mg/min—milligram(s) per minute
mg%—milligram(s) per 100 grammes or per 100 millilitres
1 mg%—1 milligram per 100 grammes or 100 millilitres = 10 p.p.m.
ml—millilitre(s)
mm—millimetre(s)
mmHg—millimetre(s) of mercury
mμ—millimicron(s)
m.p.—melting-point
μ—micron(s)
μg—microgram(s)
μg/l—microgram(s) per litre
μl—microlitre(s)
N—normal
oz—ounce(s)
PEG—polyethyleneglycol
pH—hydrogen ion concentration
p.p.m.—parts per million
p.v.c.—polyvinyl chloride
q.v.—*quod vide*, 'which see'
Rf—relative flow (see p. 32)
RRT—relative retention time (retention time of sample relative to that of a reference compound)
Supp.—Supplement
U.S. and U.S.A.—United States of America
U.V.—ultraviolet
viz.—*videlicet*, 'namely'
vol—volume(s)
v/v—volume in volume
w/v—weight in volume
w/w—weight in weight
wt—weight

Acknowledgements

Gifts of drugs are gratefully acknowledged from A. R. Alha, A. S. Curry, N. B. Eddy, C. Farmilo, R. C. Frost, J. J. Gordon, D. G. Harvey, H. Isbell, P. Janssen, D. K. de Jongh, E. B. May, G. West and T. D. Whittet; Abbott Laboratories Ltd, Alcon Laboratories Inc., Allen & Hanburys Ltd, Laboratoire Amido, Armour Pharmaceutical Co. Ltd, Astra-Hewlett Ltd, Asta-Werke, A.G., Ayerst Labs, Bayer Products Co., Beecham Research Laboratories, C. L. Bencard, Bengué & Co. Ltd, Berk Pharmaceuticals Ltd, Boehringer Ingleheim Ltd, Boots Pure Drug Co. Ltd, Bristol Labs, Inc., The British Drug Houses Ltd, The British Dyewood Co. Ltd, Burroughs Wellcome & Co., Camden Chemical Co. Ltd, Carlo Erba (U.K.) Ltd, Ciba Laboratories Ltd, Clay & Abraham (Mfg) Ltd, Coates & Cooper Ltd, Coutelier Frères, Cyanamid of Great Britain Ltd, Dales Pharmaceuticals Ltd, Denver Laboratories Ltd, Dista Products Ltd, The Distillers Co. Ltd, Duncan, Flockhart & Evans Ltd, Endo Laboratories Inc., Evans Medical Ltd, FBA Pharmaceuticals Ltd, Fisons Pharmaceuticals Ltd, Geigy (U.K.), Ltd, Geistlich Sons Ltd, Glaxo Laboratories Ltd, Hoechst Pharmaceutical Ltd, Hoffmann-LaRoche Inc., Hommel Pharmaceuticals Ltd, Hopkin & Williams Ltd, Horlicks Ltd, Imperial Chemical Industries Ltd, Knoll Ltd, Laboratories for Applied Biology Ltd, Laborec, Lakeside Labs Inc., Lannacher Heilmittel, Levmedic Ltd, Eli Lilly & Co. Ltd, Lincoln Labs Inc., Lloyd Anphar Ltd, Lloyd-Hamol Ltd, Macfarlan Smith Ltd, McNeil Laboratories Inc., Mallinckrodt Chemical Works, May & Baker Ltd, M.C.P. Pure Drugs Ltd, Menley & James Ltd, Merck, Sharp & Dohme Ltd, E. Merck, A.G., Merrell-National (Laboratories) Ltd, Moore Medicinal Products Ltd, National Drug Co., Nepera Laboratories, Nicholas Laboratories Ltd, Nicholas Products Ltd, Nipa Laboratories Ltd, Novocol Chem. Mfg Co. Inc., N.V. Nederlandsche Cocaine Fabriek, Organon Laboratories Ltd, Ortho Pharmaceutical Ltd, Parke Davis & Co., Pfizer Ltd, Pharmaceutical Mfg Co., Pharmaceutical Society of Great Britain, Pharmacia Laboratories Inc., Philips Roxane Inc., Pitman-Moore Co., Plant Protection Ltd, Reckitt & Sons Ltd, Reed & Carnrick, Riker Laboratories, A. H. Robins Co. Ltd, Roche Products Ltd, Rona Laboratories Ltd, Roussel Laboratories Ltd, Rybar Laboratories Ltd, Sandoz Products Ltd, Savory & Moore Ltd, Schering Corp., G. D. Searle & Co. Ltd, Seceph SA, Selpharm Laboratories Ltd, Sigurta Farmaceutici, Smith Kline & French Ltd, Smith & Nephew Pharmaceuticals Ltd, T. & H. Smith Ltd, Sojuzchimexport (USSR), E. R. Squibb & Sons Ltd, Sterling-Winthrop Laboratories, Strasenburgh Labs, Tavolek Laboratories Ltd, Upjohn Ltd, U.S. Vitamin & Pharmaceutical Corp., Veritas Drug Co. Ltd, A. Wander Ltd, Ward Blenkinsop & Co. Ltd, William R. Warner & Co. Ltd, West-Silten Pharmaceuticals Ltd, Whiffen Chemicals Ltd, White Laboratories Inc., S. S. White Co., Winthrop Laboratories Inc., Wright, Layman & Umney Ltd, and John Wyeth & Brother Ltd.

PART 1: Analytical Techniques

Screening Tests for Common Drugs

G. Higgins

During the past decade, the large increase in the use of drugs has been reflected in the number of patients admitted to hospital suffering from overdosage.

Some conception of the amount of drugs ingested is given by figures published for the year 1963 when 7000 million aspirin, 1200 million barbiturate, and 14,000 million other types of tablets were prescribed for National Health Service patients alone.

In nearly all countries, an increase in cases of drug overdosage has been reported and now constitutes a major reason for admission to the medical wards of hospitals. In one town in the south of England, in 1955, patients suffering from overdoses amounted to 13% of the cases admitted to the adult medical wards (Higgins, unpublished data) and, in a town in the Midlands, the figure was 18·9% (Ellis, Comish, and Hewer, 1966). The total number of patients taking such overdoses is difficult to obtain, since many do so in their own homes and recover without treatment, but it is estimated that the number of non-fatal poisonings, deliberate and accidental, in the U.S.A. exceeds a million per year.

Whilst in many cases the cause of a coma can be easily recognised by the discovery of tablets or capsules on the person or in the bed of the patient or by reference to the prescribing physician, in many cases no such cause is obvious. In these cases recourse must be made to the clinical biochemical laboratory. Thus the role of the hospital laboratory is becoming increasingly important in the diagnosis and treatment of such cases.

However, although sometimes the ingestion of an excessive amount of drug can be assumed, every case of coma demands expert clinical, particularly neurological, examination since the symptoms displayed in comas caused by natural causes and by drug overdosage may be very similar.

It is also recommended that the sugar and urea content of the patient's blood be estimated, modern 'filter-stick' methods such as the 'Dextrostix' and 'Urastrat' being easily applicable when laboratory facilities are not immediately available.

A review of the drugs ingested shows that in the majority of cases of drug overdosage, the drugs are limited to one or more of about a dozen types. It is the purpose of this chapter to describe a series of tests that can be rapidly applied to biological material to identify some of the drugs most commonly encountered. Even when one drug has been identified, the possibility of another drug having been ingested must be recognised since, in recent years, there has been an increase in the number of patients taking more than one drug.

The specimens generally available from the living patient are blood and gastric contents collected before the customary stomach wash-out but in many of the tests described below the use of urine is indicated, and it is suggested that a specimen of urine be obtained from all patients even if catheterisation is necessary to obtain it.

In a survey of 305 consecutive cases admitted to a hospital in the south of England in 1965 the drugs ingested were barbiturates in 48% of cases, aspirin and other mild analgesics in 32%, tranquillisers in 9%, and hypotensive drugs in 3%; carbon monoxide poisoning was responsible for 4% of the cases; 10% of the cases had ingested more than one type of drug.

In a similar survey in the Midlands in 1964 the figures were barbiturates in 36% of cases, aspirin and other mild analgesics in 39%, tranquillisers in 10%, mixtures of these drugs in 5%, and carbon monoxide in 5%.

It is apparent from these figures that examination of biological specimens for barbiturates, aspirin, and tranquillisers should elucidate the nature of the drug in about 85% of cases.

It is suggested therefore that, in any scheme devised for the identification of drugs causing coma, these drugs should be first sought for.

SCHEME FOR THE RAPID IDENTIFICATION OF SOME DRUGS COMMONLY TAKEN IN OVERDOSAGE

The tests outlined below are designed to detect drugs taken in overdosage and are not necessarily sensitive enough to detect drugs when taken in medicinal doses only. The scheme should be followed in cases where there is no clue to the identity of the drug. When there is evidence of its nature, it may be tested for directly—see Details of Screening Tests, p. 6.

Tests Performed Directly on Urine

1. *'Clinistix' test for glucose*—dip a 'Clinistix' strip into urine and read the colour after 10 seconds.
2. *Rothera's test for ketones*—saturate 3 ml of urine with ammonium sulphate crystals, add 3 drops of strong ammonia solution and a few drops of freshly prepared 5% sodium nitroprusside solution. A purple colour develops if acetone or acetoacetic acid is present.
   A 'Ketostix' strip can also be used.
3. *Dichromate test for alcohols*—to 1 ml of urine add 1 ml of 10% sodium dichromate in 50% sulphuric acid. A green colour develops if an alcohol is present.
4. *Ferric chloride test for salicylates*—to 2 ml of urine add 2 drops of ferric chloride solution. A violet colour develops if salicylate is present.
5. *'Phenistix' test for salicylates and chlorpromazine*—dip a 'Phenistix' strip into urine and read the colour within 10 seconds.
6. *FPN test for phenothiazines*—to 1 ml of urine add 1 ml of *FPN reagent*. A variety of colours ranging through pink, red, orange, violet, and blue indicates the presence of a phenothiazine derivative.
7. *Forrest test for imipramine, desipramine, and trimipramine*—to 1 ml of urine add 1 ml of *Forrest reagent*. A green colour develops if imipramine, desipramine, or trimipramine is present.
8. *Fujiwara's test for trichloro-compounds*—mix 1 ml of 10% sodium hydroxide solution and 1 ml of redistilled pyridine and heat in a boiling water-bath for 2 minutes; if no colour develops, add 2 ml of urine and repeat the heating. The

development of a pink to red colour in the pyridine layer indicates the presence of trichloro-compounds, e.g. chloroform, chloral, chlorbutol, trichloroethane, trichloroethanol, and trichloroacetic acid.

9. *Alphanaphthol–sodium nitrite test for* p-*aminophenol*—to 2 ml of urine acidified with dilute hydrochloric acid, add 3 drops of 1% sodium nitrite solution and 3 drops of freshly prepared 1% alphanaphthol in 10% sodium hydroxide solution. A red colour develops if *p*-aminophenol is present. *p*-Aminophenol is a metabolite of phenacetin and paracetamol.

NOTE. This test may be positive with any compound containing a primary aromatic amino-group.

Tests Performed Directly on Blood

1. *Estimation of sugar*—by the glucose oxidase method or, approximately, by the 'Dextrostix' method—to exclude diabetic or hypoglycaemic coma.
2. *Estimation of urea*—by a standard method or, approximately, by the 'Urastrat' method—to exclude uraemia.
3. *Carboxyhaemoglobin*—blood diluted 1 in 200 with 0·01N ammonium hydroxide is examined spectroscopically and the position of the α-band determined. Examination with the Reversion spectroscope permits direct comparison with normal blood.

Tests Performed on Extracts of Specimens

A. Tests Performed on Acid Ether Extracts

Specimens of blood (preferably 10 ml), urine (25 ml), or stomach contents (5 to 20 ml) are acidified with hydrochloric acid to pH 3 to 4 and then extracted twice with 25 ml of ether. The specimen is saved for alkaline chloroform extraction (procedure B). The ether extracts are combined, washed with 5 ml of water, dried by passing through anhydrous sodium sulphate, and evaporated just to dryness. The residue is tested for:

(1) *Barbiturates*—cobalt acetate–lithium hydroxide test (p. 9).

(2) *Carbromal*—fluorescein–hydrogen peroxide test (p. 10).

(3) *Diazepam*—ultraviolet absorption of the residue in 2N hydrochloric acid (p. 11).

(4) *Ergot Alkaloids*—(extract of stomach contents only) potassium hydroxide test (p. 12), *p*-dimethylaminobenzaldehyde test (p. 130).

(5) *Ethchlorvynol*—ethanolic phloroglucinol–hydrochloric acid test (p. 12).

(6) *Glutethimide*—cobalt acetate–lithium hydroxide test, ultraviolet absorption (p. 12).

(7) *Methaqualone*—ultraviolet absorption of ethanolic solution (p. 13).

(8) *Salicylic Acid*—ferric chloride test (p. 8).

B. Tests Performed on Alkaline Chloroform Extracts

The specimen after acid extraction (procedure A) is made alkaline (pH 10) with dilute ammonia solution and extracted twice with 25 ml of chloroform. The extracts are combined, washed with 5 ml of water, dried by passing through anhydrous sodium sulphate, and evaporated just to dryness. The residue is tested for:

(1) *Amitriptyline and Nortriptyline*—ultraviolet absorption of residue in 0·1N hydrochloric acid (p. 7).

(2) *Amphetamine*—Marquis test (p. 7).

(3) *Chlordiazepoxide*—diazotisation test on the extract hydrolysed with hydrochloric acid (p. 10).

(4) *Codeine*—Marquis test (p. 11).

(5) *Meprobamate*—ethanol–furfural test (p. 13).

(6) *Methaqualone*—ultraviolet absorption of ethanolic solution of residue (p. 13).

(7) *Phenytoin*—ultraviolet absorption of residue in bicarbonate buffer (pH 11) (p. 14).

(8) *Quinine*—fluorescence test after treatment with sulphuric acid (p. 15).

Many of the tests on the acid ether and alkaline chloroform extracts may be performed as spot tests after the residue has been spotted on filter paper.

DETAILS OF SCREENING TESTS

Alcohols—Ethanol and Methanol

Although coma due to acute ethanol overdosage is not commonly met, the synergistic action of ethanol with other drugs makes it important that its presence be detected and its role in the cause of the coma evaluated.

1. *Preliminary screening test on urine—in the absence of ketonuria*

1 ml of urine is added to 1 ml of 10% sodium dichromate in 50% sulphuric acid. In the presence of alcohol in amounts of more than 150 mg% urine, a green colour develops within 10 seconds, in amounts more than 75 mg% urine the green colour appears in 45 seconds or less. If the solution is heated, as little as 20 mg% of alcohol in urine can be detected.

Since other substances, such as other alcohols, can respond to this test, positive results should be confirmed.

2a. *Confirmation of screening test on blood or urine—Wintergreen test*

5 ml of blood or 10 ml of urine is steam-distilled and the first 5 ml of distillate is collected and tested for ethanol or methanol; 1 ml of the distillate, 1 ml of sulphuric acid, and 0·1 g of sodium salicylate are mixed and gently boiled. The odour of wintergreen (methyl salicylate) indicates the presence of ethanol or methanol.

2b. *Confirmation of ethanol—Iodoform test*

To 2 ml of the distillate is added a few drops of 10% sodium hydroxide solution then several drops of iodine until a persistent yellow colour appears. The appearance of yellow crystals of iodoform may indicate the presence of ethanol. Methanol does not interfere but acetone does.

2c. *Confirmation of methanol—Chromotropic acid test*

To 2 ml of the distillate is added acidified potassium permanganate reagent drop by drop until the solution remains pink. The excess permanganate is decolorised with a dropwise addition of 10% oxalic acid solution, added one drop at a time, and 0·1 g of chromotropic acid is added; 1·5 ml of sulphuric acid is poured down the sides of the tube so that it will underlay the distillate. A purple ring at the junction of the acid and distillate indicates the presence of methanol. The intensity of the purple colour when mixed is proportional to the amount of methanol present. This test is specific for formaldehyde and for methanol if the latter is first oxidised.

Amitriptyline and Nortriptyline

Amitriptyline and nortriptyline may be excreted unchanged or as conjugated metabolites. Both must therefore be sought in cases of poisoning.

Screening tests on urine

The unchanged drug. 25 ml of urine is made alkaline (pH 12) with 10% sodium hydroxide solution and extracted for 3 minutes with 50 ml of chloroform. The urine is saved. The chloroform extract is washed with 20 ml of 0·1N sodium hydroxide, followed by 20 ml of water. The washed extract is then extracted with 10 ml of 0·1N hydrochloric acid and the ultraviolet absorbance from 200 to 300 mμ measured and the curve compared with a curve obtained from the pure drug similarly treated. Maximum absorption occurs at 240 mμ.

Metabolites. The extracted urine from the previous test is neutralised with 6N hydrochloric acid and a further 0·2 ml of acid added. The solution is heated in a boiling water-bath for 60 minutes, cooled, and made alkaline with 10% sodium hydroxide solution. The urine is then extracted with chloroform as in the previous test. The absorbance of the acid extract is also measured from 200 to 300 mμ. In the presence of a metabolite a peak occurs at 290 mμ.

These methods can be used as the basis of quantitative methods in which case the unchanged drug is calculated on the absorbance at 240 mμ and the metabolite at 290 mμ.

Amphetamine

Amphetamine can be detected in the urine for about 60 hours after the ingestion of a large dose but, because it is slowly excreted, the concentration in the urine is low. If dilute urines are encountered, correspondingly larger volumes must be used for the analysis.

The detection of amphetamine is not easy and control urines containing no drug and added drug should always be processed in the same way as the test urine.

Screening test on urines—when the ingestion of a large dose is suspected

50 ml of urine is made acid with hydrochloric acid and extracted with 30 ml of ether. This ether extract is discarded. The urine is then made alkaline (pH 10) by the addition of ammonium hydroxide solution and extracted twice with 50 ml of chloroform or ether. The combined extracts are washed, filtered, and, after the addition of one drop of 0·1N hydrochloric acid, evaporated down to 0·5 ml. The extract must *not* be evaporated to dryness.

The residue is spotted on to filter paper impregnated with sodium citrate, dried, and tested with *Marquis reagent*—an orange colour turning to brown is given by amphetamine.

Confirmation may be made by thin-layer chromatography or gas chromatography—see under Amphetamine (p. 192) and Dexamphetamine (p. 287).

Urines of patients suspected of having had small doses of amphetamine and urines that are dilute are steam-distilled as follows:

50 ml of urine (or more, if dilute) is made alkaline with sodium hydroxide solution and steam-distilled into 5 ml of 0·5N hydrochloric acid; 10 ml of distillate is collected. The acidified distillate is made alkaline with sodium hydroxide solution, extracted with chloroform or ether, and tested as outlined above.

Aspirin and Salicylic Acid

Poisoning by aspirin is commonly encountered and may be lethal when more than 50 tablets are ingested. Many patients who have taken doses of aspirin that could be lethal may not appear to be very ill and the seriousness of their condition may not be recognised. Conversely, the ingestion of one or two aspirin tablets within the preceding 24 hours may give a positive urine test. The estimation of plasma levels of salicylate is indicated whenever positive urine tests are obtained.

1. *Preliminary screening test on urine*

To 1 ml of urine is added 3 drops of ferric chloride solution. A violet colour indicates the presence of salicylate.

2. *Confirmation of screening test on blood or urine*

0·5 ml of urine or plasma is added to 4·5 ml of 0·55% ferric nitrate in 0·04N nitric acid. A purple colour proportional to the concentration of salicylate is obtained. This test may be used as the basis of a quantitative test. *Trinder's reagent* may also be used.

Confirmation that the colour is given by salicylate and not another drug is obtained by applying the 'wintergreen test' as for alcohols (p. 6) to material extracted from the biological sample.

3. *Tests on gastric contents*

Aspirin recovered from the stomach must be hydrolysed to salicylic acid before the above tests are applied. This may be done by boiling a sample of the gastric contents with a few drops of 1N hydrochloric acid, cooling, and neutralising.

Barbiturates

Barbituric acid and its derivatives are the drugs most commonly taken in overdoses, the severity of the poisoning being related to the amount and type of the barbiturate ingested. Since patients taking phenobarbitone or barbitone may be quite conscious with blood concentrations that would be lethal if they had similar levels of, for example, quinalbarbitone or pentobarbitone, positive urinary findings of the presence of barbiturate should be evaluated by the identification of the type of barbiturate and by the estimation of the blood-level.

Since barbiturate may rapidly pass through the stomach, analysis of gastric aspirations or washings may be unreliable and should only be used when it is known that a short period has elapsed—1 or 2 hours—between the ingestion of the drug and the aspiration or wash-out of the stomach.

Screening test

50 ml of urine or stomach contents is made acid (pH 4 to 5) by the addition of a few drops of 10% sulphuric acid and extracted twice with 50 ml of ether. The combined ether extracts are washed with water and dried by filtering. If highly coloured with pigment, the extract can be shaken with 0·1 g of washed charcoal and filtered. The extract is evaporated to dryness and the residue taken up into 1 ml of chloroform.

To one half of this solution is added 2 drops of freshly prepared 1% cobalt acetate in methanol, followed by freshly prepared 1% lithium hydroxide in methanol, drop by drop. A blue ring at the junction indicates the presence of barbiturate.

Confirmation and identification of the barbiturate is established by thin-layer chromatography or by gas chromatography—see under Barbiturates, p. 208.

The severity of the poisoning should be assessed by the estimation of the amount of the barbiturate in the blood (see p. 208).

Carboxyhaemoglobin

Poisoning by carbon monoxide may occur in atmospheres which contain coal-gas or in which incomplete combustion of paraffin oil burners, coal fires, or smouldering cloth occurs. The affinity of haemoglobin for carbon monoxide is great enough for poisoning to occur even when only small quantities of the gas are present in the atmosphere.

When, however, patients are withdrawn from the carbon-monoxide contaminated atmosphere, carboxyhaemoglobin quickly disappears from the blood and only traces may remain one hour later, i.e. sometimes by the time the patient has reached hospital.

Rapid screening test—for large amounts of carboxyhaemoglobin

A sample of blood is diluted 1 in 20 with 0·01N ammonium hydroxide and compared with a sample of normal blood similarly treated. A pinkish tint suggests the presence of carboxyhaemoglobin.

Confirmation of screening test

The blood is diluted 1 in 200 with 0·01N ammonium hydroxide and examined in the Reversion spectroscope which has been previously adjusted so that the α-bands of normal haemoglobin are in alignment. A shift of the α-bands so that they are no longer in alignment when the solution of the test blood is examined confirms the presence of carboxyhaemoglobin. The shift in the position of the α-band is proportional to the concentration of carboxyhaemoglobin.

Estimation of carboxyhaemoglobin

The absorbance of the blood, diluted 1 in 200 as above, is measured at 541, 560, and 576 mμ, and the ratios 541:560 mμ and 576:560 mμ calculated. The carboxyhaemoglobin is calculated from the graph prepared by determining these ratios on blood containing known amounts of carboxyhaemoglobin.

Carbromal

Carbromal is often prescribed as Carbrital, a combination of carbromal and pentobarbitone. Acute overdosage will then simulate barbiturate poisoning and can be assessed by the estimation of blood concentrations of pentobarbitone and bromide. Chronic poisoning may take the form of bromide poisoning. Carbromal is only detected in the blood following the ingestion of very large doses.

Screening test for carbromal

Stomach contents or washings are made acid with hydrochloric acid and extracted twice with 50 ml of ether. Blood, 10 ml or 20 ml, is extracted three times with 30 ml of chloroform.

The extracts are combined, washed with water, filtered, and evaporated to dryness. The residue is spotted into a white porcelain dish with 2 drops of 5% sodium hydroxide solution and dried with gentle heat. After cooling, 2 drops of 1% fluorescein solution, 4 drops of glacial acetic acid, and 4 drops of strong hydrogen peroxide solution (100 vol.) are added and evaporated to dryness on a boiling water-bath. A red colour indicates carbromal.

Screening test for bromide

2 ml of plasma, 6 ml of water, and 2 ml of 20% trichloroacetic acid, are well mixed and filtered. To 5 ml of the filtrate is added 1 ml of 0·5% gold chloride solution. In the presence of bromide, a yellow to gold colour, dependent upon the amount present, develops.

Chlordiazepoxide

Screening test on blood or urine

5 to 10 ml of plasma or urine is made alkaline with ammonium hydroxide solution and extracted twice with 10 ml of chloroform. The combined chloroform extracts are washed with 2 ml of water and extracted with 5 ml of 6N hydrochloric acid by shaking for 5 minutes. The hydrochloric acid extract is taken off and the traces of chloroform which remain in the acid are driven off with gentle heat. When all of the chloroform has been removed, the acid extract is heated in an autoclave or in a liquid paraffin bath at 125° for 30 minutes. The volume is made up to 5 ml with water and cooled; 0·5 ml of 0·1% sodium nitrite solution is added and it is left for 3 minutes; 0·5 ml of 0·5% ammonium sulphamate solution is then added and again left for 3 minutes; finally, 0·5 ml of 0·1% *N*-1-naphthylethylenediamine dihydrochloride solution is added. A pinkish mauve colour develops on standing if chlordiazepoxide is present.

NOTE. Both chlordiazepoxide and a metabolite of diazepam yield the same product after acid hydrolysis—2-amino-5-chlorobenzophenone; hence a positive test can no longer be accepted as indicating the presence of chlordiazepoxide only.

Chlorpromazine and Other Phenothiazine Derivatives

General screening test on urine

To 1 ml of urine is added 1 ml of *FPN reagent*. A pink to red to orange colour indicates the presence of a phenothiazine.

Additional screening test on urine

To 1 ml of urine is added 1 ml of a reagent composed of 10% sulphuric acid 80 ml and 5% ferric chloride solution 20 ml. A pink to mauve colour is given by various phenothiazines, including chlorpromazine and promazine.

Screening test on urine for Thioridazine

To 1 ml of urine is added 1 ml of a reagent composed of 30% sulphuric acid 98 ml and 5% ferric chloride solution 2 ml. A pale pink colour deepening through pink to blue, depending on the amount of drug present, indicates thioridazine.

Codeine

Excessive amounts of codeine are often ingested as Compound Codeine Tablets and other mixed aspirin, phenacetin, and codeine preparations. In these cases salicylate will also be present in the urine and the finding of the latter drug should be followed by the testing of the urine for codeine.

Screening tests on urine (not specific)

50 ml of urine is made alkaline (pH 10) with ammonium hydroxide solution and extracted twice with 50 ml of chloroform. The combined extracts are washed with 3 ml of distilled water, dried with anhydrous sodium sulphate, filtered, and evaporated to dryness. The residue is taken up in 1 ml of ethanol and spotted on to filter paper. The spots are tested by (i) the addition of a drop of *Marquis reagent*—a reddish colour which turns to blue-violet develops if codeine is present, and (ii) the addition of a drop of 0·5% aqueous ammonium vanadate solution followed by a drop of sulphuric acid—a green colour which changes to blue indicates codeine.

Confirmation of the presence of codeine may be made by paper or thin-layer chromatography (p. 268).

Diazepam

Screening tests on blood, urine, and stomach contents

10 ml of urine, 5 ml of blood, or an aliquot of the stomach contents is brought to near neutral pH by the addition of an equal volume of phosphate buffer (pH 7·0). The solution is extracted twice with equal volumes of ether, being shaken each time for 5 minutes. The combined ether extract is washed twice with 2 ml of 0·1N sodium hydroxide and twice with 2 ml of water and then extracted with 3 ml of 2N hydrochloric acid by shaking for 10 minutes. The ultraviolet absorption is measured over the range of 200 to 300 mμ and compared with diazepam standards similarly treated. The acid extract of the drug has absorption maxima at 240 and 280 mμ (see note under Chlordiazepoxide, p. 10).

Ergot Alkaloids—including Ergotamine and Lysergide

Ergotamine is sometimes prescribed for the treatment of migraine and poisoning may occur through the ingestion of a large single dose or through repeated moderate doses.

No simple test is available for the detection of ergotamine or lysergide in urine. Qualitative tests can be performed on the gastric contents but unfortunately they are not very sensitive.

Screening tests on gastric contents or vomit

The gastric contents or vomit are shaken mechanically with 4 volumes of ether for 15 minutes.

The ether extract is divided into 3 portions and the following tests are performed:

1. to one portion, 5 ml of 10% potassium hydroxide solution is added and gently heated in a water-bath. Great caution must be used—ether is highly inflammable. A 'fishy' odour of trimethylamine indicates ergotamine.
2. to another portion, 3 ml of sulphuric acid is added carefully. An orange colour, turning blue at the junction of the liquids develops if ergotamine is present.
3. to the third portion, 2 g of sodium carbonate is added and mixed. A red-violet colour develops.

NOTE. Ergot alkaloids exhibit a bright blue fluorescence under ultraviolet light and give a purple colour with the *p*-dimethylaminobenzaldehyde test (p. 130).

Ethchlorvynol

A characteristic pungent odour of ethchlorvynol arising from the vomit or stomach contents often gives a clue to the ingestion of the drug.

Screening test on blood, gastric contents, and urine

The specimen is made acid with hydrochloric acid and extracted with ether. The solvent layer is dried by passing through a layer of anhydrous sodium sulphate; 2 ml of the dried solvent is transferred to a test tube and 0·4 ml of a freshly prepared 10% phloroglucinol solution in ethanol is added, followed by 3·6 ml of hydrochloric acid. The tube is heated in a boiling water-bath for 30 minutes. When ethchlorvynol is present a pale green colour forms within a few minutes and gradually changes to orange.

This test can be used as the basis of a quantitative method when the orange colour may be measured at a wavelength of 508 mμ and compared with standards similarly treated.

Glutethimide

Glutethimide can be extracted from vomit, gastric contents, blood, and urine in a manner similar to that used for barbiturate extractions.

Screening test on urine

50 ml of urine is acidified with hydrochloric acid to a pH of 4 to 5 and extracted twice with 20 ml of ether. The ether is washed, dried, and evaporated to dryness. The residue is taken up in chloroform and to a portion is added 2 drops of freshly prepared 1% cobalt acetate in methanol followed by freshly prepared 1% lithium hydroxide in methanol, drop by drop. A blue colour which quickly changes to blue-green and then to green suggests glutethimide.

The remainder of the chloroform solution is extracted with 0·5N sodium hydroxide and the ultraviolet absorption curve from 220 to 270 mμ is measured. Glutethimide has an absorption maximum at 235 mμ but this peak decreases rapidly due to hydrolysis of the piperidine ring (Curry, 1963b).

Imipramine, Desipramine, and Trimipramine

Screening test on urine—Forrest test

To 1 ml of urine is added 1 ml of *Forrest reagent.* A greenish-yellow colour darkening to dark green, depending on the amount of drug present, immediately appears. Phenothiazine derivatives give a purple colour which often fades with this test.

Estimation of blood-levels of imipramine may be misleading as the ingestion of toxic amounts may only give rise to blood-levels of 0·1 mg% or less. Blood-levels after the ingestion of toxic doses of desipramine are usually higher—1 to 2 mg%.

Meprobamate and other Carbamates

Screening test on urine

20 to 50 ml of urine made alkaline (pH 10) with ammonium hydroxide solution is extracted twice with double its volume of chloroform. The combined extracts are washed, dried with anhydrous sodium sulphate, and evaporated to dryness. The residue is taken up in 1 ml of ether and spotted on to filter paper, with a control, and the spots stained with 10% furfural in ethanol. The filter paper is dried at room temperature and then placed in hydrochloric acid fumes. In the presence of a carbamate the spots turn blue-black.

The presence of meprobamate may be confirmed by evaporating the remainder of the ether solution of the residue to dryness, taking the residue up in 1 ml of sulphuric acid, and heating in a boiling water-bath for 20 minutes. After cooling, the solution is diluted with water and the ultraviolet absorption measured from 400 to 540 mμ. The curve obtained is compared with a standard similarly treated.

Methaqualone

Methaqualone is often prescribed in combination with diphenhydramine as 'Mandrax'.

Screening test on gastric contents, vomit, blood, and urine

Since extraction of methaqualone is incomplete from either acid or alkaline solution, it is suggested that extractions should be made at acid, alkaline, and neutral pH.

A sample of the vomit, gastric contents, blood (10 ml), or urine (30 ml) is extracted with twice its volume of ether or chloroform from acid (pH 4), near neutral, and alkaline (pH 10) conditions. The extracts are combined, washed with water, dried, filtered, and evaporated to dryness. If the residue is coloured or dirty, it is dissolved in ether and treated with a minimum of charcoal to remove colouring matter, filtered, and evaporated to dryness. The residue is taken up in ethanol and the ultraviolet absorption curve is measured from 200 to 320 mμ.

Methaqualone has absorption maxima at 225, 263, 304, and 316 mμ. If the residue is dissolved in 0·5N sulphuric acid in place of ethanol, absorption peaks occur at 234 and 269 mμ.

Nitrazepam

Nitrazepam may be excreted as the unchanged drug or as the 7-amino- and 7-acetylamino-metabolites.

Screening test on urine for the unchanged drug

5 ml of urine is made alkaline (pH 10) by shaking with ammonium hydroxide solution for 30 seconds and 250 mg of sodium dithionite is added, the solution being shaken for 10 minutes and then heated at 50° for 60 minutes. After cooling, it is extracted with 10 ml of a mixture of equal parts of redistilled methylene chloride and ethyl acetate by shaking for 10 minutes. The solvent layer is washed with 10 ml of 5% aqueous borax solution and then extracted with 5 ml of 0·2N hydrochloric acid; 4 ml of the acid phase is cooled in ice and to it is added 0·2 ml of 0·4% sodium nitrite solution. After standing for 5 minutes, 0·2 ml of 2% ammonium sulphamate is added, well mixed, and allowed to stand for a further 5 minutes; 0·2 ml of 0·4% *N*-1-naphthylethylenediamine dihydrochloride solution is then added and the colour which develops on standing is compared with standards similarly treated, at a wavelength of 555 mμ.

Screening test on urine for metabolites

The procedure is as above but the reduction step (i.e. the addition of sodium dithionite) is omitted.

Paracetamol and Phenacetin

Although these drugs may be excreted partly in the unchanged form following the ingestion of large amounts, they are mostly excreted as *p*-aminophenol.

Screening test on urine for p-*aminophenol*

To 1 ml of urine is added 2 to 3 drops of 10% hydrochloric acid and the solution cooled; 2 to 3 drops of 1% sodium nitrite solution is then added followed by 2 to 3 drops of freshly prepared 1% alphanaphthol in 10% sodium hydroxide solution. A red colour indicates the presence of *p*-aminophenol. Control blanks should be set up and treated in the same way.

Excessive amounts of alkaline alphanaphthol may give false results.

Phenytoin

Phenytoin is often prescribed in combination with phenobarbitone. Acute overdosage of these drugs then simulates barbiturate poisoning. Chronic poisoning by phenytoin may result from retention of the drug during long-term therapy.

Screening test on blood

5 ml of blood is made alkaline (pH 8 to 9) with ammonium hydroxide solution and extracted with a mixture of 20 ml of cyclohexane and 1 ml of n-butanol. After centrifuging, the aqueous layer is discarded and the organic layer washed with 10 ml of 1N hydrochloric acid. Most of the phenobarbitone, if present, remains in the aqueous phases under these conditions.

The organic solvent is then extracted with 4 ml of bicarbonate buffer (pH 11). The ultraviolet absorption from 220 to 270 mμ of the bicarbonate extract is measured and compared with the curve obtained from an extract of the pure drug, similarly processed.

This procedure can be used as the basis of a quantitative measurement, based on the difference of the optical density at 240 and 260 mμ.

Quinidine and Quinine

Rapid screening test on urine for large amounts

20 ml of urine is made alkaline with ammonium hydroxide solution and extracted with an equal amount of ether or chloroform and the extract is shaken with 3 ml of 10% sulphuric acid. A blue fluorescence, more noticeable under ultraviolet light, suggests quinine or quinidine.

It can be confirmed by fluorescent emission, which occurs at 450 mμ when an exciting light of wavelength 250 mμ is applied, if a spectrofluorimeter is available.

Trichloro-compounds—Chloral Hydrate, Chlorbutol, Chloroform, Trichloroethylene, and Trichloroethane

These substances may be extracted from tissues and blood by steam distillation into a cold container or by extraction with acidified ether.

Screening test—Fujiwara's test

1 ml of urine or distillate from blood or gastric contents is made alkaline with 1 ml of 10% sodium hydroxide solution and 1 ml of pyridine is added. The tubes are shaken and placed in a boiling water-bath for 2 minutes. A pink to red colour in the pyridine layer indicates the presence of one of the group. Blank and control tubes must be treated similarly because contamination of the atmosphere with laboratory reagents may give positive results. Metabolites of carbon tetrachloride may also give a positive result with this test.

Confirmation of the presence and identification of these compounds may be established by gas chromatography.

Extraction Methods in Toxicology

J. V. Jackson

Toxicological extraction methods provide suitable concentrates or residues to which identification techniques can be applied. These methods must be capable of dealing with a wide variety of samples, efficient at low concentration levels, and applicable to a large number of different substances. Despite the increased sensitivity of modern identification techniques, successful detection is still very dependent on the efficiency of the extraction process. The toxicologist is often requested for details of his extraction procedure, the implicit assumption being that he has one particular favourite method. No single method, however, is suitable for all samples or for all the toxic compounds now available. In fact, the ability to select the most suitable extraction method is as important to the toxicologist as the choice of the best treatment for his patient is to a doctor. The choice of the method to be used is dependent on a great many factors which are considered in detail below.

It should be noted that the methods described in this chapter have no authoritative basis. The quantities and other details specified are only a guide and may be varied to suit the particular analytical problem. In most cases the main objective is detection and not quantitative estimation. Most analysts appreciate that there is no single chemical procedure which alone will detect or exclude all known poisons but many fail to realise that this applies equally both to extraction methods and to the biological sample submitted for analysis. In order to exclude the maximum number of poisons it is necessary to analyse a variety of tissues and body fluids and to employ several different extraction methods.

Factors Influencing Choice of Method

A toxicological analysis must be carefully planned to ensure success and the 'backbone' of this plan will be the type and number of extraction methods employed. Four main factors must be considered. These are (1) the analytical aim, (2) the type of material to be analysed, (3) the resources available, and (4) the nature of the substances to be extracted. Answers are required therefore to the following questions.

1. Analytical Aim. Is the analyst required to detect lethal, toxic, therapeutic, or normal concentrations? Are only unchanged drugs of interest or must he also consider metabolised, conjugated, and protein-bound compounds? Is absolute proof of identity required or will an approximate indication of the type of poison be adequate? Should he exclude as many poisons as possible or will a more limited screening suffice?

2. Type of Material. Is the amount of sample large or small? Is it simple or complex (e.g. suspected poisoned water or exhumed viscera)? How many samples require analysis? Some extraction methods are more suitable for batch analysis, others are too time-consuming if more than one or two samples are to be extracted.

3. Resources Available. What identification methods are available? How much time and what personnel can be allocated to the problem?

4. Nature of the Poison. Is a particular poison or type of poison indicated by the case history? If so, is it a common substance with many published extraction methods or a new drug requiring trial extractions to establish its behaviour when processed? Is only one substance suspected or was the intoxicant a compound preparation containing several drugs? What drugs were administered as antidotes or to control the toxic symptoms?

GENERAL AND SPECIAL METHODS

When none of the above information is available the case is usually called a 'general unknown'. This type of case presents the analyst with a dilemma, for he cannot identify the unknown poison until he has extracted it and yet he may fail to extract it unless he knows its identity. To solve this dilemma analytical schemes employing probing or spot tests and general methods of extraction have been developed by toxicologists. Most of the extraction methods described in this chapter will be of this type because these general methods are essential for the investigation of unknown poisonings and have several advantages even when the toxic agent is known or suspected.

The specialised methods, that is, procedures designed to extract an individual poison or a select group of poisons, can be made efficient, rapid, and selective, even if not specific, because of their more limited purpose, but in certain circumstances they waste both time and material and may mislead the analyst. A specialised method is wasteful, for example, when the suspected poison is not present and misleading when the poisoning was caused by the combined effects of two or more drugs.

Some specialised methods of extraction are non-selective because the extraction details have been simplified for rapid processing of case material, because they utilise a non-specific identification technique, or, more frequently, because they are designed to estimate the drug rather than to identify it. For example, many of the methods based on the Bratton–Marshall colour reaction only require the preparation of a protein-free filtrate; consequently the drugs which give this reaction are never really extracted and the only evidence of identification involves the assumption that the drug sought produced the positive colour—a dangerous assumption in many cases! These non-selective special methods should not be used unless the analyst knows the identity and dosage of the drug administered and has full control of the environmental factors of the subject supplying the analytical material, e.g. drug investigations on laboratory animals and excretion-rate or plasma concentration studies on supervised subjects. Unfortunately, this type of method is often the only one the manufacturer can supply.

References to certain specialised methods are given in the monographs in Part 2 of this book; the general methods are described below. The choice of general methods is a matter of personal preference. Every method has its good and bad points and these have been listed as far as possible but this topic is very controversial so the only real guide is personal experience. It is usually better to acquire a lot of experience with a few methods than a little experience with many.

CLASSIFICATION

For analytical purposes, most toxicologists classify poisons according to the methods used for their extraction. It is convenient to consider five main classes as follows: (1) volatile poisons, isolated by distillation or diffusion, (2) metallic poisons, isolated by oxidation of the organic matter, (3) toxic anions, isolated by dialysis or ion-exchange methods, (4) non-volatile organic poisons, isolated by solvent extraction, and (5) miscellaneous poisons, requiring special extraction techniques. This classification is not rigid as many substances can be extracted by more than one of these methods and sometimes a combination of methods is necessary for efficient extraction. It is impossible to describe all these techniques in detail in a chapter of this size; only methods of fairly general application will therefore be mentioned.

1. Volatile Poisons

Many of these compounds can be detected without extraction, either by their odour or by gas chromatography of a small air-sample taken from the container in which they have been submitted; fluid samples may also be injected directly into a gas chromatographic instrument. It is important, therefore, to allow the sample to thaw and to smell it or examine it by gas chromatography before proceeding with a distillation process which can be time-consuming.

Two distillations are generally necessary. The first from acidified material to isolate acid and neutral volatile poisons, and the second from alkaline material to separate the volatile basic compounds. The distillates can often be used directly for qualitative and quantitative examinations but additional processing (e.g. solvent extraction) is sometimes required, especially when a volatile basic substance is sought.

Very simple distillations requiring only a suitable flask, air condenser, and test-tubes to collect the distillates may be used for routine qualitative testing of blood, urine, and gastric washings suspected of containing ethanol, methanol, acetone, acetaldehyde, etc., but usually more efficient methods are needed and a steam-distillation apparatus with ground-glass joints, steam-trap and anti-froth head, straight Leibig condenser, and a receiver immersed in an ice-bath should be available. All apparatus must, of course, be scrupulously clean.

Steam Distillation of Acid and Neutral Volatiles

Between 50 and 100 g of minced frozen tissue is macerated with an equal quantity of distilled water. The slurry is then transferred to the distillation flask with another equal quantity of water. The material is acidified with tartaric acid or dilute sulphuric acid and a few drops of a silicone antifoaming agent is added. The flask is then placed in a water-bath or heating mantle and connected to the condenser and steam-generator. Steam is passed until a volume of distillate equal in volume to the original sample has been collected (first fraction), when the receiver is changed and another similar fraction is collected. Alternatively, distillation may be continued until small aliquots give a negative spot test (if the poison is known) or have no abnormal odour. These distillates are labelled 'ACID and NEUTRAL VOLATILES'.

STEAM DISTILLATION OF BASIC VOLATILES

After cooling, the tissue slurry is made alkaline with solid magnesium oxide or dilute sodium hydroxide solution and steam distillation continued—the condenser, adaptor, and receiving flask should of course be rinsed or changed. The tip of the adaptor should be immersed in 0·1N hydrochloric acid contained in the receiver to prevent loss of the more volatile organic bases as they emerge from the condenser. The volume of distillate collected will depend on the compound sought but when this is unknown a rough guide is to collect two fractions each equal to the original volume of sample taken. These fractions are labelled 'BASIC VOLATILES'.

NOTES. Care should be taken to make the slurry acid or alkaline only immediately prior to distillation. A better yield of the volatile poison can often be achieved by saturating the slurry with sodium chloride.

Units of the type where the sample flask and steam-generator are combined take less bench space and require only one source of heat but are generally less versatile and more fragile than the conventional equipment.

As many of the compounds in this class can cause rapid death, distillation of the alimentary tract and its contents frequently yields large quantities of volatile poison. Samples of brain, lung, liver, and kidney are all suitable materials for analysis, and for some poisons, e.g. cyanide, the spleen should be analysed. Blood and urine can often be analysed more easily by microdiffusion methods or by gas chromatography.

TESTING THE DISTILLATES

(*a*) *Poison Known.* The distillates are suitable for direct testing if the poison is indicated by the case history. The appropriate monograph in Part 2 of this book should be consulted for a suitable test. A negative test may indicate the need to concentrate the distillate. Several methods can be utilised depending on the nature of the poison. Redistillation is useful especially if the distillate is collected in small fractions, for the very volatile compounds often distil over completely in the first few millilitres. Fractional distillation is recommended by Umberger (1954).

The less volatile substances may be solvent-extracted. The distillate is saturated with sodium chloride (acidified in the case of the acid volatiles or made alkaline for basic volatiles) and extracted with two 25-ml portions of ether; the choice of solvent is governed by the poison suspected and by the screening method to be adopted—see table of screening methods (p. 20). The ether extracts are dried with anhydrous sodium sulphate, filtered, and concentrated to about 10 ml by evaporation. The final concentration should be carried out at room temperature.

(*b*) *Poison Unknown.* Distillates may be screened by (a) spot tests, (b) paper, thin-layer, or gas chromatography, (c) ultraviolet spectrophotometry, or (d) infrared spectrophotometry—see table of screening methods (p. 20).

The analyst should be aware of the fact that the substance found may not be the original poison ingested. Thus the presence of xylene may be due to the ingestion of commercial preparations (e.g. pesticides) containing xylene as a solvent, *p*-nitrophenol may be found after parathion poisoning, acetaldehyde

SCREENING METHODS FOR VOLATILE POISONS

Substances	*Methods*	*References*
(i) Alcohols, aldehydes, aniline, benzene, camphor, carbon disulphide, carbon tetrachloride, chloral, chloroform, cyanides, *p*-dichlorobenzene, ketones, naphthols, phosphorus, pyridine, thymol	Spot tests and ultraviolet spectrophotometry (hexane as solvent)	Kaye (1961)
(ii) Most of the above plus nearly all the common industrial organic solvents	Infra-red spectrophotometry	Stewart and Erley (1965)
(iii) As for (i) but in greater detail	Spot tests—about 30 reagents are listed for probing and confirmatory tests on distillates	Gonzales *et al.* (1954)
(iv) Benzene, naphthalene, nitrobenzene, toluene, xylenes	Steam distillation, extraction with carbon tetrachloride, nitration, and final alkaline ether extraction of the nitrated hydrocarbons, followed by colour tests and paper and thin-layer chromatography	Bonnichsen *et al.* (1966)
(v) Alcohols, aldehydes, amphetamine, cyanides, ephedrine, halogenated aliphatic hydrocarbons, ketones, methylpentynol, nicotine, parathion, phenols, phosphorus, tranylcypromine	Tests for acid, neutral, and alkaline volatiles using spot tests, ultraviolet spectrophotometry, paper chromatography, and crystal tests	Curry (1963c)

after paraldehyde poisoning, and chloroform after chloral hydrate poisoning. Other volatile metabolites and impurities are mentioned in more detail by Turner (1965).

2. Metallic Poisons

The general extraction methods for this group have not changed as radically as the methods for the other groups because the number of metallic poisons is limited, their toxicity has been recognised for centuries, and their elemental nature ensures that the toxicologist is not plagued with breakdown problems. Isolation of this group may often be achieved by a simple ashing process, though wet oxidation methods are generally preferred. The various methods have been adequately reviewed by the Analytical Methods Committee (1960), Middleton and Stuckey (1953), and Dyfverman (1963). As only a very limited number of the drugs in this book have a toxic metal component, details of these methods are not given in this chapter, though any plan for a full toxicological analysis for an unknown poison must, of course, make provision for this group.

3. Toxic Anions

Treatment with permanganates, bromides, iodides, thiocyanates, chlorates, phosphates, etc. is not so prevalent as it was in the past because better remedies are available. Nevertheless, poisonings do still occur and it is surprising how little work has been done to investigate isolation methods for this group. It is rare to find tissue levels quoted for many of these substances, the typical published account of a fatality or an overdose being confined to a clinical history, details of the treatment employed, and the subsequent pathology. This may be due to the fact that many of the toxic anions are taken in such large amounts that their presence is usually indicated by the circumstantial evidence and therefore analytical confirmation is not required or because few systematic extraction schemes have been published. The conventional inorganic analytical tests, applied to a filtered specimen of the alimentary tract contents, will often suffice to confirm the diagnosis but an attempt at isolation and determination in tissues should be worth while if only to uphold Orfila's maxim that the real toxic agent is not identified unless it has been found in the body tissues.

Method A. A portion of the alimentary tract contents is filtered through a Whatman No. 90 grade filter paper. If the contents are thick and mucoid they should be treated with distilled water to form a filterable slurry. Spot tests for chlorate, bromate, oxalate, etc. are performed on aliquots of the filtrate. If the filtrate is unsuitable, i.e. too turbid, or if the slurry will not filter, a fresh 10% w/v solution of sodium carbonate is added, and the anion tests repeated after heating and filtering.

Method B. Curry (1963c) has described a systematic method based on dialysis of the test material in Cellophane bags or Visking tubing. This provides a better solution for testing and it frequently succeeds in cases where method A fails. It is more time-consuming however, and may give low yields with tissue slurries containing borate, chlorate, and oxalate. Two dialysates are prepared, one from the untreated contents and the other after making the sample acid with hydrochloric acid. These are dialysed against two 250-ml quantities of distilled water for 2 hours using mechanical stirring. When the sample for analysis is small the Cellophane or Visking tubing bag in which it is contained may be attached to a blade of the stirrer.

Method C. Ammonium Sulphate–Methanol. Rieders and Frere (1963) found that the dialysis of borate, chlorate, and oxalate from tissue slurries gave low yields even after 16 hours. Their method consists in coagulation of the tissue slurry with ammonium sulphate, concentration of the protein-free filtrate by precipitation of the ammonium sulphate with methanol, and evaporation of the supernatant liquid.

4. Non-volatile Organic Poisons—Isolated by Solvent Extraction

At the turn of the century less than 50 drugs could be classified as organic non-volatiles, but the pharmaceutical explosion which has occurred in recent years, whereby many new drugs are marketed each year, has made this classification obsolete in the sense that 90% of the drugs and poisons to be classified now fall into this group. It is too large for convenience and must be subdivided. Isolation procedures for this group therefore are divided into two stages. STAGE 1 involves the preparation of an aqueous concentrate and STAGE 2 the fractionation of this concentrate into several subgroups which consist usually of strong acid, weak acid, neutral, basic, and amphoteric drug fractions. There are many ways of achieving this division; a typical scheme is outlined in the diagram on p. 26 and as far as possible the extractions of the drugs in this book have been classified according to this scheme.

Stage 1: Preparation of the Aqueous Phase

Most of the orthodox toxicological methods require the preparation of a protein-free aqueous filtrate before the sub-group fractionation process is carried out. Brief practical details of four of these methods are given below together with a guide to their respective merits and some useful references if additional information is required.

(*a*) *A Modified Stas–Otto Method*

About 200 g of minced frozen tissue is acidified with tartaric acid and homogenised in a blender with 400 ml of ethanol. This slurry is heated on a water-bath for about 1 hour—if heat-labile alkaloids are suspected, the temperature should be below 60° or, better, the slurry should be allowed to digest overnight. The tissue–ethanol mixture is cooled and filtered. This process is then repeated with the residue and the two filtrates are combined. The ethanol is removed by low-temperature evaporation (i.e. by using a large shallow evaporating basin on a water-bath with a warm-air fan arranged to blow across the surface) or preferably by vacuum distillation. A syrup is produced which is extracted with 100 ml of hot absolute ethanol. This should be added gradually in several small portions, each being stirred with the syrup and decanted off before the next portion is added. The residue left behind after this treatment should be dry and granular, if it is still 'sticky' further treatment with hot absolute ethanol is required. The decanted portions are filtered and evaporated as before. This final residue is extracted with 100 ml of water acidified with a few drops of sulphuric acid and allowed to stand overnight if possible. Alternatively, it is transferred to a conical flask with the acidulated water and shaken for about 1 hour. If time permits and if the residue is fatty, the aqueous extract is decanted and the residue re-extracted with 100 ml of hot acidulated water, cooled and combined with the first extract. The water extracts are filtered (fluted Whatman No. 1 paper) and the filtrate is ready for solvent extraction in accordance with the procedure described for Stage 2 (p. 25).

Comments. This is a good general method which has been used for over one hundred years and therefore a large amount of data is available in the literature. Theoretically, it should extract most of the organic poisons and only a small amount of extraneous material. Unfortunately this ideal is not always achieved. The principles are simple but the practical application is something of an art. Its main disadvantages are that it entails many time-consuming extractions, filtrations, and evaporations; the extracts are often impure and the subsequent drug yield poor, and it is inconvenient for liquid samples. Nevertheless, one has the reassuring knowledge that many drugs have been successfully extracted by this method, it is useful to those analysts who receive their samples in alcohol, and it makes the analysis of obnoxious samples, such as faeces and putrefied material, a little less unpleasant.

(*b*) *A Tungstate Method*

50 g of minced frozen tissue is homogenised in a blender with 50 ml of a 25% w/v sodium tungstate solution and 50 ml of water. The mixture is transferred to a litre beaker and the blender washed with up to a further 200 ml of water which is

added to the homogenised tissue. Sodium bisulphate solution (50 ml of a 50% w/v solution) is added and the mixture is stirred and heated until it darkens in colour and protein coagulation occurs. It is then filtered hot through two Whatman No. 5 filter papers by means of a vacuum pump. When cool, the filtrate is ready for solvent extraction in accordance with the procedure described for Stage 2 (p. 25).

COMMENTS. This modification is based on a version of the Valov (1946) method. Providing the ratios of sample to reagents are maintained, any amount of tissue or blood from 10 to 200 g may be treated. It is rapid, generally produces a clean filtrate, and is particularly good for acidic and neutral drugs, but the extraction of some basic drugs by this method is less efficient than by other methods.

(*c*) *Ammonium Sulphate Method*

200 g of minced frozen tissue is homogenised in a blender with 200 ml of water acidified with dilute hydrochloric acid. Solid ammonium sulphate is added to make a saturated solution. The mixture is warmed in a water-bath to 65° until the protein coagulates—if heat-labile compounds are known to be absent the temperature may be increased to 90°; the higher temperature gives more efficient coagulation and cleaner filtrates and residues. When coagulation is complete, the mixture is cooled slightly and filtered through a Buchner funnel with Whatman No. 5 paper. The residue is then extracted with 200 ml of hot water and filtered as before—if the tissue is very fatty, the combined filtrates are left in a refrigerator and the solidified fat subsequently removed by filtration through a fluted Whatman No. 4 paper. When cool, the combined filtrates are ready for solvent extraction in accordance with the procedure described for Stage 2 (p. 25).

COMMENTS. This is a modification of the Nickolls (1956) method. The original Daubney and Nickolls method (1938) was designed to extract basic drugs and, although subsequent modifications have made it possible to use it as a general method, the extraction of acidic and neutral drugs is generally less efficient than the tungstate method. It is more rapid than the Stas–Otto method and is particularly recommended for samples with a high protein content and for the extraction of metabolites. Organic drugs with poor solubility in ether (e.g. iproniazid, phenelzine, morphine, etc.) may, nevertheless, be extracted with ether when the aqueous phase is saturated with ammonium sulphate. Another advantage of this method is that it is suitable for a wide variety of samples—it has been used for the isolation of organic poisons from viscera, urine, blood, intestinal and gastric contents, exhumation samples, meat pies, vegetable soups, tea, coffee, and raw eggs.

(*d*) *Acid Digest Method*

A measured portion of minced tissue or blood is mixed with an equal portion of concentrated hydrochloric acid. The resulting slurry is then diluted with an equal volume of water and heated in a boiling water-bath for 1 hour—the dilution with water is omitted for urine samples. The acid slurry is cooled and filtered. The residue is washed with water. If this residue is bulky it is transferred to a beaker and extracted with a volume of water equal to the original slurry. The first filtrate plus the filtered residue washings is then ready for solvent extraction in accordance with the procedure described for Stage 2 (p. 25).

COMMENTS. This method has the advantage that it liberates protein-bound and conjugated drugs that would otherwise not be available for solvent extraction. The hydrolysis that takes place during the preparation of the aqueous filtrate by this method gives increased yields of most of the phenothiazine drugs, imipramine, amitriptyline, quinine, and morphine. Increased yield of barbiturate drugs has also been reported by some workers. Unfortunately, it will decrease the yield of any drugs that are heat-labile or sensitive to acid hydrolysis. Atropine, aconitine, and cocaine, for example, should not be extracted by this method, and paracetamol, orphenadrine, dextropropoxyphene, nitrazepam, diazepam, and chlordiazepoxide are decomposed by the treatment with hot strong acid. These latter drugs can be extracted without decomposition by using 1N acid and keeping the temperature below 40° (Stevens, 1967) but these conditions would be too mild to release some of the conjugated drugs. If the amount of sample for analysis is very limited the residue remaining after steam distillation may be extracted by this method.

(*e*) *Direct Solvent Extraction*

In the past, direct solvent extraction was rarely used by the toxicologist except for the extraction of a known drug. The Extra Pharmacopoeia (Martindale), Vol. II, 23rd Edn, 1955, for example, contains direct solvent extraction methods for barbiturates, chlorpromazine, mephenesin, and methylpentynol in blood, but most of the other drug-extraction methods mentioned favoured the preparation of a protein-free filtrate. The introduction of reliable commercial ultraviolet and infra-red spectrophotometric instruments and the development of chromatographic procedures, particularly thin-layer and gas chromatographic techniques, has led to an increased interest in direct solvent extraction. These direct extraction methods are rapid and convenient but most of the published work is concerned with the extraction of a specific drug. Some general methods have been published but again these are usually designed for a particular detection technique and often only consider one of the major groups of drugs, e.g. the alkaloids.

Direct methods may be recommended for the extraction of fresh biological fluids but most toxicologists still rely on the classic protein precipitation methods for tissue analysis, especially when the nature of the drug is unknown. The most popular solvents employed are ether and/or chloroform. If the drug is unknown, the choice is a personal one; there is no perfect solvent. Trial extractions may be performed if the drug's identity is known or suspected and if time is available; otherwise, guidance may be obtained from the quoted solubility.

One of the most serious complications of direct solvent extraction methods is the formation of emulsions. Chloroform is probably worse than ether in this respect and certainly ether emulsions are easier to break. Prevention is better than cure, however, and a good general rule is to ensure that the solvent volume is much larger than the sample volume. If possible, a ratio of 10:1 is recommended, but when large volumes of biological fluids have to be extracted this is not practical.

The 'rolling' technique is usually the best solution in these cases. The sample and the extracting solvent are transferred to a bottle which is stoppered and placed upon rotating rollers. This technique avoids emulsion formation and is remarkably efficient (Clarke and Kalayci, 1963; Moss, 1965).

A typical direct solvent extraction method for fluid samples is as follows.

A measured volume of the sample is transferred to a separating funnel and acidified with 2N hydrochloric acid, 10 volumes of ether is added, and the mixture shaken for 1 minute. The ether is decanted off—this is the Acid Ether or A fraction.

The sample remaining in the funnel is made alkaline with 2N ammonium hydroxide and extracted with 10 volumes of chloroform—this is the Basic Chloroform or D fraction.

These A and D fractions may be dried, filtered, and evaporated, or further subdivided as in the diagram on p. 26. Successful identifications can often be made on these relatively crude A and D residues, especially when the sample for analysis is not too complex, the drug sought is present at a concentration in excess of 10 p.p.m., and the test employed is very sensitive and able to tolerate a high impurity:drug ratio.

Blood samples may be extracted at physiological pH unless ammoniacal decomposition has begun. If possible, coagulation should be avoided as the main advantages of this method will be lost and drug recoveries will be low. Small homogenised tissue samples may also be extracted but often troublesome emulsions are formed.

COMMENTS. This type of method is rapid, simple, and fairly efficient, especially when it is used with chromatographic examination procedures. It does not give good coverage of drugs which are extensively metabolised to hydroxy-compounds; these need salt-saturation techniques or the use of a more polar solvent. It is not a good method for drugs which are present as conjugated metabolites or exhibit strong protein-binding, e.g. morphine, amitriptyline, and phenylbutazone, etc.

STAGE 2: FRACTIONATION OF THE AQUEOUS PHASE

The fractionation of the aqueous phase, prepared by one of the methods detailed above, depends on the fact that most organic drugs can be extracted from aqueous solutions by immiscible solvents, the neutral and acidic drugs being extracted from acid aqueous solutions, and the basic drugs from alkaline aqueous solutions.

The neutral drugs can, of course, be isolated from either acid or alkaline aqueous solutions but it is usual to co-extract them with the acidic drugs rather than the basic drugs because the acid group is smaller and usually less of a problem than the basic group. If the acid group (e.g. salicylates and barbiturates) is known to be absent and the analyst wishes to proceed directly to the extraction of the basic drugs (i.e. by making the aqueous phase alkaline and extracting with ether or chloroform), he must remember that if any neutral drugs are present they will now be co-extracted with the basic drugs.

The diagram on p. 26 outlines the usual procedure. Precise details of solvent volumes, pH values, etc. have not been given because the scheme shown is a general one (i.e. it assumes that the poison is not known) and these details will vary according to the type of sample to be analysed. The aim at this stage is to discover if any poison is present and, if so, to isolate and identify it. Quantitative recovery cannot be expected until this information is known; only then can the best extraction method be selected and only then will precise details be required so that the analyst can calculate recovery factors. The notes which follow amplify certain points about the general extraction scheme shown in the diagram and should enable the analyst to modify it to suit his particular problem.

Explanatory Notes for Diagram of Extraction Scheme

The amount of solvent employed at points (1) and (2) in the diagram (p. 26) should be greater than or equal to that of the aqueous phase if this is large (i.e. 50 ml) and two such extractions should be made. If the aqueous phase is small, however, a single extraction with a volume of solvent 5 to 10 times that of the

Extraction Scheme for Non-volatile Organic Poisons

Stage 1

Direct Extraction — *or* — *Protein Precipitation*

Direct Extraction

urine, blood, stomach washings, water, beer, minerals, spirits, tablets, capsules, crystalline powders

Liquid samples are acidified
Solid samples are extracted with acidulated water

Protein Precipitation

urine, blood, stomach contents, food, milk, tea, coffee; tissues, faeces

Aqueous filtrate is prepared by Methods (a) Stas–Otto (b) Tungstate (c) Ammonium Sulphate or (d) Acid Digest

Stage 2

Filtrate

Extract with ether (1)*

Residue

This fraction will contain drugs which are insoluble in acidulated water (see Miscellaneous Poisons, p. 28)

Ether 'A' Fraction

This is called the Acid Ether Extract and will contain all the ether-soluble acidic and neutral drugs

It may be subdivided into 3 fractions:
A1—strong acid drugs
A2—weak acid or phenolic drugs
C—neutral drugs

Aqua

Make alkaline with ammonium hydroxide and extract with $CHCl_3$ (2)*

Chloroform 'D' Fraction

This is called the Basic Chloroform Extract and will contain all the chloroform-soluble basic drugs

It may be subdivided into 3 fractions:
D1—basic drugs with chloroform-soluble salts
D2—non-amphoteric basic drugs
D3—amphoteric drugs

Aqua

This fraction will contain the water-soluble, ether-insoluble, and chloroform-insoluble drugs (see Miscellaneous Poisons, p. 28)

* See references to (1) and (2) in Explanatory Notes, p. 25.

aqueous phase is usually effective. The classic technique of extracting with three or more small volumes of solvent is usually not worth while. It often produces emulsions and frequently yields more 'muck' in the residue than extra drug.

The Acid Ether Extract (or A fraction) will contain most of the acidic and neutral drugs (e.g. salicylates, barbiturates, phenols, carbamates, pyrazolones, etc.) whilst the Basic Chloroform Extract (or D fraction) will contain most of the basic drugs (e.g. antihistamines, phenothiazine tranquillisers, antidepressants, and alkaloids). These A and D fractions may be dried with anhydrous sodium sulphate, filtered and evaporated, and examined by paper or thin-layer chromatography or they may be subdivided, as shown in the diagram, by the methods indicated below. The analyst thus has the choice of preparing two, three, four, five, or six residues. The number chosen will depend on the amount of information or clues he has available about the probable identity of the unknown poison and on the nature of the sample he has to analyse.

Tablets, simple powders (e.g. capsule contents, sugar, salt, etc.) and liquids (e.g. water, beer, minerals and spirits, and 'watery' gastric washings) often require only a two-residue fractionation (namely the production of an A and a D residue). Blood, urine, and beverages such as milk, tea, and coffee, on the other hand, generally need a three-residue fractionation, whilst foodstuffs, tissue samples, faeces, stomach and intestinal contents with a large amount of partially digested food, and exhumation material often require a four- or five-residue fractionation. The ability to recognise the necessity for further fractionation from the appearance of the filtrates, precipitates, and residues is an art which can only be acquired by practical experience.

Subdivision of the A Fraction. The Acid Ether Extract is extracted twice with 1/10th of its volume of a freshly prepared 5% w/v sodium bicarbonate solution (A1 fraction), and then with two portions of 0·1N sodium hydroxide each equivalent to about 1/10th the original volume of the ether phase—this provides the A2 fraction. The remaining ether phase constitutes the C fraction. The bicarbonate solution will contain any strong acid drugs, the sodium hydroxide solution any phenolic or weak acid drugs, and the ether any neutral drugs.

The separated sodium bicarbonate and sodium hydroxide phases are acidified with hydrochloric acid and re-extracted with ether. These ether extracts are labelled A1 and A2 respectively. All three ether phases, i.e. A1, A2, and C, are dried with anhydrous sodium sulphate, filtered, and evaporated.

Subdivision of the D Fraction. The basic drugs can be divided into those whose salts are chloroform-soluble (D1), those which are extracted by solvents from aqueous solutions made alkaline with sodium hydroxide (D2), and those which are amphoteric and are not extracted by solvents from dilute sodium hydroxide solutions (D3).

The D1 group is larger than is generally supposed and apart from the phenothiazines includes most of the antihistamines, some alkaloids like aconitine, cocaine, papaverine, and hydrastine, and the synthetic narcotics alphaprodine, pethidine, and methadone. This extraction of the alkaloidal salts into the immiscible solvent generally occurs when they are present as the hydrochlorides and the extracting solvent is chloroform, but it is interesting to note that even strychnine sulphate can be extracted by chloroform from aqueous solution at pH 4·5.

The D2 fraction contains most of the other nitrogenous bases and the D3 fraction contains amphoteric bases such as those containing a phenolic group.

To prevent the loss of volatile bases, e.g. amphetamine and pethidine, a few drops of 2N hydrochloric acid should be added to the chloroform of the D fraction before it is evaporated. The residue, containing the basic drugs as their hydrochlorides, is then extracted with water, filtered if necessary, and extracted twice with equal volumes of chloroform. This chloroform solution is the D1 fraction. The aqueous phase is then made alkaline with 2N sodium hydroxide solution and again extracted with two equal volumes of chloroform (D2 fraction). Finally, the alkaline aqueous phase is acidified, made alkaline with solid sodium bicarbonate to pH 8·5, and extracted twice with ethyl acetate or a chloroform:ethanol mixture (D3 fraction). Unless volatile bases are known to be absent, the chloroform of the D2 fraction should again be evaporated in the presence of hydrochloric acid or slowly by a cold air-stream if the base is required.

The subdivision of the D fraction is not usually necessary, although if specific identification cannot be achieved it does assist the analyst to form an opinion of the drug's possible identity if he knows in which subgroup it was found.

The initial D residue obtained from most samples requires only a simple purification step before it is submitted to chromatographic analysis. A convenient procedure is to extract the chloroform solution with 0·1N sulphuric acid. The ultraviolet spectrum of this acid extract should be recorded at this stage, if possible. The extract is then made alkaline with a few drops of 2N ammonium hydroxide solution, re-extracted twice with equal volumes of chloroform, and finally washed, dried, and evaporated. This procedure is termed a 'back extraction' and it is a very useful general method of 'clean-up'.

5. Miscellaneous Poisons

Drugs which may not be isolated in detectable amounts by any of the above methods fall into this category. The number is relatively small, which is fortunate because they vary so much in character that it is almost impossible to devise a general extraction scheme. Broadly speaking, they are drugs which are very water-soluble or extremely water-insoluble at all pH values. The group includes proteins, glycosides, and certain lipids.

(a) WATER-SOLUBLE COMPOUNDS. The water-soluble, solvent-insoluble drugs form a difficult group. They can only be eliminated by special, rather than general, extraction methods and tests. Insulin, the choline drugs, and many of the antihypertensive drugs, e.g. bretylium, guanethidine, and hexamethonium, are typical members of this group.

The antihypertensive drugs have been extracted from blood and urine by cation-exchange chromatography (Tompsett *et al.*, 1961; Tompsett, 1962) as follows. A mixture of 100 ml of urine and 10 ml of 10N hydrochloric acid is applied to a column (70 × 10 mm) containing 3 g of Dowex 50W X12 (200 to 400 mesh). The column is eluted with 100 ml of 5N hydrochloric acid and 100 ml of 8N hydrochloric acid. The eluates are combined and evaporated to dryness in a vacuum still. The residue is then identified by paper chromatography.

The aqueous phase remaining after the extraction of the D fraction (see diagram on p. 26) may be acidified with dilute acetic acid, evaporated to dryness, and extracted with methanol. The methanol extract will contain most of the quaternary ammonium compounds and may be purified by paper chromatography (Clarke, 1960b).

(b) WATER-INSOLUBLE COMPOUNDS. The best general extraction method for the water-insolubles is a continuous solvent extraction process. The continuous extractor of Curry and Phang (1960), which can extract several hundred grammes of tissue with only about one litre of ethanol at 30°, has improved the extraction efficiency for saponins, glycosides, cantharidin, and pesticides. Where this apparatus is not available the sample should be ground and dried with anhydrous sodium sulphate and sand, packed into a large Soxhlet thimble, and extracted with the appropriate organic solvent in a Soxhlet apparatus.

Freeze-drying has been used recently by Erben (1967) to prepare blood and tissues for solvent extraction. If the toxicologist could easily reduce his samples to the consistency of many of the dried food products now available, some of these extraction problems might be solved.

Many of the water-insoluble drugs are soluble in alkaline solutions, e.g. many of the hydantoin anticonvulsants, chlorothiazide-type diuretics, and sulphonamides. The direct extraction methods are therefore often more efficient for these drugs than the protein precipitation methods where much of the drug will be rejected in the protein precipitate.

Insoluble drugs with high ultraviolet extinction coefficients are not likely to be overlooked. Barbiturates, for example, which have solubilities in water of about 1 in 1000 would often be termed 'insoluble', but they usually present no problem to the toxicologist because their E(1%, 1 cm) values are relatively high. For the same reason, sulphonamides, although commonly classified as insoluble, are easily detected, even when not suspected, either by ultraviolet spectral examination or by sensitive colour reactions—see under the relevant monographs in Part 2.

The analyst is also assisted by the fact that the toxic dose of both these groups of so-called 'insoluble' drugs are relatively high compared with those of other insoluble drugs, e.g. digoxin.

Detection of the small number of drugs which are liable to be missed by efficient general extraction methods and routine residue screening must depend on adequate case histories (so that the problem is not a 'General Unknown') and by development of good spot tests.

EXTRACTION STATEMENTS IN PART 2

Where possible the statements under the heading Extraction in the monographs in Part 2 have been given with reference to the diagram Extraction Scheme for Non-volatile Organic Poisons (p. 26). However, it has proved impossible to test every drug with this extraction scheme, therefore general guiding statements have been included.

'*X* is extracted by organic solvents from aqueous acid solutions' means that from theoretical considerations or from published work one can infer that *X* should be found in the A fraction. Similarly, '*X* is extracted by organic solvents from aqueous alkaline solutions' means that *X* should be found in the D fraction. The statement '*X* is extracted by organic solvents from aqueous acid or alkaline solutions' means that *X* will be found in the C fraction provided acid extraction precedes the alkaline extraction (see p. 27). The statement '*X* is extracted by organic solvents from aqueous ammoniacal solutions' has been used in some monographs in Part 2 to emphasise the fact that phenolic compounds cannot be extracted with chloroform from solutions made alkaline with sodium or potassium hydroxide.

Paper Chromatography

R. H. Fox

Paper chromatography is a very useful aid to the separation and identification of drugs and poisons. Although the development of thin-layer chromatography has provided the advantages of speed, sensitivity, and resolution in many cases, paper chromatography has the merit of simplicity and is capable of handling much greater quantities of material. This frequently enables a separated component to be eluted from the paper and further information such as ultraviolet and infra-red absorption spectra to be obtained. The technique is of the greatest assistance in the detection and identification of drugs and poisons isolated from body fluids and viscera and it is true to say that paper chromatography has been a major factor in the advancement of the science of analytical toxicology.

With the aid of paper chromatography it is frequently possible to detect microgram amounts of drugs in extracts of tissues and body fluids, and the problems presented by the use of multiple drug therapy may often be resolved by the use of chromatographic techniques. Any analyst who has been confronted with the problem of drug identification in tissue extracts will appreciate the enormous value of a chromatographic 'clean-up' of the extracts. Another factor of the greatest value is the use of general reagents or other methods of detection, such as ultraviolet absorption or fluorescence which can provide a very rapid means of establishing the absence of groups of drugs or of drawing attention to the presence of a compound requiring further investigation.

Methods

In general, paper chromatography is performed by either upward or downward migration of substances on a sheet of filter paper, one end of which is dipping into a suitable solvent.

In the **ascending** method, the solvent is placed at the bottom of the developing chamber. The substances to be analysed are applied to the paper on a starting line, which is drawn on the paper in pencil, and the paper is suspended in the solvent so that the starting line is a few centimetres above the surface of the solvent.

In the **descending** method, the developing chamber is equipped with a solvent trough which is supported at the top of the chamber and the paper bearing the substances under investigation is hung over a glass rod so that the end on which the spots of substance have been applied dips into the solvent in the trough.

In both techniques the developing chambers are sealed by ground-glass lids during development. At the end of the development, which is usually when the solvent front has travelled almost to the end of the paper, the paper is removed, the position of the solvent front is marked, and the paper is dried before inspection by ultraviolet light and application of chromogenic sprays. Some systems require 'equilibration', i.e. the vapour phase in the developing chamber is allowed to reach equilibrium with the solvent before the run is commenced.

Rf Values

The basic measurement in paper chromatography is known as the Rf value which is simply

$$\frac{\textit{distance travelled by substance from starting point}}{\textit{distance travelled by solvent front from starting point}}$$

This value is influenced by a number of factors including the temperature, the composition of the solvent, the time of the run, the size of the tank, and the length of time the paper is equilibrated with the solvent in the developing chamber before actual chromatography (Clarke and Hawkins, 1963). Hence great care should be exercised in drawing conclusions from Rf values. Whenever possible, control substances or mixtures of substances should be run on the same chromatogram as the unknown to enable the performance of the particular system to be checked and several samples of the unknown should be run on the same paper to enable as many tests for identity as possible to be applied.

Apparatus

A large variety of commercial apparatus is available for both descending and ascending paper chromatography. For the latter, however, a suitable apparatus is a circular jar approximately 30 cm high × 18 cm in diameter equipped with a ground-glass lid. The lid has a hole 4 cm from one edge through which is inserted a cork carrying a glass rod bent at right angles from which the papers may be suspended. Reels of chromatography paper, 12·5 cm wide, are cut into lengths of about 28 cm and a hole punched centrally at one end to enable the rod to pass through.

Simple ascending chromatography may be carried out in a beaker covered with a clock glass using a piece of filter paper rolled into a cylinder and secured with a paper clip.

Application of Samples

The sample solution should be applied in such a way as to prevent diffusion over too large an area—it should be confined to a spot about 0·5 cm in diameter. If it is necessary to make several applications of a dilute solution to the same spot, the spot should be dried between applications—a hair dryer is useful for this purpose. A special device for applying solutions of samples has been described by Clarke and Sowter (1964).

Relative Advantages of Methods

The ascending method enjoys the advantage that very simple apparatus may be used. The descending method requires more elaborate apparatus but faster running is achieved and the separation of compounds of low Rf value may be enhanced by permitting the solvent to run off the end of the paper.

Two-dimensional chromatography is widely used in the field of amino-acids but has found little application in the identification of drugs and poisons. The method involves the chromatography of a single spot of the sample which is placed at one corner of the paper. The spot is first developed with one solvent system and, after drying, the partially resolved substances are developed with another solvent in a direction at right angles to the first solvent. The resultant two-dimensional pattern of components is revealed by inspection under ultraviolet light and by suitable chromogenic sprays.

Location Reagents

As most organic compounds are colourless, some method must be employed to render the separated spots visible to the naked eye. When the paper is examined under ultraviolet light (preferably of wavelength 254 mμ), many compounds are revealed as fluorescent or absorbing spots. These spots may be ringed with pencil. The paper may then be sprayed with some reagent which will react with the substance in question to give a coloured compound. Suitable location reagents are listed under the systems described in the following pages and details of their composition and use are given in Appendix 1.

Instead of being sprayed, papers may be dipped into the reagent; in the case of reagents (such as Marquis) made up in concentrated sulphuric acid it is more satisfactory to spread the paper on a sheet of opal glass and pour the reagent over it.

Elution of Samples

Spots may be cut out of the paper and the material eluted and used for further identification techniques such as spectrophotometry. With untreated paper and unsprayed spots, simple elution with any suitable solvent will be enough. Material which has been located with iodoplatinate solution may be decolorised by treatment with a drop of a freshly prepared 10% sodium sulphite solution and the free base liberated by the addition of a drop of strong ammonia solution. Spots on citrate-buffered paper should be further treated with a drop of 10% barium chloride solution to convert the sodium citrate to the insoluble barium salt (Clarke, 1960a). Clarke and Hawkins (1960) have described a micro-evaporator which enables a dry eluate to be obtained after the spots of material have been treated as described above.

Paper Chromatographic Systems

The most usual systems employ solvents consisting of a mixture of organic solvent and water, with or without acid or alkaline buffering agents, the paper sheet being untreated. Other systems employ papers treated with various buffers and use aqueous organic mixtures as solvents. Two further important variations are the use of aqueous solvents on papers treated with hydrophobic substances (e.g. liquid paraffin, tributyrin, olive oil) and the use of non-aqueous solvents on paper impregnated with aqueous buffer; the former is known as 'reversed phase' chromatography—see systems RP1a and RP1b (pp. 41–2). Details of the various systems referred to in the monographs in Part 2 are given in the following pages.

For more detailed information on the various techniques and mechanisms of paper chromatography the reader is referred to *Chromatographic and Electrophoretic Techniques* (ed. I. Smith, New York, Interscience Publishers, 1960, Vol. I), *Chromatographic Reviews* (ed. M. Lederer, Amsterdam/New York, Elsevier Publishing Company, 1959 to date, Vols. 1 to date), and *A Manual of Paper Chromatography and Paper Electrophoresis* (ed. R. J. Block, E. L. Durrum, and G. Zweig, New York, Academic Press Inc., 1955).

2

SYSTEM P1: Nitrogenous Bases—General Screening Method

(i) Curry, A. S. and Powell, H., *Nature*, 1954, **173**, 1143
(ii) Clarke, E. G. C., *Methods of Forensic Science*, ed. Frank Lundquist, New York, Interscience Publishers, 1962, Vol. 1, p. 31

PAPER. Whatman No. 1, sheet 14 × 6 in, buffered by dipping in a 5% solution of sodium dihydrogen citrate, blotting, and drying at 25° for 1 hour. It can be stored indefinitely.

SAMPLES. 2·5 μl of a 1% solution; in 2N acetic acid if possible, otherwise in 2N hydrochloric acid, 2N sodium hydroxide, or ethanol.

SOLVENT. 4·8 g of citric acid in a mixture of 130 ml of water and 870 ml of n-butanol. This may be used for several weeks if water is added from time to time to keep the specific gravity at 0·843 to 0·844.

EQUILIBRATION. None.

DEVELOPMENT. Ascending, in a tank 8 × 11 × 15½ in, 4 sheets being run at a time. Time of run, 5 hours.

LOCATION. (1) Examination under ultraviolet light (254 mμ)
(2) *Iodoplatinate spray*
(3) *Bromocresol green spray*
(4) *Bromine–starch–potassium iodide*
(5) Clarke–Kalayci test
(6) Diazotisation followed by *alkaline betanaphthol spray* or N-*1-naphthylethylenediamine spray*
(7) *Diazotised* p-*nitroaniline–sodium hydroxide spray*
(8) p-*Dimethylaminobenzaldehyde spray*
(9) *Dragendorff spray*
(10) *FPN spray*
(11) *Iodine vapour*
(12) *Marquis reagent*
(13) *Millon's reagent*
(14) *Ninhydrin spray*
(15) *Nitrogen dioxide vapour*
(16) *Paraformaldehyde–phosphoric acid test*
(17) *Potassium permanganate spray*

Rf VALUES

The conditions described above were used to obtain the Rf values given in the monographs in Part 2 and listed in Part 3.

NOTE. As this system is not equilibrated, experimental conditions must be strictly adhered to in order to obtain reproducible results.

SYSTEM P2: Barbiturates

Fox, R. H. (unpublished data)

PAPER. Whatman No. 1, sheet 16 × 7½ in, prepared by dipping in a 10% solution of trisodium orthophosphate ($Na_3PO_4,12H_2O$), blotting, and hanging over glass rods overnight to dry. The drying may be accelerated by heating in an oven.

The prepared paper keeps indefinitely. Before use, the paper is dipped in a mixture of acetone: water (3:1). While the acetone is evaporating (about 2 minutes) spots of the barbiturate solutions are applied to a line ruled 3 inches from one end of the paper.

SAMPLES. 1% solutions of barbituric acids in ethanol, chloroform, ether, or other volatile organic solvent. Aqueous solutions of barbiturate salts may also be applied direct to the paper without prior isolation of the acid. The amount applied should be 10 to 50 μg.

SOLVENT. Ethylene dichloride. For the descending method, the ethylene dichloride is placed in the trough of the tank, water being placed in the bottom of the tank to keep the atmosphere saturated with water vapour. Occasional replenishment of the ethylene dichloride and water is all that is required to maintain the system in working order.

EQUILIBRATION. None.

DEVELOPMENT. (a) Descending, allowing the solvent front to descend about 10 inches. Time of run, 1½ hours. (b) Ascending—as a rapid screening method. A small piece of the treated paper may be placed in a 600-ml beaker and the chromatogram run for 10 to 20 minutes.

LOCATION. Under ultraviolet light (254 mμ) the barbiturates show as dark spots. If a small quantity of fluorescein is dissolved in the acetone–water mixture, the paper will exhibit a yellow fluorescence and the absorbing spots will be more readily visible.

CONTROLS. Since the quantity of water left after evaporation of the acetone is variable, the Rf values are not constant. It is essential that spots of three or four different barbiturates be run as controls on each occasion.

Rf VALUES—relative to Amylobarbitone

Allobarbitone	0·09	Methylphenobarbitone	2·00
Allylbarbituric acid	0·40	Nealbarbitone	0·72
Amylobarbitone	1·00	Pentobarbitone	1·16
Barbitone	0·06	Phenobarbitone	0·09
Butobarbitone	0·52	Phenylmethylbarbituric acid	0·06
Cyclobarbitone	0·24	Probarbital	0·08
Heptabarbitone	0·58	Quinalbarbitone	1·40
Hexobarbitone	2·40	Secbutobarbitone	0·52
Ibomal	0·29	Thialbarbitone	1·80
Metharbitone	1·35	Thiopentone	1·80
Methohexitone	1·68	Vinbarbitone	0·21

SYSTEM P3: Barbiturates

Ahmed, Z. F., El-Darawy, Z. I., Aboul-Enein, M. N., Abu El-Naga, M. A., and El-Leithy, S. A., *Journal of Pharmaceutical Sciences*, 1966, **55**, 433

PAPER. Whatman No. 1, impregnated by dipping in a 20 to 30% solution of formamide in acetone for about 10 to 15 minutes and drying in air. It should be stored in the dark.

SAMPLES. 3 to 4 μl of a solution in chloroform.

SOLVENT. 5N Ammonium hydroxide: benzene: chloroform (6:3:13).

EQUILIBRATION. Tank saturated with 20 to 30% of formamide in acetone.

DEVELOPMENT. Descending. Time of run, 2 to 2½ hours.

LOCATION. *Silver nitrate spray*, which produces white spots.

Rf VALUES

Allobarbitone	0·15	Hexobarbitone	0·77
Amylobarbitone	0·31	Methylphenobarbitone	0·63
Aprobarbitone*	0·19	Pentobarbitone	0·41
Barbitone*	0·06	Phenobarbitone*	0·07
Butobarbitone	0·24	Quinalbarbitone	0·13
Cyclobarbitone*	0·18		

* No real separation is achieved between aprobarbitone and cyclobarbitone and between barbitone and phenobarbitone.

SYSTEM P4: Barbiturates

Ahmed, Z. F., El-Darawy, Z. I., Aboul-Enein, M. N., Abu El-Naga, M. A., El-Leithy, S. A., *Journal of Pharmaceutical Sciences*, 1966, **55**, 433

PAPER and SAMPLES. As for P3.

SOLVENT. 5N Ammonium hydroxide: n-butanol: chloroform: formamide (3:3:5:1).

EQUILIBRATION, DEVELOPMENT, and LOCATION. As for P3.

Rf VALUES

Allobarbitone	0·12	Hexobarbitone	0·85
Amylobarbitone	0·46	Methylphenobarbitone	0·90
Aprobarbitone	0·29	Pentobarbitone	0·64
Barbitone*	0·09	Phenobarbitone*	0·06
Butobarbitone	0·35	Quinalbarbitone	0·56
Cyclobarbitone	0·23		

* Not too good a separation

SYSTEM P5: Barbiturates

Neil, M. W. and Payton, J. E., *Medicine, Science and the Law*, 1961, **2**, 4

PAPER. Whatman No. 1 or No. 4, sheets 10 × 38 cm.

SAMPLES. 10 to 15 μg as a solution in ethanol.

SOLVENT. Light petroleum.

EQUILIBRATION. Twenty-four hours before use, a vessel containing 200 ml of 60% v/v methanol in water is placed on the bottom of the tank with a sheet of Whatman No. 1 paper, 10 × 40 cm, dipping into it to provide a solvent wick to aid equilibration. Approximately 500 ml of light petroleum is run into the bottom of the tank and the lid replaced.

DEVELOPMENT. Descending, light petroleum being placed in the solvent trough. Time of run, on No. 1 paper: overnight; on No. 4 paper: 4 hours.

LOCATION. The paper is exposed to ammonia vapour and examined under ultraviolet light (254 mμ); all the spots absorb.

Rf VALUES—relative to Quinalbarbitone

Amylobarbitone	0·66	Hexobarbitone	2·35
Barbitone	0·07	Pentobarbitone	0·70
Butobarbitone	0·39	Phenobarbitone	0·10
Cyclobarbitone	0·22	Quinalbarbitone	1·00

SYSTEM P6: Neutral Drugs—Carbamates

Moss, M. S. and Jackson, J. V., *Journal of Pharmacy and Pharmacology*, 1961, **13**, 361

PAPER. Whatman No. 1.

SAMPLES. The residue from extraction is dissolved in a small quantity of ethanol.

SOLVENT. Strong ammonia solution:pentanol (1:9).

EQUILIBRATION. None.

DEVELOPMENT. Ascending, in 200 ml of solvent. Time of run, at least 5 hours.

LOCATION. (1) Examination under ultraviolet light (254 mμ). (2) *Furfural–hydrochloric acid spray*, which produces purple to intense blue-black spots on a pale green or grey background. The colour is stable for several months. Phenazone also gives a positive reaction, but only after a time lag of half an hour.

Rf VALUES

Carbachol (pure sample in methanol)	0·00
Ethinamate (pure sample in ethanol)	0·93
Mephenesin carbamate (pure sample in acetone)	0·83
Meprobamate (pure sample in acetone)	0·86
Methylpentynol carbamate (pure sample in ethanol)	0·88
Styramate (pure sample in acetone)	0·76
Urethane (pure sample in acetone)*	0·73

* Urethane evaporates, so it must be run immediately after spotting

SYSTEM P7: Neutral Drugs—Carbamates

Moss, M. S. and Jackson, J. V., *Journal of Pharmacy and Pharmacology*, 1961, **13**, 361

PAPER. Whatman No. 1, impregnated by dipping in a 40% solution of oleic acid in acetone, blotting immediately, and drying at room temperature.

SAMPLES. The residue from extraction is dissolved in a small quantity of ethanol.

SOLVENT. Acetic acid (glacial):water (1:1), shaken with a few drops of oleic acid.

EQUILIBRATION. None.

DEVELOPMENT. Ascending. Time of run, at least 6 hours.

LOCATION. As for P6.

Rf VALUES

Carbachol (pure sample in methanol)	0·82
Ethinamate (pure sample in ethanol)	0·51
Mephenesin carbamate (pure sample in acetone)	0·64
Meprobamate (pure sample in acetone)	0·71
Methylpentynol carbamate (pure sample in ethanol)	0·72
Styramate (pure sample in acetone)	0·78
Urethane (pure sample in acetone)*	0·89

* Urethane evaporates, so it must be run immediately after spotting

SYSTEM P8: Neutral Drugs—Dicoumarol and some Related Compounds

Christensen, F., *Acta Pharmacologica et Toxicologica*, 1964, **21**, 23

PAPER. Whatman No. 1.

SAMPLES. Solutions in ethanol or in 0·1M sodium hydroxide containing 5 to 30 μg.

SOLVENT. 3M Ammonium hydroxide:n-butanol (1:1).

EQUILIBRATION. None.

DEVELOPMENT. Descending.

LOCATION. (1) Examination under ultraviolet light (360 mμ). (2) *Diazotised o-dianisidine spray*. (3) *Diazotised sulphanilic acid spray*.

Rf VALUES

Dicoumarol	0·76	Phenindione	0·77
Ethyl biscoumacetate	0·75	Salicylic acid	0·60
Nicoumalone	0·88		

SYSTEM P9: Neutral Drugs—Dicoumarol and some Related Compounds

Christensen, F., *Acta Pharmacologica et Toxicologica*, 1964, **21**, 23

PAPER and SAMPLES. As for P8.

SOLVENT. 3M Ammonium hydroxide:ethyl acetate (1:1).

EQUILIBRATION, DEVELOPMENT, and LOCATION. As for P8.

Rf VALUES

Dicoumarol	0·31	Phenindione	0·04
Ethyl biscoumacetate	0·23	Salicylic acid	0·05
Nicoumalone	0·28		

SYSTEM P10: Neutral Drugs—Dicoumarol and some Related Compounds

Christensen, F., *Acta Pharmacologica et Toxicologica*, 1964, **21**, 23

PAPER and SAMPLES. As for P8.

SOLVENT. Acetic acid (glacial):benzene:water (2:2:1).

EQUILIBRATION, DEVELOPMENT, and LOCATION. As for P8.

Rf VALUES

Dicoumarol	0·96	Phenindione	0·96
Ethyl biscoumacetate	0·96	Salicylic acid	0·82
Nicoumalone	0·80		

SYSTEM P11: Organophosphorus Pesticides

Irudayasamy, A. and Natarajan, A. R., *Analyst*, 1965, **90**, 503

PAPER. Whatman No. 1, impregnated by dipping in a 15% v/v solution of liquid paraffin in light petroleum (boiling range 60° to 80°) and drying at room temperature for 1 hour.

SAMPLES. 1 to 2 μl of a solution in ethanol.

SOLVENT. n-Butanol:dimethylformamide:water (1:14:5).

EQUILIBRATION. None.

DEVELOPMENT. Ascending, until the solvent front has advanced about 90 cm. Time of run, about 3 hours.

LOCATION. The paper is exposed for about 20 seconds to bromine vapour and then allowed to stand in air for a few minutes to remove the final traces of bromine. The paper is then sprayed with *congo red spray* which produces clear blue spots against a red background. These spots are stable for 4 days, or 10 days if protected from light.

Rf VALUES

Diazinon	0·56
Malathion	0·90
Parathion	0·71

SYSTEM P12: Salicylates

(i) Algeri, E. J. and Walker, J. T., *American Journal of Clinical Pathology*, 1952, **22**, 37
(ii) Stevens, H. M., *Medicine, Science and the Law*, 1964, **4**, 118, and 1965, **5**, 157

PAPER. Whatman No. 1.

SAMPLES. Extract dissolved in a small quantity of acetone.

SOLVENT. Strong ammonia solution:n-butanol:water (33:100:66). The top layer of this mixture is placed in the solvent trough and the lower layer at the bottom of the tank.

EQUILIBRATION. None.

DEVELOPMENT. Descending, until the solvent front has advanced about 15 cm.

LOCATION. (1) Examination under ultraviolet light (254 mμ). (2) *Ferric chloride spray*.

Rf Values

Aminosalicylic acid	0·19	Gentisic acid	0·32
Aspirin	0·52	Mefenamic acid	0·80
(Aspirin is converted to salicylic acid on the paper by the alkaline solvent)		Salicylamide	0·45
		Salicylic acid	0·52
		Sulthiame	0·55

SYSTEM P13: Steroids—Corticosteroids

Johnson, C. A. and Fowler, S., *Journal of Pharmacy and Pharmacology*, 1964, **16**, Supp. 17T

Paper. Whatman No. 1, impregnated with a 40% v/v solution of formamide in methanol, which should be prepared immediately before use.

Samples. About 25 μg in 5 μl of acetone.

Solvent. A saturated solution of formamide in chloroform.

Equilibration. The prepared paper is equilibrated for 2½ hours in a tank which has been saturated with the solvent for 24 hours.

Development. Descending, until the solvent front has advanced about 35 cm.

Location. The paper is heated at 105° for 40 minutes, rapidly passed through a shallow layer of *DPST solution*, and immediately examined in subdued light. The reagent produces a violet spot on a pale yellow background.

Rf Values

Betamethasone	0·16	Hydrocortisone	0·26
Cortisone	0·62	Prednisolone	0·15
Dexamethasone	0·21	Prednisone	0·55

SYSTEM P14: Steroids—Corticosteroids

Johnson, C. A. and Fowler, S., *Journal of Pharmacy and Pharmacology*, 1964, **16**, Supp. 17T

Paper and Samples. As for P13.

Solvent. A saturated solution of formamide in a mixture of benzene:chloroform (1:1).

Equilibration. As for P13.

Development. Descending, until the solvent front has advanced about 22 cm.

Location. As for P13.

Rf Values

Betamethasone acetate	0·44	Fluocinolone acetonide	0·40
Betamethasone 17-valerate	0·86	Hydrocortisone acetate	0·59
Betamethasone 21-valerate	0·89	Prednisolone acetate	0·49
Cortisone acetate	0·80	Prednisolone pivalate	0·89
Dexamethasone acetate	0·60	Prednisone acetate	0·74
Fludrocortisone acetate	0·45	Triamcinolone acetonide	0·52

SYSTEM P15: Steroids—Synthetic Oestrogens in Urine

Tompsett, S. L., *Journal of Pharmacy and Pharmacology*, 1964, **16**, 207

PAPER. Whatman No. 1, stapled in the form of a cylinder.

SAMPLES. Urine is refluxed with hydrochloric acid, then extracted with ether. The extract is evaporated to dryness and dissolved in ethanol so that 1 ml of ethanol solution is equivalent to 50 ml of urine; 20 μl of this solution is applied to the paper.

SOLVENT. Strong ammonia solution:isopropanol:water (1:8:1).

EQUILIBRATION. None.

DEVELOPMENT. Ascending.

LOCATION. (1) *Pauly's reagent.* (2) *Diazotised* p-*nitroaniline spray.*

Rf VALUES

Dienoestrol*	0·85
Hexoestrol*	0·85
Stilboestrol*	0·85

* No separation

SYSTEM P16: Thiazide Diuretics

Pilsbury, V. B. and Jackson, J. V., *Journal of Pharmacy and Pharmacology*, 1966, **18**, 713

PAPER. Whatman No. 1.

SAMPLES. 5 μl of an extract dissolved in acetone.

SOLVENT. Strong ammonia solution:amyl alcohol (1:9).

EQUILIBRATION. None.

DEVELOPMENT. Ascending. Time of run, 6½ hours.

LOCATION. (1) Examination under ultraviolet light (254 mμ). (2) *Sodium naphthaquinone spray,* which produces stable orange spots within 5 to 15 minutes.

Rf VALUES

Bendrofluazide	0·22	Hydrochlorothiazide	0·08
Benzthiazide	0·36	Hydroflumethiazide	0·62
Chlorothiazide	0·05	Methyclothiazide	0·73
Cyclopenthiazide	0·80	Polythiazide	0·88
Frusemide	0·75	Teclothiazide	0·72

SYSTEM RP1a: Reversed Phase—General Screening Method

Street, H. V., *Acta Pharmacologica et Toxicologica*, 1962, **19**, 312 and 325

PAPER. Whatman No. 1 or No. 3, sheet 17 × 19 cm, impregnated by dipping in a 10% solution of tributyrin in acetone and drying in air.

SAMPLES. 5 μl of 1 to 5% solutions in ethanol or chloroform.

SOLVENT. Acetate buffer (pH 4·58).

EQUILIBRATION. The beaker containing the solvent is equilibrated in a thermostatically controlled oven at 95° for about 15 minutes.

DEVELOPMENT. Ascending. The paper is folded into a cylinder and clipped, the cylinder is inserted in the beaker containing the solvent which is not removed from the oven. A plate-glass disk thickly smeared with silicone grease may serve as a cover. Time of run, 15 to 20 minutes.

LOCATION. (1) Examination under ultraviolet light (254 mμ). (2) *Iodoplatinate spray*. (3) *Bromine–starch–potassium iodide*. (4) *Furfural–hydrochloric acid spray*. (5) *Potassium permanganate spray*.

Rf VALUES. These are given in the appropriate monographs in Part 2 and are listed in Part 3.

SYSTEM RP1b: Reversed Phase—General Screening Method

(i) Street, H. V., *Journal of the Forensic Science Society*, 1962, **2**, 118
(ii) Street, H. V., *Journal of Pharmacy and Pharmacology*, 1962, **14**, 56

PAPER and SAMPLES. As for RP1a.

SOLVENT. Phosphate buffer (pH 7·4).

EQUILIBRATION. The beaker containing the solvent is equilibrated in a thermostatically controlled oven at 86° for about 15 minutes.

DEVELOPMENT and LOCATION. As for RP1a.

Rf VALUES. These are given in the appropriate monographs in Part 2 and are listed in Part 3.

Thin-layer Chromatography

A. S. Curry

The use of thin-layer chromatography for the separation and identification of drugs and other compounds has developed into an everyday analytical tool for three main reasons—speed, sensitivity, and high resolution. Adequate separations of submicrogram quantities of material may be accomplished in under half an hour.

About 1960, when toxicologists became aware of thin-layer chromatography, the increase in sensitivity of the technique over conventional paper chromatography was undoubtedly the most attractive feature. At that period, paper chromatography had come to be of inestimable value in separating such large groups of compounds as the alkaloids into smaller groups containing perhaps only a few members, but most of the methods required at least 10 to 20 μg of material. The possibility of achieving separations on perhaps 0·1 μg of material by thin-layer chromatography excited all toxicologists.

However, thin-layer chromatography has not completely replaced paper chromatography in toxicology. It has taken a natural place as an additional chromatographic aid, being used on specific problems which are not so well solved by the other techniques or when the amount of material is very small. Typical examples of this are the cases in which therapeutic doses of several basic drugs may have been ingested, and only a small volume of blood is available for analysis—this occurs on many occasions when psychiatric disorders are involved. The monoamine oxidase inhibitors (substituted hydrazine derivatives) are difficult to detect by paper chromatography, but a phosphomolybdate spray readily reveals them as blue spots on a thin-layer plate. They are often found together with amitriptyline, chlorpromazine, or imipramine, and are more easily and quickly separated by thin-layer than by paper chromatography.

A further example of the usefulness of thin-layer chromatography is the identification of cannabis and cannabis resin. The classical test is the slow formation of a violet colour with Beam's reagent which is given by cannabidiol. This test is of relatively low sensitivity when done on plant material, but if a benzene extract from the plant or resin, or even from a smoked pipe, is purified by passage through a Florisil column and then submitted to thin-layer chromatography, a violet spot appears rapidly when the plate is sprayed with Beam's reagent. The clean-up process, coupled with the chromatographic separation, means that the cannabidiol is concentrated and purer.

Technique

The main layer media used are silica gel G, aluminium oxide G, kieselguhr G, and cellulose powder. The layer is prepared by spreading a thick aqueous slurry of the adsorbent rapidly and uniformly over the surface of a suitable support such as a glass plate. Several thin-layer spreading devices, which are adjustable, are commercially available. Plates may be coated in batches if they are placed side by side on a flat surface. The coated plates are air-dried and finally activated by heating at temperatures between 100° and 250° for a given time. The prepared plates may be stored in a desiccator. An optimum layer thickness of 0·25 mm is chosen for most routine analytical work.

The mixture of components to be separated is applied in a suitable solvent as small spots at least 1 cm apart along a starting line 1·5 cm from one end of the plate. The plate is then placed in a developing chamber containing solvent to a depth of 0·5 to 1 cm, and the chamber is closed with an airtight lid. The components of the mixture separate as the solvent ascends the layer. The solvent is usually allowed to rise about 10 to 15 cm up the plate which is then removed from the chamber, dried in warm air, and examined for the positions of the separated substances.

As with paper chromatography, some thin-layer systems require 'equilibration'. This is achieved by lining the developing chamber with filter paper which dips into the solvent.

Rf Values

The basic measurement in thin-layer chromatography is the same as that in paper chromatography—the Rf value (see p. 32). In my view, thin-layer chromatography, like paper chromatography, is a comparative art rather than an absolute one. Although Rf values and their reproducibility are certainly valuable criteria of identification, the effort required to produce absolute values is not always worth the trouble.

The most important factor in the reproducibility of Rf values is the nature of the layer at the time of use—in particular, it should be of uniform thickness. Much stress is placed in the literature on using dehydrated plates and on their storage in desiccators prior to use; this is certainly necessary for some investigations but, on the whole, no disadvantages are apparent if prepared plates are left on the laboratory bench for long periods before use.

Another important factor is the amount of binder present in the layer. Calcium sulphate is itself a strong adsorbent and it is possible that variations in the amount present can affect the separation.

Temperature is not such a critical factor in thin-layer chromatography due to the comparatively short developing time.

As with paper chromatography, control substances or mixtures of substances should be run on the same chromatogram as the unknown.

Apparatus

There are many variations in the design of equipment available for thin-layer chromatography. The support for the layer is usually a square (20 × 20 cm) or oblong (5 × 20 or 10 × 20 cm) glass plate. Precoated plates, plastic films of many sizes, and specially constructed drying racks are now commercially available. The drying racks greatly facilitate the storage of prepared plates.

In most forensic science laboratories, home-made plates are the order of the day—from microscope slides to the 20 × 20 cm size. Refinements such as the use of mixed layers with concentration gradients or indeed commercial equipment for making accurately prepared layers have not been widely used in toxicology because of the necessary increase in preparation time. As far as the developing chamber is concerned, although commercial ones are in widespread use, a beaker is often preferred, especially for small plates.

Application of Samples

The solution of the sample is spotted on to the plate from a micropipette or microsyringe, and care must be taken to avoid diffusion of the spot over too wide an area. The solution should be applied in stages and the spot dried in a stream of warm air. The amount of sample applied is normally between 1 and 10 μg. The use of larger plates and thicker layers enables larger amounts of sample to be applied.

Location Reagents

The methods of detecting substances after separation are essentially the same as in paper chromatography; corrosive spray reagents may be used and the plates may be heated after spraying. Many compounds are initially detected by examination of the plate under ultraviolet light (254 mμ), and many manufacturers supply precoated plates containing a material whose fluorescence is quenched by compounds absorbing at this wavelength. Suitable location reagents are listed under the systems described in the following pages, and details of their composition and use are given in Appendix 1.

One disadvantage of thin-layer chromatography compared with paper chromatography is that thin-layer chromatograms are more difficult to store as permanent records—although, of course, photographs or tracings can be made of the developed plates. However, a method of preserving the actual layer has been developed which involves spraying the chromatogram with a solution of polyvinyl propionate (Neatan); this sets to a clear plastic film and can easily be stripped from the glass plate under water together with the adhering layer.

Elution of Samples

Because of the smaller quantities of material used and the smaller sizes of the spots obtained in thin-layer chromatography, elution of the separated substances from the thin-layer plate is more difficult than in paper chromatography. An amount of adsorbent, taken from the same plate at a corresponding Rf value and treated in exactly the same way as the section of adsorbent containing the sample, acts as a reference control. After the addition of the eluting solvent to the section of the layer, centrifugation is usually necessary to remove the adsorbent. Aqueous solvents are not suitable for elution from adsorbents containing calcium sulphate binder. Some silica gel generally dissolves in an organic solvent but this can be minimised if the solvent is evaporated and a second, less polar one substituted.

The quantity of material present may be estimated directly on the layer by measuring the intensity of colour of the spot with a densitometer or by measuring the fluorescence of the spot.

Thin-layer Chromatographic Systems

There is generally little correlation between Rf values obtained with paper and with thin-layer solvent systems, but special mention must be made of the butanol–citric acid system which can be used on citrated paper (System P1, p.

34), or on a cellulose thin-layer plate, for the separation of alkaloids. The close correspondence in Rf values so obtained is of particular value in that the vast amount of information already available for the paper system can be transposed to the more sensitive and rapid thin-layer system.

Two-dimensional thin-layer chromatography has been used quite successfully in the separation of mixtures of drugs.

Details of the various systems referred to in the monographs in Part 2 are given below.

SYSTEM T1: Nitrogenous Bases—General Screening Method

Sunshine, I., *American Journal of Clinical Pathology*, 1963, **40**, 576 (modified)

PLATES. Glass plates, 20 × 20 cm, coated with a slurry consisting of 30 g of silica gel G in 60 ml of water to give a layer 0·25 mm thick and dried at 110° for 1 hour.

SAMPLES. 1·0 μl of a 1% solution in 2N acetic acid ('Microdrops', see p. 136, may also be employed).

SOLVENT. Strong ammonia solution: methanol (1·5:100). It should be changed after two runs.

EQUILIBRATION. The solvent is allowed to stand in the tank for 1 hour.

DEVELOPMENT. Ascending, in a tank, 21 × 21 × 10 cm, the ends of the tank being covered with filter paper to assist evaporation. Time of run, 30 minutes.

LOCATION.
(1) Examination under ultraviolet light (254 mμ)
(2) *Acidified iodoplatinate spray*
(3) Diazotisation followed by *alkaline betanaphthol spray* or N-*1-naphthylethylenediamine spray*
(4) *Diazotised* p-*nitroaniline–sodium hydroxide spray*
(5) *Dragendorff spray*
(6) p-*Dimethylaminobenzaldehyde spray*
(7) *Iodine–carbon tetrachloride spray*
(8) *Marquis reagent*
(9) *Nitrogen dioxide vapour*
(10) *Potassium permanganate spray*

Rf VALUES
The conditions described above were used to obtain the Rf values given in the monographs in Part 2 and listed in Part 3.

SYSTEM T2: Antihistamines and Chlordiazepoxide

Cochin, J. and Daly, J. W., *Journal of Pharmacology and Experimental Therapeutics*, 1963, **139**, 160

PLATES. Glass plates, coated with a slurry consisting of 30 g of aluminium oxide G in 30 ml of water and dried at 80° for 45 minutes. They should be stored in a desiccator.

SAMPLES. 10 to 50 μl (about 1 to 20 μg) of the extract in ethanol.

SOLVENT. Acetic acid: butanol: butyl ether (10:40:80).

EQUILIBRATION. None.

DEVELOPMENT. Ascending, until the solvent front has advanced 10 cm.

LOCATION. *Iodoplatinate spray.*

Rf VALUES

Antazoline	0·38	Doxylamine	0·60
Bromodiphenhydramine	0·63	Hydroxyzine	0·84
Brompheniramine	0·48	Mepyramine	0·56
Carbinoxamine	0·63	Methapyrilene	0·56
Chlorcyclizine	0·49	Phenindamine	0·65
Chlordiazepoxide	0·70	Pheniramine	0·63
Chloropyrilene	0·66	Thonzylamine	0·59
Chlorpheniramine	0·52	Tripelennamine	0·62
Diphenhydramine	0·53	Triprolidine	0·81

SYSTEM T3: Antihistamines and Tranquillisers

Cochin, J. and Daly, J. W., *Journal of Pharmacology and Experimental Therapeutics*, 1963, **139**, 160

PLATES. Glass plates, coated with a slurry consisting of 25 g of silica gel G in 50 ml of water and dried at 80° for 30 minutes. They should be stored in a desiccator.

SAMPLES. As for T2.

SOLVENT. Ammonium hydroxide solution:benzene:dioxan (5:60:35).

EQUILIBRATION. None.

DEVELOPMENT. As for T2.

LOCATION. (1) *Iodoplatinate spray* detects all the compounds.
(2) *Sulphuric acid–ethanol spray* detects only the phenothiazines and related compounds.

Rf VALUES

Amitriptyline	0·74	Methapyrilene	0·83
Antazoline	0·31	Methdilazine	0·40
Bromodiphenhydramine	0·86	Methoxypromazine	0·74
Brompheniramine	0·42	Perphenazine	0·36
Carbinoxamine	0·33	Phenindamine	0·90
Chlorcyclizine	0·90	Pheniramine	0·68
Chlordiazepoxide	0·10	Prochlorperazine	0·70
Chloropyrilene	0·70	Promazine	0·62
Chlorpheniramine	0·40	Promethazine	0·70
Chlorpromazine	0·94	Pyrrobutamine	0·84
Chlorprothixene	0·80	Thiopropazate	0·97
Diphenhydramine	0·91	Thioridazine	0·97
Doxylamine	0·52	Thonzylamine	0·65
Fluopromazine	0·95	Trifluoperazine	0·69
Fluphenazine	0·34	Trimeprazine	0·96
Hydroxyzine	0·27	Tripelennamine	0·92
Imipramine	0·86	Triprolidine	0·40
Mepyramine	0·82		

SYSTEM T4: Antihistamines and Tranquillisers

Cochin, J. and Daly, J. W., *Journal of Pharmacology and Experimental Therapeutics*, 1963, **139**, 160

PLATES. As for T3.

SAMPLES. As for T2.

SOLVENT. Acetic acid: ethanol: water (30:50:20).

EQUILIBRATION and DEVELOPMENT. As for T2.

LOCATION. As for T3.

Rf VALUES

Amitriptyline	0·65	Methdilazine	0·61
Antazoline	0·72	Methoxypromazine	0·58
Bromodiphenhydramine	0·80	Pecazine	0·57
Brompheniramine	0·47, tailing	Perphenazine	0·44
Carbinoxamine	0·40, tailing	Phenindamine	0·67
Chlorcyclizine	0·68	Pheniramine	0·38, tailing
Chlordiazepoxide	0·67	Pipamazine	0·72
Chloropyrilene	0·56, tailing	Prochlorperazine	0·27
Chlorpheniramine	0·41, tailing	Promazine	0·38
Chlorpromazine	0·70	Promethazine	0·59
Chlorprothixene	0·73	Pyrrobutamine	0·82
Diphenhydramine	0·61	Thiopropazate	0·67
Doxylamine	0·38, tailing	Thioridazine	0·65
Fluopromazine	0·79	Thonzylamine	0·57
Fluphenazine	0·58	Trifluoperazine	0·33
Hydroxyzine	0·70	Trimeprazine	0·64
Imipramine	0·77	Tripelennamine	0·48, tailing
Mepyramine	0·43, tailing	Triprolidine	0·48, tailing
Methapyrilene	0·52, tailing		

SYSTEM T5: Antihistamines and Tranquillisers

Cochin, J. and Daly, J. W., *Journal of Pharmacology and Experimental Therapeutics*, 1963, **139**, 160

PLATES. As for T3.

SAMPLES. As for T2.

SOLVENT. n-Butanol: methanol (40:60).

EQUILIBRATION and DEVELOPMENT. As for T2.

LOCATION. As for T3.

Rf VALUES

Amitriptyline	0·39	Chlordiazepoxide	0·73
Antazoline	0·40	Chloropyrilene	0·29
Bromodiphenhydramine	0·33	Chlorpheniramine	0·20
Brompheniramine	0·16	Chlorpromazine	0·30
Carbinoxamine	0·17	Chlorprothixene	0·46
Chlorcyclizine	0·40	Diphenhydramine	0·25

Doxylamine	0·17	Pipamazine	0·56
Fluopromazine	0·40	Prochlorperazine	0·32
Fluphenazine	0·68	Promazine	0·37
Hydroxyzine	0·62	Promethazine	0·22
Imipramine	0·29	Pyrrobutamine	0·32
Mepyramine	0·27	Thiopropazate	0·70
Methapyrilene	0·30	Thioridazine	0·20
Methdilazine	0·16	Thonzylamine	0·32
Methoxypromazine	0·24	Trifluoperazine	0·40
Pecazine	0·29	Trimeprazine	0·30
Perphenazine	0·48	Tripelennamine	0·23
Phenindamine	0·48	Triprolidine	0·26
Pheniramine	0·19		

SYSTEM T6: Phenothiazines and their Sulphoxides

(i) Korczak-Fabierkiewicz, C., Kofoed, J., and Lucas, G. H. W., *Journal of Forensic Sciences*, 1965, **10**, 308
(ii) idem, *Nature*, 1966, **211**, 147

PLATES. Glass plates, 20 × 20 cm, coated with silica gel G or with aluminium oxide G.

SAMPLES. 2 spots of a solution of the phenothiazine are applied at the lower left and right corners of the plate.

SOLVENT. 3 g of ammonium acetate in a mixture of 20 ml of distilled water and 100 ml of methanol.

EQUILIBRATION. None.

DEVELOPMENT. Ascending, until the solvent front has advanced to 3 to 4 cm from the top of the plate.

LOCATION. Examination under ultraviolet light.

Conversion to the sulphoxide derivative. The right hand spot is wetted lightly with small drops of hydrogen peroxide solution and dried in a stream of hot air (about 60°). The plate is replaced in the tank, the treated spot being at the bottom and development being allowed to proceed in a direction at right angles to the initial one.
Location of the sulphoxide derivative. Examination under ultraviolet light.

ELUTION. The areas around the spots are removed, the material eluted with distilled water, and examined spectrophotometrically.

Rf VALUES. (a) of original drug; (b) of sulphoxide

	a	b
Acepromazine	0·58	0·39
Acetophenazine	0·69	0·16
Carphenazine	0·71	0·16
Chlorpromazine	0·62	0·48
Chlorprothixene	0·66	0·45
Diethazine	0·69	0·44
Dimethoxanate	0·56	0·41

Ethopropazine	0·70	0·47
Fluopromazine	0·69	0·50
Fluphenazine	0·75	0·59
Isothipendyl	0·64	0·41
Methdilazine	0·64	0·43
Methoxypromazine	0·67	0·35
Perphenazine	0·65	0·45
Phenothiazine	0·69	0·37
Pipamazine	0·83	0·53
Prochlorperazine	0·55	0·15
Promazine	0·51	0·37
Promethazine	0·66	0·38
Propiomazine	0·77	0·54
Prothipendyl	0·69	0·48
Thiethylperazine	0·47	0·28
Thiopropazate	0·77	0·25
Thioproperazine	0·43	0·26
Thioridazine	0·71	0·46
Trifluoperazine	0·63	0·41
Trimeprazine	0·71	0·50

SYSTEM T7: Narcotic Analgesics

Mulé, S. J., *Analytical Chemistry*, 1964, **36**, 1907

PLATES. Glass plates, 20 × 20 cm, coated with a slurry consisting of 30 g of silica gel G in 60 ml of double-distilled water.

SAMPLES. 1 to 5 μl (about 1 to 25 μg) of the extract in 25 to 100 μl of methanol.

SOLVENT. Strong ammonia solution:benzene:dioxan:ethanol (5:50:40:5).

EQUILIBRATION. None.

DEVELOPMENT. Ascending, in a tank, $8\frac{1}{2} \times 4\frac{1}{2} \times 8\frac{1}{2}$ in, containing 100 ml of the solvent, until the solvent front advances 10 cm. After the plate has been air-dried for 10 minutes, it is dried in an oven at 100° for 15 minutes.

LOCATION. *Iodoplatinate spray.*

Rf VALUES

Alphaprodine	0·93	Levomethorphan	0·91
Codeine	0·39	Levorphanol	0·80
Dextropropoxyphene	0·97	Methadone	0·99
Dextrorphan	0·80	6-Monoacetylmorphine	0·64
Diamorphine	0·76	Morphine	0·11
Dihydromorphine	0·10	Nalorphine	0·35
Ethylmorphine	0·46	Norcodeine	0·13
Hydrocodone	0·41	Normorphine	0·04
Hydromorphone	0·17	Pethidine	0·97
Ketobemidone	0·47	Phenazocine	0·97
Levallorphan	0·98	Piminodine	0·99

SYSTEM T8: Narcotic Analgesics

Mulé, S. J., *Analytical Chemistry*, 1964, **36**, 1907

PLATES and SAMPLES. As for T7.

SOLVENT. Acetic acid (glacial): ethanol: water (30:60:10).

EQUILIBRATION, DEVELOPMENT, and LOCATION. As for T7.

Rf VALUES

Alphaprodine	0·40	Levomethorphan	0·43
Codeine	0·29	Levorphanol	0·47
Dextropropoxyphene	0·68	Methadone	0·59
Dextrorphan	0·47	6-Monoacetylmorphine	0·40
Diamorphine	0·35	Morphine	0·27
Dihydromorphine	0·21	Nalorphine	0·55
Ethylmorphine	0·25	Norcodeine	0·50
Hydrocodone	0·25	Normorphine	0·48
Hydromorphone	0·21	Pethidine	0·41
Ketobemidone	0·39	Phenazocine	0·87
Levallorphan	0·70	Piminodine	0·73

SYSTEM T9: Ergot Alkaloids

(i) Genest, K. and Farmilo, C. G., *Journal of Pharmacy and Pharmacology*, 1964, **16**, 250
(ii) French, W. N. and Wehrli, A., *Journal of Pharmaceutical Sciences*, 1965, **54**, 1515
(iii) Clarke, E. G. C., *Journal of the Forensic Science Society*, 1967, **7**, 46

PLATES. For (i): glass plates coated with a slurry consisting of 30 g of silica gel G (Merck) in 60 ml of 0·1N sodium hydroxide to give a layer 0·25 mm thick. For (ii): glass plates coated with a slurry consisting of 5 g of silica gel G (Merck) in 10 ml of 0·1N sodium hydroxide; the plates are activated before use by heating at 110° for 30 minutes.
For (iii): as for (i) followed by activation before use by heating at 110° for 30 minutes.

SAMPLES. For (i): 1 to 10 μg in water.
For (ii): about 5 μg in ethanol.
For (iii): 1 μl of a 1% solution in 2N acetic acid.

SOLVENT. For (i), (ii), and (iii): chloroform: methanol (9:1).

EQUILIBRATION. For (ii) and (iii): the solvent is allowed to stand in the tank for 1 hour.

DEVELOPMENT. For (i) and (iii): Ascending, about 20 cm. Time of run, about 10 minutes.
For (ii): Ascending. Time of run, about 33 minutes.

LOCATION. (1) Examination under ultraviolet light (254 mμ). (2) p-*Dimethylaminobenzaldehyde spray* which produces blue spots.

Rf VALUES	for (i)	for (ii)	for (iii)
Dihydroergotamine	0·35	0·45	0·56
Ergocristine	0·71	—	—
Ergometrine maleate	0·18	0·19	0·23
Ergotamine tartrate	0·52	0·51	0·58

Ergotoxine	0·45–0·69–0·81	—	0·78
Lysergamide	—	—	0·18
Lysergic acid	0·05	—	0·01
Lysergide	0·60	0·61	0·63
Methylergometrine	—	0·23	0·30
Methysergide	—	0·35	0·49

SYSTEM T10: Barbiturates; Glutarimides, Bromoureides, and Hydantoins

Bogan, J., Rentoul, E., and Smith, H., *Journal of the Forensic Science Society*, 1964, **4**, 147

PLATES. Glass plates coated with a slurry consisting of 30 g of silica gel G (Merck) in 60 ml of water to give a layer 0·25 mm thick and dried at 120° for 30 minutes. The plates should be used immediately.

SAMPLES. The extracted residue in 200 µl of chloroform is spotted on the plate 0·5 cm above the level of the solvent, the diameter of the spots being not more than 2 mm and the spots not less than 0·5 cm apart. The chloroform is removed by infra-red heat.

SOLVENT. Acetone:chloroform (1:9).

EQUILIBRATION. In the bottom of a gas jar lined with filter paper, the solvent is placed to a depth of 1 cm and the plates equilibrated above it.

DEVELOPMENT. Ascending, until the solvent front advances 10 cm. Time of run, about 17 minutes.

LOCATION. (1) *Fluorescein spray*, which produces pink spots. (2) *Mercurous nitrate spray*, which produces black spots, fading rapidly. (3) *Potassium permanganate spray*, which produces yellow-brown spots on a purple background. (4) *Zwikker's reagent spray*, which produces pink or green spots.

Rf VALUES

Allobarbitone	0·27	Metharbitone	0·55
Allylbarbituric acid	0·36	Methohexitone	0·67
Amylobarbitone	0·33	Methylphenobarbitone	0·59
Aprobarbitone	0·30	Nealbarbitone	0·38
Barbitone	0·22	Pentobarbitone	0·33
Bemegride	0·39	Phenobarbitone	0·24
Bromvaletone	0·26	Phenylmethylbarbituric acid	0·12
Butallylonal	0·28	Phenytoin	0·20
Butobarbitone	0·33	Probarbital	0·24
Carbromal	0·50	Quinalbarbitone	0·44
Cyclobarbitone	0·32	Thialbarbitone	0·69
Glutethimide	0·52	Thiopentone	0·68
Heptabarbitone	0·31	Vinbarbitone	0·28
Hexobarbitone	0·50		

SYSTEM T11: Barbiturates; Glutethimide, Ethinamate, Ethchlorvynol, and Methyprylone

Cochin, J. and Daly, J. W., *Journal of Pharmacology and Experimental Therapeutics*, 1963, **139**, 154

PLATES. Glass plates coated with a slurry consisting of 25 g of silica gel G in

50 ml of water and dried at 80° for 30 minutes. They should be stored in a desiccator.

SAMPLES. 5 to 10 μl of a chloroform or methanol solution containing 1 to 20 μg of extracted residue.

SOLVENT. Acetic acid (glacial): benzene (1:9).

EQUILIBRATION. None.

DEVELOPMENT. Ascending, until the solvent front has advanced 10 cm.

LOCATION. (1) *Mercurous nitrate spray*, which produces white spots on a grey background. This spray allows detection of 1 to 5 μg of barbiturates and of glutethimide but is less sensitive towards ethinamate, ethchlorvynol, and methyprylone for which 10 to 20 μg of sample is required. (2) *Potassium permanganate spray*, which produces yellow spots on a purple background for barbiturates containing an unsaturated side-chain or a 2-mercapto-substituent. The spray may be used independently or following the mercurous nitrate spray. It detects 5 to 10 μg amounts of ethinamate, ethchlorvynol, or methyprylone and should be used for confirmation.

Rf VALUES

Allobarbitone	0·43	Metharbitone	0·53
Allylbarbituric acid	0·48	Methohexitone	0·75
Amylobarbitone	0·42	Methylphenobarbitone	0·85
Barbitone	0·38	Methyprylone	0·81
Cyclobarbitone	0·55	Pentobarbitone	0·40
Ethchlorvynol	0·32	Phenobarbitone	0·36
Ethinamate	0·65	Quinalbarbitone	0·46
Glutethimide	0·54	Secbutobarbitone	0·49
Hexobarbitone	0·49	Thiopentone	0·73

SYSTEM T12: Barbiturates; Glutethimide, Ethinamate, Ethchlorvynol, and Methyprylone

Cochin, J. and Daly, J. W., *Journal of Pharmacology and Experimental Therapeutics*, 1963, **139**, 154

PLATES and SAMPLES. As for T11.

SOLVENT. Strong ammonia solution: benzene: dioxan (5:75:20).

EQUILIBRATION, DEVELOPMENT, and LOCATION. As for T11.

Rf VALUES

Allobarbitone	0·48	Metharbitone	0·66
Allylbarbituric acid	0·50	Methohexitone	0·78
Amylobarbitone	0·52	Methylphenobarbitone	0·60
Barbitone	0·40	Methyprylone	0·45
Cyclobarbitone	0·38	Pentobarbitone	0·49
Ethchlorvynol	0·95	Phenobarbitone	0·26
Ethinamate	0·55	Quinalbarbitone	0·54
Glutethimide	0·99	Secbutobarbitone	0·52
Hexobarbitone	0·58	Thiopentone	0·70

SYSTEM T13: Barbiturates; Glutethimide, Ethinamate, Ethchlorvynol, and Methyprylone

Cochin, J. and Daly, J. W., *Journal of Pharmacology and Experimental Therapeutics*, 1963, **139**, 154

PLATES and SAMPLES. As for T11.

SOLVENT. Acetone:chloroform (1:9).

EQUILIBRATION, DEVELOPMENT, and LOCATION. As for T11.

Rf VALUES

Allobarbitone	0·55	Metharbitone	0·85
Allylbarbituric acid	0·67	Methohexitone	0·92
Amylobarbitone	0·60	Methylphenobarbitone	0·98
Barbitone	0·50	Methyprylone	0·50
Cyclobarbitone	0·68	Pentobarbitone	0·57
Ethchlorvynol	0·95	Phenobarbitone	0·50
Ethinamate	0·81	Quinalbarbitone	0·64
Glutethimide	0·80	Secbutobarbitone	0·62
Hexobarbitone	0·77	Thiopentone	0·94

SYSTEM T14: Cardiac Glycosides

Johnston, E. J. and Jacobs, A. L., *Journal of Pharmaceutical Sciences*, 1966, **55**, 531

PLATES. Glass plates, coated with a slurry of silica gel G (Merck) to give a layer 0·25 mm thick, air-dried for 10 minutes, and activated in an oven at 120° for 45 minutes. They should be stored in a desiccator.

SAMPLES. 1 to 100 μg, usually in methanol.

SOLVENT. Benzene:ethanol (7:3 v/v).

EQUILIBRATION. None.

DEVELOPMENT. Ascending.

LOCATION. (1) *Perchloric acid spray*, which produces spots fluorescing under ultraviolet light (366 mμ) and a charring effect after the sprayed plate has been in an oven at 100° for a few minutes. (2) p-*Anisaldehyde spray*, which produces blue spots (ouabain, yellow spot) after the sprayed plate has been heated at 100° for a few minutes.

Rf VALUES

Acetyldigitoxin	0·82	Digoxin	0·62
Deslanoside	0·27	Lanatoside C	0·36
Digitoxin	0·72	Ouabain	0·09

SYSTEM T15: Organophosphorus Pesticides

Pejković-Tadić, I., Ćelap, M. B., Janjić, T. J., and Vitorović, S. Lj., *Analyst*, 1966, **91**, 595

PLATES. Glass plates, 20 × 20 cm, coated with a slurry of silica gel G to give a layer 0·2 mm thick.

SAMPLES. 1 to 3 μl of a standard chloroform solution.

SOLVENT. Acetone:hexane (1:4).

EQUILIBRATION. None.

DEVELOPMENT. Ascending, until the solvent front has advanced 14 cm. Time of run, about 30 minutes.

LOCATION. *Palladium chloride spray.*

Rf VALUES

Azinphos-methyl	0·14
Diazinon	0·50
Malathion	0·29

SYSTEM T16: Organophosphorus Pesticides

Bunyan, P. J., *Analyst*, 1964, **89**, 615

PLATES. Glass plates, 20 × 20 cm, coated with a slurry of silica gel H (Merck) to give a layer 0·25 mm thick. They are activated in an oven at 125° for 30 minutes.

SAMPLES. Spotted in a row 2 cm from the bottom of the plates.

SOLVENT. Acetone:benzene (1:9).

EQUILIBRATION. None.

DEVELOPMENT. Ascending, until the solvent front has advanced 10 cm.

LOCATION. *Bromophenol blue spray*, which produces blue or mauve spots after drying the sprayed plates at 80° for 10 minutes and removing the background with *5% aqueous acetic acid spray*. The colour of the spots is heightened by exposing the plates to ultraviolet irradiation for several minutes—the background becomes brown.

Rf VALUES

Azinphos-methyl	0·40	Diazinon	0·38
Demeton-O	0·60	Dimethoate	0·03
Demeton-S	0·19	Malathion	0·45

SYSTEM T17: Aspirin and Metabolites in Urine

Cummings, A. J. and King, M. L., *Nature*, 1966, **209**, 620 (after Gänshirt, H. and Malzacher, A., *Archiv. der Pharmazie*, 1960, **293**, 925)

PLATES. Glass plates, 20 × 20 cm, coated with a slurry consisting of silica gel GF254 (Merck).

SAMPLES. Spots of urine direct or of ether extract from acidified urine.

SOLVENT. Acetic acid (glacial):benzene:ether:methanol (18:120:60:1).

EQUILIBRATION. None.

DEVELOPMENT. Ascending.

LOCATION. Ultraviolet light (254 mμ).

Rf VALUES (approximate)
Aspirin 0·50; Salicylic acid 0·57; Gentisic acid 0·34.

SYSTEM T18: Corticosteroids

Hall, A., *Journal of Pharmacy and Pharmacology*, 1964, **16**, Supp. 9T

PLATES. Glass plates, 20 × 20 cm, coated with silica gel G (Machery, Nagel) slurry to give a layer 0·25 mm thick and dried at 110° for 1 hour.

SAMPLES. 1 μl of a solution in 1 ml of chloroform:methanol (1:1). Cortisone acetate is run as a control.

SOLVENT. Dichloroethane:methyl acetate:water (100:50:50). Shake together, then allow to separate. Run the lower layer through a filter paper into a tank, lined with Whatman No. 4 filter paper, to a depth of 1·5 cm.

EQUILIBRATION. None.

DEVELOPMENT. Ascending, until the solvent front has advanced to 3 cm from the top of the plate. The plate is air-dried for 5 minutes then heated at 105° for 5 minutes.

LOCATION. *DPST spray*, which is sensitive to less than 1 μg of corticosteroid.

Rf VALUES—relative to Cortisone acetate

Betamethasone	0·26	Hydrocortisone	0·19
Betamethasone 17-valerate	0·71	Hydrocortisone acetate	0·66
Deoxycortone acetate	1·92	Prednisolone acetate	0·53
Deoxycortone pivalate	2·22	Prednisolone pivalate	1·10
Dexamethasone acetate	0·79	Prednisone acetate	0·79
Fludrocortisone acetate	0·87	Triamcinolone acetonide	0·50
Fluocinolone acetonide	0·53		

SYSTEM T19: Corticosteroids

Hall, A., *Journal of Pharmacy and Pharmacology*, 1964, **16**, Supp. 9T

PLATES and SAMPLES. As for T18. Hydrocortisone is run as a control.

SOLVENT. Methylene chloride:dioxan:water (100:50:50). Shake together then allow to separate. The lower layer is run through filter paper into a tank to a depth of 1·5 cm.

EQUILIBRATION, DEVELOPMENT, and LOCATION. As for T18.

Rf VALUES—relative to Hydrocortisone

Betamethasone	1·00	Prednisolone	0·83
Cortisone acetate	1·88	Prednisone	1·21
Dexamethasone	1·00	Triamcinolone	0·59
Fluocinolone acetonide	1·40	Triamcinolone acetonide	1·39
Hydrocortisone hydrogen succinate	0·18		

SYSTEM T20: Separation of Oestradiol, Oestriol, and Oestrone

Jacobsohn, G. M., *Analytical Chemistry*, 1964, **36**, 275

PLATES. Glass plates, 8 × 8 in, coated uniformly with a slurry consisting of 30 g of silica gel H (Merck) in 70 ml of distilled water to give a layer 0·25 mm thick. After drying in air for 1 hour, the plates are activated in an oven at 100° for at least 2 hours. They should be used immediately after cooling or kept in the oven for no longer than 2 days.

SOLVENT. Ethanol (99%):methylene chloride (7·5:100) in a tank to a depth of 1·5 cm.

EQUILIBRATION. None.

DEVELOPMENT. Ascending, until the solvent front has advanced 15 cm from the original line of samples. Time of run, about 40 minutes.

LOCATION. (1) Examination under ultraviolet light (256 mμ), which produces a greenish-yellow fluorescence with, in the case of oestriol, a purple tinge. (2) *50% Sulphuric acid spray.* Pink (oestradiol and oestrone) or purple (oestriol) spots are produced when the sprayed plates are heated in an oven at 100° for 13 minutes.

Rf VALUES

Oestradiol	0·37	Oestrone	0·58
Oestriol	0·07		

SYSTEMS T21a, 21b, and 21c: Vitamin D Compounds

Norman, A. W. and DeLuca, H. F., *Analytical Chemistry*, 1963, **35**, 1247

PLATES. Glass plates coated uniformly with a slurry consisting of Cab-O-Sil silica gel (Research Specialties Co., Richmond, Calif.) to give a layer 0·25 mm thick. The plates are activated at 140° for at least 16 hours before use.

SAMPLES. 10 to 20 μg in 2 μl of ether applied 2·8 cm from the bottom of the plate.

SOLVENT. (a) Acetone:Skellysolve B (10:90 v/v)
(b) Chloroform 100%
(c) Acetone:Skellysolve B (5:95 v/v)

NOTE. Skellysolve B (Phillips Petroleum Co.) is essentially n-hexane.

The solvent is placed in a glass chamber to a depth of 1 cm.

EQUILIBRATION. None.

DEVELOPMENT. Ascending, until the solvent front has advanced 10 cm. Time of run, about 35 minutes.

LOCATION. *0·2M Sulphuric acid spray.* After spraying, the spots are developed by heating the plates with two 250-watt lamps for 15 minutes.

Rf VALUES for solvents:	(a)	(b)	(c)
Calciferol	0·33	0·44	0·15
Cholecalciferol	0·32	0·44	0·15
Cholesterol	0·30	0·41	—

SYSTEM T22: Sulphonamides (unsubstituted)

Klein, S. and Kho, B. T., *Journal of Pharmaceutical Sciences*, 1962, **51**, 966

PLATES. Glass plates, 20 × 20 cm, coated with a slurry consisting of 30 g of silica gel G (Merck) mixed with 60 ml of distilled water and air-dried for 5 minutes. They should be stored in a desiccator over silica gel. The plates should be activated at 105° for 30 minutes and cooled before use.

SAMPLES. 5 μl, containing about 1 μg, of a solution in acetone.

SOLVENT. Chloroform:ethanol:heptane (1:1:1) containing 1·5% of water.

EQUILIBRATION. Tank equilibrated with the solvent for at least 3 hours.

DEVELOPMENT. Ascending, until the solvent front has advanced about 15 cm.

LOCATION. Diazotisation followed by N-*1-naphthylethylenediamine spray*, which produces reddish-purple spots.

Rf VALUES

Sulphacetamide	0·42	Sulphanilamide	0·53
Sulphadiazine	0·47	Sulphaquinoxaline	0·66
Sulphadimidine	0·64	Sulphathiazole	0·50
Sulphamerazine	0·57		

SYSTEM T23: Sulphonamides (N,4-substituted)

Kho, B. T. and Klein, S., *Journal of Pharmaceutical Sciences*, 1963, **52**, 404

PLATES. Glass plates, 20 × 20 cm, coated with a slurry consisting of 30 g of silica gel G (Merck) mixed with 60 ml of distilled water and air-dried for 5 minutes. They should be stored in a desiccator over silica gel. The plates should be activated at 105° for 30 minutes and cooled before use.

SAMPLES. 2 μl of an approximately 0·05% solution in acetone, spotted in a line 15 mm from the edge of the plate.

SOLVENTS. (a) Ethanol:methanol (1:1). Mix 60 ml each of anhydrous ethanol and analytical grade methanol and put into an unlined tank. (b) 0·05N Hydrochloric acid:n-propanol (1:4). Mix 100 ml of n-propanol in 25 ml of water and 0·1 ml of concentrated hydrochloric acid and put into a tank lined with filter paper.

EQUILIBRATION. The two tanks are allowed to equilibrate overnight.

DEVELOPMENT. The plate is notched at 5 cm and 10 cm from the starting line. Ascending, until the solvent front (a) has advanced 5 cm. The plate is removed, dried at 100° for 5 minutes, allowed to cool, then placed in solvent (b) until the solvent front has advanced to 10 cm. The plate is removed and again dried at 100° for 5 minutes.

LOCATION. (1) Examination under ultraviolet light (254 mμ). (2) *Bromocresol purple spray*, which produces blue or purple spots on a yellow background.

Rf VALUES

Phthalylsulphacetamide	0·51	Succinylsulphathiazole	0·43
Phthalylsulphathiazole	0·61		

Gas Chromatography

H. Leach

Gas chromatography is essentially a method of separating mixtures of substances of analytical interest. Although the equipment can vary from very simple, often home-made, apparatus to very complex and sophisticated assemblies, the principle is a simple one and is analogous to other forms of chromatography.

The basic instrument consists of a tubular column containing a packing of finely powdered material which, for gas–liquid chromatography, has been coated with a suitable substance. This substance, a liquid at operating temperatures, is the stationary phase of the system. At the entrance to the column is a port through which the sample can be introduced and at the exit is a device, which may be either chemical or electrical, to detect substances emerging from the column. The column, and often the detector, is enclosed in a thermostatically controlled oven. If a stream of gas is passed through the column the components of the sample mixture travel along the column in the gas stream. The speed of their progress is dependent on the absorption and adsorption of the components by the very large surface area of the stationary phase. By a choice of a suitable stationary phase the partition between gas and stationary phase will be different for each component of the sample mixture so that by the time the sample is beginning to reach the end of the column the components will be separated and emerge into the detector as individual compounds. The response of the detector to the emerging compounds is amplified and the resulting signal fed to a chart recorder.

The procedure is therefore similar to other forms of chromatography except that the mobile phase and the sample are in the vapour state. The gas used as the mobile phase contributes little to the efficiency of the chromatographic process although it is of importance from the point of view of the detector efficiency. It is the column which determines the efficiency of the separation and the correct choice of both support material and stationary phase is of prime importance.

COLUMNS

The columns used for analytical work can be of metal or glass. The usual sizes are $\frac{1}{8}$ or $\frac{1}{4}$ inch, outside diameter, with a bore of from 1·5 mm to 3 mm. Lengths can vary greatly from very short columns of about 1 foot to many feet for difficult separations but the usual column length is about 5 to 6 feet. Metal columns are convenient to fill since they can be packed when straight and later bent into a helix or 'U' shape to fit the instrument. For some labile materials metal columns are unsuitable and decomposition of the sample may occur, possibly due to catalytic action. Copper columns are rather prone to produce this effect. Aluminium is better but high-grade stainless steel tubing is the material of choice if metal columns are to be used.

Glass columns, apart from their fragility and the necessity of bending to shape before packing, are the most suitable for analytical work at microgram and sub-microgram ranges. Even glass may still require treatment with a silanising agent such as hexamethyldisilazane or dimethyldichlorosilane to reduce decomposition and tailing of peaks to a minimum.

Glass columns have the further advantage of allowing inspection of the packing both when the column is prepared and during its life. Separation of parts of the packing or channelling can often be found in columns which have shown some change in their performance and the possibility of detecting column packing changes by simple inspection is a great advantage.

Capillary Columns are narrow bore (0·01 inch) stainless steel or glass tubes from 30 to hundreds of feet in length. The stationary phase is deposited on the inner wall. The length allows very high efficiencies to be obtained but only very minute samples can be analysed.

STATIONARY PHASES

Gas chromatography is frequently divided into Gas–Solid Chromatography (GSC) and Gas–Liquid Chromatography (GLC). The distinction is made on the basis of the stationary phase.

Stationary Phase in Gas–Solid Chromatography

In gas–solid chromatography, the stationary phase is an active solid. For most purposes only three solid adsorbents are in common use and this form of chromatography is almost entirely restricted to the analysis of permanent gases. The three solids used are molecular sieve, silica gel, and activated charcoal. These can be used for the following types of separation.

Molecular Sieve (4A, 5A, 13X) gives good general separation of inorganic gases. Carbon dioxide is irreversibly adsorbed below 160°. Oxygen and nitrogen are well separated.

Silica Gel gives good separation of inorganic gases. Carbon dioxide, carbon monoxide, hydrogen, and nitrogen are all separated. Oxygen and nitrogen are not resolved.

Molecular sieve and silica gel columns can be used in parallel for the analysis of respiratory gases where resolution of oxygen, nitrogen, and carbon dioxide is of importance.

Activated Charcoal separates inorganic and light organic gases.

All the above materials can be used at temperatures up to 250°. Most gas analyses, however, can be conducted at room temperature.

In addition to their use as stationary phases in GSC both molecular sieve and activated charcoal are often used in combination with a filter in the gas lines for gas chromatography to remove trace contaminants from the gases. Short cylindrical columns sufficiently robust to withstand the line gas pressure and about 6 inches long by 1 inch in diameter will be sufficient to remove trace impurities from hydrogen and the carrier gases.

Molecular sieve and charcoal can be used in the form of 1/16th-inch pellets for the packing of columns but better results may be obtained if used in the form of powder. This should be free from fines; a size of about 40 to 60 mesh will give good results.

Porous Polymer Beads. The introduction of cross-linked porous polymer beads has provided a new type of active solid with very extensive capabilities. These can be used not only for the separation of gases but also for many organic substances, particularly volatile liquids. However, the use of porous-bead packings of this type is more closely related to gas–liquid chromatography separations and they are dealt with in that section (p. 65).

Stationary Phase in Gas–Liquid Chromatography

The stationary phase in gas–liquid chromatography is a liquid which is coated on an inert, finely particulate support so that a large surface area of the liquid is available for partition.

Support Materials

Although the behaviour of the column is largely dependent on the liquid phase, the support material can play a very important role, particularly when a low concentration of liquid phase is used. The choice of a suitable support can be as critical as the choice of the stationary phase, and a number of factors must be considered if satisfactory results are to be obtained.

A good support material should have the following properties:

(i) it should have a very large surface area;
(ii) it should be chemically inert and without adsorptive effects;
(iii) it should be physically robust so that a graded powder does not break up into fine powder with normal handling;
(iv) when coated with stationary phase it should pack easily and uniformly into the column.

For their original work, James and Martin (1952), used Celite 545 as a support material; later workers introduced crushed firebrick for this purpose. With the appreciation of the importance of the role of the support in the efficiency of the chromatographic separation came the demand for more uniform materials tailored for the purpose and a number of commercial supports are now available.

The basic material for the supports most commonly used is diatomaceous earth. This is calcined, usually with a flux, and then crushed and graded into a number of screened particle sizes. The sizes in general use are 60–80, 80–100, and 100–120 mesh. Grades finer than 120 mesh are very seldom used due to the great resistance to gas flow produced by the finer powders. It is of great importance that the material used should be of as uniform a particle size as possible and entirely free from fines.

Some of the common support materials are:

Chromosorb P. Processed firebrick. The 'P' denotes the pink colour which is due to the presence of iron oxide. A relatively dense material with a packed density of about 0·5 g per cm^3. Surface area is about 4 m^2 per g. A relatively hard robust material.

Chromosorb W. Diatomaceous earth calcined with the addition of sodium carbonate. The 'W' denotes the white colour. It is less dense than P with a packed density of approximately 0·3 g per cm^3. The surface area is about 1 m^2 per g. It is softer than P and has a greater tendency to produce fines.

Chromosorb G. Calcined diatomaceous earth. The density is similar to that of P but the surface area is much less (about 0·5 m^2 per g). It is the least reactive of the Chromosorbs. The high resistance to mechanical damage together with the density and inertness makes it very suitable for low loaded columns. The amount of stationary phase should not exceed 5% (this is the equivalent of 10% on usual supports).

Celite 545. A flux calcined diatomaceous earth from the same origin as Chromosorb W. The manufacturing process is similar but not identical. The properties are very similar to those of Chromosorb W.

Teflon. Powdered polytetrafluoroethylene. It is inert to almost all substances and is a useful support for the analysis of polar compounds which tail badly. The low density of this type of support gives columns of low efficiency. Coated supports are very difficult to pack into columns and should be cooled below the transition point of 19° before handling.

Glass Beads. Non-absorbent and only suitable for very low column loadings. They have a low surface area and produce columns of low efficiency.

A very useful review of support materials is given by Palframan and Walker (1967). These authors also review the methods of deactivating support materials.

Further Treatment of Support Materials

Ideally the support should be totally inert and used only to hold the liquid phase. With diatomaceous support materials this ideal is never completely realised and, in general, the cruder the support material the more common will be undesirable effects. Firebrick, for example, is sufficiently reactive to give some separation in the absence of any stationary phase and adsorption effects are about 10 times greater with Chromosorb P than with W. Even with highly efficient materials such as Chromosorb W it is usually necessary to treat the material further to reduce undesirable properties to a minimum. A considerable number of the commercially available support materials, such as the Gas–Chroms S, A, P, and Z, also Anakrom and Diatoport, are calcined diatomaceous earths which have been treated to reduce adsorptive or catalytic effects.

Deactivation of Support Materials

The common initial method of treatment is by washing the graded material with acid and this is often followed by a base wash. The object of this treatment is to remove metallic impurities from the material and there is no doubt that acid washing frequently improves the performance of the support although it can be shown that the composition of the material is very little altered by acid treatment and while a little aluminium and iron is removed this is only a small proportion of that present in the material.

Deactivation can also be achieved by coating the active sites on the support with a liquid phase having polar functional groups and if the stationary phase is non-polar it may be necessary to add a small quantity of a strongly polar substance to produce deactivation. Polyethylene glycol 400, sorbitan mono-oleate (Span 80), and other surface-active agents at concentrations of about 0·2% have been used for this purpose but unfortunately they often cause some temperature limitation of the column.

The most common and satisfactory method of deactivation is by reaction at the active sites of the support. This is most conveniently done by *silanisation.* The washed and dried support is treated with a solution of dimethyldichlorosilane or hexamethyldisilazane. These substances react with any hydroxyl groups on the surface of the particles. The great advantage of this method of treatment is that it imposes no temperature limitation on the column and is simple to perform.

Commercial support materials which have been further treated by the above procedures are available and are usually designated by a suffix to the name, e.g. AW, AWHMDS.

Purification of Support Materials

To 50 to 100 grammes of the graded material, e.g. 80–100 mesh Chromosorb W, add 4 to 6 times the powder volume of concentrated hydrochloric acid. Allow to stand for several hours with gentle stirring at intervals to suspend the material. Decant the acid and wash with several quantities of distilled water until the washings are neutral.

For each wash the material should be suspended in about 10 volumes of water and, after settling for a sufficient time for the bulk of the material to deposit, the supernatant should be poured off so that it carries the finely particulate material with it. This removal of fines is of great importance.

After the final wash, drain the material as completely as possible and wash twice with 2 volumes of methanol. If desired it can then be base washed by treatment with 2% potassium hydroxide in methanol and finally washed again with methanol until the base is completely removed.

After the last methanol wash, transfer the material to a large evaporating basin and dry in an oven at 110° overnight.

Transfer the dry support to a large Buchner flask, add 5 volumes of a 1 to 2% solution of dimethyldichlorosilane or hexamethyldisilazane in toluene or carbon tetrachloride and apply a vacuum to facilitate penetration of the reagent into the particles. Swirl the flask gently from time to time. After 20 to 30 minutes, filter the suspension by vacuum and wash the material in the funnel with 2 lots of toluene and then with methanol. The last methanol wash should be done by sucking dry, suspending the material in methanol in a beaker, and, after pouring off any fines produced by the manipulation, finally filtering under vacuum, washing once with methanol, and drying at 100° to 120°.

Throughout the process the greatest care should be taken to avoid rough handling of the support. This is particularly important after the silanisation process, for abrasion of the particles will not only produce fines which are themselves objectionable but will also expose fresh active areas of the particles.

Stationary Phase Materials

The total number of substances which have been used as stationary phases in gas–liquid chromatography runs into hundreds. Many of these have been reported, particularly in the early days of gas chromatography, as having particular advantages for the separation of related groups of compounds.

At the present time the tendency has been in the direction of restricting the use of stationary phases to a minimum and, apart from a few specialised applications, the number of stationary phases in common use is comparatively small.

Stationary phases are usually classified on the basis of their polarity or selectivity towards some feature of the material to be separated such as molecular weight or shape, boiling-point, or the presence of particular functional groups in the molecule.

For general use in the toxicological field the following stationary phases will enable all but a few difficult substances to be adequately chromatographed.

NON-POLAR PHASES

SE-30 Silicone Gum Rubber. Maximum operating temperature 250°.
Probably the most widely used of all materials. Separates on the molecular size and shape and generally in order of molecular weight.

A recent phase, very similar to SE-30 in separating ability but with a much higher maximum working temperature, is OV-1.

Apiezon L Hydrocarbon Grease. Maximum operating temperature, 250°.
Very useful at moderately high loadings (about 10%) for hydrocarbons, essential oils, barbiturates, and neutral drugs.

POLAR PHASES

Polyethylene Glycol 400 (PEG 400; macrogol 400). Maximum operating temperature, 100°.
Very useful for alcohols, ethers, aldehydes, and other 'low boiling' compounds. Formerly the most widely used phase for alcohols, etc., but has now been superseded by the Porapak type of polymer bead.

Carbowax 1500 and *1540* (polyethylene glycols 1500 and 1540; macrogols 1500 and 1540).
These are similar in separating efficiency and behaviour to PEG 400 but have a greater temperature stability—up to 150°.

Carbowax 20M (polyethylene glycol 20,000). Maximum operating temperature, 250°.
The general characteristics of this high molecular weight material are broadly similar to those of the polyethylene glycols of lower molecular weight and Carbowax 20M is generally used as a polar material for 'high boiler' separations. For this purpose, low-loaded columns are required if retention times are not to be unduly long and concentrations of about 2% are usually used. Carbowax 20M can be used for alkaloid and other basic drug separations and, unless phenolic substances are likely to be present, it is often used on a modified support made by coating the support material with potassium hydroxide to give a concentration of about 5% before the Carbowax coating is applied.

Fluorosilicone Polymers

The most common polymer of this type is QF-1. The maximum operating temperature is 250°. The recent OV-17 is stable up to 350°. It is a more polar material than SE-30 but is not so selective as Carbowax. Generally used for the separation of high molecular weight material; the usual column loadings are up to 3%. It is a useful complementary column to SE-30.

Silicone Nitrile Polymers: XF-1105, XF-1150, and *XE-60*

The last of these is the most widely used of the cyanosilicone polymers and it has been widely used for steroid separations. It is a moderately polar material which shows selective retention for hydroxyl groups. Like the fluorosilicone polymer QF-1 it can be used as a complement to SE-30 columns for high molecular weight compounds at loadings of about 3%. The maximum operating temperature is 250°.

Polyesters

A large number of polyesters are available with differing degrees of polarity. These include neopentyl glycol succinate, adipate, and sebacate, cyclohexanedimethanol adipate and succinate, and ethylene glycol esters. Neopentyl glycol succinate is probably the most widely used and has an upper temperature limit of 225°.

Porous Polymer Beads

Polymer beads as a phase material for gas chromatography were first described by Hollis (1966). They consist of divinyl-benzene cross-linked polystyrene. They probably represent the first phase material to be specifically tailored for gas chromatographic separations. A number of types of polymer bead are available at the moment with similar but slightly different characteristics. They are available as Porapak (P, Q, R, S, and T), Polypak (types 1 and 2), and Chromosorb 101 and 102.

These substances can be used up to a temperature of 250° and, being homogeneous solids, there is no bleed of stationary phase such as is found with conventional stationary phases.

The versatility of these substances is very great and they can be used for the separation of permanent gases, organic acids, glycols, amines, and many substances which are extremely difficult or impossible to analyse on other columns. They are widely used for the separation of volatile solvents, particularly alcohols. The tailing which is often a feature of chromatograms of highly polar substances is eliminated or very much diminished.

A variety of mesh sizes is available corresponding to the usual support sizes. For most work, 80–100 or 100–120 mesh will be found suitable in columns of 1·5 to 2 metres. Finer cuts than these require a rather high inlet pressure in long columns.

Although the polymer bead phases are usually employed in the natural state, it is possible, for some applications, to modify their properties by coating with some other stationary phase. Silanising the beads can also be used to improve performance in very difficult separations.

The materials at present available may be considered as the first generation of an entirely new type of column packing and within their own limitations they have produced an enormous improvement in analytical capability for many substances which were a serious analytical problem. It is not too much to expect that later generations of specially made column packings will bring even greater improvements and that the days of the conventional 'inert' support and liquid phase may be numbered.

Coating the Support Material

The two basic methods of applying the stationary phase material to the support material use either evaporation or filtration. There are many modifications of these basic procedures which can be used but all are variations on these methods.

Evaporation

The amount of support material required is weighed into a flask which is sufficiently robust to withstand a vacuum. The flask capacity should be at least twenty times the *volume* of the support material. In general, not more than 25 to 50 grammes of support material should be coated. Too large a quantity makes it difficult to produce a uniform product.

The correct amount of stationary phase to give the desired concentration is dissolved in a suitable solvent; chloroform, dichloromethane, or hexane will cope with the majority of materials.

The solution is added to the support material in the flask and sufficient solvent should be present to give a thin slurry. A gentle vacuum is applied and the flask agitated, very gently, in a hot water-bath. This requires careful attention in the early stages to avoid foaming and loss of solution. The heating under vacuum is continued until the material is dry. With concentrations up to 10% it should appear as a free-flowing powder when the vacuum is released. When dry, the powder is transferred to a dish and final drying is done overnight at 100°. If a rotary vacuum evaporator is available this can be used to advantage but the speed of rotation should be kept low to avoid abrasive damage to the particles of support material.

Filtration

The correct amount of support material is weighed (usually 25 g) and is suspended in a solution of the stationary phase. The concentration of the solution should be approximately half the desired concentration on the support material. A vacuum is applied to assist penetration and after standing for a few minutes the slurry is filtered on a Buchner funnel by vacuum. The cake of coated support material is transferred to a dish and dried at 100°. If 25 g of support material and 100 ml of solution is used, the concentration on the support will be approximately twice that of the solution when Celite or Chromosorb W is used as a support. The exact amount can be determined either by evaporating the filtered solution and weighing the residue or by taking a small portion of the coated material and exhaustively extracting by Soxhlet.

This method of coating is only suitable for low-loaded supports and, with coatings of the order of 1 or 2%, generally gives a more even thin film than can be produced by the evaporation method. The difficulty of obtaining accurate and reproducible concentrations unless a number of trial runs are made is the main disadvantage.

Choice of Column

The choice of a suitable column is, in many cases, a matter of personal preference and will also depend on the type of work which is undertaken. For toxicological screening procedures it is obviously desirable to keep the number of columns to a minimum and for general purposes the following four columns will be found capable of coping with the majority of toxicological problems:

(1) 2·5% SE-30 or OV-1—for 'high boilers' and some more volatile compounds;
(2) 3% XE-60 or 1% QF-1—a more polar general-purpose column;
(3) 10% Apiezon L—for barbiturates, neutral drugs, and many 'low boilers';
(4) Porapak Q or PEG 400—for alcohols and other volatiles.

Apart from the separating characteristics of the columns themselves there are other considerations which are often of considerable practical relevance. For example, if only one instrument is available but has an oven which will take two columns, it is convenient to run an Apiezon and an SE-30 column together at the same temperature of about 225°. The Apiezon column can be used for barbiturate and neutral drug screening and the SE-30 for basic drugs without the necessity to shut down to change columns.

Again, if a Porapak column is used for volatiles, it can be left in the oven when the instrument is used at high temperature, whereas a PEG 400 column would not only be ruined by this procedure but the decomposition products would contaminate the pipework and the detector.

Maximum Operating Temperatures of Columns

The maximum operating temperatures which have been given are those which will show negligible bleed of the stationary phase when columns are used with a flame ionisation detector (p. 69). All phases will bleed very slightly at high temperatures although normally this is unnoticeable. When an electron capture detector (p. 70) is used the effect of the bleed may be enough to prevent efficient operation and it is often necessary to fix much lower maximum temperature limits for this detector.

Columns are conditioned, when new or after being out of use, by heating to about 25° to 50° above the normal working temperature. Care should be taken that this does not lead to the maximum operating temperature being exceeded. It is of paramount importance to ensure that there is a flow of gas through any column which is in the instrument oven. If the column is idle the gas flow need only be a few millilitres per minute but neglect of this will lead to column deterioration and possibly to decomposition of the stationary phase with detector contamination.

From time to time, when columns have been in use for some time, it is often advantageous to clean them up by the injection of successive small amounts of water. Columns which are giving a noisy record can often be restored to good condition by this treatment and in bad cases numerous 10-μl aliquots of water should be injected at close to the maximum working temperature of the column. When a 'clean' recording is produced the temperature should be reduced to about 150° and two or three 10-μl aliquots of hexamethyldisilazane injected. Needless to say, this silanisation procedure should not be used with Carbowax (polyethylene glycol) columns.

If numbers of dirty samples have been injected, the top portion of the column may show marked discoloration, even to the point of pyrolised material being present. The top few inches of packing should be removed and the column refilled with new coated support. Any glass wool or string should be replaced with new material and the column reconditioned for about 48 hours.

During the conditioning of a new column or during the water 'clean-up' of an old column, the column should be disconnected from the detector to avoid the possible condensation of very high boiling material within the detector. This type of contamination can be very difficult to remove.

DETECTORS

Thermal Conductivity Detectors

Katharometers, or thermal conductivity detectors, at present in use consist of a metal block of high thermal capacity drilled with channels to carry the sample stream and also a reference gas stream. In the channels are electrically heated filaments or thermistors. The sample and reference stream elements are connected in a Wheatstone bridge configuration so that the resistance of the two elements can be balanced with carrier gas flowing. When a sample component emerges into the sample stream the thermal conductivity of the system is changed and the resulting change in temperature of the wire causes a change in resistance. This change unbalances the bridge and the change in signal can be displayed on a chart recorder.

This type of detector is attractive for use where the amount of sample is not limited and requires only a chart recorder, a simple bridge circuit, and a stable power supply. It is still the most common detector for permanent gas analysis.

The disadvantages of this type of detector include a rather low sensitivity and a critical dependence on stable temperature and gas flow conditions.

Although hydrogen is theoretically the ideal gas for use as a carrier, the hazard involved has led to the use of helium for this type of detector. Nitrogen or argon can also be used but with loss of sensitivity and peak reversal with some substances.

The katharometer will respond to all gases and vapours with a different thermal conductivity to the carrier gas.

Gas Density Balance

This detector uses thermal elements similar to the katharometer but is designed to detect the change in density which takes place when a sample component is carried in the gas stream. The principle allows the detector to produce a predictable response and calibration is minimised. The detector can also be used for the determination of molecular weights. The sensitivity of this form of detector is comparable with that of a katharometer and this comparatively low sensitivity together with the complexities of manufacture has resulted in its being little used in the gas chromatography of drugs.

Ionisation Detectors

The thermal conductivity detectors measure a common property of both carrier gas and component vapour and for stable operation require a constant gas flow and power supply. The ultimate sensitivity of such detectors is limited by the need to keep the control of these factors within very fine limits. If sensitivity is to be increased it is necessary to use a detector which will respond only to some specific property of the sample components and which is not responsive to the carrier gas. Ionisation detectors are of this type and are capable of sensitivities about 10^4 times as great as the katharometer.

(1) FLAME IONISATION DETECTOR. This detector was introduced by McWilliam and Dewar (1958) and apart from some minor refinements in construction the same basic detector is probably the most widely used of all the ionisation detectors.

The carrier gas stream from the column is mixed with a supply of hydrogen and the mixture burned at a small jet in a flow of air sufficient for combustion and for the removal of the combustion products. Above the jet is an electrode which may be simply a wire or an annular ring around the jet. The polarising voltage of about 150 volts is applied between the jet and the electrode. When a component appears in the flame the ionisation allows the current between the electrodes to increase. The increase in current is detected by measuring the voltage drop across a very high resistance in the circuit using a very high impedance amplifier.

Although the detector need not be physically small the reaction volume is approximately that of the flame and is usually only a few cubic millimetres. The background current of this detector is very low (10^{-12}A) as is the noise level (10^{-14}A).

The design of the detector is not critical providing that the electrodes do not become hot enough to lead to thermionic emission effects. Any of the usual carrier gases can be used with this detector and minor changes in gas flow are without effect. The flow of hydrogen should be approximately equal to the carrier and an air supply of about 10 times the combined gas volumes is necessary to give adequate purging of the detector body.

Sensitivity is very high and less than 10^{-11}g of component per ml of carrier gas can be detected. The limit of detection is dependent on a minimum noise level and the gases and particularly the air supply must be effectively filtered.

The lower ionisation efficiency when compared with an argon detector (see p. 70) formerly required a more sensitive and stable amplifier for flame detectors than was required with an argon detector. The improvements in amplifier design with the increasing use of flame detectors now means that there is little to choose in terms of sensitivity between the most sensitive of the argon detectors and the flame detector.

The response of the flame detector is roughly dependent on the number of carbon atoms in the substance but the response is much lower if oxygen or nitrogen is present in the molecule. Apart from considerations of operating conditions it is necessary to calibrate for the individual substances if the detector is to be used quantitatively.

The insensitivity of the detector to water is a most useful feature which allows aqueous solutions to be used if desired. It will respond to all organic compounds with the exception of formic acid.

Recently a new detector combining a flame ionisation detector and a halogen and phosphorus sensitive detector has become commercially available. After burning in the flame of the hydrogen detector the combustion products pass into the second part of the device where they are in contact with a spiral containing alkali salts and the increase in ionisation current as a result of the presence of halogen or phosphorus is detected. Sensitivity is less than 5 nanograms for P, Cl, Br, and I.

(2) ARGON IONISATION DETECTOR. The argon detector was first introduced by Lovelock (1958a and 1958b) and consists of a cylindrical cell with inlet and exit ports and an insulated central electrode. Within the cell is a source of radioactivity which is commonly strontium-90 for high temperature use or tritium for temperatures up to about 200°.

A high potential is applied between the cell body and the electrode. The radioactivity excites the argon atoms of the carrier gas to a metastable state. When an argon atom collides with a component molecule, energy is transferred and ionisation occurs and the electrical field accelerates the liberated electron which excites further argon atoms. The increase in ionisation current is amplified and recorded.

This type of detector has undergone numerous modifications with the aim of reducing the effective cell volume and increasing the sensitivity and linear range. Argon detectors were formerly the most popular choice for work at high sensitivities but the necessity to restrict the carrier gas to argon and the short linear range and sensitivity to water vapour has led to their gradual fall from favour with the increasing use of flame detectors.

(3) CROSS SECTION DETECTOR. This is a modified argon detector and indeed for many purposes the argon and cross section detectors can be used interchangeably. This detector is used with an ionisation potential of about 100 volts. Although of low sensitivity it has a very wide working range of up to 100% component and was formerly widely used for detection in preparative gas chromatography. It is an unselective detector and responds to all gases and vapours and like the katharometer the carrier gas contributes the largest part of the signal.

(4) ELECTRON CAPTURE DETECTOR. This detector was described by Lovelock and Lipsky (1960) and the theoretical basis for its use was explained by Lovelock (1961) in a paper discussing the ionisation detectors generally. It is a selective detector with a very high sensitivity for compounds with a high affinity for electrons. Halogens, nitro-compounds, carbonyl compounds, and acids and esters are detected at very high sensitivities. The response of the detector can be made selective for different types of compounds by changing the operating conditions. Suitable changes in electron energy may be made by changing the potential across the cell or by changing the carrier gas.

The early forms of this detector consist of a small chamber with two electrodes at the ends of the cell parallel to each other. A source of radioactivity, usually tritiated metal foil, is placed close to the cathode electrode. This source ionises the carrier gas and a sufficient potential is applied to the electrodes (2 to 30 volts) to collect all the electrons at the anode where they produce a steady background current. When an electron capturing substance appears in the chamber some of the electrons are removed and a fall in the detector current is produced. It will be seen that this type of detector gives an indication by loss of signal rather than the increase in signal given by other forms of ionisation detectors.

More recent designs of the detector use a concentric electrode instead of the parallel plate and advantages are claimed for such designs. Maggs and Swan (1966) and Hartmann and Oaks (1965) have described in detail the design and operation of two commercial concentric electrode detectors.

Although the electron capture detector can be polarised from a suitable low-voltage direct-current supply, there are some advantages in using a pulsed power supply. The voltage is applied for a period of 0·5 to 10 μseconds and with an interval between the pulses of 5 to 500 μseconds. This form of operation has been found to be almost essential with parallel plate detectors although concentric detectors can be operated under direct-current conditions.

If a small amount of a gas such as carbon dioxide or methane is added to the carrier gas, the usefulness of the detector is increased. The quenching agent helps to maintain thermal equilibrium and assists the capture of electrons. If argon is used, the addition of a quenching agent is essential if reversal of the response is to be avoided.

The quenching agent is often added, mixed with carrier gas, by introduction directly into the detector. It then serves a dual function, for, in addition to the quenching action, the increased gas flow through the detector purges the detector body and also reduces the concentration of the components to give an extended range of detection. With low column gas flows, particularly when capillary columns are used, it may be necessary to add quench gas in order to give a suitable gas flow through the detector and avoid the peak widening and distortion which occurs at suboptimal flow rates.

The selectivity of the electron capture detector is a marked disadvantage so far as its use as a general detector is concerned, for at amplifier sensitivities sufficient to give a good response to halogen-containing solutes, for example, there will be a low and often undetectable response to many other substances with low electron capturing properties.

By running an electron capture and a flame ionisation detector simultaneously, however, a versatile and highly informative detection system is produced. The emerging gas can be passed first through the electron capture detector and then into a flame detector but because the sensitivity of the two is so high that there is generally ample reserve of sensitivity in hand, it is more usual to run them in parallel. The gas from the column is split into two streams, each going to a detector. By varying the split ratio, it is possible to introduce even more selectivity, and the simultaneous recording of the signals from the two channels by the use of a two-pen recorder allows the relative response of the two detectors to be immediately compared.

If the source of radioactivity in the electron capture detector is tritiated metal foil, the maximum working temperature is about 200° and if operation at higher temperatures is required it is necessary to use a detector fitted with a more heat stable source such as ^{63}Ni. In practice, the temperature limitation of tritium is not as disadvantageous as it might appear, for at high temperatures the column bleed, which may be undetectable with a flame ionisation detector, may be so severe that operation of the electron capture detector is impractical. The recently introduced OV series of silicone polymer materials are particularly useful for electron capture work when high column temperatures must be used to achieve separations.

AMPLIFIERS AND RECORDERS

Since both of these instruments form the terminal part of the detection system they can be considered together. Ionisation amplifiers usually comprise an electrometer input unit followed by a solid state power amplifier. The essential feature is a very high input impedance and although Field Effect Transistors have suitable characteristics, it is more usual to find an electrometer valve. Improvement in reliability is, however, leading to the increasing use of solid state input units.

The input impedance of an amplifier should exceed 10^{11} ohms and this is essential for high sensitivity. The detector current passes through a very high resistance of about 10^{10} ohms and the voltage drop is measured by the amplifier.

As the detector is effectively in parallel with the input resistor it is of the utmost importance that the insulation of the detector be as high as possible or the sensitivity of the system will be decreased. Detector insulators must be kept clean and all connexions to the detector electrodes must be constructed to maintain an almost infinite resistance to earth. The very small currents which pass through the leads require connexions of the highest quality and the number of plugs and sockets in the input circuitry should be minimal. Even one plug and socket connexion can contribute a considerable noise level and, ideally, soldered connexions between detector and amplifier are desirable.

The amplifier also has provision for attenuating the input signal to give a number of ranges. These may be expressed as fractions of full sensitivity or in terms of detector current giving a full-scale signal to the recorder. The range of sensitivities in a typical amplifier is between 10^{-11} and 10^{-7} A.

Backing-off controls are also provided. These control circuitry which injects a signal in opposition to the detector signal so that the standing current of the detector can be suppressed.

The output of the amplifier is connected to the recorder and it is customary to find a number of output voltages between 1 millivolt and 100 millivolts provided so that the amplifier will be compatible with recorders of differing sensitivity. Almost all the recorders in use are the potentiometric type and use a null-balancing system. Care should be taken that the range of the recorder is matched to the output of the amplifier.

There is little to choose between the many makes of recorder but examination of the chart drive mechanism should ensure that the paper movement is entirely dependent on the positive drive top roller and that the paper take-up spool contributes nothing to the paper movement. One or two recorders which are available depend on the paper being taut between the drive roller and the take-up spool. This type of recorder is not suitable, because, if slackness of the paper develops, the drive speed varies and this makes accurate calculation of retention times impossible.

Recorders in which the case can be left open and the paper allowed to fall free have many advantages for this type of work and in this case the paper drive should be positive without the necessity to weight the free end of the paper.

For most work, a chart drive speed in the range 10 to 15 inches per hour is quite adequate although many recorders are fitted with variable speeds. Except for special purposes, there is no advantage in a large number of chart speeds for it is seldom that speeds below 6 inches per hour or above 24 inches per hour are necessary or even desirable.

INTRODUCTION OF SAMPLES

1. Gases and Vapours. If qualitative or semi-quantitative gas analysis is required it is sufficient to introduce the sample by injection through the inlet port septum using a gas-tight syringe. The amount will depend on the sensitivity of the detection system and also on whether trace components are to be detected. Usual volumes are in the range 0·2 to 10 ml. Conventional hypodermic syringes with gas-tight barrels and plungers are available but are very expensive. Cheap and satisfactory alternatives are plastic disposable syringes. These can be used for almost all gas samples and are only unsuitable when the gas or vapour will attack the plastic material. The plastic is usually polystyrene but polypropylene syringes are available at little extra cost.

For accurate quantitative work a calibrated gas loop is desirable. This is a length of tubing of known capacity connected to a four-way valve. Sample gas is passed through the loop to flush it and then the valve is turned to connect one end of the loop to the carrier gas and the other end to the chromatograph inlet. The gas sample is then swept into the instrument by the flow of carrier gas.

2. Volatile Liquids. These can be introduced by injection using a microsyringe of 1 to 10 μl capacity but with sensitive detection systems it is often necessary to dissolve the sample in a suitable solvent to reduce the sample size and avoid overloading the detector. The technique is then identical to that used with solid samples.

HEAD-SPACE GAS ANALYSIS. For the detection of volatile substances this technique is very valuable; if a 'dirty' sample such as stomach or intestinal contents is to be examined it can be done without contaminating the column.

The sample is placed in a bottle closed by a serum cap or a perforated metal cap with a rubber wad. If a rubber solvent is likely to be present the rubber wad should be replaced by silicone rubber or a disk of polythene below the rubber.

The bottle is warmed to about 50° in a water-bath and then 1 ml of the gas above the liquid sample is removed with a disposable syringe and injected. It is desirable to keep the sample small to leave a reasonable head-space in the bottle. 'Bijou' bacteriological bottles are very suitable and a 0·5-ml amount of sample material will permit a number of repeated injections.

3. Solids. Solid samples are dissolved in a suitable solvent and injected with a microsyringe. It is better to keep the solution as concentrated as possible to reduce the size of the 'solvent peak'. Even with very small amounts of material it is possible to use a 0·1 or 1% solution by keeping the volume of solvent to a minimum. The small glass conical-bottomed tubes used for bacteriological agglutination tests (Dreyer's tubes) are very cheap and will allow a large number of injections to be made from 0·05 ml of solution. If the amount of material is very small and much more dilute solutions have to be used it is necessary to inject the same amount of solvent alone to check that spurious peaks from the solvent will not interfere.

SOLID INJECTION. When solvent interference is serious, the sample can be injected as a solid. Solid injection devices are available from many of the accessory manufacturers but a solid injector can be improvised by inserting a narrow-bore hypodermic needle down the lumen of a wider and shorter needle. The fine needle should protrude from the end of the wider needle for about 5 mm. The narrow needle passes through a silicone rubber plug in the hub of the wide needle to make a gas-tight seal and the hub of the narrow needle is also plugged.

The length of the outer needle must be great enough to be within the heated injection zone of the instrument when it is inserted through the septum.

The solution of sample is evaporated on to the end of the finer needle by adding successive small amounts while heating the end of the needle under an infra-red lamp. The needle is then withdrawn so that it is within its outer sheath formed by the other needle. After inserting through the inlet septum the inner needle is pushed forward to expose the sample and allow it to be carried off into the column. An added refinement is to arrange for a slow flow of carrier gas through the inner needle during the injection to assist in transferring the sample.

Injection-port Heating and On-column Injection

Many instruments allow a portion of the inlet system near to the injection port to be separately heated. This aids volatilisation of the sample and the temperature of the heated zone is usually set about 50° above the column. This method allows the use of short needles and also permits the inlet port to be fitted with a removable glass liner to prevent charred material from blood and similar samples appearing on the column. For very volatile substances like alcohols this method of injection gives good results and the flash vaporisation ensures that the sample appears on the column as a narrow plug of vapour. It is also suitable for many substances which are usually regarded as non-volatile, but unstable materials may be decomposed by the temperature of the injection system; this is particularly pronounced when the system is constructed of metal.

For labile substances, the most satisfactory method is by the use of on-column injection. This requires that the injection port and the column are in a straight line so that a long needle on the syringe can just enter the top of the column packing. This is the method of choice for many drugs, but clean extracts should be used to minimise column contamination.

SPECIAL TECHNIQUES AND ACCESSORIES

Temperature Programming

For some complex mixtures with a number of components of widely varying retention characteristics it is sometimes very difficult or impractical to choose a column temperature which will allow all the components to be resolved. In these circumstances it is necessary to vary the column temperature throughout the analysis. In its simplest form this can be done by injecting the sample into the instrument at room temperature and then switching on the heaters with the thermoregulator set to the highest temperature which is required. By using a thermometer to measure the rise in temperature and plotting a graph of temperature against time, satisfactory results can be obtained for occasional runs. This system can be improved by using a Variac transformer in the heater supply circuit so that the power to the heaters can be adjusted to give varying rates of rise.

When reproducibility is necessary it is essential to use more sophisticated methods of temperature control and most manufacturers make suitable temperature programming units for their equipment. These units allow an initial temperature to be set, followed by a steady rise in temperature at a pre-set gradient up to a maximum. Some of these units will also hold the column at the maximum temperature for a selected time and then cut the heater power and apply a cold air blast to reduce the oven temperature ready for the next run. The main problem of temperature programming is the increase in gas viscosity with increasing temperature; ideally, the gas flow should be controlled on a mass basis rather than by simple pressure control. To minimise gas flow effects two columns are often run in parallel with their individual detectors connected in parallel to one amplifier.

Gas Pressure and Flow Controllers

Although the gas flow to the instrument can be controlled by the gas regulators at the cylinders it is better to provide some means of control at the instrument. The simplest way is by the use of needle valves, which are not expensive. A better method is by small pressure regulators. The gas-cylinder regulator is set to about 10 lb per square inch above the highest required pressure and the small regulators are then used to give the fine control. The best method of all, although rather expensive, is by the use of mass flow controllers. These can be set to deliver a fixed flow of gas and this will not vary appreciably even with changes in pressure or with variation in the viscosity of the gas at the column temperatures.

Some form of flow indication is also very desirable. It is possible to measure the gas flow by connecting a graduated tube containing soap solution to the outlet of the column and measuring the time for a bubble to pass between two calibration marks but it is very much simpler to incorporate a 'spinning float' type of flow meter in the gas supply line to the column. This allows the gas flow to be continuously monitored without the necessity of partially dismantling the detector to make connexions.

At the very least, some form of fine gas control should be provided at the instrument. In addition, some visual indication of the flow rate through the column is highly desirable.

On-column Derivative Formation

This is a very simple and useful technique for substances which can be converted to simple derivatives such as acetates or methyl derivatives. The sample containing the substance is injected as usual but this injection is immediately followed by the injection of the reagent. For acetylation, acetic anhydride can be used—morphine, for example, can be converted to diacetylmorphine by the injection of acetic anhydride; a second small peak due to the monoacetyl derivative can often also be seen. Barbiturates can be methylated by the injection of a methanol solution of tetramethylammonium hydroxide.

Fraction Collection

It is useful to be able to use the separating ability of gas chromatography as a prelude to some more specific method of identification and, of these, mass spectrometry or infra-red spectrophotometry are the most useful. For mass spectrometry it is now possible to use time-of-flight instruments fitted with a sample introduction system which can be connected to the outlet of the gas chromatograph.

Since it is usually necessary to be able to monitor the appearance of peaks by the gas chromatograph detector, the gas stream is split at a point between the column outlet and the detector. The sensitivity of a flame ionisation detector will usually be great enough to allow a 1 : 10 or 1 : 100 split with the bulk of the sample going, via a heated line, to the outside of the instrument. For mass spectrometry the heated effluent line goes first to an enrichment device which partially separates the bulk of the carrier gas before the sample stream is introduced into the ion source. It is desirable to keep to an optimum peak shape for mass spectrometry and so temperature programming is necessary to avoid both the very sharp peaks at the beginning and the broad peaks at the end of isothermal runs.

This technique is becoming more and more popular and with the advent of low-cost mass spectrometers it will be more widely used. As the gas chromatograph is not usually used for compounds of very high molecular weight, a mass spectrometer designed specifically for the purpose could have a relatively restricted mass range. For the majority of substances which are studied by gas chromatography this need not exceed 600, and perhaps with an instrument designed specifically for gas chromatography, low-cost mass spectrometers will be almost as common as their infra-red counterparts.

When the sample is required for infra-red or ultraviolet spectrophotometry it must be collected in a trap. This presents a number of practical problems, for the sudden cooling of the carrier gas can leave the sample component in aerosol form and it will pass through the trap. This can be avoided, if argon is used, by cooling the trap in liquid nitrogen to condense the carrier gas and leave a solution in liquid argon.

A simple and effective means of trapping is to pass the effluent into a short glass or metal column of coarse Celite or other support material. This may be cooled if necessary in CO_2-acetone. When the peak has emerged, the tube can be quickly changed and the trapped material eluted later with a suitable solvent.

A number of special pieces of apparatus are available for the trapping of fractions for infra-red examination. These employ special cells and handling equipment so that the sample can be transferred straight into the spectrophotometer (see p. 108).

EVALUATION

A number of mathematical studies have been done on gas chromatography and these have contributed a great deal of useful information on the various factors which affect performance. Although the practical gas chromatographer may not require the information which has come from the more detailed studies it is essential that he has an understanding of some of the important factors which govern performance. There is also some considerable variation in the terms which are used in evaluating separations. The terms described here are those most commonly employed.

The gas chromatogram shown in the diagram below is an actual chromatogram of a number of barbiturates run on a 10% Apiezon column. The abscissa represents time and the ordinate is the detector response.

GAS CHROMATOGRAM OF A MIXTURE OF BARBITURATES

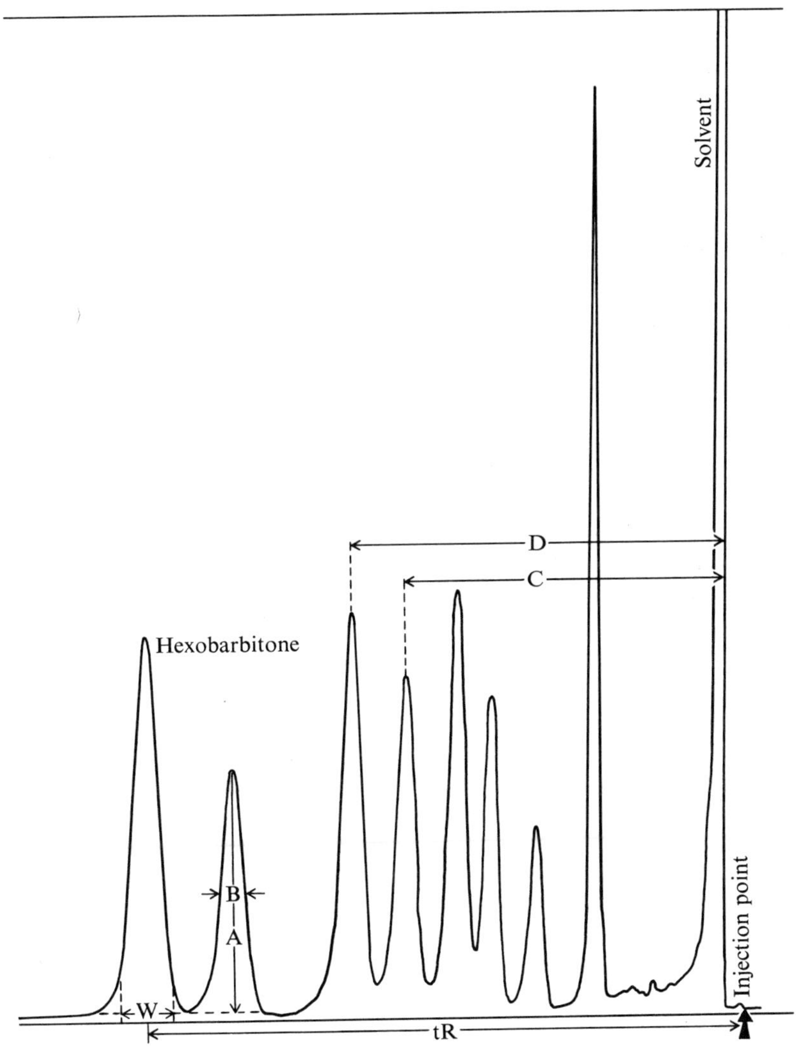

Retention Time. The uncorrected retention time is the dimension *tR* and is the time elapsed from the injection of the sample to the point of maximum detector response for the substance. It is this parameter which is used for the calculation of column efficiency.

Relative Retention Time (RRT). This is the retention time of the sample calculated with respect to the retention time of a reference compound.

Retention Volume. This is also used instead of retention time but not usually for column efficiency calculation. It is the volume of carrier gas required, from the injection point to the point of maximum response. It may be obtained by multiplying the retention time by the average flow rate. Unfortunately, the flow rate is usually measured at room temperature and at atmospheric pressure (column outlet) and these figures must be corrected for the average temperature and pressure of the column if errors are to be avoided.

Corrected or Adjusted Retention Time. This is the retention time corrected for the dead space in the column and may be represented as $tR - t(gas)$, where the second term is the time for the emergence of the front. In the diagram (p. 77) the front is indicated by the emergence of the solvent peak and, if a volatile solvent is used at elevated temperatures, the time taken for the solvent to emerge closely approximates $t(gas)$.

Corrected Retention Volumes are calculated on the same basis.

Column Efficiency. Efficiencies are calculated using the concept of a number of discrete discontinuous separations as though the column instead of performing a continuous separation was behaving as a number of units each undertaking a distinct step of separation. The analogy is drawn between the process of fractional distillation and the column is treated as though composed of a series of theoretical 'plates'. By this concept, efficiency can be expressed either as the total number of theoretical plates in the column or as the height equivalent to a theoretical plate.

It can be calculated as follows

$$N = 16\left(\frac{tR}{W}\right)^2$$

where W is the peak width as shown in the diagram (p. 77). This formula gives the total number of theoretical plates and the height equivalent to a theoretical plate can be calculated from this.

It will be seen that the plate number will depend on the peak chosen for the measurement and the substance used must be stated.

For the purpose of calculation the measurement of the actual time to the appearance of the peak is too cumbersome and the dimensions tR, W, etc. are measured in millimeters. Providing that uniformity in the units of measurement is maintained it is possible, of course, to use any suitably small units for the calculations.

Resolution. This depends upon the narrowness of the peaks and the distance of separation of the peak maxima. As in other calculations using peak widths these are calculated from the extrapolation of tangents to the baseline as shown in the diagram (p. 77).

A simple index of resolution may be given as the separation factor and this is the ratio of the corrected retention time of the two peaks: D/C—see diagram, p. 77. The resolution can be calculated more exactly by dividing the distance between two peak maxima by the average peak width:

$$\text{Resolution} = \frac{2(tR_1 - tR_2)}{W_1 + W_2}$$

For satisfactory separations, resolution should be greater than unity.

Peak Areas. For quantitative work, the most satisfactory measurement is peak area and this may be defined as the product of the peak height (A) and the width at half the peak height (B)—see diagram, p. 77. For this kind of calculation a suitable chart speed should be chosen to give easily measured peak widths.

SOME PRACTICAL POINTS

Determination of the correct carrier gas flow for maximum efficiency must be undertaken for any column. It is unwise to use a published gas flow as anything more than a general guide. For best results run a number of chromatograms of a standard substance and calculate the column efficiency. This should always be done with a new column; the efficiency can then be checked at intervals to detect changes in the column leading to loss of efficiency.

It is also unwise to assume that published column temperatures are invariably correct. They may be accurate; on the other hand they may be no more accurate than the calibration of the thermostat setting on the particular instrument which was used. Small changes in column temperatures can produce very noticeable changes not only in retention times but also in sensitivity.

For a particular separation use the lowest temperature compatible with a reasonable analysis time. If the time is excessive it is generally better to reduce the stationary phase loading than to increase the column temperature.

The column length could also be increased if efficiency is low but this is often impractical since a doubling of efficiency requires that the length be increased by a factor of 4.

To ensure even packing of the column the size of particle should not exceed one-twentieth of the column diameter or there may be some loss of efficiency from undesirable diffusion effects. The range of particle size should be within 20%.

If very small mesh sizes are used or if there is a heavy loading of stationary phase on the smaller mesh supports, there will be an excessive pressure drop along the column. This means that the linear gas velocity will vary and only part of the column will be operating at the optimum gas flow.

The column outlet is usually at about atmospheric pressure and if a high inlet pressure is required to obtain a satisfactory rate of gas flow it is unlikely that high efficiencies will be realised. For the best results the inlet:outlet pressure ratio should not exceed 2:1.

Do not forget that as there is a maximum temperature at which a column can be operated there is also a minimum temperature below which the efficiency will drop sharply. The stationary phase must be a liquid at the temperature of operation, and if a column is run at too low a temperature in an effort to obtain longer retention times, the stationary phase may still be in the solid or semisolid form.

If trace impurities are sought in the presence of a preponderating component, a number of stationary phases of differing polarities should be tried. Trace impurities are easily seen if they emerge before the main component of a mixture, while they may be completely lost in the tail if they come just after the large peak. Early peaks are also sharper and thus, for the same peak area, will be higher—this effect can contribute enormously to the successful detection of trace substances.

Remember that the solvent used for the sample can sometimes produce unsuspected derivatives and give different retention times. Try to use an inert non-polar solvent if possible but be wary of acetone and other ketones. These readily form derivatives with primary amines and can produce very surprising results.

GAS CHROMATOGRAPHIC DATA

The relative retention times given in Part 3 and in the monographs in Part 2 must be used with caution. The figures given in the monographs have, for the most part, been determined in duplicate and with the maximum stability in operating conditions. The operational variables, however, between different instruments and different laboratories may give figures which can show substantial variation. A number of factors may be responsible, including changes in column packings, slight changes in temperature—especially where these are in terms of thermostat calibrations and are not directly measured—and variations in gas flow rates, which can give quite different retention times even on one instrument. The use of relative retention times can minimise these effects but cannot always eliminate them.

In common with other methods of chromatography it is desirable that each worker determine for himself the relative retention times for the substances he expects to find.

The figures given in Part 3 and in the monographs in Part 2 should be used as a guide and not as constants. They can give a useful indication of possible identity. For example, if a basic drug is chromatographed on 2·5% SE-30 at 225° and its relative retention time to codeine is approximately 2·0, a very large number of bases with relative retention times below, say, 1·8 and above 2·2 can be eliminated. If other evidence suggests that it might be a morphine derivative, then a strong possibility exists that it is either diamorphine (2·08) or phenazocine (2·15). Comparison of the retention times given for these substances, or even one of them, will give strong confirmation of probable identity. By using a number of columns, the criteria of identity can match so closely that the correct identity can be ascribed to the unknown with a high degree of certainty.

Although a large number of compounds have been examined in the compilation of the data these can only be a fraction of the numbers which have been reported in the literature. In many cases when duplication has occurred the correspondence between reported values and the ones which have been determined has been very close. Unfortunately, this has not always been the case and even when the operating conditions have been reproduced as accurately as possible there have been marked changes in the retention times.

Minor variations in column packings and possible errors in reported temperatures and gas flows may be responsible for some of these discrepancies which make direct comparison very difficult. This emphasises the importance of determining one's own data and restricting the number of stationary phases to a minimum. Even if there is gross variation in individual retention times when compared with published data, especially if the method of coating the support has resulted in an unusual amount of stationary phase being used in the column, the published data can still save a great deal of work. The order of emergence of a series of compounds on a particular column packing will be the same, despite great variation in concentration or operating conditions, and frequently this may be sufficient information to lead to a close approximation of identity. Confirmation is then a fairly simple matter.

Although it would be desirable to use a number of columns in the collection of data, a great deal of useful information can be obtained from one column, and two columns greatly increase the usefulness of the method.

In compiling the data for this book the number of compounds to be examined was so great that work was restricted to the minimum number of columns. Because the retention data in the monographs in Part 2 are intended to be used for the screening of an unknown and not for final identification, the operating temperature has been restricted to one or two values. Obviously, for mixtures of substances with widely differing behaviour, the temperature may be far from the optimum. On SE-30 at 225° (system G2) a drug like amphetamine will come off in the solvent while a substance such as deserpidine will not emerge in a reasonable period of time. In these circumstances, either the literature should be consulted or the operating conditions changed by lowering the temperature for 'low boilers' or by increasing the temperature or reducing the amount of stationary phase for the 'high boilers' to enable a retention time relative to a reference substance with a similar retention to the unknown to be determined.

For convenience, the term 'relative retention time' has been used. Many of the figures given in the literature are in terms of retention time and these have been calculated with respect to some reference substance to give relative retention times.

For the substances included in the data given for systems G2, G4, and G5, the figures given are 'adjusted relative retention times' and have been calculated with respect to the reference substance by using the start of the solvent peak rather than the injection point as the point from which the peak distance has been measured. At high temperatures the time of emergence for the solvent can be taken as equivalent to the gas hold-up of the column and by using the solvent peak as a datum the figures give results closely approximating to the adjusted relative retention time. It has been found that this method of calculation gives better reproducibility.

Variation in the size of sample injected can give rise to considerable variation in retention times. Some stationary phases are more susceptible to this effect than others and SE-30 low loaded columns, for example, often exhibit this behaviour. To avoid this effect as far as possible, the data for the substances with systems G2, G4, and G5 have been determined with a sample size of approximately 2 μg in 0·5 μl of solvent.

It is advisable to test the columns in use by injecting varying amounts of sample and noting the magnitude of any shift in retention time with varying sample size.

System Numbers

The system numbers indicate the stationary phase and when different concentrations of the same phase have been used a different system number is used for each.

In the monographs in Part 2, the retention times given are relative to the stated reference compound; when only a single column temperature has been used the system number is followed by the relative retention time but if more than one column temperature has been employed the relevant temperature is given after the system number.

SYSTEM G1

COLUMN. 1% SE-30 on 100–120 mesh Anakrom ABS. 6 ft × 4 mm internal diameter borosilicate glass columns.
COLUMN TEMPERATURES. 180° and 250°.
CARRIER GAS. Argon.
GAS FLOW. 65 ml per minute at 180° and 80 ml per minute at 250°.
DETECTOR. Argon ionisation detector or flame ionisation detector.

This system is described by Kazyak and Knoblock (1963) who first used an argon ionisation detector and later a flame ionisation detector (hydrogen flow 50 ml per minute, air flow 300 ml per minute). Kazyak and Knoblock (1963) published their results as retention times and for the monographs in Part 2 these have been recalculated as retention times relative to codeine or diphenhydramine.

SYSTEM G2

COLUMN. 2·5% SE-30 on 80–100 mesh Chromosorb W AWHMDS. 5 ft × 4 mm internal diameter glass columns.
COLUMN TEMPERATURES. 120° and 225°.
CARRIER GAS. Nitrogen.
GAS FLOW. 50 ml per minute.
DETECTOR. Flame ionisation detector, hydrogen 50 ml per minute, air flow 300 ml per minute.

The results given at a column temperature of 120° are largely based on the work of Beckett *et al.* (1967), but the figures given in the monographs in Part 2 have been recalculated with reference to ephedrine, and those given at a column temperature of 225° are relative to codeine or diphenhydramine.

SYSTEM G3

COLUMN. 3% QF-1 on 100–120 mesh Anakrom ABS.
COLUMN TEMPERATURE. 200°.
CARRIER GAS. Argon.
GAS FLOW. 80 ml per minute.

This is a second system reported by Kazyak and Knoblock (1963). All the other conditions are as for system G1. The data given by these authors has been recalculated for the monographs in Part 2 to give retention times relative to diphenhydramine.

SYSTEM G4

COLUMN. 3% XE-60 silicone nitrile polymer on 100–120 mesh Chromosorb W.
COLUMN TEMPERATURE. 225°.

All the other operating conditions are as for system G2. The retention times given in the monographs in Part 2 are relative to codeine or diphenhydramine.

SYSTEM G5

COLUMN. 10% Apiezon L on 80–100 mesh Chromosorb W AWHMDS.
COLUMN TEMPERATURE. 210°.
CARRIER GAS. Argon or nitrogen.
GAS FLOW. 50 ml per minute.
DETECTOR. Flame ionisation detector, hydrogen 50 ml per minute, air flow 300 ml per minute.

The retention times given in the monographs in Part 2 are relative to barbitone. Results very similar to those obtained on this system have been obtained with 4% Apiezon L on Chromosorb G.

SYSTEM G6

COLUMN. 5% SE-30 on 60–80 mesh Chromosorb W AW. 5 ft × $\frac{1}{8}$ in internal diameter stainless steel columns.
COLUMN TEMPERATURE. 230°.
CARRIER GAS. Nitrogen.
GAS FLOW. 30·7 ml per minute.
DETECTOR. Flame ionisation detector, hydrogen 22 ml per minute.

This system is described by Parker *et al.* (1963). The authors used a number of column temperatures. The best separations were achieved at a temperature of 230° and this system was used at this temperature. The figures given in the monographs in Part 2 are the retention times relative to codeine.

SYSTEM G7

COLUMN. 5% SE-30 on 60–80 mesh Chromosorb W AW. 4 ft × 5 mm internal diameter glass columns.
COLUMN TEMPERATURE. 180°.
CARRIER GAS. Argon.
GAS FLOW. 28·6 ml per minute.
DETECTOR. Argon ionisation detector.

This system is described by Parker and Kirk (1961). The retention times given in the monographs in Part 2 are relative to barbitone.

SYSTEM G8

COLUMN. Porapak Q polymer beads 80–100 mesh. 5 ft × 4 mm internal diameter glass columns.
COLUMN TEMPERATURES. 100° and 160°.

All the other operating conditions are as for system G2. The retention times given in the monographs in Part 2 are relative to n-propanol.

Ultraviolet Absorption Spectrophotometry

C. Daglish

Absorption spectrophotometry was first used early in the century as an analytical tool in the identification and estimation of natural products. As instrumentation improved and quartz optics replaced those of glass the available spectrum was extended more and more into the ultraviolet. With this extension a theoretical approach to the subject became possible and absorption spectrophotometry has become an essential part of theoretical chemistry. However, much of the original empiricism remains—particularly is this so in the analytical laboratory where a collection of unrelated absorption data of the compounds likely to be met is of greater value than the theoretical reasons why individual molecules exhibit selective absorption of light. It is mainly with this practical aspect of the subject that we are concerned in the application of the technique to the measurement of drugs, but some understanding of the principles involved is necessary if pitfalls are to be avoided.

1. Units and Definitions

The absorption of radiant energy by an organic compound gives rise to electronic transitions within the molecule, the frequency of absorption being related to the difference in energy of the orbital originally occupied by the electron and that of the excited one to which it is promoted. Since these electron transitions are accompanied by changes in both vibrational and rotational energies, the subsequent absorption band will be considerably broader than it would be if only the electron were involved. These broad bands are characteristic of ultraviolet absorption, particularly in solution, although in certain cases, especially in non-polar solvents, some fine vibrational structure may be discernible.

The properties of light, in which frequency (ν) and wavelength (λ) are interrelated such that

$$\lambda\nu = c$$

and

$$E = h\nu$$

(where c is the velocity, E is the energy of the transition, and h is Planck's constant) allow the absorption data to be plotted in terms of the more familiar wavelength scale used in practice. It should be remembered, however, that frequency is a much more fundamental property of radiation than is wavelength. As such it can be measured in electronvolts (eV) or in kcal/mole, and for the ultraviolet region the following correlations exist:

λ	200	300	400 mμ
ν	50,000	33,333	25,000 cm^{-1}
eV	6·2	4·11	3·12
E	143	95	72 kcal/mole

Thus the wavelength of an absorption band can be correlated with frequency and the energy difference of the electronic transition in the molecule. This is measured in millimicrons where

$$1 \text{ m}\mu = 10 \text{ Å} = 10^{-7} \text{ cm}$$

Using this nomenclature the region of the electromagnetic spectrum with which we shall be concerned is usually divided into the visible (400 to 800 mμ), the ultraviolet (200 to 400 mμ), and below this, the vacuum or far ultraviolet.

2. The Intensity of Absorption

When light is passed through a solution of an absorbing entity, part is reflected at the interfaces, part is absorbed, and the remainder transmitted. The amount of light absorbed is proportional to the concentration and to the path length such that

$$\log_e \frac{I_o}{I} = kn$$

where I_o is the intensity of incident light, I is the intensity of transmitted light, and n is proportional to concentration and path length.

Changing from natural logarithms, one obtains

$$\log_{10} \frac{I_o}{I} = \text{optical density} = \epsilon cl$$

where ϵ is the molecular coefficient of absorption (molecular extinction coefficient), c is the concentration, and l is the path length) and the specific absorption (specific extinction coefficient)

$$E^{1\%}_{1\text{ cm}} = \log_{10} \frac{I_o}{I} \quad \text{when } c = l = 1$$

and

$$\epsilon = E^{1\%}_{1\text{ cm}} \times 0{\cdot}1 \text{ molecular weight}$$

If the instrument is calibrated in terms of transmittance or % transmittance, then

$$\log_{10} \frac{I_o}{I} = \log_{10} \frac{100\%}{\% \text{ transmittance}}$$

$$= \frac{2}{\log_{10} \% \text{ transmittance}}$$

and $$\text{optical density} = \log_{10} \frac{I_o}{I} = 2 - \log_{10} \% \text{ transmittance}$$

These are forms of the well-known Beer–Lambert Law upon which most of the practical measurements of spectroscopy depend. Thus, given the information that the E(1%, 1 cm) at 276 mμ for aspirin is 65·5, then it follows that a 0·005% solution measured in a 1-cm cell will give a reading of 0·328. Doubling the concentration or the cell length will double this value. The intensity of absorption (or extinction coefficient) is controlled by the number and size of the molecules of the absorbing species and the probability of the transition. For unit probability, the molecular extinction coefficient (ϵ) has a limiting value of 10^5. In practice, values of 10^4 are regarded as high. With such values, very small concentrations may be estimated and such measurements may be made in the presence of other molecules which do not absorb light of the same wavelength. Herein lies the value of absorption spectrophotometry.

3. Types of Transition

Having established that the wavelength of maximum absorption is related to the energy change of an electronic transition and that the intensity of this absorption is controlled by the number and size of absorbing molecules in the light path, it is not out of place to consider the types of transition likely to be encountered. These are as follows:

Type	*Wavelength*	*Occurrence*
$\pi \rightarrow \pi^*$	190 mμ	Compounds with conventional double or triple bonds
$n \rightarrow \pi^*$	280 mμ	Compounds in which the electron from a lone pair is excited to an antibonding orbital, i.e. in those compounds containing C=O, C=S, C=N, N=O, etc.
$n \rightarrow \sigma^*$	190–200 mμ	Saturated compounds containing heteroatoms
Electron-Transfer		This has been applied by Longuet-Higgins and Murrell (1955) to describe the transitions involving the conjugation of unlike chromophores and of those of the new intense bands which appear in the spectrum of benzenoid compounds on introduction of a substituent with available *p*-electrons or one with electron-withdrawing properties

As can be seen from this list of transitions, the electrons involved are those of particular groups. It was to these groups which were considered to be responsible for light absorption, that the name *chromophore* was given. Similarly, those groups, which, whilst not exhibiting ultraviolet absorption themselves, greatly influenced that of the molecule to which they were attached were called *auxochromes*. Such groups are those containing unshared electrons, i.e. OH, NH_2, SH, halogens, etc.

4. Factors Affecting Absorption Measurements

(a) The Beer–Lambert Law

This law, which states that light absorption is proportional to both concentration and path length of the absorbing species, is regarded as fundamentally true although its application is not so general as was once believed. It is true when only one species gives rise to the observed absorption. Unfortunately, as most work is done in solution this condition is rarely met because of

(i) solute-solvent interaction with complex formation;
(ii) the presence of different species such as ionic forms;
(iii) thermal effects;
(iv) fluorescent effects.

(b) SOLVENT EFFECTS

It follows therefore that absorption measurements are greatly influenced by the solvent. This is noticeable on changing from a non-polar to a more polar one, e.g. cyclohexane to ethanol, and becomes pronounced in aqueous solution where, with change of pH, various ionic absorbing species may be formed. This is illustrated in FIG. 1, below, for the absorption of phenol in cyclohexane, in ethanol, and in alkaline solution, in the last of which no longer is the phenol the absorbing entity but the differently absorbing phenate ion.

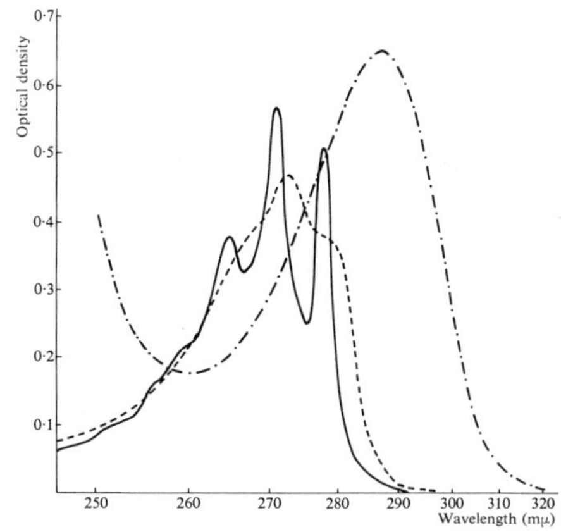

FIG. 1. EFFECTS OF SOLVENTS ON ULTRAVIOLET ABSORPTION OF PHENOL
——— = cyclohexane
- - - - = ethanol
·—·— = 0·1N sodium hydroxide

Use can be made of this change of absorption with pH or polarity of solvent in the examination of mixtures where one component can be made to ionise and its absorption shifted to a more readily accessible region of the spectrum—see under 5(d) Mixtures, p. 88.

(c) INSTRUMENTAL EFFECTS

A review of the effects of instrument adjustment on the absorption intensity measurements, particularly the effect of the slit-width used, has recently been written by Rogers (1966). It can be shown also that when photoelectric detecting devices are being used, optimal instrumental accuracy is obtained at measurements approaching 0·434 optical density, i.e. 36·7% transmission. Instrumental errors increase rapidly with optical density readings below 0·2 and above 0·7. One should therefore test the validity of the Beer–Lambert Law at constant instrumental reading by varying both the concentration and path length rather than by keeping the path length constant and varying only the concentration.

5. Applications of Ultraviolet Absorption Spectrophotometry

It follows from what has been said that electronic transitions in a molecule give rise to specific absorption bands at definite wavelengths which can be used for the identification of the molecule. The intensity of absorption is a measure of the concentration of the absorbing entity present. Since, however, ultraviolet absorption bands are, in general, broad there can be considerable overlap of these for different compounds and in order to identify more positively an unknown, one should consider both the wavelength and the specific absorption (E 1%, 1 cm).

Because of the quantitative nature of the technique, other physical properties can be determined which may help in identification. These are solubility, partition coefficient, dissociation constant (in compounds capable of yielding differently absorbing ions with change of pH), and, in some cases, molecular weight.

(a) Solubility

Since the optical density of a solution is directly proportional to concentration, then if the specific absorption is known or determined, this can be used to calculate the amount of solute present in a large number of solvents.

(b) Partition Coefficient

The partition coefficient is the ratio of the concentration of solute in immiscible solvents, therefore the determination of the optical density of a solution before and after shaking with such a solvent gives a ready measure of the coefficient. Let d_1 and d_2 be two such optical density readings then $(d_1 - d_2)$ is proportional to the amount of solute transferred to the second solvent. If the volume of the solvents used is the same, the partition coefficient is equal to $d_2/(d_1 - d_2)$.

(c) Molecular Weight

Provided that substituents in a molecule have the same or similar effects on the absorption, it is possible to calculate the molecular weight of unknown derivatives by comparing the absorption of these with that of known compounds since the molecular extinction coefficients are essentially constant. Thus, an unidentified compound isolated from walnuts hydrolysed to give α-hydrojuglone (Daglish, 1950). Its absorption spectrum closely resembled that of 5-acetoxy-1,4-dihydroxynaphthalene. By measuring the absorption of each of these and knowing the molecular weight of the 5-acetate, values of 329, 341, and 343 were found at three different wavelengths for the molecular weight of the unknown. This suggested that it was 1,4,5-trihydroxynaphthalene substituted with a hexose sugar at the 5-position with a theoretical value for the molecular weight of 338.

(d) Mixtures

The measurements so far described can be made quite accurately since only simple solutions are involved. In practice, however, it is more common to meet mixtures the analysis of which introduces certain difficulties and reduces the accuracy. The difficulties are not insurmountable once it is realised that, provided there is no interaction in solution, the absorption of a mixture is the sum of the separate absorptions of the components. For the quantitative estimation of these components it is necessary to know the absorption characteristics of each. In many cases, however, the components of a mixture other than that in which one is interested give rise to non-specific or background absorption only and the problem reduces to one of correcting for this.

(i) *Mixtures with a single absorbing entity present.* The simplest case of a mixture is that in which only the compound under test shows selective absorption. With pharmaceutical preparations, e.g. tablets, the problem reduces then merely to the use of a selective solvent, usually ethanol, which will dissolve the active ingredient away from inert excipients. Since this is extremely rapid the method is used extensively in quality control work. Even with apparently intractable material such as plants, it is often possible to obtain spectroscopically acceptable solutions if the desired component is volatile. Thus allyl isothiocyanate can be readily determined in mustard by distilling with a mixture of ethanol and water and trapping the distillate in ethanol. The isothiocyanate can be measured by using a value of 90 for the E(1%, 1 cm) at 246 mμ. By adding a few drops of ammonia to the distillate and allowing to stand until the reaction is complete (4 hours at room temperature) the resulting allyl thiourea has E(1%, 1 cm) 1192 at 240 mμ. This in effect increases the sensitivity of the estimation twelvefold such that it is possible to carry out this assay on as little as 4 mustard seeds.

(ii) *Mixtures of two or more absorbing components.* In those cases where the absorption curve of the substance to be measured is affected by background or irrelevant absorption, such as the determination of the phenol in Chloroxylenol Solution or of hexachlorophane in toilet preparations, there are several ways of improving the accuracy of the analysis.

First, in the case of phenols, changing the solvent to an alkaline one shifts the absorption to longer wavelength and increases the intensity of absorption by at least 50%. At the new longer wavelength, one can expect background absorption to be less since such absorption usually increases from long to short wavelengths. Since the extinction coefficient of the phenol has been increased relative to the background, the accuracy of the determination is improved.

Secondly, it is possible to improve the assay by examining the extract in two solvents. Hexachlorophane (FIG. 2) in ethanol exhibits an absorption maximum at 300 mμ at which E(1%, 1 cm) is 152, with no or little absorption at 320 mμ. In potassium hydroxide solution the wavelength of the maximum shifts to 320 mμ at which the E(1%, 1 cm) is 303. Therefore, by making separate dilutions of the original extract into ethanol and potassium hydroxide and reading these both at 320 mμ, the difference between readings is a measure of hexachlorophane present, in which case the concentration is estimated by using E(1%, 1 cm) 299 for calculation.

Thirdly, for those cases where the absorption of the compound under investigation cannot be shifted by change of pH, one can use the method of Morton and Stubbs (1946). This depends upon a geometrical calculation using measurements at three wavelengths, at two of which the intensity of absorption of the pure compound is the same and upon the assumption that the irrelevent absorption is linear over this wavelength range.

When two or more components of a mixture are to be determined, the absorption of each at two or more wavelengths is measured. Then, assuming that no interaction takes place, the mixture at these various wavelengths will have absorptions

$$d_1 = c_1a_1 + c_2b_1 + \cdots$$
$$d_2 = c_1a_2 + c_2b_2 + \cdots$$

where d_1 and d_2 are the measured optical densities at λ_1 and λ_2 respectively; c_1 and c_2 are the concentrations of the components; a_1 and a_2 are the absorptions of component a at λ_1 and λ_2; and b_1 and b_2 are the absorptions of component b at λ_1 and λ_2.

Then
$$c_1 = \frac{d_1b_2 - d_2b_1}{(a_1b_2 - a_2b_1)}$$

and
$$c_2 = \frac{d_1a_2 - d_2a_1}{(a_2b_1 - a_1b_2)}$$

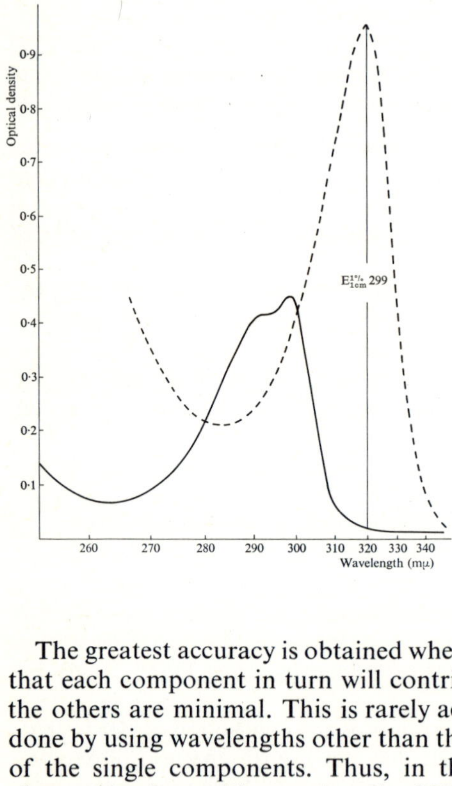

FIG. 2. ULTRAVIOLET ABSORPTION OF HEXACHLOROPHANE IN ETHANOL AND POTASSIUM HYDROXIDE SOLUTION
——— = ethanol
- - - - = 0·1N potassium hydroxide

The greatest accuracy is obtained when the wavelengths λ_1 and λ_2 are so chosen that each component in turn will contribute largely to the total absorption and the others are minimal. This is rarely accomplished in practice but much can be done by using wavelengths other than those normally used for the determination of the single components. Thus, in the analysis of mixtures of aspirin and phenacetin, the aspirin wavelength of 276 mμ normally used has to be abandoned in favour of the 229 mμ peak, as shown by the following absorption figures:

	$E^{1\%}_{1cm}$ at		
Wavelength (λ)	229	244	276 mμ
Aspirin	484	144	65·5
Phenacetin	444	639	128

(iii) *Determination of dissociation constants* (pK_a). Compounds capable of dissociating in solution show absorption curves which are greatly influenced by change of pH. As this is changed, so the absorption passes from that of the undissociated molecule to that of the fully dissociated ion and at any intermediate value of pH the curve is that of a mixture. This is illustrated for hexachlorophane in FIG. 2. The determination of the pK_a value of such a compound is only that of the analysis of a two-component system, the composition of which can be altered by changing the pH. This is normally done by measuring the absorption at the wavelength of the ionic absorption in strongly acidic and strongly alkaline solution and also in buffer of the approximate pK_a value.

Then $$pK_a = pH + \log \frac{b - e}{e - a}$$

where e is the absorption in buffer of known pH, a is the absorption in acid solution, and b is the absorption in alkaline solution.

(iv) *Hydrolysis.* The removal of a substituent group from a molecule usually has a dramatic effect upon the absorption characteristics, e.g. aspirin and its hydrolysis product, salicylic acid—λ 276 mμ E(1%, 1 cm) 65·5 and λ 302 mμ E(1%, 1 cm) 259 respectively in 0·1N sulphuric acid. Consequently, hydrolysis can be followed by absorption measurements and the extent calculated by the method described for two-component systems (p. 89).

(e) IDENTIFICATION OF UNKNOWN SUBSTANCES

Rarely is one called upon to identify an unknown compound solely by the use of ultraviolet absorption spectrophotometry. However, considerable inroads into the solution of the problem can be made from a study of the wavelength and intensity of absorption and the effect on these of changing the solvent or its pH. In order to facilitate the reference of experimental with published data, lists in ascending wavelength order of the absorptions of drugs recorded in neutral, aqueous, or ethanolic solutions and in alkaline and acidic solutions are set out in Part 3 of this book. More can be achieved, however, by subdividing these into types of absorption such as (i) no specific absorption in the region 200 to 400 mμ, (ii) specific absorption unaltered by change of pH, and (iii) specific absorption altered by change of pH.

(i) *No Specific Absorption in the Region 200 to 400 mμ*

In section 3 (p. 86), mention is made of the electronic transitions responsible for absorption in this region. It follows that if no specific absorption is observed then the compound under investigation is incapable of undergoing these transitions and pertinent groups, such as those involving double bonds or heteroatoms, are absent. Thus hydrocarbons and the simple aliphatic alcohols and their esters are devoid of ultraviolet absorption. All will give rise, however, to nonspecific absorption which increases at shorter wavelength.

(ii) *Specific Absorption Unaltered by Change in pH*

Here one must differentiate between the inevitable slight changes in absorption characteristics brought about by change of solvent from those large differences observed with the compounds to be discussed in group (iii). This lack of change may group together large numbers of chemically unrelated compounds, but it does at least eliminate the possibility of the presence of barbiturates and of compounds possessing readily ionisable groups such as the phenols.

Naturally, the spectrophotometry of this group will vary as much as its chemistry so that one can at least differentiate a number of groups of chemically related compounds by the similarity of their absorptions.

The first of such groups is that of the steroidal drugs listed in TABLE 1, all of which show a single strong absorption band at 240 mμ which is due to the

TABLE 1. STEROIDAL DRUGS WITH ABSORPTION AT 240 mμ

Compound	$E^{1\%}_{1cm}$	*Compound*	$E^{1\%}_{1cm}$
Cortisone	390	Methyltestosterone	535
Deoxycortone	440	Norethisterone	571
Dexamethasone	355	Norethynodrel	560
Dimethisterone	467	Prednisolone	415
Ethisterone	520	Prednisone	430
Fludrocortisone	405	Progesterone	540
Fluocinolone Acetonide	360	Testosterone	560
Hydrocortisone	435	Triamcinolone (238 mμ)	380

TABLE 2. COMPOUNDS EXHIBITING BENZENOID ABSORPTION WITH λ_{max} AT 257 mμ

Dose-Volume Relationship for Ultraviolet Measurements of Single Dosage Forms

Volume (ml) of Solvent per Single Dosage Form	*Amount of Single Dosage Form per 100 ml*	*Optical Density*	λ_{max}	$E^{1\%}_{1cm}$	*Drug*
1000	0·1	0·550	259	11·0	Ethotoin
1000	0·1	0·540	256	18·0	Methsuximide
1000	0·1	0·464	259	11·6	Phenprobamate
1000	0·1	0·460	257·5	18·4	Glutethimide
500	0·2	0·436	257	10·9	Styramate
400	0·25	0·435	256·5	8·7	Hydroxyphenamate
250	0·4	0·600	257·5	6·0	Primidone
250	0·4	0·540	257	9·0	Benzathine Penicillin
250	0·4	0·500	258	10·0	Aletamine
250	0·4	0·486	257·5	8·1	Trimetaphan Camsylate
200	0·5	0·400	259	16·0	Chlorphenoxamine
200	0·5	0·350	258	14·0	Piperidolate
100	1	0·600	257·5	8·0	Ethoheptazine
100	1	0·468	258	18·7	Benzphetamine
100	1	0·452	257	11·3	Methylephedrine
100	1	0·450	257	18·0	Diphenhydramine
100	1	0·400	257	8·0	Etafedrine
100	1	0·390	257·5	13·0	Adiphenine
100	1	0·375	257	15·0	Tolazoline
100	1	0·372	257	12·4	Dextropropoxyphene
100	1	0·340	259	17·0	Azacyclonol
100	1	0·332	257	8·3	Alphaprodine
50	2	0·570	257	9·5	Ephedrine
50	2	0·563	257	5·6	Tricyclamol Chloride
50	2	0·560	258·5	14·0	Doxapram
50	2	0·550	255	11·0	Phenmetrazine

Volume (ml) of Solvent per Single Dosage Form	*Amount of Single Dosage Form per 100 ml*	*Optical Density*	λ_{max}	$E^{1\%}_{1cm}$	*Drug*
50	2	0·535	257·5	10·7	Phenformin
50	2	0·525	256·5	7·5	Phendimetrazine
50	2	0·500	258	5·0	Amprotropine
50	2	0·452	257	11·3	Pseudoephedrine
50	2	0·385	257	7·7	Pethidine
50	2	0·364	259	13·0	Chlophedianol
50	2	0·360	258·5	9·0	Alverine
50	2	0·360	256	18·0	Pemoline
25	4	0·640	259	16·0	Phenadoxone
25	4	0·620	259	15·5	Dipipanone
25	4	0·600	257	10·0	Phenelzine
25	4	0·450	256·5	9·0	Phenylpropanolamine
25	4	0·440	258	11·0	Benzilonium Bromide
25	4	0·420	258	4·2	Hexocyclium Methylsulphate
25	4	0·400	257	10·0	Bethanidine
25	4	0·400	258	10·0	Racemoramide
20	5	0·525	258·5	10·5	Fencamfamin
20	5	0·475	259	19·0	Ambutonium Bromide
20	5	0·443	258	17·7	Methadone
20	5	0·368	257·5	14·7	Phenglutarimide
20	5	0·365	258	7·3	Prolintane
20	5	0·360	257	14·4	Methylamphetamine
20	5	0·345	258	6·9	Mephentermine
10	10	0·600	258	4·0	Carbetapentane
10	10	0·555	258	11·1	Pipenzolate Bromide
10	10	0·540	259	5·4	Valethamate Bromide
10	10	0·530	257	10·6	Amphetamine
10	10	0·500	258	10·0	Diphenylpyraline
10	10	0·495	259	9·9	Dextromoramide
10	10	0·410	258·5	4·1	Oxeladin
10	10	0·400	258	4·0	Butethamate
10	10	0·375	258	6·0	Caramiphen
10	10	0·360	258	12·0	Pipethanate
10	10	0·300	258	12·0	Clidinium Bromide
10	10	0·300	257	6·0	Procyclidine
5	20	0·540	257·5	5·4	Oxyphenonium Bromide
5	20	0·480	259	12·0	Benztropine
5	20	0·440	258	11·0	Poldine
5	20	0·348	257	2·9	Atropine
5	20	0·326	256	8·2	Benzhexol
5	20	0·300	258	15·0	Pipradrol
2·5	40	0·480	258	12·0	Benactyzine
2	50	0·390	257·5	7·8	Glycopyrronium Bromide
2	50	0·375	256·5	6·0	Cycrimine
1	100	0·550	259	11·0	Aminopentamide
0·3	333	0·550	257·5	5·0	Hyoscine Hydrobromide
0·2	500	0·340	257·5	13·7	Fentanyl

presence in each of a carbonyl group conjugated with an unsaturated bond in ring A of the steroidal nucleus.

Two further groups that can be recognised are those with (a) *benzenoid absorption with λ_{max} at 257 mμ* and (b) *benzenoid absorption with λ_{max} at 262 to 268 mμ*.

Benzenoid absorption is that of an aromatic compound substituted such that the auxochromic groups ($-NH_2$, $-OH$, etc.) are not conjugated with the aromatic ring, consequently the absorption is similar to that of the parent, benzene, which in ethanol shows at least 5 bands, the major one of which is at 255 mμ. Since the chromophore, in this case the benzene ring, is being diluted as it were by the ultraviolet inactive substituent groups, the specific absorption, E(1%, 1 cm), will necessarily be less than that of benzene, i.e. about 20. This is illustrated by the values found for the compounds, such as amphetamine, ephedrine, etc., in TABLE 2 (pp. 92–3), most of which are considerably below 20.

It follows that if all the compounds of TABLE 2 exhibit not only the same type of absorption, but also almost the same specific intensity, difficulties are likely to be encountered in differentiating the members of such a group. Particularly is this so if these are met as plain white tablets or as colourless single-dose injections. However, since the amount of drug present in these dosage forms will vary with the dose of that particular drug, from the 0·3 mg of hyoscine hydrobromide to the 500 mg of ethotoin, there will be enormous differences in the intensity of absorption of solutions containing the amount present in a single dosage form in a fixed volume of solvent, usually 0·1N sulphuric acid.

One can thus make use of a combination of the amount of the dosage form and the E(1%, 1 cm) of the compound to differentiate the different members of the groups. In order to obtain solutions with optical density readings within the range of the instrument, one can either vary the volume of solvent per single dosage form or vary the amount of the dosage form per fixed volume of solvent. These correlations are set out in TABLE 2 for those compounds exhibiting benzenoid absorption with the maximum occurring at a wavelength of 257 mμ and in TABLE 3 for those with the maximum at 262 to 268 mμ. In each table *Column 1* shows the volume of solvent that will be required if one whole tablet, capsule, or single-dose injection or suspension is used for the assay, and *Column 2* the amount of such dosage forms necessary to be dissolved in 100 ml of solvent to give the same optical density reading.

Thus for our two extreme examples one would have to dissolve one tablet of ethotoin in 1000 ml of solvent or take 0·1 tablet per 100 ml of solvent to give approximately the same reading as one tablet of hyoscine hydrobromide in 0·3 ml or 333 tablets per 100 ml.

(iii) *Specific Absorption Altered by Change in pH*

Large reversible bathochromic shift with increase in intensity on making alkaline. This type of absorption is essentially that of phenols but it can be demonstrated by non-phenolic compounds, such as ascorbic acid and other enediols. It is not given by the ionisable hydroxyl group of carboxylic acids which tend to show a hypsochromic shift. It has been mentioned both with regard to the estimation of hexachlorophane and the determination of pK_a values and is shown in FIG. 2. It is so readily demonstrated, by the addition of a drop of strong alkali to a neutral solution with a re-run of the absorption curve, that it is extremely useful in

TABLE 3. COMPOUNDS EXHIBITING BENZENOID ABSORPTION WITH λ_{max} AT 262 TO 268 mμ

Dose-Volume Relationship for Ultraviolet Measurement of Single Dosage Forms

Volume of Solvent per Single Dosage Form	*Amount of Single Dosage Form per 100 ml*	*Optical Density*	λ_{max}	$E_{1cm}^{1\%}$	*Drug*
2500	0·04	0·520	262	26·0	Tolbutamide
2500	0·04	0·390	268	39·0	Phenoxymethyl-penicillin
1000	0·1	0·460	265	23·0	Chlormezanone
500	0·2	0·480	264	24·0	Orphenadrine
250	0·4	0·560	262·5	28·0	Cyclizine
200	0·5	0·450	264	18·0	Bretylium Tosylate
200	0·5	0·425	265·5	34·0	Meclozine
100	1	0·625	263·5	25·0	Chlorcyclizine
100	1	0·436	263·5	21·8	Fenfluramine
100	1	0·400	261	16·0	Pargyline
100	1	0·325	267	12·9	Chlorphentermine
50	2	0·520	262	13·0	Debrisoquine
25	4	0·516	263	12·9	Hydroxyzine
0·5	200	0·535	262·5	10·7	Phencyclidine

identification. It is completely reversible and therefore readily distinguished from alkaline hydrolysis of esters of phenols (aspirin to salicylic acid).

Since the absorption changes smoothly from that of the undissociated molecule to that of the ion with change of pH, a plot of the absorption will give a family of curves passing through at least one point, the *isosbestic point*, at which both the wavelength and intensity are independent of pH. As such, it is a further means of identification and can be determined simply by adding alkali and acid to a neutral solution and noting the intercept of the two curves.

It is impossible to list here all the compounds showing such change in absorption with pH, but, besides the phenols *per se*, such as chlorocresol, chloroxylenol, etc., it occurs with those compounds not normally regarded as phenols, e.g. the salicylate and hydroxybenzoate esters, coumarin, eugenol, and vanillin, etc. Several of these are listed in TABLE 4 (p. 96).

A variant of this method of identification consists in determining the absorption in alkaline relative to that in neutral or acid solution by placing the alkaline solution in the sample beam and the acid one in the reference beam. The difference curve so obtained is a much more positive means of identification. Unfortunately, with those instruments without optical density scales extending into the negative region, the cells have to be transposed at each isosbestic point. It is possibly because of this instrument difficulty that the difference curve has not found as much favour with analysts as it has with biochemists.

Shift, either bathochromic or hypsochromic but without an increase in intensity accompanying the former, on changing the pH. What may be regarded as the

TABLE 4. COMPOUNDS SHOWING BATHOCHROMIC SHIFT AND INCREASE IN INTENSITY ON MAKING THE SOLUTION ALKALINE

	Neutral or Acidic		*Alkaline*	
Compound	λ_{max}	$E^{1\%}_{1cm}$	λ_{max}	$E^{1\%}_{1cm}$
Aloin	351	217	388	239
Ascorbic Acid	245	560	265	860
Chlortetracycline	319	150	346	267
Chlorzoxazone	279	300	287·5	420
Cyprenorphine	287	36	301	60
Etorphine	287	36	301	63
Hexoestrol	280	140	295	175
Levallorphan	281·5	51·5	299	70
Morphine	285	40	296	87
Nalorphine	283·5	40	296	67·3
Phenylephrine	273	96	291	158
Salicylamide	302	295	328	435
Thiopentone	287	900	302	1080

converse behaviour of that just described for phenols, is shown by aromatic aminogroups when the amine is attached directly to the ring, in that ionisation suppresses completely the contribution of the auxochrome and the resultant absorption is that of the parent, benzene. Thus aniline in ethanol has strong absorption with λ_{max} 286 mμ, E(1%, 1 cm) 179. In acid solution this is changed to typical benzenoid absorption with three peaks at 249, 255, and 261 mμ with E(1%, 1 cm) 16 at 255 mμ.

Rarely in the study of the absorption of drugs does one meet with examples as simple as aniline. Its derivative, aminosalicylic acid, shows considerable change of absorption on altering the pH, which is only to be expected since one is dealing with three ionisable groups, the amine, phenol and carboxylic acid. Nevertheless, even with complex molecules, considerable information as to identity can be gathered by observing the change in absorption with pH. Some of these effects are listed in TABLES 5, 6, and 7. TABLE 5 lists those compounds exhibiting bathochromic shifts and TABLE 6 those with hypsochromic shifts on acidification. Sometimes the alteration of the curve is such that one peak moves bathochromically and the other hypsochromically or a single peak may be split into subsidiary ones. Compounds showing such behaviour are listed in TABLE 7.

TABLE 5. COMPOUNDS SHOWING BATHOCHROMIC SHIFT ON MAKING THE SOLUTION ACID

	Neutral		*Acid*	
	λ_{max}	$E^{1\%}_{1cm}$	λ_{max}	$E^{1\%}_{1cm}$
Aconitine	228	180	234	230
Carbinoxamine	260	144	263	320
Diethylpropion	246	460	253	580
Emetine	230	251	240	350
Hydroxychloroquine	233	410	257	390
	253	400	329	430
	329	270	343	470
Quinine	236	920	250	833
	278	110	316	128
	332	135	340	156
Sulphafurazole	253	780	268	480
Sulphanilamide	254	1402	263	1106

TABLE 6. COMPOUNDS SHOWING HYPSOCHROMIC SHIFT ON MAKING THE SOLUTION ACID

	Neutral		*Acid*	
	λ_{max}	$E^{1\%}_{1cm}$	λ_{max}	$E^{1\%}_{1cm}$
Amidopyrine	265	450	256	530
Aniline	286	179	255	16
			261	12·5
Benzocaine	294	1340	272	101
			278	100
Captodiame	271	550	263·5	400
Chlordiazepoxide	260	1080	244	1100
Chloropyrilene	243	410	238	398
	308	90	312	180
Hydrochlorothiazide	274	500	272	650
	320	90	314	100
Isocarboxazid	272	320	~240	180
Isothipendyl	249	870	244·5	850
Mepyramine	248·5	435	239	450
	311	100	316	205
Methotrimeprazine	255	1110	251·5	987
	310	219	302	176
Phenindamine	262·5	250	259	225
Phenylbutazone	264	660	235·5	460
Prothipendyl	249	810	242	740
Thioridazine	276	840	261	1120
Thonzylamine	241	680	235	800
Tripelennamine	248·5	520	238·5	460

TABLE 7. COMPOUNDS SHOWING CHANGES IN ABSORPTION ON ACIDIFICATION

	Neutral		*Acid*	
	λ_{max}	$E^{1\%}_{1cm}$	λ_{max}	$E^{1\%}_{1cm}$
Chlorpheniramine	261·5	150	264	240
	268	110		
Clemizole	253	230	274	300
	267	170		
	274	190		
Doxylamine	260	100	262	210
	268	75		
Imipramine	253·5	300	251	265
Iproniazid	240	150	265·5	200
	272	150		
	305	200		
Nikethamide	255	840	262	1200
	260	860		
Pheniramine	261	140	264	230
	268	110		
Phenyramidol	240	620	236·5	580
	297	170	308	300
Thenyldiamine	246	940	238·5	940
	310	150	313	330

Absorption in alkaline solution which disappears on acidification. The *barbiturates* as a group are of interest spectrophotometrically because they only exhibit ultraviolet absorption in alkaline solution, the wavelength, intensity, and stability of which is dependent on pH. In acid solution practically no absorption is noted.

This phenomenon is shown by a number of other compounds, but because of the high incidence of poisoning by barbiturates, their identification and determination is of great importance to toxicologists. Consequently, considerable time has been devoted to using spectrophotometric measurements to this end as shown by the papers of Curry (1963b), Goldbaum (1952), Stevenson (1961), and Stainier *et al.* (1963).

The absorption of the barbiturates of general formula I is due to the ionisation in alkaline solution to the absorbing species II and III. Substitution on N^1-nitrogen prevents the ionisation going beyond stage II^1:

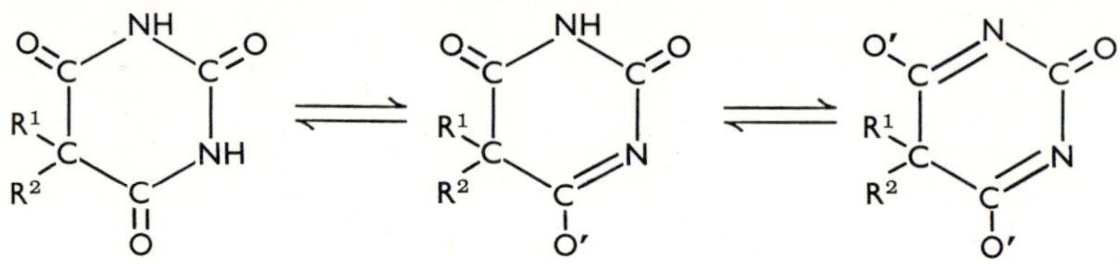

I II III

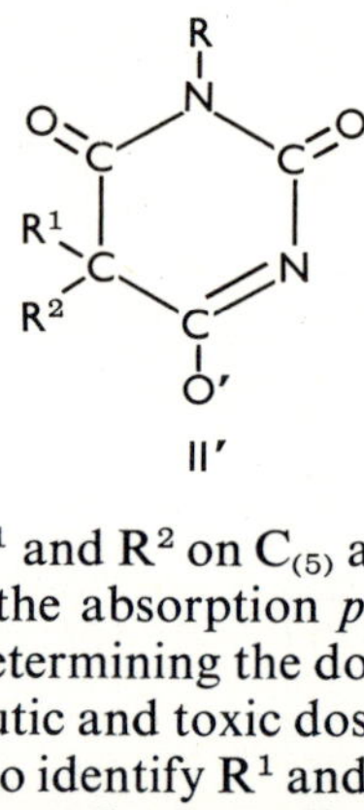

II′

Since the substituent groups R^1 and R^2 on $C_{(5)}$ are not conjugated with this chromophore, they will not effect the absorption *per se*. The nature of R^1 and R^2 does play a very large part in determining the dosage, duration of action, and the safety margin between therapeutic and toxic doses. Methods have therefore been evolved which have attempted to identify R^1 and R^2 by their effect on the stability of the absorption, by the difference in absorption at two pH levels, and by partition experiments prior to absorption measurements.

Ionisation of the molecule starts at pH levels above 9·5. None is apparent at pH 8·6, the pH of sodium bicarbonate solution, which can therefore be used to separate aspirin from a chloroform solution of aspirin and barbiturate in the analysis of tablets of such mixtures. In 0·05M borax buffer, about pH 10, all barbiturates show absorption with λ_{max} 240 mμ (TABLE 8). Above this pH level, the absorption shifts to λ_{max} about 255 mμ in 0·45N or 1N sodium hydroxide except for *N*-substituted compounds whose λ_{max} rarely exceeds 244 mμ (see FIG. 3). In these strongly alkaline solutions the absorption intensity falls with time due to hydrolysis of the molecule. Consequently in the analysis of these compounds, solutions should not be kept alkaline for longer than is necessary and the components stabilised by making acid and extracting into ether.

Since the molecule exists in solution below pH 8·6 in the undissociated form, it shows no specific absorption, only that of a general curve increasing in intensity towards the shorter wavelengths. The difference in intensity between the curves of the ionised and unionised forms is usually used for quantitative estimation, the wavelength being 240 mμ and the solvents, buffer pH 10 and pH 2, whence most barbiturates have an E(1%, 1 cm) of about 450, or as Curry (1963b) suggests, a solution of 1 mg in 45 ml gives an optical density difference of 1·0. Because of the change of wavelength and intensity with pH it is essential that the pH is kept constant for each reading.

FIG. 3. EFFECT OF pH ON ULTRAVIOLET ABSORPTION OF AMYLOBARBITONE
——— = pH 10
– – – – = 0·5N sodium hydroxide
·—·— = pH 2

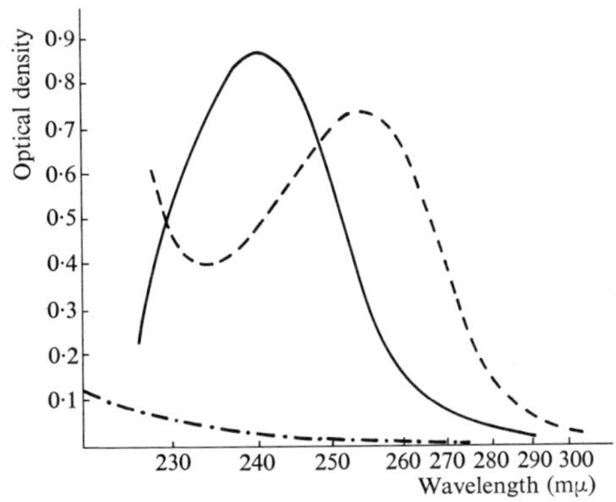

TABLE 8. $E_{1cm}^{1\%}$ VALUES FOR BARBITURATES AT 240 mμ IN BORAX (pH 10) BUFFER
(after Stevenson, 1961)

Allobarbitone	442	Methylphenobarbitone	458
Allylbarbituric Acid	415	Narcobarbital	320
Amylobarbitone	424	Pentobarbitone	411
Aprobarbitone	438	Phenobarbitone	431
Barbitone	538	Probarbital	452
Butallylonal	280	Quinalbarbitone	374
Butobarbitone	453	Secbutobarbitone	439
Cyclobarbitone	423	Talbutal	401
Heptabarbitone	400	Vinbarbitone	446
Ibomal	301		

This method then gives a quantitative estimate for all barbiturates. In order to differentiate the individual members of the group the following techniques have been applied. Goldbaum (1952) plotted the difference in intensity at fixed wavelengths for solutions in pH 10 buffer and 0·45N sodium hydroxide. The ratio of the optical-density difference at different wavelengths to that at 260 mμ was then used as a means of identification. Stevenson (1961) introduced a partition step to separate by polarity the different types of barbiturate before measuring these in borax buffer and 1N sodium hydroxide. Blood samples were shaken with butyl ether which removed all barbiturates. This in turn was shaken twice with borax buffer then with 1N sodium hydroxide. In this way the low potency compounds including phenobarbitone appeared in the borax extract whilst the high potency ones, amylobarbitone, pentobarbitone, and quinalbarbitone, appeared in the alkali extract. These last were estimated at 255 mμ in the strong alkali and at 240 mμ after the addition of ethylenediamine dihydrochloride solution which reduced the pH to 10. Stainier and his colleagues (1963) measured the fall with time of the extinction of solutions in 1N sodium hydroxide and showed that the rate varied with the nature of the substituents. A summary of their results is given in TABLE 9.

TABLE 9. TIME TAKEN FOR THE DISAPPEARANCE OF THE ABSORPTION PEAK IN 1N SODIUM HYDROXIDE SOLUTION (after Stainier *et al.*, 1963)

Hexobarbitone	30 minutes
Methylphenobarbitone	1 hour
Phenylmethylbarbituric Acid	1 hour
Metharbitone	24 hours
Narcobarbital	more than 48 hours

In the procedure advocated by Curry (1963b), blood which is deproteinated by tungstic acid is extracted by ether. Acidic substances are removed by shaking with bicarbonate, then the barbiturates are extracted by shaking with 3% sodium hydroxide solution. Since this will also extract glutethimide and bemegride with absorption bands at 235 mμ and 230 mμ respectively, which may interfere with the barbiturate estimation, the alkaline extract is re-acidified, extracted with ether, and this solvent then removed. The residue is dissolved in 0·45N sodium hydroxide and readings taken at 235 and 255 mμ immediately and after 5 minutes. If glutethimide is present the 235 mμ reading will fall by about 50% in this time. The addition of ammonium chloride to the solution readjusts the pH to 10 and the barbiturates are read at 240 mμ with no longer any interference from the glutethimide. This of course gives only total barbiturates. Separation of these from an ether extract is achieved by paper or thin-layer chromatography.

(f) COLORIMETRIC PROCEDURES

Colour Tests for the identification of drugs are described on pp. 123–34. These may be carried out as spot tests on single crystals or on drops of solution on an opalescent tile or by spraying various reagents on paper or thin-layer chromatograms or by the normal test-tube reactions. Many of these last are capable of being developed into colorimetric reactions which can be measured quantitatively either by making visual comparison of the colour of the unknown with that of solutions of known composition or by measuring the intensity of colour in a spectrophotometer.

The factors effecting measurement are essentially those applicable in the ultraviolet region. The instrumental difficulties are that the dispersion of quartz is such that in the visible region (400 to 700 mμ) the wavelengths tend to be crowded together and the accuracy of determining these is not as great as in the ultraviolet region. This can be overcome by using a glass-prism instrument or one fitted with a diffraction grating. If filter colorimeters are used then care must be exercised in the selection of the filter, the one of choice being that which transmits a band identical to the absorption band of the test solution.

The difficulties of measurement are those involving the chemistry of the reaction and the stability of the colour. Such factors as time, pH, light, temperature, concentration, and the effect of added substances must all be investigated if any degree of accuracy is to be attained. Once these are controlled and a reasonably stable colour produced this can be measured in a number of ways depending upon the use to be made of the test and the instrument available.

The simplest quantitative colorimetric procedures are those of the limit tests of the *British Pharmacopoeia*, an example of which is that of salicylic acid in aspirin. Solutions of iron (ferric) salts give a violet colour with the former but not with the latter. Hence by dissolving the aspirin under test in ethanol, diluting with water, and adding acid ferric ammonium sulphate solution, a violet colour is produced. The intensity of the colour is compared with and should not exceed that of a standard solution of salicylic acid. Instead of using a single limit test concentration, a series of salicylic acid solutions of known concentration may be used and the colour of the test solution compared with these for a determination of the actual salicylic acid content.

This development of the limit test can be used to plot a calibration curve. The intensity of colour of a number of standards is determined and plotted as a function of concentration. The intensity of the unknowns is then determined and the concentration read off from the graph. For highly reproducible procedures the graph may only require checking at intervals by including a standard with a series of unknowns. For less stable colours it is necessary to run standards and unknowns for each determination. This difficulty can be circumvented by the use of 'internal standards'. In this case, for each unknown, three aliquots are taken and to two of these are added known amounts of standard, such that the solutions now contain x, $x + s$, and $x + 2s$. The colour reaction is performed and the intensity of colour measured. A plot is then made of added standard against intensity and the plot extrapolated to $-x$, the amount in the unknown.

Provided the colour is stable, spectrophotometric measurements can be converted into E(1%,1 cm) values and these used for the calculation of concentration of unknown solutions just as for other absorbing substances. In this way there is no difference between the measurement of the colour of a naturally occurring substance such as β-carotene and that of chemically produced colours. Thus colorimetric procedures can range from quantitative limit tests in Nessler glasses to measurement procedures which are indistinguishable from those normal to absorption spectrophotometric procedures.

The reasons for using colorimetry are various, not least of which are increased sensitivity and specificity. Frequently these are interdependent. In the case of salicyclic acid in aspirin the colour reaction is a specific one for the breakdown product. Also it is much more sensitive than direct ultraviolet absorption measurements. In complex mixtures, time may be saved in avoiding tedious extraction procedures by performing a colorimetric reaction for the desired component under investigation. This is particularly true of biological systems and also those of crude drugs where mixtures of closely related chemical compounds may exist but only one gives the colour test. However, it must be remembered that many colour tests are those produced by the chemical reaction of a particular group in the molecule, such as the diazotisation of an amino-group followed by coupling with a phenol in alkali, and hence are only specific for this group and not the whole molecule. However, by selecting chromogenic reagents and coupling the colour reaction with a solvent extraction of the final colour, increased specificity may be obtained.

Presentation of Ultraviolet Spectral Data

Considerable variation can occur between instruments in the measurement of optical densities and the derived E(1%, 1 cm) values. Consequently, for quantitative work, these constants should be determined on the pure substance with the instrument to be used. The ultraviolet spectral data quoted in Part 2 of this book have been collected from confirmed spectra run in two laboratories and from various reputable literature sources. Wherever possible, and whenever the literature has quoted the use of a salt, the E(1%, 1 cm) values have been recalculated with reference to the active moiety, i.e. the free base or acid. Exceptions to this are the quaternary ammonium compounds and those salts in which the acid moiety itself has an ultraviolet absorption, e.g. closylates (*p*-chlorobenzene-sulphonates) and tosylates (toluene-*p*-sulphonates). In this connexion it should also be noted that some of the tables in this chapter record the results of analyses of commercially available compounds in their standard dosage forms and consequently do not necessarily correspond directly to the recalculated values given in Part 2.

Infra-red Absorption Spectrophotometry

D. I. Chapman and M. S. Moss

Infra-red spectrophotometry is an extremely useful technique in the identification of drugs since, with a few reservations, every compound produces a different spectrum. This means that the infra-red spectrum is equivalent to a 'fingerprint' of the drug being examined. In this respect it is quite different from an ultraviolet absorption spectrum, which is rarely specific for any one compound.

When radiant energy passes through a transparent medium it may be reflected, absorbed, or transmitted. Infra-red spectrophotometry is the study of the transmitted or absorbed radiant energy in that region of the electromagnetic spectrum from wavelength (λ) 0·8 to 1000 μ, where μ is the micron and 1 μ = 10^4 Å = 10^{-4} cm. An alternative and more commonly used measurement is the frequency, which is the number of waves per unit length, and is usually expressed in terms of wavenumbers ($\tilde{\nu}$), the units of which are reciprocal centimetres (cm^{-1}). A simple relationship exists between wavenumber in cm^{-1} and wavelength in microns:

$$\tilde{\nu} = \frac{10^4}{\lambda}$$

The 'true' frequency (ν) is the number of waves per second and is rarely encountered in analytical applications of infra-red spectrophotometry: $\nu = c/\lambda$ where c is the velocity of light.

The infra-red spectrum is commonly divided into three regions, namely, the near infra-red from 12,500 to 5000 cm^{-1} (0·8 to 2·0 μ), the mid infra-red, which is usually simply referred to as the infra-red, from 5000 to 400 cm^{-1} (2 to 25 μ), and the far infra-red from 400 to 10 cm^{-1} (25 to 1000 μ). Only the mid infra-red region of the spectrum from 4000 to 650 cm^{-1} (2·5 to 15·4 μ) will be considered in this chapter, since this has been more widely used in the identification of compounds than either the remainder of the region or the far and near infra-red regions.

When a compound is subjected to infra-red radiation, transitions take place between rotational and vibrational energy levels of the *ground* electronic energy state. These transitions give rise to an absorption spectrum characteristic of the compound. This is in contrast to ultraviolet radiation which, because of its greater energy, also causes transitions between rotational and vibrational energy levels of higher electronic energy states. However, in the infra-red, absorption occurs only where a change of the dipole of a molecule can take place. Therefore, diatomic molecules such as hydrogen, nitrogen, and oxygen, in which there is no resultant dipole, do not absorb in the infra-red.

Total symmetry about a bond between two atoms will eliminate certain absorption bands; for example, the symmetrical ethane molecule gives no carbon–carbon stretching absorption bands. Particular bonds or functional groups in a molecule have specific absorption bands at a given wavelength. Changes in the wavelength of a band have been correlated with changes in either the structural environment or the physical state of the compound. These correlations form the basis of modern qualitative analytical work in infra-red spectrophotometry. Such correlations are discussed in detail by Bellamy (1962a) and a useful summary is provided by Cross (1960). However, many bands in the complex region from 1600 to 650 cm^{-1} (6·25 to 15·4 μ), which is often referred to as the 'fingerprint' region, are still of unconfirmed origin.

A large proportion of the bands are characteristic of the molecule as a whole and cannot be assigned to particular functional groups. Three main types of absorption band occur, namely fundamental, overtone, and combination. Fundamental bands are the primary absorption bands for each mode of vibration, overtone bands occur at multiples of the fundamental band wavelength, and combination bands occur at wavelengths which are the sum or difference of two or more fundamental bands. Overtone and combination bands are normally much weaker than fundamental bands.

INSTRUMENTATION

A large number of infra-red spectrophotometers are available commercially; many of them are robust and can be used in an ordinary analytical laboratory. In many instruments the number of controls has been reduced to a minimum and, consequently, they are simple and easy to use. Nowadays the main problems are the preparation of the sample and the interpretation of the spectrum.

The basic components of an infra-red spectrophotometer are shown diagrammatically in FIG. 1.

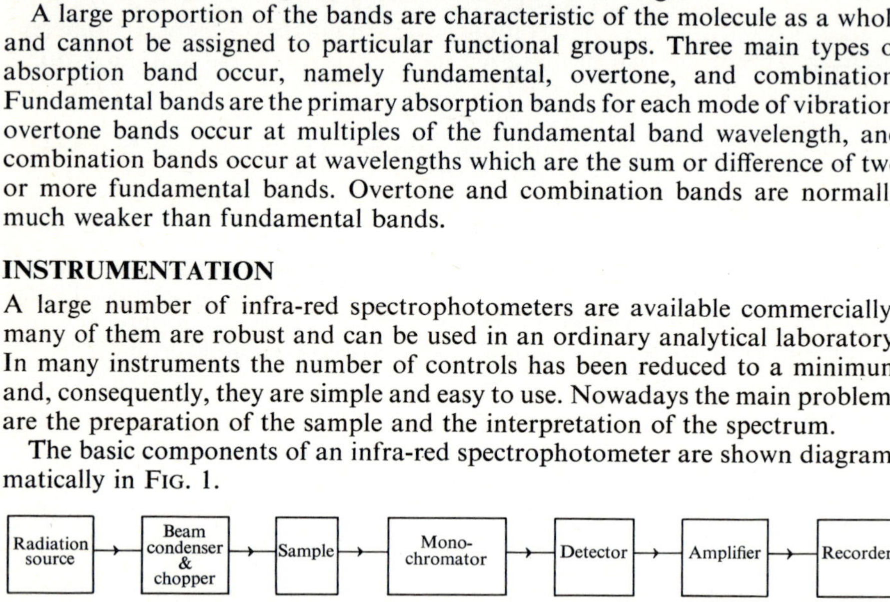

FIG. 1. SCHEMATIC DIAGRAM OF AN INFRA-RED SPECTROPHOTOMETER

The source of infra-red radiation is usually either a Nernst or a Globar filament. The Nernst filament is a thin rod of rare earth oxides, which must be heated to about 1000° before it becomes electrically conducting and which is maintained at about 1500°. The Globar is a silicon carbide rod, which is electrically conducting when cold and is maintained at about 1200°. The intensity of radiation from both these sources declines rapidly with increasing wavelength. In instruments which operate over a wide frequency, this loss in energy is compensated by programming the opening of the slits in the monochromator.

Infra-red spectrophotometers can be either single or double beam instruments. In double beam instruments the beam of radiation is switched alternately through the sample and through a reference cell at about 10 cycles per second. The use of a reference cell enables unwanted absorption, such as that of solvents, to be compensated for. Most modern instruments are of the double beam type.

The monochromator consists of either a prism or a grating to disperse the radiation arriving from either the sample or the reference beam and a collimator and narrow slits to produce radiation of a very narrow range of wavelength (approximating to monochromatic light). So far no prism material has been found which is ideal throughout the infra-red region. The best and most widely used material is sodium chloride which can be used from 3700 to 600 cm^{-1}. However, its power of dispersion decreases towards 3700 cm^{-1} and it is also rather poor at low frequencies. Potassium bromide is preferred at lower frequencies and can be used from 1000 to 400 cm^{-1}.

The detector is either a thermocouple or a Golay cell and is coupled through an amplifier to a recorder.

The infra-red spectrum of a compound represents the variation of absorption, or transmittance, with changing wavelength. Some spectrophotometers record *absorption* whereas others record *transmittance*. The difference between these two types of spectra is that one is the mirror image of the other about the abscissa, e.g. a 90% absorption is the same as a 10% transmittance. Another difference in spectrophotometers is that some employ a linear wavelength scale whilst others employ linear wavenumber. The resulting spectra appear quite different and some practice is required in comparing the two types—see FIG. 2 and FIG. 3 (p. 106). In the past, most instruments employed a linear wavelength scale because it was easier to achieve with prism optics. Nowadays, the tendency is to employ linear wavenumber and scale expansion beyond 2000 cm^{-1}.

PURIFICATION OF SAMPLES

An infra-red spectrum can be of more value in identification than any other single test recorded in this work. Unfortunately, the difficulties in obtaining such a spectrum are proportionately great. The problem is twofold; firstly, the substance to be identified must be as pure as possible, and secondly, the quantity must be sufficient to absorb the infra-red radiation sufficiently to produce a spectrum. The main difficulty regarding quantity is not so much the insensitivity of the spectrophotometer, since 50 μg of material is ample for most instruments, but the difficulty of purifying and handling such small quantities without substantial losses in the many stages before placing in the infra-red beam.

This section is designed to give some practical advice on suitable procedures. It is assumed that the starting material is a residue from the evaporation of a solvent extract of viscera or other material. The drug in this residue has been concentrated probably several thousand times by this extraction process but it is in a chemical sense very impure in that it will still contain a great deal of extraneous matter co-extracted from the starting material.

Despite the many purification techniques available, such as microdistillation, recrystallisation, etc., for the toxicologist no method is generally so suitable as some form of chromatography, followed by elution of the compound to be identified. The technique of gas–liquid chromatography is probably the most useful of all chromatographic methods.

(i) Paper and Thin-layer Chromatography

Suitable systems of chromatography are dealt with in the chapters on pp. 31–42 and 43–58. Any of these systems are potentially useful where it is required to elute a spot, but it is worth mentioning that systems which employ a stationary phase absorbed onto the paper or thin-layer plate are to be avoided, due to the fact that it is difficult to remove the spot without the stationary phase, which will

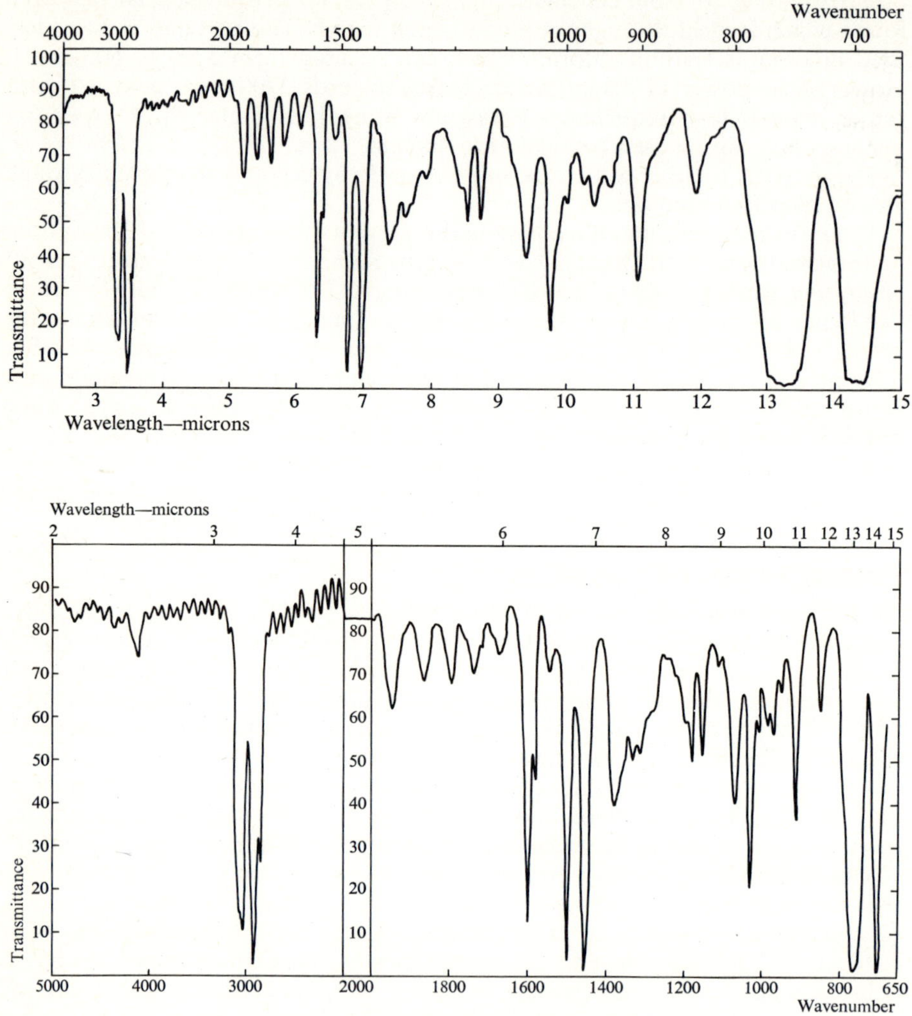

FIG. 2 & 3. TYPES OF INFRA-RED SPECTRA

interfere with the infra-red spectrum. The otherwise excellent reversed phase system of Street (1962) is a good example. Furthermore, location reagents must be chosen with care and a destructive reagent, such as the Marquis reagent for alkaloids, is best avoided. The chemist would be well advised to use a non-destructive reagent such as iodoplatinate, the colour complex being decomposable to yield the original compound unchanged.

Experience of elution techniques has shown that on the whole, paper systems are preferable to silica-gel thin-layer chromatography. The principal objection to thin-layer chromatography is that recoveries of drug, especially at low levels, can sometimes be surprisingly poor. Difficulties associated with elution from thin-layer plates have also been reported by Snavely and Grasselli (1964), Spencer and Beggs (1966), and Idler, Kimball, and Truscott (1966). Against this objection there are of course the advantages that a thin-layer chromatographic system is speedier and will often give better resolution of spots. In addition, thin-layer powders are available with fluorescent additives which facilitate location of spots without altering them chemically. Only experience can determine the best chromatographic system and eluting solvent for any particular drug or group.

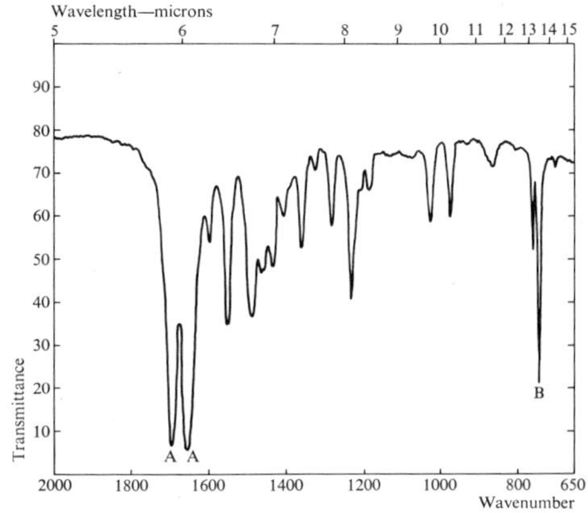

FIG. 4. SPECTRUM OF PURE CAFFEINE

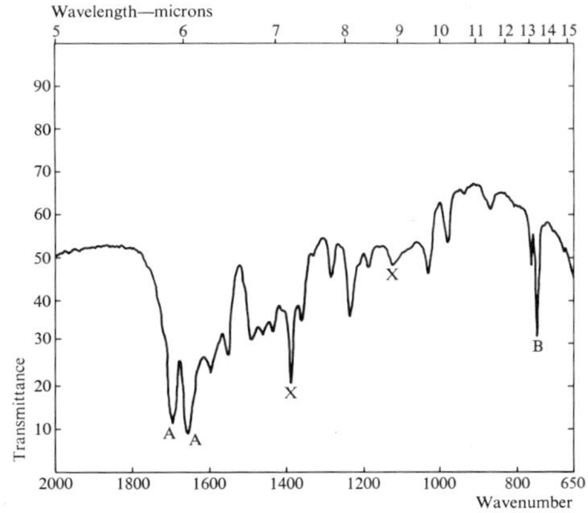

FIG. 5. SPECTRUM OF CAFFEINE ELUTED FROM A THIN-LAYER CHROMATOGRAPHY PLATE (Note: the bands marked X are not present in the spectrum of pure caffeine)

FIG. 4 and FIG. 5 show two infra-red spectra of caffeine, one of the pure drug and the other of an eluate from a thin-layer platc. The eluate was obtained from a two-dimensional thin-layer chromatogram of an extract of urine from a horse that had previously been given caffeine. In this case, thin-layer chromatography proved quite suitable for a satisfactory purification of the extract, and the eluate contained sufficient caffeine for infra-red spectrophotometry, notwithstanding the above objections. The spectra shown are typical of the small differences obtained between eluates and pure drugs under these conditions.

In the case described, the plate was run in the two-dimensional system described for steroids by Moss and Rylance (1966). The caffeine spot was located under ultraviolet light and the powder in this area scraped from the plate with a spatula. The powder was then shaken with 2 ml of methanol for 10 minutes in a stoppered tube, the tube centrifuged, and the supernatant solvent removed with a Pasteur pipette. The solvent was evaporated in a beaker containing about 100 mg of potassium bromide under vacuum at room temperature and a disk prepared from the powder. James (1967) has suggested that for steroids better recoveries are obtained by the addition of 2 or 3 drops of water to the thin-layer chromatography powder before adding the eluting solvent.

Similar elution techniques can be applied to paper chromatograms, the area of paper removed being cut into small pieces before shaking with solvent.

To avoid overloading the paper or thin-layer plate, the solution for chromatography can be applied as a line (as usually employed for electrophoresis) rather than as a spot. Elution from a paper strip of this kind can be done by descending chromatography.

Chromatographic materials are relatively inert to eluting solvents, but eluted material almost always includes unwanted extraneous matter co-extracted from the paper or thin-layer chromatography film. Although it is advisable to use an elution of a 'blank' area as a reference solution for ultraviolet spectrophotometry, we have not found it necessary for infra-red work. However, it is advisable to obtain an infra-red spectrum of any stationary phase from which elutions are made, as this can account for certain minor differences between the spectrum of an eluate of a compound and that of the pure compound.

(ii) Gas–Liquid Chromatography

Gas–liquid chromatography provides a very convenient method of obtaining pure samples for infra-red spectrophotometry. Unlike paper and thin-layer chromatography it is not necessary to elute the sample from the solid support after the chromatogram has been developed. However, the sample can still be contaminated with impurities eluted from the stationary phase. The effluent from the chromatograph is usually a vapour at an elevated temperature, and the problem is to trap efficiently small quantities in a form suitable for presentation to the spectrophotometer. The method used will depend on whether the compound to be collected is a solid or liquid and, if the latter, on its volatility. The chapter on Gas Chromatography (pp. 59–83) deals with the collection of fractions from a gas chromatograph by trapping. The spectra of the fractions obtained can be determined by the standard techniques, which are discussed below, provided enough sample is available. In many cases, however, the amount of material will be too small to enable the compound to be collected and transferred to standard cells. Therefore this section will be limited to a brief summary of the ways in which small samples can be obtained from a gas chromatograph in a form suitable for presentation to the spectrophotometer.

(a) *Silver chloride microcells*

Microcells extruded from silver chloride and known as 'Extrocells' (*Research & Industrial Instruments Company*) can be fitted with a silicone rubber serum cap and connected to the outlet of the chromatograph by means of a hypodermic needle. The sample collects in the neck of the cell which is then centrifuged in order to force the sample into the main body of the cell. Solvents can be added if solution spectra are required and are, of course, necessary if the compound is a solid. The cells can be used either at room temperature or they can be cooled in freezing mixtures or liquid nitrogen and can be used many times provided that they are stored in the dark. The cells are available with path lengths from 0·1 to 0·01 mm and volumes of 2 to 0·2 μl respectively. Their main disadvantage is that they have to be centrifuged for cleaning as well as for filling and emptying.

(b) *Membrane filters* [*Millipore (U.K.) Limited*]

Membrane filters composed of pure esters of cellulose can be used to collect samples from a chromatograph. The filters, which are about 25μ thick, are supplied in matched pairs so that by using a double beam spectrophotometer, it is possible to compensate for the absorption of the filter. The filter is placed in a specially designed metal and Teflon holder. The Teflon inlet section reduces condensation of the effluent before it reaches the filter and the metal outlet section allows the filter to be cooled. The filter holder, which has a female Luer taper in the Teflon inlet, is connected to the outlet of the chromatograph just before the sample emerges. When the sample has been collected, the filter is then removed and placed in the beam of the spectrophotometer, the matching filter being placed in the reference beam. The method is simple and easy to use and is capable of giving extremely good results. The main difficulty, which is common to all these methods of collecting fractions, is to determine the optimum temperature of the outlet tube from the chromatograph and the temperature of the collecting device. This problem can only be solved by trial and error.

(c) *Alkali halide tubes*

The idea of using an alkali halide as a medium for collecting fractions from a gas chromatograph was first proposed by Leggan (1961). A straight tube containing a plug of powdered alkali halide can be connected to the outlet of the chromatograph. The effluent condenses on the halide which can then be pressed into a disk. This technique is most useful for compounds which are solid at room temperature. An automated version of this technique has been developed and has been described by Gray, Metcalfe, and Leslie (1963).

(iii) Microsublimation

This simple technique can be highly effective in purifying certain compounds for infra-red spectrophotometry. The apparatus used is illustrated (FIG. 6 on p. 110). Drugs may be sublimed from an evaporated solvent extract in the tube onto the cold finger of the apparatus and transferred to the potassium bromide powder simply by grinding the powder gently with the cold finger.

SAMPLE PREPARATION

Infra-red spectra can be determined in the solid, liquid, and vapour phases. As most drugs are solid at room temperature, the determination of spectra in this phase has been used most widely. The various techniques will be outlined briefly; full experimental details are given by Miller (1965). Quantitative methods will not be considered.

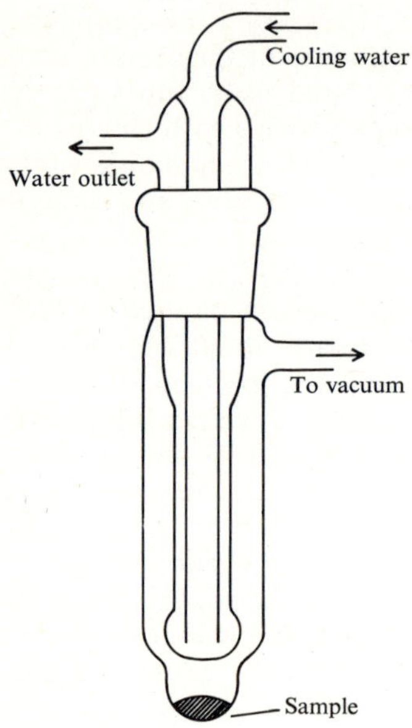

FIG. 6. APPARATUS FOR MICROSUBLIMATION

(i) Solids

The infra-red spectra of finely powdered solids cannot be readily determined since most of the radiation will be scattered and lost. Consequently solids are generally examined either as thin films or as dispersions in either liquids or solids.

(a) *Alkali halide disks*

The technique of dispersing the compound in an alkali halide has been widely used in the identification of drugs and is probably the most useful method available.

The finely powdered dry compound, about 1 mg, is mixed with an alkali halide, about 250 mg, ground either mechanically in an agate ball mill or by hand in an agate mortar, and pressed into a thin disk. If the sample is insufficiently ground, the formation of asymmetrical bands, which vary in position and intensity from the accepted values, may be obtained. This phenomenon, which is known as the Christiansen effect, may give the impression of impurities in the sample.

Originally, potassium bromide was used as the alkali halide and the technique is still often referred to as the 'KBr technique'. Potassium chloride has also been widely used and is often considered to be superior to potassium bromide because it is less hygroscopic. If only small quantities of the drug are available, a thin cardboard mask with a slot in the centre can be used. It is placed in the die and the slot filled with the drug–alkali halide mixture before pressing. About 0·2 mg of compound is required when a mask is used and, with special equipment, spectra can be obtained from as little as 0·01 mg. The use of a mask is often employed routinely because it proves a support for the alkali halide and so enables it to be handled more readily.

These disks can be stored in Cellophane envelopes and give good spectra several years after preparation. A well-prepared disk should have over 80% transmittance in regions where the sample does not absorb, although it will not necessarily be visually clear. It is not always easy to obtain a good disk when a very small amount of a recovered drug is available. In these instances, attenuation of the reference beam can 'sharpen' the spectrum. Another technique is to heat the alkali halide disk to about 80° for 30 to 60 minutes by means of an infra-red lamp. This evaporates any absorbed water and often results in an improvement of the spectrum. However, the high temperature accentuates the disadvantages of the alkali halide disk technique; in addition, the following artefacts have been observed:

(i) formation of anhydrides from carboxylic acids;
(ii) ketals and cyanohydrins reverting to the parent ketone;
(iii) loss of water from secondary alcohols.

There are several disadvantages inherent in the alkali halide disk technique; some of these have been discussed by Duyckaerts (1959).

The alkali halides which are generally used are hygroscopic and it is very difficult to exclude all traces of water. This results in a hydroxyl band often being found in the spectrum. A number of compounds containing hydroxyl groups either form hydrogen bonds with the alkali halide or are adsorbed on its surface, so the method is unsuitable if the hydroxyl band is to be examined. In such cases, polytetrafluoroethylene (PTFE; Teflon) powder can sometimes be used in place of the alkali halide. Polymorphism occurs in many compounds and the grinding and pressing can alter the crystal form and consequently the spectrum. Cleverley and Williams (1959) have reported this phenomenon in barbiturates. Splitting of bands also frequently occurs. Another disadvantage is the possibility of chemical changes occurring during the preparation of the disk. For example, double decomposition can occur:

$$\text{Base HCl} + \text{KBr} \longrightarrow \text{Base HBr} + \text{KCl}$$

Hydrochlorides should, therefore, always be examined in potassium chloride and not potassium bromide. Other changes which have been observed are:

(i) hydration of compounds not containing water;
(ii) saponification of acid chlorides;
(iii) decomposition of unstable compounds, e.g. azides and compounds containing bromine and iodine.

Despite these disadvantages the technique is still probably the most useful one for the identification of solid drugs. The advantages are that, besides being easy to use, the absorption of the alkali halide is very low and the quantity of compound required is small. The disks can easily be stored for reference purposes or the compound can be recovered if required.

(b) *Mulls*

Solid compounds can also be dispersed in liquids and one of the most widely used is liquid paraffin (Nujol). The finely powdered drug (2 to 3 mg) is mixed with one drop of the liquid and ground in an agate mortar. Sufficient liquid is then added so that the final mull is the consistency of a thin cream. The mull is spread on an alkali halide plate, usually sodium chloride or potassium bromide, and another plate placed on top. The film between the plates should be free of air bubbles.

A disadvantage of this method over the previous one is that the spectrum of the liquid will be superimposed upon that of the sample. Consequently, liquid paraffin cannot be used if the carbon–hydrogen stretching frequencies are to be examined and a halogenated liquid such as 'Fluorolube' (a fluorinated hydrocarbon) or hexachlorobutadiene must be employed. The disadvantages of changes in polymorphic forms and consequent changes in spectra also occur with this method.

(c) *Films*

This method is of use where it is necessary to obtain spectra free from dispersing media. The film can be prepared either by melting the solid and pouring it onto a suitable surface or by evaporation of a solution. This method is not widely used in drug analysis and will not be considered further.

(ii) Liquids

The determination of spectra of compounds in solution as well as that of pure liquids will be considered in this section. A wide range of various types of cell are available for determining spectra in the liquid phase. These cells usually consist of two parallel transparent windows separated by a spacing gasket and fitted with inlet and outlet ports. The width between the windows is usually between 0·1 and 0·01 mm. Variable path length cells in which one window on a piston moves in relation to the other window are also available. This type of cell is particularly useful where spectra of concentrated solutions are being recorded since the solvent can be placed in the reference beam of the spectrophotometer and the solvent peaks cancelled. The spectra of viscous non-volatile liquids can also be determined by simply sandwiching a thin film between two alkali halide plates.

The number of suitable solvents is limited and the most widely used are carbon tetrachloride and carbon disulphide because they have relatively few absorption bands in the infra-red region. Other solvents which have been used include chloroform, ethylene dichloride, methylene dichloride, benzene, cyclohexane, and n-heptane. The concentration of the compound is usually about 5 to 10% but concentrations up to 20% w/v have been employed. These high concentrations mean that hydroxyl and amino-compounds often exhibit bands due to inter-molecular hydrogen bonding.

A disadvantage of this method is that interactions between the compound and the solvent can occur. This may result in quite considerable changes in frequency of certain bands occurring in different solvents. Another disadvantage is that because most of the solvents used are highly volatile, the heat of the infra-red radiation can cause appreciable losses and consequent changes in concentration by evaporation.

(iii) Gases

Determination of infra-red spectra in the gaseous phase is very rarely used in routine analytical work unless, of course, the substance being examined is a gas at room temperature. The method may become more widely used with the advent of infra-red spectrophotometers coupled directly to gas–liquid chromatographs. Special long-path, air-tight cells are required for this method, which will not be considered further.

METHODS OF USING THE INFRA-RED DATA

The index of infra-red peaks on pp. 688–723 is designed to enable the operator to identify a drug from its infra-red spectrum. Provided the spectrum is reproduced in Part 3 (pp. 727–793), the index will enable retrieval of the appropriate standard spectrum.

The 444 infra-red spectra which have been reproduced in Part 3 have been chosen because it is believed that these compounds are the ones most likely to be encountered in pharmaceutical and toxicological investigations. Spectra from 2000 to 650 cm^{-1} only are depicted in Part 3 even though a wider region is discussed in this chapter. If the region from 4000 to 650 cm^{-1} had been depicted in full, it would have meant either a very compressed spectrum with a consequent loss of clarity or a large increase in the cost of publication. It was therefore decided to reproduce only the most useful part of the spectrum, viz. the 'fingerprint' region. When trying to identify compounds, the entire spectrum can, of course, be determined and compared with that of known compounds. The spectra have been indexed according to the wavenumber of the most strongly absorbing bands—a modification of the scheme proposed by Curry (1963a).

On each infra-red spectrum reproduced in Part 3, certain major bands have been marked. These bands, or 'peaks', have been labelled 'A', 'B', and 'C' in decreasing order of intensity. Theoretically, it should have been possible to index all the spectra reproduced here according to the major band, with the second and third intensities as confirmation. In practice, however, this was not possible because quite often there is more than one band in some spectra with the same absorption intensity or with intensity so close that the relative values could not be relied upon to be reproducible. For this reason we have frequently labelled more than three major bands, though never more than six. Where bands have the same or nearly the same intensities, they have been ascribed the same letters. The choice of whether two bands, close together in intensity, should be given the same letter or different ones has been fairly arbitrary and the letters used are only a guide to their intensity. Most infra-red spectrophotometers are not sufficiently accurate to justify a closer criterion. It will not affect the use of the index if the operator ascribes intensities 'A' and 'B' to two bands both of which we have labelled 'A'.

Every band marked on the spectra in Part 3 has been listed in sequential order of wavenumber in the index on pp. 688–723, the category of band being listed 'A', 'B', or 'C' in parentheses. Opposite each wavenumber is a list of all compounds having a band of this value marked on the spectra. The spectrum of the unknown compound should be examined and the frequency of the most strongly absorbing bands noted. These bands may then be correlated with those in the index and the spectrum identified in accordance with the method outlined on p. 688.

INTERPRETATION

We describe here the method of using the spectra and the procedure to be followed if the spectrum of the unknown compound does not match any of those reproduced in Part 3. Interpretation, in the usual sense of allocating bands to various types of structures, will not be dealt with in detail because of the vast number of widely different compounds involved. Besides which, for many compounds this detailed information is not available.

Infra-red spectrophotometers, particularly the type used in analytical laboratories, do not always give the correct frequency of the absorption bands. There are a number of reasons why the frequency recorded can differ from the correct value. Among these are errors inherent in the instrument, errors of adjustment, and errors in fitting the paper to the recorder and in the printing of the paper. The error in the frequency is greater at higher wavenumbers than at lower ones. At 5000 cm^{-1} the error inherent in the instrument alone can easily be as large as ± 50 cm^{-1}. Therefore it is essential to calibrate each spectrum *before* it is removed from the recorder.

For qualitative analytical work calibration is best done with a thin film of polystyrene. After the spectrum of the sample has been recorded, the polystyrene film is placed in the sample beam and a few of the main bands are recorded. The bands recorded are those whose frequency is known and which do not coincide with the main bands in the spectrum of the unknown. The differences between the recorded and correct frequency of the band are then calculated and these will probably vary in different regions of the spectrum. In order to calculate the correct frequency of a band, the difference between the recorded and correct frequency of a close polystyrene band is either added to or subtracted from the recorded frequency. The spectrum of bromvaletone calibrated with polystyrene is shown in FIG. 7 and the recorded and corrected frequencies are given in the table below. An alternative approach is to prepare a calibration graph. The spectrum of polystyrene is recorded and the differences (+ or −) between the observed and correct frequencies are plotted against wavenumber. The error at any particular frequency can then be obtained from the graph.

The method employed to identify the spectrum will depend very largely on how much information about the compound is already available. In many cases the separation procedure and behaviour on paper and thin-layer chromatography, e.g. Rf values and colour reactions, will have indicated the type of compound present if not its specific identity. In cases where the identity of the compound is believed to be known, one can simply compare the spectrum with that obtained from an authentic sample.

If this procedure fails, and in cases where the type of compound is unknown or can only be allocated to a certain class, e.g. a phenothiazine or a barbiturate, then reference must be made to the infra-red index (pp. 688–723). Comparison of the spectrum of the unknown with that of the suspected compound should either confirm or dispute the tentative identification. If the two spectra have been recorded under similar conditions on the same type of instrument then they should be very similar in appearance. If the spectra have been recorded on

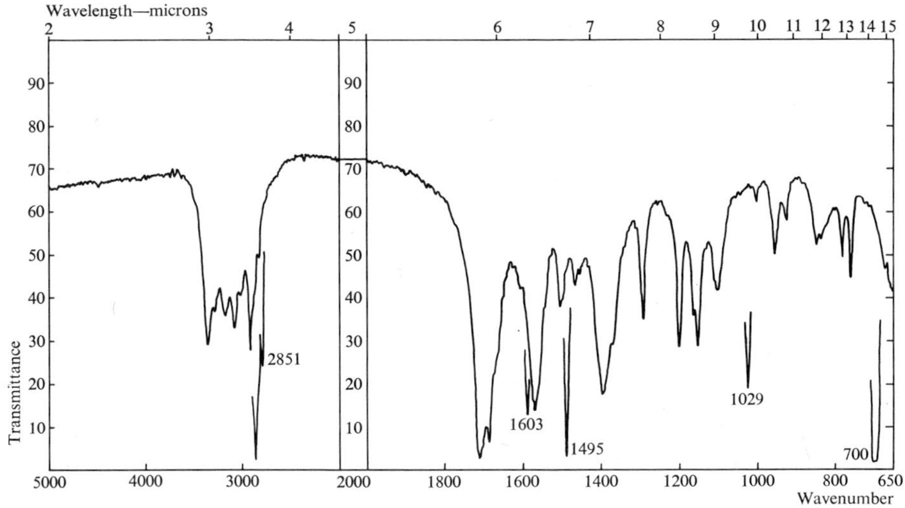

FIG. 7. SPECTRUM OF BROMVALETONE CALIBRATED WITH POLYSTYRENE

RECORDED AND CORRECTED WAVENUMBER OF CERTAIN BANDS IN THE INFRA-RED SPECTRUM OF BROMVALETONE

Recorded Wavenumber	*Correction*	*Corrected Wavenumber*
3460	+56	3516
2910	+56	2966
1712	+13	1725
1688	+13	1701
1570	+13	1583
1505	+ 5	1510
1397	+ 5	1402
1103	+ 2	1105
958	+ 2	960
762	0	762

different instruments then they may, superficially at least, appear very different. In this case a more detailed study of band frequencies and relative intensities must be undertaken.

The final stage in the process of identification must always be the comparison of the spectrum of the unknown with that of the pure drug obtained under as near identical conditions as possible and on the *same* instrument. If infra-red spectrophotometry is used frequently then the compilation of a collection of spectra of pure compounds is worth while.

If the spectrum does not agree with any of the spectra reproduced in Part 3 then reference must be made either to one's own collection of spectra, if this contains additional compounds, or to the literature. If the type of compound is known then the appropriate literature can be consulted, whereas if it is unknown an attempt must be made to interpret the spectrum. Most types of functional groups exhibit absorption bands in particular regions of the spectrum. For example, the hydroxyl group of alcohols, phenols, and acids exhibits an O—H stretching band in the region from 3700 to 2500 cm^{-1}. The carbonyl group of ketones, aldehydes, acids, and esters exhibits a C=O stretching band in the region from 1870 to 1535 cm^{-1}. The precise location of the band will often give an indication of the structural environment of the group, though no attempt will be made here to interpret in the conventional sense the spectra of all the drugs and related compounds which may be encountered. The ability to deduce the type of compound, e.g. a cyclic ureide, from an infra-red spectrum is useful when the occasional unusual compound occurs. However, in the large majority of cases this procedure is completely unnecessary because the preliminary examinations will have provided the information. The correlation of frequency with functional groups has been discussed in detail by Bellamy (1962a).

The method of interpreting spectra in a conventional sense will be illustrated by reference to the barbiturates and ureides, both groups of compounds being derivatives of urea. It is, of course, comparatively easy to interpret a spectrum when the structure of the compound is known and a large number of similar compounds are available for study. The infra-red spectra of barbiturates and of their complexes with various compounds have been studied by Umberger and Adams (1952), Price, Bradley, Fraser, and Quilliam (1954), Levi and Hubley (1956), and Chatten and Levi (1957). The following interpretation is based on their work and on an examination of 28 barbiturate spectra and 9 ureide spectra which are reproduced, in part, in this book. It is hoped that this examination will give the reader some idea of the approach to the interpretation of the infra-red spectrum of an unknown drug.

The barbiturates, which form a large and important class of drugs, are derivatives of malonyl urea (barbituric acid) and all of them have two substituents in position 5.

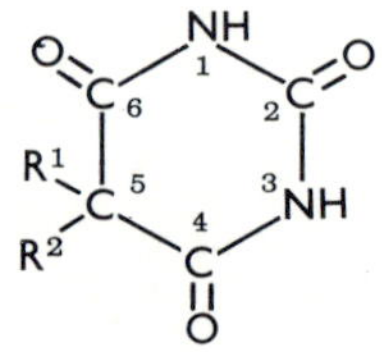

In addition, some of them are also substituted in position 1 and in others the oxygen atom attached to position 2 is replaced by sulphur to form thiobarbiturates. The barbiturates can be classified chemically into three classes:

(i) 5,5-disubstituted barbituric acids,
(ii) 1,5,5-trisubstituted barbituric acids, and
(iii) 5,5-disubstituted thiobarbituric acids.

These groups can be further divided depending on whether the substituents in position 5 are alkyl, alkenyl, aryl, or cycloalkenyl. In most common types of barbiturate one of the 5-substituents is either ethyl or allyl and the other is either a straight or branched chain alkyl or alkenyl group with five or fewer carbon atoms. Some barbiturates are marketed as sodium salts.

The infra-red spectrum of a barbiturate will depend on the class of compound, the nature of the substituents, and whether it is the free acid or the sodium salt. Barbiturates appear to be particularly susceptible to changes in crystal form when they are ground. Therefore, the method of preparation of alkali halide disks, whether by grinding mechanically or by hand, can cause profound changes in the infra-red spectrum. The phenomenon is illustrated by Cleverley and Williams (1959) for the regions 1800–1600 and 900–700 cm^{-1}.

The free barbiturates, with the exception of phenobarbitone and barbituric acid, do not absorb appreciably above 3300 cm^{-1}, a feature which distinguishes them from the ureides; a weak band of unknown origin occurs sometimes between 3500 and 3400 cm^{-1}. All the barbiturates have two bands which occur near 3200 and 3100 cm^{-1} and are due to N—H stretching vibrations. In the 5,5-disubstituted compounds the relative intensity of the two bands is similar although that at 3100 cm^{-1} is usually slightly less intense. In compounds having a substituent other than hydrogen on the nitrogen atom at position 1, the intensity of the band at 3100 cm^{-1} may be greatly reduced and is often present only as a shoulder on the band at 3200 cm^{-1}, e.g. metharbitone. Methylphenobarbitone appears to be an exception in that the band at 3100 cm^{-1} is the most intense one in the region. The spectrum of this compound published by Levi and Hubley (1956) also exhibits this band. A similar phenomenon occurs with the sodium salts since here again one of the hydrogen atoms in either position 1 or 3 has been replaced.

A series of up to four medium to intense bands occurs in the region 3000 to 2800 cm^{-1} and is due to alkyl C—H stretching vibrations of the substituents in positions 1 and 5. The intensity of the bands gives a very approximate indication of the number of C—H bonds and hence the number of carbon atoms in the chain. This does not appear to apply to the sodium salts, in which the band occurring at 3000 to 2950 cm^{-1} is usually increased in intensity, compared to that of the free acid, and becomes the strongest band. Compare, for example, the spectra of barbitone (FIG. 8) and barbitone sodium (FIG. 9)—p. 118.

The barbiturates have up to three strongly absorbing bands in the region 1765 to 1670 cm^{-1}. These bands are due to the C=O stretching vibrations and have been studied in detail by Price, Bradley, Fraser, and Quilliam (1954). A knowledge of the origin of these bands is useful in helping to understand the differences in the spectra of the various types of barbiturate. The band occurring at the highest frequency, about 1760 to 1740 cm^{-1}, is due to C=O vibrations at positions 4 and 6 which are perpendicular to the axis of symmetry of the molecule. The next band, occurring at about 1720 to 1700 cm^{-1} is also due to C=O vibrations at positions 4 and 6 but is affected by the C=O vibration at position 2. The band at the lowest frequency, about 1700 to 1670 cm^{-1}, is due to the C=O vibration at position 2. The free barbiturates have three bands in this region and in symmetrical molecules they are all of similar intensity. In asymmetrical molecules the band at the highest frequency is often less intense than the other two and this is particularly so when the molecule is substituted in position 1—compare the spectrum of phenobarbitone (p. 754) with that of methylphenobarbitone (p. 746).

The sodium salts of the barbiturates have only two bands in this region, since the molecule is no longer symmetrical, and these occur at a lower frequency,

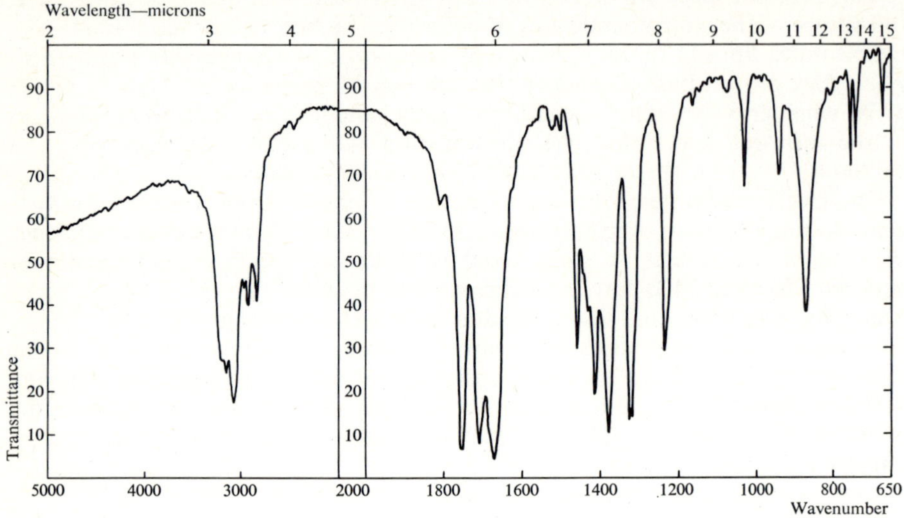

FIG. 8. SPECTRUM OF BARBITONE

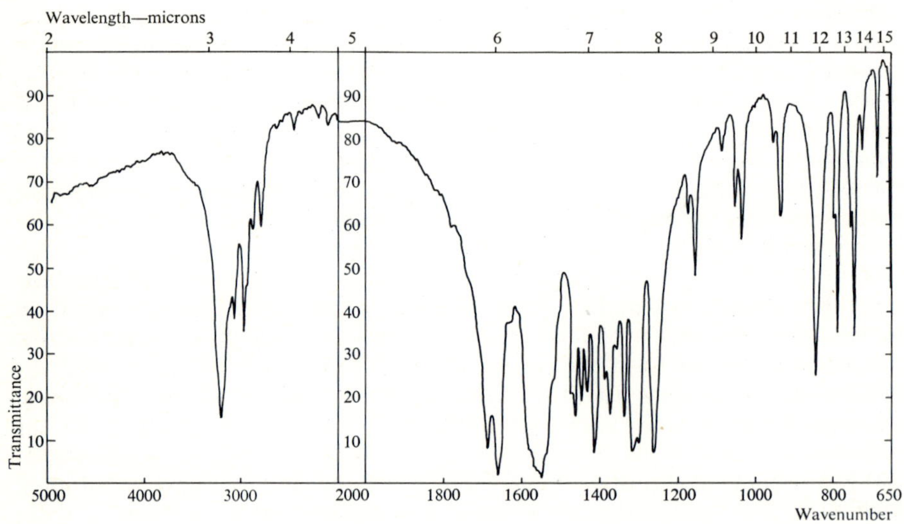

FIG. 9. SPECTRUM OF BARBITONE SODIUM

between 1700 to 1650 cm^{-1}. In addition, a broad strongly absorbing band occurs between 1600 and 1550 cm^{-1}; the free barbiturates show practically no absorption in this region. The sodium salts of the thiobarbiturates exhibit only the lowest of the three C=O vibrations and this occurs in the region 1700 to 1680 cm^{-1}. They do, however, exhibit the broad, strongly absorbing band, which occurs between 1650 and 1600 cm^{-1}. It can be seen, therefore, that the number, position, and intensity of the bands between 1800 and 1500 cm^{-1} give a very good indication of whether the barbiturate is in the form of the free acid or the salt or whether it is a salt of a thiobarbiturate.

Most barbiturates have a number of strongly absorbing bands between 1460 and 1250 cm^{-1} and some of these are due to C—H deformation and C—N stretching vibrations. The sodium salts of the thiobarbiturates have a broad strongly absorbing band between 1500 and 1480 cm^{-1} which is believed to be due to C—N stretching vibrations in which the carbon atom is also attached to sulphur. This band is not present in ordinary barbiturates and therefore provides another means of distinguishing those containing sulphur. Many barbiturates exhibit a few weak to medium intense absorption bands in the region 1150 to 900 cm^{-1}. The l-substituted barbiturates exhibit a greater number of sharp bands of medium intensity. Those compounds which contain an allyl group exhibit bands at about 1000 to 960 cm^{-1} which are due probably to C—H deformation vibrations. The sodium salts of the thiobarbiturates show a band of medium intensity between 1020 and 1000 cm^{-1}. Finally, many barbiturates, but not the thiobarbiturates, exhibit a broad band of medium to strong intensity between 900 and 800 cm^{-1}.

The ureides, which form a smaller and less important class of drugs than the barbiturates, are monosubstituted ureas in which one of the hydrogen atoms has been replaced by an acyl group. Chemically they can be divided into three types depending on whether the acyl group is (i) alkyl or alkenyl, (ii) halogenated, or (iii) aryl–alkyl, and can be represented as: $R \cdot CO \cdot NH \cdot CO \cdot NH_2$.

All the ureides have three N—H stretching bands and these absorb strongly in the region 3450 to 3250 cm^{-1}, features which distinguish them from the barbiturates. The third band is due presumably to the presence of a second hydrogen atom on one of the nitrogen atoms. The three bands of medium intensity which usually occur between 3000 and 2800 cm^{-1} are due to various alkyl C—H stretching vibrations. The reduction in intensity of these bands indicates a reduced number of alkyl C—H bonds in the molecule. This may be seen by comparing the spectrum of pheneturide (FIG. 10) containing six alkyl C—H bonds with that of phenacemide (FIG. 11) containing only two alkyl C—H bonds. In the latter compound the bands have almost disappeared. The bands in the region 3500 to 2800 cm^{-1} give, therefore, a good indication of whether the compound is a ureide or a barbiturate and also some indication of the amount of alkyl substitution.

Two strongly absorbing bands occur in the region 1720 to 1660 cm^{-1} and are due to C=O stretching vibrations. The position and intensity of these bands are quite different from those found in the free barbiturates but are similar to those found in the sodium salts. However, the latter class of compounds is readily distinguished by the very strong, broad band at 1600 to 1550 cm^{-1}. The ureides also absorb in this area but the bands usually occur at a slightly higher frequency, 1620 to 1580 cm^{-1}, and are only of medium intensity.

A broad band of medium intensity occurs in all ureides in the 1400 cm^{-1} region and is probably due to the amide group. The band may either have a shoulder as in ethylbutyrylurea or become a doublet, as in carbromal.

The remainder of the ureide spectrum varies a great deal from compound to

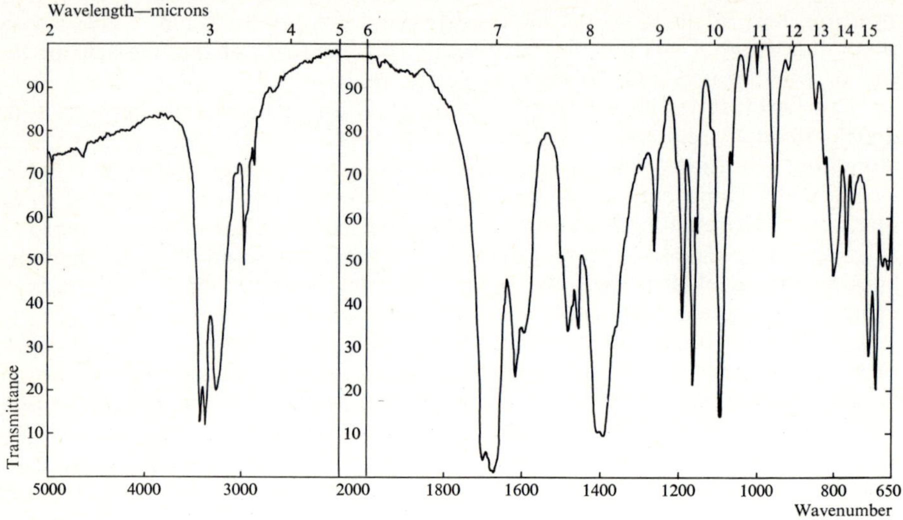

FIG. 10. SPECTRUM OF PHENETURIDE

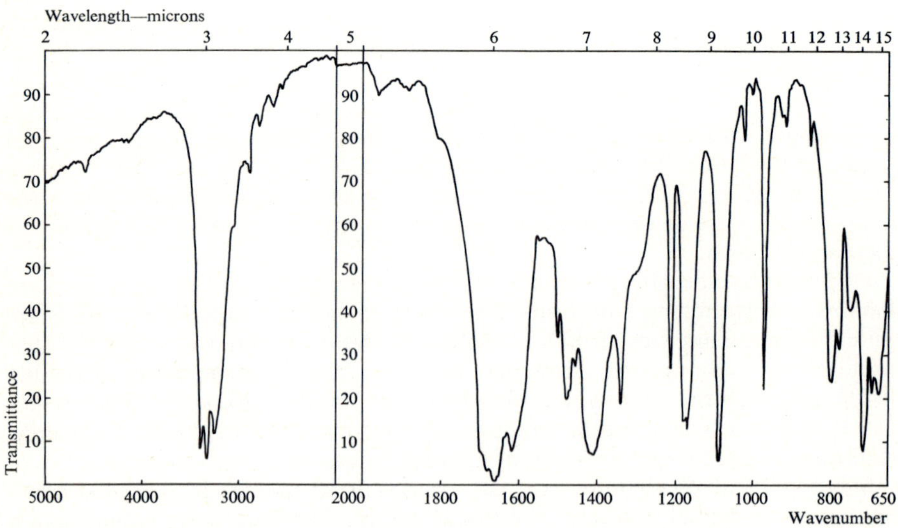

FIG. 11. SPECTRUM OF PHENACEMIDE

compound because of the wide variation in the nature of the substituents. Very little work has been done on the interpretation of the spectra of ureides and because of the small number of compounds commercially available it is not possible to assign bands to particular groups with certainty.

PUBLISHED SPECTRA

There are several useful indexes of infra-red spectra as well as collections of published spectra. An index to the spectra of about 36,000 compounds published between 1945 and 1962 has been compiled by Hershenson (1959 and 1964). The American Society for Testing Materials (ASTM) (1962 and 1963) has published an index to 43,500 spectra and a supplement has also been issued. Another index containing about 10,000 references has been published by the Ministry of Aviation (1960). Szymanski (1963) has published a monograph listing over 8500 band positions of organic and inorganic compounds and these are tabulated according to wavelength. Clark and Chianta (1957) have published an index of spectra of biochemicals. The most comprehensive collection of published spectra is that of the Sadtler Research Laboratories; over 33,000 spectra of pure compounds and 850 spectra of pharmaceuticals have been published, in addition to 2000 spectra of biochemicals and 12,500 spectra of commercial products. Since 1956 Butterworth & Co. (Publishers) Ltd and Verlag Chemie, GmbH (London and Weinheim) have published over 13,000 spectra on punched cards under the title 'Documentation of Molecular Spectroscopy'. Smaller collections of published spectra include 466 surface-active agents (Hummel, 1962), 335 compounds of pharmaceutical interest (Sammul, Brannon, and Hayden, 1964), 150 drugs and related compounds (Sunshine and Gerber, 1963), and 44 compounds of toxicological interest (Hubley, Levi, and Eagleson, 1960).

Information on the infra-red spectra of groups of compounds which are thought to be of particular interest to the pharmacist and toxicologist is reviewed in the following section. The review is not intended to be comprehensive but rather to give guidance on location and interpretation of spectra not reproduced in this book. The application of infra-red spectrophotometry to toxicology has been described by Hubley and Levi (1960a and b) and by Alha and Tamminen (1965). The detection of volatile organic compounds and gases in man by infra-red spectrophotometry has been reviewed by Stewart and Erley (1965). Bellamy (1962b) has produced a useful review on the infra-red spectra of compounds of biological interest and has included a section on interpretation.

Alkaloids. The spectra of 400 alkaloids, together with numerous other physical data, have been published by Holubek and Strouf (1967). The spectra of opium alkaloids and related compounds have been catalogued by Levi, Hubley, and Hinge (1955) and other collections of spectra have been published by Marion, Ramsay, and Jones (1951), Pleat, Harley, and Wiberley (1951) and Manning (1955).

Barbiturates. The spectra of barbiturates have been discussed in detail in this chapter (pp. 116–19). Sublimation of the residue from a chloroform extraction onto an alkali halide disk has been used when identifying barbiturates from tissue extracts on the 5 to 50 μg scale (Bonnichsen, Maehly, and Nordlander, 1960).

Carbohydrates. Spedding (1964) has reviewed the infra-red spectra of carbohydrates and the use of this technique in the determination of structure has been described by Barker, Bourne, and Whiffen (1956). Kuhn (1950) has published the infra-red spectra of 79 carbohydrates.

Hormones. The infra-red analysis of hormones has been reviewed by Rosenkrantz (1957).

Narcotics and related bases. A comprehensive collection of spectra has been published by Levi, Hubley, and Hinge (1955) and the frequency of their functional groups has been tabulated by Farmilo and Genest (1963).

Nucleic acids. The infra-red spectra of nucleic acids and related compounds have been reviewed by Shimanouchi, Tsuboi, and Kyogoku (1964).

Penicillins. The infra-red spectra of 14 penicillins have been published by Ovechkin (1963).

Phenothiazines. The infra-red spectra of 19 phenothiazines have been published by Scapini and Gardini (1964) and of 6 phenothiazine sulphoxides by Turner (1963). The attenuated total reflectance infra-red spectra of chlorpromazine and 14 possible metabolites have been described by Warren, Thompson, Zarembo, and Eisdorfer (1967).

Steroids. An atlas of steroid spectra has been produced by Neudert and Roepke (1965) and spectra have also been published by Dobriner, Jones, and Katzenellenbogen (1953) and Roberts, Jones, and Gallagher (1958). The 'fingerprint' region between 1350 and 650 cm^{-1} is of particular interest in steroid spectra and has been reviewed by Cole (1956). The analysis of steroids has also been reviewed by Rosenkrantz (1955) and the occurrence of polymorphism in pharmaceutically important steroids has been discussed by Mesley and Johnson (1965).

Ureides. The spectra of ureides have been discussed on pp. 119–21.

Vitamins. The infra-red spectra of vitamins have been reviewed by Rosenkrantz (1957).

Colour Tests

H. M. Stevens

Many substances give distinct colours when brought into contact with various chemical reagents. Sometimes the colour reaction with a particular reagent is not confined to a single compound but is produced by most of the compounds in a given class or even by substances not in that class. This type of test is called a 'general test' and can only be used as a preliminary guide to the nature of the substance to be identified.

The second type of colour test is the 'special test', where a colour produced with a certain reagent is specific for the compound under investigation. The special tests help considerably in identifying substances but absolute and final identification is usually only possible if some physical characteristic such as an infra-red spectrum can be obtained from the material. Special tests are described in detail in the relevant monographs in Part 2 and will not be dealt with further at this stage.

Many colour tests, both 'general' and 'special', can be carried out as 'micro' tests by using the techniques introduced by Clarke and Williams (1955). These techniques, which are described at the end of this chapter under the heading Microtests (p. 133), enable the identification of compounds to be effected on the microgram scale.

The compounds cited below have in the main been restricted to those for which monographs appear in Part 2; it must be realised, however, that many other organic compounds will give similar responses to these tests.

GENERAL TESTS

In the following paragraphs the 'general' tests are described, the various substances which respond being listed under the heading of the colour(s) obtained. These colours are set down in order of the spectrum from violet/purple through green and red to brown and black.

The tests have been classified according to the main component of the reagent and subdivided on the basis of the subsidiary components.

I Sulphuric Acid

A drop of the cold concentrated acid is brought into contact with a smear (if a liquid) or a few fragments (if a solid) of the test material on a white tile. In many instances this test may be carried out on the microscale.

PURPLE: Lymecycline, oxytetracycline, rolitetracycline, tetracycline.

BLUE: Chlortetracycline, demethylchlortetracycline, thioridazine.

GREEN: Strophanthin-K—sulphuric acid: water (4:1) must be used.

YELLOW: Bromodiphenhydramine, cyclizine, diphenhydramine, diphenylpyraline, ethyl biscoumacetate, griseofulvin, oestradiol, orphenadrine, pipradrol, prednisone.

ORANGE: Amitriptyline, chlorprothixene, cortisone, ethinyloestradiol, hydrocortisone, methacycline, spironolactone (50% sulphuric acid must be used; when heated the solution turns red).

RED: Caramiphen (if heated), hexamine (if heated), methylprednisolone (after 1 minute), ouabain, phenothiazines (but not trifluoperazine), prednisolone (after 1 minute).

BROWN: Methylpentynol.

I A **Sulphuric Acid**—with nitrous acid; Liebermann's reagent

This reagent (see Appendix 1) is prepared by dissolving 1 g of potassium nitrite in 10 ml of sulphuric acid. The reagent was originally developed for giving intense colours with phenols. The test is carried out as for Sulphuric Acid (I).

VIOLET: *o*-Aminophenol, methocarbamol, paracetamol, phenacetin, resorcinol.

BLUE: *p*-Aminophenol, diphenylamine, mefenamic acid, phenol (changing to red), yohimbine.

GREEN: Alphanaphthol, betanaphthol, chlorotrianisene (changing to pink on the addition of water), colchicine, hydrastine.

YELLOW: Benzathine penicillin, benzoic acid, benzylpenicillin, cocaine, *o*-, *m*-, and *p*-hydroxybenzoic acid, physostigmine, tropacocaine.

ORANGE: Compounds generally containing a *mono*-substituted benzene group not attached directly to a carbonyl group—acetanilide, amphetamine, aniline, atropine, caramiphen, ephedrine, glutethimide, hyoscine, methoin, methylphenobarbitone, pethidine, phenacemide, phenobarbitone, phenylmethylbarbituric acid, phenytoin, sulphinpyrazone, warfarin.

RED: Acepromazine (brownish-pink), brucine, oxytetracycline.

BROWN: *m*-Aminophenol, chlortetracycline, cotarnine, cresols, ethinamate, methylpentynol, noscapine, tetracycline, veratrine.

BLACK: Codeine, diamorphine, emetine, morphine, narceine, papaverine.

I B **Sulphuric Acid (60%)**—containing potassium dichromate (0·5%)

This test is carried out as for Sulphuric Acid (I) unless any modifications are mentioned.

PURPLE: Strychnine (changing to red), yohimbine (fades rapidly to slate blue).

BLUE: Aniline, desipramine, imipramine, thioridazine.

RED: Brucine, griseofulvin (5 mg is dissolved in 1 ml of sulphuric acid and 5 mg of powdered potassium dichromate added).

BROWN: Warfarin.

NOTE. The above tests are carried out in the cold. However, when alcohols and other reducing agents are warmed with a solution of potassium dichromate in dilute sulphuric acid (*acidified potassium dichromate solution*, p. 804) the potassium dichromate is reduced to the green chromium salt.

I C **Sulphuric Acid**—with chromotropic acid (see also under Screening Tests, p. 6)

RED: Formaldehyde. A few drops of a solution are added to a dilute solution of chromotropic acid in sulphuric acid.

I D Sulphuric Acid—with resorcinol

VIOLET: Formaldehyde. A little resorcinol is shaken with the test solution and some sulphuric acid is run down the inside of the tube to form a layer under the mixed solution—a reddish-violet ring appears at the junction of the 2 layers.

GREEN: Saccharin. A little is heated with an excess of resorcinol in sulphuric acid to *just* below the boiling point of the mixture—green. When the solution is cooled, diluted, and made alkaline with sodium hydroxide a green fluorescence is produced.

RED: Tartaric acid. A little is warmed with resorcinol and a few drops of sulphuric acid.

I E Sulphuric Acid—with vanillin

VIOLET: Menthol. About 10 mg is dissolved in 1 ml of sulphuric acid and 1 ml of a 1% solution of vanillin in sulphuric acid is added—orange-yellow; the addition of 1 ml of water gives a violet colour which distinguishes menthol from thymol.

I F Sulphuric Acid—with pyrocatechol

VIOLET: Metaldehyde. One drop of sulphuric acid is added to a small amount of solid followed by a trace of pyrocatechol—violet-red.

I G Sulphuric Acid—with betanaphthol

GREEN: Tartaric acid. The substance is heated with an equal bulk of betanaphthol and a few drops of sulphuric acid.

YELLOW: Malic acid (the test is carried out as above).

RED: Oestradiol. About 0·05 mg is heated at 100° with 1 ml of a 2·5% solution of betanaphthol in sulphuric acid for 2 minutes. The mixture is cooled and 1 ml of water is added—orange-yellow which changes to red when the solution is heated at 100° for 90 seconds.

I H Sulphuric Acid—with phenol

GREEN: Sulphonal. A little of the substance is heated with a few drops of sulphuric acid containing a trace of phenol.

NOTE. The colour tests using sulphuric acid in conjunction with formaldehyde (Marquis test), ammonium vanadate (Mandelin's test), and ammonium molybdate (Fröhde's test) are described under Microtests, p. 133.

II Nitric Acid

One of the most important tests using this reagent is Vitali's test (p. 133). Drugs which give a colour when treated with concentrated nitric acid, in the same way as with sulphuric acid in test I, p. 123, include:

BLUE: Desipramine, imipramine, thioridazine (with 50% nitric acid).

YELLOW: Phenols and phenolic substances (warming with the acid is sometimes necessary).

RED: Antazoline, bialamicol (100 mg is dissolved in 2 ml of water and 2 ml of concentrated nitric acid added), brucine, hexylresorcinol

(1 ml of 70% nitric acid is added to 1 ml of a saturated aqueous solution).

II A **Nitric Acid**—with ceric ammonium sulphate

VIOLET: Primaquine. 10 mg is dissolved in 5 ml of water and 1 ml of a 5% solution of ceric ammonium sulphate in dilute nitric acid is added.

II B **Nitric Acid**—with mercuric nitrate; Millon's reagent

This reagent consists of 1 part of metallic mercury dissolved in 1 part of fuming nitric acid (w/w), the solution being diluted with 2 parts of water (v/v). A small quantity of the test material or a few drops of the test solution is warmed with a few drops of the reagent.

RED: Phenolic compounds.

III **Hydrochloric Acid**

YELLOW: Chlordiazepoxide. A few fragments are moistened with 2N hydrochloric acid and evaporated to dryness on a water-bath. Triacetyloleandomycin. 10 mg of the substance is heated with 5 ml of the acid on a water-bath—greenish-yellow.

III A **Hydrochloric Acid**—with wood shavings

ORANGE: Sulphonamides. The substance is acidified with 2N hydrochloric acid and the mixture placed on wood shavings or newspaper. This test produces a positive response with many substances containing an aromatic amino-group.

III B **Hydrochloric Acid**—with furfuraldehyde

VIOLET: Allantoin. A solution of the substance in ethanol is treated with a concentrated furfuraldehyde solution in ethanol to which a little of the concentrated acid is added.

BLACK: Carbamates—carbachol, ethinamate, mephenesin carbamate, meprobamate, methylpentynol carbamate, styramate, urea, urethane. A spot of an acetone or ethanol solution of the substance is placed on filter paper. After drying, the paper is sprayed lightly with a 10% v/v solution of furfuraldehyde in ethanol. The paper is then exposed to hydrochloric acid fumes.

III C **Hydrochloric Acid**—with potassium dichromate

VIOLET: Paracetamol. A few mg of the test material is boiled gently with 2 to 3 ml of the concentrated acid for 3 minutes. The solution is cooled, diluted with water to about 3 times its volume, and a few drops of a cold dilute solution of potassium dichromate added to it. The violet colour persists; this is in contradistinction to phenacetin which also gives a violet colour that soon turns red.

III D **Hydrochloric Acid**—with sodium nitrite

VIOLET: Amidopyrine. To a dried spot, or a few fragments on a white tile, is added a drop of water and a small droplet of the dilute acid.

A few small crystals of sodium nitrite are added and the mixture stirred.

GREEN: Phenazone (details as for Amidopyrine).

ORANGE: Sulphaphenazole and sulphasomizole. The substance is treated with the dilute acid, followed by a few crystals of sodium nitrite—a bright orange precipitate.

III E **Hydrochloric Acid**—with potassium chlorate; amalic acid test

A few fragments of the substance under test are placed on a watch-glass and mixed with 2 to 3 drops of concentrated hydrochloric acid. A few crystals of potassium chlorate are added and, after stirring, the mixture on the watch-glass is evaporated to dryness on a boiling water-bath. The glass is cooled and the residue moistened with a drop or two of 2N ammonium hydroxide. The colour of the residue becomes purple.

PURPLE: Acepifylline, bamifylline, bufylline, caffeine, diprophylline, etamiphylline, proxyphylline, theobromine, theophylline.

IV **Sodium Hydroxide** or **Potassium Hydroxide**

VIOLET: Santonin. About 10 mg is warmed with 1 ml of a solution of potassium hydroxide in ethanol.

BLUE: *m*-Dinitrobenzene, 2,4-dinitrotoluene. A drop of 2N alkali is added to an acetone solution of the substance. The blue colour changes to violet-red on addition of acetic acid.

YELLOW: Acetaldehyde. One or two drops are added to a large excess (1 to 2 ml) of 40% sodium hydroxide solution and the mixture is heated to boiling—yellow turbid solution with a characteristic smell.

Nicotinamide. A little dry material is heated with 5% sodium hydroxide solution.

p-Nitrophenol. A drop of sodium hydroxide solution is added to a little dry material.

ORANGE: *m*-Nitrophenol (the test is carried out as for *p*-Nitrophenol).

ORANGE-RED: Chloramphenicol. A little dry material is heated with 5% sodium hydroxide solution; ammonia vapour may be evolved.

Nitrofurantoin. 5 mg is dissolved in 5 ml of 0·1N sodium hydroxide—deep yellow changing to deep orange-red.

Nitrofurazone. 10 mg of the compound is dissolved in 10 ml of 20% sodium hydroxide solution.

RED: *o*-Nitrophenol and phenolphthalein. A drop of sodium hydroxide solution is added to a little dry material.

2,4,6-Trinitrotoluene. A drop of sodium hydroxide solution is added to an acetone solution.

IV A **Sodium Hydroxide**—with iodine

VIOLET: Alphanaphthol. The substance is added to a mixture of equal volumes of iodine solution in potassium iodide and 2N sodium hydroxide. The reagent mixture must contain a small excess of alkali. Betanaphthol does not react.

IV B Sodium Hydroxide or **Potassium Hydroxide**—with chloroform

BLUE: Alphanaphthol and betanaphthol. A little of the substance is heated with 2N sodium hydroxide and a few drops of chloroform.

RED: Hydroquinone. A solution in chloroform is warmed with a small amount of solid potassium hydroxide. The mixture changes colour through yellow to red or red-brown.

IV C Sodium Hydroxide—with alphanaphthol or betanaphthol

BLUE: Chloroform. A drop of the liquid is heated with a small quantity of the naphthol in 2N sodium hydroxide.

IV D Sodium Hydroxide—with phenol

BLUE: *p*-Aminophenol. The substance is shaken with a solution of phenol in 2N sodium hydroxide.

IV E Sodium Hydroxide—with resorcinol

RED: Chloroform. A drop of the liquid is heated with a small amount of resorcinol in 2N sodium hydroxide.

IV F Sodium Hydroxide—with potassium mercuric iodide; Nessler's reagent

The potassium mercuric iodide present in the reagent (see Appendix 1) reacts with ammonia to yield an orange flocculent mercuric complex. Substances which are hydrolysed in alkaline solution to yield ammonia give a positive response with this test. Equal volumes of the reagent and the test solution (aqueous) are mixed and heated gently.

ORANGE-BROWN: Bromvaletone, chloramphenicol, and nicotinamide (all 3 yield the precipitate on heating above 40°), carbromal (on heating to 40°).

DARK BROWN: Paracetamol (on heating to about 80°).

IV G Sodium Hydroxide—with sodium nitroprusside

One or two drops of a test solution is added to a dilute aqueous solution of sodium nitroprusside and 1 or 2 drops of 2N sodium hydroxide is then added.

ORANGE-RED: Ketones.

RED: Acetaldehyde.

IV H Sodium Hydroxide—with pyridine; Fujiwara's test

A little of the solid or a drop of a test solution is added to a mixture of pyridine (1 ml) and 20% sodium hydroxide solution (2 ml). The mixture is heated on a boiling water-bath for 3 to 5 minutes with vigorous periodic shaking. A control test must be carried out. The colour appears in the pyridine layer.

RED: Chloral hydrate, chloramphenicol, chlorbutol, chloroform, trichloroethane, trichloroethanol, trichloroethylene.

NOTE. Chloralose does not respond to this test unless it is first heated to 100° with an equal volume of sulphuric acid to hydrolyse it.

IV I Potassium Hydroxide—with dimethylformamide

BLUE: Furazolidone. 1 mg is dissolved in 1 ml of dimethylformamide and 0·05 ml of 1N ethanolic potassium hydroxide.

V Sodium Hypochlorite

VIOLET: Aniline. Aqueous sodium hypochlorite solution is added drop by drop to an aqueous solution of aniline. The initial colour is brown but this is very transient and rapidly becomes violet. The test is sensitive to 1 part of aniline in 66,000 parts of solution.

ORANGE: Aminoguanidine, guanidine, sulphanilamide, sulphanilic acid (these compounds are treated as for Aniline, above).

VI Ammonia

YELLOW: Nitrazepam. A drop of an acetone solution is spotted on filter paper and exposed to ammonia vapour. The bright yellow colour fades when the vapour is withdrawn. Solutions of nitrazepam and its salts are turned yellow by the addition of ammonium hydroxide solution.

Aloin. 5 ml of dilute ammonia solution is added to 5 mg of the substance; the mixture turns yellow, green, and finally brown. The solution exhibits a yellow fluorescence in ultraviolet light.

VI A Ammonia—with copper sulphate

PURPLE: Proguanil. To 10 ml of a saturated solution of proguanil hydrochloride is added 1 drop of 10% copper sulphate solution and 2·5 ml of dilute ammonia solution and the mixture is shaken well. 5 ml of benzene is then added and the mixture is again shaken. The upper benzene layer is coloured purplish-red.

VII Ferric Chloride

Usually 1 or 2 drops of a 5% aqueous solution is added to a solution of the substance under test in ethanol or acetone. Water may be used as a solvent but only when the test material is readily soluble, since dissociation of the coloured iron complex may rapidly occur and the colour will not be seen.

VIOLET: Salicylates—aminosalicylic acid (in water), salicylaldehyde, salicylamide, salicylic acid, salicyluric acid; also amidopyrine, dipyrone (the ferric chloride solution is added to fragments on a tile), hexachlorophane (transient).

m- and *p*-Nitrophenol. The solution in water is boiled and cooled before the ferric chloride solution is added to it.

Saccharin. This substance is kept for ½ minute in a molten mixture with potassium hydroxide. The melt is then dissolved in water, acidified, and treated with the reagent.

Streptomycin. A little streptomycin sulphate is boiled with 1N sodium hydroxide, then *just* acidified with hydrochloric acid and treated with ferric chloride solution.

BLUE: Alphanaphthol, gentisic acid (ink-blue), guaiacol, morphine, paracetamol, parachlorophenol, phenol.

GREEN: Betanaphthol, hexylresorcinol, hydroquinone (transient), hydroxyquinoline, paraphenylenediamine (in water).
Adrenaline, ethylnoradrenaline, isoetharine, isoprenaline, noradrenaline, and nordefrin (solutions on the gradual addition of 5% sodium bicarbonate solution turn from green to blue-violet and then red).

YELLOW: Gluconic acid (in water), glucuronic acid (in water), lactic acid (in water), pantothenic acid (after boiling with a few drops of sodium hydroxide and making *just* acid before adding the reagent).

ORANGE: *m*-Aminophenol (in water).

ORANGE-RED: Acetates and propionates. A few drops of ferric chloride solution is added to neutral solutions of the substances. The colour due to propionate will pass into amyl alcohol on shaking but that due to acetate remains in the lower aqueous layer.

RED: Pentachlorophenol, phenazone, thiourea (after keeping the solid molten for $\frac{1}{2}$ minute).

BROWN: *o*- and *p*-Aminophenol (in water).

VIII *p*-Dimethylaminobenzaldehyde

The test is usually carried out by spraying dried spots of the test solution on filter paper or chromatographic paper with a 1% solution of the reagent in a mixture of ethanol:hydrochloric acid (1:1). Heating the substance under test with a 1% solution of *p*-dimethylaminobenzaldehyde in sulphuric acid is sometimes used as a colour test.

NOTE. Most of these reactions can be carried out as Microtests—see p. 133.

PURPLE: Ergot alkaloids including lysergide and dimethyltryptamine and its derivatives (including psilocybin). The colour appears on warming the paper in hot air.
Chlordiazepoxide. Heating the paper in a closed dish on a boiling water-bath for 30 to 40 minutes is necessary to bring up the colour.

YELLOW: Most compounds containing a primary aromatic amino-group, e.g. aminosalicylic acid, anileridine, aniline, procaine, and sulphanilamide, respond to this test.
Bromvaletone and carbromal. The colour develops overnight but is pale.
Carbamates.
Phenacetin. The colour develops on standing overnight.
Phenacemide. The colour develops on warming.
Sulthiame. The paper is dried in warm air and the background faded by dipping the paper in 2N ammonium hydroxide.

ORANGE: Paracetamol. The colour forms on standing overnight.

RED: Cannabis extracts. The material is warmed in a tube with 1 or 2 drops of ethanol and a few drops of a solution of *p*-dimethylaminobenzaldehyde in sulphuric acid.
Phenazone. The colour appears on warming the paper in hot air.

IX **Copper Sulphate**—Copper sulphate test

If one drop of a 1% solution of copper sulphate is added to a 1% solution of the substance under test in 0·1N sodium hydroxide, the following colours are obtained.

BLUE: Phthalylsulphacetamide, sulphacetamide (pale blue), sulphaguanidine, sulphanilamide, sulphaphenazole (greyish-blue).

GREEN: Phthalylsulphathiazole, succinylsulphathiazole (greyish-green), sulphadimethoxine and sulphaquinoxaline (yellowish-green), sulphadimidine (turning to reddish-brown), sulphaethidole, sulphafurazole, sulphamerazine (turning dark brown), sulphamethizole, sulphamethoxazole, sulphamoprine (turning dull orange), sulphapyridine (turning brownish-green), sulphasomidine, sulphormethoxine (pale green).

BROWN: Sulphadiazine (turning purplish-brown), sulphamethoxydiazine (purplish-brown), sulphamethoxypyridazine (greenish-brown), sulphasalazine (orange-brown), sulphathiazole (purplish-brown), sulphasomizole.

IX A **Copper Sulphate**—with sodium hydroxide; Chen's test

To one drop of a 1% solution of the compound in 1% acetic acid add 1 drop of 1% copper sulphate solution followed by 1 drop of 2N sodium hydroxide. This test can be carried out on the microscale but the technique is not very satisfactory.

PURPLE: Bamethan, clorprenaline, ephedrine, metanephrine, metaraminol, methylephedrine, normetanephrine, norpseudoephedrine, orciprenaline (changing to green), oxedrine, phenylephrine, phenylpropanolamine, pseudoephedrine.

GREEN: Adrenaline (changing to greenish-brown), adrenolone (changing to orange then yellow-brown), ethylnoradrenaline (grey-green), isoetharine (grey-green changing to red-brown and then to yellow-brown), isoprenaline (changing to brown), noradrenaline (changing to greenish-brown), nordefrin.

IX B **Copper Sulphate**—with sodium nitrite; McNally's test

About 1 mg of the substance is dissolved in a few drops of acetone and 1 to 2 ml of water is added. One or two drops of a 0·5% solution of copper sulphate in 10% acetic acid is added, followed by a pinch of solid sodium nitrite. The mixture is shaken, heated gradually to boiling, and maintained at boiling for a few minutes.

RED: Aspirin and salicyclic acid.

NOTE. Other salicylates, such as salicyluric acid and salicylamide, give only a yellowish-orange colour, which is not diagnostic. Aminosalicylic acid gives a chocolate-brown precipitate.

X **Bromine** and **Ammonia**—Thalleioquin test

A drop of an aqueous solution of the substance is placed on a white tile and mixed with a drop of bromine solution. When the orange colour of the bromine has disappeared and the solution is *just* tinted yellow, the mixture is exposed to ammonia vapour. The test can be carried out on the microscale (see p. 133).

GREEN: Hydroquinidine, hydroquinine, quinidine, quinine.
Cinchonidine and cinchonine do *not* give a positive reaction with this test.

NOTE. A test involving the use of bromine and ammonia is also used for the identification of purines on paper chromatograms—see the Clarke–Kalayci test, Appendix 2.

XI **Alkaline Cobalt Test**—Zwikker's test

This is a well-established presumptive test for barbiturates and structurally similar compounds. In essence it consists in mixing solutions of a cobalt salt (acetate or nitrate) with a solution of the substance under test in the absence of water and then making the mixture alkaline without introducing water. The colour produced by a positive response is a deep violet-blue. With barbiturates the colour is fairly persistent (i.e. it is retained for several minutes) but with certain other compounds it rapidly fades to a dirty slate-blue. The solvent medium used in this test is usually anhydrous ethanol or methanol and the alkalinising agent may be ammonia vapour, sodium hydroxide, lithium hydroxide, or even barium hydroxide.

Two methods have been found to be generally useful for rapid testing in a small tube. (1) Ethanolic solutions of cobalt acetate or nitrate and the substance under test are mixed and then shaken with a pellet of sodium hydroxide. The test produces better results when the cobalt solution is fairly weak and the barbiturate is in slight excess. (2) To a pinch of the powdered substance, 1 ml of 0·2% cobalt acetate solution in methanol is added and, after agitation to dissolve the solid, 1 ml of a 1% solution of lithium hydroxide in methanol is added.

VIOLET-BLUE: Amylobarbitone and the other barbiturates (the colour persists for 5 to 10 minutes), bemegride (the colour persists for 1 to 2 minutes), glutethimide (the colour persists for a few minutes), phenytoin (the colour fades in 30 to 60 seconds), primidone (the colour is only transient).

The formation and persistence of the violet-blue colour with Zwikker's test is therefore a good indication of the presence of a barbiturate.

XII **Iodoform Test**

To 2 ml of a dilute solution of the test material is added a few drops of 2N sodium hydroxide; several drops of a 0·1N solution of iodine in potassium iodide is then added until a persistent yellow colour appears. The appearance of yellow crystals of iodoform on gentle heating indicates the presence of acetaldehyde, acetone, or ethanol. A positive response is also given by ethyl methyl ketone, isopropanol, lactic acid, and a number of quinones, quinols, and *m*-dihydric phenols.

XIII **Paraformaldehyde–Phosphoric Acid Test**

A drop of 1% paraformaldehyde in 90% phosphoric acid is added to a small crystal placed on a white tile. The test may also be carried out on the microscale and the reagent may be used to detect spots on paper chromatograms. The test is very specific for solanidine and solanine.

PURPLE: Phenothiazines.
STEEL-BLUE: Solanidine, solanine.
GREY: Deserpidine, yohimbine.
YELLOW: Colchicine, demecolcine.
ORANGE: Ergotamine, pentaquin, propantheline, thebaine.

MICROTESTS

Many colour tests may be carried out on the microgram scale using the method developed by Clarke and Williams (1955) which involves a technique similar to that described for Microcrystal Tests (p. 135). Microrods are made by heating pieces of glass rod, each about 20 cm long and 0·5 cm in diameter, in the middle and pulling them out until the diameter at the thinnest point is about 0·1 cm. They are then broken at this point, and the ends ground flat (FIG. 1a, p. 136). When the narrow end of such a rod is allowed to touch the surface of a liquid, and then removed, it brings away a small drop adhering to the glass. This pendant drop (FIG. 1b, p. 136) is known as a microdrop, and is the standard quantity used for all the microcrystal and microcolour tests which are described in this book. It has a volume of about 0·1 μl (Hawkins, 1959); a conventional drop (0·05 ml) will thus provide material for 500 different tests. It is imperative that the end of the rod should only touch the surface of the liquid and not penetrate it, as in the latter case there may be several droplets of indefinite size adhering to the sides of the rod and none to its end.

Tests are carried out by transferring a microdrop of the test solution to a small piece of opal glass and adding a microdrop of the appropriate reagent. The residue left after evaporation of the drop may be almost invisible; it is therefore advisable to indicate the location of the first drop on the glass with a pencil mark.

Sulphuric Acid–Formaldehyde Test (Marquis Test). A microdrop of the test solution is placed on the glass, allowed to evaporate to dryness, and a microdrop of *Marquis reagent* is added.

Ammonium Molybdate Test (Fröhde's Test). A microdrop of a 0·5% aqueous ammonium molybdate solution is added to a microdrop of the test solution and the residue after evaporation is moistened with sulphuric acid.

Ammonium Vanadate Test (Mandelin's Test). A microdrop of a 0·5% aqueous solution of ammonium vanadate is added to a microdrop of the test solution and the residue after evaporation is moistened with sulphuric acid.

Diazotisation Test. This test detects compounds containing a primary aromatic amino-group. To a microdrop of the test solution are added successively micro-drops of 1N hydrochloric acid, a 1% aqueous sodium nitrite solution, and a 4% solution of betanaphthol in 2N sodium hydroxide.

Vitali's Test. A microdrop of the test solution is allowed to dry and a microdrop of fuming nitric acid is added. The colour (A) is noted; the drop is evaporated to dryness on a boiling water-bath and the colour (B) is noted; the residue is moistened with freshly prepared ethanolic potassium hydroxide solution and the colour (C) is noted. The colours are recorded as A/B/C. It should be noted that many compounds give various shades of yellow, orange, and brown which are of little diagnostic value.

OTHER TESTS

The following tests have been designated as MICRO tests in the monographs in Part 2 but they may also be performed on the macro scale. They are described in the General Tests section—*p*-dimethylaminobenzaldehyde test (VIII, p. 130), ferric chloride test (VII, p. 129), paraformaldehyde-phosphoric acid test (XIII, p. 132), sulphuric acid test (I, p. 123), and thalleioquin test (X, p. 131).

Treatment of Bromides and Iodides

The colours recorded in Part 2 for the microtests with sulphuric acid are those obtained with the free base. In the case of a salt these may be modified by the nature of the acid radical present; bromides and iodides, for example, usually give a green or blue colour with the ammonium molybdate test. In the case of a compound extracted from biological material no difficulty will arise, as it will be extracted as the base, but care must be taken in applying colour tests directly to pharmaceutical preparations. These may, of course, be converted to the free base but it is often quicker to convert bromide or iodide to nitrate, which gives the same colour as the base. This may be done as follows. To 0·5 ml of a 1% solution of the salt in dilute acetic acid add 1 drop of an 8% solution of silver nitrate. Centrifuge off the precipitated silver halide, decant the supernatant liquid, and add to it 1 drop of a 2% solution of sodium chloride in order to remove excess silver. Centrifuge again, and use the supernatant liquid for the colour tests.

SENSITIVITY OF MICROTESTS

As the volume of a microdrop is 0·1 μl, it follows that a microdrop of a 1% solution will contain 1 μg, a microdrop of a 0·5% solution 0·5 μg, and so on. The sensitivity of a test refers to the smallest quantity of a substance that will give a positive result in that test. This may be stated as the concentration of the solution used or the actual weight of the test material present in a microdrop of such a solution. Thus, if the most dilute solution to give a positive result is 1 in 1000, the sensitivity may be recorded as 1 in 1000 or as 0·1 μg. The former convention has been adopted for Microcrystal Tests (p. 135) which are carried out in solution, the latter for colour tests which are usually performed on the solid material.

Microcrystal Tests

E. G. C. Clarke

The crystal, or microcrystal, test is one of the oldest, the simplest, and the most sensitive tests used in toxicology. Although nowadays it has fallen into disfavour and been very largely replaced by instrumental methods, it remains of considerable value for confirmatory purposes.

It is not proposed to deal here with the history of the development of this test or with the various ways in which it has been adapted to meet special needs. This has been done admirably in a recent work by Fulton (1969). It is, however, necessary to explain that the 'microcrystal' test which we are describing here is quite different from the 'crystallographic' test. The microcrystal test is a 'matching' test, identification being achieved by comparing the microscopic appearance of the crystals formed when the test solution is mixed with a certain reagent with those formed when the same reagent is mixed with a solution of a known substance. The crystallographic test is a physical test in which identification is carried out by the measurement of various optical properties, such as the refractive index and the extinction, of crystals of the test substance itself or of some suitable derivative. This procedure is of limited use in toxicology as it needs more material than is usually available.

The microcrystal test is unsuitable as a primary method of identification of an unknown compound, as it does not lend itself to form the basis of an identification scheme. Its real value is as a means of final identification to confirm a provisional diagnosis made from chromatographic or spectrophotometric evidence, its extreme simplicity, the rapidity with which it may be performed, and its high degree of specificity, rendering it ideal for this purpose. Its most common application is to basic nitrogenous drugs of the alkaloidal type, although it may also be adapted for use with neutral and acidic compounds.

In its simplest form the test consists in mixing a drop of a solution of the test material with a drop of the reagent on a microscope slide and observing the crystals formed under the microscope. This is quite adequate if sufficient material is available and if the crystals of the derivative appear at once; but if they form only slowly, or if attempts are made to increase the sensitivity of the test by decreasing the size of the drop used, loss of water due to evaporation will cause the drop to become saturated with the reagent, which will be deposited as crystals and mask the crystals of the derivative. Evaporation may be avoided by the use of a cover-slip, but in this case the crystals, formed in the two-dimensional environment of a thin film, will be grossly distorted and in no way characteristic.

Hanging Microdrop Technique

In order to overcome these difficulties and to provide a method that should be sensitive enough to be used with the quantity of material that could be eluted from a paper chromatogram, Clarke and Williams (1955) introduced the 'hanging microdrop' technique. This is the method that has been used to obtain the crystals described under the subheading 'Crystal Tests' and preceded by the word 'MICRO' in the various monographs in Part 2 of this book.

The procedure is as follows. A supply of 'microrods' is prepared by heating pieces of glass rod, each about 20 cm long and 0·5 cm in diameter, in the middle and pulling them out until the diameter at the thinnest point is about 0·1 cm. They are then broken at this point and the ends are ground flat (FIG. 1a). When the narrow end of such a rod is allowed to touch the surface of a liquid and then removed, it brings away a small drop adhering to the glass. This pendant drop (FIG. 1b) is known as a microdrop and is the standard quantity used for all the microcrystal and microcolour tests (see p. 133) to be described. It has a volume of about 0·1 µl (Hawkins, 1959); a conventional drop (0·05 ml) will thus provide material for 500 different tests. It is imperative that the end of the rod should

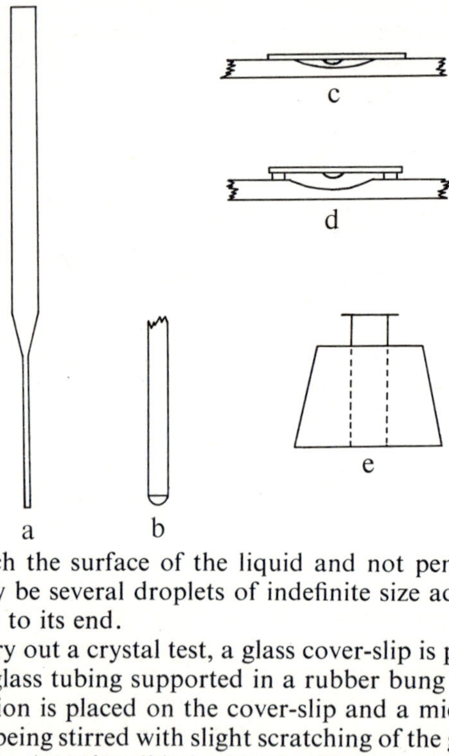

FIG. 1. MICRODROP TECHNIQUE

only touch the surface of the liquid and not penetrate it, as in the latter case there may be several droplets of indefinite size adhering to the sides of the rod and none to its end.

To carry out a crystal test, a glass cover-slip is placed on a stand made from a piece of glass tubing supported in a rubber bung (FIG. 1e). A microdrop of the test solution is placed on the cover-slip and a microdrop of the reagent added, the drop being stirred with slight scratching of the glass to promote the formation of crystals. A cavity slide is ringed with gum arabic solution, inverted over the cover-slip, and re-inverted so as to leave a 'hanging drop' (FIG. 1c). In this, crystals are free to form slowly in a three-dimensional environment, evaporation being prevented, or at least very greatly retarded, by the gum arabic seal. They thus form in regular, reproducible shapes.

The drop is examined at once under low magnification by both ordinary and polarised light and the appearance of any precipitate (amorphous, oil droplets, or crystals) noted. In the absence of crystals, it is re-examined at intervals for the next 24 hours. Many crystals do not form until after a lapse of twelve hours or more, indicated in the monographs in Part 2 as 'overnight'. This delay is partly an intrinsic characteristic of the particular crystals and partly due to the fact that the drop slowly becomes more concentrated owing to evaporation and diffusion of water vapour through the gum arabic seal. Should it be necessary to preserve a specimen (e.g. as an exhibit for forensic purposes) this evaporation may be stopped and the drop prevented from drying out by painting a solution of bitumen in toluene over the gum arabic. Such a slide may be preserved for several months, if it is handled with care and kept horizontal.

If, on the other hand, it is desired to promote evaporation so as to concentrate the drop more rapidly and so obtain a quicker result in a case of urgency, use may be made of a 'pedestal' slide. This is made by cementing small pieces of broken cover-slip to act as distance pieces on opposite sides of the depression of an ordinary cavity slide. The microdrops of test solution and reagent are mixed on the cover-slip as described above. The distance pieces are moistened with a little of the gum arabic solution and the cover-slip is picked up by inverting the slide over it and pressing the distance pieces against its edges.It is re-inverted as before (FIG. 1d) and examined at frequent intervals. Evaporation takes place fairly rapidly through the gap between the cover-slip and the slide. As soon as any precipitate is visible, the gap is closed by ringing it with the gum arabic solution. In this way tests which might take 12 hours by the ordinary method may sometimes be carried out in a tenth of the time.

Crystal Forms and Habit

When definite crystals have been formed, their form and habit (i.e. the positions which they occupy relative to one another—rosettes, sheaves, and so on) should be noted. They may also be sketched or photographed for the purposes of record. It may be mentioned here that certain crystals are unstable and disappear in an hour or two. They may then be compared with the descriptions given for crystals formed from the various compounds described in the monographs in Part 2. It must, however, be emphasised that descriptions of crystals, or for that matter drawings or photographs, can only enable a tentative identification to be made. Final identification must depend on the comparison of the crystals formed from the unknown with those prepared from an authentic sample of the drug and the same reagent.

Descriptive Terms

To help with the making of a provisional identification, a glossary of the various terms used in describing crystals is given below. Such descriptions cannot be exact, as the different forms merge imperceptibly into one another.

A *needle* is a long thin crystal with pointed ends, a *rod* being similar but with the ends square-cut. A *blade* is a broad needle, becoming a *plate* when length and breadth are of the same order of magnitude. A *tablet* is a plate with appreciable thickness, becoming a *prism* as the thickness increases. *Splinters* are small irregular rods and needles, and *grains* are very small lenticular crystals.

A *rosette* is a collection of crystals radiating from a single point, while a *tuft* or *fan* is a sector of such a rosette, a double tuft being called a *sheaf*. A *burr* or *hedgehog* is a rosette which is so dense that only the tips of the needles show. A *star* is a rosette with only four to six components, while a *cross* usually denotes a single cruciform crystal. A *cluster* is a loose complex of crystals, being called a *bundle* or *bunch* when the majority of the crystals lie in one direction. *Dendrites* are multibrachiate branching crystals.

The terms wedges, dumb-bells, and combs are used to denote similarity with these objects. *Smudge rosettes* and *gelatinous rosettes* are reproducible assemblies which are possibly not truly crystalline.

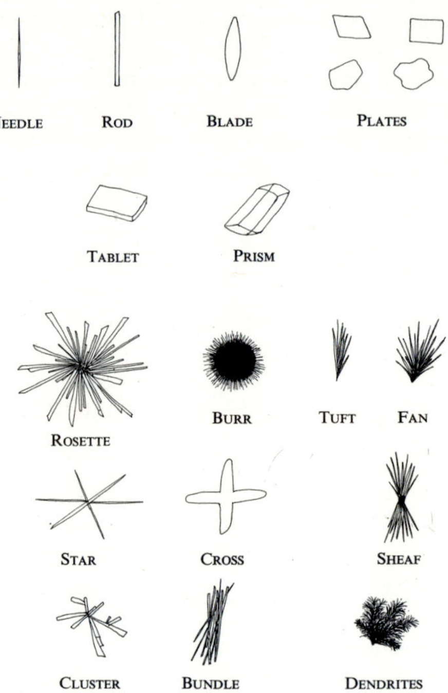

FIG. 2. MICROCRYSTALS

Irregular Forms

Difficulties in obtaining an exact match between the crystals of the unknown and those of the control may arise from a number of causes. Impurities in the test solution may lead to the formation of deformed and irregular crystals, but this may usually be overcome by using material eluted from paper or thin-layer chromatograms. Polymorphism is occasionally a source of trouble. Under different conditions of temperature, pH, etc., a compound may crystallise in entirely different forms. This may usually be obviated by ensuring that the test crystals and those of the control are prepared under identical conditions. Finally, the difficulty most commonly encountered arises from the fact that the appearance of the crystals may depend very much on the concentration of the solution from which they are formed. A substance which may form a mass of small irregular plates from a concentrated solution may crystallise as beautiful regular rosettes from a more dilute one. The answer to this problem is to use test and control solutions of approximately the same concentration. There is some slight difficulty here, as the concentration of the test solution will usually be a matter of guess-work, but if the control drop appears to be more crowded with crystals than the test drop the former may be repeated with a more dilute solution.

Reagents

As a general rule, solutions for crystal tests should be in the range 1 to 0·1%, although a few compounds need more concentrated solutions than this and many give excellent crystals at far greater dilution. The best solvent to use is 2N acetic acid and, unless otherwise stated, this has been used for the crystal tests described in Part 2. Crystals form more readily from solution in dilute hydrochloric acid, but this has the disadvantage that it may hydrolyse unstable compounds. They form more readily still in more concentrated mineral acids, and this has led Fulton (1969) to introduce a series of reagents made up in moderately concentrated sulphuric and phosphoric acids instead of in water. Solutions may be made up in 50% ethanol, acidified if necessary, but a higher proportion of alcohol than this is undesirable as it tends to precipitate the reagent.

In the past, several hundred solutions have been used as reagents for microcrystal tests. These include halides of the heavy metals, double halides of cadmium, bismuth, and mercury, various solutions of iodine, alkalis, and sundry organic acids. For the purposes of this book the number has been reduced to thirty. Details of these are given in Appendix 1. In selecting these, preference has been given to those which remain stable for long periods, most of those listed being usable for a year or more. The necessity to make up a solution specially whenever it is needed detracts greatly from the inherent simplicity of the microcrystal test.

Specific Applications of the Tests

As has been said above, the microcrystal test is of little use in the general search for an unknown drug. Its value comes later, particularly in differentiating between compounds of very similar constitution, when the field has been considerably narrowed by chromatographic or spectrophotometric screening. Consider, as an example, the case of phenmetrazine (p. 486) and phendimetrazine (p. 481). Their Rf values for both paper chromatography (system P1) and thin-layer chromatography (system T1) are too close together to permit differentiation, their ultraviolet spectra are very similar, and neither gives any colour reactions of value, yet they may be distinguished from one another in a few moments by means of a crystal test, phenmetrazine giving dense rosettes with a solution of picrolonic acid and phendimetrazine giving masses of small needles.

A particular instance where the microcrystal test is practically the only method of distinguishing between compounds is that of the optical isomers. If a reasonable quantity of the pure compound is available this may, of course, be done by measurement of the optical rotation, but this is impracticable when it comes to microgram quantities. There is usually little difficulty in distinguishing between the racemic form of a drug on the one hand and its optically active isomers on the other, as although the crystals formed with many of the reagents will be similar, there are usually one or two cases where they are markedly different, although crystals given by the (+)- and (−)-forms are identical. Indeed, one can usually find a reagent with which the racemic form gives crystals and the optically active ones an amorphous precipitate. Differentiation may then be achieved by the following method, taking as an example the case of the three forms of the analgesic drug 3-hydroxy-*N*-methylmorphinan.

The (−)-isomer, levorphanol, and (±)-isomer, racemorphan, are proscribed narcotic drugs under International control, but the (+)-isomer, dextrorphan, is without analgesic or addictive properties and is not controlled. Differentiation between these compounds is therefore a matter of considerable forensic interest. Its achievement depends on the fact that when a solution of racemorphan in 2N hydrochloric acid is treated with sodium carbonate solution by the microdrop technique described above, bunches of small plates are formed within half an hour, while under similar conditions levorphanol and dextrorphan give only amorphous precipitates which do not crystallise even after standing for 48 hours. To distinguish between levorphanol and dextrorphan the following procedure is used: place a microdrop of the test solution on a cover-slip; add a microdrop of a solution of, say, levorphanol, made from an authentic sample; then add a microdrop of sodium carbonate solution; seal, invert, and examine under the microscope in the usual way. If the test solution is levorphanol, then addition of more levorphanol will not affect it and the precipitate formed will be amorphous. But if it is dextrorphan, the test drop will now contain both (+)- and (−)-isomers, and crystals typical of the racemic compound will be formed.

This method is of general application, provided that one can find a reagent that will give crystals with the racemic form but not with the (+)- or (−)-isomers and that a sample of one of these enantiomorphs is available for cross testing. Some other examples: trinitrobenzoic acid gives rosettes of crystals with racemethorphan but oily amorphous precipitates with dextromethorphan and levomethorphan; ammonium thiocyanate solution gives large plates (best seen under polarised light) with racemoramide but oily droplets with dextromoramide and levomoramide; gold chloride solution gives small, curved, irregular needles almost at once with racemic propoxyphene but no crystals with dextropropoxyphene and levopropoxyphene for several hours, when large straight needles may form.

Differentiation between the (+)-, (−)-, and racemic forms of amphetamine is not easy but can usually be carried out by adding platinic bromide solution to a 1% solution of the drug. The (+)- and (−)-forms give a mixture of hexagonal and rhomboidal plates and prisms, which polarise brightly, while the racemic form gives masses of thin irregular plates which polarise hardly at all. A drop of dexamphetamine mixed with a drop of levamphetamine gives the same crystals as the racemate and this enables differentiation to be made.

Atropine may be distinguished from hyoscyamine by the crystals given with potassium tri-iodide solution (3), the former giving irregular hexagons in clusters and bundles, the latter small plates and prisms, often in crosses and arrow-heads. The concentration of the alkaloidal solution should be in the range 1 in 200 to 1 in 800.

The antihistamine drug pheniramine and its halogen derivatives chlorpheniramine, dexchlorpheniramine, brompheniramine, and dexbrompheniramine, provide another example of the way in which microcrystal tests may be used in conjunction with other methods of analysis to distinguish between closely related compounds. Pheniramine itself may be distinguished from its chloro- and bromo-derivatives by paper chromatography (system P1) as it has a much lower Rf value (0·27). The halogenated pheniramines all have the same Rf value (0·45) but the chloro-derivatives may be distinguished from the bromo-derivatives by the fact that the former show a blue fluorescence in ultraviolet light, the latter a strong absorption. Crystal tests may be used to differentiate between the racemic and the optically active forms, as chlorpheniramine and brompheniramine give dense rosettes with lead iodide solution, while dexchlorpheniramine and dexbrompheniramine give feathery rosettes and sheaves which polarise brightly. This test is also best carried out with solutions in the range 1 in 200 to 1 in 800.

Sensitivity

The sensitivity of microcrystal tests is expressed in terms of the concentration of the solution used—see under Sensitivity of Microtests, p. 134.

The Metabolism of Drugs

R. L. Smith

The majority of drugs and other organic compounds that are considered foreign to the body undergo metabolic changes *in vivo*. These changes are brought about by a system of enzymes of low substrate specificity requirement which are present mainly in the liver and which are capable of metabolising a diversity of organic substances along a number of pathways. A teleological significance has been attributed to these enzymes since their function appears to be the detoxication of potentially harmful substances taken in from the environment. This view has developed since the urinary and biliary metabolites of most foreign organic compounds are usually polar water-soluble substances of low toxicity or of lower toxicity than their precursors. This is not strictly true, however, since instances are now known in which a foreign compound is converted in the body to a more toxic substance.

Many drugs of forensic interest, such as barbiturates, phenothiazine derivatives, and narcotics, suffer chemical alteration in the body and are excreted mainly in the form of metabolites. Therefore, the metabolic fate of drugs is of concern to the toxicologist since the detection of the metabolites in biological media may allow the identification of the precursor drug.

THE GENERAL PATTERN OF DRUG METABOLISM

Drugs can undergo many different types of biochemical reactions. These reactions can, however, be divided into 4 main types, namely, **oxidations**, **reductions**, **hydrolyses**, and **syntheses**. The oxidations, reductions, and hydrolyses are many and varied whereas the synthetic reactions, or conjugation processes, appear to be relatively few in number. In the conjugation reactions the foreign compound or a metabolite formed by a preliminary oxidative, reductive, or hydrolytic reaction is combined with a substance provided by the body (the conjugating agent) and this is frequently derived from a carbohydrate or an amino-acid.

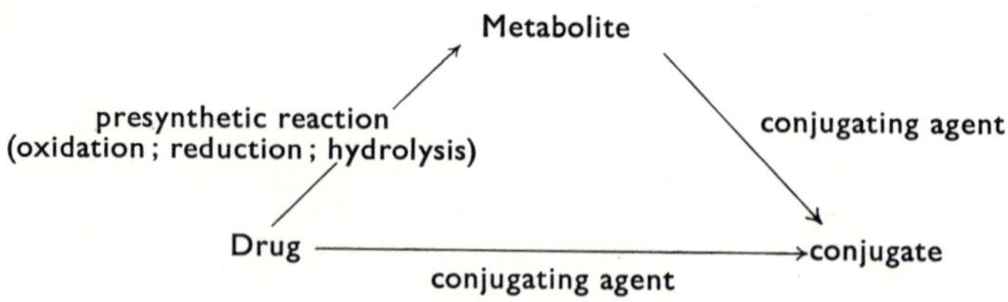

For a conjugation reaction to occur directly, the drug must possess in its structure a suitable centre for conjugation (e.g. an amino-, carboxyl, or hydroxyl group). If such a group is absent then the compound may acquire one by undergoing a preliminary oxidative, reductive, or hydrolytic reaction. These preliminary reactions which serve to introduce conjugation centres are sometimes referred to as presynthetic reactions since they precede the conjugation reaction. Most of the presynthetic and conjugative reactions of foreign compounds are catalysed by enzymes present mainly in the liver, particularly in the endoplasmic reticulum.

THE BIOCHEMICAL REACTIONS OF FOREIGN COMPOUNDS

Oxidations

Oxidation is one of the most general reactions of foreign compounds and includes such reactions as hydroxylation of alkyl, aryl, and heterocyclic groups, oxidation of alcohols and aldehydes, oxidative deamination of amines, oxidative dealkylation, oxidation of sulphur compounds to sulphoxides and sulphones, *N*-oxide formation, oxidative splitting of rings, dehalogenation, and other processes—see accompanying table of Oxidative Reactions of Drugs. The oxidation reaction results usually in the compound acquiring a group, e.g. a hydroxyl or carboxyl group, which can act as a centre for conjugation. The enzymes responsible for the oxidative reactions of drugs are found mainly in the liver and have a requirement for reduced triphosphopyridine nucleotide ($NADH_2$).

OXIDATIVE REACTIONS OF DRUGS

Type of Oxidation	*Example*	*Metabolite*
Hydroxylation of aromatic compound	acetanilide	paracetamol
Hydroxylation of alkyl groups	pentobarbitone	hydroxypentobarbitone
Oxidation of alkyl groups to carboxylic acids	thiopentone	thiopentone carboxylic acid
Oxidative deamination	amphetamine	phenylacetone
O-Dealkylation	codeine	morphine
N-Dealkylation	imipramine	desipramine
Sulphoxidation	chlorpromazine	chlorpromazine sulphoxide
Replacement of sulphur by oxygen	parathion	paraoxon

Reductions

Reduction is usually less common than oxidation but for several types of compound it is a general reaction. Thus, aldehydes or ketones may be reduced to primary and secondary alcohols respectively and nitro- and azo-groups to amines—see accompanying table of Reductive Reactions of Drugs.

REDUCTIVE REACTIONS OF DRUGS

Type of Reduction	*Example*	*Metabolite*
Conversion of aldehyde to primary alcohol	chloral	trichloroethanol
Reduction of ketone to hydroxyl group	menaphthone	1,4-dihydroxy-2-methylnaphthalene
Reduction of nitro-group to amine	picric acid	picramic acid
Reductive splitting of azo-group to amine	prontosil	sulphanilamide
Conversion of disulphides to sulphydryl derivatives	disulfiram	diethyldithiocarbamic acid

Hydrolyses

Hydrolysis is a metabolic pathway *in vivo* for some esters and amides. Plasma and the liver contain esterases which will hydrolyse drugs such as procaine, succinylcholine, cocaine, and pethidine.

Syntheses

In the synthetic (conjugation) reactions the compound or a metabolite formed by an oxidation, reduction, or hydrolysis combines with an endogenous substance which is frequently derived from a carbohydrate or an amino-acid. The metabolite so formed is sometimes referred to as a conjugate. These are frequently highly polar water-soluble substances which are readily excreted in the urine and/or bile. The conversion of an organic substance to a conjugate usually results in a reduction in its toxicity; hence the conjugation reactions are sometimes called detoxication mechanisms. The enzymes responsible for these synthetic reactions are located mainly in the liver but they may occur in other tissues. In man, seven conjugation reactions are known—see accompanying table. Generally speaking these mechanisms and sometimes others are present to a greater or lesser extent in other species.

CONJUGATION REACTIONS

Reaction	*Conjugate Formed*	*Precursors*
Glucuronide synthesis	β-glucuronide	hydroxy- and amino-compounds
Sulphate conjugation	sulphate ester	hydroxy-compounds
	sulphamate	amines
Glycine conjugation	glycine	aromatic carboxylic acids
Glutamine conjugation	glutamine	certain arylacetic acids
Acetylation	*N*-acetyl	aromatic amines, hydrazines
Methylation	*O*-, *N*-methyl derivative	phenols and amines
Thiocyanate synthesis	thiocyanate	cyanides

(a) GLUCURONIDE SYNTHESIS. The glucuronic acid conjugation is the most widespread and versatile of the various conjugation mechanisms probably because the intermediates and enzymes involved in their synthesis are present in many tissues and also because of the wide variety of chemical groups to which glucuronic acid can be transferred. Thus glucuronide synthesis generally represents an important pathway of metabolism for alcohols (primary, secondary, and tertiary), phenols, carboxylic acids, primary amines, certain sulphonamides, hydroxylamines, certain *N*-heterocyclic compounds, and thiols.

CLASSES OF COMPOUND FORMING GLUCURONIDES

Class of Compound	*Glucuronide Type*	*Structure*
alcohol	ether	$R{\cdot}O{\cdot}C_6H_9O_6$
phenol	ether	$Ar{\cdot}O{\cdot}C_6H_9O_6$
hydroxylamine	hydroxylaminic	$Ar{\cdot}NH{\cdot}O{\cdot}C_6H_9O_6$
carboxylic acid	ester	$Ar{\cdot}CO{\cdot}O{\cdot}C_6H_9O_6$
primary amine	*N*-glucuronide	$Ar{\cdot}NH{\cdot}C_6H_9O_6$
sulphonamide	*N*-glucuronide	$p\text{-}NH_2{\cdot}C_6H_4{\cdot}SO_2{\cdot}NR^1{\cdot}C_6H_9O_6$
thiol	thioether	$R{\cdot}S{\cdot}C_6H_9O_6$

R = alkyl group; Ar = aryl group; R^1 = heterocyclic group

$C_6H_9O_6$ = glucuronic acid

The glucuronides formed by the various classes of compound are similar in that they are polar, water-soluble compounds readily excreted by the kidneys or liver. However, the various types of glucuronides differ markedly in their chemical stability. Thus, ether glucuronides require hot concentrated acid for hydrolysis whereas ester glucuronides are readily hydrolysed by warm dilute acid; both are attacked by β-glucuronidase. The stability of *N*-glucuronides varies; some are decomposed on contact with dilute acid whereas others need more vigorous conditions. *N*-Glucuronides appear to be relatively stable to β-glucuronidase.

(b) SULPHATE CONJUGATION. This pathway of drug metabolism converts phenols and alcohols to sulphate esters and certain aromatic amines to sulphamates (*N*-sulphates). These conjugates are also strong acids which are readily excreted. They are hydrolysed by warm dilute mineral acid and by sulphatase enzymes.

$$\mathrm{R{-}X{-}H} + \underset{\text{sulphate}}{\mathrm{HO{\cdot}SO_2{\cdot}OH}} \longrightarrow \mathrm{R{-}X{-}SO_2{\cdot}OH} + \mathrm{H_2O}$$

[X = —O— in alcohols or phenols or —NH— in amines]

(c) GLYCINE AND GLUTAMINE CONJUGATION. Glycine conjugation is a common reaction of carboxylic acids, particularly aromatic acids or those containing aromatic residues. It is rarely seen with aliphatic acids since they are readily oxidised in the body.

$$\mathrm{R{\cdot}COOH} \xrightarrow{\text{glycine}} \mathrm{R{\cdot}CO{\cdot}NH{\cdot}CH_2{\cdot}COOH}$$

The glutamine conjugation is a reaction of relatively restricted occurrence and has been found only in man and certain other primates. Furthermore, it is confined to particular arylacetic acids, e.g. phenylacetic and indolyl-3-acetic acid and 3,4-dihydroxy-5-methoxyphenylacetic acid (a metabolite of mescaline, p. 404).

(d) ACETYLATION. Acetylation is a biochemical reaction of compounds containing the amino-group. Thus it occurs with aromatic amines and with hydrazine and its derivatives. The process consists in the acetylation of the amino-group to give the monoacetyl compound; diacetylation rarely occurs. Acetylation is a common reaction of sulphonamide drugs, thus:

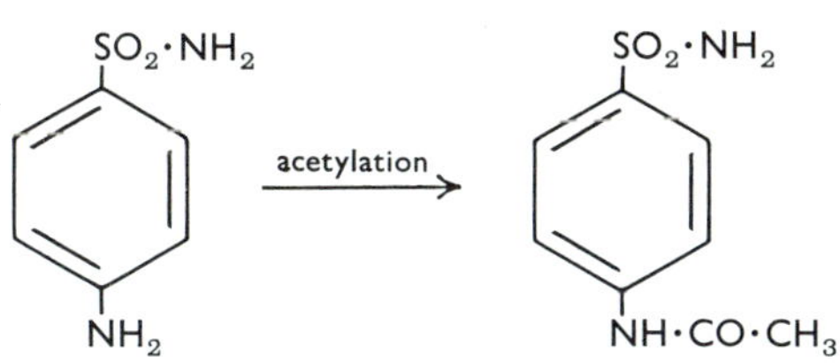

sulphanilamide $\quad$ N^4-acetylsulphanilamide

(e) METHYLATION. Biological methylation is a reaction of many foreign compounds particularly certain *N*-heterocyclic compounds and phenols. Thus, pyridine, quinoline, and isoquinoline and some of their derivatives undergo *N*-methylation, e.g. nicotinic acid; similarly, phenolic compounds, particularly catechols, undergo *O*-methylation, e.g. adrenaline—see overleaf.

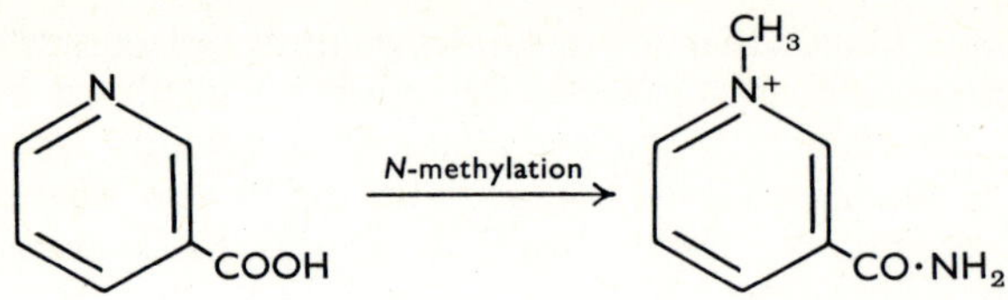

nicotinic acid → *N*-methylnicotinamide

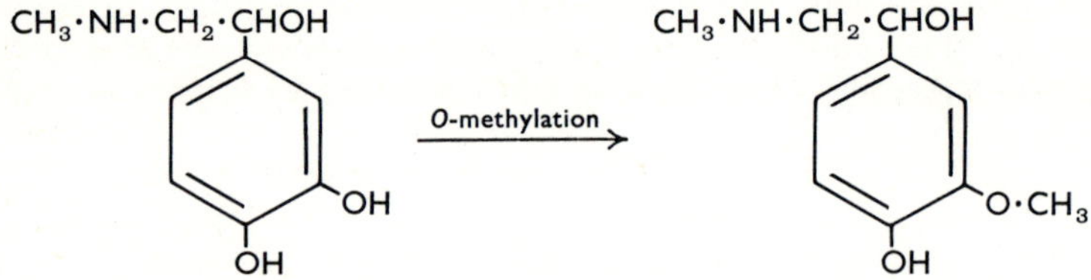

adrenaline → metanephrine

(f) THIOCYANATE SYNTHESIS. See under Cyanide Derivatives, p. 154.

METABOLICALLY INERT COMPOUNDS

A number of compounds are not metabolised *in vivo* and are excreted unchanged. These appear to be of two kinds: (a) highly ionised acids and bases and (b) relatively neutral compounds containing biochemically unreactive groups. Examples of the first type are sulphonic acid derivatives, sulphamic acid derivatives (e.g. cyclamates), and strong bases such as the polymethylene α-ω-bistrimethylammonium salts (e.g. hexamethonium and decamethonium). Examples of the second type are barbitone, acetazolamide, tolazoline, streptomycin, and some sulphones. In general, it appears that the following groups are not biochemically reactive or are metabolised only with difficulty: highly ionised carboxyl (—COOH) and sulphonic acid ($—SO_2 \cdot OH$) groups; quaternary ammonium ($—N^+(R)_3$); sulphonamide ($—SO_2 \cdot NH_2$); guanidino ($—NH \cdot C(:NH) \cdot NH_2$); sulphone ($—SO_2—$). Compounds possessing these groups are not metabolised unless they have other groups capable of undergoing metabolic change.

In some cases the biochemical reactivity of a group may depend upon its situation. Thus, the sulphone group of the diarylsulphones (e.g. dapsone) is metabolically inert whereas the sulphone group of several aliphatic sulphone drugs (e.g. sulphonal) undergoes oxidation.

METABOLIC FATE OF DRUGS

In this section the main metabolic reactions of various types of drugs are outlined. The emphasis is on principles rather than detail.

Alcohols

A diverse range of alcohols find application in medicine and pharmacy including ethanol, n-propanol, n-butanol, and chloramphenicol (primary alcohols), isopropanol and its 1,1,1-trichloro-derivative (secondary alcohols), and chlorbutol and methylpentynol (tertiary alcohols). In addition, many drugs, e.g. chloral and its derivatives, numerous barbiturates, and glutarimide derivatives, are metabolised in the body to form metabolites containing an alcoholic group.

In general, the alcoholic hydroxyl group is capable of being metabolised along two pathways, namely, conjugation with glucuronic acid and by oxidation. The extent to which these two reactions occur depends upon the structure of the alcohol and in particular on whether the structure is primary, secondary, or tertiary, and on the presence of substituents in the molecule.

Primary aliphatic alcohols undergo the two general reactions *in vivo*, namely, direct conjugation with glucuronic acid and oxidation to a carboxylic acid (via an aldehyde). The carboxylic acid may be oxidised to CO_2 or conjugated to give an ester glucuronide.

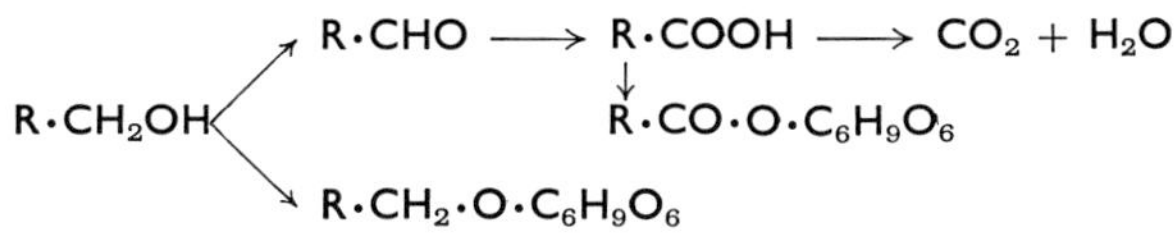

The extent to which primary alcohols undergo direct conjugation appears to depend upon the speed of oxidation. If this is rapid, little ether glucuronide is formed. Simple aliphatic alcohols, e.g. ethanol, are largely metabolised to CO_2 but substitution of the alkyl group tends to inhibit complete oxidation. Substituted alcohols undergo direct conjugation with glucuronic acid and oxidation as far as the corresponding carboxylic acid which is excreted unchanged or conjugated. Thus trichloroethanol, which is a metabolite of chloral and is partly responsible for the hypnotic action of the drug, undergoes direct conjugation and also some oxidation to trichloroacetic acid.

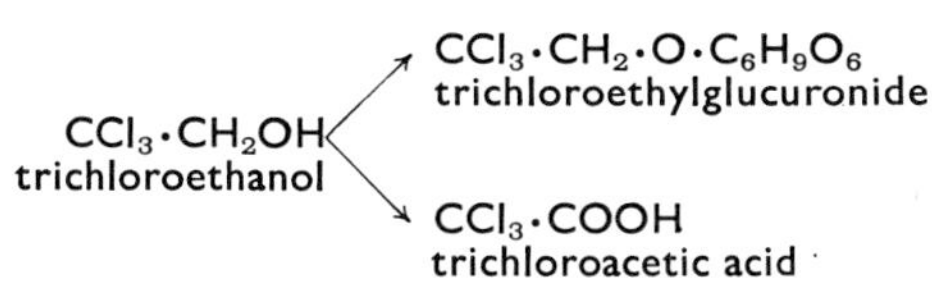

Tribromoethanol and 2,2,3-trichlorobutanol (a metabolite of butylchloral hydrate) are both metabolised mainly by direct conjugation with glucuronic acid.

$CBr_3{\cdot}CH_2{\cdot}O{\cdot}R$
tribromoethanol (R=H)
tribromoethylglucuronide (R=—$C_6H_9O_6$)

$CH_3{\cdot}CHCl{\cdot}CCl_2{\cdot}CH_2{\cdot}O{\cdot}R$
2,2,3-trichlorobutanol (R=H)
2,2,3-trichlorobutylglucuronide (R=—$C_6H_9O_6$)

Primary aromatic alcohols may also undergo direct conjugation with glucuronic acid or oxidation (to benzoic acid or phenylacetic acid according to whether there are an even or odd number of carbon atoms in the side-chain).

Generally, aromatic primary alcohols which are substituted on the carbon next to the functional group tend to resist oxidation and are conjugated. Thus, chloramphenicol is extensively conjugated in man to give the 3-glucuronide (see overleaf).

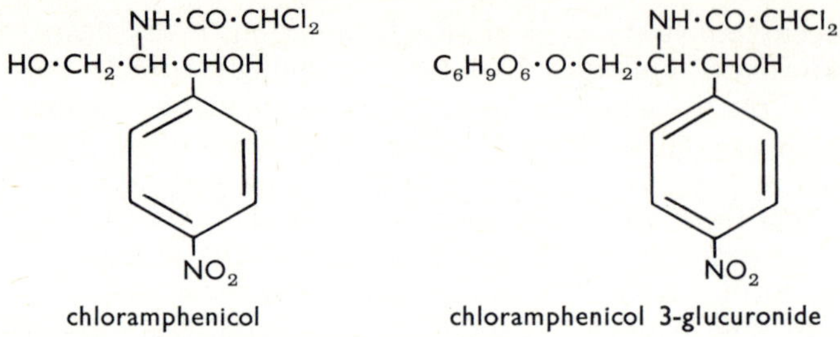

Secondary aliphatic alcohols can undergo two types of reaction, namely, conjugation with glucuronic acid and oxidation to a ketone which may be further oxidised or reduced back to the alcohol.

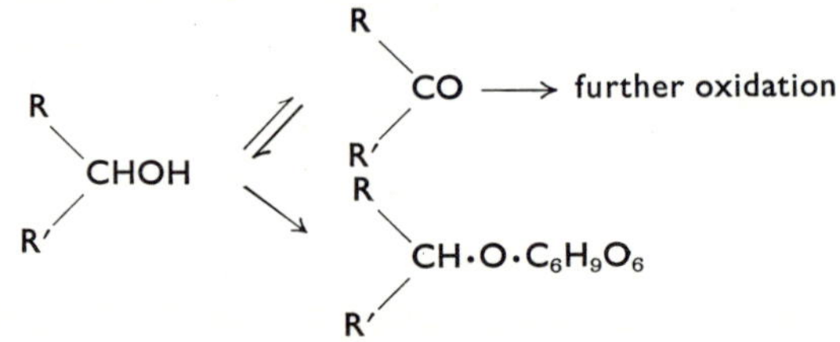

Simple secondary aliphatic alcohols are largely oxidised to their respective ketones. Substitution, particularly with halogens, lowers the extent of oxidation and increases conjugation as in the case of 1,1,1-trichloroisopropanol which is highly conjugated *in vivo*.

Secondary aromatic alcohols are metabolised mainly by direct conjugation with glucuronic acid. Thus, benzhydrol, a metabolite of the antihistamine drug diphenhydramine, is metabolised by direct conjugation with glucuronic acid.

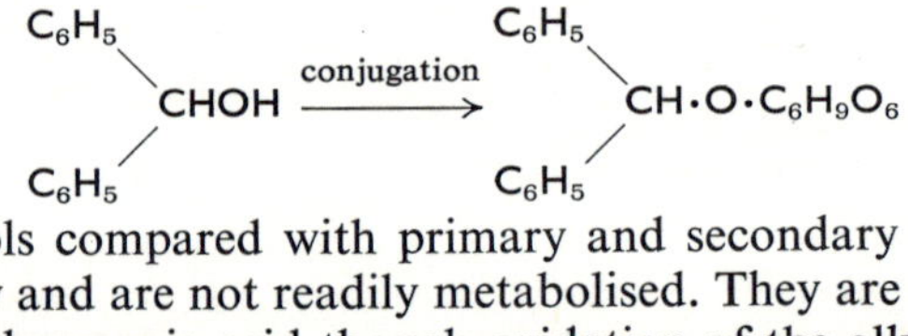

Tertiary alcohols compared with primary and secondary alcohols are more stable biologically and are not readily metabolised. They are usually extensively conjugated with glucuronic acid though oxidation of the alkyl groups attached to the carbinol group can occur. The two hypnotic drugs chlorbutol and methylpentynol are both tertiary alcohols and are highly conjugated *in vivo* though oxidation of the latter drug appears to occur in man.

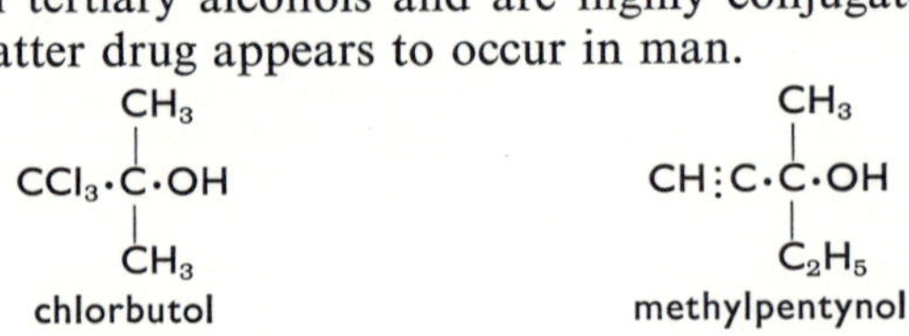

Aldehydes

Simple aliphatic aldehydes, e.g. formaldehyde and acetaldehyde, are readily oxidised in the body to the corresponding fatty acid which undergoes β-oxidation to give CO_2 and water. Halogenated aldehydes, e.g. chloral and butylchoral hydrates, are less readily oxidised and mainly suffer reduction to the corresponding primary alcohol which then undergoes conjugation with glucuronic acid.

Aromatic aldehydes (e.g. benzaldehyde) are oxidised to the corresponding carboxylic acids which are then excreted as conjugates.

$$\mathrm{Ar{\cdot}CHO} \longrightarrow \mathrm{Ar{\cdot}COOH}$$

Ketones

Simple aliphatic ketones are not readily metabolised in the body and are partly eliminated unchanged in the expired air. Apart from acetone, most ketones are probably also reduced to a variable extent and the secondary alcohol formed excreted combined with glucuronic acid.

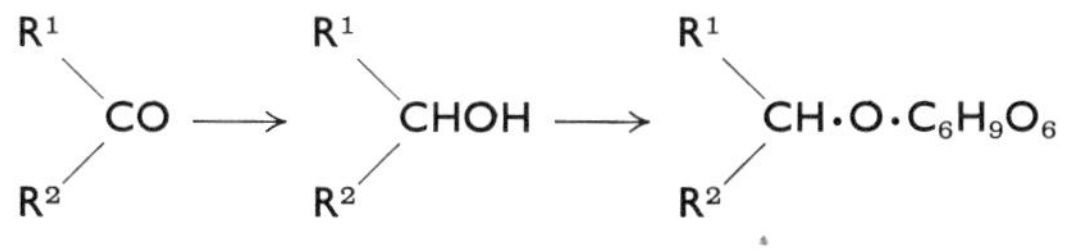

Aliphatic Amines

A large number of potent drugs both natural (e.g. the catecholamines, ephedrine) and synthetic (e.g. amphetamine, dibenamine) are β-derivatives of ethylamine. As far as the primary amine group of compounds of this type is concerned, three possible fates may obtain. The compound may be deaminised to the aldehyde which is then oxidised to the corresponding carboxylic acid; it may be acetylated; it may be biologically stable and excreted unchanged.

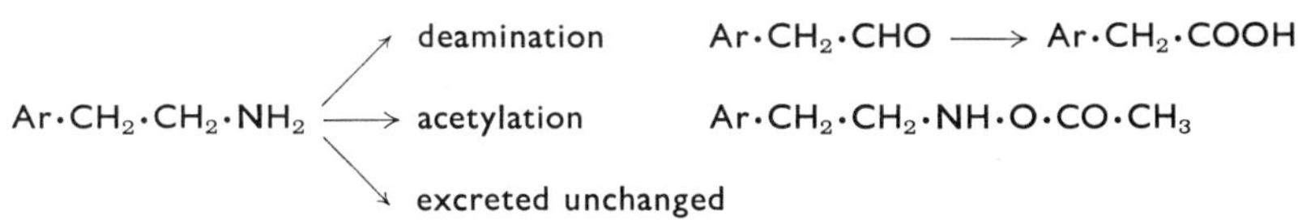

Histamine, for example, undergoes oxidative deamination to imidazoleacetic acid and acetylation to *N*-acetylhistamine as well as a number of other reactions not involving the amino-group.

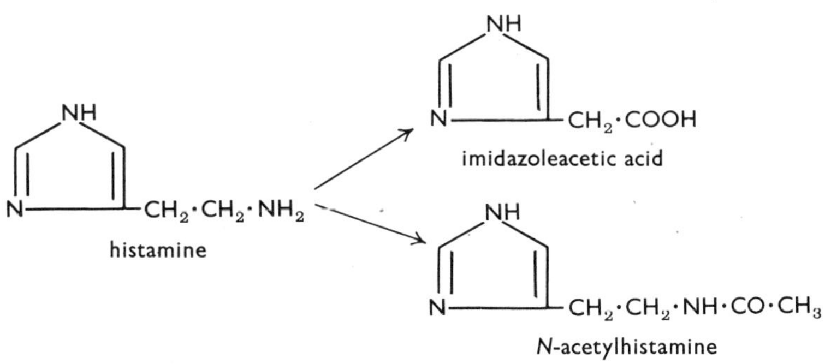

Noradrenaline, mescaline (3,4,5-trimethoxyphenethylamine), and amphetamine are similarly metabolised at least in part by oxidative deamination. Thus, in man, one of the several metabolites of mescaline has been identified as 3,4,5-trimethoxyphenylacetic acid formed by deamination and oxidation. Similarly, the major urinary metabolite of amphetamine is hippuric acid derived from deamination and oxidation of the side-chain (see overleaf).

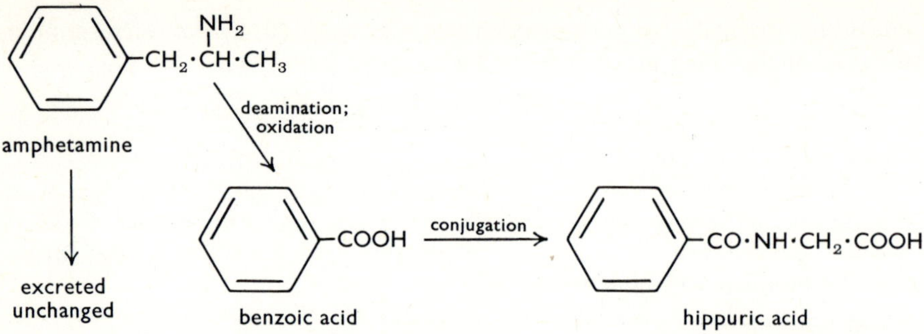

Ephedrine is a secondary amine and its main metabolic reaction involving the side-chain appears to be *N*-demethylation to the primary amine, norephedrine. This is excreted unchanged in some species though in others it is further oxidised.

Carbamates

Carbamate esters are used as tranquillising drugs and as cholinesterase inhibitors. They appear to undergo three types of metabolic change, namely, oxidation of substituent alkyl groups, hydrolysis of the carbamate linkage, and direct conjugation with glucuronic acid to give *N*-glucuronides. Dicarbamate esters of 2,2-disubstituted propanediols, e.g. meprobamate, are metabolised mainly by $(\omega-1)$-oxidation of one of the $C_{(2)}$-substituents and by *N*-glucuronide formation.

METABOLITES OF MEPROBAMATE AND COGENERS

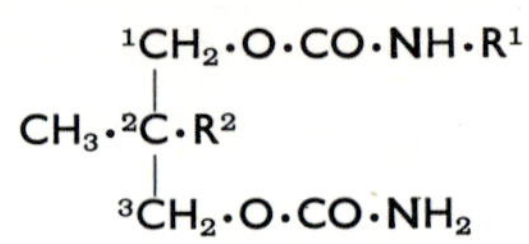

	R^1	R^2	*Structure of R^2 in oxidation product*
Meprobamate	H	$—CH_2·CH_2·CH_3$	$—CH_2·CHOH·CH_3$
Mebutamate	H	$—CH(CH_2·CH_3)(CH_3)$	$—CH(CHOH·CH_3)(CH_3)$
Carisoprodol	$—CH(CH_3)_2$	$—CH_2·CH_2·CH_3$	$—CH_2·CHOH·CH_3$

The oxidation products are excreted both free and conjugated with glucuronic acid. In the case of the carbamate anticholinesterases, e.g. neostigmine, pyridostigmine, and physostigmine, hydrolysis of the ester linkage occurs, though for neostigmine administered parenterally much of the dose is excreted in the urine unchanged but not when given orally.

Hydrazine Derivatives

Hydrazine derivatives find application as antihypertensives (hydrallazine) and monoamine oxidase inhibitors (phenelzine, isocarboxazid) and for the treatment of tuberculosis (isoniazid). Chemically, therapeutic hydrazines are of three types, namely, acyl, aryl, and arylalkyl hydrazine derivatives. Acyl hydrazines are all hydrolysed *in vivo* to some extent and they may also undergo acetylation. Thus isoniazid is hydrolysed partly to isonicotinic acid which is excreted as its glycine conjugate and it is also acetylated to *N*-acetylisoniazid.

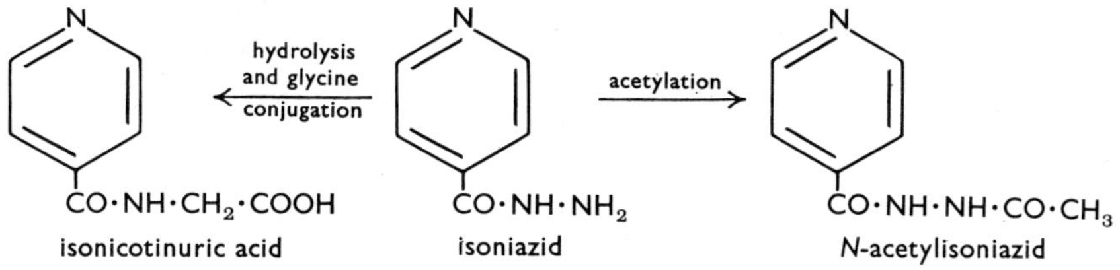

Both iproniazid and isocarboxazid are similarly hydrolysed, the former also undergoing dealkylation.

Salicylhydrazide, however, is largely metabolised by direct conjugation with glucuronic acid but some hydrolysis to salicylic acid occurs. Aryl hydrazines, e.g. phenylhydrazine and hydrallazine, are metabolised by oxidation of the aryl group or by acetylation of the hydrazine residue. Thus, phenylhydrazine is *p*-hydroxylated and the phenol produced is excreted as its glucuronide while hydrallazine is acetylated to form *N*-acetylhydrallazine.

Guanidines

The guanidine group is found in a number of important drugs, e.g. streptomycin, proguanil, guanethidine, and sulphaguanidine. As far as is known, this structure is not metabolised *in vivo*. Streptomycin and its dihydro-derivative are excreted by man largely unchanged while sulphaguanidine is eliminated as its *N*-acetyl conjugate containing an intact guanidine residue. Proguanil, a diguanide, is excreted by man partly unchanged and as a triazine metabolite formed by a cyclisation reaction. This metabolite is mainly responsible for the antimalarial activity of the parent drug.

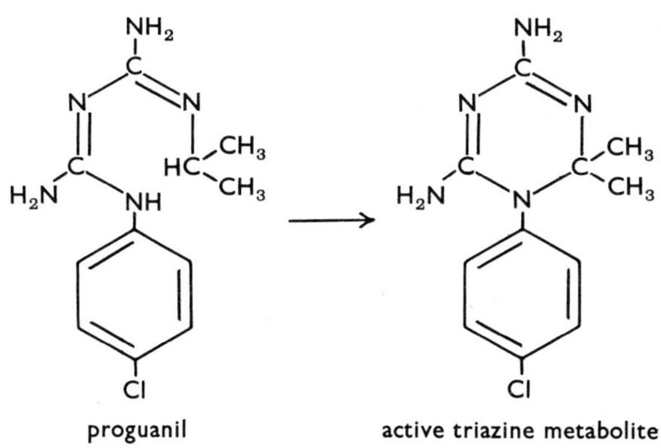

Aromatic Amines

Aromatic amines can undergo the following metabolic reactions: acetylation; conjugation of the amino-group with glucuronic acid and sulphate; and hydroxylation of the aromatic nucleus. Acetylation is a general reaction of aromatic amines and occurs for example with most sulphonamide drugs. Conjugation with glucuronic acid and with sulphate to form *N*-glucuronides and

N-sulphates, however, are usually minor reactions. Hydroxylation of the nucleus of aromatic amines commonly occurs unless a substituent which is capable of an alternative metabolic reaction, is present in the ring. Usually the hydroxyl group is entered ortho and/or para to the amino-group (or a group derived from this, e.g. acetamido-). Acetanilide, for example, is hydroxylated in the para position to give *p*-acetamidophenol (paracetamol) which is an active analgesic and is excreted in the urine as the corresponding glucuronic acid and sulphate conjugates. The related drug, phenacetin, contains in its structure a group capable of being metabolised, i.e. the ethoxy-group, and in fact this group is metabolised and aromatic hydroxylation does not occur. Thus phenacetin undergoes de-ethylation *in vivo* to give the same metabolite as acetanilide, namely, *p*-acetamidophenol (paracetamol).

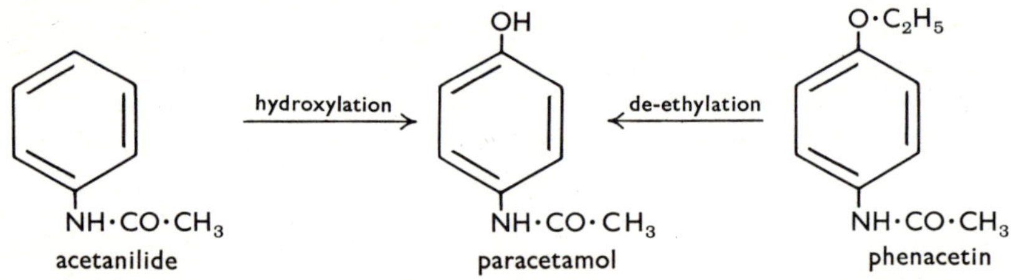

A number of local anaesthetic drugs contain an aromatic amino-group since they are ester derivatives of *p*-aminobenzoic acid, e.g. procaine, benzocaine, butethamine, and amethocaine. These drugs, however, are not metabolised as aromatic amines but suffer hydrolysis in the ester group. Procaine, for example, is rapidly hydrolysed *in vivo* to *p*-aminobenzoic acid and diethylaminoethanol:

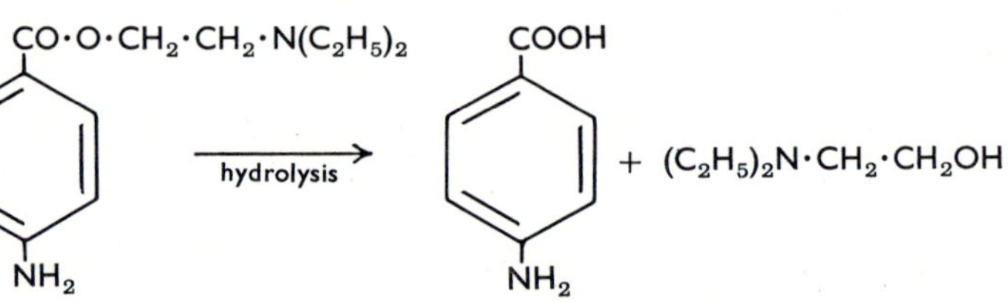

Phenols

Numerous phenols of diverse types find application as drugs. Their structural complexity ranges from that of the simple phenolic antiseptics (e.g. chlorocresol, chloroxylenol, thymol, and resorcinol) to complex phenolic substances such as synthetic sex hormones, morphine, and the tetracyclines. In addition, phenols are intermediary metabolites of many drugs, e.g. amphetamine, phenobarbitone, phenytoin, codeine, and papaverine.

The two major biochemical reactions of phenols are conjugation of the hydroxyl group with glucuronic acid to form aryl glucosiduronic acids and with sulphate to give ethereal sulphates. In addition, some phenols may undergo a third minor reaction, namely, hydroxylation to form a dihydric phenol. The orientation of the new phenolic hydroxyl group depends upon the groups already present in the molecule; usually it is introduced ortho and/or para to the existing hydroxyl group.

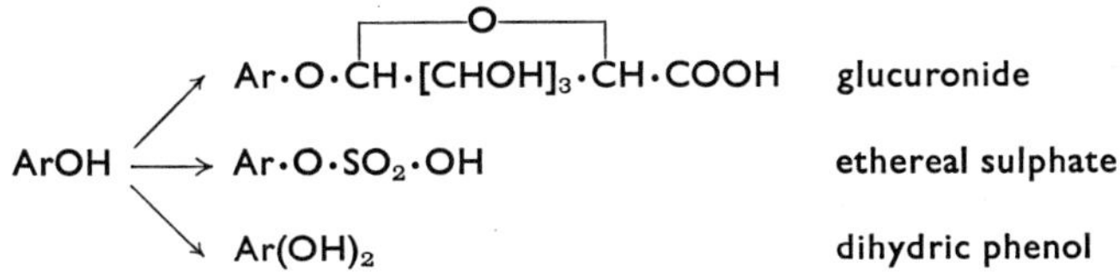

Phenol itself, for example, undergoes conjugation reactions to form mainly phenylglucuronide and phenylsulphate and a small part is oxidised to catechol and quinol which then also undergo conjugation.

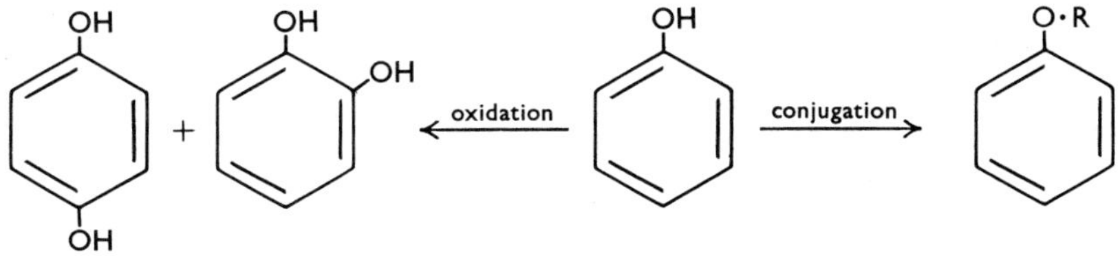

quinol catechol phenol phenylglucuronide ($R = -C_6H_9O_6$)

phenylsulphate ($R = -SO_2{\cdot}OH$)

The relative extent to which glucuronic acid and sulphate conjugation of a phenol occurs is influenced by its structure and pK_a. Thus, high glucuronic acid conjugation and almost negligible sulphate conjugation appears to be characteristic of phenols containing in their structures two or more isolated aromatic rings, e.g. stilboestrol, hexoestrol, phenolphthalein, and thyroxine. The acidity of the phenolic group is important since phenols of pK_a < 7 do not readily conjugate with sulphate but do so with glucuronic acid.

Methylation and dehydroxylation of phenols are reactions of relatively restricted occurrence. Methylation has been observed with certain mono-, di-, and tri-hydric phenols, particularly with catechol derivatives. Dehydroxylation, i.e. the removal of phenolic hydroxyl groups, occurs particularly with certain catechol acids and appears to be a reaction carried out by the gut bacteria.

Aromatic Acids

In general, aromatic carboxylic acids can undergo two biochemical reactions, namely, conjugation with glycine and with glucuronic acid.

$$Ar{\cdot}CO{\cdot}NH{\cdot}CH_2{\cdot}COOH \xleftarrow{\text{glycine}} Ar{\cdot}COOH \xrightarrow{\text{glucuronic acid}} Ar{\cdot}CO{\cdot}O{\cdot}C_6H_9O_6$$

Thus, both salicylic acid and *p*-aminosalicylic acid are metabolised at least in part to their respective glycine and glucuronic acid conjugates:

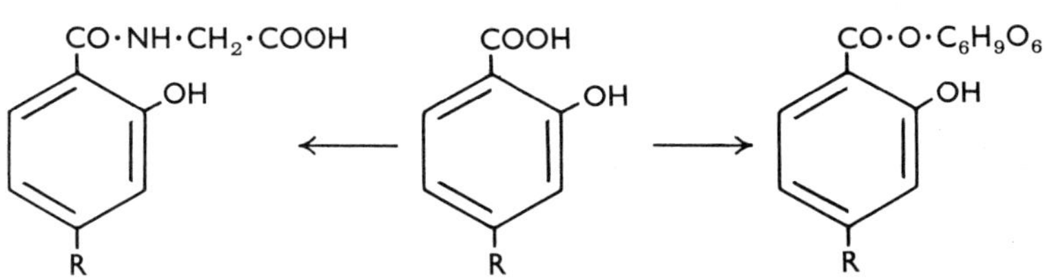

(salicylic acid, R = H; *p*-aminosalicylic acid, $R = -NH_2$)

For some carboxylic acids, e.g. the anti-inflammatory drug, indomethacin, and the oral cholecystographic medium, iopanoic acid, glucuronic acid conjugation appears to be more important and these drugs are excreted mainly as their ester glucuronides.

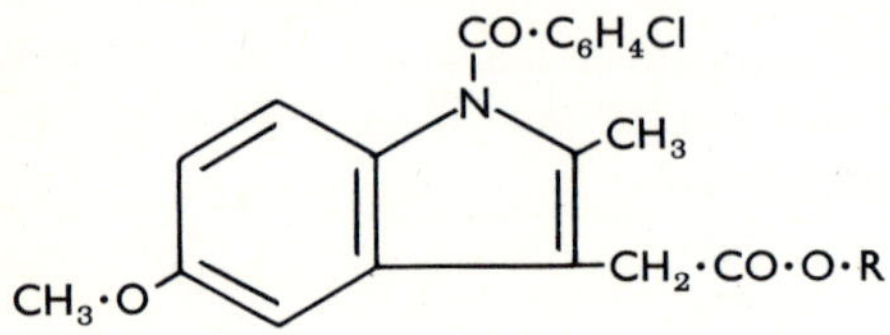

indomethacin (R = H)
indomethacin glucuronide
($R = -C_6H_9O_6$)

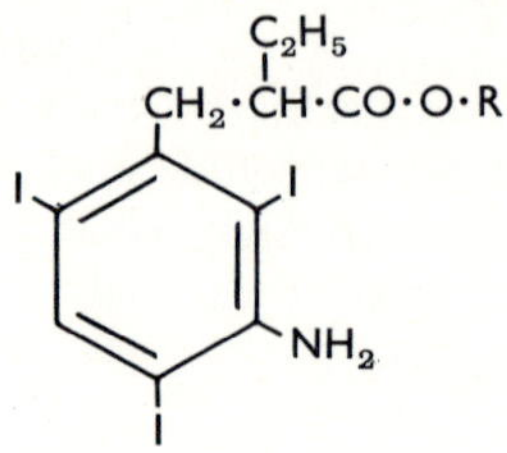

iopanoic acid (R = H)
iopanoic acid glucuronide
($R = -C_6H_9O_6$)

Esters of carboxylic acids are frequently extensively hydrolysed in the body. Thus, methyl salicylate and acetylsalicylic acid (aspirin) are largely hydrolysed *in vivo* to salicylic acid. Hydrolysis of ester links occurs in the metabolism of the following drugs: pethidine, heroin, cocaine, atropine, and the synthetic esters of antibiotics, e.g. erythromycin propionate and the mono- and di-succinic acid esters of chloramphenicol.

Cyanide Derivatives

A few cyanide derivatives find application in therapeutics, e.g. the tuberculostatic agent, cyacetazide, the tranquilliser, pericyazine, and the vitamin, cyanocobalamin. In addition, bitter almonds and cherry-laurel, preparations of which are occasionally used medicinally, both contain cyanogenetic glycosides.

Cyanide in organic combination is not toxic unless it can be metabolised to cyanide ions. Alkyl cyanides are readily metabolised to CN^- *in vivo* and their high toxicity is largely ascribable to this reaction. In these circumstances the cyanide formed is ultimately metabolised like inorganic cyanide to thiocyanate which appears in the urine.

$$CN^- + S \longrightarrow CNS^-$$

By contrast the cyanide group attached to an aromatic ring is to a large extent metabolically stable and alternative reactions, e.g. hydroxylation of the nucleus, may occur.

Sulphones

Aliphatic sulphones, such as sulphonal and methylsulphonal (trional), are largely metabolised by oxidation of the sulphone group to unknown metabolites, possibly sulphonic acids. By contrast the sulphone group of diarylsulphones, e.g. dapsone and its derivatives, appears to be metabolically stable and metabolism occurs in other parts of the molecule. Dapsone, in part, forms a water-soluble *N*-glucuronide:

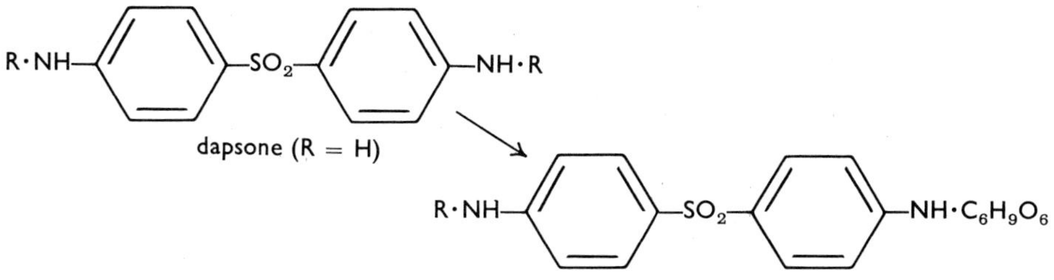

dapsone *N*-glucuronide

A number of disubstituted derivatives of dapsone are similarly used as antileprotic drugs, e.g. sulfoxone (R = $—CH_2·SO_2Na$), glucosulphone [R = —CH-$(SO_3Na)·(CHOH)_4·CH_2OH$], and solapsone [R = —$CH(SO_3Na)·CH_2·CH$-$(SO_3Na)·C_6H_5$]. They are metabolised at least in part to the parent drug.

Sulphonic Acids

The sulphonic acid group ($—SO_2·OH$) appears to be biologically stable and is not readily metabolised and simple aliphatic and aromatic sulphonic acids are usually excreted unchanged. However, more complex sulphonic acids, e.g. sulphobromophthalein and amaranth, undergo metabolism but in other parts of the molecule.

Sulphonamides

The most important metabolic reactions of the sulphonamide drugs involve the N^4- and N^1-amino-groups shown in the following general structure.

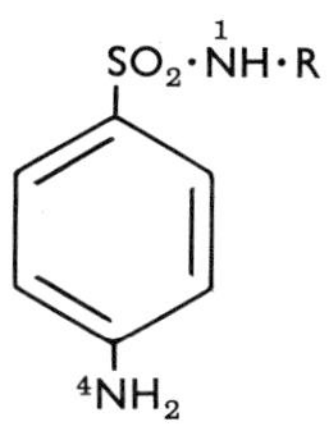

R = H (sulphanilamide);
$-CO·CH_3$ (sulphacetamide) or
a heterocyclic group

Metabolism of the N^4-amino-group is usually the more important and this group can undergo three reactions, namely, acetylation, N^4-glucuronide formation, and N^4-sulphate synthesis.

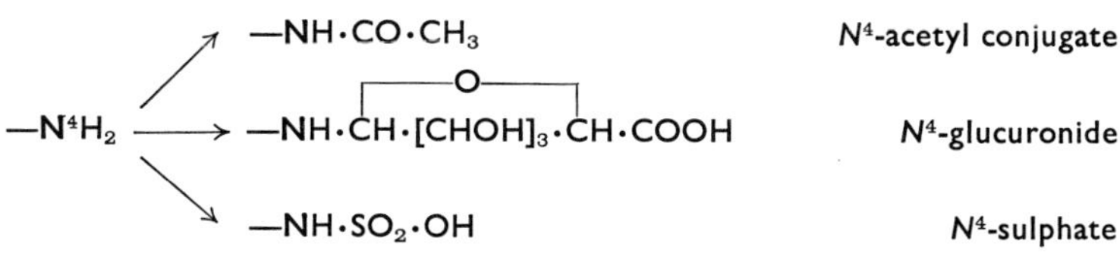

Of these reactions N^4-acetylation is the most extensive but the extent to which it occurs varies with the sulphonamide, species, and individual. The acetylated derivative is therapeutically inactive but because of its low solubility it may cause kidney damage. N^4-Glucuronides and N^4-sulphates of sulphonamides are usually relatively minor products. The former, which are acid labile, appear to be formed by spontaneous combination of the sulphonamide with free glucuronic acid. Metabolic reactions involving the N^1-amino-group appear to occur haphazardly. Thus, N^1-acetylation is so far known to occur only in the case of sulphanilamide and N^1-glucuronide formation in man occurs only with sulphathiazole and sulphadimethoxine. Oxidative metabolism of the heterocyclic R group of a number of sulphonamides occurs, the products being excreted as conjugates (e.g. sulphasomizole and sulphapyridine).

Barbiturates

Metabolism is an important factor controlling the pharmacological activity of barbiturates. Their potency and duration of action depends upon their rate of metabolism. The chemical changes which barbiturates undergo are of four types, namely, (1) oxidation of the groups at $C_{(5)}$, (2) *N*-dealkylation, (3) splitting of the barbiturate ring, and (4), in the case of thiobarbiturates, exchange of the sulphur for oxygen. Hexobarbitone is, for example, metabolised along pathways (1), (2), and (3) as follows:

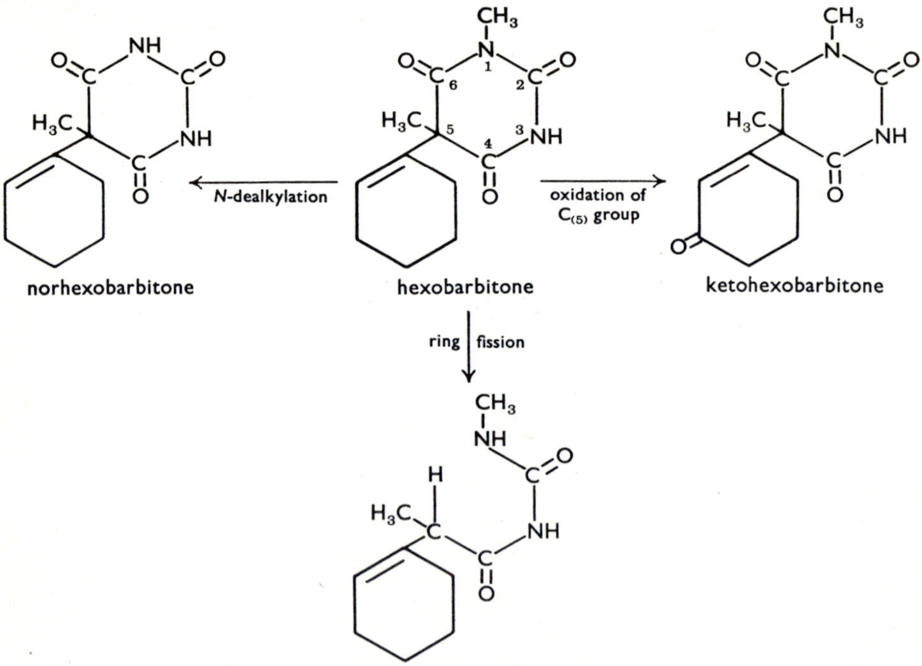

(1) OXIDATION OF GROUP AT $C_{(5)}$. This is the more important metabolic pathway of most barbiturates. The larger of the two groups at $C_{(5)}$ usually suffers oxidation and the products are alcohols, ketones, phenols, or carboxylic acids which may be excreted both free and conjugated—see table opposite.

(2) *N*-DEALKYLATION. This reaction occurs with *N*-alkylated barbiturates to a variable extent. Both *N*-methylbarbitone and *N*-methylphenobarbitone are

OXIDATIVE METABOLISM OF THE 5-SUBSTITUENT OF SOME BARBITURATE DRUGS

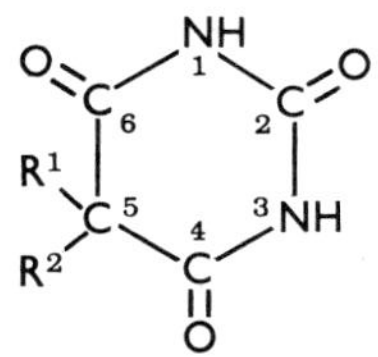

R^1 = ethyl, except in the case of quinalbarbitone (=—$CH_2 \cdot CH{:}CH_2$), and, for thiopentone, oxygen at $C_{(2)}$ is replaced by sulphur

Barbiturate	*R^2*	*Metabolite*	*Structure of oxidised R^2 group*
Phenobarbitone	—C_6H_5	*p*-hydroxyphenobarbitone	—C_6H_4OH
Butobarbitone	—$CH_2 \cdot CH_2 \cdot CH_2 \cdot CH_3$	hydroxybutobarbitone	—$CH_2 \cdot CH_2 \cdot CHOH \cdot CH_3$
Secbutobarbitone	—$CH(CH_3) \cdot CH_2 \cdot CH_3$	secbutobarbitone carboxylic acid	—$CH(CH_3) \cdot CH_2 \cdot COOH$
Amylobarbitone	—$CH_2 \cdot CH_2 \cdot CH(CH_3)_2$	hydroxyamylobarbitone	—$CH_2 \cdot CH_2 \cdot COH(CH_3)_2$
Pentobarbitone	—$CH(CH_3) \cdot CH_2 \cdot CH_2 \cdot CH_3$	hydroxypentobarbitone	—$CH(CH_3) \cdot CH_2 \cdot CHOH \cdot CH_3$
		pentobarbitone carboxylic acid	—$CH(CH_3) \cdot CH_2 \cdot CH_2 \cdot COOH$
Quinalbarbitone	—$CH(CH_3) \cdot CH_2 \cdot CH_2 \cdot CH_3$	hydroxyquinalbarbitone	—$CH(CH_3) \cdot CH_2 \cdot CHOH \cdot CH_3$
		quinalbarbitone carboxylic acid	—$CH(CH_3) \cdot CH_2 \cdot CH_2 \cdot COOH$
Cyclobarbitone	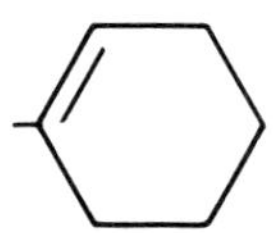	hydroxycyclobarbitone	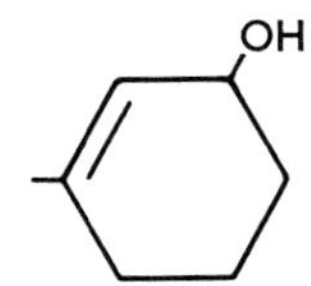
		ketocyclobarbitone	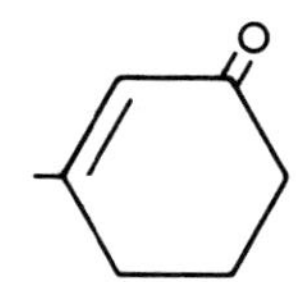
Thiopentone	—$CH(CH_3) \cdot CH_2 \cdot CH_2 \cdot CH_3$	thiopentone carboxylic acid	—$CH(CH_3) \cdot CH_2 \cdot CH_2 \cdot COOH$

largely demethylated to their nor-analogues but this reaction is less significant with hexobarbitone.

(3) RING FISSION. The barbituric acid ring is relatively stable and its fission to substituted urea derivatives appears to be a minor reaction. Small quantities of metabolites arising from splitting of the ring have been reported to occur in the urine of animals dosed with the following barbiturates: hexobarbitone, pentobarbitone, amylobarbitone, thiopentone, and thialbarbitone.

(4) DESULPHURATION. This is a general reaction of thiobarbiturates but variable in extent. The products are the corresponding oxygen analogues.

Glutarimides

Glutarimide based drugs have the following general structure:

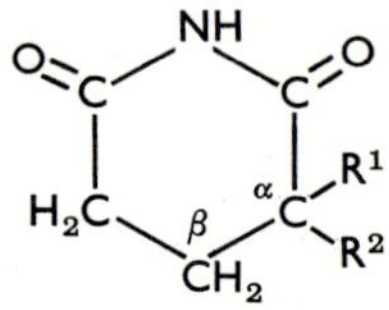

(where R^1 and R^2 are alkyl, aryl, or acyl groups; for bemegride R^1 and R^2 are in the β-position). The metabolic reactions of the glutarimides are: (a) oxidation of the α- (or β-) substituents, the hydroxylated products being excreted free and conjugated, (b) hydroxylation of the ring, and (c) ring-fission. Generally, the glutarimide ring is metabolically stable and little if any splitting occurs. However, in the case of thalidomide (α-phthalimidoglutarimide) the amide bonds are unstable and spontaneous hydrolysis of the glutarimide and phthalimide rings occur. The glutarimide rings of glutethimide, aminoglutethimide, and bemegride are not split and oxidative changes occur in the side-chain and in the ring. Glutethimide is hydroxylated in the glutarimide ring (I) and in the ethyl side-chain (II) and the metabolites formed are excreted as conjugates; II can also lose the oxidised ethyl group to form α-phenylglutarimide (III).

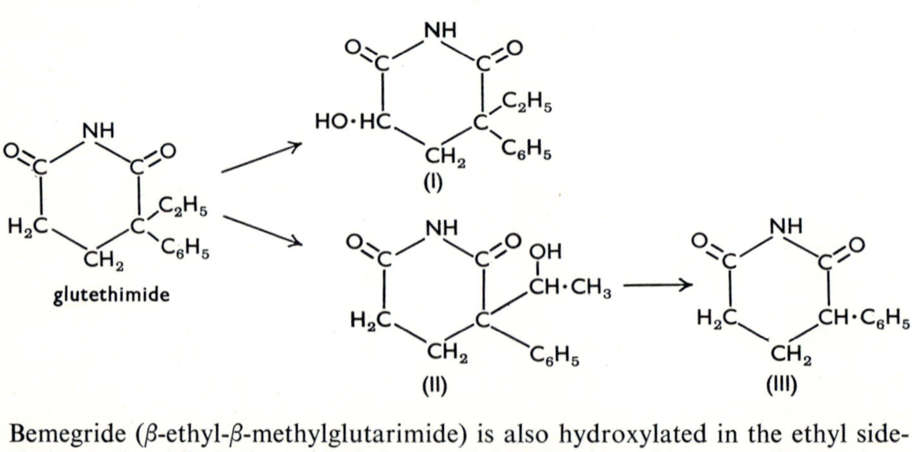

Bemegride (β-ethyl-β-methylglutarimide) is also hydroxylated in the ethyl side-chain to give β-(1-hydroxyethyl)-β-methylglutarimide and is excreted as such.

Hydantoins

The hydantoin drugs are metabolised by two mechanisms, namely, oxidation of the aromatic group at $C_{(5)}$ and by ring-fission. Phenytoin (5,5-diphenyl-hydantoin) for example undergoes aromatic hydroxylation to give 5-*p*-hydroxy-phenyl-5-phenylhydantoin and hydrolysis of the hydantoin ring to afford α-aminodiphenylacetic acid. Methoin, which is methylated at $N_{(3)}$, is largely *N*-dealkylated to 5-ethyl-5-phenylhydantoin which is then metabolised in the same way as phenytoin, that is, by aromatic hydroxylation and ring-fission.

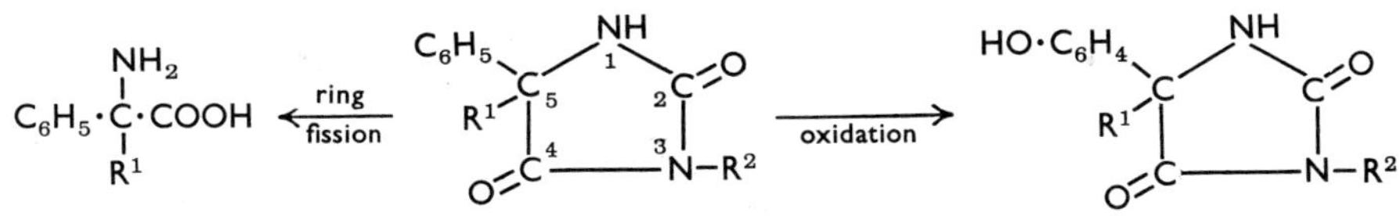

phenytoin (R^1 = $-C_6H_5$, R^2 = H)
methoin (R^1 = $-C_2H_5$, R^2 = $-CH_3$)

Oxazolidine Derivatives

Some oxazolidine derivatives are used as anti-epileptic drugs, e.g. troxidone and paramethadione. The main metabolic reaction of these drugs is dealkylation at $N_{(3)}$. The metabolites formed probably play a role in the therapeutic action of these drugs.

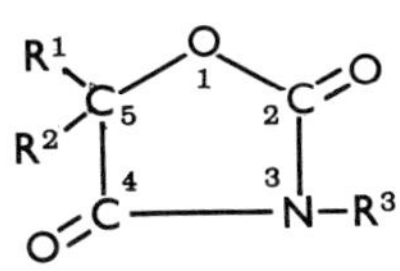

troxidone (R^1 = R^2 = R^3 = $-CH_3$)
paramethadione (R^1 = R^3 = $-CH_3$, R^2 = $-C_2H_5$)

Pyrazole Derivatives

Pyrazole derivatives are used as analgesics and antipyretics (phenazone, amido-pyrine, and dipyrone) and for the treatment of rheumatoid conditions (phenyl-butazone and oxyphenbutazone).

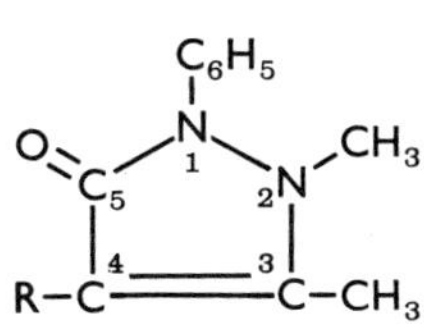

(I)

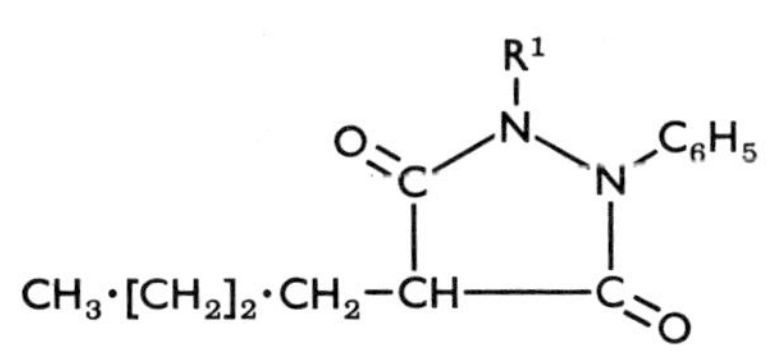

(II)

(a) phenazone (R = H)
(b) amidopyrine (R = $-N(CH_3)_2$)
(c) dipyrone (R = $-NCH_3 \cdot CH_2 \cdot SO_3Na$)

(a) phenylbutazone (R^1 = $-C_6H_5$)
(b) oxyphenbutazone (R^1 = $-C_6H_4OH$-*p*)

Pyrazole derivatives are metabolised mainly by oxidation of the substituent group at positions 1 and 4. It is not known whether the pyrazole ring itself is metabolised or not. Phenazone is hydroxylated to give 4-hydroxyphenazone (R = —OH in Ia) which is excreted mainly as its glucuronide conjugate (R =

—O·$C_6H_9O_6$). Amidopyrine (Ib) undergoes oxidative demethylation to 4-aminophenazone (R = —NH_2) which is excreted free and as its *N*-acetyl conjugate.

The antirheumatic drug phenylbutazone (IIa) undergoes oxidation in the aromatic nucleus to give oxyphenbutazone (IIb) which also has antirheumatic properties and is used in its own right as a drug; phenylbutazone also forms a second metabolite by ($\omega-1$)-hydroxylation of the butyl side-chain.

Coumarins

The metabolic fate of the clinically used coumarins has not been fully established.

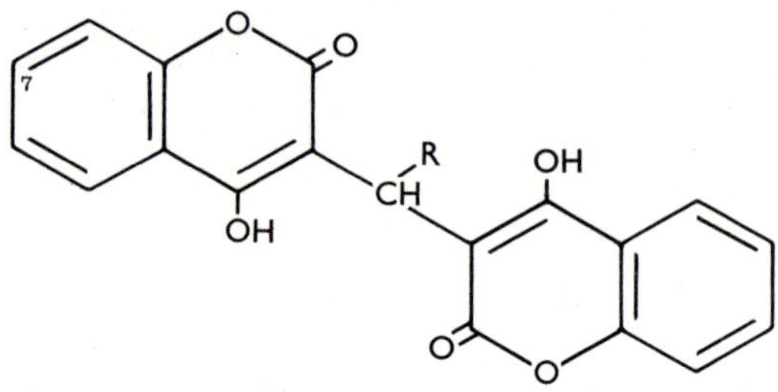

dicoumarol (R = H); ethyl biscoumacetate (R = $-CO\cdot O\cdot C_2H_5$)

Both dicoumarol and ethyl biscoumacetate are extensively metabolised in man. Ethyl biscoumacetate is hydroxylated in the 7-position and other reactions, such as fission of the coumarin ring and the ester link, probably occur but have not yet been adequately demonstrated.

Quinolines

A number of important drugs, both naturally occurring and synthetic, are quinoline derivatives. The two metabolic reactions of quinoline itself are hydroxylation and methylation; the latter is a minor reaction. The quinoline ring appears to be stable but there is evidence that ring-fission may occur with halogenated 8-hydroxyquinolines and this might be important in the sensitisation shown by some patients to these drugs. Generally, quinoline based drugs are metabolised by hydroxylation of the ring followed by conjugation or by metabolism of the ring substituents.

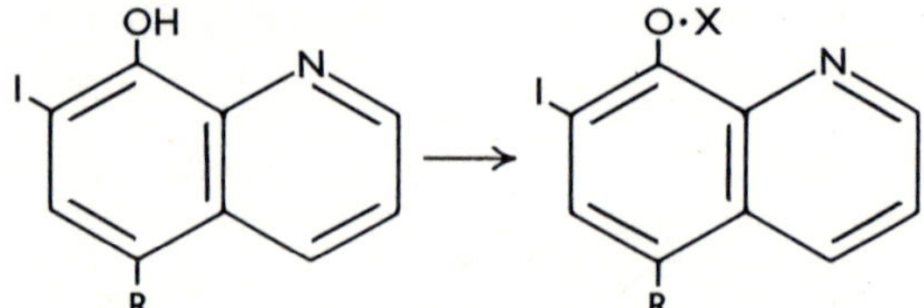

clioquinol (R = Cl); di-iodohydroxyquinoline (R = I); chiniofon (R = $-SO_2\cdot OH$); X = $-C_6H_9O_6$ (glucuronide) or $-SO_2\cdot OH$ (sulphate)

Halogenated quinolinols (hydroxyquinolines) are used as amoebicides and are metabolised in part by direct conjugation with glucuronic acid and sulphate. 8-Aminoquinoline forms the basis of an important group of synthetic antimalarial drugs. These are extensively metabolised in man and their antimalarial activity is due to metabolite formation. They are metabolised by two general

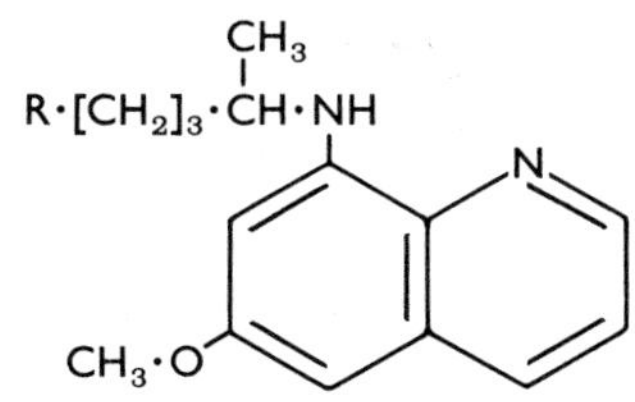

primaquine (R = $-NH_2$)
pamaquin (R = $-N(C_2H_5)_2$)

reactions, namely, by oxidation to a quinone which has antimalarial activity and by *N*-dealkylation. Quinone formation occurs by oxidation of the 5,6-diol formed by hydroxylation at $C_{(5)}$ and *O*-demethylation at $C_{(6)}$.

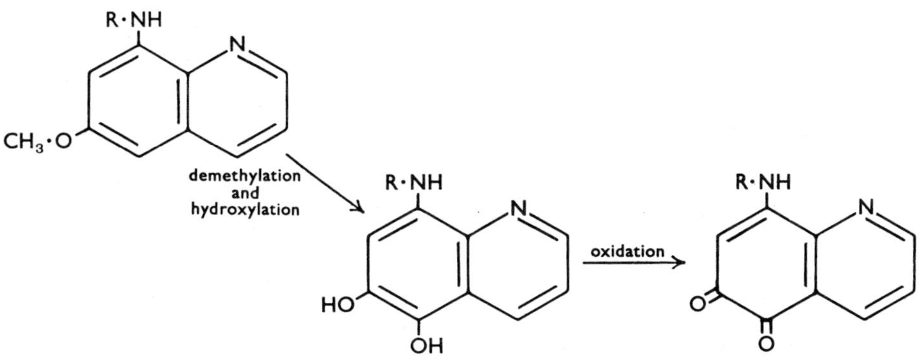

Several antimalarial drugs are based on 4-aminoquinoline, e.g. chloroquine [R = $-CHCH_3\cdot(CH_2)_3\cdot N(C_2H_5)_2$] and hydroxychloroquine [R = $-CHCH_3\cdot(CH_2)_3\cdot NC_2H_5\cdot CH_2\cdot CH_2OH$]. Chloroquine is metabolised by oxidative dealkylation to the corresponding mono-*N*-de-ethyl compound.

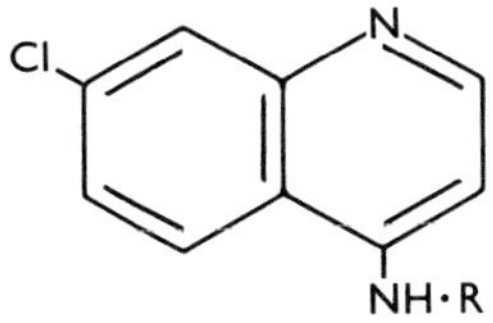

The cinchona alkaloids, quinine and quinidine, are derivatives of quinoline. Both drugs are metabolised by hydroxylation at the 2-position of the quinuclidine nucleus and also, but to a smaller extent, at the 2′-position of the quinoline ring (see overleaf).

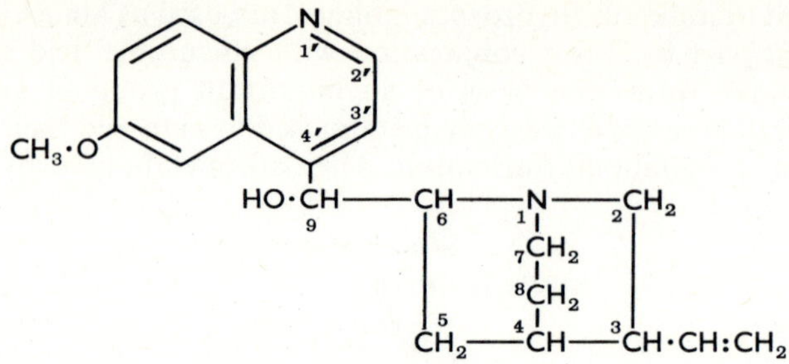

quinine

Quinidine differs from quinine in its configuration about atoms 6 and 9

Isoquinolines

The isoquinoline structure is found in the opium derivative papaverine. In man, the drug undergoes a selective demethylation to give 4-hydroxypapaverine which is then excreted in the urine almost entirely as a glucuronide.

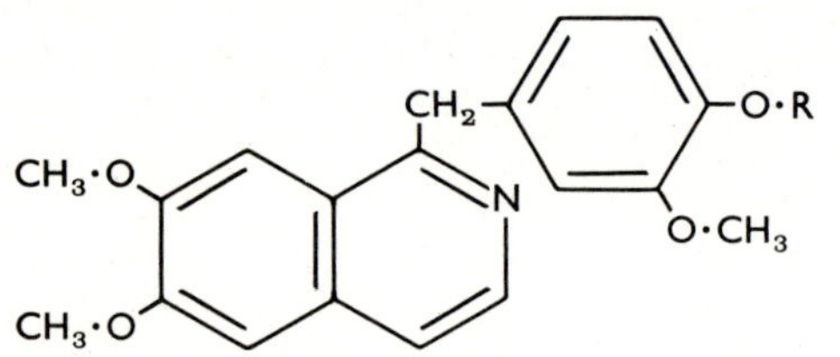

papaverine (R = $-CH_3$)
4-hydroxypapaverine (R = H)
4-hydroxypapaverine glucuronide (R = $-C_6H_9O_6$)

The curare alkaloids are derivatives of isoquinoline. One of these alkaloids, *d*-tubocurarine, is excreted by man partly unchanged and partly as unknown metabolites.

Indoles

A number of important drugs, particularly the ergot and rauwolfia alkaloids, are indole derivatives. Because of their chemical complexity, their metabolic fate is not fully established. Both lysergide (LSD) and ergometrine appear to undergo

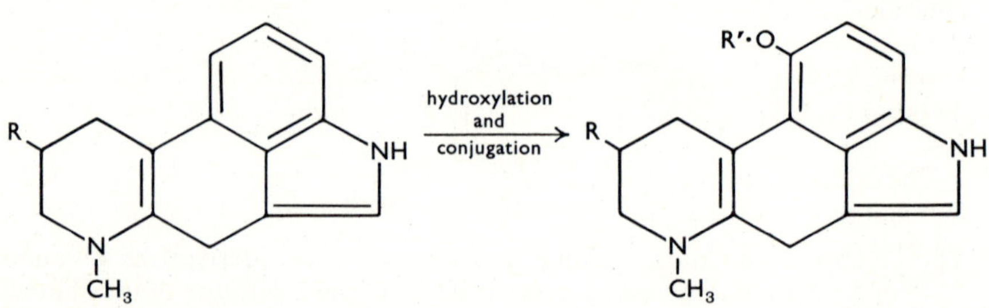

lysergide (R = $-CO \cdot N(C_2H_5)_2$)
ergometrine (R = $-CO \cdot NH \cdot CH(CH_3) \cdot CH_2OH$)

R′ = H or $-C_6H_9O_6$

hydroxylation in the 12-position and the hydroxy-derivatives formed are excreted in the bile as glucuronides.

Reserpine probably undergoes a number of reactions *in vivo* but the only ones so far demonstrated to occur are *O*-demethylation and hydrolysis of the trimethoxybenzoyl ester group.

HYDROLYSIS OF RESERPINE

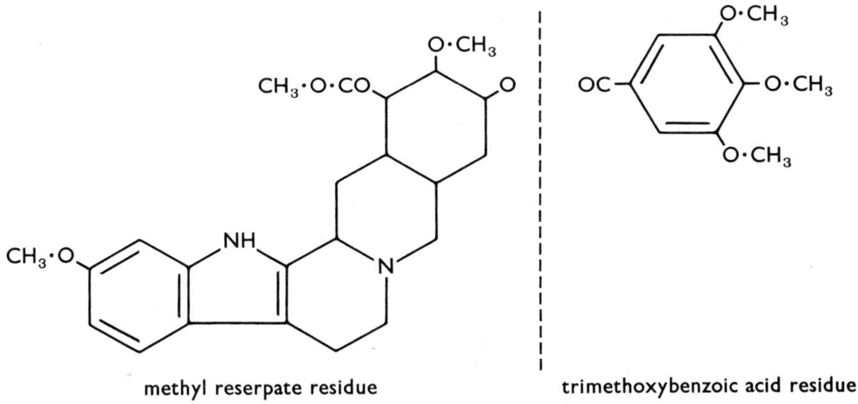

Phenothiazine Derivatives

Therapeutically useful phenothiazine derivatives have the following general formula:

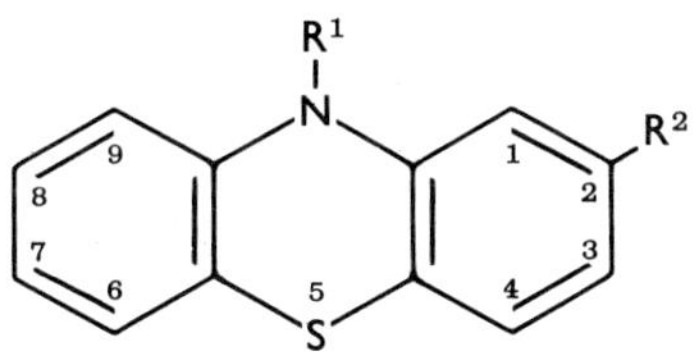

where R^1 is usually a dialkylaminoalkyl group or an alkyl group containing a heterocyclic residue and R^2 is Cl, —CF_3, or —$S{\cdot}CH_3$. The known metabolic reactions of phenothiazines are: (a) sulphoxidation to a sulphoxide or sulphone, (b) dealkylation of the dialkylamino-group, (c) ring hydroxylation followed by conjugation, and (d) oxidation of the dialkylamino-group to an *N*-oxide. Combinations of these reactions occur giving rise to numerous metabolites so that the metabolic fate of these compounds is complex and at present incompletely known. Chlorpromazine, for example, is metabolised to at least 20 urinary metabolites; the structures of the more important are given in the table on p. 164.

The most important of these pathways for chlorpromazine is hydroxylation and conjugation with glucuronic acid. Promethazine, pecazine, promazine, and thioridazine undergo sulphoxidation and the last two also suffer dealkylation. Thioridazine is also extensively metabolised to phenolic metabolites and their glucuronide conjugates. Generally, metabolites of the phenothiazines are excreted in both the urine and bile but in some cases biliary elimination may be more important, e.g. thioridazine.

PRINCIPAL URINARY METABOLITES OF CHLORPROMAZINE

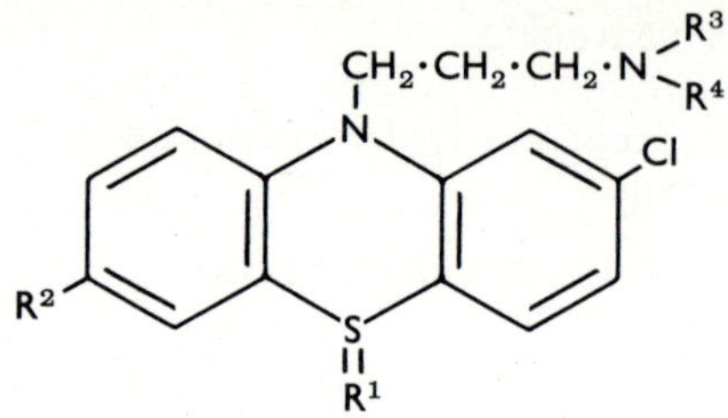

Metabolite	*R*[1]	*R*[2]	*R*[3]	*R*[4]
chlorpromazine 5-oxide	O	H	$-CH_3$	$-CH_3$
demonomethylchlorpromazine	—	H	H	$-CH_3$
dedimethylchlorpromazine	—	H	H	H
demonomethylchlorpromazine 5-oxide	O	H	H	$-CH_3$
dedimethylchlorpromazine 5-oxide	O	H	H	H
7-hydroxychlorpromazine	—	$-OH$	$-CH_3$	$-CH_3$
7-hydroxydemonomethylchlorpromazine	—	$-OH$	H	$-CH_3$
7-hydroxydedimethylchlorpromazine	—	$-OH$	H	H
7-hydroxychlorpromazine 5-oxide	O	$-OH$	$-CH_3$	$-CH_3$

[the hydroxylated metabolites are excreted free ($R^2 = -OH$) and conjugated with glucuronic acid ($R^2 = -C_6H_9O_7$)]

Morphine and Related Compounds

The narcotic analgesics are of four types, namely, (1) the naturally occurring opium alkaloids (morphine and codeine) and their synthetic derivatives (heroin, hydromorphone, hydrocodone, and nalorphine), (2) morphinans (levorphanol, dextromethorphan, and levallorphan), (3) methadones (methadone, acetylmethadol, and dextropropoxyphene), and, (4) the phenylpiperidines (pethidine, alphaprodine, and anileridine).

OPIUM ALKALOIDS

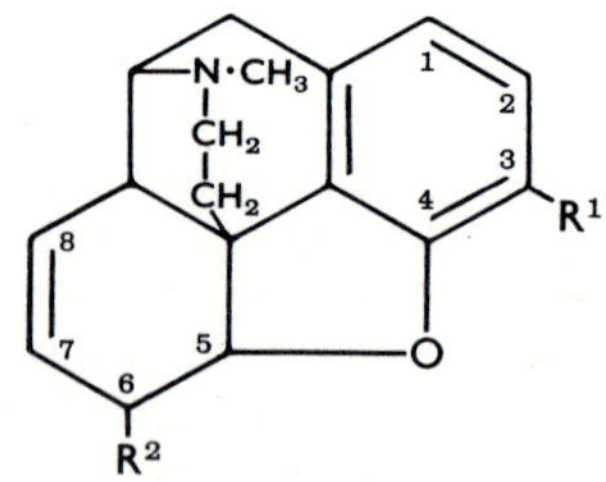

	R[1]	*R*[2]
morphine	$-OH$	$-OH$
codeine	$-O\cdot CH_3$	$-OH$
heroin	$-O\cdot CO\cdot CH_3$	$-O\cdot CO\cdot CH_3$

In the dihydro-derivatives of morphine and codeine the $\Delta^{7,8}$-double bond is absent and there is a keto-group at $C_{(6)}$.

Morphine is metabolised along three pathways, namely, by conjugation with glucuronic acid to give 'bound' morphine, by *N*-dealkylation to normorphine, and by *O*-methylation to yield codeine.

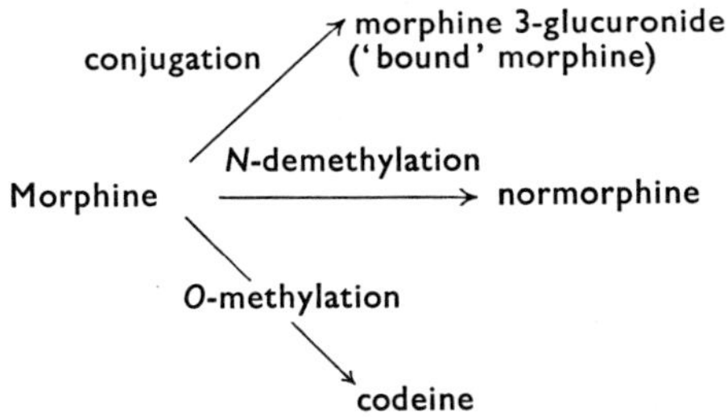

Heroin (diacetylmorphine) is largely metabolised as morphine since this is rapidly formed *in vivo* by hydrolysis of the acetyl groups. Codeine is metabolised by conjugation with glucuronic acid and by *N*-demethylation to norcodeine; it also suffers *O*-demethylation to a small extent to give morphine.

MORPHINANS. Little is known about the metabolic fate of the morphinans except that they are largely metabolised. They appear to undergo at least two reactions, namely, conjugation with glucuronic acid and *N*-dealkylation.

METHADONES. Similarly, little is known about the metabolic fate of these drugs except that little unchanged material is excreted. *N*-Demethylation is a metabolic pathway for methadone, acetylmethadol, and dextropropoxyphene.

PHENYLPIPERIDINES. Of the various narcotic analgesics based on phenylpiperidine only the metabolism of pethidine and anileridine has been established in any detail. Both analgesics are metabolised by hydrolysis of the ester group to give pethidinic acid and anileridinic acid respectively. In addition, pethidine is extensively *N*-demethylated to norpethidine which is excreted free and as its hydrolysis product norpethidinic acid. Anileridine and anileridinic acid are also acetylated in the aromatic amino-group to give their respective acetyl conjugates.

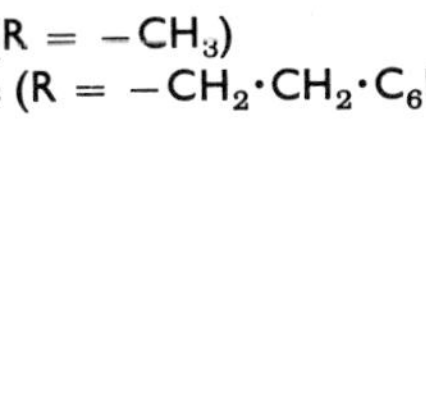

pethidine (R = $-CH_3$)
anileridine (R = $-CH_2{\cdot}CH_2{\cdot}C_6H_4{\cdot}NH_2$-*p*)

PART 2: Monographs
Analytical and Toxicological Data

ACEPIFYLLINE *Xanthine Derivative*

Synonym: Piperazine Theophylline Ethanoate.
Proprietary Names: Étaphylline; Etophylate. It is an ingredient of Heptonal.

Piperazine 1,3-dimethylxanthin-7-ylacetate
$C_4H_{10}N_2,C_9H_{10}N_4O_4 = 324{\cdot}3$

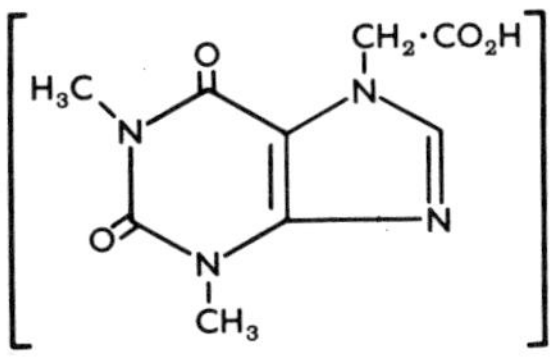

A white powder.
Solubility. Very soluble in water.

Extraction. Acepifylline is extracted by organic solvents from aqueous alkaline solutions.

Chromatography. PAPER: system P1—Rf 0·28 (location under ultraviolet light, weak absorption; location by the Clarke–Kalayci test, reddish-purple).
THIN-LAYER: system T1—Rf 0·04 (location reagents: *strongly acid iodoplatinate spray*, positive reaction; *iodine–carbon tetrachloride spray*, positive reaction).

Colour Test. Amalic acid test—purple.

Crystal Tests. MICRO: *platinic chloride solution* —small plates, often rectangular (*sensitivity:* 1 in 1000); *styphnic acid*—small plates or needles (*sensitivity:* 1 in 1000).

Ultraviolet Absorption Spectrum. Acepifylline in 0·1N sulphuric acid, maxima at 205 mμ (E1%, 1cm 846) and 274 mμ (E1%, 1cm 329).

Infra-red Absorption Spectrum. Potassium bromide disk. The principal peaks are: A 1660 or 1700, B 1370 (p. 771).

Dose. Up to 4 g daily.

ACEPROMAZINE *Tranquilliser*

Synonym: Acetylpromazine.

2-Acetyl-10-(3-dimethylaminopropyl)phenothiazine
$C_{19}H_{22}N_2OS = 326{\cdot}5$

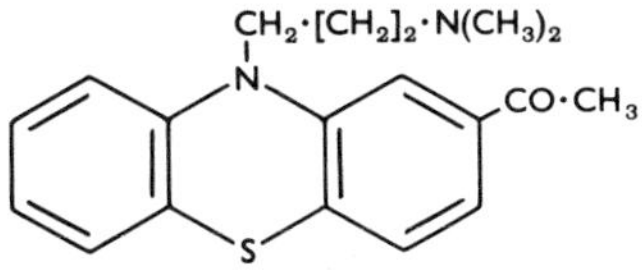

An orange-coloured oil which boils between 220° and 240° at 0·5 mm Hg.

ACEPROMAZINE MALEATE

Proprietary Name: Notensil.

A yellow crystalline powder. M.p. 135° to 138°.
Solubility. Soluble 1 in 23 of water, 1 in 40 of ethanol, and 1 in 3 of chloroform; slightly soluble in ether.

Screening Test. *FPN reagent* with urine—orange-red (see p. 10).

Extraction. Acepromazine may be isolated in the D1 fraction (see p. 27); hydrolysis of biological material is required in order to improve the yield.

Chromatography. PAPER: system P1—Rf 0·55 (location under ultraviolet light, yellow fluorescence; location reagents: *iodoplatinate spray*, strong reaction; *bromocresol green spray*, weak reaction); system RP1a—Rf 0·54 (location under ultraviolet light, orange fluorescence; location reagent *iodoplatinate spray*, positive reaction); system RP1b—Rf 0·07 (location under ultraviolet light, yellow fluorescence; location reagent *iodoplatinate spray*, positive reaction).
THIN-LAYER: system T1—Rf 0·40 (location reagent *acidified iodoplatinate spray*, positive reaction); system T6—Rf 0·58 (the spot may be converted on the plate to the sulphoxide, Rf 0·39; location of both spots under ultraviolet light).
GAS: system G2/225—retention time 2·44 relative to codeine.

Colour Tests. MICRO: sulphuric acid–formaldehyde test—yellow-green → red (*sensitivity:* 0·1 μg); ammonium molybdate test—brown → purple (*sensitivity:* 0·1 μg); ammonium vanadate test—green → red (*sensitivity:* 0·1 μg); Vitali's test—purple → yellow/yellow/yellow (*sensitivity:* 0·1 μg).

Crystal Tests. MICRO: *gold chloride solution*—masses of very small rods (*sensitivity:* 1 in 1000); *potassium tri-iodide solution* (*1*)—small plates from hydrochloric acid solution (*sensitivity:* 1 in 1000).

Ultraviolet Absorption Spectrum. Acepromazine in 0·1N sulphuric acid, maxima at 243 mμ (E1%, 1cm 503), 278 mμ (E1%, 1cm 366), and 374 mμ (E1%, 1cm 36·5).

Infra-red Absorption Spectrum. Acepromazine (base). Potassium bromide disk. The principal peaks are: A 1455, B 1410 or 1675, C 1220 (p. 771).

Dose. Up to 100 mg daily may be given in major psychotic disturbances.

Toxicity. The acute lethal dose of phenothiazine tranquillisers in man appears to be in the range 15 to 150 mg/kg, although severe toxic symptoms have occurred with doses of less than 1 mg/kg.
LD50 (oral): in rats 130 mg/kg.

ACETALDEHYDE

Synonyms: Acetic Aldehyde; Aldehyde; Ethanal; Ethyl Aldehyde.

$CH_3{\cdot}CHO = 44{\cdot}05$

A colourless inflammable liquid. B.p. 20·2°. Refractive index, at 20°, 1·3316.

Solubility. Soluble in water, ethanol, and ether.

Extraction. Acetaldehyde is volatile and may be isolated by distillation (see p. 18).

Chromatography. GAS: system G8/160—retention time 2·80 relative to n-propanol.

Colour Tests. *Acidified potassium dichromate solution*—green, on warming; iodoform test—positive reaction; *Schiff's reagent*—purple.

Quantitative Estimation. Clancy and Kramm (1963) have described a colorimetric method of estimation of acetaldehyde.

Metabolism. Acetaldehyde is oxidised *in vivo* to acetic acid which is eventually oxidised to carbon dioxide and water. A minor pathway involves condensation with pyruvic acid to yield acetoin. Acetaldehyde is a major intermediary metabolite of ethanol.

Toxicity. The maximum permissible atmospheric concentration is 200 p.p.m. Acetaldehyde is more toxic than ethanol and acetic acid.
LD50 (oral): in rats 1·9 g/kg.

ACETANILIDE *Analgesic and Antipyretic*

Synonym: Antifebrin.

N-Phenylacetamide

$C_6H_5{\cdot}NH{\cdot}CO{\cdot}CH_3 = 135{\cdot}2$

Colourless shining lamellar crystals or white crystalline powder. M.p. 113° to 115°.

Solubility. Soluble 1 in 200 of water, 1 in 20 of boiling water, 1 in 3·5 of ethanol, 1 in 50 of ether, and 1 in 8 of chloroform.

Extraction. Acetanilide is extracted by organic solvents from aqueous acid or alkaline solutions.

Ultraviolet Absorption Spectrum. Acetanilide in ethanol, maximum at 242 mμ (E 1%, 1 cm 1129).

Infra-red Absorption Spectrum. Potassium bromide disk. The principal peaks are: A 752 or 1598 or 1660 (p. 727).

Quantitative Estimation. See under Paracetamol, p. 465.

Metabolism. Acetanilide is rapidly hydroxylated to paracetamol (*p*-hydroxyacetanilide) through which the analgesic and antipyretic effects of the drug are chiefly exerted; paracetamol is excreted mainly as glucuronic and sulphuric acid conjugates and may be hydrolysed to *p*-aminophenol which is excreted entirely as conjugates; following the administration of 2 g of acetanilide in man, 0·1% of the dose was excreted in 24 hours as unchanged drug, 0·04% as aniline, 3% as free paracetamol, and 82% as conjugated paracetamol (Brodie and Axelrod, 1948).
The main toxic effect of acetanilide, the formation of methaemoglobin, seems to be related to the concentration of aniline in the blood; it is thought to be formed by an oxidation product of the amine (Brodie and Axelrod, 1949; Kiese, 1965).

Acetanilide is completely absorbed from the gastro-intestinal tract and maximum plasma levels are attained within 1 to 2 hours. It is distributed fairly rapidly and evenly throughout the body. It penetrates the red blood-cells and tends to concentrate there (Lester and Greenberg, 1947). After reaching its peak, the plasma level of acetanilide falls almost to zero in 7 hours.

Dose. Up to 1 g daily has been given but it has been superseded by safer analgesics.

Toxicity. The acute lethal dose in man is between 5 and 20 g. Fatalities have occurred in children and in aged and very sick patients following the ingestion of 0·66 to 2 g.
LD50 (oral): in rats 800 mg/kg.

ACETAZOLAMIDE *Diuretic*

Synonym: Acetazoleamide.
Proprietary Name: Diamox.

5-Acetamido-1,3,4-thiadiazole-2-sulphonamide

$C_4H_6N_4O_3S_2 = 222{\cdot}2$

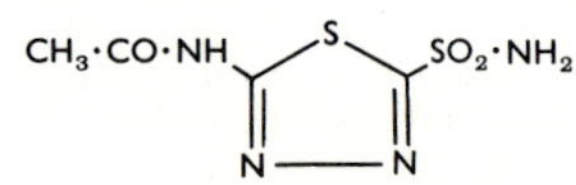

A white crystalline powder. M.p. about 258°.

Solubility. Soluble 1 in 1400 of water and 1 in 166 of ethanol; insoluble in ether and chloroform.

ACETAZOLAMIDE SODIUM
Synonym: Sodium Acetazolamide.
Proprietary Name: Diamox Sodium.
Solubility. Soluble in water.

Extraction. Acetazolamide is extracted by organic solvents from aqueous acid solutions.

Ultraviolet Absorption Spectrum. Acetazolamide in 0·1N hydrochloric acid, maximum at 265 mμ (E 1%, 1 cm 474).

Infra-red Absorption Spectrum. Acetazolamide (base). Potassium bromide disk. The principal peaks are: A 1167, B 1363, C 1316 or 1548 (p. 727).

Quantitative Estimation. Acetazolamide may be estimated by its inhibitory effect on the action of carbonic anhydrase (Maren *et al.*, 1954).

Metabolism. Acetazolamide is a powerful carbonic anhydrase inhibitor and, after administration, the urine of patients may be found to inhibit carbonic anhydrase. Following oral administration in man and dogs in doses of 20 mg/kg or less, acetazolamide is rapidly absorbed and over 70% of the dose is excreted unchanged in the urine in 24 hours (Maren *et al.*, 1954).

Dose. Up to 1·5 g daily has been given.

Toxicity. Fatal cases of thrombocytopenic purpura and agranulocytosis have been reported in elderly patients treated with 250 mg of acetazolamide daily over 7 to 9 weeks.

ACETIC ACID

Synonyms: Concentrated Acetic Acid; Glacial Acetic Acid (99% w/w).

$CH_3 \cdot CO_2H = 60 \cdot 05$

A clear, colourless, strongly acid liquid. M.p. not lower than 14·8°. B.p. about 117°. Refractive index 1·3718.

Solubility. Miscible with water, ethanol, ether, and chloroform.

Extraction. Acetic acid is volatile and may be isolated by distillation (see p. 18).

Chromatography. GAS: simple aliphatic acids can be chromatographed on Porapak Q under the conditions of system G8; the retention time is approximately 2·0 relative to propionic acid, but sensitivity for acetic acid is low if flame ionisation detectors are used.

Colour Test. *Ferric chloride solution,* after neutralisation with ammonium hydroxide solution—red.

Quantitative Estimation. Acetic acid may be isolated from blood and other tissues by vacuum distillation, and estimated by subsequent gas chromatography (Lester, 1964).

Metabolism. Acetic acid is incorporated into many tissues. It has been demonstrated to be a metabolite of ethanol in man, following the oxidation of ethanol to acetaldehyde, and it is eventually oxidised to carbon dioxide and water.

Toxicity. The estimated maximum safe concentration of acetic acid in air is 10 p.p.m. and the estimated lethal dose in man is 20 ml.

LD50 (oral): in rats 3·31 g/kg.

ACETOMENAPHTHONE

Vitamin-K Analogue

Synonyms: Acetomenadione; Menadiol Diacetate.
Proprietary Names: Prokayvit Oral; Vitavel K.

1,4-Diacetoxy-2-methylnaphthalene

$C_{15}H_{14}O_4 = 258 \cdot 3$

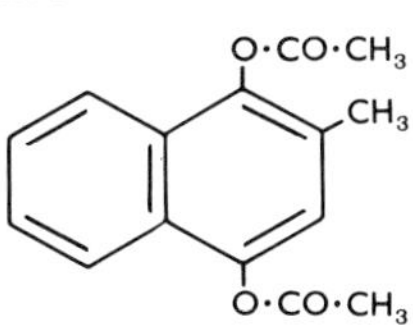

A white crystalline powder. M.p. 112° to 115°.

Solubility. Almost insoluble in water; slightly soluble in cold ethanol; soluble 1 in 3·3 of boiling ethanol; soluble in acetic acid.

Extraction. Biological material must be dehydrated and extracted with ethanol (see p. 29).

Ultraviolet Absorption Spectrum. Acetomenaphthone in ethanol, maximum at 285 mμ (E1%, 1cm 230 to 260).

Infra-red Absorption Spectrum. Potassium bromide disk. The principal peaks are: A 1200, B 1151, C 1740 (p. 727).

Dose. Up to 20 mg daily.

ACETONE

Industrial Solvent

Synonyms: Dimethyl Ketone; 2-Propanone.

$CH_3 \cdot CO \cdot CH_3 = 58 \cdot 08$

A volatile colourless inflammable liquid which must be stored in a cool place. B.p. 56°. Refractive index 1·3591.

Solubility. Miscible with water, ethanol, ether, and chloroform.

Screening Tests. Rothera's test on urine—purple (indicative of a ketone); iodoform test—yellow crystals (see p. 6).

Extraction. Acetone is volatile and may be isolated by distillation (see p. 18).

Chromatography. GAS: system G8/100—retention time 0·59 relative to n-propanol; system G8/160—retention time 0·70 relative to n-propanol.

Colour Test. Iodoform test—positive reaction.

Ultraviolet Absorption Spectrum. Acetone in ethanol, maxima at 233 mμ (E1%, 1cm 2·0) and 271 mμ (E1%, 1cm 2·7).

Quantitative Estimation. Stewart *et al.* (1961b) have described a rapid infra-red method for the determination of acetone in blood, following extraction into carbon disulphide, and in expired air; the sensitivity of detection in blood is 1·5 mg% and in air 10 μg/l. Following microdiffusion from blood, urine, and tissue homogenates, acetone may be determined spectrophotometrically (Klendshoj and Feldstein, 1955).

Metabolism. Acetone may be absorbed through the lungs or skin; inhalation of the vapour at high concentrations may lead to narcosis and unconsciousness. Large doses of acetone are excreted mainly unchanged but small doses, between 1 and 7 mg/kg, are almost completely metabolised in rats by oxidation; at this dose level in rats, about 7% is exhaled unchanged and 50% is oxidised to carbon dioxide which is exhaled within 24 hours.

Acetone is the main metabolite of isopropanol and it can be detected in the urine in one hour and in the expired air in 15 minutes after the ingestion of isopropanol (Kemal, 1927).

Acetone is often detectable in the blood and urine of diabetics.

Toxicity. The estimated maximum safe concentration in air for acetone is 1000 p.p.m. and the estimated lethal dose in man is 50 g.

LD50 (oral): in rats 9·75 g/kg.

ACETOPHENAZINE *Tranquilliser*

Synonym: Sch 6673.

2-Acetyl-10-{3-[4-(2-hydroxyethyl)piperazin-1-yl]propyl}phenothiazine

$C_{23}H_{29}N_3O_2S = 411{\cdot}6$

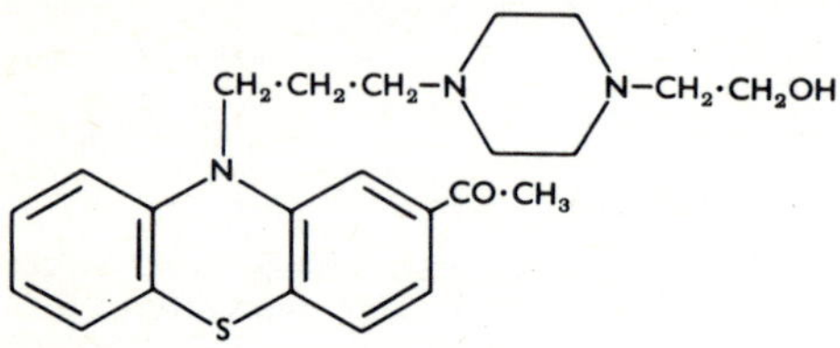

ACETOPHENAZINE MALEATE

Synonym: Acetophenazine Dimaleate.

Proprietary Name: Tindal.

Screening Test. *FPN reagent* with urine—red-violet (see p. 10).

Extraction. Acetophenazine is extracted by organic solvents from aqueous alkaline solutions.

Chromatography. PAPER: system P1—Rf 0·23 (location under ultraviolet light, yellow fluorescence; location reagents: *iodoplatinate spray*, strong reaction; *potassium permanganate spray*, strong reaction; *bromocresol green spray*, weak reaction); system RP1a—tailing (location under ultraviolet light, yellow fluorescence; location reagent *iodoplatinate spray*, positive reaction); system RP1b—Rf 0·00 (location as for RP1a).

THIN-LAYER: system T1—Rf 0·51 (location reagent *acidified iodoplatinate spray*, positive reaction); system T6—Rf 0·69 (the spot may be converted on the plate to the sulphoxide, Rf 0·16; location of both spots under ultraviolet light).

Colour Tests. MICRO: sulphuric acid–formaldehyde test—(yellow) red-purple (*sensitivity:* 0·1 μg); ammonium molybdate test—(yellow) deep purple (*sensitivity:* 0·1 μg); Vitali's test—(yellow) yellow/yellow/yellow (*sensitivity:* 0·5 μg).

Crystal Tests. MICRO: *picric acid*—feathery rosettes or rosettes of needles (*sensitivity:* 1 in 200); *potassium chromate solution*—bunches of plates (*sensitivity:* 1 in 1000).

Ultraviolet Absorption Spectrum. Acetophenazine in ethanol, maxima at 243 mμ (E1%, 1 cm 670) and 280 mμ (E1%, 1 cm 545); in 0·1N sulphuric acid, maxima at 243 mμ (E1%, 1 cm 469), 278 mμ (E1%, 1 cm 331), and 374 mμ (E1%, 1 cm 31).

Infra-red Absorption Spectrum. Acetophenazine (base). Potassium bromide disk. The principal peaks are: A 1408 or 1455, B 1670, C 1220 (p. 771).

Dose. Up to 80 mg daily.

Toxicity. The acute lethal dose in man of phenothiazine tranquillisers appears to be in the range 15 to 150 mg/kg, although severe toxic symptoms have occurred with doses of less than 1 mg/kg.

ACETORPHINE *Narcotic Analgesic*

Synonyms: 3-*O*-Acetyl-19-propylorvinol; M 183.

*O*³-Acetyl-7,8-dihydro-7α-[1(*R*)-hydroxy-1-methylbutyl]-*O*⁶-methyl-6,14-*endo*ethenomorphine

$C_{27}H_{35}NO_5 = 453{\cdot}6$

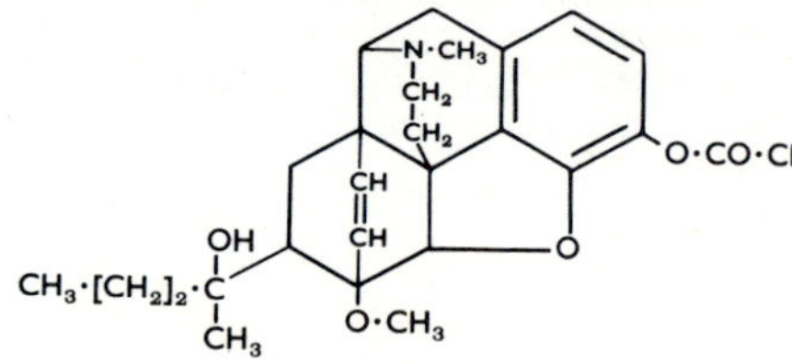

Acetorphine melts at 193°.

CAUTION. *It is dangerous to smell or taste this material.*

Solubility. Soluble 1 in 4000 of water; readily soluble in ethanol, ether, and chloroform.

ACETORPHINE HYDROCHLORIDE

A white crystalline hygroscopic powder. M.p. 204°. It is hydrolysed in solution to etorphine and acetic acid.

Solubility. Soluble 1 in 50 of water and 1 in 10 of ethanol.

Extraction. Acetorphine is extracted by organic solvents from aqueous alkaline solutions.

Chromatography. PAPER: system P1—Rf 0·68 (location under ultraviolet light, absorption; location reagents: *iodoplatinate spray*, strong reaction; *Dragendorff spray*, strong reaction).

THIN-LAYER: system T1—Rf 0·72 (location reagents: *acidified iodoplatinate spray*, positive reaction; *Marquis reagent*, grey; *potassium permanganate spray*, positive reaction).

Colour Tests. MICRO: sulphuric acid–formaldehyde test—bluish-grey → yellow-brown (*sensitivity:* 0·5 μg); ammonium molybdate test—bluish-purple → blue → dull green (*sensitivity:* 0·1 μg); Vitali's test— –/–/faint orange (*sensitivity:* 1·0 μg).

Crystal Tests. MICRO: *potassium cadmium iodide solution*—rosettes of rods (*sensitivity:* 1 in 1000); *potassium permanganate solution*—rosettes of blades (*sensitivity:* 1 in 400).

Ultraviolet Absorption Spectrum. Acetorphine in 0·1N sulphuric acid, maximum at 283 mμ (E1%, 1 cm 45).

Toxicity. LD50 (subcutaneous): in rats 7·0 mg/kg.

NOTE. Acetorphine is a highly potent analgesic and narcotic which has been tried as a sedative to assist in the control of large animals. Its effects may be antagonised by cyprenorphine or nalorphine.

ACETYLCARBROMAL *Sedative*

Synonym: Acetcarbromal.

Proprietary Name: Abasin.

N-Acetyl-*N'*-(α-bromo-α-ethylbutyryl)urea
$C_9H_{15}BrN_2O_3 = 279{\cdot}1$

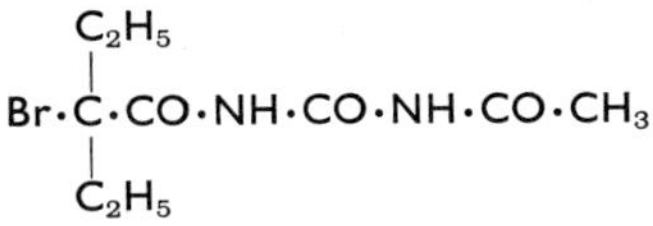

A white crystalline powder, which is decomposed by boiling water. M.p. 109°.
Solubility. Soluble 1 in 1000 of water; soluble in ethanol, ether, and chloroform.

Extraction. Acetylcarbromal is extracted by organic solvents from aqueous acid or alkaline solutions.

Chromatography. GAS: system G5—retention time 0·22 relative to barbitone.

Ultraviolet Absorption Spectrum. Acetylcarbromal in ethanol:water (1:1), maximum at 210 mμ (E1%, 1 cm 480); in 0·1N sodium hydroxide, maximum at 237 mμ (E1%, 1 cm 325).

Infra-red Absorption Spectrum. Potassium bromide disk. The principal peaks are: A 1484, B 1755, C 1696 (p. 727).

Dose. Up to 1·5 g daily.

ACETYLCHOLINE *Parasympathomimetic*

(2 - Acetoxyethyl)trimethylammonium hydroxide
$C_7H_{17}NO_3 = 163{\cdot}2$

$$[CH_3{\cdot}CO{\cdot}O{\cdot}[CH_2]_2{\cdot}N(CH_3)_3]^+ \, OH^-$$

A white hygroscopic crystalline powder which is readily hydrolysed in alkaline solution.
Solubility. Soluble in water.

ACETYLCHOLINE BROMIDE
Deliquescent colourless crystals or white powder hydrolysed by hot water and alkalis. M.p. 143°.
Solubility. Very soluble in cold water; soluble in ethanol; insoluble in ether.

ACETYLCHOLINE CHLORIDE
A white, very hygroscopic, crystalline powder; solutions are unstable. Protect from light and water.
Solubility. Very soluble in water; soluble in ethanol and chloroform; insoluble in ether.

Extraction. Acetylcholine is a quaternary ammonium compound (see p. 29).

Chromatography. PAPER: system P1—Rf 0·04 (location reagent *iodoplatinate spray*, strong reaction); system RP1b—Rf 0·57 (location under ultraviolet light, absorption).
THIN-LAYER: system T1—Rf 0·02 (location reagent *acidified iodoplatinate spray*, positive reaction).

Crystal Tests. MICRO: *mercuric chloride solution* —rhomboids (*sensitivity:* 1 in 1500); *potassium bismuth iodide solution*—rods (*sensitivity:* 1 in 3000).

Infra-red Absorption Spectrum. Acetylcholine chloride. Potassium bromide disk. The principal peaks are: A 950, B 955, C 1088 or 1475 (p. 771).

Metabolism. When injected intravenously its action is very transient as it is hydrolysed by cholinesterase; when given orally, it is broken down in the gut.

Dose. Up to 200 mg, subcutaneously or intramuscularly.

ACETYLDIGITOXIN *Cardiac Glycoside*

Synonym: Acetyldigitoxoside.
Proprietary Name: Acylanid(e).

α-Acetyldigitoxin, the acetyl group being attached to the terminal glucose residue of the digitoxose moiety.
$C_{43}H_{66}O_{14} = 807{\cdot}0$

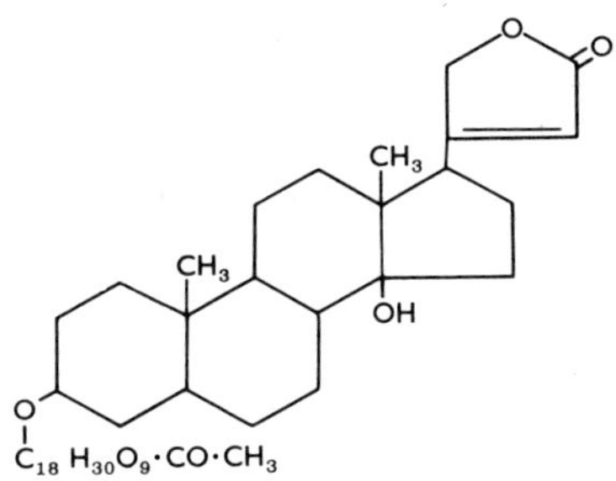

A white crystalline powder. M.p. 217° to 221°.
Solubility. Sparingly soluble in water, ether, and chloroform.

Extraction. Acetyldigitoxin may be isolated by continuous extraction under reduced pressure with ethanol (see p. 29).

Chromatography. THIN-LAYER: system T14—Rf 0·82 (location reagents: *perchloric acid spray*, followed by examination under ultraviolet light, red fluorescence; p-*anisaldehyde spray*, blue).

Metabolism. Studies in rats have indicated that acetyldigitoxin is extensively metabolised; the urine contained acetyldigitoxin, digitoxin, digoxin, and a metabolite of digoxin; the bile contained acetyldigitoxin and digoxin. Metabolites were also detected in the blood, liver, heart, and kidneys. It was only slowly excreted by rats, about 5% of the dose being present in the urine after 12 hours and 9% in the bile after 6 hours (Martin and Wright, 1960). About 60% of an oral dose of acetyldigitoxin is absorbed from the gastro-intestinal tract and it takes effect within 2 to 4 hours of administration but, since it is more rapidly metabolised than digitoxin, its effect is of shorter duration.

Dose. Up to 4 mg in 24 hours.

Toxicity. LD50 (intravenous): in cats 0·5 mg/kg.

ACETYLDIHYDROCODEINE
Narcotic Analgesic

6-Acetoxy-4,5-epoxy-3-methoxy-*N*-methylmorphinan

$C_{20}H_{25}NO_4 = 343{\cdot}4$

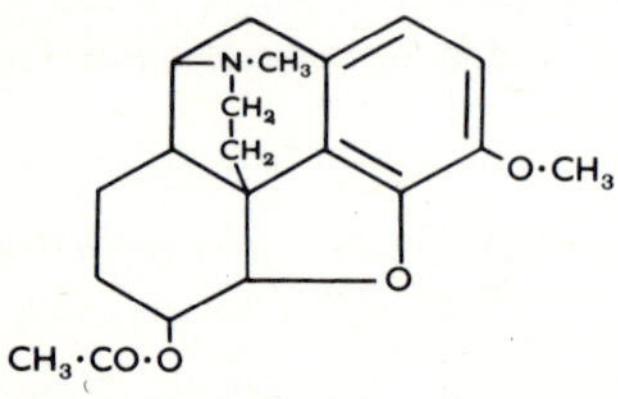

Extraction. Acetyldihydrocodeine is extracted by organic solvents from aqueous alkaline solutions.

Chromatography. PAPER: system P1—Rf 0·34 (location under ultraviolet light, strong absorption; location reagents: *iodoplatinate spray*, strong reaction; *bromocresol green spray*, weak reaction); system RP1a—Rf 0·89 (location reagent *iodoplatinate spray*, positive reaction); system RP1b—Rf 0·10 (location as for RP1a).
THIN-LAYER: system T1—Rf 0·26 (location reagent *acidified iodoplatinate spray*, positive reaction).

GAS: system G2/225—retention time 1·27 relative to codeine.

Colour Tests. MICRO: sulphuric acid–formaldehyde test—purple (*sensitivity:* 0·25 μg); ammonium molybdate test—green → blue (*sensitivity:* 0·25 μg); Vitali's test—faint yellow/–/orange (*sensitivity:* 1·0 μg).

Crystal Tests. MICRO: *picric acid*—gelatinous rosettes (*sensitivity:* 1 in 1000); *picrolonic acid*—bunches of serrated needles, forming overnight (*sensitivity:* 1 in 400).

Ultraviolet Absorption Spectrum. Acetyldihydrocodeine in ethanol, maximum at 284·5 mμ and minimum at 264 mμ; in 0·5N sodium hydroxide, maximum at 283 mμ and minimum at 263 mμ; in 0·1N sulphuric acid, maximum at 283 mμ (E1%, 1cm 43).

ACINITRAZOLE *Antiprotozoal (Veterinary)*

Synonym: Aminitrozole.
Proprietary Names: Entramine A; Trichorad; Tritheon.

2-Acetamido-5-nitrothiazole

$C_5H_5N_3O_3S = 187{\cdot}2$

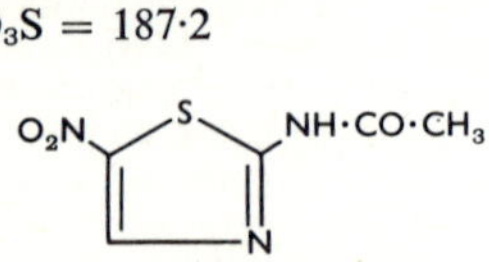

A cream-coloured crystalline powder. M.p. 264° to 265°; slight decomposition may occur.
Solubility. Very slightly soluble in water; soluble 1 in 300 of ethanol and 1 in 900 of chloroform; slightly soluble in ether; soluble in aqueous solutions of sodium hydroxide and ammonia.

Extraction. Acinitrazole is extracted by organic solvents from aqueous acid solutions.

Chromatography. PAPER: system P1—Rf 0·90 (location under ultraviolet light, absorption; location reagent *potassium permanganate spray*, weak reaction); system RP1a—Rf 0·39 and 0·66 (location under ultraviolet light, absorption).

THIN-LAYER: system T1—Rf 0·80 (location reagent *potassium permanganate spray*, positive reaction).

Ultraviolet Absorption Spectrum. Acinitrazole in ethanol, maxima at 235 mμ and 341 mμ (E1%, 1cm 590); in 0·1N sulphuric acid, maxima at 237 mμ (E1%, 1cm 282) and 345 mμ (E1%, 1cm 435).

Infra-red Absorption Spectrum. Potassium bromide disk. The principal peaks are: A 1345, B 1210, C 1485 (p. 771).

Quantitative Estimation. The determination of acinitrazole in animal feeds by extraction with dimethylformamide, chromatographic purification on an alumina column, and subsequent differential spectrophotometry is described (Report by the Prophylactics in Animal Feeds Subcommittee of the Analytical Methods Committee, 1966).

Dose. In turkeys, 100 to 300 mg.

ACONITINE *Depressant and Diaphoretic*

Acetylbenzoylaconine

$C_{34}H_{47}NO_{11} = 645{\cdot}8$

An alkaloid present in species of *Aconitum*, including monkshood, *A. anglicum*, and *A. napellus* agg. (Ranunculaceae).
Colourless crystals. M.p. 196°, with decomposition.
Solubility. Soluble 1 in 4500 of water, 1 in 40 of ethanol, 1 in 70 of ether, and 1 in 3 of chloroform.

ACONITINE NITRATE
A white crystalline powder or colourless crystals. M.p. about 200°, with decomposition.
Solubility. Soluble in water and ethanol.

Extraction. Aconitine may be isolated in the D1 fraction (see p. 27).

Chromatography. PAPER: system P1—Rf 0·62 (location under ultraviolet light, absorption; location reagent *iodoplatinate spray*, weak reaction).

THIN-LAYER: system T1—Rf 0·71 (location reagent *acidified iodoplatinate spray*, positive reaction).

GAS: system G6—retention time 1·08 relative to codeine.

Crystal Tests. MICRO: *sodium carbonate solution*—rosettes (*sensitivity:* 1 in 400); *potassium per-*

manganate solution—dense rosettes of rods (*sensitivity:* 1 in 400).

Ultraviolet Absorption Spectrum. Aconitine in ethanol:water (1:1), maxima at 228 mμ (E1%, 1 cm 180) and 270 mμ (E1%, 1 cm 20); in 0·1N sulphuric acid, maxima at 234 mμ (E1%, 1 cm 235) and 275 mμ (E1%, 1 cm 18).

Infra-red Absorption Spectrum. Aconitine (base). Potassium bromide disk. The principal peaks are: A 1092 or 1273, B 1713 (p. 771).

Dose. Up to 0·3 mg has been given.

Toxicity. Aconitine affects both the heart and the central nervous system and is one of the most potent and quick-acting poisons. It is well absorbed from the gastro-intestinal tract and death may occur within a few minutes. If the poisoning does not prove fatal within 8 to 10 hours, recovery is to be expected. The estimated lethal dose in man is 2 mg; as little as 5 ml of aconite tincture (0·05% total alkaloids) may prove fatal.

CASE EXAMPLES. 1 to 1·5 mg caused serious but non-fatal poisoning (Merchant *et al.*, 1963); two students who accidentally ingested between 5 and 10 mg recovered without treatment (Fiddes, 1958).

ACRIFLAVINE *Antiseptic*

A mixture of 3,6-diamino-10-methylacridinium chloride hydrochloride and 3,6-diaminoacridine dihydrochloride, in the ratio of approximately 2:1.

$C_{14}H_{14}ClN_3,HCl$ = 296·2; $C_{13}H_{11}N_3,2HCl$ = 282·2

An orange-red crystalline powder; a precipitate may form on dilution or standing of aqueous solutions.

Solubility. Soluble 1 in 3 of water and 1 in 40 of ethanol; almost insoluble in ether and chloroform.

Extraction. Acriflavine is very soluble in water; special extraction methods are required (see p. 28).

Chromatography. PAPER: system P1—Rf 0·23 (location under ultraviolet light, yellow-green fluorescence; location reagents: *iodoplatinate spray*, weak reaction; *bromocresol green spray*, weak reaction).

THIN-LAYER: system T1—Rf values were obtained at 0·07, 0·22, 0·28, 0·62 (location under ultraviolet light, yellow-green fluorescence).

Colour Tests. MICRO: sulphuric acid–formaldehyde test—(orange) yellow → red (*sensitivity:* 1·0 μg); ammonium molybdate test—(orange) pale yellow (*sensitivity:* 1·0 μg); Vitali's test—(orange) orange/orange-brown/brown (*sensitivity:* 1·0 μg).

Crystal Tests. MICRO: *ammonium thiocyanate solution*—small oily needles (*sensitivity:* 1 in 1000); *trinitrobenzoic acid solution*—long needles and smudge rosettes (*sensitivity:* 1 in 1000).

Ultraviolet Absorption Spectrum. Acriflavine in 0·1N hydrochloric acid, maxima at 238 mμ (E1%, 1 cm 720), 262 mμ (E1%, 1 cm 1522), and 450 mμ (E1%, 1 cm 1192).

Metabolism. Acriflavine is excreted as glucuronides and ethereal sulphates; it may be oxidised but the oxidation products have not been characterised.

ADIPHENINE *Parasympatholytic*

2-Diethylaminoethyl diphenylacetate

$C_{20}H_{25}NO_2$ = 311·4

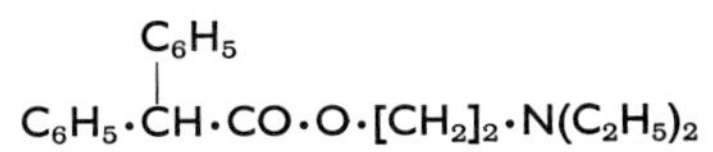

ADIPHENINE HYDROCHLORIDE

Synonym: Spasmolytine.

Proprietary Name: Trasentin.

White crystals. M.p. 113° to 114°.

Solubility. Readily soluble in water; sparingly soluble in ethanol and ether.

Extraction. Adiphenine is extracted by organic solvents from aqueous alkaline solutions.

Chromatography. PAPER: system P1—Rf 0·74 (location reagents: *iodoplatinate spray*, strong reaction; *bromocresol green spray*, weak reaction); system RP1a—Rf 0·32 (location reagent *iodoplatinate spray*, positive reaction); system RP1b—Rf 0·00.

THIN-LAYER: system T1—Rf 0·61 (location reagent *acidified iodoplatinate spray*, positive reaction).

Colour Tests. MICRO: ammonium vanadate test—green → blue (*sensitivity:* 0·1 μg); Vitali's test— -/-/blue-purple (*sensitivity:* 0·025 μg).

Ultraviolet Absorption Spectrum. Adiphenine in 0·1N sulphuric acid, maxima at 248 mμ (E1%, 1 cm 9), 253 mμ (E1%, 1 cm 11), 257·5 mμ (E1%, 1 cm 13), and 264 mμ (E1%, 1 cm 10).

Infra-red Absorption Spectrum. Adiphenine (base). Potassium bromide disk. The principal peaks are: A 1736, B 1145, C 700 (p. 771).

Metabolism. Adiphenine is a synthetic parasympatholytic drug used principally for its antisecretory and spasmolytic actions. It is relatively non-toxic and cumulation does not occur. The effect is exerted about 30 minutes after oral administration and within 10 to 15 minutes of intramuscular injection.

Dose. Up to 450 mg daily.

Toxicity. The lethal dose in man is probably between 10 and 100 mg/kg.

ADRENALINE *Sympathomimetic*

Synonyms: Epinephrine; Epirenamine; Levorenin; Suprarenin.

Proprietary Names: Adrenaline is an ingredient of many proprietary preparations—see Extra Pharmacopoeia (Martindale), 25th Edn, pp. 55–6.

(−) - 1 - (3,4 - Dihydroxyphenyl) - 2 - methylaminoethanol
$C_9H_{13}NO_3 = 183{\cdot}2$

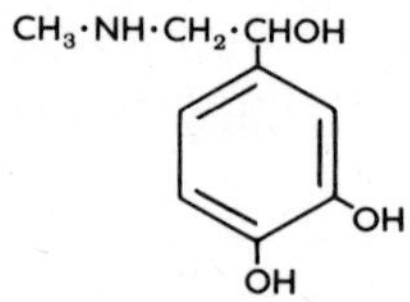

A white crystalline powder which slowly darkens on exposure to air and light. M.p. about 212°, with decomposition.

Solubility. Very slightly soluble in water; insoluble in ethanol, ether, and chloroform. It is readily soluble in solutions of mineral acids and in solutions of alkalis but is unstable in neutral or alkaline solution.

ADRENALINE ACID TARTRATE
Synonym: Adrenaline Bitartrate.

A white crystalline powder which slowly darkens on exposure to air and light. M.p. about 150°, with decomposition.

Solubility. Soluble 1 in 3 of water and 1 in 520 of ethanol; almost insoluble in ether and chloroform.

NOTE. It is the form of adrenaline generally used for preparing adrenaline injections and solutions.

Chromatography. PAPER: system P1—Rf 0·06 (location under ultraviolet light, absorption; location reagents: *bromocresol green spray*, weak reaction; *potassium permanganate spray*, strong reaction).

THIN-LAYER: system T1—Rf 0·18, streaking (location reagent *potassium permanganate spray*, positive reaction).

GAS: chromatography of adrenaline and related amines is given by Fales and Pisano (1962).

Colour Tests. Chen's test—green → greenish-brown.

MICRO: sulphuric acid–formaldehyde test—orange → dull purple; ammonium molybdate test—(orange-brown) dull green; Vitali's test—yellow/yellow/orange.

Crystal Tests. MICRO: *gold bromide solution*—small dense rosettes, forming overnight; *mercuric chloride solution*—very small rosettes, forming overnight.

Ultraviolet Absorption Spectrum. Adrenaline in 0·01N hydrochloric acid, maximum at 280 mμ (E1%, 1 cm 150).

Infra-red Absorption Spectrum. Adrenaline (base). Potassium bromide disk. The principal peaks are: A 1253 or 1274 or 1500 (p. 727).

Quantitative Estimation. Adrenaline and noradrenaline may be estimated spectrofluorimetrically in urine following column chromatographic separation (Pekkarinen and Pitkänen, 1955); Choulis (1967) describes a method of separation of adrenaline from dopamine and noradrenaline, involving thin-layer chromatography and subsequent determination by spectrophotometry.

Metabolism. Adrenaline is an active principle of the suprarenal gland. It is the typical stimulant of the sympathetic nervous system with a rapid onset and short duration of action. It is not absorbed from the gastro-intestinal tract but when injected it disappears rapidly from the circulation into the tissues. When infused intravenously, only 0·5 to 2% is excreted in the urine unchanged, the remainder being deactivated by oxidative deamination or *O*-methylation. The resulting compounds, 3,4-dihydroxymandelic acid and the 3-*O*-methylated amine, metanephrine, being excreted free, as sulphate or glucuronide conjugate, or as a further metabolite, 3-methoxy-4-hydroxymandelic acid. It has been suggested that there is a significant difference in the post-mortem adrenaline blood-levels following cases of violent and natural sudden death (Lund, 1964).

Dose. Up to 0·5 mg (base), subcutaneously, as a single dose.

Toxicity. The minimum subcutaneous lethal dose for an adult appears to be about 4 mg and the maximum tolerated dose 7 to 8 mg (Freedman, 1955). The lethal oral dose in rats is 30 mg/kg.

CASE EXAMPLES. A report of 12 fatal and 4 non-fatal cases of accidental adrenaline overdosage, many of which occurred through the injection of over-concentrated solutions (Freedman, 1955).

(1) A 36-year-old woman died very shortly after receiving 40 ml of a solution containing 0·1% of adrenaline and 0·5% of procaine hydrochloride, whereas the solution should have contained only 0·002% of adrenaline. (2) A 29-year-old pregnant woman was diagnosed to have a breech presentation. The surgeon injected 6 ml of adrenaline in mistake for 6 ml of 2% procaine. A living child was delivered but the mother died. Attempts to recover adrenaline from specimens of blood and perineal skin were unsuccessful (Johnson, 1960).

Report of survival following the subcutaneous injection of an overdose, 16 mg, of adrenaline. With appropriate treatment the patient gradually recovered over a period of 3 to 4 days (Lewis, 1967).

ADRENALONE *Local Haemostatic*

1 - (3′,4′ - Dihydroxy) - 2 - methylaminoacetophenone
$C_9H_{11}NO_3 = 181{\cdot}2$

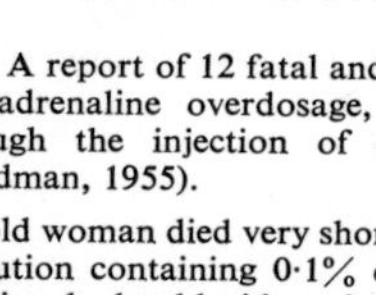

Adrenalone occurs as needles. M.p. 235° to 236°, with decomposition.

Solubility. Sparingly soluble in water, ethanol, and ether.

ADRENALONE HYDROCHLORIDE
Proprietary Names: Haemodan; Kephrine; Stryphnon.

A white crystalline powder. M.p. 243°.

Solubility. Soluble 1 in 8 of water and 1 in 45 of ethanol; almost insoluble in ether and in chloroform.

Extraction. Adrenalone should be extracted by organic solvents from aqueous alkaline solutions.

Chromatography. PAPER: system P1—Rf 0·11 (location under ultraviolet light, pale blue fluorescence; location reagents: *bromocresol green spray*, weak reaction; *potassium permanganate spray*, strong reaction); system RP1a—Rf 0·79 (location under ultraviolet light, blue fluorescence).

Colour Tests. Chen's test—green → orange → yellow-brown.
MICRO: sulphuric acid–formaldehyde test—greenish-yellow; ammonium molybdate test—(brown) green; ammonium vanadate test—(grey) orange; Vitali's test—deep orange/brown/brown.

Crystal Tests. MICRO: *sodium carbonate solution*—coarse blades or small irregular plates (*sensitivity:* 1 in 100); *sodium phosphate solution*—irregular crystals (*sensitivity:* 1 in 100).

AJMALINE *Myocardial Depressant*

Synonym: Rauwolfine.

$C_{20}H_{26}N_2O_2 = 326·4$

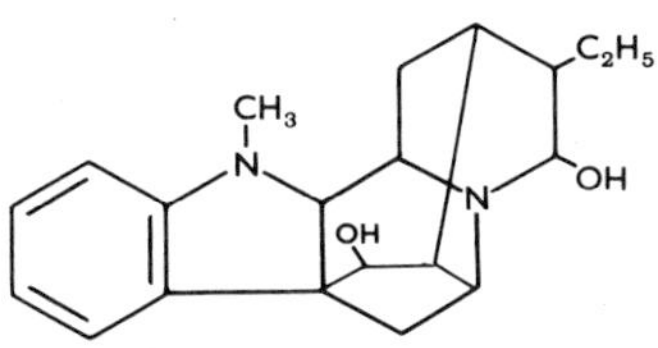

An alkaloid obtained from the root of *Rauwolfia serpentina* (Apocynaceae).
Pale amber, solvated, tetragonal prisms from methanol. M.p. 160°.
Solubility. Soluble in ethanol, ether, chloroform, and methanol.

Extraction. Ajmaline is extracted by organic solvents from aqueous alkaline solutions.

Chromatography. PAPER: system P1—Rf 0·79 (location under ultraviolet light, blue fluorescence; location reagents: *iodoplatinate spray*, strong reaction; *potassium permanganate spray*, weak reaction).
THIN-LAYER: system T1—Rf 0·62 (location reagent *potassium permanganate spray*, positive reaction).

Colour Tests. MICRO: sulphuric acid–formaldehyde test—purple (*sensitivity:* 1·0 μg); ammonium molybdate test—faintly purple → red (*sensitivity:* 0·1 μg); ammonium vanadate test—red (*sensitivity:* 0·25 μg); Vitali's test—red/yellow/yellow (*sensitivity:* 0·1 μg).

Ultraviolet Absorption Spectrum. Ajmaline in 0·1N hydrochloric acid, maxima at 245 mμ (E1%, 1 cm 181) and 290 mμ. No change is observed in alkaline solution.

Metabolism. Ajmaline is closely related chemically and pharmacologically to quinidine. It has been used in the treatment of cardiac arrhythmias. It may be detected in the urine several hours after ingestion of extracts and tinctures of rauwolfia.

Toxicity. The estimated lethal dose in man is within the range 100 to 500 mg/kg.

CASE EXAMPLE. A 56-year-old woman died 2½ hours after ingesting fifty 50-mg tablets of ajmaline and sixty 5-mg tablets of diazepam. Post-mortem levels of ajmaline: blood, about 1 mg%; liver, about 5 mg%; stomach contents, 470 mg%; urine, 4·4 mg%. Diazepam and its acid hydrolysis product, 2-methylamino-5-chlorobenzophenone, were identified in the stomach contents. A blood-alcohol level of 159 mg% was also determined (Alha, 1966).

ALCURONIUM CHLORIDE *Muscle Relaxant*

Synonyms: Allnortoxiferin Chloride; Diallylnortoxiferine Dichloride; Diallyltoxiferine Chloride; Ro 4-3816.
Proprietary Name: Alloferin.

Diallyldinortoxiferin dichloride pentahydrate
$C_{44}H_{48}N_4O_2,2HCl,5H_2O = 827·9$

No characteristic melting-point; a brown colour appears at 220°; still not melted at 350°.
Solubility. Soluble 1 in 4 of water, 1 in 36 of ethanol, and 1 in 5 of methanol.

Extraction. Alcuronium chloride is a quaternary ammonium compound (see p. 29).

Chromatography. PAPER: system P1—Rf 0·14 (location under ultraviolet light, absorption; location reagents: *iodoplatinate spray*, strong reaction; *potassium permanganate spray*, strong reaction).
THIN-LAYER: system T1—Rf 0·01 (location reagent *potassium permanganate spray*, positive reaction).

Colour Tests. MICRO: sulphuric acid–formaldehyde test—greenish-brown (*sensitivity:* 0·5 μg); ammonium molybdate test—dull purple (*sensitivity:* 0·1 μg); ammonium vanadate test—blue-purple (*sensitivity:* 0·1 μg); Vitali's test—brown/yellow/brown (*sensitivity:* 0·5 μg).

Crystal Tests. MICRO: *potassium iodide solution*—small dense rosettes (*sensitivity:* 1 in 200); *zinc chloride solution*—small dense rosettes (*sensitivity:* 1 in 200).

Ultraviolet Absorption Spectrum. Anhydrous solid in water, maximum at 293 mμ (E1%, 1 cm 659) and minimum at 237 mμ; a shoulder at 320 mμ.

Infra-red Absorption Spectrum. Potassium bromide disk. The principal peaks are: A 1495, B 1592, C 1283 or 1462 or 1650 (p. 727).

Dose. Up to 15 mg intravenously.

ALDRIN *Pesticide*

Synonym: HHDN.
Proprietary Name: Octalene.

Aldrin usually contains 95% w/w HHDN

[1,2,3,4,10,10-Hexachloro-1,4,4a,5,8,8a-hexahydro-1,4(*exo*):5,8(*endo*)-dimethanonaphthalene] and 5% w/w active related compounds.

$C_{12}H_8Cl_6 = 364{\cdot}9$

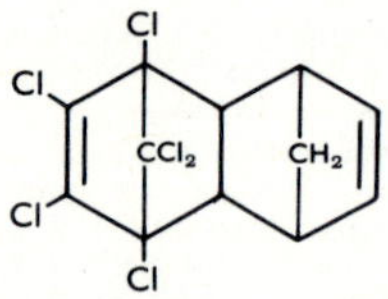

White crystals. Stable in air and light; when heated to decomposition it evolves highly toxic fumes of phosgene and hydrogen chloride. M.p., pure grade 104° to 104·5°, technical grade about 90°.

Solubility. Insoluble in water; soluble 1 in 20 of ethanol, 1 in 1 of acetone, 1 in 0·55 of benzene, and 1 in 0·33 of carbon tetrachloride.

Extraction. Aldrin is extracted by organic solvents from aqueous acid or alkaline solutions.

Chromatography. PAPER: Mitchell (1956) has described 2 systems for the separation of chlorinated pesticides including aldrin.

Colour Test. Johnson (1956) has described a colour test which detects aldrin in the presence of dieldrin and endrin.

Ultraviolet Absorption Spectrum. Aldrin in ethanol, maximum at 290 to 310 mμ (E1%, 1 cm 2).

Quantitative Estimation. Aldrin may be determined spectrophotometrically (Garhart *et al.*, 1952; Friestad, 1963), from blood by gas chromatography (Jain *et al.*, 1965), and from biological tissues by gas chromatography (Hamence *et al.*, 1965).

Metabolism. Aldrin is poorly absorbed from the gastro-intestinal tract but when dissolved in oils or other lipids it is readily absorbed by the skin and gastro-intestinal tract. It is stored in the body fat and persists for several weeks after the cessation of exposure.

Aldrin is rapidly metabolised in the body by epoxidation to dieldrin, p. 299.

Toxicity. The estimated lethal dose in man is 5 g. Severe symptoms may follow absorption of 1 to 3 g.

LD50 (oral): in cattle 25, in dogs 65 to 95, in rabbits 50 to 80, in rats about 50, and in sheep 15 mg/kg.

CASE EXAMPLES. The body fat of a 23-year-old man, poisoned by aldrin whilst engaged in its manufacture, contained 6 mg% dieldrin 15 days after the last exposure and 0·01 mg% 4 months later. The blood-levels of two men exposed to aldrin in the same plant were 0·028 and 0·013 mg% dieldrin respectively. In 2 further cases of poisoning the levels in the body fat were 14·9 mg% dieldrin 3 weeks after the last exposure and 4·4 mg% 5 weeks after exposure; the blood-levels were 0·053 mg% and 0·013 mg% respectively (Kazantzis *et al.*, 1964).

ALETAMINE *Analgesic*

Synonym: NDR 5061A.

α-Allylphenethylamine

$C_{11}H_{15}N = 161{\cdot}2$

$$C_6H_5{\cdot}CH_2{\cdot}\underset{}{\overset{NH_2}{\overset{|}{C}}}H{\cdot}CH_2{\cdot}CH{:}CH_2$$

ALETAMINE HYDROCHLORIDE

White crystals.

Solubility. Soluble in water.

Extraction. Aletamine is extracted by organic solvents from aqueous alkaline solutions.

Chromatography. PAPER: system P1—Rf 0·65 (location reagents: *iodoplatinate spray*, white; *bromocresol green spray*, strong reaction).

THIN-LAYER: system T1—Rf 0·63 (location reagents: *acidified iodoplatinate spray*, positive reaction; *potassium permanganate spray*, positive reaction).

GAS: system G2/120—retention time 0·62 relative to ephedrine.

Colour Tests. MICRO: sulphuric acid–formaldehyde test—orange (*sensitivity:* 0·5 μg); ammonium molybdate test—faint blue (*sensitivity:* 1·0 μg).

Crystal Tests. MICRO: *platinic chloride solution*—plates (*sensitivity:* 1 in 200); *styphnic acid*—branching needles, forming overnight (*sensitivity:* 1 in 400).

Ultraviolet Absorption Spectrum. Aletamine in 0·1N sulphuric acid, maxima at 247·5 mμ (E1%, 1 cm 6), 252·5 mμ (E1%, 1 cm 9), 258 mμ (E1%, 1 cm 10), and 264 mμ (E1%, 1 cm 8).

ALLANTOIN *Dermatological Agent*

Synonyms: Alyoxyldiureide; Cordianine.

5-Ureidohydantoin

$C_4H_6N_4O_3 = 158{\cdot}1$

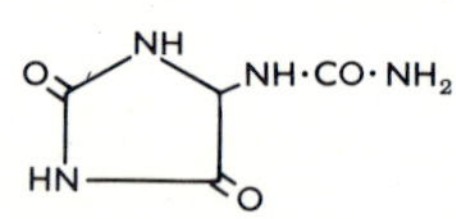

A white crystalline powder. M.p. 235°.

Solubility. Soluble 1 in 130 of water and 1 in 500 of ethanol; more soluble in hot water and hot ethanol; almost insoluble in ether.

Colour Test. Treat a solution with concentrated furfuraldehyde solution to which a little hydrochloric acid is added—violet.

Ultraviolet Absorption Spectrum. Allantoin in solution at pH 9·4, maximum at 224 mμ (E1%, 1 cm 350).

Infra-red Absorption Spectrum. Potassium bromide disk. The principal peaks are: A 1710, B 1652, C 1530 (p. 728).

ALLOBARBITONE *Barbiturate*

Synonyms: Allobarbital; Diallylbarbitone; Diallylbarbituric Acid; Diallylmalonylurea.
Proprietary Name: Dial.

5,5-Diallylbarbituric acid
$C_{10}H_{12}N_2O_3 = 208{\cdot}2$

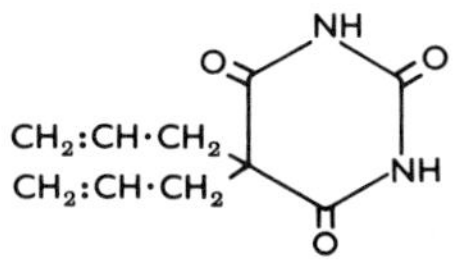

A white crystalline powder. M.p. 172° to 174°.
Solubility. Soluble 1 in 800 of water, 1 in 20 of ethanol, and 1 in 30 of ether; soluble in alkali solutions.

Screening Tests. See under Barbiturates, p. 208.

Extraction. Allobarbitone may be isolated in the A2 fraction (see p. 27).

Chromatography. PAPER: system P2—Rf 0·09 relative to amylobarbitone (location under ultraviolet light, dark spot); system P3—Rf 0·15 (location reagent *silver nitrate spray*, white); system P4—Rf 0·12 (location as for P3); system RP1b—Rf 0·51 (location under ultraviolet light after exposure to ammonia; location reagent *potassium permanganate spray*, yellow on pink).

THIN-LAYER: system T10—Rf 0·27 (location reagents: *mercurous nitrate spray*, black; *potassium permanganate spray*, yellow-brown on purple); system T11—Rf 0·43 (location reagents: *mercurous nitrate spray*, white on grey; *potassium permanganate spray*, yellow on purple).

GAS: system G5—retention time 1·47 relative to barbitone; retention time 0·21 relative to phenobarbitone; system G7—retention time 1·30 relative to barbitone.

Colour Test. Zwikker's test—violet-blue.

Ultraviolet Absorption Spectrum. Allobarbitone is a 5,5-derivative—see Screening Test 3 under Barbiturates, p. 208.

Infra-red Absorption Spectrum. Potassium bromide disk. The principal peaks are: A 1687, B 1375, C 1437 (p. 728).

Quantitative Estimation. See under Barbiturates, p. 208.

Metabolism. Allobarbitone is an intermediate-acting barbiturate—see under Barbiturates, p. 208. It may persist unchanged in the body for as long as a week; between 10 and 35% of the unchanged drug may be excreted relatively slowly in the urine.

Dose. Up to 300 mg, as a hypnotic.

Toxicity. The estimated lethal dose in man is about 2·5 g; the blood-level associated with severe poisoning is 1 to 4 mg%. The lethal oral dose in rabbits is 50 mg/kg.

ALLOPURINOL *Uricosuric Agent*

Synonyms: BW 56-158; HPP; Isopurinol.
Proprietary Names: Zyloprim; Zyloric.

4-Hydroxy-1*H*-pyrazolo[3,4-*d*]pyrimidine
$C_5H_4N_4O = 136{\cdot}1$

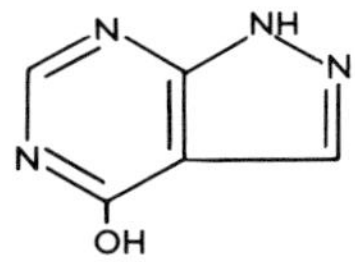

A slightly creamy-white powder. It does not have a definite melting point; it is unchanged up to 300°, after which it begins to darken and at an indefinite high temperature it chars and decomposes.
Solubility. Sparingly soluble in water and ethanol; insoluble in chloroform and ether; soluble in solutions of alkali hydroxides.

Colour Test. Shake a few mg with about 5 ml of 0·1N sodium hydroxide, add 3 ml of *Folin–Ciocalteu reagent* and 5 ml of 20% sodium carbonate solution—grey-blue.

Ultraviolet Absorption Spectrum. Allopurinol in 0·1N hydrochloric acid, maxima at 231 mμ (E1%, 1 cm about 320) and 250 mμ (E1%, 1 cm 563).

Metabolism. Allopurinol is of value in the treatment of gout because it is an inhibitor of xanthine oxidase, the enzyme responsible for converting xanthine and hypoxanthine to uric acid. Xanthine and hypoxanthine are more easily excreted than uric acid. Allopurinol is metabolised to alloxanthine which is also an inhibitor of xanthine oxidase; it is rapidly excreted in the urine but alloxanthine is only slowly excreted. Allopurinol also inhibits the metabolism of mercaptopurine to 6-thiouric acid and it will therefore potentiate the activity of mercaptopurine.

Dose. Up to 600 mg daily.

ALLYLBARBITURIC ACID *Barbiturate*

Synonyms: Butalbital; Itobarbital; Tetrallobarbital.
NOTE. The name Butalbital has also been applied to talbutal (p. 560), the s-butyl analogue.
Proprietary Name: Sandoptal.

5-Allyl-5-isobutylbarbituric acid
$C_{11}H_{16}N_2O_3 = 224{\cdot}3$

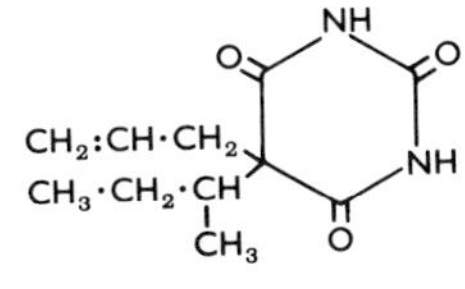

A white crystalline powder. M.p. 138° to 139°.
Solubility. Slightly soluble in cold water; more soluble in boiling water; freely soluble in ethanol, ether, and chloroform; soluble in aqueous solutions of alkalis.

Screening Tests. See under Barbiturates, p. 208.

Extraction. Allylbarbituric acid may be isolated in the A2 fraction (see p. 27).

Chromatography. PAPER: system P2—Rf 0·40 relative to amylobarbitone (location under ultraviolet light, dark spot).
THIN-LAYER: system T10—Rf 0·36 (location reagents: *mercurous nitrate spray*, black; *potassium permanganate spray*, yellow-brown on purple); system T11—Rf 0·48 (location reagents: *mercurous nitrate spray*, white on grey; *potassium permanganate spray*, yellow on purple).
GAS: system G7—retention time 1·47 relative to barbitone.

Colour Test. Zwikker's test—violet-blue.

Ultraviolet Absorption Spectrum. Allylbarbituric acid is a 5,5-derivative—see Screening Test 3 under Barbiturates, p. 208.

Infra-red Absorption Spectrum. Potassium bromide disk. The principal peaks are: A 1688 or 1716, B 1428 or 1740 (p. 728).

Quantitative Estimation. See under Barbiturates, p. 208.

Metabolism. Allylbarbituric acid is an intermediate-acting barbiturate—see under Barbiturates, p. 208.
According to Staub (1950), 20% of the ingested dose may be excreted unchanged in man.

Dose. Up to 800 mg has been given as a hypnotic.

ALLYLPRODINE *Narcotic*

3-Allyl-1-methyl-4-phenyl-4-propionyloxypiperidine

$C_{18}H_{25}NO_2 = 287{\cdot}4$

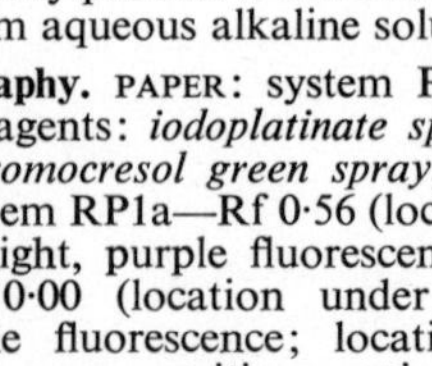

Extraction. Allylprodine is extracted by organic solvents from aqueous alkaline solutions.

Chromatography. PAPER: system P1—Rf 0·75 (location reagents: *iodoplatinate spray*, strong reaction; *bromocresol green spray*, strong reaction); system RP1a—Rf 0·56 (location under ultraviolet light, purple fluorescence); system RP1b—Rf 0·00 (location under ultraviolet light, purple fluorescence; location reagent *iodoplatinate spray*, positive reaction).

Colour Tests. MICRO: sulphuric acid–formaldehyde test—blue-black (*sensitivity:* 0·1 μg); ammonium vanadate test—grey-olive; ammonium molybdate test—grey → green; Vitali's test— -/-/grey-purple → brown.

Crystal Tests. MICRO: *picric acid*—small rectangular needles and plates (*sensitivity:* 1 in 1000); *styphnic acid*—very small irregular needles (*sensitivity:* 1 in 1000).

Ultraviolet Absorption Spectrum. Allylprodine in 0·1N sulphuric acid, maxima at 251·5 mμ (E1%, 1cm 9), 257·5 mμ (E1%, 1cm 10), and 263·5 mμ (E1%, 1cm 8·3).

ALOIN *Purgative*

A crystalline substance obtained from aloes. It consists almost entirely of barbaloin:

$C_{21}H_{22}O_9,H_2O = 436{\cdot}4$

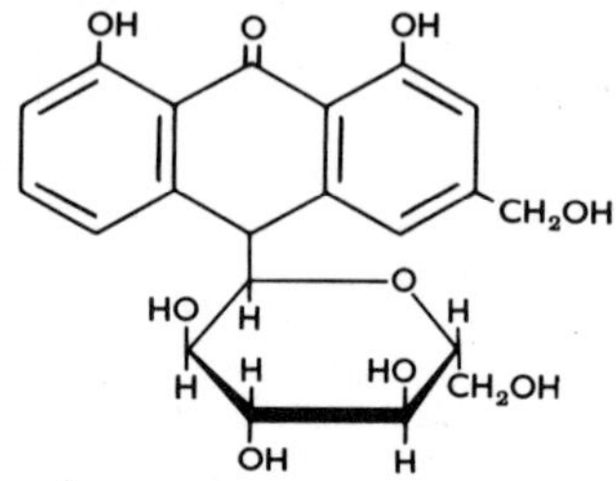

A dull yellow crystalline powder which darkens on exposure to light. Stable in neutral or acid solutions, but not in alkaline solutions. M.p. of barbaloin 146° to 148°.

Solubility. Almost entirely soluble 1 in 130 of water; soluble 1 in 20 of ethanol; very slightly soluble in ether and chloroform.

Extraction. Aloin is extracted by organic solvents from aqueous acid solutions.

Colour Tests. To 5 mg, add 5 ml of *dilute ammonia solution*—yellow → green → brown. The solution gives a yellow fluorescence in ultraviolet light.

Ultraviolet Absorption Spectrum. Aloin in water, maxima at 268 mμ (E1%, 1cm 164), 295·5 mμ (E1%, 1cm 194), and 351 mμ (E1%, 1cm 217).

Quantitative Estimation. A quantitative assay procedure involving paper and thin-layer chromatography and subsequent spectrophotometry is described by Böhme and Kreutzig (1964).

Dose. Up to 60 mg.

Toxicity. Purgative doses of aloin may cause renal irritation. The urine, if alkaline, is coloured red.

ALPHACETYLMETHADOL *Narcotic*

Synonyms: α-Acetylmethadone; Alphacéméthadone; α-Amidon Acetate; α-Methadol Acetate.

α-6-Dimethylamino-4,4-diphenyl-3-acetoxyheptane

$C_{23}H_{31}NO_2 = 353{\cdot}5$

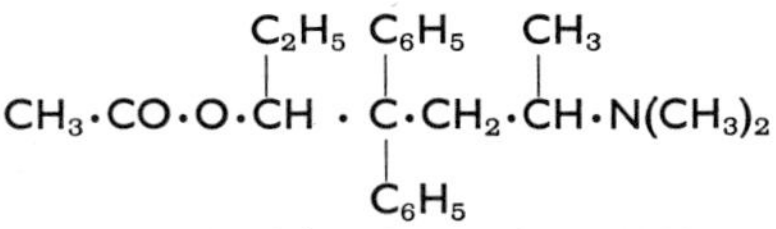

Alphacetylmethadol melts at about 130°.

Three isomers of alphacetylmethadol are obtainable, (+), (−), and (±). The Chromatography, Colour Tests, and Crystal Tests given below were performed on (±)-alphacetylmethadol hydrochloride.

ALPHACETYLMETHADOL HYDROCHLORIDE
Synonym: NIH 2953.
White crystals which melt at 213° to 214°.
Solubility. Soluble in water.

Extraction. Alphacetylmethadol is extracted by organic solvents from aqueous alkaline solutions.

Chromatography. PAPER: system P1—Rf 0·75 (location under ultraviolet light, absorption; location reagent *iodoplatinate spray*, weak reaction).

THIN-LAYER: system T1—Rf 0·59 (location reagent *acidified iodoplatinate spray*, positive reaction).

GAS: system G2/225—retention time 2·70 relative to diphenhydramine; system G4—retention time 2·20 relative to diphenhydramine.

Colour Tests. MICRO: sulphuric acid–formaldehyde test—purple-brown → grey-green; ammonium molybdate test—brown-purple → green; ammonium vanadate test—grey-green.

Crystal Tests. MICRO: *potassium chromate solution*—small rosettes of plates (*sensitivity:* 1 in 1000); *potassium iodide solution*—small rods and plates (*sensitivity:* 1 in 400).

Ultraviolet Absorption Spectrum. Alphacetylmethadol in ethanol:water (1:1), maximum at 259 mμ (E1%, 1cm 11·2).

Metabolism. After oral or subcutaneous administration, alphacetylmethadol is slowly metabolised by most tissues and since its excretion in the rat is negligible even after it has virtually disappeared from the tissues, it may be concluded that alphacetylmethadol is disposed of essentially by degradation (Way and Adler, 1962); *N*-demethylation is one metabolic pathway.

Toxicity. LD50 (subcutaneous): in mice 40 mg/kg.

ALPHAMEPRODINE *Narcotic*

α-3-Ethyl-1-methyl-4-phenyl-4-propionyloxypiperidine

$C_{17}H_{25}NO_2 = 275{\cdot}4$

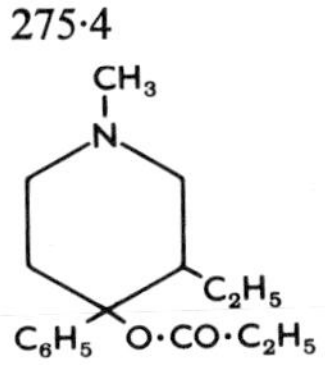

ALPHAMEPRODINE HYDROCHLORIDE
White crystals.
Solubility. Soluble in water.

Extraction. Alphameprodine is extracted by organic solvents from aqueous alkaline solutions.

Chromatography. PAPER: system P1—Rf 0·75 (location reagents: *iodoplatinate spray*, strong reaction; *bromocresol green spray*, weak reaction); system RP1a—Rf 0·57 (location reagent *iodoplatinate spray*, positive reaction); system RP1b—Rf 0·00 (location under ultraviolet light, purple fluorescence).

THIN-LAYER: system T1—Rf 0·50, streaking (location reagent *acidified iodoplatinate spray*, positive reaction).

GAS: system G2/225—retention time 1·0 relative to diphenhydramine; system G4—retention time 0·48 relative to diphenhydramine.

Colour Tests. MICRO: sulphuric acid–formaldehyde test—brownish-red (*sensitivity:* 0·25 μg); ammonium molybdate test—blue-grey → green with blue rim (*sensitivity:* 0·5 μg); ammonium vanadate test—grey (*sensitivity:* 0·5 μg).

Crystal Tests. MICRO: *platinic bromide solution*—bunches of rods or plates (*sensitivity:* 1 in 1000); *platinic chloride solution*—plates, often in rosettes or bunches (*sensitivity:* 1 in 1000).

Ultraviolet Absorption Spectrum. Alphameprodine in 0·1N sulphuric acid, maxima at 247 mμ (E1%, 1cm 5·4), 251·5 mμ (E1%, 1cm 6·9), 257 mμ (E1%, 1cm 8·3), and 263 mμ (E1%, 1cm 6·6).

ALPHAMETHADOL *Narcotic*

α-6-Dimethylamino-4,4-diphenylheptan-3-ol

$C_{21}H_{29}NO = 311{\cdot}5$

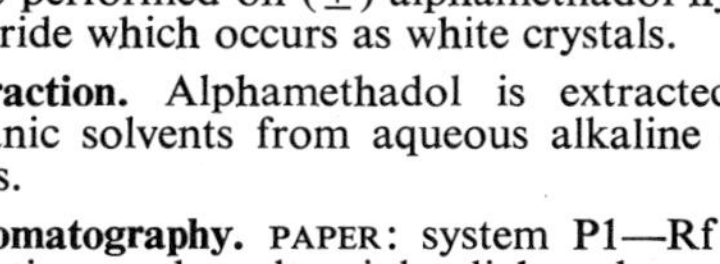

Three isomers of alphamethadol are obtainable, (+), (−), and (±). The Chromatography, Colour Tests, and Crystal Tests given below were performed on (±)-alphamethadol hydrochloride which occurs as white crystals.

Extraction. Alphamethadol is extracted by organic solvents from aqueous alkaline solutions.

Chromatography. PAPER: system P1—Rf 0·74 (location under ultraviolet light, absorption; location reagent *iodoplatinate spray*, strong reaction).

THIN-LAYER: system T1—Rf 0·57 (location reagent *acidified iodoplatinate spray*, positive reaction).

GAS: system G2/225—retention time 2·55 relative to diphenhydramine; system G4—retention time 2·44 relative to diphenhydramine; system G5—retention time 0·69 relative to barbitone.

Colour Tests. MICRO: sulphuric acid–formaldehyde test—purple-brown → grey-green (*sensitivity:* 0·25 μg); ammonium molybdate test—brown-purple → green (*sensitivity:* 0·25 μg); ammonium vanadate test—grey-green (*sensitivity:* 0·25 μg).

Crystal Tests. MICRO: *potassium chromate solution*—fans of small needles (*sensitivity:* 1 in 200); *zinc chloride solution*—rods or plates, often in bunches (*sensitivity:* 1 in 200).

Ultraviolet Absorption Spectrum. Alphamethadol in 0·1N sulphuric acid, maxima at 253·5 mμ (E1%, 1cm 17·5) and 259 mμ (E1%, 1cm 20·2).

ALPHAPRODINE *Narcotic Analgesic*

Synonyms: NU 1196; Prisilidene.

α-1,3-Dimethyl-4-phenyl-4-propionyloxypiperidine

$C_{16}H_{23}NO_2$ = 261·4

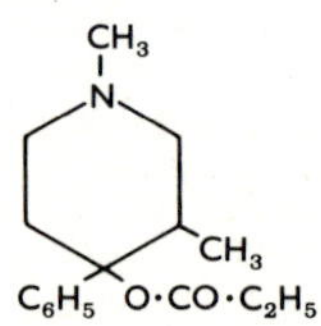

B.p. 70° to 75° at 0·02 mm Hg.

Solubility. Insoluble in water; soluble in chloroform.

ALPHAPRODINE HYDROCHLORIDE

Proprietary Name: Nisentil Hydrochloride.

A white crystalline powder which is stable to air, light, and heat. M.p. 218° to 220°.

Solubility. Soluble 1 in about 1 of water; freely soluble in ethanol and chloroform; very slightly soluble in ether.

Extraction. Alphaprodine is extracted by organic solvents from aqueous alkaline solutions.

Chromatography. PAPER: system P1—Rf 0·58 (location reagents: *iodoplatinate spray*, strong reaction; *bromocresol green spray*, weak reaction); system RP1a—Rf 0·86 (location reagent *iodoplatinate spray*, positive reaction).

THIN-LAYER: system T1—Rf 0·45 (location reagent *acidified iodoplatinate spray*, positive reaction); system T7—Rf 0·93 (location as for T1); system T8—Rf 0·40 (location as for T1).

GAS: system G2/225—retention time 0·84 relative to diphenhydramine; system G4—retention time 0·91 relative to diphenhydramine.

Colour Tests. MICRO: sulphuric acid–formaldehyde test—brownish-red (*sensitivity:* 0·5 μg); ammonium molybdate test—blue-grey → green with blue rim (*sensitivity:* 0·25 μg); ammonium vanadate test—blue-grey (*sensitivity:* 0·5 μg).

Crystal Tests. MICRO: *picric acid*—small serrated plates, often in bunches (*sensitivity:* 1 in 400); *styphnic acid*—very small crystals, best viewed under polarised light (*sensitivity:* 1 in 1000).

Ultraviolet Absorption Spectrum. Alphaprodine in ethanol, maxima at 252 mμ, 258 mμ, and 264 mμ; minima at 240 mμ, 255 mμ, and 262 mμ. Alphaprodine hydrochloride in water, maxima at 251 mμ, 257 mμ, and 263 mμ; minima at 236 mμ, 254 mμ, and 261 mμ.

Dose. Up to 60 mg subcutaneously.

Toxicity. Alphaprodine resembles pethidine but its action is more rapid in onset and of shorter duration. It has little cumulative effect but tolerance and drug dependence can develop. The estimated minimum lethal dose in man is between 60 and 120 mg.

LD50 (intravenous): in mice 43 and in rabbits 20 mg/kg; (subcutaneous): in rats 50 mg/kg.

ALVERINE *Parasympatholytic*

Synonyms: Dipropyline; Gamatran; Phenpropamine.

Proprietary Names: Kalmadol; Sestron; Spasmaverine; Supavan.

N-Ethyl-3,3′-diphenyldipropylamine

$C_{20}H_{27}N$ = 281·4

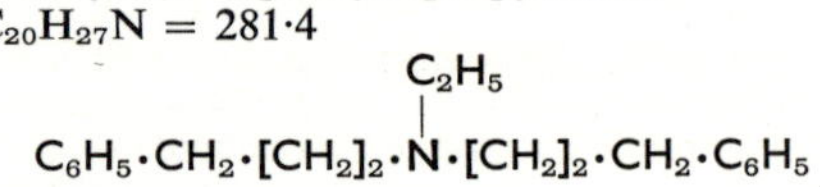

ALVERINE CITRATE

Proprietary Names: Profenil; Spacolin.

White powder. M.p. 100° to 102°.

Solubility. Slightly soluble in water and chloroform; sparingly soluble in ethanol; very slightly soluble in ether.

Extraction. Alverine is extracted by organic solvents from aqueous alkaline solutions.

Chromatography. PAPER: system P1—Rf 0·86 (location reagent *iodoplatinate spray*, strong reaction); system RP1b—Rf 0·00 (location under ultraviolet light, absorption).

THIN-LAYER: system T1—Rf 0·58 (location reagent *potassium permanganate spray*, positive reaction).

Colour Tests. MICRO: sulphuric acid–formaldehyde test—orange-red (*sensitivity:* 0·25 μg); ammonium vanadate test—grey-green (*sensitivity:* 0·25 μg).

Ultraviolet Absorption Spectrum. Alverine in 0·1N sulphuric acid, maxima at 252·5 mμ (E1%, 1cm 6), 258·5 mμ (E1%, 1cm 9), 264 mμ (E1%, 1cm 7), and 268 mμ (E1%, 1cm 6).

Infra-red Absorption Spectrum. Alverine (base). Potassium bromide disk. The principal peaks are: A 695, B 742 or 1188 or 1448 (p. 771).

Dose. Up to 40 mg by slow intravenous injection; up to 1 g daily by mouth.

AMBAZONE *Bacteriostatic*

Proprietary Name: Iversal.

1,4-Benzoquinone amidinohydrazone thiosemicarbazone monohydrate

$C_8H_{11}N_7S,H_2O = 255{\cdot}3$

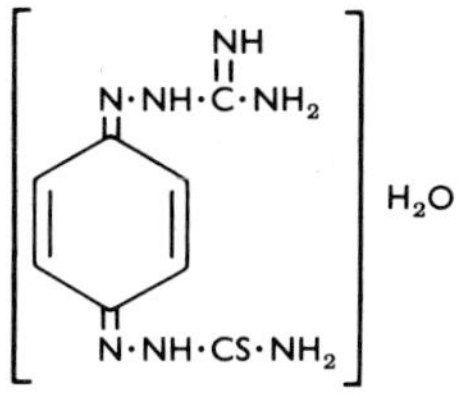

Brown or copper-coloured crystals. M.p. 192° to 194°, with decomposition.
Solubility. Sparingly soluble in water; moderately soluble in ethanol; freely soluble in dilute acids.

Extraction. Ambazone is extracted by organic solvents from aqueous alkaline solutions.

Chromatography. PAPER: system P1—Rf 0·08 (yellow) (location under ultraviolet light, brown fluorescence; location reagent *potassium permanganate spray*, strong reaction); system RP1a—Rf 0·43 (location under ultraviolet light, brownish-orange fluorescence; location reagent *iodoplatinate spray*, positive reaction); system RP1b—Rf 0·28 (location as for RP1a).
THIN-LAYER: system T1—Rf 0·66 (location reagent *potassium permanganate spray*, positive reaction).

Crystal Tests. MICRO: *ammonium thiocyanate solution*—small needles (*sensitivity:* 1 in 400); *picric acid*—small rosettes (*sensitivity:* 1 in 1000).

Ultraviolet Absorption Spectrum. Ambazone in 0·1N sulphuric acid, maximum at 398·5 mμ (E1%, 1cm 2330).

Infra-red Absorption Spectrum. Potassium bromide disk. The principal peaks are: A 1090 or 1120 or 1160 (p. 772).

Dose. Up to 50 mg daily.

AMBENONIUM CHLORIDE

Anticholinesterase

Synonyms: Ambestigmine Chloride; Oxazyl; Win 8077.
Proprietary Name: Mytelase.

2,2′-Oxamidobis[*o*-(chlorobenzyl)triethylammonium chloride]
$C_{28}H_{42}Cl_4N_4O_2 = 608{\cdot}5$

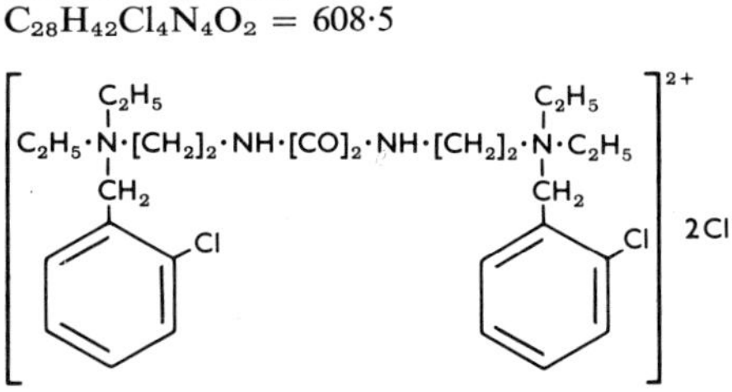

A white crystalline powder. M.p. 184°.
Solubility. Soluble 1 in 5 of water.

Extraction. Ambenonium chloride is a quaternary ammonium compound (see p. 29).

Chromatography. PAPER: system P1—Rf 0·10 (location under ultraviolet light, absorption; location reagents: *iodoplatinate spray*, strong reaction; *bromocresol green spray*, weak reaction); system RP1a—Rf 0·94 (location reagent *iodoplatinate spray*, positive reaction); system RP1b—Rf 0·86 (location under ultraviolet light, absorption; location reagent *iodoplatinate spray*, positive reaction).
THIN-LAYER: system T1—Rf 0·02 (location reagent *acidified iodoplatinate spray*, positive reaction).

Crystal Tests. MICRO: *platinic chloride solution*—bunches of serrated blades (*sensitivity:* 1 in 1000); *potassium permanganate solution*—dendrites (*sensitivity:* 1 in 1000).

Ultraviolet Absorption Spectrum. Ambenonium chloride in 0·1N sulphuric acid, maxima at 271·5 mμ (E1%, 1cm 37), 278 mμ (E1%, 1cm 39), and 292 mμ (E1%, 1cm 24).

Infra-red Absorption Spectrum. Potassium bromide disk. The principal peaks are: A 1675, B 1505, C 767 or 1465 (p. 772).

Dose. Up to 100 mg daily.

Toxicity. The estimated minimum lethal dose in man is 60 mg.

AMBUTONIUM BROMIDE

Parasympatholytic

Synonym: BL 700B.
Proprietary Name: it is an ingredient of Aludrox SA.

(3-Carbamoyl-3,3-diphenylpropyl)ethyldimethylammonium bromide
$C_{20}H_{27}BrN_2O = 391{\cdot}4$

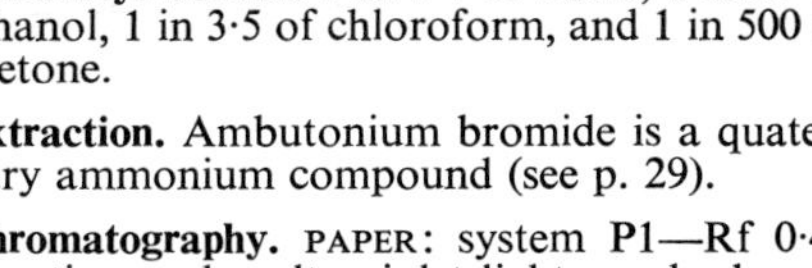

White crystals. M.p. 209° to 220°, with decomposition.
Solubility. Soluble 1 in 1·4 of water, 1 in 27 of ethanol, 1 in 3·5 of chloroform, and 1 in 500 of acetone.

Extraction. Ambutonium bromide is a quaternary ammonium compound (see p. 29).

Chromatography. PAPER: system P1—Rf 0·43 (location under ultraviolet light, weak absorption; location reagent *iodoplatinate spray*, strong reaction); system RP1a—Rf 0·95 (location reagent *iodoplatinate spray*, positive reaction); system RP1b—Rf 0·85 (location as for RP1a).
THIN-LAYER: system T1—Rf 0·03 (location reagent *acidified iodoplatinate spray*, positive reaction).

Crystal Tests. MICRO: *lead iodide solution*—rosettes of curving needles (*sensitivity:* 1 in 1000); *platinic iodide solution*—long plates and needles (*sensitivity:* 1 in 1000).

Ultraviolet Absorption Spectrum. Ambutonium bromide in ethanol, maxima at 253 mμ, 259 mμ, and 265 mμ; minima at 251 mμ, 256 mμ, and 263 mμ; in 0·1N sulphuric acid, maxima at 253 mμ (E1%, 1 cm 18), 259 mμ (E1%, 1 cm 19), and 265 mμ (E1%, 1 cm 16).

Dose. Up to 25 mg.

Toxicity. The lethal dose in man is probably between 10 and 100 mg/kg.

AMETAZOLE *Gastric Secretion Indicator*

Synonym: Betazole.

3-(2-Aminoethyl)pyrazole

$C_5H_9N_3$ = 111·2

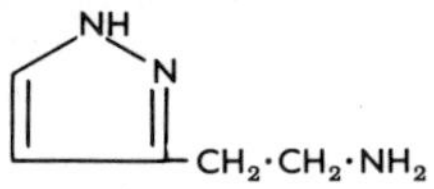

A viscous liquid. B.p. 118° to 123° at 0·5 mm Hg.

AMETAZOLE HYDROCHLORIDE

Proprietary Name: Histalog.

A white crystalline powder. Softens at about 215° and finally melts at about 240°.

Solubility. Soluble in water; almost insoluble in chloroform.

Extraction. Ametazole is extracted by organic solvents from aqueous alkaline solutions.

Chromatography. PAPER: system P1—Rf 0·08 (location reagents: *iodoplatinate spray*, white; *bromocresol green spray*, weak reaction); system RP1a—Rf 0·95 (location under ultraviolet light, pale blue fluorescence; location reagent *iodoplatinate spray*, positive reaction); system RP1b—Rf 0·87 (location as for RP1a).

THIN-LAYER: system T1—Rf 0·24 (location reagent *potassium permanganate spray*, positive reaction).

Crystal Tests. MICRO: *platinic chloride solution*—gelatinous rosettes, forming overnight (*sensitivity:* 1 in 1000); *platinic iodide solution*—masses of splinters (*sensitivity:* 1 in 1000).

Dose. Usually 50 mg subcutaneously.

AMETHOCAINE *Local Anaesthetic*

Synonym: Tetracaine.

2-Dimethylaminoethyl *p*-butylaminobenzoate

$C_{15}H_{24}N_2O_2$ = 264·4

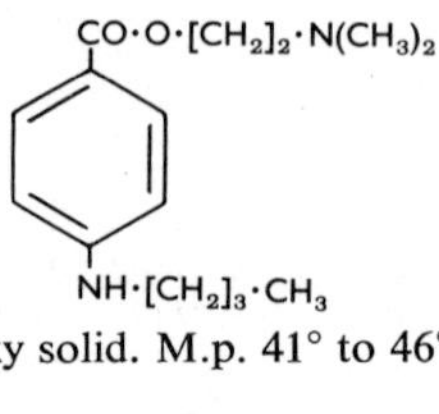

White waxy solid. M.p. 41° to 46°.

Solubility. Very slightly soluble in water; soluble in ethanol, ether, and chloroform.

AMETHOCAINE HYDROCHLORIDE

Synonyms: Butethanol; Dicaine; Pantocaine; Pontocaine.

Proprietary Names: Anethaine; Dynexan; Meethobalm; Rexocain.

A white hygroscopic crystalline powder. M.p. 147° to 150°. Amethocaine hydrochloride may occur as 2 other polymorphic forms, melting at about 134° and about 139°; mixtures may melt within the range 134° to 147°.

Solubility. Soluble 1 in 8 of water, 1 in 40 of ethanol, and 1 in 22 of chloroform; insoluble in ether.

Extraction. Amethocaine is extracted by organic solvents from aqueous alkaline solutions.

Chromatography. PAPER: system P1—Rf 0·48 (location under ultraviolet light, blue fluorescence; location reagent *iodoplatinate spray*, strong reaction); system RP1a—Rf 0·56 (location under ultraviolet light, blue fluorescence; location reagent *iodoplatinate spray*, positive reaction); system RP1b—Rf 0·00 (location as for RP1a).

THIN-LAYER: system T1—Rf 0·57 (location reagent *acidified iodoplatinate spray*, positive reaction).

GAS: system G1/180—retention time 3·95 relative to diphenhydramine; system G2/225—retention time 3·04 relative to diphenhydramine; system G3—retention time 5·06 relative to diphenhydramine; system G4—retention time 0·69 relative to codeine.

Colour Test. MICRO: Vitali's test—-/pale yellow/red (*sensitivity:* 1·0 μg).

Crystal Tests. MICRO: *gold bromide solution*—fine irregular crystals (*sensitivity:* 1 in 3000); *potassium chromate solution*—sheaves of long needles (*sensitivity:* 1 in 1500).

Ultraviolet Absorption Spectrum. Amethocaine in 0·1N sulphuric acid, maxima at 229 mμ, 281 mμ, and 312 mμ.

Infra-red Absorption Spectrum. Amethocaine (base). Potassium bromide disk. The principal peaks are: A 1598, B 1270, C 1166 (p. 772).

Quantitative Estimation. Porush *et al.* (1965) describe a spectrophotometric method of estimation of amethocaine in blood following tracheal instillation.

Metabolism. Amethocaine is rapidly hydrolysed in the blood, by the esterase enzymes, to *p*-aminobenzoic acid; it is completely destroyed within an hour of injection. It can rarely be isolated from blood even within a few minutes of administration. The rate of hydrolysis is more rapid in human than in canine blood (Porush *et al.*, 1965).

Toxicity. The maximum amount that may be administered safely by injection is probably 10 ml of a 1% solution. When used topically the maximum safe amount is 100 mg.

LD50 (intravenous): in mice and in rabbits 8 mg/kg.

AMICARBALIDE *Antiprotozoal (Veterinary)*
NN'-Di(3-amidinophenyl)urea
$C_{15}H_{16}N_6O = 296{\cdot}3$

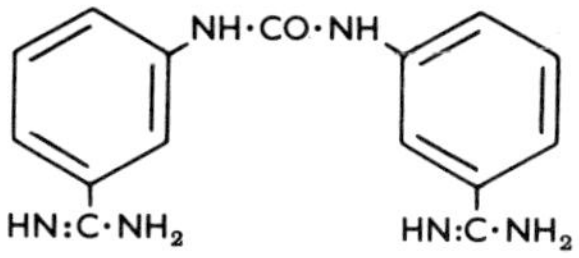

AMICARBALIDE ISETHIONATE
Synonym: M&B 5062 A.
Proprietary Name: Diampron.

A white powder. M.p. 200° to 204°.
Solubility. Soluble 1 in 1 of water and 1 in 250 of ethanol; insoluble in ether and chloroform.

Extraction. Amicarbalide is extracted by organic solvents from aqueous alkaline solutions.

Chromatography. PAPER: system P1—Rf 0·03 (location under ultraviolet light, blue fluorescence; location reagents: *iodoplatinate spray*, weak reaction; *bromocresol green spray*, weak reaction); system RP1a—tailing (location under ultraviolet light, blue fluorescence; location reagent *iodoplatinate spray*, positive reaction); system RP1b—tailing (location under ultraviolet light, blue fluorescence).
THIN-LAYER: system T1—Rf 0·05, streaking (location reagent *acidified iodoplatinate spray*, positive reaction).

Colour Test. MICRO: Vitali's test—pale yellow/pale yellow/red (*sensitivity:* 0·25 μg).

Crystal Tests. MICRO: *gold bromide solution*—blades in crosses (*sensitivity:* 1 in 3000); *potassium bismuth iodide solution*—fans of needles or dendrites (*sensitivity:* 1 in 3000).

Ultraviolet Absorption Spectrum. Amicarbalide in 0·1N sulphuric acid, maximum at 232 mμ (E1%, 1 cm 128) and an inflexion at about 257 mμ.

Infra-red Absorption Spectrum. Amicarbalide (base). Potassium bromide disk. The principal peaks are: A 1195, B 1590 or 1672 (p. 772).

Dose. In cattle, 5 to 10 mg/kg body-weight, by injection.

AMIDOPYRINE *Analgesic and Antipyretic*
Synonyms: Aminophenazone; Aminopyrine; Dimethylaminoantipyrine; Dimethylaminophenazone.
Proprietary Name: Pyramidon.

4-Dimethylamino-1,5-dimethyl-3-oxo-2-phenylpyrazoline
$C_{13}H_{17}N_3O = 231{\cdot}3$

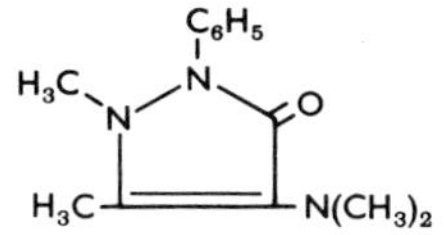

A white crystalline powder. M.p. 107° to 109°.
Solubility. Soluble 1 in 20 of water, 1 in 2 of ethanol, 1 in 13 of ether, and 1 in 1 of chloroform.

AMIDOPYRINE CAMPHORATE
A white crystalline powder.
Solubility. Soluble 1 in 15 of water and 1 in 2 of ethanol.

Extraction. Amidopyrine is extracted by organic solvents from aqueous acid or alkaline solutions.

Chromatography. PAPER: system P1—Rf 0·62 (location under ultraviolet light, dark blue fluorescence; location reagent *iodoplatinate spray*, weak reaction); system RP1a—Rf 0·68 (location under ultraviolet light, absorption); system RP1b—Rf 0·53 (location under ultraviolet light, absorption; location reagent *bromine–starch–potassium iodide*).
THIN-LAYER: system T1—Rf 0·66 (location reagent *acidified iodoplatinate spray*, positive reaction).
GAS: system G3—retention time 3·0 relative to diphenhydramine.

Colour Tests. MICRO: ferric chloride test—blue-purple; Vitali's test— -/brown/brown-orange (*sensitivity:* 1·0 μg).

Crystal Tests. MICRO: *mercuric chloride solution*—clusters of curved needles (*sensitivity:* 1 in 1000); *potassium iodide solution*—small stout rods (*sensitivity:* 1 in 1000).

Ultraviolet Absorption Spectrum. Amidopyrine in 0·1N sulphuric acid, maximum at 256 mμ (E1%, 1 cm 530), minimum at 228 mμ, and a shoulder at 242 mμ.

Infra-red Absorption Spectrum. Amidopyrine (base). Potassium bromide disk. The principal peaks are: A 1660, B 1315, C 1126 (p. 728).

Metabolism. In man, amidopyrine is completely metabolised at the rate of 10 to 30% per hour, only about 3% of the ingested dose being excreted unchanged. About 50% of a 500-mg dose is excreted in 3 days as 4-aminophenazone and its acetyl derivative, 4-acetamido-aminophenazone, the latter being the major metabolite. Several other metabolites may also be found in the urine, including a demethylated derivative, methylaminophenazone, and 2 red pigments, rubazonic acid and methylrubazonic acid. The last 2 are responsible for the reddish coloration of the urine (Pechtold, 1964; Smith *et al.*, 1964; Schüppel and Soehring, 1965). Three further metabolites have been isolated and described by Vecerkova *et al.* (1967).

Toxicity. The use of amidopyrine is now discouraged owing to the risk of fatal agranulocytosis which has followed doses as small as 1 g. The estimated acute lethal dose in man is in the range 5 to 30 g.
LD50 (oral): in rats 1·7 g/kg.

AMINACRINE *Antiseptic*
Synonym: 5-Aminoacridine.

9-Aminoacridine
$C_{13}H_{10}N_2$ = 194·2

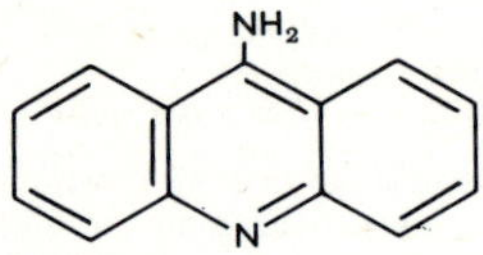

Yellow needles. M.p. 241°.
Solubility. Freely soluble in ethanol; slightly soluble in chloroform; soluble in acetone.

AMINACRINE HEXYLRESORCINATE
Synonyms: Acrisorcin; Aminacrine 4-Hexylresorcinate.
Proprietary Name: Akrinol.

A yellow crystalline powder.
Solubility. Slightly soluble in water and ethanol.

AMINACRINE HYDROCHLORIDE
Synonyms: Acramine Yellow; Aminoacridine Hydrochloride.

A pale yellow crystalline powder. M.p. about 235°.
Solubility. Soluble 1 in 300 of water; a saturated solution is pale yellow with a greenish-blue fluorescence; soluble 1 in 150 of ethanol; almost insoluble in ether and chloroform.

Extraction. Aminacrine is extracted by organic solvents from aqueous alkaline solutions.

Chromatography. PAPER: system P1—Rf 0·58 (location under ultraviolet light, bright blue fluorescence; location reagent *iodoplatinate spray*, strong reaction); system RP1a—Rf 0·45 (location under ultraviolet light, blue fluorescence; location reagent *iodoplatinate spray*, positive reaction); system RP1b—Rf 0·38 (location as for RP1a).
THIN-LAYER: system T1—Rf 0·54 (location reagent *acidified iodoplatinate spray*, positive reaction).

Colour Test. MICRO: Vitali's test—(yellow)-/-/bright purple.

Crystal Tests. MICRO: *potassium iodide solution*—needles (*sensitivity:* 1 in 1000); *potassium permanganate solution*—small needles (*sensitivity:* 1 in 1000).

Ultraviolet Absorption Spectrum. Aminacrine in 0·1N sulphuric acid, maxima at 260 mμ (E1%, 1 cm 3290), 313 mμ (E1%, 1 cm 58), 326 mμ (E1%, 1 cm 63), 381 mμ (E1%, 1 cm 217), 400 mμ (E1%, 1 cm 325), and 422 mμ (E1%, 1 cm 256).

Infra-red Absorption Spectrum. Aminacrine (base). Potassium bromide disk. The principal peaks are: A 760 or 1556 or 1645 or 1655, B 750 (p. 772).

Toxicity. LD50 (oral): in mice 78 mg/kg.

AMINOBENZOIC ACID
Synonyms: Amben; 4-Aminobenzoic Acid; PAB; PABA; Vitamin H′.
Proprietary Name: it is an ingredient of Pabamin.

p-Aminobenzoic acid
$C_7H_7NO_2$ = 137·1

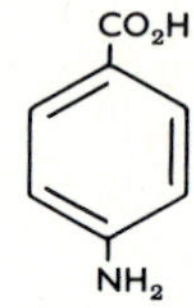

A white crystalline powder which discolours on exposure to air and light. M.p. 186° to 189°.
Solubility. Soluble 1 in 170 of cold water, 1 in 10 of boiling water, 1 in about 8 of ethanol, and 1 in about 50 of ether; slightly soluble in chloroform.

Extraction. Aminobenzoic acid is extracted by organic solvents from aqueous acid solutions.

Chromatography. PAPER: system P1—Rf 0·83 (location under ultraviolet light, blue fluorescence; location reagents: diazotisation followed by *alkaline betanaphthol spray*, red; *potassium permanganate spray*, weak reaction).
THIN-LAYER: system T1—Rf 0·58 (location reagent p-*dimethylaminobenzaldehyde spray*, yellow).

Colour Tests. MICRO: diazotisation test—red; Vitali's test—-/-/faint orange (*sensitivity:* 1·0 μg).

Crystal Tests. MICRO: *gold bromide solution*—needles (*sensitivity:* 1 in 100); *gold bromide–hydrochloric acid solution*—small needles, forming overnight (*sensitivity:* 1 in 100).

Ultraviolet Absorption Spectrum. Aminobenzoic acid in ethanol, maxima at 228 mμ (E1%, 1 cm 340) and 289 mμ (E1%, 1 cm 1256).

Infra-red Absorption Spectrum. Potassium bromide disk. The principal peaks are: A 1597, B 1168, C 1290 (p. 728).

Metabolism. Aminobenzoic acid is absorbed and excreted rapidly. In several animal species aminobenzoic acid is metabolised by acetylation at its amino-group and by conjugation with glucuronic acid or glycine at its carboxyl group; it may also be decarboxylated. In man, following a dose of about 6 g, the main urinary metabolites are *p*-aminobenzoylglucuronide and *p*-aminohippuric acid with smaller amounts of *p*-acetamidobenzoylglucuronide and very little *p*-acetamidohippuric acid, *p*-acetamidobenzoic acid, and unchanged aminobenzoic acid (Tabor *et al.*, 1951). Aminobenzoic acid may often be detected in the urine as the breakdown product of many of the procaine-type local anaesthetics.

Dose. Doses of up to 12 g daily have been given.

Toxicity. Toxic symptoms may occur when the blood-level of aminobenzoic acid is in excess of 60 to 80 mg%.
LD50 (oral): in rabbits 1·83 and in rats 6 g/kg.

AMINOGLUTETHIMIDE *Anticonvulsant*

Synonym: Ciba 16038.
Proprietary Name: Elipten.

α-p-Aminophenyl-*α*-ethylglutarimide
$C_{13}H_{16}N_2O_2 = 232{\cdot}3$

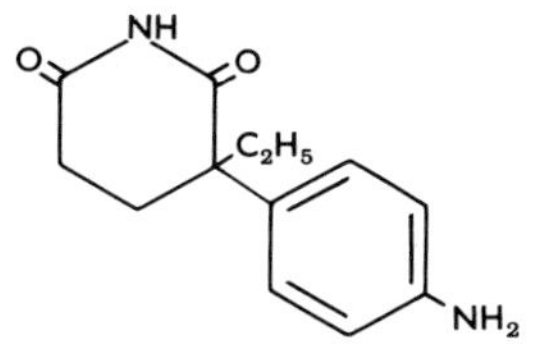

A white crystalline powder. M.p. about 151°.
Solubility. Very slightly soluble in water; freely soluble in organic solvents.

Extraction. Aminoglutethimide is extracted by organic solvents from aqueous acid or alkaline solutions.

Chromatography. Douglas and Nicholls (1965) have described a paper chromatographic system which determines aminoglutethimide in urine.

Quantitative Estimation. Douglas and Nicholls (1965) have described a spectrophotometric method of estimating aminoglutethimide in urine samples.

Metabolism. In contrast to glutethimide which is extensively metabolised, aminoglutethimide is excreted unchanged to a considerable extent in the urine. Forty-eight hours after oral administration the average total excretion represents 39% of a 250-mg dose and 54% of a 500-mg dose (Douglas and Nicholls, 1965).

Dose. Up to 1·5 g daily.

Toxicity. The estimated minimum lethal dose is 5 g. Because aminoglutethimide produces sexual precocity, masculinisation of young females, and other untoward effects, it was withdrawn from the U.S. market in February, 1966.

AMINOHIPPURIC ACID *Diagnostic Agent*

Synonyms: PAHA; *p*-Aminobenzoylglycine; Para-aminohippuric Acid.
Proprietary Name: Nephrotest.

N-p-Aminobenzoylaminoacetic acid
$C_9H_{10}N_2O_3 = 194{\cdot}2$

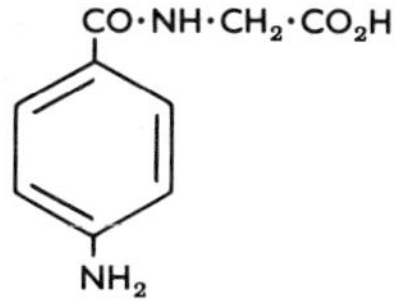

A white crystalline powder which hydrolyses in alkaline solution. M.p. 198°.
Solubility. Soluble 1 in 45 of water, 1 in 50 of ethanol, and 1 in 5 of dilute hydrochloric acid; sparingly soluble in ether and chloroform.

Extraction. Aminohippuric acid is extracted by organic solvents from aqueous acid solutions.

Chromatography. PAPER: system P1—Rf 0·41 (location under ultraviolet light, blue fluorescence; location reagents: diazotisation followed by *alkaline betanaphthol spray*, red; *potassium permanganate spray*, weak reaction). THIN-LAYER: system T1—Rf 0·55 (location reagent p-*dimethylaminobenzaldehyde spray*, yellow).

Colour Tests. MICRO: diazotisation test—red; Vitali's test— –/–/faint orange (*sensitivity:* 1·0 μg).

Ultraviolet Absorption Spectrum. Aminohippuric acid in methanol, maximum at 280 mμ (E1%, 1 cm 880); in 0·1N hydrochloric acid, maximum at 223 mμ (E1%, 1 cm 555).

NOTE. Aminohippuric acid is employed in the form of an injection of the sodium salt to measure kidney function, the usual dose being 2 g intravenously. Aminohippuric acid is a major metabolite of aminobenzoic acid.

AMINOMETRADINE *Diuretic*

Synonyms: Aminometramide; SC 3497.
Proprietary Names: Mictine; Mincard.

1-Allyl-6-amino-3-ethyl-1,2,3,4-tetrahydro-2,4-dioxopyrimidine
$C_9H_{13}N_3O_2 = 195{\cdot}2$

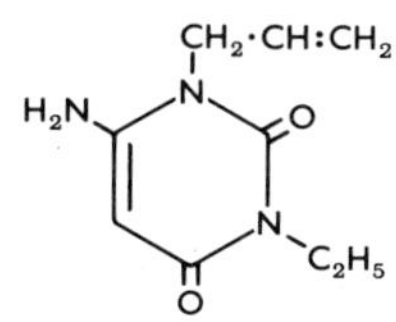

A white crystalline powder. M.p. of the anhydrous substance, about 142°.
Solubility. Soluble 1 in 50 of water, 1 in 2·5 of ethanol, and 1 in 8 of chloroform.

Extraction. Biological material must be dehydrated and extracted with ethanol (see p. 29).

Ultraviolet Absorption Spectrum. Aminometradine in ethanol, maximum at 267 mμ (E1%, 1 cm 1120).

Infra-red Absorption Spectrum. Potassium bromide disk. The principal peaks are: A 1608, B 1642, C 1508 (p. 728).

Dose. Up to 800 mg daily.

AMINOPENTAMIDE *Parasympatholytic*

Synonyms: BL 139; Dimevamide; Valemeramide.

γ-Dimethylamino-*αα*-diphenylvaleramide
$C_{19}H_{24}N_2O = 296{\cdot}4$

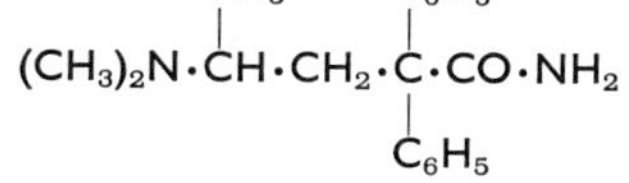

The (±)-form crystallises as long prisms from dilute ethanol which melt at 183° to 184°.
Solubility. Practically insoluble in water.

AMINOPENTAMIDE SULPHATE

Proprietary Name: Centrine.

A white crystalline powder. The (±)-form is normally used in medicine. It is a white crystalline powder which melts at 178° to 181°.

Solubility. Soluble in water and ethanol.

Extraction. Aminopentamide is extracted by organic solvents from aqueous alkaline solutions.

Chromatography. PAPER: system P1—Rf 0·47 (location under ultraviolet light, weak absorption; location reagent *iodoplatinate spray*, strong reaction).

THIN-LAYER: system T1—Rf 0·30 (location reagent *acidified iodoplatinate spray*, positive reaction).

Crystal Tests. MICRO: *potassium tri-iodide solution (3)*—small plates or needles (*sensitivity:* 1 in 1000); *sodium carbonate solution*—oily needles or fans of rods (*sensitivity:* 1 in 1500).

Ultraviolet Absorption Spectrum. Aminopentamide in 0·1N sulphuric acid, maxima at 253 mμ (E1%, 1cm 9), 259 mμ (E1%, 1cm 11), and 265 mμ (E1%, 1cm 9); minimum at about 249 mμ.

Infra-red Absorption Spectrum. Aminopentamide (base). Potassium bromide disk. The principal peaks are: A 695, B 750 or 1370 (p. 772).

Dose. Up to 2 g daily.

AMINOSALICYLIC ACID *Tuberculostatic*

Synonyms: 4-Aminosalicylic Acid; PAS; Para-aminosalicylic Acid.

Proprietary Names: Parapas; Parasal.

4-Amino-2-hydroxybenzoic acid

$C_7H_7NO_3 = 153{\cdot}1$

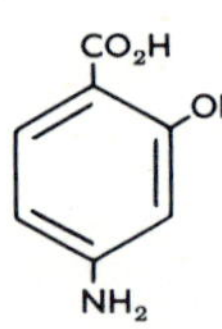

A white powder which darkens on exposure to light and air. It is unstable in aqueous solution. M.p. 150° to 151°, with effervescence.

Solubility. Soluble 1 in 600 of water, 1 in 20 of ethanol, 1 in 50 of ether, 1 in 4000 of chloroform, and 1 in 6 of acetone.

NOTE. Aminosalicylic acid is used as Calcium Aminosalicylate (*Proprietary Name:* Aminacyl), Isoniazid Aminosalicylate (p. 383), Phenyl Aminosalicylate (*Proprietary Names:* Dantyl; Neotebanyl), Potassium Aminosalicylate (*Proprietary Name:* PASkalium), and Sodium Aminosalicylate (*Proprietary Names:* Aminacyl; Entepas; Paramisan Sodium; Pasade).

Screening Test. *Ferric chloride solution* with urine—reddish-violet, after hydrolysis (see p. 4).

Extraction. Aminosalicylic acid may be isolated in the A1 fraction (see p. 27).

Chromatography. PAPER: system P1—Rf 0·80 (location under ultraviolet light, blue fluorescence; location by diazotisation followed by *alkaline betanaphthol spray*; location reagent *ferric chloride spray*, red-violet); system P12—Rf 0·19 (location under ultraviolet light, blue fluorescence; location reagent *ferric chloride spray*, reddish-violet).

THIN-LAYER: system T1—Rf 0·70 (location reagent p-*dimethylaminobenzaldehyde spray*, yellow).

Colour Tests. *Trinder's reagent*—purple; McNally's test—chocolate brown precipitate; *p*-dimethylaminobenzaldehyde test—yellow.

Ultraviolet Absorption Spectrum. Aminosalicylic acid in ethanol, maxima at 239 mμ (E1%, 1cm 545), 281 mμ (E1%, 1cm 949), and 304 mμ (E1%, 1cm 101); in 0·1N hydrochloric acid, maxima at 234 mμ (E1%, 1cm 417) and 300 mμ (E1%, 1cm 277); in 0·1N sodium hydroxide, maxima at 265 mμ (E1%, 1cm 797) and 298 mμ (E1%, 1cm 520).

Infra-red Absorption Spectrum. Potassium bromide disk. The principal peaks are: A 1392, B 1301 or 1363, C 1638 (p. 729).

Quantitative Estimation. Aminosalicylic acid may be spectrophotometrically determined in blood and urine as the nitritopentacyanocobaltate complex (Caccia, 1957).

Metabolism. Aminosalicylic acid is rapidly and completely absorbed from the gastro-intestinal tract in man. Peak plasma levels are reached 1 to 2 hours after oral administration and about 70% is present in the plasma within 15 minutes of absorption. Excretion is also rapid, about 85% of a 10-g oral dose being eliminated in 10 hours. The following compounds may be found in the urine: 14 to 33% of unchanged drug, 28 to 63% of *p*-acetamidosalicylic acid and 0 to 26% of p-aminosalicyluric acid (Way *et al.*, 1955). In addition, *p*-acetamidosalicylglucuronide, *p*-aminosalicylglutamine, and *m*-aminophenol may be detected in small quantities.

Dose. Up to 16 g daily may be given.

Toxicity. Prolonged administration may give rise to the toxic symptoms of the salicylates.

LD50 (oral): in mice 4 g/kg.

CASE EXAMPLE. A patient who was treated with 12 g of aminosalicylic acid daily for 29 days (total 348 g) suddenly developed severe toxic symptoms from which he did not recover. On the 20th day after cessation of treatment the blood-level of aminosalicylic acid was 2 mg% (Loubeyre and Farkas, 1951).

AMIPHENAZOLE *Analeptic*

Synonym: DAPT.

2,4-Diamino-5-phenylthiazole

$C_9H_9N_3S = 191{\cdot}3$

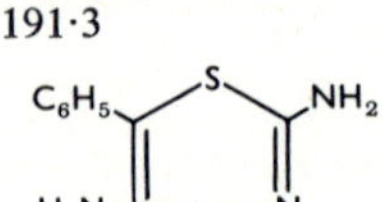

Amiphenazole occurs as flakes from water or

dilute ethanol which turn brown on exposure to light and air. M.p. 163° to 164°, with decomposition.

AMIPHENAZOLE HYDROCHLORIDE
Proprietary Name: Daptazole.

A white crystalline or granular powder; aqueous solutions are stable at room temperature for 24 hours. M.p. 236°.
Solubility. Soluble 1 in 16 of water and 1 in 50 of ethanol; slightly soluble in ether and chloroform.

Extraction. Amiphenazole is extracted by organic solvents from aqueous alkaline solutions.

Chromatography. PAPER: system P1—Rf 0·45 (location under ultraviolet light, absorption; location reagents: *iodoplatinate spray*, weak reaction; *iodine vapour*, weak reaction; *potassium permanganate solution*, weak reaction); system RP1a—Rf 0·75 (location under ultraviolet light, absorption); system RP1b—Rf 0·34 (location as for RP1a).
THIN-LAYER: system T1—Rf 0·71 (location reagent *acidified iodoplatinate spray*, positive reaction).

Colour Test. MICRO: Vitali's test— –/light brown/light brown.

Crystal Tests. MICRO: *picric acid*—dense rosettes (*sensitivity:* 1 in 200); *sodium carbonate solution* —bunches of irregular needles (*sensitivity:* 1 in 400).

Ultraviolet Absorption Spectrum. Amiphenazole in 0·1N sodium hydroxide, an inflexion at 232 mμ and a maximum at 312 mμ (E 1%, 1 cm 419); in 0·1N sulphuric acid, maxima at 228 mμ (E 1%, 1 cm 907) and 261 mμ (E 1%, 1 cm 374).

Infra-red Absorption Spectrum. Amiphenazole (base). Potassium bromide disk. The principal peaks are: A 1495, B 1637, C 688 or 1346 (p. 729).

Dose. Up to 800 mg daily.

AMISOMETRADINE *Diuretic*

Synonym: Aminoisometradine.
Proprietary Name: Rolicton.

6-Amino-1,2,3,4-tetrahydro-3-methyl-1-methylallyl-2,4-dioxopyrimidine
$C_9H_{13}N_3O_2 = 195{\cdot}2$

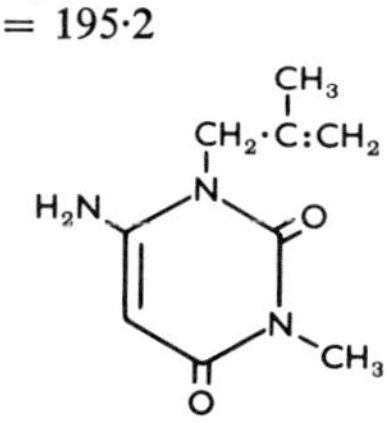

Amisometradine is a structural isomer of aminometradine. A white crystalline powder. M.p. 175°.
Solubility. Slightly soluble in cold water, the solubility increasing rapidly on heating; freely soluble in ethanol and acetone; insoluble in ether.

Extraction. Amisometradine is extracted by organic solvents from aqueous acid or alkaline solutions.

Chromatography. PAPER: system P1—Rf 0·84 (location under ultraviolet light, absorption; location reagents: *iodine vapour*, weak reaction; *potassium permanganate spray*, weak reaction); system RP1a—Rf 0·78 (location under ultraviolet light, absorption); system RP1b—Rf 0·75 (location as for RP1a).
THIN-LAYER: system T1—Rf 0·68 (location reagent *potassium permanganate spray*, positive reaction).

Crystal Tests. MICRO: *gold bromide solution*—bunches of blades or prisms (*sensitivity:* 1 in 1000); *platinic chloride solution*—star-shaped crystals (*sensitivity:* 1 in 200).

Ultraviolet Absorption Spectrum. Amisometradine in methanol, maximum at 267 mμ (E 1%, 1 cm 1060); in 0·1N sulphuric acid, maximum at 268·5 mμ (E 1%, 1 cm 1030).

Infra-red Absorption Spectrum. Potassium bromide disk. The principal peaks are: A 1639, B 1492 or 1604, C 1680 (p. 729).

Dose. Up to 1·6 g daily.

Toxicity. LD50 (oral): in mice 610 mg/kg.

AMITRIPTYLINE *Antidepressant*

10,11 - Dihydro - 5 - (3 - dimethylaminopropylidene)-5*H*-dibenzo[*a*,*d*]cycloheptene
$C_{20}H_{23}N = 277{\cdot}4$

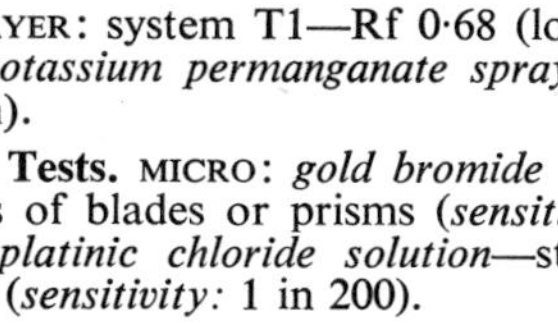

A colourless oil which becomes yellow on standing due to oxidation to a ketonic product. This product has not yet been detected in the urine but the presence of a substantial amount of a neutral metabolite is indicated (Henwood, 1967).

AMITRIPTYLINE HYDROCHLORIDE
Proprietary Names: Elavil; Laroxyl; Saroten; Tryptanol; Tryptizol.

Colourless crystals or a white powder. M.p. about 197°.
Solubility. Soluble 1 in 1 of water, 1 in 1·5 of ethanol, and 1 in 1·2 of chloroform; insoluble in ether.

Screening Test. See under Screening Tests, p. 7.

Extraction. Amitriptyline may be isolated in the D2 fraction (see p. 28); hydrolysis of biological material is required in order to improve the yield.

Chromatography. PAPER: system P1—Rf 0·77 (location under ultraviolet light, absorption;

location reagent *iodoplatinate spray*, strong reaction); system RP1a—Rf 0·32 (location under ultraviolet light, absorption; location reagent *iodoplatinate spray*, positive reaction); system RP1b—Rf 0·00.

THIN-LAYER: system T1—Rf 0·49 (location reagent *acidified iodoplatinate spray*, positive reaction); system T3—Rf 0·74 (location reagent *iodoplatinate spray*, positive reaction).

GAS: system G2/225—retention time 0·58 relative to codeine; system G4—retention time 0·29 relative to codeine.

Colour Tests. MICRO: sulphuric acid–formaldehyde test—brown-orange (*sensitivity:* 0·1 µg); ammonium molybdate test—orange → green (*sensitivity:* 0·25 µg); ammonium vanadate test —brown (not always seen) → green (*sensitivity:* 0·25 µg); Vitali's test—brown flash/–/–/pale brown (*sensitivity:* 1·0 µg).

Ultraviolet Absorption Spectrum. Amitriptyline in ethanol, maximum at 242 mµ (E1%, 1 cm 260); in 0·1N sulphuric acid, maximum at 240 mµ (E1%, 1 cm 500). Amitriptyline hydrochloride in methanol, maximum at 239 mµ (E1%, 1 cm about 450).

Infra-red Absorption Spectrum. Amitriptyline (base). Potassium bromide disk. The principal peaks are: A 752, B 765, C 775 (p. 772).

Quantitative Estimation. Forbes *et al.* (1965) have described a method for the quantitative estimation of amitriptyline in urine involving extraction with chloroform, purification by thin-layer chromatography, followed by elution in ethanol, and subsequent spectrophotometric determination. Wallace and Dahl (1967) describe a rapid and specific spectrophotometric method of determination of amitriptyline and its principal metabolites in biological materials; the procedure involves extraction into n-hexane and oxidation of the compounds with alkaline potassium permanganate to yield carbonyl derivatives which have a characteristic ultraviolet spectrum.

Metabolism. Amitriptyline is rapidly absorbed from the gastro-intestinal tract and is largely bound to plasma proteins. The serum concentration is never high as amitriptyline accumulates rapidly in various tissues. Metabolism and excretion in the urine are rapid and very little drug can be found in the tissues 24 hours after the administration of medium doses. Three metabolites have been detected in human urine. Demethylation, hydroxylation, and conjugation with glucuronic acid are thought to occur in the liver. Analysis of the urine collected for 2 days after a volunteer had ingested 50 mg and for 4 days after he had ingested 100 mg indicated an excretion of 1% of unchanged drug; the level in the urine following the 50-mg dose was not measurable on the second day and after the 100-mg dose the level was no longer measurable by the fourth day (Forbes *et al.*, 1965).

Dose. Usually 25 mg thrice daily; doses of up to 300 mg daily have been given.

Toxicity. Recoveries have taken place after ingestion of 1 to 1·8 g of amitriptyline.

LD50 (oral): in mice 280 mg/kg.

CASE EXAMPLES. A 25-year-old man died fairly soon after ingesting between 1·25 and 2·5 g of amitriptyline. Semi-quantitative post-mortem levels of amitriptyline (w/w) after extraction involving hydrolysis: blood, about 0·04 mg%; brain, about 5 mg%; kidney, 0·5 to 1 mg%; liver, about 1·5 mg%; urine, about 1·3 mg%. The stomach contents which were not hydrolysed were found to contain between 20 and 100 mg% (w/w). A probable metabolite of amitriptyline was detected in the blood, kidney, liver, and urine (Sunshine and Bäumler, 1963).

(1) A 26-year-old woman took 2 g of amitriptyline with suicidal intent. A salt and water emetic which she was given was ineffective since she was found dead 7 hours later. At post-mortem examination the urine contained 49·5 mg% of amitriptyline and traces of a metabolite; the blood, kidneys, and liver contained traces of amitriptyline and a metabolite. (2) A 47-year-old woman was found dead after ingesting an unknown quantity of amitriptyline. Post-mortem levels: urine, 6 mg%; traces of amitriptyline in the blood, kidneys, and liver (Forbes *et al.*, 1965).

(1) An 8-year-old girl died about 12 hours after the alleged ingestion of 1·4 g of amitriptyline and 112 mg of perphenazine; she vomited before death. Post-mortem levels: blood, 1·3 mg%; liver, 3·0 mg%; urine, 1·0 mg%. The stomach contents contained 24 mg of amitriptyline and 112 mg of perphenazine. (2) A 33-year-old man was found dead 10 days after being given a prescription for 90 tablets containing in total 2·25 g of amitriptyline and 360 mg of perphenazine. At post-mortem examination the blood contained 1·1 mg% of amitriptyline and the stomach contents 200 mg of amitriptyline and 25 mg of perphenazine (McBay, 1967).

AMODIAQUINE *Antimalarial*

Synonyms: Amodiachin; SN 10751.

7-Chloro-4-(3-diethylaminomethyl-4-hydroxy-anilino)quinoline

$C_{20}H_{22}ClN_3O = 355{\cdot}9$

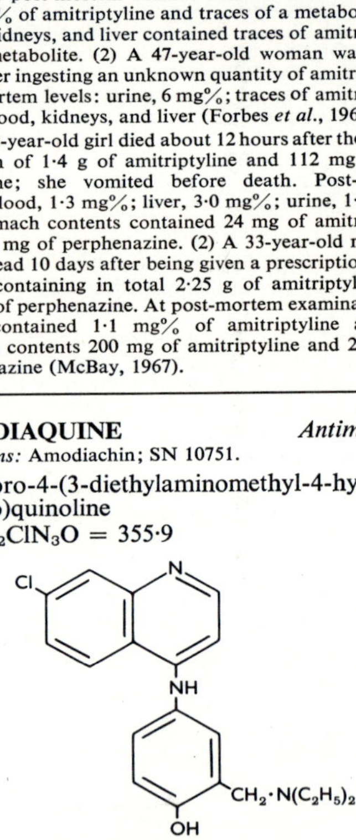

White crystals. M.p. 208°.

AMODIAQUINE HYDROCHLORIDE

Proprietary Name: Camoquin.

A yellow crystalline powder. M.p. 158° to 160°.

Solubility. Soluble 1 in 22 of water and 1 in 70 of ethanol; almost insoluble in ether and chloroform.

Extraction. Amodiaquine is extracted by organic solvents from aqueous alkaline solutions.

Chromatography. PAPER: system P1—Rf 0·19

(location under ultraviolet light, yellow fluorescence; location reagents: *iodoplatinate spray*, strong reaction; *bromocresol green spray*, strong reaction; system RP1a—Rf 0·60 (location under ultraviolet light, yellow fluorescence; location reagent *iodoplatinate spray*, positive reaction); system RP1b—Rf 0·00.

THIN-LAYER: system T1—Rf 0·61 (location reagent *acidified iodoplatinate spray*, positive reaction).

Colour Tests. To 1 ml of a 2% solution, add 0·5 ml of *cobalt thiocyanate solution*—green precipitate.

MICRO: ammonium molybdate test—green (*sensitivity:* 0·25 μg); Vitali's test—orange/brown/red-brown.

Crystal Tests. MICRO: *gold cyanide solution*—snowflake rosettes or burrs (*sensitivity:* 1 in 1000); *potassium cadmium iodide solution*—burrs (*sensitivity:* 1 in 1000).

Ultraviolet Absorption Spectrum. Amodiaquine in 0·1N sulphuric acid, maxima at 224 mμ (E1%, 1cm 1014), 238 mμ (E1%, 1cm 600), and 342 mμ (E1%, 1cm 440).
Amodiaquine hydrochloride in 0·1N hydrochloric acid, maximum at 343 mμ (E1%, 1cm about 436).

Infra-red Absorption Spectrum. Amodiaquine (base). Potassium bromide disk. The principal peaks are: A 1565, B 1480, C 815 or 1255 or 1535 (p. 772).

Dose. Up to 600 mg (base) daily for 3 days.

Toxicity. A 2½-year-old child recovered within 3 or 4 days after ingesting between 1 and 1·6 g of amodiaquine (Reid, 1960).

AMOLANONE *Local Anaesthetic*

Synonym: AP 43.

γ-Diethylamino-α-*o*-hydroxyphenyl-α-phenylbutyrolactone

$C_{20}H_{23}NO_2 = 309·4$

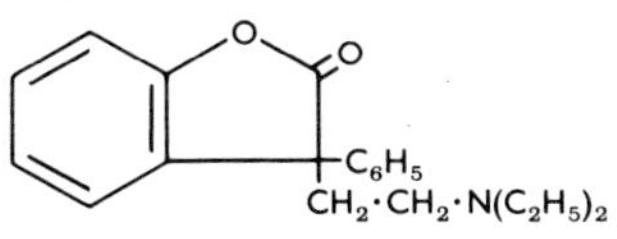

White crystals. M.p. 43° to 44°. B.p. 192° to 194°.

AMOLANONE HYDROCHLORIDE

Proprietary Name: Amethone Hydrochloride.

White crystals. M.p. 152° to 153°.

Solubility. Soluble in water.

Extraction. Amolanone is extracted by organic solvents from aqueous alkaline solutions.

Chromatography. PAPER: system P1—Rf 0·72 (location under ultraviolet light, absorption; location reagents: *iodoplatinate spray*, strong reaction; *bromocresol green spray*, weak reaction).

THIN-LAYER: system T1—Rf 0·71 (location reagent *acidified iodoplatinate spray*, positive reaction).

GAS: system G2/225—retention time 0·66 relative to codeine; system G4—retention time 0·43 relative to codeine.

Colour Test. MICRO: Vitali's test— –/pale brown/yellow (*sensitivity:* 0·25 μg).

Crystal Tests. MICRO: *gold bromide–hydrochloric acid solution*—plates and blades, forming overnight (*sensitivity:* 1 in 1000); *gold chloride solution*—serrated plates (*sensitivity:* 1 in 1000).

Ultraviolet Absorption Spectrum. Amolanone hydrochloride in 0·1N sulphuric acid, maxima at 265 mμ, 269 mμ (E1%, 1cm 55), and 276·5 mμ.

Infra-red Absorption Spectrum. Amolanone (base). Potassium bromide disk. The principal peaks are: A 1795, B 1025, C 750 or 1455 (p. 773).

Toxicity. Amolanone has been used for local anaesthesia of the lower urinary tract, a 0·33% solution being instilled intra-urethrally. The maximum safe amount for topical use is stated to be 30 ml of a 0·33% solution.

AMOPYROQUINE *Antimalarial*

Synonym: PAM 780.

7 - Chloro - 4 - (4 - hydroxy - 3 - pyrrolidin - 1′ - ylmethylanilino)quinoline

$C_{20}H_{20}ClN_3O = 353·9$

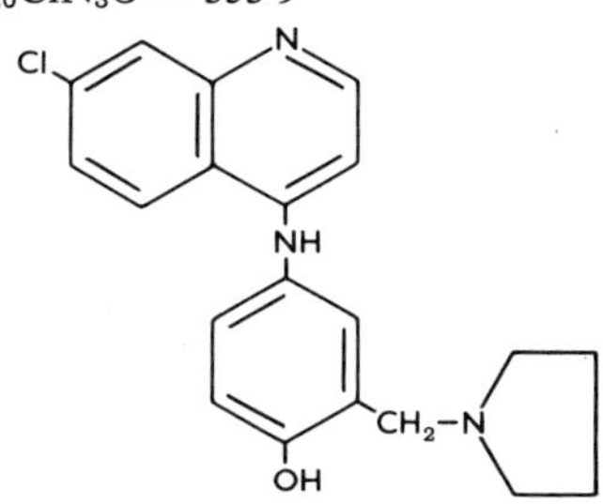

AMOPYROQUINE HYDROCHLORIDE

Proprietary Name: Propoquin.

A yellow crystalline powder.

Extraction. Amopyroquine is extracted by organic solvents from aqueous alkaline solutions.

Chromatography. PAPER: system P1—Rf 0·16 (location under ultraviolet light, pale yellow fluorescence; location reagents: *iodoplatinate spray*, strong reaction; *bromocresol green spray*, strong reaction); system RP1a—tailing (location under ultraviolet light, pale green fluorescence; location reagent *iodoplatinate spray*, positive reaction); system RP1b—Rf 0·06 (location as for RP1a).

THIN-LAYER: system T1—Rf 0·45 (location reagent *acidified iodoplatinate spray*, strong reaction).

Colour Tests. MICRO: ammonium molybdate test—(yellow) blue-black → green (*sensitivity:* 0·1 μg); Vitali's test—(yellow) orange/yellow/ brown (*sensitivity:* 0·1 μg).

Crystal Tests. MICRO: *gold cyanide solution*—rosettes (*sensitivity:* 1 in 1000); *trinitrobenzoic acid solution*—gelatinous rosettes, best viewed under polarised light (*sensitivity:* 1 in 1000).

Ultraviolet Absorption Spectrum. Amopyroquine in 0·1N sulphuric acid, maxima at 224 mμ (E1%, 1 cm 1040), 238 mμ (E1%, 1 cm 598), and 342 mμ (E1%, 1 cm 441).

Infra-red Absorption Spectrum. Amopyroquine (base). Potassium bromide disk. The principal peaks are: A 1563, B 1490, C 1252 (p. 773).

AMPHETAMINE *Central Stimulant*

Synonyms: Isomyn; Phenopromine; Phenylisopropylamine; Racemic Desoxynorephedrine.
Proprietary Name: Benzedrine.

(±)-α-Methylphenethylamine
$C_9H_{13}N = 135{\cdot}2$

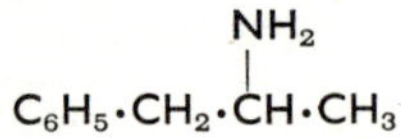

A colourless, mobile, slowly volatile liquid, which absorbs carbon dioxide from the air to form a volatile compound. B.p. 200° to 203°.
Solubility. Soluble 1 in 50 of water; freely soluble in ethanol, ether, and chloroform.

NOTE. For the (+)-isomer see under Dexamphetamine, p. 287. For a microcrystalline method of differentiation of amphetamine from dexamphetamine and levamphetamine, see Microcrystal Tests, p. 140.

AMPHETAMINE PHOSPHATE
Synonym: Monobasic Racemic Amphetamine Phosphate.

A white crystalline powder which decomposes at about 300° and sinters at about 150°.
Solubility. Freely soluble in water; slightly soluble in ethanol; almost insoluble in ether and chloroform.

AMPHETAMINE SULPHATE
Synonyms: Phenamine; Psychedrinum.

A white powder. M.p. about 300°, with decomposition.
Solubility. Soluble 1 in 9 of water and 1 in 515 of ethanol; insoluble in ether and chloroform.

Screening Test. See under Screening Tests, p. 7.

Extraction. Amphetamine is extracted by organic solvents from aqueous alkaline solutions; it is volatile and may be isolated by distillation from alkaline solutions (see p. 18).

Chromatography. PAPER: system P1—Rf 0·51 (location reagents: *iodoplatinate spray*, white; *bromocresol green spray*, strong reaction).

THIN-LAYER: system T1—Rf 0·48 (location reagent *potassium permanganate spray*, positive reaction).

GAS: system G2/120—retention time 0·28 relative to ephedrine.

Colour Test. MICRO: sulphuric acid–formaldehyde test—orange → brown.

Crystal Tests. MICRO: *platinic bromide solution*—masses of irregular plates, weakly birefringent (*sensitivity:* 1 in 200); *platinic iodide solution*—masses of irregular plates (*sensitivity:* 1 in 400).

Ultraviolet Absorption Spectrum. Amphetamine in 0·1N sulphuric acid, maxima at 251·5 mμ (E1%, 1 cm 5·5), 257 mμ (E1%, 1 cm 15), and 263 mμ (E1%, 1 cm 8).

NOTE. The ultraviolet absorption spectra of pethidine (p. 476) and phenethylamine (p. 482) bear many points of resemblance to that of amphetamine. However, the 3 compounds may be separated by paper or thin-layer chromatography.

Infra-red Absorption Spectrum. Amphetamine (base). Liquid film. The principal peaks are: A 695, B 737, C 1452 (p. 729).

Metabolism. Amphetamine is well absorbed from the gastro-intestinal tract. In dogs, low plasma levels seem to indicate rapid accumulation in the tissues. The excretion of unchanged amphetamine is influenced by the urinary pH, being as much as 54% at pH 5 and as low as 2·9% at pH 8 (Beckett *et al.*, 1965b). Between 30 and 40% of amphetamine is usually excreted unchanged in the urine within 48 hours, mostly in the first 24 hours after ingestion; after treatment involving large doses, amphetamine may be detected in the urine up to 7 days after the cessation of treatment (Alles and Wisegarver, 1961). Following oral administration in small doses in man, 66% of the dose was excreted in the first 24 hours and 91% by the third day, none being found in the faeces; in addition to 30% of the dose excreted as unchanged drug, the urine contained 3% as conjugated *p*-hydroxyamphetamine, 3% as conjugated benzylmethyl ketone, benzoic acid (16% as hippuric acid and 4% as benzoylglucuronide), and traces of conjugated 1-phenylpropan-2-ol; hence, deamination through phenylacetone to benzoic acid appears to be the major metabolic pathway although unchanged amphetamine is the main excretory product (Dring *et al.*, 1966).

Dose. Up to 20 mg as a single dose.

Toxicity. Continued use of amphetamine may cause addiction, and ingestion of up to 10 times the usual therapeutic dose is common among addicts. The estimated minimum lethal dose in children is 20 mg and that for adults may be 10 times as great; however, fatalities are rare. One common and alarming result of acute amphetamine poisoning may be the development of an acute psychosis and severe cases often present as an acute mental disturbance.

LD50 (oral): in mice 22 and in rabbits 85 mg/kg.

CASE EXAMPLES. A 23-year-old man was admitted to hospital very shortly after continuously inhaling from a Benzedrine inhaler for 5 hours. He had one psychotic episode but recovered within 3 days. The urine passed over the 3 days contained a total of 36 mg amphetamine base (corresponding to an oral dose of 72 to 130 mg amphetamine) and the inhaler, on analysis after the patient's admission, contained only 60 mg of amphetamine instead of the original 325 mg. A 32-year-old man recovered 3 days after consuming 17 pints of beer and chewing the contents of 1½ Benzedrine inhalers (487·5 mg of amphetamine) (Greenwood and Peachey, 1957).

NOTE. Amphetamine has been used to stimulate the performance of racehorses.

AMPICILLIN *Antibiotic*

Synonyms: BRL 1341; P 50; Anhydrous Ampicillin; [D-(−)-α-Aminobenzyl]penicillin.
Proprietary Name: Penbritin.

6-[D(−)-α-Amino-α-phenylacetamido]penicillanic acid

$C_{16}H_{19}N_3O_4S = 349{\cdot}4$

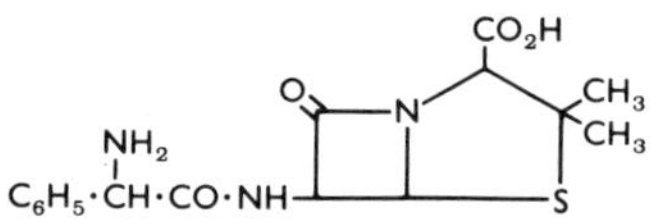

A white microcrystalline powder.
Solubility. Soluble 1 in 170 of water; almost insoluble in ethanol, ether, and chloroform.

AMPICILLIN SODIUM
A white hygroscopic crystalline powder. Aqueous solutions containing 10% or more deteriorate rapidly on storage.
Solubility. Soluble 1 in 2 of water and 1 in 50 of acetone; slightly soluble in chloroform; insoluble in ether.

AMPICILLIN TRIHYDRATE
A white microcrystalline powder.
Solubility. Soluble 1 in 150 of water; almost insoluble in ethanol, ether, and chloroform.

Extraction. Ampicillin is soluble in water; special extraction methods are required (see p. 28).

Colour Test. Suspend 10 mg in 1 ml of water and add 2 ml of a mixture of 2 ml of *potassium cupri-tartrate solution* and 6 ml of water—magenta-violet.

Metabolism. Ampicillin is excreted in high concentration in the bile and therefore may be used in the treatment of infections of the biliary and intestinal tracts. During treatment involving 2 to 3 g of ampicillin daily for 14 days, blood-levels ranged from 0·2 to 3·2 mg%, and urine levels from 25·6 to 204·8 mg% (Kennedy *et al.*, 1963). After doses of 250 mg to 1 g, peak serum-levels from 0·219 to 0·679 mg% were apparent within 2 hours. Some 30% of the dose was excreted in the urine within 6 hours (Knudsen *et al.*, 1961). Excretion begins within 3 hours and ceases after 48 hours (Stewart *et al.*, 1961a).

Dose. Ampicillin, up to 6 g daily, by mouth; ampicillin sodium, up to 3 g, intramuscularly.

AMPROLIUM HYDROCHLORIDE *Anticoccidial (Veterinary)*

Proprietary Names: Amprol; Amprolmix; Pancoxin.

1-(4-Amino-2-propylpyrimidin-5-ylmethyl)-2-methylpyridinium chloride hydrochloride

$C_{14}H_{20}Cl_2N_4 = 315{\cdot}2$

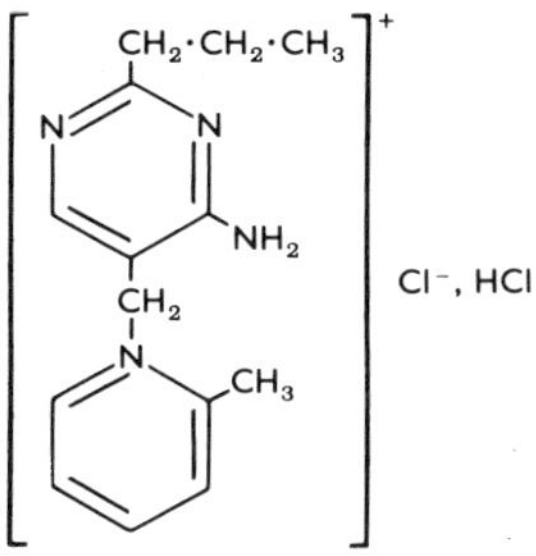

A white powder. M.p. 247°, with decomposition.
Solubility. Soluble 1 in 2 of water and 1 in 170 of ethanol; very slightly soluble in ether; insoluble in chloroform.

Extraction. Amprolium hydrochloride is extracted by organic solvents from aqueous alkaline solutions.

Chromatography. PAPER: system P1—Rf 0·03 (location under ultraviolet light, pale blue fluorescence; location reagents: *iodoplatinate spray*, strong reaction; *bromocresol green spray*, weak reaction; *potassium permanganate spray*, weak reaction); system RP1a—Rf 0·89 location reagent *iodoplatinate spray*, positive reaction); system RP1b—Rf 0·88 (location as for RP1a).

THIN-LAYER: system T1—Rf 0·02 (location reagent *acidified iodoplatinate spray*, positive reaction).

Colour Test. MICRO: Vitali's test— –/–/faint yellow (*sensitivity:* 1·0 μg).

Crystal Tests. MICRO: *picric acid*—bunches of prisms (*sensitivity:* 1 in 1000); *platinic bromide solution*—small rods in bunches, best viewed under polarised light (*sensitivity:* 1 in 1000).

Ultraviolet Absorption Spectrum. Amprolium hydrochloride in 0·1N sulphuric acid, maxima at 246 mμ (E1%, 1 cm 592) and about 263 mμ (E1%, 1 cm 563).

Infra-red Absorption Spectrum. Potassium bromide disk. The principal peaks are: A 1638, B 1488 or 1522 or 1593 (p. 773).

Quantitative Estimation. Amprolium hydrochloride may be estimated by colorimetric determination of the orange-coloured complex which it forms with 2,7-naphthalenediol (Schulz and Szalkowski, 1961; Report by the Prophylactics in Animal Feeds Subcommittee of the Analytical Methods Committee, 1964).

AMPROTROPINE *Parasympatholytic*
3-Diethylamino-2,2-dimethylpropyl(±)-tropate
$C_{18}H_{29}NO_3 = 307{\cdot}4$

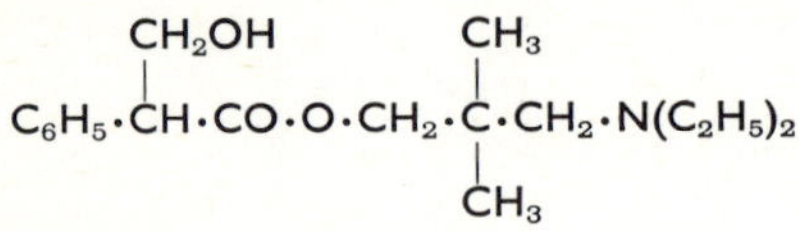

AMPROTROPINE PHOSPHATE
Proprietary Name: Syntropan.

A white crystalline powder. M.p. 142° to 145°.
Solubility. Soluble in water; slightly soluble in ethanol; insoluble in ether and chloroform.

Extraction. Amprotropine is extracted by organic solvents from aqueous alkaline solutions.

Chromatography. PAPER: system P1—Rf 0·61 (location reagents: *iodoplatinate spray*, weak reaction; *bromocresol green spray*, weak reaction).
THIN-LAYER: system T1—Rf 0·71 (location reagent *acidified iodoplatinate spray*, positive reaction).
GAS: system G2/225—retention time 1·7 relative to diphenhydramine; system G4—retention time 2·4 relative to diphenhydramine.

Colour Test. MICRO: ammonium molybdate test —blue (*sensitivity:* 1·0 μg).

Crystal Test. MICRO: *lead iodide solution*—hexagonal plates.

Infra-red Absorption Spectrum. Amprotropine (base). Potassium bromide disk. The principal peaks are: A 1730, B 1162, C 1060 or 1195 or 1378 (p. 773).

Dose. Up to 400 mg daily.

AMYDRICAINE *Local Anaesthetic*
1,1-Di(dimethylaminomethyl)propyl benzoate
$C_{16}H_{26}N_2O_2 = 278{\cdot}4$

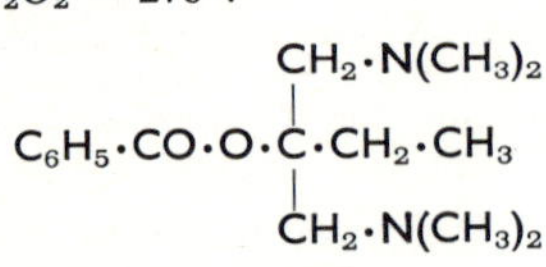

AMYDRICAINE HYDROCHLORIDE
Proprietary Name: Alypin Hydrochloride.

A white hygroscopic crystalline powder. M.p. about 169°.
Solubility. Soluble 1 in 1 of water and 1 in 4 of ethanol; soluble in chloroform; insoluble in ether.

Extraction. Amydricaine is extracted by organic solvents from aqueous alkaline solutions.

Chromatography. PAPER: system P1—Rf 0·40 (location under ultraviolet light, dark blue fluorescence; location reagent *iodoplatinate spray*, strong reaction); system RP1a—Rf 0·79 (location reagent *iodoplatinate spray*, positive reaction); system RP1b—Rf 0·00.
THIN-LAYER: system T1—Rf 0·41 (location reagent *acidified iodoplatinate spray*, positive reaction).

Crystal Tests. MICRO: *potassium bismuth iodide solution*—blades and needles (*sensitivity:* 1 in 3000); *potassium tri-iodide solution* (*1*)—blades and plates (*sensitivity:* 1 in 3000).

Ultraviolet Absorption Spectrum. Amydricaine in 0·1N sulphuric acid, maxima at 236·5 mμ (E1%, 1 cm 437) and 277 mμ (E1%, 1 cm 40); amydricaine hydrochloride in water, maximum at about 234 mμ (E1%, 1 cm 450).

Infra-red Absorption Spectrum. Amydricaine (base). Potassium bromide disk. The principal peaks are: A 1282, B 1715, C 710 (p. 773).

Toxicity. Amydricaine is as toxic as cocaine. The minimum subcutaneous lethal dose in dogs is 70 and in rats 200 to 430 mg/kg.

AMYL ACETATE *Industrial Solvent*
Consists of a mixture of isomeric acetates
$CH_3{\cdot}CO_2(C_5H_{11}) = 130{\cdot}2$

A colourless, mobile, neutral, inflammable liquid. B.p. 135° to 145°. Refractive index 1·1400.
Solubility. Very slightly soluble in water; miscible with ethanol and ether.

Extraction. Amyl acetate is volatile and may be isolated by distillation (see p. 18).

Toxicity. The suggested maximum allowable atmospheric concentration of amyl acetate is 100 p.p.m. and the estimated lethal dose in man is 50 g. Amyl acetate may cause irritation of the skin and mucous membranes.

AMYL ALCOHOL *Industrial Solvent*
Consists mainly of a mixture of isopentan-1-ol $[(CH_3)_2CH{\cdot}CH_2{\cdot}CH_2OH]$, with some 2-methylbutan-1-ol $[CH_3{\cdot}CH_2{\cdot}CH(CH_3)CH_2OH]$
$C_5H_{12}O = 88{\cdot}15$

A colourless liquid. B.p. 128° to 132°. Refractive index 1·4075.
Solubility. Slightly soluble in water; miscible with ethanol, ether, and chloroform.

Screening Tests. See under Screening Tests, p. 6.

Extraction. Amyl alcohol is volatile and may be isolated by distillation (see p. 18).

Chromatography. GAS: system G8/160—retention time 5·1 relative to n-propanol.

Metabolism. Studies in rats have shown that the 2 constituents of amyl alcohol are mainly metabolised by oxidation. Upon injection in rats they disappear from the blood in 3 to 9 hours and about 1 to 7% of the dose is eliminated unchanged in the expired air and urine. In rabbits between 7 and 10% is excreted as glucuronide conjugates.

Toxicity. Amyl alcohol has an action similar to that of ethanol but it is a more pronounced local irritant, its vapours rapidly producing intense irritation of the nose, eyes, and throat. Exposure to excessive concentrations causes headache and nausea. It is fairly toxic when ingested orally. The estimated lethal dose in man is stated to be 30 g, and the maximum permissible atmospheric concentration is 100 p.p.m.

AMYL NITRITE *Coronary Vasodilator*

Synonym: Isoamyl Nitrite.

Consists chiefly of the nitrites of 3-methylbutan-1-ol and 2-methylbutan-1-ol

$C_5H_{11}NO_2 = 117{\cdot}1$

A clear, yellow, volatile, inflammable liquid, which must be protected from air and light, in a cool place. B.p. 90° to 100°. Refractive index 1·3871.

CAUTION. *Amyl nitrite forms an explosive mixture with air or oxygen. It is very inflammable and must not be used where it may be ignited.*

Solubility. Insoluble in water; miscible with ethanol, ether, and chloroform.

Extraction. Amyl nitrite is volatile and may be isolated by distillation (see p. 18).

Colour Tests. To 0·2 ml of amyl nitrite, add 2 ml of a 2% ferrous sulphate solution and 5 ml of dilute hydrochloric acid—greenish-brown; to 0·2 ml of amyl nitrite, add 0·5 ml of aniline and 5 ml of glacial acetic acid—deep orange-red.

Metabolism. When inhaled, amyl nitrite is rapidly absorbed, the onset of its effect is immediate, and its action lasts from 2 to 8 minutes. It is probably metabolised by hydrolysis to nitrite and amyl alcohol. When given by mouth it is pharmacologically inactive, probably being rapidly hydrolysed in the gastro-intestinal tract to nitrous acid. Recovery has occurred after the ingestion of 12 ml.

Dose. 0·12 to 0·3 ml, by inhalation.

AMYLMETACRESOL *Antiseptic*

5-Methyl-2-pentylphenol

$C_{12}H_{18}O = 178{\cdot}3$

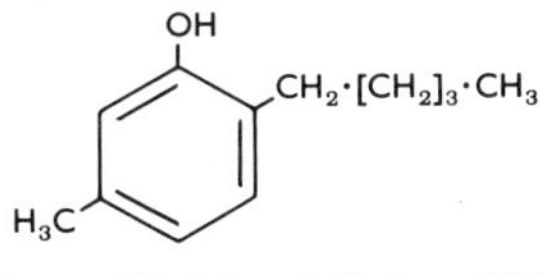

A colourless solid. M.p. 24°. B.p. 137° to 139°, at 15 mm Hg.

Solubility. Almost insoluble in water; soluble in ethanol and ether.

Extraction. Amylmetacresol is extracted by organic solvents from aqueous acid solutions.

Ultraviolet Absorption Spectrum. Amylmetacresol in ethanol, maximum at about 277 mμ (E1%, 1cm about 121); minimum at about 245 mμ (E1%, 1cm about 9).

Metabolism. Amylmetacresol is rapidly absorbed and excreted in the urine.

Toxicity. LD50 (oral): in rats 2·5 to 4·5 g/kg.

AMYLOBARBITONE *Barbiturate*

Synonyms: Amobarbital; Pentymalum.
Proprietary Name: Amytal.

5-Ethyl-5-isopentylbarbituric acid

$C_{11}H_{18}N_2O_3 = 226{\cdot}3$

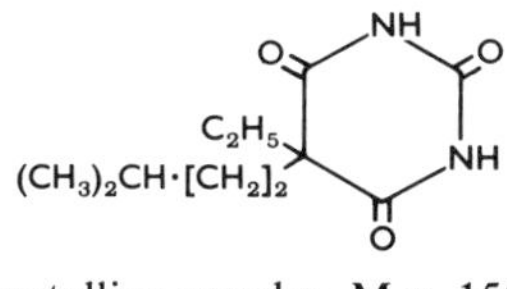

A white crystalline powder. M.p. 155° to 158°.

Solubility. Soluble 1 in 1500 of water, 1 in 5 of ethanol, 1 in 6 of ether, and 1 in 20 of chloroform; soluble in aqueous solutions of alkali hydroxides and carbonates.

AMYLOBARBITONE SODIUM

Synonyms: Barbamyl; Sodium Amobarbital; Soluble Amylobarbitone.
Proprietary Name: Sodium Amytal.

A white hygroscopic granular powder.

Solubility. Soluble 1 in less than 1 of water and 1 in 2 of ethanol; insoluble in ether and chloroform.

Screening Tests. See under Barbiturates, p. 208.

Extraction. Amylobarbitone may be isolated in the A2 fraction (see p. 27).

Chromatography. PAPER: system P2—Rf 1·00 (location under ultraviolet light, dark spot); system P3—Rf 0·31 (location reagent *silver nitrate spray*, white); system P4—Rf 0·46 (location as for P3); system P5—Rf 0·66 relative to quinalbarbitone (location under ultraviolet light after exposure to ammonia, absorption); system RP1b—Rf 0·15 (location under ultraviolet light after exposure to ammonia; location reagent *potassium permanganate spray*, yellow on pink).

THIN-LAYER: system T10—Rf 0·33 (location reagents: *mercurous nitrate spray*, black; *Zwikker's reagent spray*, pink); system T11—Rf 0·42 (location reagent *mercurous nitrate spray*, white on grey).

GAS: system G1/180—retention time 0·69 relative to diphenhydramine; system G3—retention time 2·0 relative to diphenhydramine; system G5—retention time 2·14 relative to barbitone; retention time 0·31 relative to phenobarbitone; system G7—retention time 2·0 relative to barbitone.

Gas chromatography of the hydroxylated metabolite (see under Metabolism): system G7—retention time 4·40 relative to barbitone.

Colour Test. Zwikker's test—violet-blue.

Ultraviolet Absorption Spectrum. Amylobarbitone is a 5,5-derivative—see Screening Test 3 under Barbiturates, p. 208.

Infra-red Absorption Spectrum. Amylobarbitone. Potassium bromide disk. The principal peaks are: A 1716, B 1689, C 1745 (p. 729).

Quantitative Estimation. See under Barbiturates, p. 208. Kamm and Van Loon (1966) have described a gas chromatographic method for the estimation of microgram quantities of the hydroxylated metabolite of amylobarbitone in urine, and Moy and Wetherell (1967) have described a differential spectrophotometric method of determination of amylobarbitone when present together with quinalbarbitone.

Metabolism. Amylobarbitone is an intermediate-acting barbiturate—see under Barbiturates, p. 207. In man, it is excreted in the urine partly unchanged and partly as the hydroxylated metabolite, 5-ethyl-5-(3-hydroxy-3-methylbutyl) barbituric acid (Cochin and Daly, 1963a). Forty-five per cent of the dose is excreted in the urine as this hydroxylated metabolite in 3 days and small amounts of the metabolite are detectable for as long as 5 days following the ingestion of a single 180-mg dose (Kamm and Van Loon, 1966).
Jackson and Moss (1961) isolated the metabolite in the urine of a woman who had died 30 hours after ingesting an unknown quantity of amylobarbitone and quinalbarbitone; they describe its isolation by paper chromatography. About 44% of the amylobarbitone present in blood post mortem appears to be protein-bound (Turner, 1964b).

Dose. Up to 600 mg daily.

Toxicity. The estimated minimum lethal dose in man is 1·5 g; the blood-level associated with severe poisoning is 2 to 4 mg%. When the blood-level is in the region of 1·5 to 2 mg% recovery is possible.
LD50 (oral): in rabbits 575 mg/kg.

CASE EXAMPLES. A 51-year-old man swallowed 20 g of amylobarbitone. Twelve hours after ingestion the blood-level was 16 mg%. He recovered after dialysis (Terplan and Unger, 1966).
A 77-year-old woman was found dead after ingesting about fifty-five 200-mg (11 g) amylobarbitone capsules in 4 days. Post-mortem levels were: blood, 16·3 mg%; brain, 11·9 mg%; liver, 36·2 mg%; stomach contents, 3030 mg; urine, 0·7 mg%. The blood-level is stated to be one of the highest ever recorded (Shanahan, 1967).

AMYLOCAINE *Local Anaesthetic*

1-Dimethylaminomethyl-1-methylpropyl benzoate
$C_{14}H_{21}NO_2 = 235{\cdot}3$

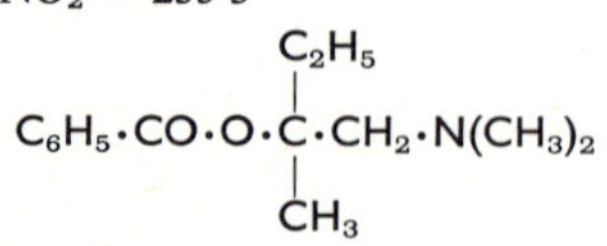

AMYLOCAINE HYDROCHLORIDE
Proprietary Name: Stovaine.

A white crystalline powder. M.p. 177° to 179°.
Solubility. Soluble 1 in 2 of water and 1 in 3 of dehydrated ethanol; almost insoluble in ether.

Extraction. Amylocaine may be extracted by organic solvents from aqueous alkaline solutions.

Chromatography. PAPER: system P1—Rf 0·60 (location under ultraviolet light, absorption; location reagents: *iodoplatinate spray*, strong reaction; *bromocresol green spray*, weak reaction).
THIN-LAYER: system T1—Rf 0·66 (location reagent *acidified iodoplatinate spray*, positive reaction).

Crystal Tests. MICRO: *gold chloride solution*—serrated plates (*sensitivity:* 1 in 1500); *picric acid*—bunches of rods and plates (*sensitivity:* 1 in 1500).

Ultraviolet Absorption Spectrum. Amylocaine in 0·1N sulphuric acid, maxima at 234 mμ (E1%, 1 cm 580) and 275 mμ (E1%, 1 cm 43).

Infra-red Absorption Spectrum. Amylocaine (base). Potassium bromide disk. The principal peaks are: A 1275, B 1710, C 710 or 1110 (p. 773).

Toxicity. Amylocaine has only about half the systemic toxicity of cocaine but is much more irritant. The minimum lethal subcutaneous dose in mice is 350 and in rabbits 178 mg/kg.

ANDROSTERONE *Androgen*

3α-Hydroxy-5α-androstan-17-one
$C_{19}H_{30}O_2 = 290{\cdot}5$

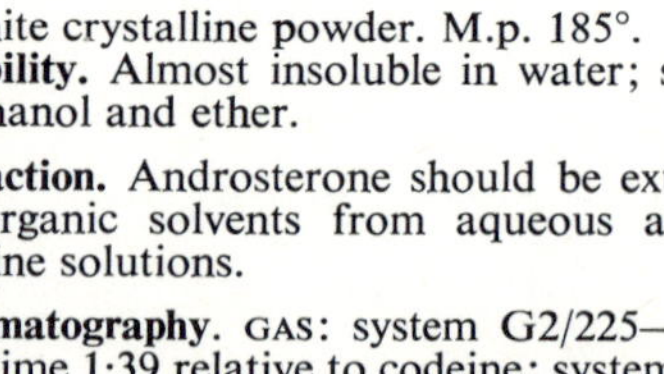

A white crystalline powder. M.p. 185°.
Solubility. Almost insoluble in water; soluble in ethanol and ether.

Extraction. Androsterone should be extracted by organic solvents from aqueous acid or alkaline solutions.

Chromatography. GAS: system G2/225—retention time 1·39 relative to codeine; system G4—retention time 1·7 relative to codeine.

Crystal Test. MICRO: *potassium tri-iodide solution (3)*—bundles of fine needles.

Quantitative Estimation. Androsterone may be estimated in urine by spectrophotometry (Pontius, 1962) and by gas chromatography (Sparagana *et al.*, 1962).

NOTE. Androsterone is a naturally occurring androgen which may be isolated from male urine. It is a major metabolite of testosterone.

ANILERIDINE *Narcotic Analgesic*

Proprietary Names: Alidine; Leritine.

Ethyl 1-*p*-aminophenethyl-4-phenylpiperidine-4-carboxylate

$C_{22}H_{28}N_2O_2 = 352{\cdot}5$

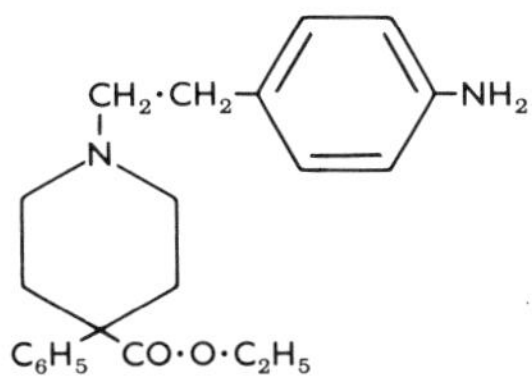

A white crystalline powder which oxidises and darkens in colour when exposed to light and air. It is polymorphic; one form melts at about 80° and another at about 89°.

Solubility. Very slightly soluble in water; soluble 1 in 2 of ethanol and 1 in 1 of chloroform; soluble in ether.

ANILERIDINE HYDROCHLORIDE

A white crystalline powder. M.p. about 270°, with decomposition.

Solubility. Freely soluble in water; sparingly soluble in ethanol; practically insoluble in ether and chloroform.

ANILERIDINE PHOSPHATE

A white crystalline powder.

Solubility. Freely soluble in water; solutions are unstable above pH 4.

Extraction. Anileridine may be isolated in the D2 fraction (see p. 27).

Chromatography. PAPER: system P1—Rf 0·22 (location under ultraviolet light, pale green fluorescence; location reagents: *iodoplatinate spray*, weak reaction; *potassium permanganate spray*, weak reaction).

THIN-LAYER: system T1—Rf 0·73 (location reagent *acidified iodoplatinate spray*, positive reaction).

GAS: system G1/250—retention time 2·44 relative to codeine.

Colour Tests. MICRO: sulphuric acid–formaldehyde test—orange, slowly (*sensitivity:* 1·0 μg); diazotisation test—red (*sensitivity:* 0·1 μg); *p*-dimethylaminobenzaldehyde test—yellow.

Ultraviolet Absorption Spectrum. Anileridine in 0·1N sulphuric acid, maximum at 258 mμ (E 1%, 1 cm 12·6); anileridine hydrochloride in *phosphate buffer* (pH 7·0), maxima at 234 mμ and 285 mμ.

Infra-red Absorption Spectrum. Anileridine (base). Potassium chloride disk. The principal peaks are: A 1700, B 1120, C 1179 or 1512 (p. 729).

Metabolism. In man, anileridine has been shown to be metabolised by two routes; it may be hydrolysed to anileridinic acid which undergoes acetylation and is excreted as acetylanileridinic acid and it may conjugate with acetic acid to yield acetylanileridine, part of which is excreted and part de-esterified to yield acetylanileridinic acid; in addition, an unidentified diazotisable substance has been found unconjugated in human urine. The following urinary excretion pattern of anileridine has been found in man after oral administration: 5% of the dose was excreted unchanged, 7 to 14% as free anileridinic acid, 1 to 2% as acetylanileridinic acid and 15 to 35% was accounted for as unidentified diazotisable substances (Way and Adler, 1962).

Dose. Up to 100 mg (base) by mouth, daily.

Toxicity. The estimated minimum lethal dose in man is 0·5 g but it may be up to 10 times greater in addicts. Anileridine has greater addiction-producing properties than pethidine.

ANILINE

Phenylamine

$C_6H_5{\cdot}NH_2 = 93{\cdot}13$

A colourless or slightly brown, oily liquid, which darkens on exposure to light and air. F.p. −6°. B.p. about 183°. Refractive index 1·5863.

Solubility. Soluble 1 in 40 of water; miscible with ethanol, ether, and chloroform.

Screening Test. See screening test for the metabolite, *p*-aminophenol, p. 14.

Extraction. Aniline is volatile and may be isolated by distillation.

Chromatography. PAPER: system P1—Rf 0·61 (location reagents: diazotisation followed by *alkaline betanaphthol spray*, red; p-*dimethylaminobenzaldehyde spray*, faint yellow).

THIN-LAYER: system T1—Rf 0.72 (location reagents: p-*dimethylaminobenzaldehyde spray*, bright yellow; *potassium permanganate spray*, positive reaction).

Colour Tests. Extract the aniline-containing distillate with ether, evaporate the latter at room temperature and mix the residue with 4 to 5 drops of *sulphuric acid.* Add 1 drop of a 7% aqueous solution of potassium dichromate —blue. Add aqueous calcium hypochlorite or sodium hypochlorite solution, drop by drop, to the test solution—violet-blue; sensitivity of this test 1 in 66,000.

MICRO: diazotisation test—red (*sensitivity:* 0·1 μg); Vitali's test—yellow/brown/brown (*sensitivity:* 0·5 μg).

Crystal Tests. MICRO: *gold bromide solution*—branching rods, forming overnight (*sensitivity:* 1 in 200); *picrolonic acid*—fine needles (*sensitivity:* 1 in 1000).

Ultraviolet Absorption Spectrum. Aniline in ethanol, maxima at 235 mμ (E 1%, 1 cm 1007) and 286 mμ (E 1%, 1 cm 179); in 0·1N hydrochloric acid, maxima at 249 mμ (E 1%, 1 cm 13), at 255 mμ (E 1%, 1 cm 16), and 261 mμ (E 1%, 1 cm 12·5).

Quantitative Estimation. Aniline may be estimated by the method of Bratton and Marshall (1939).

Metabolism. In man, the 2 major metabolites of aniline are *p*-aminophenol and paracetamol (*p*-acetamidophenol) which are both excreted in the urine in conjugated form. In rabbits, 3 to 4 days after administration of a dose of aniline, the following urinary excretion products have been found: 1% of the dose as free aniline, 6% as conjugated aniline, probably an *N*-glucuronide, 0·2% as acetanilide, 40% as conjugated *p*-aminophenol, and 7% as conjugated *o*-aminophenol; over 60% of the dose was excreted in the urine, only 3% being excreted in the faeces. The bulk of the metabolites was excreted 2 to 3 days after administration but traces of aniline and its metabolites remained in the body for a considerable length of time. The main toxic effect of aniline, the formation of methaemoglobin, is thought to be caused not by aniline itself but by an oxidation product (Brodie and Axelrod, 1949; Kiese, 1965). In cases of poisoning, both the blood and urine may become brownish-black in colour, due to the formation of methaemoglobin.

Aniline is readily absorbed from the skin and mucous membranes.

Toxicity. The lethal dose in man may be as low as 1 g, although recovery has followed the ingestion of 30 g. Serious disturbances may occur after exposure for about 1 hour to atmospheric concentrations of 100 to 160 p.p.m. The maximum permissible atmospheric concentration of aniline is 5 p.p.m.

LD50 (oral): in dogs 0·5 and in guinea-pigs 2·5 g/kg.

CASE EXAMPLE. A 21-year-old woman ingested about 80 ml of aniline. The blood and urine were chocolate-coloured. Nine hours after ingestion, haemodialysis was instituted and continued for about 7½ hours; just before dialysis the blood-level of aniline was 2·52%. Dialysis removed 1·3 g of aniline; 357 mg appeared in the urine over 4 days. The patient gradually recovered (Lubash *et al.*, 1964).

ANTAZOLINE *Antihistamine*

Synonyms: Imidamin; Phenazolinum.

2-(*N*-Benzylanilinomethyl)imidazoline

$C_{17}H_{19}N_3 = 265{\cdot}4$

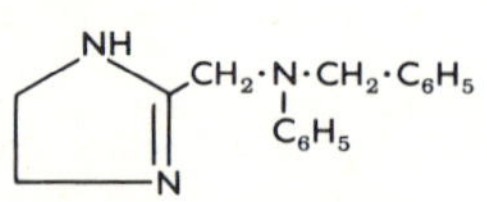

Antazoline melts at about 121°.

ANTAZOLINE HYDROCHLORIDE

Proprietary Names: Antistin; Histostab.

A white crystalline powder. M.p. about 240°, with decomposition.

Solubility. Soluble 1 in 50 of water and 1 in 16 of ethanol; almost insoluble in ether; slightly soluble in chloroform.

ANTAZOLINE MESYLATE

A white powder. M.p. 165° to 168°.

Solubility. Soluble 1 in 6 of water, 1 in 7 of ethanol, and 1 in 12 of chloroform; insoluble in ether.

ANTAZOLINE PHOSPHATE

A white crystalline powder. M.p. 194° to 198°, with decomposition.

Solubility. Soluble in water; almost insoluble in ether; sparingly soluble in methanol.

Extraction. Antazoline is extracted by organic solvents from aqueous alkaline solutions.

Chromatography. PAPER: system P1—Rf 0·74 (location under ultraviolet light, absorption; location reagents: *iodoplatinate spray*, strong reaction; *bromocresol green spray*, strong reaction); system RP1a—Rf 0·85 (location under ultraviolet light, absorption; location reagent *iodoplatinate spray*, positive reaction); system RP1b—Rf 0·52 (location under ultraviolet light, absorption).

THIN-LAYER: system T1—Rf 0·23 (location reagent *acidified iodoplatinate spray*, positive reaction); system T2—Rf 0·38 (location reagent *iodoplatinate spray*, positive reaction); system T3—Rf 0·31 (location as for T2).

GAS: system G1/250—retention time 0·89 relative to codeine; system G2/225—retention time 3·8 relative to diphenhydramine; system G3—retention time 6·60 relative to diphenhydramine; system G4—retention time 1·2 relative to diphenhydramine.

Colour Tests. MICRO: ammonium vanadate test—reddish-purple (*sensitivity:* 0·1 μg); Vitali's test—deep red/yellow-brown/brown-orange (*sensitivity:* 0·05 μg).

Crystal Tests. MICRO: *sodium carbonate solution*—needles (*sensitivity:* 1 in 100); *potassium cyanide solution*—needles and rods (*sensitivity:* 1 in 200).

Ultraviolet Absorption Spectrum. Antazoline hydrochloride in 0·1N hydrochloric acid, maxima at 241 mμ (E 1%, 1 cm 570) and 291 mμ (E 1%, 1 cm 76). Antazoline phosphate in water, maxima at about 241 mμ (E 1%, 1 cm about 410) and at about 292 mμ (E 1%, 1 cm about 50).

Dose. Usually 200 to 400 mg, but doses up to 600 mg have been given for short periods.

Toxicity. The estimated acute lethal dose in man is 25 to 250 mg/kg.

LD50 (oral): in mice 0·25 to 1 g/kg.

APOATROPINE

Synonyms: Atropamine; Atropoyltropeine.

Tropyl atropate

$C_{17}H_{21}NO_2 = 271{\cdot}4$

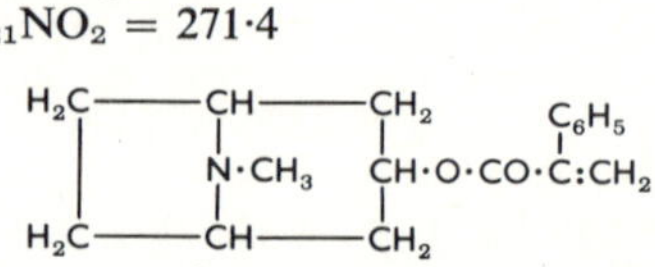

An alkaloid which has been obtained from the root of *Atropa belladonna* (Solanaceae). Apoatropine is formed during the racemisation of hyoscyamine to atropine.

It occurs as prisms from chloroform. M.p. 60° to 62°.
Solubility. Almost insoluble in water; freely soluble in ethanol, ether, and chloroform; soluble in dilute acetic acid.

Extraction. Apoatropine is extracted by organic solvents from aqueous alkaline solutions.

Chromatography. PAPER: system P1—Rf 0·51 (location under ultraviolet light, absorption; location reagent *iodoplatinate spray*, strong reaction).

THIN-LAYER: system T1—Rf 0·18 (location reagent *acidified iodoplatinate spray*, positive reaction).

GAS: system G2/225—retention time 1·75 relative to diphenhydramine; system G4—retention time 2·18 relative to diphenhydramine.

Colour Test. MICRO: Vitali's test— –/–/purple (*sensitivity:* 0·1 μg).

Crystal Tests. MICRO: *platinic chloride solution*—small blades and plates, often cruciform and serrated (*sensitivity:* 1 in 1000); *potassium triiodide solution* (*2*)—shell-like crystals (*sensitivity:* 1 in 400).

Infra-red Absorption Spectrum. Potassium bromide disk. The principal peaks are: A 1190 or 1710, B 1025 (p. 773).

Toxicity. Similar to Atropine, p. 203.
LD50 (oral): in mice 160 mg/kg.

APOMORPHINE *Emetic and Expectorant*

$C_{17}H_{17}NO_2$ = 267·3

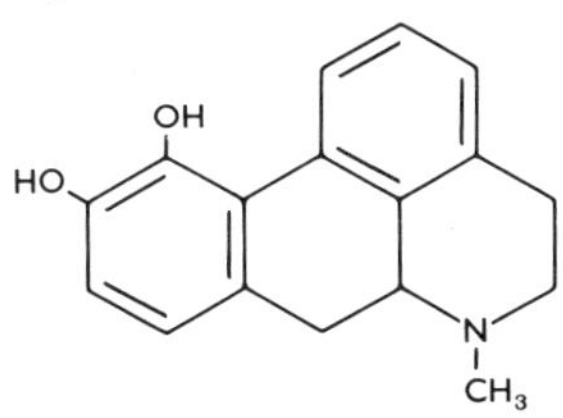

It occurs as hexagonal plates from chloroform and petroleum ether. The crystals and aqueous solutions oxidise rapidly in light and air, turning green. M.p. about 195°, with decomposition.
Solubility. Slightly soluble in water and ether; soluble in ethanol and chloroform.

APOMORPHINE HYDROCHLORIDE
Colourless glistening microcrystals. Decomposes between 225° and 236°.
Solubility. Soluble 1 in 50 of water and 1 in 50 of ethanol; sparingly soluble in ether and chloroform.

Extraction. Apomorphine may be isolated in the D3 fraction (see p. 27); hydrolysis of biological material is required in order to improve the yield.

Chromatography. PAPER: system P1—Rf 0·33 (location under ultraviolet light, blue fluorescence; location reagents: *iodoplatinate spray*, strong reaction; *bromocresol green spray*, strong reaction); system RP1a—Rf 0·55 (location under ultraviolet light, bluish-brown fluorescence; location reagent *iodoplatinate spray*, positive reaction); system RP1b—Rf 0·11 (location as for RP1a).

THIN-LAYER: system T1—Rf 0·57 (location reagent *acidified iodoplatinate spray*, positive reaction).

GAS: system G6—retention time 1·28 relative to codeine.

Colour Tests. MICRO: sulphuric acid–formaldehyde test—purple → black (*sensitivity:* 0·05 μg); ammonium molybdate test—deep green → blue-green (*sensitivity:* 0·1 μg).

Crystal Tests. MICRO: *gold bromide solution*—serrated crosses (*sensitivity:* 1 in 5000); *potassium bismuth iodide solution*—rosettes of dark needles (*sensitivity:* 1 in 5000).

Ultraviolet Absorption Spectrum. Apomorphine in 0·1N sulphuric acid, maximum at 273 mμ (E1%, 1 cm 741) and an inflexion at about 305 mμ (E1%, 1 cm 144).

Infra-red Absorption Spectrum. Apomorphine (base). Potassium bromide disk. The principal peaks are: A 1265, B 1460, C 752 or 790 or 985 (p. 773).

Quantitative Estimation. Apomorphine is usually excreted as a conjugate; therefore, prior to estimation, urine or homogenised tissue must be refluxed with 9N hydrochloric acid for 20 minutes. The solution is then neutralised, extracted with ethyl acetate, and back-extracted with 0·05N hydrochloric acid. An aliquot of the extract is oxidised at pH 6 with saturated mercuric chloride solution and the green oxidation product is extracted into isoamyl acetate where it turns violet. The product is determined spectrophotometrically at 330 mμ. The method gives 70 to 90% recoveries; as little as 0·01 mg% may be determined (Kaul *et al.*, 1961a).

Metabolism. Following injection into horses, rabbits, and rats, apomorphine is excreted in the urine largely as conjugates which yield the free drug on hydrolysis. The excretion of a small percentage in the free form appears to be dependent on the pH of the urine (Kaul *et al.*, 1961a). The conjugates have been found to be 2 glucuronides, 70% being apomorphine-3-*O*-*β*-glucuronide and 30% being apomorphine-4-*O*-*β*-glucuronide. The former conjugate has an ultraviolet maximum at 270 mμ instead of 272 mμ and in alkali this maximum shifts to 330 mμ; the latter conjugate has an ultraviolet maximum at 267 mμ and undergoes the same shift of maximum in alkali (Kaul *et al.*, 1961b).

Dose. Up to 8 mg, subcutaneously or intramuscularly.

Toxicity. The estimated minimum lethal dose in man is 100 mg.

LD50 (intravenous): in dogs 60 to 100 mg/kg.

APROBARBITONE *Barbiturate*

Synonyms: Allylisopropylmalonylurea; Allypropymal; Aprobarbital.
Proprietary Names: Allonal; Alurate; Numal.

5-Allyl-5-isopropylbarbituric acid

$C_{10}H_{14}N_2O_3 = 210{\cdot}2$

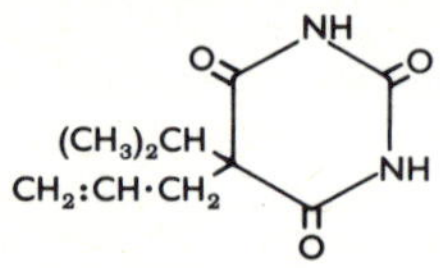

A fine white crystalline powder. M.p. 141·5° to 143·5°.

Solubility. Soluble 1 in 350 of water, 1 in 30 of boiling water, 1 in 2·5 of ethanol, 1 in 5 of ether, and 1 in 40 of chloroform.

APROBARBITONE SODIUM
Proprietary Name: Alurate Sodium.

A white hygroscopic microcrystalline powder.
Solubility. Very soluble in water; very slightly soluble in ethanol; almost insoluble in ether.

Screening Test. See under Barbiturates, p. 208.

Extraction. Aprobarbitone may be isolated in the A2 fraction (see p. 27).

Chromatography. PAPER: system P4—Rf 0·29 (location reagent *silver nitrate spray*, white); system RP1b—Rf 0·24 (location under ultraviolet light after exposure to ammonia; location reagent *potassium permanganate spray*, yellow on pink).

THIN-LAYER: system T10—Rf 0·30 (location reagents: *mercurous nitrate spray*, black; *potassium permanganate spray*, yellow-brown on purple; *Zwikker's reagent spray*, pink).

GAS: system G5—retention time 1·62 relative to barbitone; system G7—retention time 1·54 relative to barbitone.

Colour Test. Zwikker's test—violet-blue.

Ultraviolet Absorption Spectrum. Aprobarbitone is a 5,5-derivative—see Screening Test 3 under Barbiturates, p. 208.

Infra-red Absorption Spectrum. Aprobarbitone. Potassium bromide disk. The principal peaks are: A 1689 or 1715, B 1439, C 1376 (p. 730).

Quantitative Estimation. See under Barbiturates, p. 208.

Metabolism. Aprobarbitone is an intermediate-acting barbiturate—see under Barbiturates, p. 207. It is slowly eliminated from the body. Maximum plasma concentrations were reached 3 to 9 hours after a single 750-mg oral dose of aprobarbitone; the plasma level decreased by 40 to 70% within the first 24 hours; between 55 and 70% of aprobarbitone in the plasma was estimated to be protein-bound; after 4 to 8 days a total of 9 to 18% of the dose had been excreted unchanged in the urine (Lous, 1954). Following a single 150-mg oral dose of aprobarbitone, 1·1% of the dose was excreted unchanged after 9 hours, 2·3% after 24 hours, and 8·1% after 48 hours; these low recoveries indicate that a major portion of aprobarbitone may be metabolised to substances which have not yet been detected (Svendsen and Brochmann-Hanssen, 1962).

Dose. Maximum single or daily dose 300 mg.

Toxicity. The estimated minimum lethal dose in man is 2 g.

LD50 (subcutaneous): in rats 100 mg/kg.

CASE EXAMPLES. Fifty cases of severe acute aprobarbitone poisoning are reported. An ingested dose of 100 mg/kg gave an average serum concentration of 12 to 14 mg% of aprobarbitone after 24 hours; a serum concentration of 10 mg% 24 hours after ingestion was found to lead to unconsciousness for about 100 hours (Lous, 1954).

APRONAL *Hypnotic*

Synonyms: Allylisopropylacetylurea; Apronalide.
Proprietary Name: Sedormid.

N-(2-Isopropylpent-4-enoyl)urea

$C_9H_{16}N_2O_2 = 184{\cdot}2$

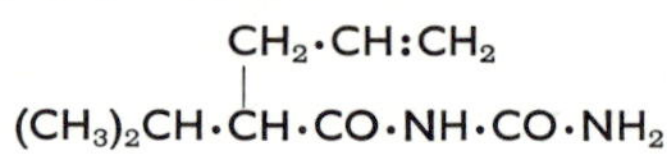

Colourless crystals or white crystalline powder. M.p. 194°.

Solubility. Soluble 1 in 4000 of cold water, 1 in 250 of boiling water, 1 in 40 of ethanol, 1 in 80 of ether, and 1 in 60 of chloroform.

Extraction. Apronal is extracted by organic solvents from aqueous acid or alkaline solutions.

Chromatography. PAPER: system RP1b—Rf 0·35 (location reagent *bromine–starch–potassium iodide*).

GAS: system G5—retention time 0·37 relative to barbitone.

Ultraviolet Absorption Spectrum. Apronal in 0·1N sodium hydroxide, inflexion at 232 mμ (E1%, 1 cm 16); in 0·1N sulphuric acid, inflexion at 227 mμ (E1%, 1 cm 240).

Infra-red Absorption Spectrum. Potassium bromide disk. The principal peaks are: A 1676, B 1416 or 1704, C 1092 (p. 730).

Dose. Maximum daily dose 750 mg.

Toxicity. The estimated minimum lethal dose in man is 15 g but death has occurred after ingestion of 13 g.

LD50 (oral): in mice 600 mg/kg.

ARECOLINE *Purgative/Taenifuge (Veterinary)*
Methyl 1-methyl-1,2,5,6-tetrahydropyridine-3-carboxylate
$C_8H_{13}NO_2$ = 155·2

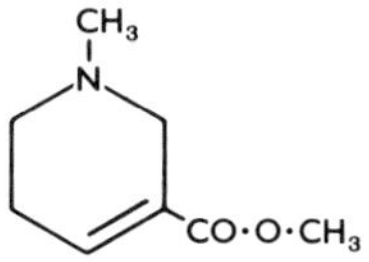

An alkaloid obtained from the seeds of *Areca catechu* (Palmae).
An oily liquid which is a strong base. B.p. 209°.
Solubility. Miscible with water, ethanol, ether, and chloroform.

ARECOLINE HYDROBROMIDE
A white crystalline powder, unstable in light. M.p. 172° to 175°.
Solubility. Soluble 1 in 1 of water and 1 in 10 of ethanol; slightly soluble in ether and chloroform.

Extraction. Arecoline is volatile and may be isolated by distillation from alkaline solutions (see p. 19).

Chromatography. PAPER: system P1—Rf 0·15 (location under ultraviolet light, absorption; location reagent *iodoplatinate spray*, strong reaction).
THIN-LAYER: system T1—Rf 0·53 (location reagent *potassium permanganate spray*, positive reaction).

Crystal Tests. MICRO: *picric acid*—small dense rosettes (*sensitivity:* 1 in 400); *potassium bismuth iodide solution*—red rhomboids (*sensitivity:* 1 in 3000).

Ultraviolet Absorption Spectrum. Arecoline in ethanol, maximum at 214 mμ (E 1%, 1 cm 444).

Infra-red Absorption Spectrum. Arecoline (base). Potassium chloride disk. The principal peaks are: A 1712, B 1262, C 1135 (p. 774).

Dose. In horses, up to 60 mg subcutaneously; in dogs, up to 15 mg by mouth.

Toxicity. The use of arecoline as a veterinary anthelmintic has caused numerous fatalities in cats and dogs.
LD50 (subcutaneous): in dogs 5 and in mice 100 mg/kg.

ASCORBIC ACID *Vitamin*
Synonyms: L-Ascorbic Acid; Cevitamic Acid; Vitamin C.
Proprietary Names: Ascorvel; Proscorbin; Redoxon.

Enolic form of 3-oxo-L-gulofuranolactone
$C_6H_8O_6$ = 176·1

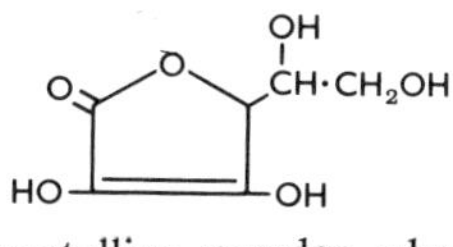

A white crystalline powder whose solutions deteriorate rapidly in air, particularly those in an alkaline medium. M.p. 190° to 192°, with decomposition.
Solubility. Soluble 1 in 4 of water and 1 in 30 of ethanol; insoluble in ether and chloroform.

Colour Tests. A solution decolorises *2,6-dichlorophenolindophenol solution*; a solution immediately reduces a 5% silver nitrate solution to a black precipitate.

Ultraviolet Absorption Spectrum. Ascorbic acid in water, maximum at 264 mμ (E 1%, 1 cm 579); ascorbic acid in 0·01 N sulphuric acid, maximum at 245 mμ (E 1%, 1 cm 560).

Quantitative Estimation. Ascorbic acid may be estimated by the reduction of the redox dye, 2,6-dichlorophenolindophenol (Hughes, 1964) or by the reduction of mercuric chloride to mercurous chloride (Kum-Tatt and Leong, 1964).

Metabolism. Ascorbic acid is readily absorbed and metabolised. However, after oral administration of large quantities, only small amounts are excreted in the urine while there is a steady rise in the level of ascorbic acid in the plasma. If the oral ingestion is continued for a sufficient period, the plasma concentration rises to a maximum, after which a rapid urinary excretion of a large part of the ingested ascorbic acid occurs (FAO/WHO Expert Committee on Food Additives, Sixth Report, 1962).

Human Requirements. The minimum daily requirement of ascorbic acid in adults is estimated to be between 10 and 30 mg daily, the normal blood-level being 0·4 to 1·5 mg%. It is estimated that the daily dietary intake is between 30 and 100 mg. The usual therapeutic dose is 200 to 500 mg daily.

Toxicity. LD50 (oral): in mice, rats, and guinea-pigs, greater than 5 g/kg.
The safety of large doses of ascorbic acid over long periods of time has not been unequivocally demonstrated.

ASPIRIN *Analgesic and Antipyretic*
Synonym: Acetylsalicylic Acid.
Proprietary Names: Asagran; Aspro; Genasprin. Aspirin is an ingredient of many proprietary preparations—see Extra Pharmacopoeia (Martindale), 25th Edn, p. 32.

o-Acetoxybenzoic acid
$C_9H_8O_4$ = 180·2

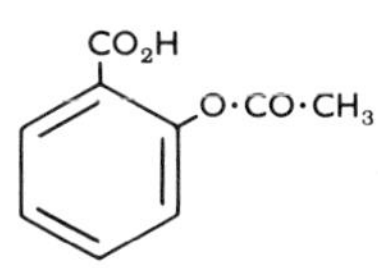

A white crystalline powder which is stable in dry air but hydrolysed by water to salicylic and acetic acids. M.p. 136°.
Solubility. Soluble 1 in 300 of water, 1 in 7 of ethanol, 1 in 20 of ether, and 1 in 17 of chloroform.

Screening Test. *Ferric chloride solution* with urine—blue-violet, after hydrolysis (see p. 8).

Extraction. Aspirin is found, usually as salicylic acid, in the A1 fraction (see p. 27).

Chromatography. PAPER: system P12—Rf 0·52 (aspirin is hydrolysed by the alkaline solvent system to salicylic acid; location under ultraviolet light, moderate blue fluorescence; location reagent *ferric chloride spray*, violet).

THIN-LAYER: system T17—Rf 0·50 (location under ultraviolet light).

GAS: system G5—retention time 0·36 relative to barbitone.

Colour Tests. *Trinder's reagent*—purple, after hydrolysis. McNally's test—red.

Ultraviolet Absorption Spectrum. Aspirin in 0·1N sulphuric acid, maxima at 229 mμ (E1%, 1 cm 484) and 276 mμ (E1%, 1 cm 65·5).

Infra-red Absorption Spectrum. Potassium bromide disk. The principal peaks are: A 1183, B 1688, C 1305 (p. 730).

Quantitative Estimation. Aspirin may be estimated as salicylic acid by the spectrophotometric methods of Trinder (1954) or Stevenson (1960)—see under Salicylic Acid, p. 539. Cotty and Ederma (1966) have described a spectrofluorimetric method of determination of aspirin in the presence of salicylic acid directly applicable to blood samples. Rowland and Riegelman (1967) have described a gas chromatographic method.

Metabolism. Aspirin appears to be absorbed intact from the gastro-intestinal tract and persists in the blood for a short time in the unhydrolysed form; 10 minutes after ingestion 50% of the blood-salicylate is in the acetylated form; after 20 minutes this has dropped to 30% (Cotty *et al.*, 1965).

Normal therapeutic blood-levels do not usually exceed 5 mg%; a dosage of 4 to 8 g daily will give a serum salicylate level of 18 to 20 mg% but the high doses given in the treatment of rheumatoid arthritis may give rise to a level of 25 mg%. A single dose of 12 g may produce a level of 35 mg% together with symptoms of acute poisoning within a few hours. The rate of excretion of aspirin varies with the pH of the urine, increasing as the pH rises. One and a half hours after ingestion, 1·5% of the dose may be found unchanged in the urine. The remainder is hydrolysed to salicylic acid which is excreted partly unchanged, partly as glucuronide conjugates and partly after conversion to salicyluric and gentisic acids; these metabolites may be separated by the chromatographic systems P12 and T17 (see pp. 39 and 55).

Dose. Usually up to 1 g; in acute rheumatism, up to 8 g daily.

Toxicity. The estimated lethal dose in man is in the range 5 to 15 g. A serum salicylate level above 30 mg% is usually indicative of poisoning by aspirin. An important toxic effect which may occur even with small doses is irritation of the gastric mucosa leading to gastro-duodenal bleeding.

LD50 (oral): in guinea-pigs 1·2, in mice 1·2, and in rats 1·2 g/kg.

CASE EXAMPLES. *Chronic Salicylate Intoxication.* (1) A 59-year-old man estimated that within 15 days he had taken 227 g of aspirin; on examination on the 15th day, the serum salicylate level was 61 mg%; he recovered. (2) A 31-year-old woman, who admitted to taking 20 to 25 aspirin tablets daily for several months and to having increased the intake to as much as 16 g per day several weeks prior to admission to hospital, was found to have a serum salicylate level, 49 hours after the last possible ingestion of salicylates, of 48 mg%; she recovered (Greer, 1965).

ATROPINE *Parasympatholytic*

Synonym: (±)-Hyoscyamine.

(±)-Tropyl tropate

$C_{17}H_{23}NO_3 = 289{\cdot}4$

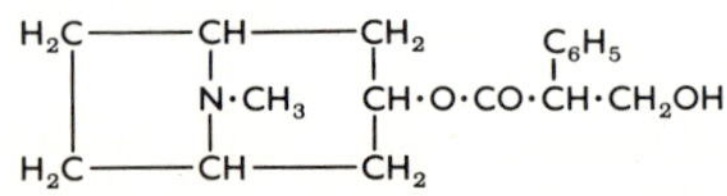

An alkaloid obtained from various solanaceous plants or prepared synthetically. It may be differentiated from hyoscyamine by the shape of the crystals obtained with *potassium triiodide solution* (*3*)—see Microcrystal Tests, p. 140.

A white crystalline powder. M.p. 115° to 118°.

Solubility. Soluble 1 in 400 of water, 1 in 50 of boiling water, 1 in 3 of ethanol, 1 in 60 of ether, and 1 in 1 of chloroform.

ATROPINE SULPHATE

Colourless crystals or a white crystalline powder which effloresces in dry air. M.p. of the anhydrous salt, 191° to 196°.

Solubility. Soluble 1 in less than 1 of water and 1 in 4 of ethanol; insoluble in ether and chloroform.

Extraction. Atropine may be isolated in the D2 fraction (see p. 27).

Chromatography. PAPER: system P1—Rf 0·37 (location under ultraviolet light, absorption; location reagents: *iodoplatinate spray*, strong reaction; *bromocresol green spray*, weak reaction); system RP1a—Rf 0·94 (location reagent *iodoplatinate spray*, positive reaction).

THIN-LAYER: system T1—Rf 0·18 (location reagent *acidified iodoplatinate spray*, positive reaction).

GAS: system G1/180—retention time 3·22 relative to diphenhydramine; system G3—retention time 3·80 relative to diphenhydramine; system G6—retention time 0·59 relative to codeine.

Colour Test. MICRO: Vitali's test— –/–/purple (*sensitivity:* 0·025 μg).

Crystal Tests. MICRO: *picric acid*—bunches of plates (*sensitivity:* 1 in 400); *potassium triiodide solution* (*3*)—irregular hexagons in clusters and bundles (*sensitivity:* 1 in 1000).

Ultraviolet Absorption Spectrum. Atropine in 0·1N sulphuric acid, maxima at 252 mμ (E 1%, 1 cm 5), 258 mμ (E 1%, 1 cm 6), and 264 mμ (E 1%, 1 cm 5).

Infra-red Absorption Spectrum. Atropine (base). Potassium bromide disk. The principal peaks are: A 1720, B 1035, C 1153 (p. 730).

Metabolism. Atropine is readily absorbed from mucous membranes, the skin, and the intestinal tract, but not from the stomach; absorption from the intestinal tract is complete in 2 hours. About one-half of the atropine circulates in the free form in the blood and the other half is bound by the plasma proteins. The metabolism of atropine varies considerably from one species to another. Hydrolysis to tropine and tropic acid is not thought to be a major metabolic route since only traces of tropic acid are recovered in the urine.

Following the intramuscular administration of single 2-mg doses of ^{14}C-labelled atropine in man, 85 to 88% of the radioactivity was excreted in the urine within 24 hours, no activity was found in the expired air, and only a trace could be extracted from the faeces; about 50% of the dose appeared in the urine unchanged, over 30% was excreted as unknown metabolites, and less than 2% appeared as free tropic acid (Gosselin *et al.*, 1960).

Dose. Up to 2 mg by mouth or by injection.

Toxicity. As little as 3 mg of atropine sulphate has proved fatal in susceptible individuals; 50 mg may be fatal in an average case, although recovery has occurred even after 1 g.

ATROPINE METHOBROMIDE

Parasympatholytic

Synonyms: Atropine Methylbromide; Methylatropine Bromide; Methylatropinium Bromide; Mydriasine.

N-Methylatropine bromide

$C_{18}H_{26}BrNO_3 = 384{\cdot}3$

A white crystalline powder. M.p. 222° to 223°.

Solubility. Soluble 1 in 1 of water and 1 in 8 of ethanol (90%); almost insoluble in ether and chloroform.

Extraction. Atropine methobromide is a quaternary ammonium compound (see p. 29).

Chromatography. As for Atropine Methonitrate.

Colour Test. As for Atropine Methonitrate.

Crystal Tests. As for Atropine Methonitrate.

Ultraviolet Absorption Spectrum. As for Atropine Methonitrate.

Infra-red Absorption Spectrum. Potassium bromide disk. The principal peaks are: A 1377, B 1718, C 1104 or 1150 (p. 774).

ATROPINE METHONITRATE

Parasympatholytic

Synonyms: Atropine Methylnitrate; Methylatropine Nitrate; Methylatropinium Nitrate.

Proprietary Names: Eumydrin; Harvatrate; Metanite; Metropine; Pylostropin.

N-Methylatropine nitrate

$C_{18}H_{26}N_2O_6 = 366{\cdot}4$

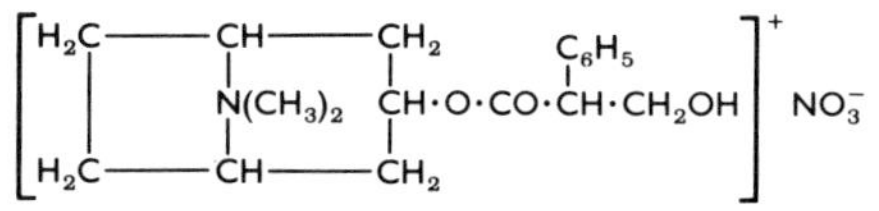

Colourless crystals. Aqueous solutions are unstable but alcoholic solutions are stable for 12 months. M.p. 166° to 168°.

Solubility. Soluble 1 in less than 1 of water and 1 in 13 of ethanol; insoluble in ether and chloroform.

Extraction. Atropine methonitrate is a quaternary ammonium compound (see p. 29).

Chromatography. PAPER: system P1—Rf 0·25 (location under ultraviolet light, absorption; location reagent *iodoplatinate spray*, strong reaction); system RP1a—Rf 0·98 (location reagent *iodoplatinate spray*, positive reaction); system RP1b—Rf 0·95 (location as for RP1a). THIN-LAYER: system T1—Rf 0·02 (location reagent *acidified iodoplatinate spray*, positive reaction).

Colour Test. MICRO: Vitali's test— -/-/purple (*sensitivity:* 0·025 μg).

Crystal Tests. MICRO: *gold chloride solution*—leaflike plates, best viewed under polarised light (*sensitivity:* 1 in 3000); *mercuric chloride solution*—plates and prisms (*sensitivity:* 1 in 1000).

Ultraviolet Absorption Spectrum. Atropine methonitrate in 1N sulphuric acid, maxima at 251 mμ (E 1%, 1 cm 4·3), 257 mμ (E 1%, 1 cm 5·2), and 263 mμ (E 1%, 1 cm 3·9).

ATROPINE *N*-OXIDE *Parasympatholytic*

Proprietary Name: Genatropine is the hydrochloride.

$C_{17}H_{23}NO_4 = 305{\cdot}4$

Chromatography. PAPER: system P1—Rf 0·40 (location reagent *iodoplatinate spray*, strong reaction).

THIN-LAYER: system T1—Rf 0·21 (location reagent *acidified iodoplatinate spray*, positive reaction).

Colour Test. MICRO: Vitali's test— -/-/purple (*sensitivity:* 0·025 μg).

Crystal Test. MICRO: *potassium bismuth iodide solution*—rectangular plates (*sensitivity:* 1 in 3000).

Ultraviolet Absorption Spectrum. Atropine *N*-oxide in 0·1N sulphuric acid, maxima at 252 mμ, 258 mμ, and 264 mμ.

Toxicity. Atropine *N*-oxide is stated to be much less toxic and better tolerated than atropine.

AZACOSTEROL *Anticholesteraemic*

Synonym: SC 12937.

17β-{[3-(Dimethylamino)propyl]methylamino} androst-5-en-3β-ol

$C_{25}H_{44}N_2O = 388{\cdot}6$

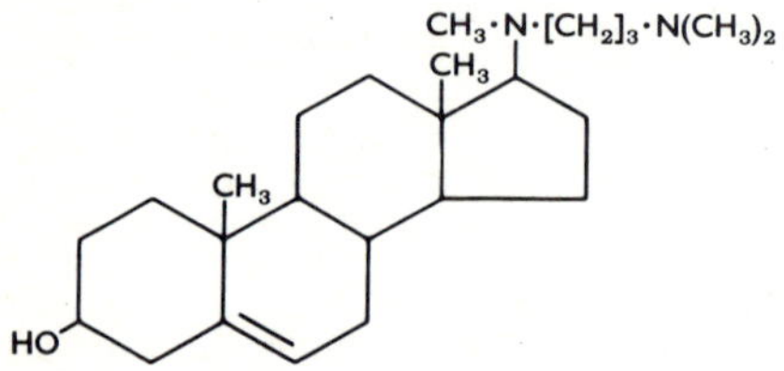

Extraction. Azacosterol is extracted by organic solvents from aqueous alkaline solutions.

Chromatography. PAPER: system P1—Rf 0·18 (location reagents: *iodoplatinate spray*, strong reaction; *bromocresol green spray*, weak reaction; *potassium permanganate spray*, weak reaction); system RP1a—Rf 0·72 (location reagent *iodoplatinate spray*, positive reaction); system RP1b—Rf 0·00 (location as for RP1a). THIN-LAYER: system T1—Rf 0·12 (location reagent *acidified iodoplatinate spray*, positive reaction).

Colour Tests. MICRO: sulphuric acid–formaldehyde test—brown-orange (*sensitivity:* 0·1 μg); ammonium molybdate test—dull orange → green (*sensitivity:* 0·1 μg); ammonium vanadate test—orange → blue (*sensitivity:* 0·1 μg).

Crystal Test. MICRO: *gold cyanide solution*—rosettes of plates (*sensitivity:* 1 in 1000).

Infra-red Absorption Spectrum. Potassium bromide disk. The principal peaks are: A 1065, B 1455, C 1345 (p. 774).

AZACYCLONOL *Tranquilliser*

Synonym: MER-17.

αα-Diphenyl-α-piperid-4-ylmethanol

$C_{18}H_{21}NO = 267{\cdot}4$

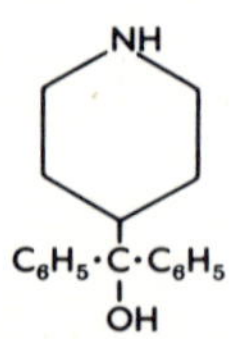

AZACYCLONOL HYDROCHLORIDE

Proprietary Name: Frenquel.

Small white crystals or powder. M.p. 270° to 281°.
Solubility. Soluble 1 in 200 of water and 1 in 1000 of ethanol; almost insoluble in ether and chloroform.

Extraction. Azacyclonol is extracted by organic solvents from aqueous alkaline solutions.

Chromatography. PAPER: system P1—Rf 0·60 (location reagents: *iodoplatinate spray*, weak reaction; *bromocresol green spray*, weak reaction). THIN-LAYER: system T1—Rf 0·15 (location reagent *acidified iodoplatinate spray*, positive reaction). GAS: system G2/225—retention time 0·70 relative to codeine.

Colour Tests. MICRO: sulphuric acid–formaldehyde test—deep yellow; ammonium molybdate test—deep yellow → green; Vitali's test—yellow flash/–/–.

Crystal Tests. MICRO: *picric acid*—dendrites (*sensitivity:* 1 in 400); *potassium iodide solution*—blades (*sensitivity:* 1 in 400).

Ultraviolet Absorption Spectrum. Azacyclonol in 0·1N sulphuric acid, maxima at 253·5 mμ (E1%, 1cm 16) and 259 mμ (E1%, 1cm 17).

Infra-red Absorption Spectrum. Azacyclonol (base). Potassium bromide disk. The principal peaks are: A 700, B 745, C 1445 (p. 774).

Dose. Up to 300 mg daily.
Azacyclonol does not produce any sedative or hypnotic effects even in large doses.

Toxicity. The lethal dose in man is probably between 100 and 500 mg/kg.

AZAMETHONIUM BROMIDE *Antihypertensive*

Synonyms: Ciba 9295; Pentamethazene Bromide; Pentamin.
Proprietary Name: Pendiomide.

3-Methyl-3-azapentamethylenebis(ethyldimethylammonium bromide)

$C_{13}H_{33}Br_2N_3 = 391{\cdot}3$

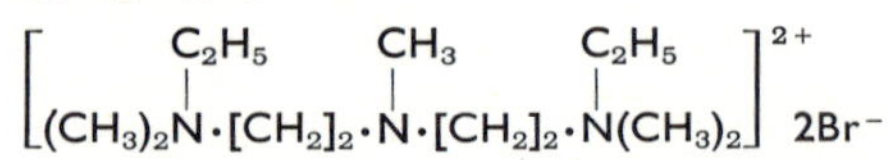

A white hygroscopic crystalline powder. M.p. 212° to 215°.
Solubility. Soluble in water and ethanol; almost insoluble in ether.

Extraction. Azamethonium bromide is a quaternary ammonium compound (see p. 29).

Chromatography. PAPER: system P1—Rf 0·02 (location under ultraviolet light, absorption; location reagents: *iodoplatinate spray*, strong reaction; *bromocresol green spray*, weak reaction; *potassium permanganate spray*, weak reaction); system RP1a—Rf 1·00 (location reagent *iodoplatinate spray*, positive reaction); system RP1b—Rf 1·00 (location as for RP1a). THIN-LAYER: system T1—Rf 0·00 (location reagent *acidified iodoplatinate spray*, positive reaction).

Crystal Tests. MICRO: *mercuric chloride solution*—small needles (*sensitivity:* 1 in 1000); *trinitrobenzoic acid solution*—fans of needles (*sensitivity:* 1 in 1000).

Infra-red Absorption Spectrum. Potassium bromide disk. The principal peaks are: A 1477, B 1014, C 968 or 1620 (p. 774).

Toxicity. LD50 (oral): in mice 2·5 g/kg.

AZAPETINE *Vasodilator*

Synonyms: Azephine; Azepine; Ro 2-3248.

6-Allyl-6,7-dihydro-5*H*-dibenz[*c,e*]azepine

$C_{17}H_{17}N = 235{\cdot}3$

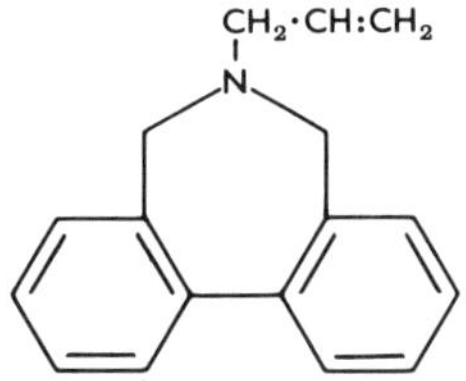

AZAPETINE PHOSPHATE

Proprietary Name: Ilidar.

Solubility. Soluble at least 1 in 100 of water.

Extraction. Azapetine is extracted by organic solvents from aqueous alkaline solutions.

Chromatography. PAPER: system P1—Rf 0·64 (location under ultraviolet light, blue fluorescence; location reagent *iodoplatinate spray*, strong reaction); system RP1a—Rf 0·20 (location under ultraviolet light, pale blue fluorescence; location reagent *iodoplatinate spray*, positive reaction); system RP1b—Rf 0·00.
THIN-LAYER: system T1—Rf 0·72 (location reagent *acidified iodoplatinate spray*, positive reaction).
GAS: system G2/225—retention time 1·30 relative to diphenhydramine.

Colour Tests. MICRO: ammonium molybdate test—blue-green (*sensitivity:* 0·1 μg); ammonium vanadate test—brown (*sensitivity:* 0·1 μg).

Crystal Tests. MICRO: *platinic bromide solution*—bunches of leaflike plates (*sensitivity:* 1 in 1000); *trinitrobenzoic acid solution*—dense rosettes (*sensitivity:* 1 in 1000).

Ultraviolet Absorption Spectrum. Azapetine in 0·1N sulphuric acid, maximum at 248 mμ (E1%, 1 cm 482).

Infra-red Absorption Spectrum. Azapetine (base). Potassium bromide disk. The principal peaks are: A 748, B 918, C 1440 (p. 774).

Dose. Up to 300 mg (base) daily.

Toxicity. LD50 (intravenous): in dogs 50, in mice 26, and in rabbits 26·5 mg/kg.

AZATHIOPRINE *Antineoplastic*

Synonym: BW 57322.
Proprietary Name: Imuran.

6-(1-Methyl-4-nitroimidazol-5-ylthio)purine

$C_9H_7N_7O_2S = 277{\cdot}3$

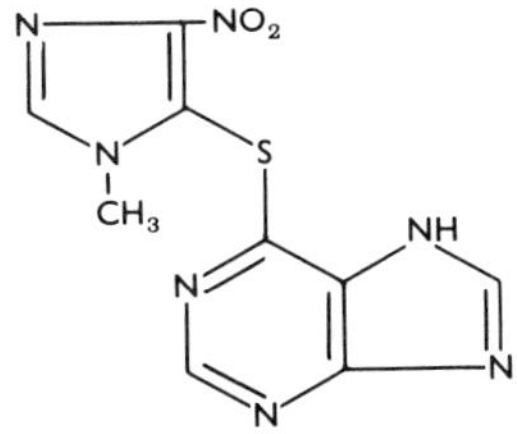

Azathioprine melts at about 246°.

Solubility. Insoluble in water; soluble in sodium hydroxide solution; slightly soluble in dilute hydrochloric acid.

Ultraviolet Absorption Spectrum. Azathioprine in 0·1N hydrochloric acid, maximum at 281 mμ (E1%, 1 cm 602); minimum at 246 mμ.

Metabolism. Azathioprine is split readily *in vitro* by sulphydryl compounds such as glutathione, and by strong alkali, to form 6-mercaptopurine. This transformation also takes place *in vivo*. About half the dose is excreted in the urine within 24 hours as the original compound and its metabolites, including 6-mercaptopurine.

Dose. Usually 2 to 5 mg/kg daily; up to 12 mg/kg daily has been given.

AZINPHOS-METHYL *Pesticide*

Synonyms: Bayer 17147; DBD.
Proprietary Names: Gusathion; Guthion.

S-(3,4-Dihydro-4-oxo-1,2,3-benzotriazin-3-ylmethyl)dimethyl phosphorothiolothionate

$C_{10}H_{12}N_3O_3PS_2 = 317{\cdot}3$

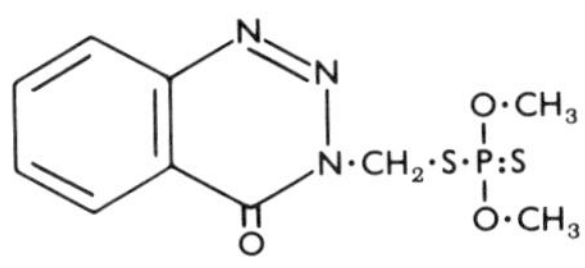

Azinphos-methyl occurs as crystals. M.p. 73° to 74°.

Solubility. Soluble 1 in 30,000 of water; soluble in ethanol.

Chromatography. THIN-LAYER: system T15—Rf 0·14 (location reagent *palladium chloride spray*); system T16—Rf 0·40 (location reagent *bromophenol blue spray* followed by *5% aqueous acetic acid spray*, blue).

Toxicity. LD50 (oral): in rats 20 mg/kg.

BAMETHAN *Vasodilator*
2-Butylamino-1-*p*-hydroxyphenylethanol
$C_{12}H_{19}NO_2 = 209{\cdot}3$

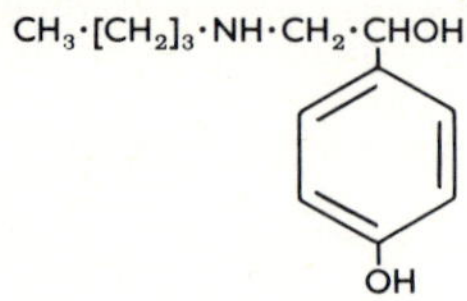

Bamethan melts at 123·5° to 125°.

BAMETHAN SULPHATE
Proprietary Names: Vasculat; Vasculit.
Solubility. Soluble in water.

Extraction. Bamethan is extracted by organic solvents from aqueous alkaline solutions.

Chromatography. PAPER: system P1—Rf 0·60 (location under ultraviolet light, absorption).
THIN-LAYER: system T1—Rf 0·58 (location reagent *potassium permanganate spray*, positive reaction).

Colour Tests. Chen's test—purple.
MICRO: ammonium molybdate test—greenish-brown (*sensitivity:* 1·0 µg); ammonium vanadate test—blue → green (*sensitivity:* 1·0 µg); Vitali's test—faint yellow/yellow/bright orange (*sensitivity:* 0·5 µg).

Crystal Test. MICRO: *gold bromide solution*—stout needles (*sensitivity:* 1 in 400).

Infra-red Absorption Spectrum. Bamethan (base). Potassium bromide disk. The principal peaks are: A 832 or 1228, B 1066, C 1108 or 1264 or 1494 (p. 774).

Dose. Usually up to 125 mg daily.

Toxicity. LD50 (subcutaneous): in mice 300 mg/kg.

BAMIFYLLINE *Xanthine Derivative*
8 - Benzyl - 7 - [2 - (*N* - ethyl - *N* - 2 - hydroxyethylamino)ethyl]-1,3-dimethylxanthine
$C_{20}H_{27}N_5O_3 = 385{\cdot}5$

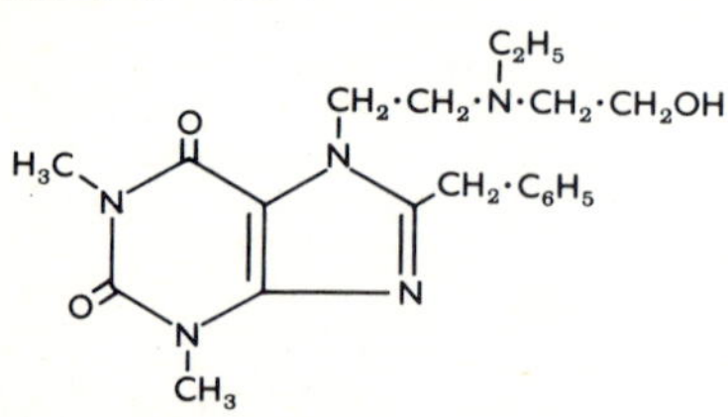

BAMIFYLLINE HYDROCHLORIDE
Proprietary Name: Trentadil.
Solubility. Soluble in water.

Extraction. Bamifylline is extracted by organic solvents from aqueous alkaline solutions.

Chromatography. PAPER: system P1—Rf 0·47 (location under ultraviolet light, strong absorption; location reagents: *iodoplatinate spray*, weak reaction; *bromocresol green spray*, weak reaction).
THIN-LAYER: system T1—Rf 0·68 (location reagent *acidified iodoplatinate spray*, positive reaction).

Colour Tests. Amalic acid test—purple (see p. 127).
MICRO: Vitali's test— –/–/blue-purple (*sensitivity:* 0·1 µg).

Crystal Tests. MICRO: *gold bromide solution*—dendrites (*sensitivity:* 1 in 1000); *lead iodide solution*—rosettes of rods, or dense rosettes (*sensitivity:* 1 in 1000).

Ultraviolet Absorption Spectrum. Bamifylline in 0·1N sulphuric acid, maximum at 278 mµ (E1%, 1 cm 303).

Infra-red Absorption Spectrum. Bamifylline (base). Potassium bromide disk. The principal peaks are: A 1650, B 1698, C 1416 or 1538 (p. 774).

Dose. 1·8 g daily.

BAMIPINE *Antihistamine*
4-(*N*-Benzylanilino)-1-methylpiperidine
$C_{19}H_{24}N_2 = 280{\cdot}4$

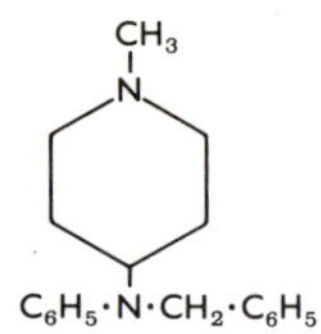

Bamipine occurs as crystals from dibutyl ether. M.p. about 115°.
Solubility. Soluble 1 in 75 of water.

BAMIPINE HYDROCHLORIDE
Proprietary Name: Soventol.
A white crystalline powder. M.p. 208° to 209°.

Extraction. Bamipine is extracted by organic solvents from aqueous alkaline solutions.

Chromatography. PAPER: system P1—Rf 0·63 (location under ultraviolet light, absorption; location reagents: *iodoplatinate spray*, strong reaction; *bromocresol green spray*, weak reaction); system RP1a—Rf 0·41 (location under ultraviolet light, absorption; location reagent *iodoplatinate spray*, positive reaction); system RP1b—Rf 0·00.
THIN-LAYER: system T1—Rf 0·46 (location reagent *acidified iodoplatinate spray*, positive reaction).

Colour Tests. MICRO: ammonium vanadate test—yellow with violet rim (*sensitivity:* 0·5 µg); Vitali's test— –/yellow/yellow (*sensitivity:* 0·5 µg).

Crystal Tests. MICRO: *potassium chromate solution*—long plates (*sensitivity:* 1 in 1000);

sodium carbonate solution—segmented rods (*sensitivity:* 1 in 1000).

Ultraviolet Absorption Spectrum. Bamipine hydrochloride in water (pH 5·5) maximum at 250 mμ; minimum at 225 mμ.

Infra-red Absorption Spectrum. Bamipine (base). Potassium bromide disk. The principal peaks are: A 725 or 745 or 1495 or 1593, B 690 or 1238 or 1275 or 1347 or 1445 (p. 775).

Dose. Up to 300 mg daily.

Toxicity. LD50 (oral): in dogs 189 and in rats 460 mg/kg.

BARBITONE *Barbiturate*

Synonyms: Barbital; Barbiton; Diemalum; Diethylmalonylurea; Malonal; Malonurea.
Proprietary Name: Veronal.

5,5-Diethylbarbituric acid
$C_8H_{12}N_2O_3 = 184{\cdot}2$

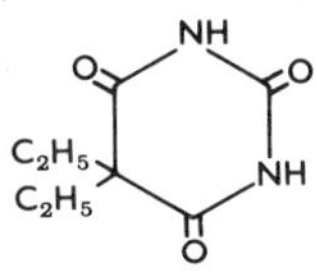

A white crystalline powder. M.p. 189° to 192°.
Solubility. Soluble 1 in 160 of water, 1 in 12 of boiling water, 1 in 15 of ethanol, 1 in 40 of ether, and 1 in 75 of chloroform; soluble in solutions of alkali carbonates and hydroxides.

BARBITONE SODIUM
Synonyms: Barbital Sodium; Diemalnatrium; Soluble Barbitone.
Proprietary Name: Medinal.

A white crystalline powder; a solution in water slowly decomposes.
Solubility. Soluble 1 in 5 of water and 1 in 600 of ethanol; insoluble in ether and chloroform.

Screening Tests. See under Barbiturates, p. 208.

Extraction. Barbitone may be isolated in the A2 fraction (see p. 27).

Chromatography. PAPER: system P2—Rf 0·06 relative to amylobarbitone (location under ultraviolet light, dark spot); system P3—Rf 0·06 (no real separation occurs between barbitone and phenobarbitone on this system; location reagent *silver nitrate spray*, white); system P5—Rf 0·07 relative to quinalbarbitone (location under ultraviolet light after exposure to ammonia, absorption); system RP1b—Rf 0·70 (location under ultraviolet light after exposure to ammonia; location reagent *potassium permanganate spray*, yellow on pink).

THIN-LAYER: system T10—Rf 0·22 (location reagents: *mercurous nitrate spray*, black; *Zwikker's reagent spray*, pink); system T11—Rf 0·38 (location reagent *mercurous nitrate spray*, white on grey).

GAS: system G1/180—retention time 0·37 relative to diphenhydramine; system G3—retention time 1·20 relative to diphenhydramine; system G5—retention time 0·14 relative to phenobarbitone.

Colour Test. Zwikker's test—violet-blue.

Ultraviolet Absorption Spectrum. Barbitone is a 5,5-derivative—see Screening Test 3 under Barbiturates, p. 208.

Infra-red Absorption Spectrum. Barbitone. Potassium bromide disk. The principal peaks are: A 1674, B 1754, C 1380 or 1707 (p. 730).

Quantitative Estimation. See under Barbiturates, p. 208.

Metabolism. Barbitone is a long-acting barbiturate—see under Barbiturates, below. It is excreted slowly and is cumulative in action. Following a single oral dose of 300 mg, 2·2% was excreted unchanged in the urine in the first 8 hours; 32 hours after administration, only 16·4% had been excreted; even after 16 days detectable amounts were still present in the urine; no metabolites or conjugates were found (Svendsen and Brochmann-Hanssen, 1962).
After a single oral dose of 1·5 g in 4 healthy subjects, the peak plasma-level was attained after 4 to 8 hours; it decreased by 19 to 24% within 24 hours; about 33% was excreted in the first 48 hours and 75 to 95% in 11 to 13 days (Lous, 1954).

Dose. Up to 900 mg daily.

Toxicity. The estimated minimum lethal dose in man is 2 g and the blood-level associated with severe poisoning is 5 to 8 mg% or higher.
LD50 (oral): in mice 600 mg/kg.

CASE EXAMPLES. A 22-year-old woman took 22 g of barbitone. Ten hours later, on admission to hospital, the barbitone plasma-level was 50 mg% and the urine level 24 mg%. She recovered (Yatzidis *et al.*, 1965).
In six cases of severe acute barbitone poisoning the amounts ingested ranged from 5 to about 25 g. Death occurred in 2 cases 150 and 160 hours after intake when the serum levels were about 10 and about 17 mg% respectively. In the 4 other cases the barbitone serum concentrations were 7 to 15 mg% on awakening from coma (Lous, 1954).

BARBITURATES

The barbiturates are derivatives of barbituric acid (malonylurea; 2,4,6-trioxohexahydropyrimidine) formed by the replacement of both hydrogen atoms on the carbon at position 5 by alkyl, aryl, or alicyclic groups. The nitrogen atom at position 1 may also be alkylated, while substitution by sulphur for oxygen on position 2 gives rise to the thiobarbiturates. Chemically, they are weak acids and form stable sodium and calcium salts.

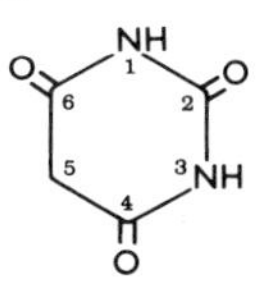

The barbiturates find extensive use as hypnotics,

sedatives, and anaesthetics. They are roughly classified as *long-acting* (e.g. phenobarbitone), *intermediate-acting* (e.g. amylobarbitone), *short-acting* (e.g. pentobarbitone), and *very short-acting* (e.g. thiopentone). This classification is, however, mainly based on pharmacological studies in animals and its relevance to therapy with the barbiturates in man is considered by some authorities to be doubtful because of the great variability in the response of individual patients. Broadly, the duration of action of barbiturates, in therapeutic doses, varies from 8 to 24 hours (long-acting), 4 to 10 hours (intermediate- to short-acting), and 3 to 4 hours (very short-acting).

Extraction. The barbiturates are extracted from biological material in the A2 fraction (see p. 27).

Screening Tests. Since the barbiturates account for nearly 50% of all cases of poisoning in the United Kingdom, their rapid recognition is a matter of considerable importance. A number of screening procedures are available.

1. To 1 to 2 ml of a solution of the test material in ethanol add 1 to 2 ml of a 1% solution of cobalt nitrate in ethanol, followed by one or two pellets of sodium hydroxide. The formation of a blue colour indicates the presence of a barbiturate. Bemegride, glutethimide, phenytoin, and primidone also give a positive reaction with this test. The use of lithium hydroxide instead of sodium hydroxide makes the test specific for barbiturates (see test 4).

2. Acidify a solution of the test material, extract with a small volume of ether, concentrate the ether, and spot on filter paper. Then (a) examine the spot under ultraviolet light (254 mμ)—an absorbing spot, whose area is increased after exposure to ammonia vapour, indicates the presence of a barbiturate; and (b) dip the filter paper in a 1% solution of cobalt chloride in dry acetone, allow to dry in air, and expose to ammonia vapour—a violet colour indicates the presence of a barbiturate. Bemegride, glutethimide, and primidone give a weak reaction. Phenytoin gives a pink colour.

3. Dissolve a portion of a tablet or the residue from the A2 fraction in 5 ml of water. Filter the solution, add one drop of 2N ammonium hydroxide solution (about pH 10), and plot the ultraviolet absorption curve: 5,5- and 1,5,5-substituted barbiturates show a peak at 240 mμ, methohexitone shows a peak at 250 mμ, and the thiobarbiturates show two peaks, the major peak at 305 mμ, the minor at 255 mμ. Add one drop of 2N sulphuric acid (about pH 2): for the 5,5- and 1,5,5- derivatives the peak disappears, for methohexitone there is a peak shift to 228 mμ, and for the thiobarbiturates a shift to 290 mμ and 239 mμ. Finally, add one drop of 4N sodium hydroxide solution (about pH 13): for the 1,5,5-derivatives the peak reappears at 240 mμ, but for the 5,5-derivatives a peak appears at 255 mμ; for methohexitone the peak returns to 250 mμ; for the thiobarbiturates the major peak returns to 305 mμ, while the smaller peak disappears.

4. In urine
Acidify 50 ml of urine to pH 4 to 5 by the addition of a few drops of 10% sulphuric acid. Extract twice with 50 ml of ether, combine the ether extracts, wash with water, and dry by filtering. Evaporate to dryness and take up the residue in 1 ml of chloroform. To this solution add 2 drops of a freshly prepared 1% solution of cobalt acetate in methanol, followed by a freshly prepared 1% solution of lithium hydroxide in methanol, added drop by drop. A blue ring at the junction indicates the presence of a barbiturate.

5. In blood
The following is a *quantitative method.* Place 1 ml of plasma or whole blood, 3 ml of *phosphate buffer* (pH 6·95), and 25 ml of chloroform in a 50-ml beaker and stir magnetically for 4 minutes. Remove the aqueous layer by suction and wash the chloroform layer with two 15-ml portions of water, being careful not to remove any chloroform. Stir the chloroform layer for two minutes with 1 ml of *mercuric bicarbonate solution*, add 15 ml of water, quickly remove the aqueous layer, add 3 ml of 0·5 N ammonium hydroxide solution, and titrate rapidly with *dithizone solution*. The chloroform layer becomes orange if a barbiturate is present. The end-point is indicated by a colour change from orange → orange-green → green, the aqueous layer becoming pink. Each ml of *dithizone solution* corresponds to 1 mg% of barbiturate in the blood (Curry, 1964a; Clow and Smith, 1967).
Quantitative estimation may also be carried out by measuring the ultraviolet absorption in *borax buffer* (0·05M) (Stevenson, 1961).
For (E 1%, 1 cm) values of barbiturates, see p. 99.

Chromatography. Identification of individual barbiturates may be carried out by paper chromatography (systems P2, P3, P4, and P5, pp. 34 to 36), thin-layer chromatography (systems T10, T11, T12, and T13, pp. 52 to 54), and gas chromatography (systems G5 and G7, p. 83).

Infra-red Absorption Spectrum. Barbituric acid. Potassium bromide disk. The principal peaks are: A 1710, B 1734, C 1350 or 1412 (p. 730).

Interpretation. In order to evaluate the significance of barbiturate blood-levels it is useful to know the duration of action of the barbiturate. With long-acting barbiturates blood-levels of 5 mg% and above may give rise to fatal poisoning and for intermediate- to short-acting barbiturates blood-levels from 1 to 3 mg% may be fatal.

Metabolism. The potency and duration of action of the barbiturates depend to a large extent upon their metabolism—see under The

Metabolism of Drugs, p. 156. They are metabolised by four routes:
(1) oxidation of the substituents at position 5 of the barbiturate ring—e.g. phenobarbitone is oxidised to 5-ethyl-5-*p*-hydroxyphenylbarbituric acid;
(2) *N*-dealkylation—e.g. methylphenobarbitone is *N*-demethylated to phenobarbitone;
(3) hydrolytic splitting of the barbiturate ring; this ring is relatively stable but small quantities of metabolites arising from ring fission have been detected;
(4) desulphurisation of the thiobarbiturates—e.g. thiopentone is partially converted to pentobarbitone.

NOTE. Bogan and Smith (1967) have published a comprehensive review of analytical investigations into barbiturate poisoning; they describe extraction procedures, thin-layer and gas chromatographic detection methods, and spectrophotometric quantitative estimation; case examples are also presented.

BEMEGRIDE *Central Stimulant*

Synonym: Methetharimide.
Proprietary Name: Megimide.

β-Ethyl-β-methylglutarimide
$C_8H_{13}NO_2 = 155{\cdot}2$

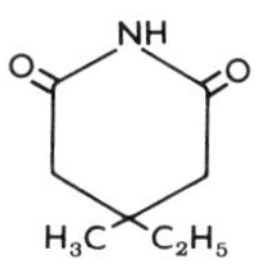

A white crystalline powder. M.p. 126° to 128°.
Solubility. Soluble 1 in 170 of water, 1 in 30 of ethanol, 1 in 100 of ether, and 1 in 4 of chloroform; soluble in solutions of alkali hydroxides.

BEMEGRIDE SODIUM
A fine white powder.
Solubility. Soluble 1 in 11 of water and 1 in 20 of ethanol; insoluble in ether.

Screening Tests. For 2 tests which may be used to detect bemegride see Screening Tests 1 and 2 under Barbiturates, p. 208.

Extraction. Bemegride is extracted by organic solvents from aqueous acid solutions.

Chromatography. PAPER: system RP1b—Rf 0·60 (location reagent *bromine–starch–potassium iodide*).
THIN-LAYER: system T10—Rf 0·39 (location reagent *mercurous nitrate spray*, black).
GAS: system G5—retention time 0·62 relative to barbitone.

Colour Test. Zwikker's test—violet-blue.

Ultraviolet Absorption Spectrum. Bemegride in 0·1N sodium hydroxide, inflexion at 250 mμ (E1%, 1 cm 8).

NOTE. The ultraviolet absorption spectrum of bemegride in the region of 240 mμ is very similar to that of the barbiturates, the absorption decreasing between pH 11 and pH 2. However, a distinction may be made if the spectrum is plotted at pH 11·5 and at pH 10 when the spectrum of bemegride undergoes radical changes (Curry, 1957).

Infra-red Absorption Spectrum. Bemegride. Potassium bromide disk. The principal peaks are: A 1668, B 1272, C 1718 (p. 731).

Metabolism. The effect of bemegride is rapid and lasts for 10 to 20 minutes. Bemegride is excreted in the urine partly unchanged and partly as a hydroxy-derivative in which the hydroxylation is thought to occur on the 1-position in the β-ethyl side-chain (McCallum, 1955). The hydroxy-derivative may also interfere with the detection of barbiturates (Curry, 1957).

Dose. 50 mg, repeated as necessary.

BENACTYZINE *Tranquilliser*

2-Diethylaminoethylbenzilate
$C_{20}H_{25}NO_3 = 327{\cdot}4$

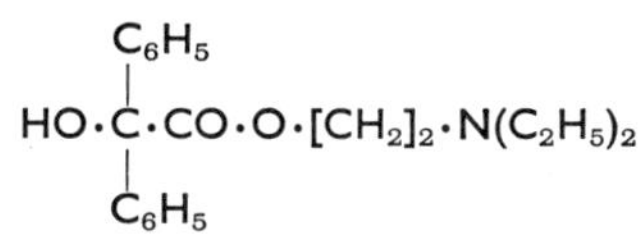

Benactyzine melts at 51°.

BENACTYZINE HYDROCHLORIDE
Proprietary Names: Cafron; Cevanol; Lucidil; Nutinal; Phobex; Suavitil.

A white crystalline powder. M.p. 177° to 181°.
Solubility. Soluble 1 in 7 of water and 1 in 22 of ethanol; insoluble in ether.

Extraction. Benactyzine is extracted by organic solvents from aqueous alkaline solutions.

Chromatography. PAPER: system P1—Rf 0·64 (location under ultraviolet light, absorption; location reagents: *iodoplatinate spray*, strong reaction; *bromocresol green spray*, weak reaction).
THIN-LAYER: system T1—Rf 0·60 (location reagent *acidified iodoplatinate spray*, positive reaction).

Colour Tests. MICRO: sulphuric acid–formaldehyde test—orange → green → blue (*sensitivity:* 0·1 μg); ammonium molybdate test—orange → olive-brown (*sensitivity:* 0·25 μg).

Ultraviolet Absorption Spectrum. Benactyzine hydrochloride in ethanol, maxima at 252 mμ (E1%, 1 cm 11), 258 mμ (E1%, 1 cm 12), and 265 mμ (E1%, 1 cm 10); in 0·1N sulphuric acid, maxima at 252 mμ (E1%, 1 cm 11), 258 mμ (E1%, 1 cm 13), 262 mμ (E1%, 1 cm 11), and 264 mμ (E1%, 1 cm 11), and an inflexion at 268 mμ.

Infra-red Absorption Spectrum. Benactyzine (base). Potassium bromide disk. The principal peaks are: A 795 or 1723, B 1231, C 1054 (p. 775).

Metabolism. Benactyzine is rapidly metabolised and excreted, resulting in a relatively brief duration of action.

Dose. Up to 8 mg daily.

Toxicity. LD50 (intraperitoneal): in mice and rats 100 to 130 mg/kg.

BENDROFLUAZIDE *Diuretic*

Synonyms: Bendroflumethiazide; FT 81.
Proprietary Names: Aprinox; Berkozide; Centyl; Naturetin; Naturine; Neo-NaClex.

3 - Benzyl - 3, 4 - dihydro - 7 - sulphamoyl - 6 - trifluoromethyl - 2*H* - benzo - 1, 2, 4 - thiadiazine 1,1-dioxide
$C_{15}H_{14}F_3N_3O_4S_2 = 421{\cdot}4$

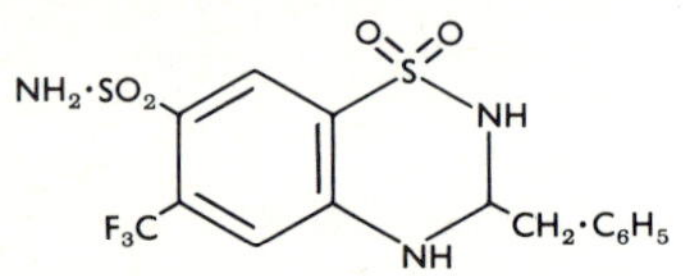

A white crystalline powder.
Solubility. Almost insoluble in water; soluble 1 in 17 of ethanol and 1 in 500 of ether; insoluble in chloroform; soluble 1 in 1·5 of acetone.

Extraction. Bendrofluazide may be isolated in the A2 fraction (see p. 27). It may be distinguished from the barbiturates by chromatography (see below), and by the presence of additional ultraviolet maxima in the region 270 to 330 mμ.

Chromatography. PAPER: system P16—Rf 0·22 (location under ultraviolet light, fluorescence; location reagent *sodium naphthaquinone spray*, strong reaction); system RP1b—Rf 0·64 (location as for P16).

Ultraviolet Absorption Spectrum. Bendrofluazide in 0·01N sodium hydroxide, maxima at 273 mμ (E1%, 1 cm 413) and 329 mμ (E1%, 1 cm 80).

Infra-red Absorption Spectrum. Potassium bromide disk. The principal peaks are: A 1162, B 1340, C 1302 or 1512 (p. 731).

Dose. Up to 10 mg daily.

BENZALDEHYDE *Flavouring Agent*

$C_6H_5{\cdot}CHO = 106{\cdot}1$

A colourless, strongly refractive liquid which becomes yellowish on keeping and oxidises in air to benzoic acid. B.p. about 179°. Refractive index, at 20°, 1·544 to 1·5465.
Solubility. Soluble 1 in 350 of water; miscible with ethanol and ether.

Extraction. Benzaldehyde is volatile and may be isolated by distillation (see p. 18).

Ultraviolet Absorption Spectrum. Benzaldehyde in ethanol, maxima at 245 mμ (E1%, 1 cm 1294), 279 mμ (E1%, 1 cm 126), and 289 mμ (E1%, 1 cm 105).

Metabolism. In several animal species benzaldehyde is metabolised to benzoic acid and its conjugate, hippuric acid.

Toxicity. The estimated lethal dose in man is 50 g. The subcutaneous lethal dose in rats is about 5 g/kg.

BENZALKONIUM BROMIDE *Antiseptic Detergent*

Proprietary Name: Morpan BB.

A mixture of alkylbenzyldimethylammonium bromides of the general formula $[C_6H_5{\cdot}CH_2{\cdot}N(CH_3)_2{\cdot}R]Br$ in which R represents a mixture of the alkyls from C_8H_{17} to $C_{18}H_{37}$.
An aqueous solution containing the equivalent of 50% of $[C_6H_5{\cdot}CH_2{\cdot}N(CH_3)_2{\cdot}C_{13}H_{27}]Br$ is a colourless or pale yellow syrupy liquid, which is miscible with water, ethanol, and acetone.

Extraction, Ultraviolet Absorption Spectrum, and **Toxicity.** As for Benzalkonium Chloride.

BENZALKONIUM CHLORIDE *Antiseptic Detergent*

Proprietary Names: Empiquat BAC; Hyamine 3500; Marinol; P.R.Q. Antiseptic; Roccal; Zephiran; Zephirol.

A mixture of alkylbenzyldimethylammonium chlorides of the general formula $[C_6H_5{\cdot}CH_2{\cdot}N(CH_3)_2R]Cl$, where R is usually $n\text{-}C_{12}H_{25}$, $n\text{-}C_{14}H_{29}$, and $n\text{-}C_{16}H_{33}$.
A white or yellowish-white, thick gel or gelatinous pieces. A solution in water gives a clear, colourless or pale yellow, syrupy liquid.
Solubility. Very soluble in water, ethanol, and acetone; soluble 1 in 100 of ether.

Extraction. Benzalkonium chloride is a quaternary ammonium compound (see p. 29).

Ultraviolet Absorption Spectrum. Benzalkonium chloride in water, maxima at about 250 mμ, 256 mμ, and 262 mμ; minima at about 232 mμ, 259 mμ, and 266 mμ.

Toxicity. Benzalkonium chloride is non-toxic at the concentrations normally used (1 in 40,000 to 1 in 1000) and it does not irritate the skin, although continuous use may cause defatting of the skin. Concentrated solutions are readily absorbed and may interfere with many cellular functions. The estimated lethal dose in man is 1 to 3 g. Daily doses of 25 mg/kg given to dogs are fatal within a few weeks.

CASE EXAMPLES. A 51-year-old woman died 14 days after a subcutaneous infiltration of the left cheek had been performed with about 20 ml of a 10% solution of benzalkonium chloride in error for procaine hydrochloride (Laves, 1960).
A woman, aged 20 years, died 3 to 4 hours after ingesting about 350 ml of a 10% benzalkonium chloride solution. The stomach contents contained 0·027 mg% (w/w) (Tiess, 1966b).

BENZAMINE *Local Anaesthetic*

Synonyms: Betacaine; Racemic Benzamine.

4-Benzoyloxy-2,2,6-trimethylpiperidine
$C_{15}H_{21}NO_2 = 247{\cdot}3$

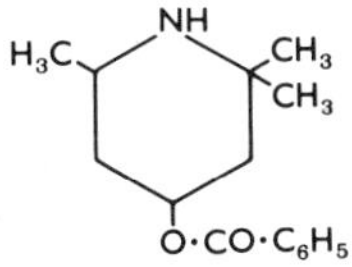

BENZAMINE HYDROCHLORIDE
Synonyms: Beta-eucaine Hydrochloride; Eucaine Hydrochloride.

A white crystalline powder. M.p. 274°, with decomposition.

Solubility. Soluble 1 in 30 of water, 1 in 35 of ethanol, and 1 in 30 of chloroform.

BENZAMINE LACTATE
A white crystalline powder. M.p. 152°.
Solubility. Soluble 1 in 5 of water and 1 in 8 of ethanol.

Extraction. Benzamine is extracted by organic solvents from aqueous alkaline solutions.

Chromatography. PAPER: system P1—Rf 0·75 (location under ultraviolet light, absorption; location reagents: *iodoplatinate spray*, weak reaction; *bromocresol green spray*, weak reaction). THIN-LAYER: system T1—Rf 0·57 (location reagent *acidified iodoplatinate spray*, positive reaction).

Crystal Tests. MICRO: *picric acid*—clusters of plates and rods (*sensitivity:* 1 in 1500); *trinitrobenzoic acid solution*—hedgehogs or bunches of needles (*sensitivity:* 1 in 400).

Ultraviolet Absorption Spectrum. Benzamine in 0·1N sulphuric acid, maxima at 233 mμ (E1%, 1 cm 511) and 274 mμ (E1%, 1 cm 29).

Infra-red Absorption Spectrum. Benzamine (base). Potassium bromide disk. The principal peaks are: A 1714, B 1276, C 711 or 1108 (p. 775).

Dose. Up to 30 mg.

Toxicity. The minimum intravenous lethal dose in rats is 15 to 25 mg/kg.

BENZATHINE PENICILLIN *Antibiotic*

Synonyms: Benzathine Benzylpenicillin; Benzathine Penicillin G; Benzethacil; Dibenzylamine Penicillin G; Penzaethinum G.

Proprietary Names: Bicillin; Dibencil; Neolin; Penditan; Penidural; Permapen.

NN'-Dibenzylethylenediamine 6-phenylacetamidopenicillanate
$C_{16}H_{20}N_2(C_{16}H_{18}N_2O_4S)_2 = 909{\cdot}1$

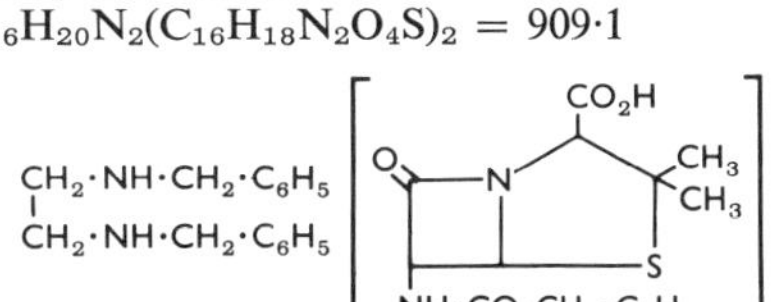

A white powder. M.p. 129° to 133°, with decomposition.

Solubility. Soluble 1 in 6000 of water and 1 in 1000 of ethanol; almost insoluble in ether and chloroform.

Ultraviolet Absorption Spectrum. Benzathine penicillin in methanol, maxima at 251 mμ (E1%, 1 cm 9), 257 mμ (E1%, 1 cm 9), 263 mμ (E1%, 1 cm 6), 266 mμ (E1%, 1 cm 4), and 320 mμ.

Metabolism. Benzathine penicillin is relatively stable in the presence of gastric juice or serum, and penicillin is slowly released following oral or intramuscular administration. When benzathine penicillin is given by mouth, the maximum concentration of penicillin in the blood is obtained less rapidly than after a comparable dose of a soluble salt of penicillin by injection but the level is maintained for a longer period; doses of 225 mg usually give effective blood-levels for 6 hours. When given by intramuscular injection, benzathine penicillin forms a depot from which penicillin is released over several days, and following a single dose of 450 mg an effective concentration in the blood may be maintained for a week or even longer.

Dose. Usually up to 900 mg daily by mouth; up to 1·8 g intramuscularly, as a single dose.

Toxicity. Allergic reactions may occur.

BENZENE *Industrial Solvent*

$C_6H_6 = 78{\cdot}11$

A clear, colourless, mobile, inflammable liquid, which burns with a luminous smoky flame. B.p. 80°.

Solubility. Insoluble in water; miscible with dehydrated ethanol, ether, acetone, glacial acetic acid, light petroleum, and oils.

Screening Test. A rapid screening test involving the detection of phenolic metabolites of benzene in urine by condensation with 2,6-dichloroquinone-4-chloroimine to give a blue colour has been described by Rainsford and Davies (1965).

Extraction. Benzene is volatile and may be isolated by distillation (see p. 18).

Chromatography. PAPER and THIN-LAYER: Bonnichsen *et al.* (1966) describe a paper system and a thin-layer system, both of which detect the nitration products of benzene, following steam distillation into carbon tetrachloride and subsequent nitration.

GAS: system G8/160—retention time 2·9 relative to n-propanol.

Ultraviolet Absorption Spectrum. Benzene in ethanol, maximum at 255 mμ (E1%, 1 cm 28).

Quantitative Estimation. Benzene may be estimated in biological fluids and tissues by steam distillation into carbon tetrachloride, nitration, and subsequent spectrophotometric determination at 570 mμ (Bonnichsen *et al.*, 1966); it may be estimated in blood by aeration of samples and subsequent infra-red spectrophotometry (Feldstein, 1965); it may be estimated in urine as its phenol metabolite (Walkley *et al.*, 1961) and by determination as organic sulphate (Ilich *et al.*, 1964).

Metabolism. Benzene is absorbed from the gastro-intestinal tract, through the skin, and from the lungs. In men exposed for 5 hours to an atmosphere containing 0·34 mg/l, about 46% of the benzene inhaled is retained; eventually, about 12% of this is exhaled, only very small amounts appearing unchanged in the urine; 10 to 40% of the retained benzene is excreted as phenol, about 3% as catechol, and 1% as quinol. The excretion of phenol and catechol is highest in the first 24 hours and is complete within 48 hours of the exposure. The excretion of quinol is slower but is usually complete in 48 hours.

The phenolic metabolites of benzene are excreted mainly in the conjugated form as ethereal sulphates and glucuronides. Two minor metabolites may also be found, L-phenylmercapturic acid and *trans-trans*-muconic acid; the latter appears to be further metabolised to carbon dioxide. The toxic effects of benzene are probably related to the formation of phenols.

Toxicity. The maximum permissible concentration of benzene in air is stated to be 25 p.p.m. Chronic poisoning may result from exposure over a period to low concentrations; 1500 p.p.m. for an hour causes marked depression and 7500 p.p.m. for half an hour or 20,000 p.p.m. for a few minutes may cause death. Fairly large doses are tolerated by mouth; 30 ml has proved fatal. LD50 (oral): in rats 5·7 g/kg.

CASE EXAMPLES. A 23-year-old woman died almost immediately after being given a slow intravenous injection of about 8 ml of benzene in mistake for a thiopentone sodium injection (Laves, 1960).

In a chronic alcoholic aged 51, who had also ingested benzene, the post-mortem ethanol levels were: blood, 0·19%; brain, 0·16%; kidneys, 0·2%; urine, 0·22%; the benzene levels were: stomach contents, 2·4 mg%, and traces in the blood. The urine also contained 0·3 mg% of acetone. It could not be established whether alcoholism, aromatic hydrocarbons, and/or a previously undetected diabetes was responsible for death. Histological investigation of the pancreas was inconclusive, due to putrefaction.

In another alcoholic aged 37 who died from accidental benzene poisoning, the post-mortem benzene levels were: brain, 1·4 mg%; kidneys, 1·8 mg%; stomach contents, 4 g%. In a third man aged 29, who died after a drinking bout, the stomach contents contained 0·6 to 0·7 mg% benzene and 1·9% ethanol. Analyses for methanol, halogenated hydrocarbons, cyanide, nicotine, pyridine, and barbiturates were negative (Bonnichsen *et al.*, 1966).

A 16-year-old youth died after 'sniffing' rubber cement containing low percentages of benzene. At post-mortem examination there was striking cerebral oedema, acute bilateral pulmonary oedema, and congestion of spleen, liver, and mucosal surfaces of the stomach and duodenum. Analyses of the tissues and blood were positive only for benzene; the blood contained 0·094 mg% of benzene and the kidneys 0·55 mg% (Winek *et al.*, 1967).

BENZENE HEXACHLORIDE *Pesticide*

Synonyms: BHC; HCH; Hexachlorocyclohexane; Technical Benzene Hexachloride.

$C_6H_6Cl_6 = 290{\cdot}8$

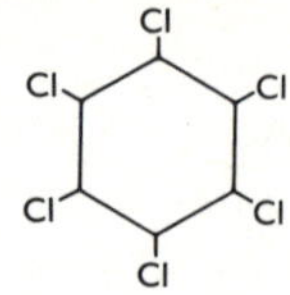

Benzene hexachloride consists of a mixture of the several isomers of 1,2,3,4,5,6-hexachlorocyclohexane, containing not less that 12% of the gamma-isomer. Benzene hexachloride has 5 known isomers, designated alpha, beta, gamma, delta, and epsilon; of these, only the gamma-isomer (see Gamma Benzene Hexachloride, p. 352) is outstandingly active as an insecticide. It occurs as white to light brown granules, flakes, or powder, with a characteristic musty odour.

Solubility. Insoluble in water; its solubility in organic solvents depends upon the proportions of the various isomers present.

Extraction. Benzene hexachloride is extracted by organic solvents from aqueous acid or alkaline solutions.

Chromatography. PAPER: Bridges *et al.* (1956) describe a method of separating the isomers of benzene hexachloride on paper impregnated with paraffin, and Cohen (1957) describes a method for distinguishing benzene hexachloride from its gamma-isomer.

Quantitative Estimation. See under Gamma Benzene Hexachloride, p. 352.

Toxicity. Benzene hexachloride is used for purposes where the musty odour associated with the mixed isomers is not objectionable. It is the form most frequently used in the manufacture of veterinary dips and sprays. The beta-isomer is absorbed selectively from the bowel and retained like dicophane, so the chronic toxicity of benzene hexachloride is greater than that of the pure gamma-isomer. Ingestion of 20 to 30 g of benzene hexachloride may produce serious toxic symptoms but death is unlikely unless this amount is dissolved in an organic solvent.

Benzene hexachloride is extremely toxic to fish.

BENZETHIDINE *Narcotic Analgesic*

Synonyms: Benzyloxyethylnorpethidine; TA 28.

Ethyl - 1 - (2 - benzyloxyethyl) - 4 - phenylpiperidine-4-carboxylate

$C_{23}H_{29}NO_3 = 367{\cdot}5$

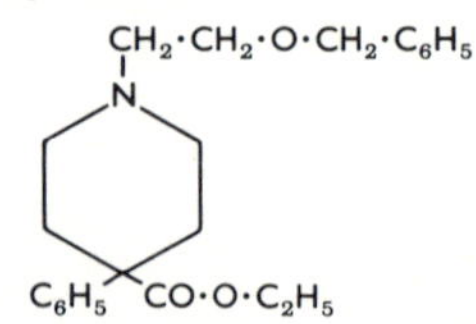

Extraction. Benzethidine is extracted by organic solvents from aqueous alkaline solutions.

Chromatography. PAPER: system P1—Rf 0·91 (location reagent *iodoplatinate spray*, strong reaction); system RP1b—Rf 0·00 (location reagent *iodoplatinate spray*, positive reaction).
THIN-LAYER: system T1—Rf 0·73 (location reagent *acidified iodoplatinate spray*, positive reaction).
GAS: system G2/225—retention time 2·53 relative to codeine; system G4—retention time 1·70 relative to codeine.

Colour Tests. MICRO: sulphuric acid–formaldehyde test—dull orange (*sensitivity:* 0·5 μg); ammonium molybdate test—orange-brown (*sensitivity:* 0·5 μg).

Crystal Tests. MICRO: *gold chloride solution*—small plates, forming overnight (*sensitivity:* 1 in 1000); *styphnic acid*—masses of blades, forming overnight (*sensitivity:* 1 in 200).

Ultraviolet Absorption Spectrum. Benzethidine in 0·1N sulphuric acid, maxima at 252 mμ (E1%, 1 cm 8·1), 257·5 mμ (E1%, 1 cm 10·2), and 263·5 mμ (E1%, 1 cm 8·4), and an inflexion at 267 mμ.

BENZETHONIUM CHLORIDE

Antiseptic Detergent

Proprietary Names: Hyamine 1622; Phemeride; Phemerol Chloride.

Benzyldimethyl-2-{2-[*p*-(1,1,3,3-tetramethylbutyl)phenoxy]ethoxy}ethylammonium chloride

$C_{27}H_{42}ClNO_2$ = 448·1

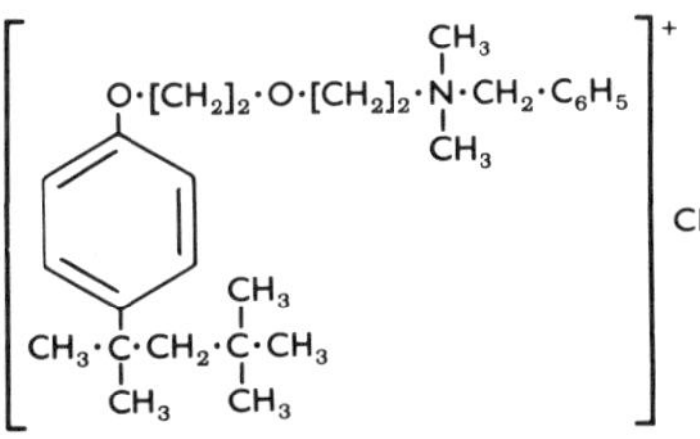

Colourless crystals. M.p. 160° to 165°.
Solubility. Soluble in water, ethanol, and chloroform; slightly soluble in ether. Store in airtight light-resistant containers.

Extraction. Benzethonium chloride is a quaternary ammonium compound (see p. 29).

Chromatography. PAPER: system P1—Rf 0·76 (location reagent *iodoplatinate spray*, strong reaction).
THIN-LAYER: system T1—Rf 0·03 (location reagent *acidified iodoplatinate spray*, positive reaction).

Colour Tests. MICRO: sulphuric acid–formaldehyde test—faint orange (*sensitivity:* 1·0 μg); Vitali's test— -/-/blue (*sensitivity:* 0·1 μg).

Crystal Test. MICRO: *zinc chloride solution*—clusters of needles, forming overnight (*sensitivity:* 1 in 400).

Ultraviolet Absorption Spectrum. Benzethonium chloride in 0·1N sulphuric acid, maxima at 265 mμ (E1%, 1 cm 19), 270·5 mμ (E1%, 1 cm 24), and 277 mμ (E1%, 1 cm 24), and an inflexion at about 278 mμ (E1%, 1 cm 19).

Infra-red Absorption Spectrum. Potassium bromide disk. The principal peaks are: A 1240, B 1505, C 1120 (p. 793).

Toxicity. Benzethonium chloride is non-toxic at the concentrations normally used (1 in 5000 to 1 in 750). The estimated lethal dose in man is 1 to 3 g.
LD50 (oral): in rats 420 mg/kg.

BENZHEXOL

Parasympatholytic

Synonym: Trihexyphenidyl.

1-Cyclohexyl-1-phenyl-3-piperidinopropan-1-ol

$C_{20}H_{31}NO$ = 301·5

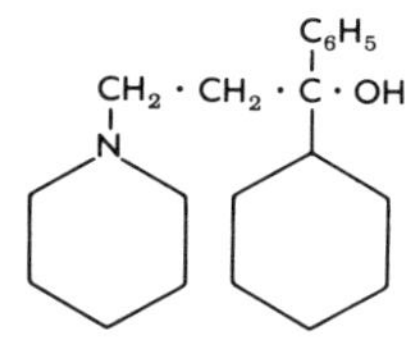

Benzhexol melts at 114°.

BENZHEXOL HYDROCHLORIDE

Proprietary Names: Artane; Pipanol.

A white crystalline powder. M.p. about 250°, with decomposition.
Solubility. Soluble 1 in 100 of water, 1 in 22 of ethanol, and 1 in 15 of chloroform; very slightly soluble in ether.

Extraction. Benzhexol is extracted by organic solvents from aqueous alkaline solutions.

Chromatography. PAPER: system P1—Rf 0·85 (location reagents: *iodoplatinate spray*, strong reaction; *bromocresol green spray*, weak reaction); system RP1a—Rf 0·29 (location reagent *iodoplatinate spray*, positive reaction); system RP1b—Rf 0·00.
THIN-LAYER: system T1—Rf 0·68 (location reagent *acidified iodoplatinate spray*, positive reaction).
GAS: system G2/225—retention time 0·74 relative to codeine; system G3—retention time 2·10 relative to diphenhydramine; system G4—retention time 2·56 relative to diphenhydramine.

Colour Tests. MICRO: sulphuric acid–formaldehyde test—faint grey-purple (*sensitivity:* 1·0 μg); ammonium vanadate test—dull grey-green (*sensitivity:* 0·25 μg).

Crystal Tests. MICRO: *potassium permanganate solution*—curved irregular plates (*sensitivity:* 1 in 1000); *gold cyanide solution*—bunches of plates (*sensitivity:* 1 in 1500).

Ultraviolet Absorption Spectrum. Benzhexol in 0·1N sulphuric acid, maxima at 247 mμ (E1%, 1 cm 6), 252 mμ (E1%, 1 cm 7), 258 mμ (E1%, 1 cm 8), and 264 mμ (E1%, 1 cm 6).

Infra-red Absorption Spectrum. Benzhexol (base). Potassium bromide disk. The principal peaks are: A 696, B 1112, C 760 (p. 775).

Dose. Up to 20 mg daily.

Toxicity. The lethal dose in man is probably between 10 and 100 mg/kg.

BENZILONIUM BROMIDE *Anticholinergic*

Synonym: PU 239.
Proprietary Name: Portyn.

3-Benziloyloxy-1,1-diethylpyrrolidinium bromide

$C_{22}H_{28}BrNO_3 = 434{\cdot}4$

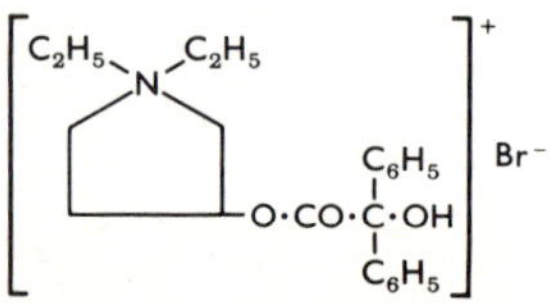

A white crystalline powder.
Solubility. Readily soluble in water.

Extraction. Benzilonium bromide is a quaternary ammonium compound (see p. 29).

Chromatography. PAPER: system P1—Rf 0·52 (location reagent *iodoplatinate spray*, strong reaction); system RP1a—Rf 0·87 (location reagent *iodoplatinate spray*, positive reaction); system RP1b—Rf 0·90 (location as for RP1a).
THIN-LAYER: system T1—Rf 0·03 (location reagent *acidified iodoplatinate spray*, positive reaction).

Colour Tests. MICRO: the following tests are performed on benzilonium nitrate (see p. 134): sulphuric acid–formaldehyde test—orange → green → blue (*sensitivity:* 0·5 μg); ammonium molybdate test—orange → green (*sensitivity:* 0·5 μg).

Ultraviolet Absorption Spectrum. Benzilonium bromide in 0·1N sulphuric acid, maxima at 252 mμ (E1%, 1 cm 10), 258 mμ (E1%, 1 cm 11), and about 264 mμ (E1%, 1cm 9), and an inflexion at 268 mμ.

Infra-red Absorption Spectrum. Potassium bromide disk. The principal peaks are: A 1728, B 1220, C 1190 (p. 731).

Dose. 30 mg daily, increasing as necessary.

BENZOCAINE *Local Anaesthetic*

Synonyms: Éthoforme; Ethyl Aminobenzoate; Norcainum.
Proprietary Name: Anaesthesin.

Ethyl *p*-aminobenzoate

$C_9H_{11}NO_2 = 165{\cdot}2$

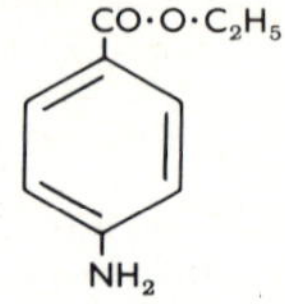

A white crystalline powder. M.p. 88° to 91°.
Solubility. Soluble 1 in 2500 of water, 1 in 8 of ethanol, 1 in 4 of ether, 1 in 2 of chloroform, and in dilute acids.

Extraction. Benzocaine is extracted by organic solvents from aqueous acid or alkaline solutions.

Chromatography. PAPER: system P1—Rf 0·90 (location under ultraviolet light, blue fluorescence; location reagents: diazotisation followed by *alkaline betanaphthol spray*, positive reaction; *ninhydrin spray*, orange).
THIN-LAYER: system T1—Rf 0·73 (location reagents: *acidified iodoplatinate spray*, positive reaction; p-*dimethylaminobenzaldehyde spray*, bright yellow).
GAS: system G5—retention time 1·48 relative to barbitone.

Colour Tests. MICRO: diazotisation test—red; Vitali's test— –/faint yellow/faint yellow (*sensitivity:* 1·0 μg).

Crystal Tests. MICRO: *mercuric chloride solution*—long rods (*sensitivity:* 1 in 1000); *picric acid*—dendrites (*sensitivity:* 1 in 1500).

Ultraviolet Absorption Spectrum. Benzocaine in ethanol, maxima at 221 mμ (E1%, 1cm 553) and 294 mμ (E1%, 1cm 1340); in 0·1N hydrochloric acid, maxima at 227 mμ (E1%, 1cm 788), 272 mμ (E1%, 1cm 101), and 278 mμ (E1%, 1cm 99).

Infra-red Absorption Spectrum. Potassium bromide disk. The principal peaks are: A 1280, B 1598 or 1680, C 1170 (p. 731).

Metabolism. Benzocaine is metabolised by hydrolysis to *p*-aminobenzoic acid.

Toxicity. At the concentrations normally used (2 to 10%), benzocaine is comparatively non-irritant and non-toxic, having only about one-tenth the toxicity of cocaine. The maximum safe amount for topical use is stated to be 5 g or 25 ml of a 20% solution.

CASE EXAMPLE. A horse weighing 480 kg received 18 g of benzocaine. Unchanged drug was still detected in the urine 5½ hours later; all saliva samples were negative. Benzocaine was isolated in this case in the C extract. *p*-Aminobenzoic acid was detected in the urine by paper chromatography (Moss, 1964).

BENZOIC ACID *Preservative*

Synonyms: Benzenecarboxylic Acid; Phenylformic Acid.

$C_6H_5{\cdot}COOH = 122{\cdot}1$

Colourless light feathery crystals. M.p. 121·5° to 123·5°.

Solubility. Soluble 1 in 350 of water, 1 in 20 of boiling water, 1 in 3 of ethanol, 1 in 3 of ether, and 1 in 8 of chloroform; soluble in sodium bicarbonate solution.

Extraction. Benzoic acid may be isolated in the A1 fraction (see p. 27).

Chromatography. GAS: system G5—retention time 0·32 relative to barbitone.

Ultraviolet Absorption Spectrum. Benzoic acid in ethanol, maxima at 228 mμ (E1%, 1cm 116), 266 mμ (E1%, 1cm 60), and 272 mμ (E1%, 1cm 72); in 0·5N hydrochloric acid, maximum at 229 mμ (E1%, 1cm 910); in 0·5N sodium hydroxide, maximum at 225 mμ (E1%, 1cm 665).

Infra-red Absorption Spectrum. Potassium bromide disk. The principal peaks are: A 708 or 1686, B 1294, C 1330 (p. 731).

Metabolism. Benzoic acid is rapidly and completely excreted in the urine; cumulation does not occur. The 2 main urinary metabolites of benzoic acid are hippuric acid and benzoylglucuronic acid. In man, rat, and rabbit, benzoic acid is almost entirely excreted as hippuric acid whereas in dogs more is excreted as a conjugate with glucuronic acid. Normal urinary excretion of hippuric acid in man may be 1 to 2·5 g daily, equivalent to 0·7 to 1·7 g of benzoic acid. The maximum rate of the hippuric acid excretion after ingestion of benzoic acid was observed to be about 17 mg/min (24 g daily) calculated as benzoic acid (FAO/WHO Expert Committee on Food Additives, Sixth Report, 1962). Benzoic acid may be found in the urine as a metabolite of benzaldehyde.

Dose. Doses of up to 4 g daily have been given therapeutically. The estimated acceptable daily intake for man is up to 5 mg/kg.

Toxicity. LD50 (oral): in dogs 2 and in rats 2·7 g/kg.

BENZOYLECGONINE *Alkaloid*

$C_{16}H_{19}NO_4$ = 289·3

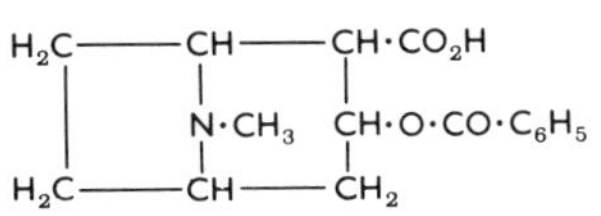

An alkaloid obtained from coca, the leaves of *Erythroxylum coca* and other species of *Erythroxylum* (Erythroxylaceae).

The hydrated form occurs as crystals and melts at 86°. The anhydrous form melts at 195°, with decomposition.

Solubility. Very soluble in hot water; soluble in ethanol and dilute acids and alkalis; insoluble in ether.

Extraction. Benzoylecgonine is extracted by organic solvents from aqueous alkaline solutions.

Chromatography. PAPER: system P1—Rf 0·40 (location under ultraviolet light, absorption; location reagents: *iodoplatinate spray*, weak reaction; *bromocresol green spray*, weak reaction).

THIN-LAYER: system T1—Rf 0·21 (location reagent *acidified iodoplatinate spray*, positive reaction).

Colour Test. MICRO: ammonium molybdate test—faint blue.

Crystal Tests. MICRO: *gold chloride solution*—long plates and needles (*sensitivity:* 1 in 200); *potassium permanganate solution*—branching needles (*sensitivity:* 1 in 400).

Ultraviolet Absorption Spectrum. Benzoylecgonine in 0·1N sulphuric acid, maxima at 234 mμ (E1%, 1cm 392) and 275 mμ (E1%, 1cm 26·4).

Metabolism. Benzoylecgonine is the first hydrolysis product formed when cocaine is metabolised in animals; it is then further hydrolysed to ecgonine and benzoic acid.

BENZPHETAMINE *Anorectic*

(+)-*N*-Benzyl-*N*-α-dimethylphenethylamine

$C_{17}H_{21}N$ = 239·4

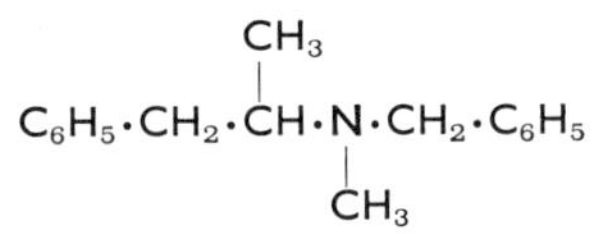

B.p. 127° at 0·2 mmHg.

BENZPHETAMINE HYDROCHLORIDE

Proprietary Name: Didrex.

Benzphetamine hydrochloride melts at 131° to 132°.
Solubility. Soluble in water.

Extraction. Benzphetamine is extracted by organic solvents from aqueous alkaline solutions.

Chromatography. PAPER: system P1—Rf 0·75 (location under ultraviolet light, absorption; location reagents: *iodoplatinate spray*, strong reaction; *bromocresol green spray*, weak reaction); system RP1a—Rf 0·17 (location reagent *iodoplatinate spray*, positive reaction); system RP1b—Rf 0·00.

THIN-LAYER: system T1—Rf 0·73 (location reagent *acidified iodoplatinate spray*, positive reaction).

GAS: system G2/120—retention time 8·8 relative to ephedrine; system G4—retention time 0·85 relative to diphenhydramine.

Colour Test. MICRO: sulphuric acid–formaldehyde test—orange (*sensitivity:* 0·25 μg).

Crystal Tests. MICRO: *gold bromide solution*—small plates or needles (*sensitivity:* 1 in 3000); *gold chloride solution*—oily rods (*sensitivity:* 1 in 3000).

Ultraviolet Absorption Spectrum. Benzphetamine in 0·1N sulphuric acid, maxima at 253 mμ

(E1%, 1 cm 18·8), 258 mμ (E1%, 1 cm 21·6), 263 mμ (E1%, 1 cm 19·4), and 268 mμ (E1%, 1 cm 13·4).

Dose. Not exceeding 150 mg daily.

Toxicity. LD50 (intraperitoneal): in mice 100 to 120 mg/kg.

BENZQUINAMIDE *Tranquilliser*

Synonym: P 2647.
Proprietary Name: Quantril (U.S.A.).
NOTE. In Great Britain, Quantril is the proprietary name of a preparation of Caffeine Citrate.

2 - Acetoxy - 1,3,4,6,7,11b - hexahydro - 9,10 - dimethoxy - 2*H* - benzo[*a*]quinolizine - 3 - carboxydiethylamide
$C_{22}H_{32}N_2O_5 = 404{\cdot}5$

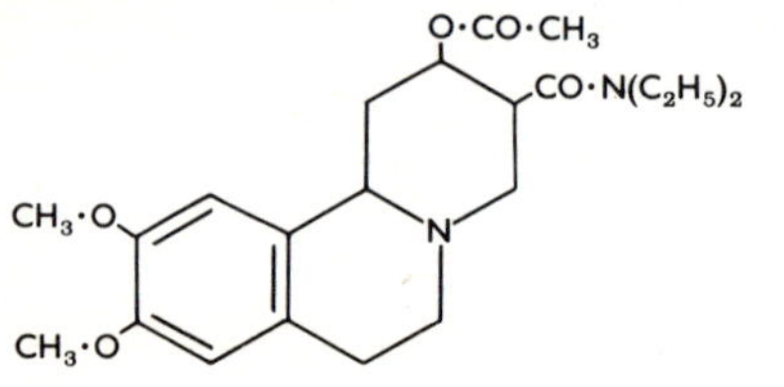

A yellowish crystalline powder.
Solubility. Soluble in dilute acetic acid.

Extraction. Benzquinamide is extracted by organic solvents from aqueous alkaline solutions.

Chromatography. PAPER: system P1—Rf 0·60 (location under ultraviolet light, white fluorescence; location reagents: *iodoplatinate spray*, weak reaction; *bromocresol green spray*, weak reaction).
THIN-LAYER: system T1—Rf 0·69 (location reagent *acidified iodoplatinate spray*, positive reaction).

Colour Tests. MICRO: sulphuric acid–formaldehyde test—yellow (*sensitivity:* 0·1 μg); ammonium molybdate test—dull green (*sensitivity:* 1·0 μg); Vitali's test—yellow/orange/brown (*sensitivity:* 0·25 μg).

Crystal Tests. MICRO: *picric acid*—smudge rosettes (*sensitivity:* 1 in 1000); *styphnic acid*—feathery rosettes (*sensitivity:* 1 in 1000).

Infra-red Absorption Spectrum. Potassium bromide disk. The principal peaks are: A 1244, B 1633 or 1733, C 1204 (p. 775).

Metabolism. Benzquinamide is rapidly and completely absorbed after oral administration and slowly and incompletely absorbed when given rectally. The total urinary excretion as unchanged benzquinamide was 3 to 7% following oral administration, 3 to 15% following intramuscular administration, and 0 to 3% when given as a suppository (Cahn *et al.*, 1963).
Six crystalline metabolites and unchanged benzquinamide were characterised in the urine of dogs following the administration of benzquinamide. Five other metabolites were recovered as crude preparations and evidence for a further 6 metabolites of unknown structure was obtained. Benzquinamide is metabolised by at least 3 pathways: *O*-deacetylation, *O*-demethylation and conjugation, and *N*-de-ethylation. The *N*-de-ethylated compounds appear to be the major metabolites in urine. Some of these metabolites have been found in man (Koe and Pinson, 1964).

Dose. Up to 1·2 g daily has been given.

BENZTHIAZIDE *Diuretic*

Synonym: P 1393.
Proprietary Names: Exna; Fovane; NaClex.

3-Benzylthiomethyl-6-chloro-7-sulphamoyl-2*H*-benzo-1,2,4-thiadiazine 1,1-dioxide
$C_{15}H_{14}ClN_3O_4S_3 = 431{\cdot}9$

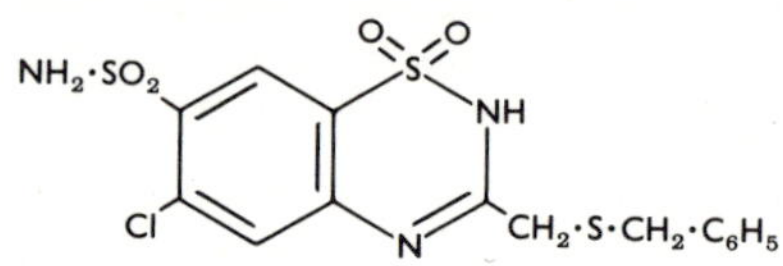

A white crystalline powder. M.p. 241° to 243°.
Solubility. Insoluble in water, ether, and chloroform; soluble 1 in 260 of ethanol and 1 in 100 of acetone.

Extraction. Benzthiazide may be isolated in the A2 fraction (see p. 27); it is distinguished from the barbiturates by chromatography (see below) and by the presence of additional ultraviolet maxima in the region 270 to 330 mμ.

Chromatography. PAPER: system P16—Rf 0·36 (location under ultraviolet light, absorption; location reagent *sodium naphthaquinone spray*, weak reaction); system RP1b—Rf 0·56 (location as for P16).

Ultraviolet Absorption Spectrum. Benzthiazide in 0·01N ethanolic hydrochloric acid, maximum at 283 mμ (E1%, 1 cm 284).

Infra-red Absorption Spectrum. Potassium bromide disk. The principal peaks are: A 1175, B 1155, C 1311 (p. 731).

Dose. Up to 200 mg daily.

BENZTROPINE *Parasympatholytic*

Synonym: Benzatropine.

3-(Diphenylmethoxy)tropane
$C_{21}H_{25}NO = 307{\cdot}4$

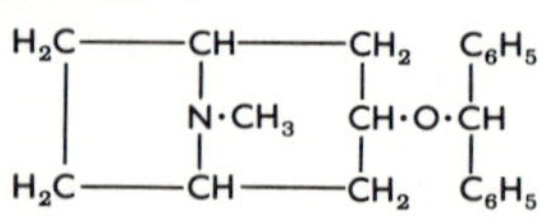

Solubility. Soluble in chloroform.

BENZTROPINE MESYLATE
Synonyms: Benztropine Methanesulphonate; Tropine Diphenylmethyl Ether.
Proprietary Name: Cogentin.

A white slightly hygroscopic crystalline powder. M.p. 142° to 144°.
Solubility. Soluble 1 in 0·7 of water and 1 in 1·5 of ethanol; insoluble in ether.

Extraction. Benztropine is extracted by organic solvents from aqueous alkaline solutions.

Chromatography. PAPER: system P1—Rf 0·76 (location reagents: *iodoplatinate spray*, strong reaction; *bromocresol green spray*, weak reaction); system RP1a—Rf 0·72 (location reagent *iodoplatinate spray*, positive reaction); system RP1b—Rf 0·08 (location as for RP1a).

THIN-LAYER: system T1—Rf 0·12 (location reagent *acidified iodoplatinate spray*, positive reaction).

GAS: system G2/225—retention time 0·92 relative to codeine; system G4—retention time 0·42 relative to codeine.

Colour Tests. MICRO: sulphuric acid–formaldehyde test—yellow (*sensitivity:* 0·025 μg); ammonium molybdate test—yellow (*sensitivity:* 0·025 μg); ammonium vanadate test—yellow (*sensitivity:* 0·1 μg).

Crystal Tests. MICRO: *potassium chromate solution*—long plates or blades (*sensitivity:* 1 in 1000); *potassium iodide solution*—fine dendrites (*sensitivity:* 1 in 400).

Ultraviolet Absorption Spectrum. Benztropine in water, maximum at 258 mμ (E1%, 1 cm 14); in 0·1N sulphuric acid, maxima at 253 mμ (E1%, 1 cm 11) and 259 mμ (E1%, 1 cm 12), and inflexions at 248 mμ and 265 mμ.

Infra-red Absorption Spectrum. Benztropine (base). Potassium chloride disk. The principal peaks are: A 1054, B 700, C 742 or 1191 (p. 775).

Dose. Up to 6 mg daily.

Toxicity. The lethal dose in man is in the range 10 to 100 mg/kg.

BENZYDAMINE *Analgesic*

Synonym: Benzindamine.

1 - Benzyl - 3 - (3 - dimethylaminopropoxy) - 1*H*-indazole

$C_{19}H_{23}N_3O$ = 309·4

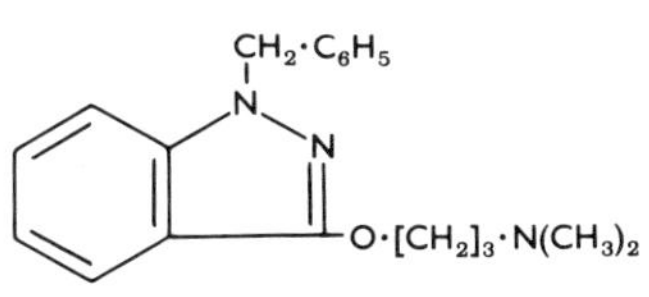

Benzydamine melts at 38° to 39°.

BENZYDAMINE HYDROCHLORIDE
Proprietary Name: Tantum.

A white crystalline powder. M.p. 157° to 159°.
Solubility. Soluble 1 in 1 of water; soluble in ethanol and chloroform; very sparingly soluble in ether.

Extraction. Benzydamine is extracted by organic solvents from aqueous alkaline solutions.

Chromatography. PAPER: system P1—Rf 0·58 (location under ultraviolet light, blue fluorescence; location reagents: *iodoplatinate spray*, weak reaction; *potassium permanganate spray*, weak reaction).

THIN-LAYER: system T1—Rf 0·40 (location reagent *acidified iodoplatinate spray*, positive reaction).

Colour Tests. MICRO: ammonium vanadate test—brownish-green (*sensitivity:* 1·0 μg); Vitali's test— –/pale yellow/dull orange (*sensitivity:* 1·0 μg).

Crystal Tests. MICRO: *lead iodide solution*—dense rosettes (*sensitivity:* 1 in 1000); *styphnic acid*—irregular blades and needles (*sensitivity:* 1 in 1000).

Ultraviolet Absorption Spectrum. Benzydamine in 0·1N sulphuric acid, maximum at 307·5 mμ (E1%, 1 cm 107); benzydamine hydrochloride in water, maximum at about 310 mμ (E1%, 1 cm about 173) and minimum at about 275 mμ.

Metabolism. The administration of benzydamine in man in oral doses of 1 mg/kg produces significant and prolonged blood-levels; a fraction is bound to the plasma proteins. About 50% of the dose is excreted unchanged in the urine; no metabolites have yet been identified. Following intravenous injection in rats, benzydamine passes into the gastro-intestinal tract but is not excreted in the faeces (Catanese *et al.*, 1966).

Dose. Usually 150 to 200 mg daily.

Toxicity. LD50 (oral): in mice 0·54; in rats over 1 g/kg.

BENZYL BENZOATE *Acaricide*

Proprietary Name: Ascabiol.

$C_{14}H_{12}O_2$ = 212·3

$$C_6H_5 \cdot CO \cdot O \cdot CH_2 \cdot C_6H_5$$

Colourless crystals or a colourless oily liquid. F.p. not below 17°. B.p. 320°.
Solubility. Insoluble in water; soluble in ethanol, ether, and chloroform.

Extraction. Benzyl benzoate is extracted by organic solvents from aqueous acid or alkaline solutions.

Ultraviolet Absorption Spectrum. Benzyl benzoate in ethanol, maximum at 230 mμ (E1%, 1 cm 843).

Metabolism. Benzyl benzoate is rapidly hydrolysed *in vivo* to benzoic acid and benzyl alcohol; the latter is then oxidised to benzoic acid.

Toxicity. LD50 (oral): in rats 1·7 mg/kg.

BENZYL NICOTINATE *Vasodilator*

Benzyl pyridine-3-carboxylate

$C_{13}H_{11}NO_2 = 213{\cdot}2$

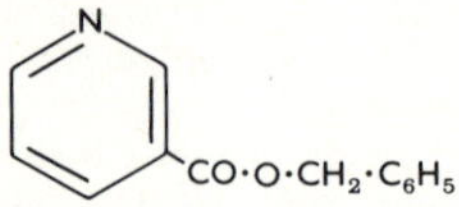

Chromatography. PAPER: system P1—Rf 0·91 (location under ultraviolet light, absorption; location reagent *iodoplatinate spray*, white spot).

THIN-LAYER: system T1—Rf 0·70 (location reagent *potassium permanganate spray*, positive reaction).

Colour Test. MICRO: ammonium molybdate test—pale grey (*sensitivity:* 1·0 μg).

Crystal Tests. MICRO: *picric acid*—irregular blades (*sensitivity:* 1 in 400); *potassium mercuric iodide solution*—branching rods (*sensitivity:* 1 in 400).

Infra-red Absorption Spectrum. Potassium chloride disk. The principal peaks are: A 1278 or 1724, B 1108, C 740 (p. 775).

BENZYLMORPHINE *Narcotic*

3-Benzyloxy-7,8-dehydro-4,5-epoxy-6-hydroxy-*N*-methylmorphinan

$C_{24}H_{25}NO_3 = 375{\cdot}5$

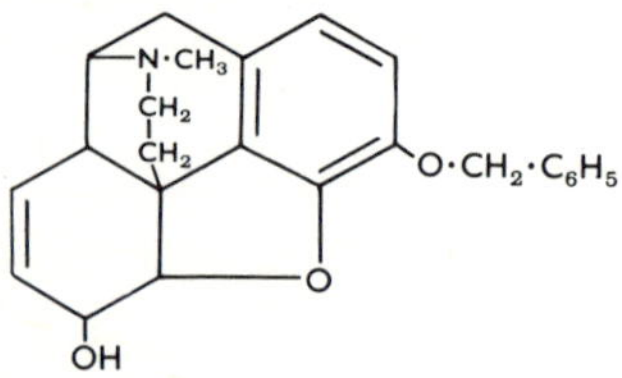

BENZYLMORPHINE HYDROCHLORIDE

A colourless microcrystalline powder.

Solubility. Soluble 1 in 200 of water and 1 in 160 of ethanol; insoluble in ether and chloroform.

Extraction. Benzylmorphine may be isolated in the D3 fraction (see p. 27).

Chromatography. PAPER: system P1—Rf 0·40 (location under ultraviolet light, absorption; location reagent *iodoplatinate spray*, strong reaction); system RP1a—Rf 0·56 (location under ultraviolet light, absorption; location reagent *iodoplatinate spray*, positive reaction); system RP1b—Rf 0·00 (location as for RP1a).

THIN-LAYER: system T1—Rf 0·37 (location reagent *acidified iodoplatinate spray*, positive reaction).

GAS: system G2/225—retention time 5·98 relative to codeine.

Colour Tests. MICRO: sulphuric acid–formaldehyde test—red → purple (*sensitivity:* 0·025 μg); ammonium molybdate test—purple → green (*sensitivity:* 0·05 μg); Vitali's test—faint yellow/faint yellow/orange (*sensitivity:* 1·0 μg).

Crystal Tests. MICRO: *potassium iodide solution*—rosettes of needles and plates (*sensitivity:* 1 in 3000); *sodium carbonate solution*—rosettes of rods (*sensitivity:* 1 in 1500).

Ultraviolet Absorption Spectrum. Benzylmorphine in ethanol, maximum at 282 mμ, minimum at 262 mμ; in 0·1N sulphuric acid, maximum at 284 mμ (E1%, 1cm 48·2); benzylmorphine hydrochloride in water, maximum at 284 mμ, minimum at 264 mμ.

Dose. Up to 30 mg.

BENZYLPENICILLIN *Antibiotic*

Synonyms: Crystalline Penicillin G; Penicillin; Penicillin G.

Proprietary Names: Crystapen; Falapen; Hyasorb; Pondets; Solupen; Tabillin.

Potassium or sodium 6-phenylacetamidopenicillanate

$C_{16}H_{17}KN_2O_4S = 372{\cdot}5$

or $C_{16}H_{17}N_2NaO_4S = 356{\cdot}4$

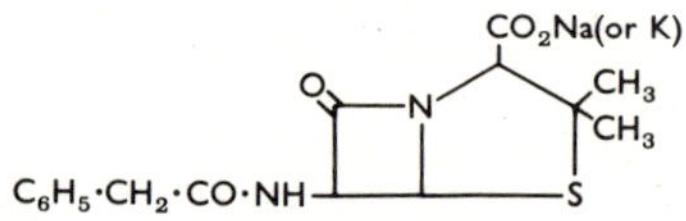

A fine white crystalline powder.

Solubility. Very soluble in water; soluble in ethanol; almost insoluble in ether and chloroform.

Ultraviolet Absorption Spectrum. Benzylpenicillin in water, maxima at 263 mμ and 280 mμ.

Metabolism. When administered by mouth, benzylpenicillin is inactivated fairly rapidly by gastric secretions and is only poorly absorbed from the upper part of the gastro-intestinal tract; maximum serum levels may not be attained for about an hour. Following intramuscular injection, benzylpenicillin appears rapidly in the blood, maximum levels being reached in 20 to 30 minutes; following a single injection of about 200 mg, a therapeutic blood-level is maintained for about 5 hours. The minimum effective serum penicillin level is about 0·0018 to 0·003 mg%; a level of 0·003 to 0·006 mg% is usually desirable. Benzylpenicillin is rapidly excreted in the urine; up to 60% of a single intramuscular dose may appear in the urine within 1 hour of administration and 95% within 4 hours. Small amounts are excreted in the bile but, as it is destroyed by enzymes in the lower gastro-intestinal tract, little or none appears in the faeces. Between 30 and 60% of the dose is excreted unchanged, most of the remainder being excreted as a fission product, penicilloic acid; the latter may be further split at its peptide linkage to give phenylacetic acid which is excreted as its glycine conjugate, phenaceturic acid.

Dose. In severe infections, as much as 24 g may be given daily.

Toxicity. Most of the deaths which occur following the administration of benzylpenicillin are due to allergic reactions or to overgrowth of resistant organisms.

BEPHENIUM HYDROXYNAPHTHOATE

Anthelmintic

Proprietary Name: Alcopar.

Benzyldimethyl(2-phenoxyethyl)ammonium 3-hydroxynaphthalene-2-carboxylate

$C_{28}H_{29}NO_4 = 443{\cdot}5$

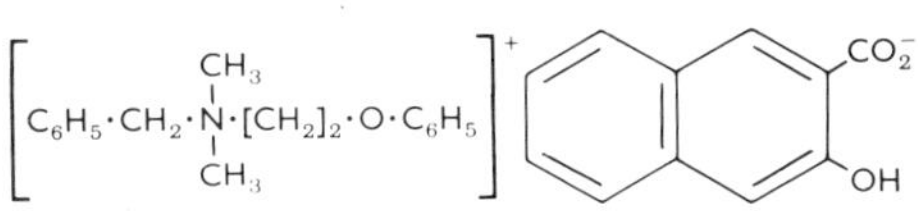

A yellow crystalline powder which gives a green fluorescence when examined under ultraviolet light. M.p. about 170°, with decomposition.

Solubility. Insoluble in water; soluble 1 in 50 of ethanol.

NOTE. Bephenium embonate has also been used.

Chromatography. PAPER: system P1—Rf 0·66 (location under ultraviolet light, yellow fluorescence; location reagent *iodoplatinate spray*, strong reaction); system RP1a—Rf 0·83 (location reagent *iodoplatinate spray*, positive reaction); system RP1b—Rf 0·84 (location as for RP1a).

THIN-LAYER: system T1—Rf 0·77 (location reagent *potassium permanganate spray*, positive reaction).

Colour Tests. MICRO: sulphuric acid–formaldehyde test—red-purple (*sensitivity:* 0·1 μg); ammonium molybdate test—green (*sensitivity:* 0·25 μg); ammonium vanadate test—green (*sensitivity:* 0·25 μg); Vitali's test—light brown/light brown/red (*sensitivity:* 0·5 μg).

Ultraviolet Absorption Spectrum. Bephenium embonate in 0·1N sodium hydroxide, maxima at about 269 mμ (E 1%, 1 cm 10), 275 mμ (E 1%, 1 cm 9), 288 mμ (E 1%, 1 cm 8), 300 mμ (E 1%, 1 cm 6), and 365 mμ (E 1%, 1 cm 6); in 0·1N sulphuric acid, maxima at 263 mμ (E 1%, 1 cm 27), 269 mμ (E 1%, 1 cm 31), and 275 mμ (E 1%, 1 cm 21).

Infra-red Absorption Spectrum. Potassium bromide disk. The principal peaks are: A 755 or 1445, B 1225 or 1348 or 1382 (p. 775).

Quantitative Estimation. Rogers (1958) describes a spectrophotometric method of determination of bephenium in urine which is a modification of the methyl orange dye-lake procedure.

Metabolism. When administered by mouth, only a small fraction of the dose is absorbed from the gastro-intestinal tract. Very little unchanged bephenium or its metabolites are excreted in the urine in man. Following ingestion of 1 g of the hydroxynaphthoate, 0·25 to 0·52% of the dose expressed as the base was recovered in the urine in 24 hours and, after the ingestion of 3 g, recovery was 0·18 to 0·22% (Rogers, 1958).

Dose. Usually 5 g as a single dose.

Toxicity. LD50 (oral): in mice 2 and in rats 5 g/kg.

BERBERINE

Alkaloid

$C_{20}H_{19}NO_5 = 353{\cdot}4$

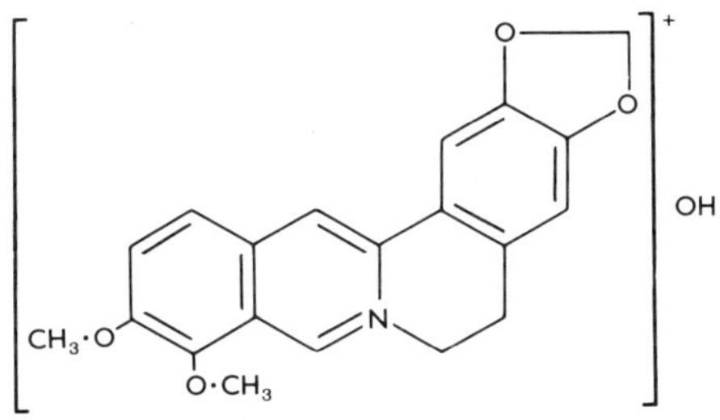

An alkaloid present in various species of *Berberis* (Berberidaceae) and many other plants. Yellow crystals. M.p. 144°.

Solubility. Soluble 1 in 4·5 of water and 1 in 100 of ethanol; very slightly soluble in ether.

BERBERINE HYDROCHLORIDE

Bright yellow crystals or powder.

Solubility. Soluble 1 in 400 of water; freely soluble in boiling water; soluble in ethanol; insoluble in ether and chloroform.

BERBERINE SULPHATE

Synonyms: Berberine Acid Sulphate; Berberine Bisulphate.

Yellow crystals or powder.

Solubility. Soluble 1 in 150 of water; slightly soluble in ethanol.

Extraction. Berberine may be isolated in the D2 fraction (see p. 27).

Chromatography. PAPER: system P1—Rf 0·25 (location under ultraviolet light, faint yellow fluorescence; location reagent *iodoplatinate spray*, weak reaction); system RP1a—Rf 0·27 (location under ultraviolet light, greenish-yellow fluorescence); system RP1b—Rf 0·35 (location as for RP1a).

THIN-LAYER: system T1—Rf 0·07 (location reagent *acidified iodoplatinate spray*, positive reaction).

GAS: system G6—retention time 0·41 relative to codeine.

Colour Tests. MICRO: sulphuric acid–formaldehyde test—(yellow) green (*sensitivity:* 0·05 μg); ammonium molybdate test—brown → green (*sensitivity:* 0·025 μg); ammonium vanadate test—blue-green → brown → purple (*sensitivity:*

0·025 μg); Vitali's test—brown/brown/dark brown (*sensitivity:* 0·025 μg).

Crystal Tests. MICRO: *gold cyanide solution*—feathery rosettes (*sensitivity:* 1 in 3000); *picric acid*—curved needles (*sensitivity:* 1 in 3000).

Ultraviolet Absorption Spectrum. Berberine in ethanol, maxima at 267 mμ (E1%, 1 cm 769), 347 mμ (E1%, 1 cm 580), and 426 mμ (E1%, 1 cm 125); in 0·1N sulphuric acid, maxima at 228 mμ (E1%, 1 cm 578), 264 mμ (E1%, 1 cm 554), and 345 mμ (E1%, 1 cm 500).

Infra-red Absorption Spectrum. Berberine (base). Potassium bromide disk. The principal peaks are: A 1505, B 1271, C 1360 (p. 776).

BETAMEPRODINE *Narcotic*

Synonym: β-Meprodine.

β-3-Ethyl-1-methyl-4-phenyl-4-propionyloxypiperidine

$C_{17}H_{25}NO_2 = 275{\cdot}4$

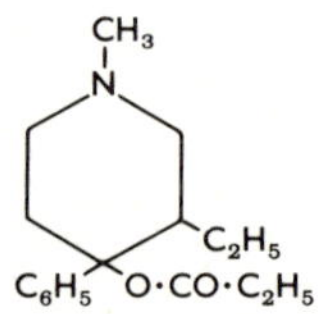

Extraction. Betameprodine is extracted by organic solvents from aqueous alkaline solutions.

Chromatography. PAPER: system P1—Rf 0·61 (location reagents: *iodoplatinate spray*, strong reaction; *bromocresol green spray*, weak reaction); system RP1a—Rf 0·60 (location reagent *iodoplatinate spray*, positive reaction); system RP1b—Rf 0·00 (location reagent *iodoplatinate spray*, positive reaction).

THIN-LAYER: system T1—Rf 0·64 (location reagent *acidified iodoplatinate spray*, positive reaction).

GAS: system G2/225—retention time 0·92 relative to diphenhydramine; system G4—retention time 0·40 relative to diphenhydramine.

Colour Tests. MICRO: sulphuric acid–formaldehyde test—reddish-purple (*sensitivity:* 0·25 μg); ammonium molybdate test—blue-grey → green (*sensitivity:* 0·5 μg); ammonium vanadate test—blue-grey (*sensitivity:* 0·5 μg).

Crystal Tests. MICRO: *picric acid*—bunches of rods (*sensitivity:* 1 in 1000); *styphnic acid*—blades, sometimes in rosettes (*sensitivity:* 1 in 200).

BETAMETHASONE *Corticosteroid*

Synonym: 9α-Fluoro-16β-methylprednisolone.

Proprietary Names: Betnelan; Celestone.

9α-Fluoro-11β,17α,21-trihydroxy-16β-methylpregna-1,4-diene-3,20-dione

$C_{22}H_{29}FO_5 = 392{\cdot}5$

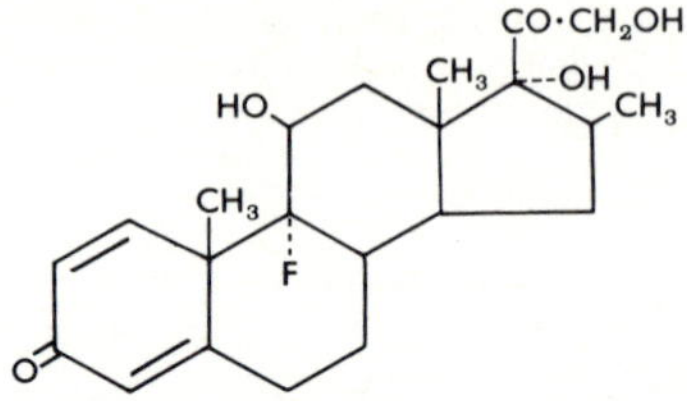

A white powder. M.p. about 246°, with decomposition. Specific rotation of a 0·5% solution in dioxan, +115° to +121°.

Solubility. Almost insoluble in water; soluble 1 in 75 of ethanol and 1 in 1100 of chloroform; very slightly soluble in ether; sparingly soluble in acetone and methanol.

BETAMETHASONE SODIUM PHOSPHATE

Synonym: Betamethasone Disodium Phosphate.

Proprietary Names: Beta-Corlan; Betnesol.

A white crystalline hygroscopic powder. Specific rotation of a 1% aqueous solution +99° to +105°.

Solubility. Soluble 1 in 2 of water and 1 in 350 of ethanol; insoluble in chloroform.

BETAMETHASONE VALERATE

9α - Fluoro - 11β,21 - dihydroxy - 16β - methyl - 17α - valeryloxypregna-1,4-diene-3,20-dione

Synonym: Betamethasone 17-Valerate.

Proprietary Name: Betnovate.

A white crystalline powder. M.p. about 193°; it may occur in a lower melting form.

Solubility. Insoluble in water; soluble 1 in 12 of ethanol, 1 in 2 of chloroform, and 1 in 50 of isopropanol.

NOTE. In alkaline media betamethasone 17-valerate undergoes a rearrangement to betamethasone 21-valerate.

Extraction. Betamethasone is extracted from neutral solutions with freshly distilled ethyl acetate.

Chromatography. PAPER, for betamethasone and betamethasone sodium phosphate: system P13—Rf 0·16 (location reagent *DPST solution*, violet on yellow); for betamethasone valerate: system P14—Rf 0·86 (location as for P13).

THIN-LAYER, for betamethasone: system T18—Rf 0·26 (location reagent *DPST spray*); for betamethasone valerate: system T18—Rf 0·71 (location reagent *DPST spray*); for betamethasone: system T19—Rf 1·00 (location reagent *DPST spray*).

Ultraviolet Absorption Spectrum. Betamethasone in ethanol, maximum at 240 mμ (E1%, 1 cm 390); betamethasone sodium phosphate in water, maximum at 241 mμ (E1%, 1 cm 297).

Infra-red Absorption Spectrum. Betamethasone. Potassium bromide disk. The principal peaks are: A 1648, B 1608, C 1697 (p. 732).

Dose. Up to 5 mg (base) daily.

NOTE. Betamethasone is a synthetic glucocorticoid and an isomer of dexamethasone.

BETANAPHTHOL *Parasiticide*

Synonyms: β-Naftol; β-Naphthol.

Naphth-2-ol

$C_{10}H_8O = 144{\cdot}2$

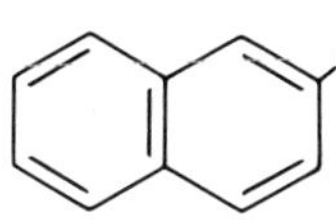

A white crystalline powder which darkens on exposure to light. M.p. 120°. B.p. 285° to 286°.

Solubility. Soluble 1 in 1000 of cold water, 1 in 80 of boiling water, 1 in 1 of ethanol, and 1 in 1·5 of ether; soluble in chloroform.

Extraction. Betanaphthol may be isolated in the A2 fraction (see p. 27).

Colour Tests. To 200 mg add 2 ml of a 8% sodium hydroxide solution and 1 drop of chloroform, then warm—blue.

MICRO: coupling with *diazotised* p-*nitroaniline solution*—red.

Ultraviolet Absorption Spectrum. Betanaphthol in ethanol, maxima at 226 mμ (E1%, 1 cm 4980), 274 mμ (E1%, 1 cm 326), 285 mμ (E1%, 1 cm 230), 322 mμ (E1%, 1 cm 120), and 330 mμ (E1%, 1 cm 140).

Metabolism. Betanaphthol is rapidly absorbed and may be absorbed through the intact skin. It is locally irritant to mucous membranes and especially irritant to the kidneys. It is excreted chiefly in combination with glucuronic acid. The urine may acquire a brownish-red tint.

Toxicity. The estimated lethal dose in man is between 2 and 5 g. Severe nephritis and fatalities have occurred following its absorption through the skin.

BETAPRODINE *Narcotic*

β-1,3-Dimethyl-4-phenyl-4-propionyloxypiperidine

$C_{16}H_{23}NO_2 = 261{\cdot}4$

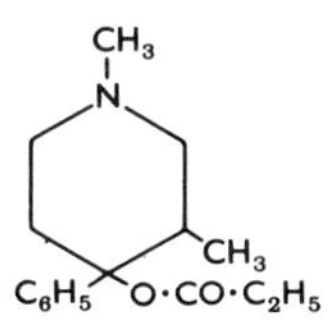

BETAPRODINE HYDROCHLORIDE

Synonym: NU 1779.

It occurs as crystals from acetone:methanol. M.p. 190° to 192°.

Extraction. Betaprodine is extracted by organic solvents from aqueous alkaline solutions.

Chromatography. PAPER: system P1—Rf 0·30, tailing (location reagent *iodoplatinate spray*, strong reaction); system RP1a—Rf 0·78 (location reagent *iodoplatinate spray*, positive reaction); system RP1b—Rf 0·04 (location under ultraviolet light, purple fluorescence; location reagent *iodoplatinate spray*, positive reaction).

THIN-LAYER: system T1—Rf 0·61 (location reagent *acidified iodoplatinate spray*, positive reaction).

GAS: system G2/225—retention time 0·84 relative to diphenhydramine; system G4—retention time 0·41 relative to diphenhydramine.

Colour Tests. MICRO: sulphuric acid–formaldehyde test—reddish-purple (*sensitivity:* 0·25 μg); ammonium molybdate test—blue-green → green with blue rim (*sensitivity:* 0·5 μg); ammonium vanadate test—blue-grey (*sensitivity:* 0·5 μg).

Crystal Tests. MICRO: *lead iodide solution*—rosettes or bunches of irregular rods (*sensitivity:* 1 in 1000); *styphnic acid*—plates, often in rosettes (*sensitivity:* 1 in 1000).

Ultraviolet Absorption Spectrum. Betaprodine in 0·1N sulphuric acid, maxima at 248 mμ (E1%, 1 cm 5), 252·5 mμ (E1%, 1 cm 6·3), 258 mμ (E1%, 1 cm 7·6), 264 mμ (E1%, 1 cm 6·3), and 268 mμ (E1%, 1 cm 4·2).

BETHANECHOL CHLORIDE *Parasympathomimetic*

Synonym: Carbamylmethylcholine Chloride.

Proprietary Names: Mechothane; Urecholine Chloride.

(2-Carbamoyloxypropyl)trimethylammonium chloride

$C_7H_{17}ClN_2O_2 = 196{\cdot}7$

$$\left[(CH_3)_3N{\cdot}CH_2{\cdot}\underset{}{\overset{CH_3}{\overset{|}{C}}}H{\cdot}O{\cdot}CO{\cdot}NH_2\right]^+ \quad Cl^-$$

A white crystalline hygroscopic powder. It occurs in two crystalline forms, one melting at about 211° and the other at about 219°.

Solubility. Soluble 1 in 1 of water and 1 in 10 of ethanol; insoluble in ether and chloroform.

Extraction. Bethanechol chloride is a quaternary ammonium compound (see p. 29).

Chromatography. PAPER: system P1—Rf 0·05 (location reagent *iodoplatinate spray*, strong reaction).

THIN-LAYER: system T1—Rf 0·02 (location reagent *acidified iodoplatinate spray*, positive reaction).

Crystal Tests. MICRO: *gold bromide solution*—plates and needles (*sensitivity:* 1 in 400); *platinic iodide solution*—plates and rods (*sensitivity:* 1 in 400).

Infra-red Absorption Spectrum. Potassium bromide disk. The principal peaks are: A 1712, B 1014 or 1340, C 1300 (p. 776).

Metabolism. Bethanechol chloride is a parasympathomimetic agent which is not destroyed by cholinesterase; it is stable in the bloodstream and in tissues.

Toxicity. The maximum safe oral dose is usually 30 mg and the maximum safe subcutaneous dose is usually 10 mg. Bethanechol chloride should never be administered intravenously or intramuscularly; the estimated minimum lethal dose in man by intravenous or intramuscular injection is 20 mg.

BETHANIDINE *Antihypertensive*

N-Benzyl-*N′N″*-dimethylguanidine

$C_{10}H_{15}N_3 = 177{\cdot}3$

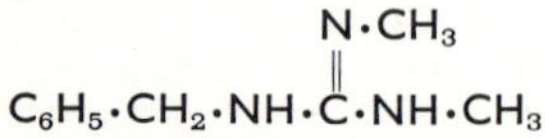

BETHANIDINE SULPHATE

Proprietary Name: Esbatal.

A white crystalline powder. M.p. 280°.

Solubility. Soluble in water; insoluble in ethanol.

Extraction. Bethanidine is extracted by organic solvents from aqueous alkaline solutions.

Chromatography. PAPER: system P1—Rf 0·62 (location under ultraviolet light, absorption; location reagents: *iodoplatinate spray*, strong reaction; *bromocresol green spray*, strong reaction).

THIN-LAYER: system T1—Rf 0·11 (location reagent *Dragendorff spray*, positive reaction).

Colour Tests. MICRO: sulphuric acid–formaldehyde test—orange-red (*sensitivity:* 0·5 μg); ammonium molybdate test—grey (*sensitivity:* 0·1 μg); Vitali's test— –/–/grey → yellow (*sensitivity:* 1·0 μg).

Crystal Tests. MICRO: *gold cyanide solution*—branching needles; *potassium cadmium iodide solution*—blades and plates (*sensitivity:* 1 in 400).

Ultraviolet Absorption Spectrum. Bethanidine in water, maxima at 251 mμ (E1%, 1 cm 10) and 257 mμ (E1%, 1 cm 13), and inflexions at 246 mμ and 262 mμ; bethanidine sulphate in water, maxima at 252 mμ (E1%, 1 cm 7·1), 258 mμ (E1%, 1 cm 8·8), and 263 mμ (E1%, 1 cm 6·7); minima at 233 mμ, 254 mμ, and 262 mμ.

Quantitative Estimation. Bethanidine may be estimated in urine by treatment with alkaline hypobromite, extraction of the bromo-derivative with carbon tetrachloride, and spectrophotometric estimation of the iodine liberated from acidified potassium iodide (McCoubrey, 1962).

Metabolism. Bethanidine is well absorbed from the gastro-intestinal tract and, in therapeutic doses, starts to take effect in 1 to 2 hours, reaching its peak in 4 to 5 hours and lasting for about 12 hours. Following oral administration of ^{14}C-labelled bethanidine, practically all the radioactivity was excreted in the urine within 24 hours (Doyle and Morley, 1965); however, chemical determination detected only about 20% of the dose excreted as unchanged bethanidine during 24 hours; the fall in urinary excretion during prolonged dosage suggests that the drug may be metabolised, but no *N*-demethylated metabolites have been detected (McCoubrey, 1962).

Dose. Up to 200 mg daily.

Toxicity. LD50 (oral): in mice 520 mg/kg.

BIALAMICOL *Anti-amoebic*

Synonyms: Biallylamicol; Biethylamicol; CT 871; PAA 701; SN 6771.

3,3′-Diallyl-5,5′-di(diethylaminomethyl)-4,4′-dihydroxybiphenyl

$C_{28}H_{40}N_2O_2 = 436{\cdot}6$

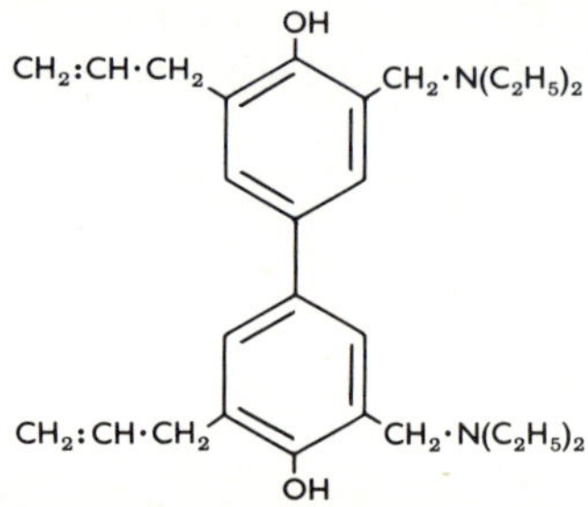

BIALAMICOL HYDROCHLORIDE

Proprietary Name: Camoform.

A white crystalline power. M.p. about 210°.

Solubility. Soluble 1 in 5 of water, 1 in 40 of ethanol, and 1 in 150 of chloroform; slightly soluble in ether.

Extraction. Bialamicol is extracted by organic solvents from aqueous ammoniacal solutions.

Colour Test. Dissolve 100 mg in 2 ml of water and add 2 ml of nitric acid—intense orange-red.

Ultraviolet Absorption Spectrum. Bialamicol in 0·01N hydrochloric acid, maximum at about 266 mμ (E1%, 1 cm about 476).

Metabolism. Bialamicol is rapidly absorbed from the gastro-intestinal tract and stored in the liver, lungs, and other tissues in high concentration. It is slowly excreted via the bile into the faeces.

Dose. Up to 1·5 g daily for 5 days.

BIBENZONIUM BROMIDE *Antitussive*

Synonyms: Diphenetholine Bromide; ES 132.

Proprietary Name: Thoragol.

[2-(1,2-Diphenylethoxy)ethyl]trimethylammonium bromide

$C_{19}H_{27}BrNO = 365{\cdot}3$

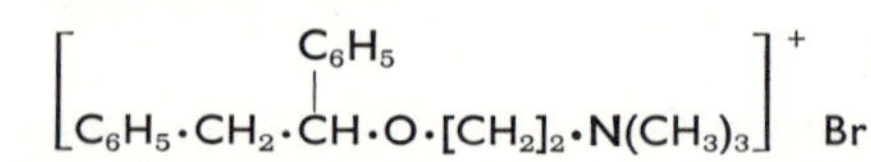

Bibenzonium bromide melts at 142° to 144°.

Solubility. Very soluble in water and ethanol; insoluble in ether.

Extraction. Bibenzonium bromide is a quaternary ammonium compound (see p. 29).

Chromatography. PAPER: system P1—Rf 0·56 (location reagent *iodoplatinate spray*, strong reaction); system RP1a—Rf 0·85 (location reagent *iodoplatinate spray*, positive reaction); system RP1b—Rf 0·84 (location as for RP1a).

THIN-LAYER: system T1—Rf 0·02 (location reagent *acidified iodoplatinate spray*, positive reaction).

Colour Tests. MICRO: the following tests are performed on bibenzonium nitrate (see p. 134): sulphuric acid–formaldehyde test—light brown; ammonium molybdate test—blue-green; ammonium vanadate test—olive; Vitali's test—-/-/purple-blue.

Crystal Tests. MICRO: *gold chloride solution*—oily brown needles, best viewed under polarised light (*sensitivity:* 1 in 1000); *lead iodide solution*—small rosettes or very small needles (*sensitivity:* 1 in 1000).

Ultraviolet Absorption Spectrum. Bibenzonium bromide in 0·1N sulphuric acid, maxima at about 247·5 mμ (E1%, 1 cm 9), 252·5 mμ (E1%, 1 cm 12), 258 mμ (E1%, 1 cm 15), 264 mμ (E1%, 1 cm 12), and 268 mμ (E1%, 1 cm 9).

Infra-red Absorption Spectrum. Potassium bromide disk. The principal peaks are: A 705, B 1095, C 749 or 759 (p. 776).

Dose. Up to 120 mg daily.

BIPERIDEN *Parasympatholytic*

1-(Bicyclo[2,2,1]hept-5-en-2-yl)-1-phenyl-3-piperidinopropan-1-ol

$C_{21}H_{29}NO = 311{\cdot}5$

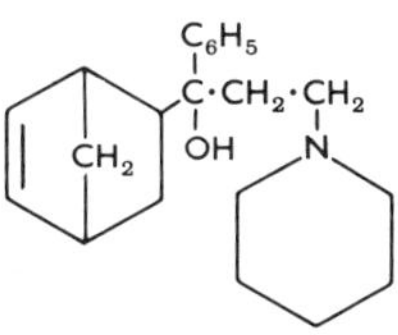

BIPERIDEN HYDROCHLORIDE

Proprietary Name: Akineton (tablets).

A white crystalline powder.

Solubility. Slightly soluble in water and ethanol.

BIPERIDEN LACTATE

Proprietary Name: Akineton (injection).

Extraction. Biperiden is extracted by organic solvents from aqueous alkaline solutions.

Chromatography. PAPER: system P1—Rf 0·87 (location reagent *iodoplatinate spray*, weak reaction).

THIN-LAYER: system T1—Rf 0·62 (location reagent *acidified iodoplatinate spray*, positive reaction).

GAS: system G2/225—retention time 0·79 relative to codeine; system G4—retention time 0·35 relative to codeine.

Colour Tests. MICRO: sulphuric acid–formaldehyde test—light red-brown (*sensitivity:* 1·0 μg); ammonium molybdate test—grey-purple → brown (*sensitivity:* 0·5 μg).

Crystal Tests. MICRO: *picrolonic acid*—sheaves of needles (*sensitivity:* 1 in 400); *zinc chloride solution*—bunches of needles (*sensitivity:* 1 in 200).

Infra-red Absorption Spectrum. Biperiden (base). Potassium bromide disk. The principal peaks are: A 697, B 733, C 1436 (p. 776).

Dose. Up to 20 mg daily.

Toxicity. The lethal dose in man is probably between 10 and 100 mg/kg.

LD50 (oral): in dogs 340, in mice 545, and in rats 750 mg/kg.

BISACODYL *Purgative*

Proprietary Names: Dulcolax; Laco.

2-(4,4′-Diacetoxydiphenylmethyl)pyridine

$C_{22}H_{19}NO_4 = 361{\cdot}4$

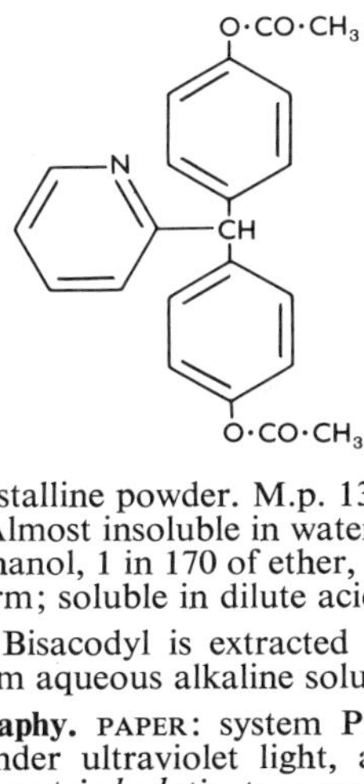

A white crystalline powder. M.p. 133° to 135°.

Solubility. Almost insoluble in water; soluble 1 in 100 of ethanol, 1 in 170 of ether, and 1 in 35 of chloroform; soluble in dilute acids.

Extraction. Bisacodyl is extracted by organic solvents from aqueous alkaline solutions.

Chromatography. PAPER: system P1—Rf 0·90 (location under ultraviolet light, absorption; location reagent *iodoplatinate spray*, very weak reaction).

THIN-LAYER: system T1—Rf 0·70 (location reagent *acidified iodoplatinate spray*, positive reaction).

Colour Tests. MICRO: sulphuric acid–formaldehyde test—purple (*sensitivity:* 0·1 μg); ammonium molybdate test—blue (*sensitivity:* 0·25 μg); ammonium vanadate test—bright purple (*sensitivity:* 0·25 μg); Vitali's test—orange/yellow/orange (*sensitivity:* 0·25 μg).

Crystal Tests. MICRO: *lead iodide solution*—blades or feathery rosettes (*sensitivity:* 1 in 1000); *sodium carbonate solution*—branching or dense rosettes or needles (*sensitivity:* 1 in 1000).

Ultraviolet Absorption Spectrum. Bisacodyl in ethanol, maxima at 259 mμ, and 263 mμ; in 0·1N methanolic potassium hydroxide, maximum at 248 mμ (E1%, 1 cm 640); in 0·1N sulphuric acid, maximum at 264·5 mμ (E1%, 1cm 266), and an inflexion at about 275 mμ (E1%, 1cm 198).

Infra-red Absorption Spectrum. Potassium bromide disk. The principal peaks are: A 1212, B 1198, C 1754 (p. 776).

Metabolism. Bisacodyl has little or no action on the small intestine and is not absorbed.

Dose. Up to 10 mg, by mouth or by rectum.

Toxicity. LD50 (oral): in rats greater than 3 g/kg.

BRETYLIUM TOSYLATE *Antihypertensive*

Proprietary Name: Darenthin.

(*o* - Bromobenzyl)ethyldimethylammonium toluene-*p*-sulphonate

$C_{18}H_{24}BrNO_3S = 414·4$

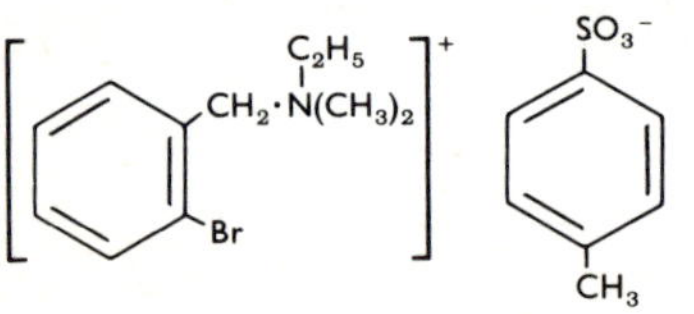

Bretylium tosylate melts at 85° to 86°.

Solubility. Soluble 1 in 1 of water and 1 in 0·4 of ethanol; insoluble in ether.

Extraction. Bretylium tosylate is a quaternary ammonium compound (see p. 29).

Chromatography. PAPER: system P1—Rf 0·44 (location under ultraviolet light, absorption; location reagent *iodoplatinate spray*, strong reaction); system RP1a—Rf 0·92 (location reagent *iodoplatinate spray*, positive reaction).

THIN-LAYER: system T1—Rf 0·01 (location reagent *acidified iodoplatinate spray*, positive reaction).

Crystal Tests. MICRO: *platinic bromide solution*—thin irregular plates, best viewed under polarised light (*sensitivity:* 1 in 1000); *potassium cadmium iodide solution*—blades, often in crosses (*sensitivity:* 1 in 1000).

Ultraviolet Absorption Spectrum. Bretylium tosylate in ethanol and in 0·1N hydrochloric acid, maxima at 256 mμ (E1%, 1cm 13), 264 mμ (E1%, 1cm 18), and 270·5 mμ (E1%, 1cm 21).

Infra-red Absorption Spectrum. Potassium bromide disk. The principal peaks are: A 1188, B 1012, C 1032 (p. 732).

Quantitative Estimation. Bretylium tosylate may be determined very rapidly in blood and urine by the formation of a complex with dipicrylamine which is extracted into benzene and measured spectrophotometrically (Johnson and Revill, 1965). Tompsett *et al.* (1961) and Tompsett (1962) describe a method of extraction from serum and urine and subsequent quantitative determination—see under Extraction Methods, Water-soluble Compounds, p. 28.

Metabolism. Following oral administration of 4·8 g of bretylium tosylate, 10·5% was recovered in the urine in 24 hours, after 400 mg, 19·3% was recovered, and after 200 mg, 27·5% was recovered (Tompsett *et al.*, 1961).

Dose. Up to 1·2 g daily.

Toxicity. LD50 (intravenous): in mice 16 mg/kg.

BROMODIPHENHYDRAMINE *Antihistamine*

Synonyms: Bromazine; Bromdiphenhydramine; Histabromamine.

2-(α-*p*-Bromophenyl-α-phenylmethoxy)-*NN*-dimethylethylamine

$C_{17}H_{20}BrNO = 334·2$

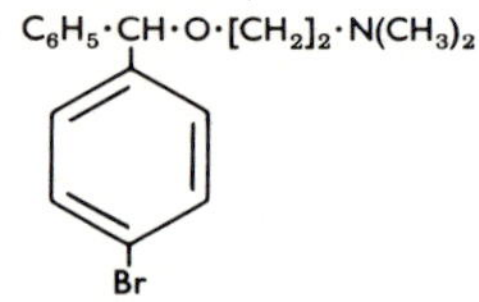

BROMODIPHENHYDRAMINE HYDROCHLORIDE

Proprietary Names: Ambodryl; Deserol.

Bromodiphenhydramine hydrochloride melts at 144° to 145°.

Solubility. Soluble in water.

Extraction. Bromodiphenhydramine is extracted by organic solvents from aqueous alkaline solutions.

Chromatography. PAPER: system P1—Rf 0·69 (location under ultraviolet light, absorption; location reagents: *iodoplatinate spray*, strong reaction; *bromocresol green spray*, weak reaction); system RP1a—Rf 0·31 (location reagent *iodoplatinate spray*, positive reaction); system RP1b—Rf 0·00.

THIN-LAYER: system T1—Rf 0·49 (location reagent *acidified iodoplatinate spray*, positive reaction); system T3—Rf 0·86 (location reagent *iodoplatinate spray*, positive reaction); system T4—Rf 0·80 (location as for T3).

GAS: system G1/180—retention time 2·82 relative to diphenhydramine.

Colour Tests. MICRO: sulphuric acid–formaldehyde test—yellow; ammonium molybdate test—yellow.

Crystal Tests. MICRO: *gold chloride solution*—plates and rods (*sensitivity:* 1 in 1000); *lead iodide solution*—plates, sometimes in small rosettes (*sensitivity:* 1 in 1000).

Ultraviolet Absorption Spectrum. Bromodiphenhydramine in 0·1N sulphuric acid, maximum at 230 mμ (E1%, 1cm 425).

Infra-red Absorption Spectrum. Bromodiphenhydramine (base). Potassium bromide disk. The principal peaks are: A 1067, B 1094 or 1483, C 696 or 1007 (p. 776).

Dose. Up to 100 mg daily.

Toxicity. Bromodiphenhydramine is about twice as potent as diphenhydramine and has a lower incidence of side-effects. The lethal dose in man is probably between 25 and 50 mg/kg.

BROMPHENIRAMINE *Antihistamine*

Synonym: Parabromdylamine.

3-*p*-Bromophenyl-*NN*-dimethyl-3-pyrid-2′-yl-propylamine

$C_{16}H_{19}BrN_2 = 319{\cdot}3$

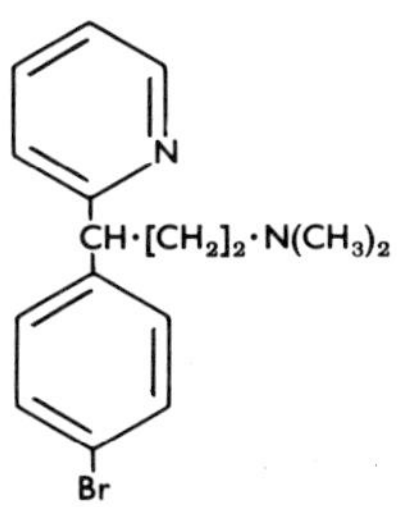

NOTE. The chromatographic data of brompheniramine are similar to those of dexbrompheniramine (p. 288) which is the (+)-isomer of brompheniramine—see also Microcrystal Tests, p. 140.

BROMPHENIRAMINE MALEATE

Proprietary Names: Dimetane; Dimotane.

A white crystalline powder. M.p. 130° to 135°.
Solubility. Soluble 1 in 5 of water, 1 in 15 of ethanol, and 1 in 15 of chloroform; slightly soluble in ether.

Extraction. Brompheniramine is extracted by organic solvents from aqueous alkaline solutions.

Chromatography. PAPER: system P1—Rf 0·45 (location under ultraviolet light, absorption; location reagents: *iodoplatinate spray*, strong reaction; *bromocresol green spray*, weak reaction).
THIN-LAYER: system T1—Rf 0·34 (location reagent *acidified iodoplatinate spray*, positive reaction); system T2—Rf 0·48 (location reagent *iodoplatinate spray*, positive reaction); system T3—Rf 0·42 (location as for T2).

Crystal Tests. MICRO: *gold bromide–hydrochloric acid solution*—plates (*sensitivity:* 1 in 100); *lead iodide solution*—dense rosettes (*sensitivity:* 1 in 1000).

Ultraviolet Absorption Spectrum. Brompheniramine in 0·1N sulphuric acid, maximum at 265 mμ (E1%, 1cm 274); minimum at 245 mμ.

Dose. Usually up to 32 mg daily.

Toxicity. The estimated lethal dose in man is between 5 and 10 mg/kg.

BROMVALETONE *Hypnotic*

Synonyms: Bromisovalerylurea; Bromisovalum; Bromylum.
Proprietary Name: Bromural.

N-(2-Bromo-3-methylbutyryl)urea

$C_6H_{11}BrN_2O_2 = 223{\cdot}1$

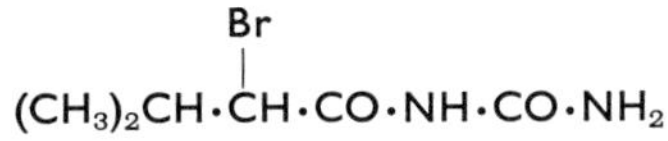

Small white crystals which sublime on heating. M.p. 147° to 150°.
Solubility. Soluble 1 in 500 of water, 1 in 15 of ethanol, 1 in 25 of ether, and 1 in 6 of chloroform; soluble in solutions of alkali hydroxides.

Extraction. Bromvaletone is extracted by organic solvents from aqueous acid or alkaline solutions.

Chromatography. THIN-LAYER: system T10—Rf 0·26 (location reagents: *fluorescein spray*, pink; *potassium permanganate spray*, yellow-brown).

Ultraviolet Absorption Spectrum. Bromvaletone in 0·1N sodium hydroxide, maximum at 228 mμ (E1%, 1cm 160).

Infra-red Absorption Spectrum. Potassium bromide disk. The principal peaks are: A 1700 or 1721, B 1581 (p. 732).

Quantitative Estimation. Goldbaum and Domanski (1966) have described a procedure involving gas chromatography for extraction and quantitative determination applicable to bromvaletone in biological fluids and tissues.

Metabolism. Bromvaletone appears to be entirely metabolised in man; none of the unchanged drug can be detected in the tissues or urine, although bromine can be found.

Dose. Usually 300 to 600 mg; maximum in 24 hours 1·5 g.

BRUCINE *Alkaloid*

Synonym: Dimethoxystrychnine.

$C_{23}H_{26}N_2O_4,4H_2O = 466{\cdot}5$

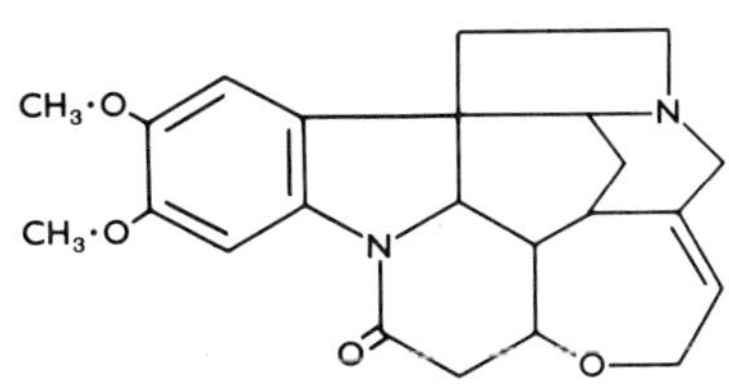

An alkaloid present in the seeds of *Strychnos nux-vomica* and other species of *Strychnos* (Loganiaceae).
Small white crystals. M.p. of the anhydrous base, 178° and m.p. of the hydrated form, 105°.
Solubility. Soluble 1 in 1320 of water, 1 in 1·3 of ethanol, 1 in 187 of ether, and 1 in 5 of chloroform.

BRUCINE SULPHATE
Small white crystals or powder.
Solubility. Soluble 1 in 75 of cold water and 1 in about 10 of boiling water; soluble 1 in 105 of ethanol and 1 in 170 of chloroform.

Extraction. Brucine may be isolated in the D1 fraction (see p. 27).

Chromatography. PAPER: system P1—Rf 0·17 (location under ultraviolet light, absorption; location reagents: *iodoplatinate spray*, weak reaction; *bromocresol green spray*, weak reaction); system RP1a—Rf 0·77 (location under ultraviolet light, absorption; location reagent *iodoplatinate spray*, positive reaction); system RP1b—Rf 0·47 (location as for RP1a).

THIN-LAYER: system T1—Rf 0·12 (location reagent *acidified iodoplatinate spray*, positive reaction).

Colour Tests. MICRO: ammonium molybdate test—blue-purple (*sensitivity:* 1·0 μg); Vitali's test—orange/red/red (*sensitivity:* 0·1 μg).

Crystal Tests. MICRO: *platinic chloride solution*—needles (*sensitivity:* 1 in 1500); *potassium chromate solution*—bunches of rods (*sensitivity:* 1 in 3000).

Ultraviolet Absorption Spectrum. Brucine in ethanol, maxima at 267 mμ (E1%, 1cm 302) and 301 mμ (E1%, 1cm 214); in 0·1N sulphuric acid, maxima at 265 mμ (E1%, 1cm 328) and 300 mμ (E1%, 1cm 219).

Infra-red Absorption Spectrum. Brucine (base). Potassium bromide disk. The principal peaks are: A 1500 or 1649, B 1190 or 1285 or 1400 or 1450 (p. 732).

Quantitative Estimation. Brucine may be determined directly in the presence of strychnine by infra-red spectrophotometry (Garratt and Marshall, 1954).

Toxicity. Brucine is less toxic than strychnine (p. 545). It causes paralysis of the peripheral nerve endings and, in doses larger than those of strychnine, violent convulsions. Lethal intravenous dose in dogs about 8 mg/kg.

BUCLIZINE *Antihistamine*

4-(*p*-Chlorodiphenylmethyl)-1-(*p*-t-butylbenzyl)piperazine

$C_{28}H_{33}ClN_2 = 433·0$

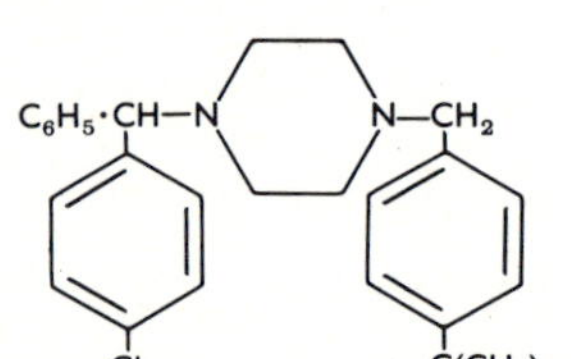

Buclizine boils between 230° and 240° at 0·001 mm Hg.

BUCLIZINE HYDROCHLORIDE
Synonym: UCB 4445.
Proprietary Names: Softran; Vibazine.

A white crystalline powder. M.p. 265° to 266°.
Solubility. Slightly soluble in water.

Extraction. Buclizine is extracted by organic solvents from aqueous alkaline solutions.

Chromatography. PAPER: system P1—Rf 0·94 (location reagents: *iodoplatinate spray*, strong reaction; *bromocresol green spray*, weak reaction).

GAS: system G2/225—retention time 16·0 relative to codeine.

Crystal Test. MICRO: *gold bromide solution*—smudge rosettes (*sensitivity:* 1 in 200).

Ultraviolet Absorption Spectrum. Buclizine in ethanol, maxima at 254 mμ (E1%, 1cm 17), 261 mμ (E1%, 1cm 17·8), about 266 mμ (E1%, 1cm 15), and an inflexion at about 278 mμ (E1%, 1cm 5).

Infra-red Absorption Spectrum. Buclizine (base). Potassium bromide disk. The principal peaks are: A 1002, B 754 or 1131 or 1482, C 1447 (p. 776).

Toxicity. The estimated lethal dose in man is 25 to 250 mg/kg.

BUFORMIN *Antidiabetic*

Synonyms: DBV; W 37.

N[1]-Butyldiguanide

$C_6H_{15}N_5 = 157·2$

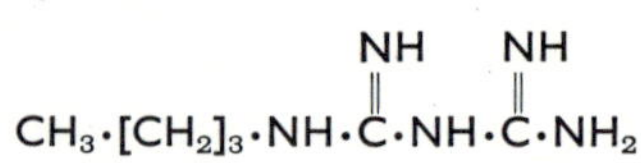

BUFORMIN HYDROCHLORIDE
Proprietary Name: Silubin.

A fine white crystalline powder. B.p. 174° to 177°.
Solubility. Soluble in water and ethanol.

Extraction. Buformin is extracted by organic solvents from aqueous alkaline solutions.

Chromatography. PAPER: system P1—Rf 0·21 (location under ultraviolet light, absorption; location reagents: *iodoplatinate spray*, white; *bromocresol green spray*, strong reaction).

Crystal Tests. MICRO: *gold bromide solution*—needles (*sensitivity:* 1 in 1000); *styphnic acid*—rosettes of needles (*sensitivity:* 1 in 200).

Ultraviolet Absorption Spectrum. Buformin in 0·1N sulphuric acid, maximum at about 300 mμ (E1%, 1cm 16).

Infra-red Absorption Spectrum. Buformin (base). Potassium bromide disk. The principal peaks are: A 1378, B 1530, C 1634 (p. 776).

Dose. Up to 300 mg daily.

Toxicity. LD50 (oral): in mice 380 and in rats 320 mg/kg.

BUFOTENINE *Hallucinogen*

Synonyms: *NN*-Dimethylserotonin; 5-Hydroxy-*N*-dimethyltryptamine; Mappine.

3-(2-Dimethylaminoethyl)-5-hydroxyindole

$C_{12}H_{16}N_2O = 204{\cdot}3$

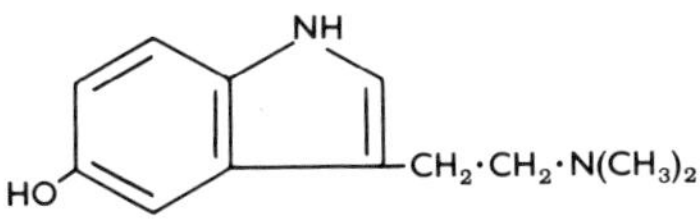

An indole alkaloid found in some species of *Piptadenia* (Mimosaceae) and *Amanita* (Agaricaceae) and in the secretions of the parotid gland of toads (*Bufo*).
A white crystalline powder. Mp. 138° to 140°.
Solubility. Almost insoluble in water; freely soluble in ethanol; slightly soluble in ether; soluble in dilute acids and alkalis.

Extraction. Bufotenine is extracted by organic solvents from aqueous alkaline solutions.

Chromatography. PAPER: system P1—Rf 0·16 (location under ultraviolet light, white fluorescence; location reagents: *iodoplatinate spray*, strong reaction; *bromocresol green spray*, weak reaction; *potassium permanganate spray*, strong reaction).
THIN-LAYER: system T1—Rf 0·32 (location reagent *p-dimethylaminobenzaldehyde spray*, purple).
GAS: system G2/225—retention time 0·37 relative to codeine.

Colour Tests. MICRO: sulphuric acid–formaldehyde test—greenish-brown (*sensitivity:* 0·5 μg); ammonium molybdate test—blue → green → yellow (*sensitivity:* 0·1 μg); Vitali's test—greenish-brown/brown/brown (*sensitivity:* 0·25 μg).

Crystal Tests. MICRO: *ammonium thiocyanate solution*—rods (*sensitivity:* 1 in 400); *gold bromide–hydrochloric acid solution*—rosettes of prisms and dense rosettes (*sensitivity:* 1 in 200).

Ultraviolet Absorption Spectrum. Bufotenine in ethanol, maxima at 223 mμ (E1%, 1 cm 1096), 277 mμ (E1%, 1 cm 302), and 300 mμ (E1%, 1 cm 224); in 0·1N hydrochloric acid, maxima at 277 mμ (E1%, 1 cm 269) and 296 mμ (E1%, 1 cm 229).

Toxicity. Bufotenine is said to have a similar hallucinogenic action to dimethyltryptamine when administered by intravenous injection in a dose of 8 to 70 mg, although it has been reported that doses of up to 20 mg intravenously and 50 mg orally do not produce a hallucinogenic effect.

BUFYLLINE *Sympathomimetic*

Synonyms: Ambuphylline; Theophylline-aminoisobutanol.
Proprietary Names: Butaphyllamine; Buthoid. It is an ingredient of Nethaprin Dospan.

2-Amino-2-methylpropan-1-ol theophyllinate

$C_{11}H_{19}N_5O_3 = 269{\cdot}3$

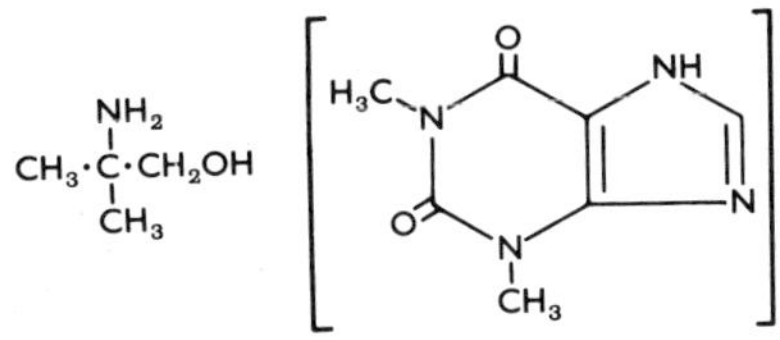

A white crystalline powder.

Extraction. Bufylline is extracted by organic solvents from aqueous alkaline solutions.

Chromatography. PAPER: system P1—Rf 0·58 (location under ultraviolet light, strong absorption); system RP1a—Rf 0·73 (location under ultraviolet light, absorption); system RP1b—Rf 0·75 (location as for RP1a).

Colour Test. Amalic acid test—purple, forming slowly (see p. 127).

Crystal Test. MICRO: *gold bromide–hydrochloric acid solution*—fine needles (*sensitivity:* 1 in 100).

Ultraviolet Absorption Spectrum. Bufylline in 0·1N sulphuric acid, inflexion at 230 mμ and maximum at 271 mμ (E1%, 1 cm 253).

Infra-red Absorption Spectrum. Potassium bromide disk. The principal peaks are: A 1665, B 1712, C 1636 (p. 777).

Dose. Up to 120 mg.

BUPHENINE *Peripheral Vasodilator*

(Distinguish from buphanine, the alkaloid of *Buphane disticha*).

Synonym: Nylidrin.

1-(*p*-Hydroxyphenyl)-2-(1-methyl-3-phenylpropylamino)propan-1-ol

$C_{19}H_{25}NO_2 = 299{\cdot}4$

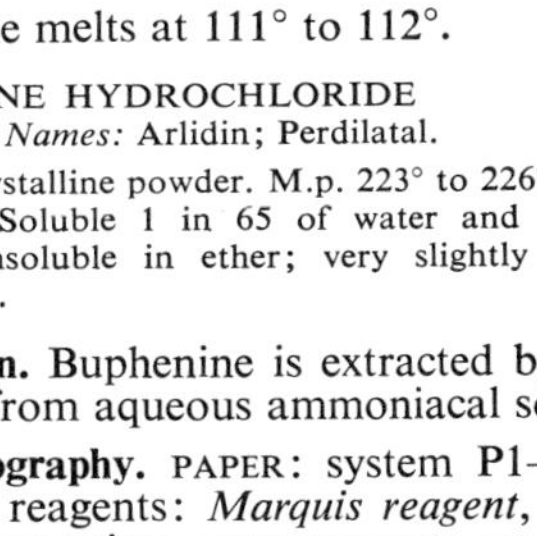

Buphenine melts at 111° to 112°.

BUPHENINE HYDROCHLORIDE

Proprietary Names: Arlidin; Perdilatal.

A white crystalline powder. M.p. 223° to 226°.
Solubility. Soluble 1 in 65 of water and 1 in 50 of ethanol; insoluble in ether; very slightly soluble in chloroform.

Extraction. Buphenine is extracted by organic solvents from aqueous ammoniacal solutions.

Chromatography. PAPER: system P1—Rf 0·80 (location reagents: *Marquis reagent*, weak reaction; *potassium permanganate spray*, weak reaction); system RP1a—Rf 0·75 (location reagent *iodoplatinate spray*, positive reaction); system RP1b—Rf 0·05 (location as for RP1a).

THIN-LAYER: system T1—Rf 0·68 (location reagent *potassium permanganate spray*, positive reaction).

GAS: system G2/225—retention time 0·91, tailing, relative to codeine.

Colour Tests. MICRO: sulphuric acid–formaldehyde test—dull red (*sensitivity:* 0·5 μg); ammonium molybdate test—blue (*sensitivity:* 0·25 μg); Vitali's test— -/yellow/orange (*sensitivity:* 0·5 μg).

Crystal Tests. MICRO: *lead iodide solution*—small dense rosettes or rosettes of plates (*sensitivity:* 1 in 200); *potassium tri-iodide solution* (*3*)—bunches of stout rods or prisms (*sensitivity:* 1 in 1000).

Ultraviolet Absorption Spectrum. Buphenine in methanol, maximum at 276 mμ (E1%, 1 cm 47); in 0·1N sulphuric acid, maximum at 274 mμ (E1%, 1 cm 39), and inflexions at 268 mμ and 279 mμ.

Dose. Up to 36 mg by mouth.

Toxicity. The estimated minimum lethal dose in adults is 2 g and in children 200 mg.

LD50 (oral): in mice greater than 0·25 and in rats greater than 4·8 g/kg.

BUPIVACAINE *Local Anaesthetic*

Synonym: Win 11318.
Proprietary Names: Carbostesin; Marcain.

1-Butyl-2′,6′-pipecoloxylidide
$C_{18}H_{28}N_2O = 288·4$

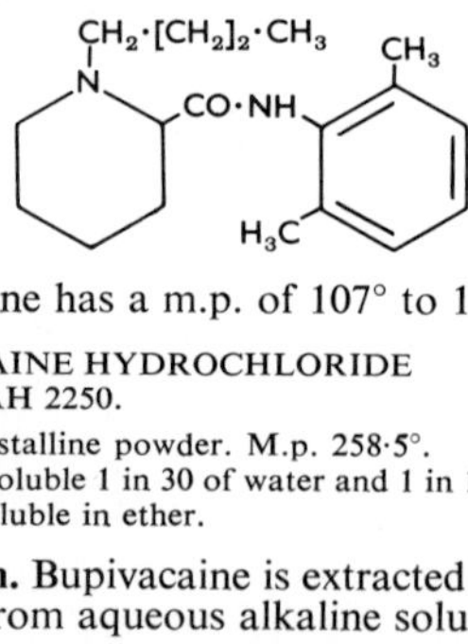

Bupivacaine has a m.p. of 107° to 108°.

BUPIVACAINE HYDROCHLORIDE
Synonym: AH 2250.

A white crystalline powder. M.p. 258·5°.
Solubility. Soluble 1 in 30 of water and 1 in 10 of ethanol; sparingly soluble in ether.

Extraction. Bupivacaine is extracted by organic solvents from aqueous alkaline solutions.

Chromatography. PAPER: system P1—Rf 0·85 (location reagents: *iodoplatinate spray*, weak reaction; *bromocresol green spray*, weak reaction).

THIN-LAYER: system T1—Rf 0·71 (location reagent *acidified iodoplatinate spray*, positive reaction).

GAS: system G2/225—retention time 0·79 relative to codeine; system G4—retention time 0·75 relative to codeine.

Crystal Tests. MICRO: *platinic bromide solution*—bundles of small needles (*sensitivity:* 1 in 1000); *sodium carbonate solution*—very small rods, best viewed under polarised light (*sensitivity:* 1 in 400).

Metabolism. When injected intravenously in man bupivacaine cannot be detected in the blood after 30 minutes.

Dose. Up to 150 mg by injection as a 0·25 to 0·5% solution.

Toxicity. Bupivacaine is more potent than prilocaine, mepivacaine, and lignocaine.

BUTACAINE *Local Anaesthetic*

3-Dibutylaminopropyl *p*-aminobenzoate
$C_{36}H_{60}N_4O_4 = 612·9$

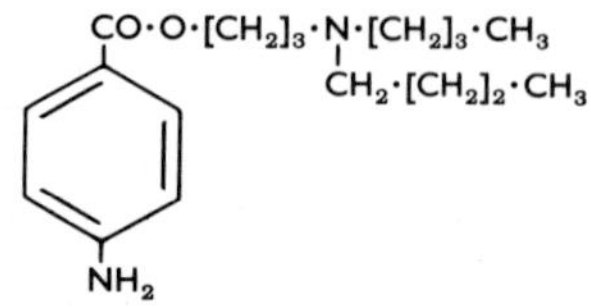

BUTACAINE SULPHATE
Proprietary Name: Butyn.

A white crystalline powder unstable to light and moisture. M.p. 100° to 103°.
Solubility. Slowly soluble 1 in less than 1 of water, more rapidly soluble on warming; soluble 1 in less than 1 of warm ethanol; insoluble in ether; slightly soluble in chloroform; soluble 1 in less than 1 of acetone.

Extraction. Butacaine is extracted by organic solvents from aqueous alkaline solutions.

Chromatography. PAPER: system P1—Rf 0·78 (location under ultraviolet light, blue fluorescence; location reagents: *iodoplatinate spray*, strong reaction; *bromocresol green spray*, weak reaction); system RP1a—Rf 0·43 (location under ultraviolet light, absorption; location reagent *iodoplatinate spray*, positive reaction); system RP1b—Rf 0·00.

THIN-LAYER: system T1—Rf 0·67 (location reagents: *acidified iodoplatinate spray*, positive reaction; p-*dimethylaminobenzaldehyde spray*, bright yellow).

Colour Tests. MICRO: diazotisation test—red; Vitali's test— -/yellow/yellow.

Crystal Tests. MICRO: *gold bromide–hydrochloric acid solution*—very small needles and plates (*sensitivity:* 1 in 3000); *potassium iodide solution*—small rods in bunches (*sensitivity:* 1 in 1500).

Ultraviolet Absorption Spectrum. Butacaine in water, maximum at 288 mμ (E1%, 1 cm 499).

Infra-red Absorption Spectrum. Butacaine (base). Potassium bromide disk. The principal peaks are: A 1165 or 1275 or 1598, B 1685 or 1702 (p. 777).

Metabolism. Butacaine has a local anaesthetic potency and a toxicity similar to those of cocaine but its action is more rapid in onset and more prolonged. It readily penetrates mucous membranes. It is hydrolysed in the serum more slowly than procaine.

Toxicity. Butacaine is usually employed topically as a 2% solution; the maximum safe amount for topical use is 100 mg or 5 ml of a 2% solution.
LD50 (oral): in rats 150 mg/kg.

BUTALLYLONAL *Barbiturate*

Synonym: Butyl-bromallyl-barbituric Acid.
Proprietary Name: Pernocton.

5-(2-Bromoallyl)-5-s-butylbarbituric acid
$C_{11}H_{15}BrN_2O_3 = 303{\cdot}2$

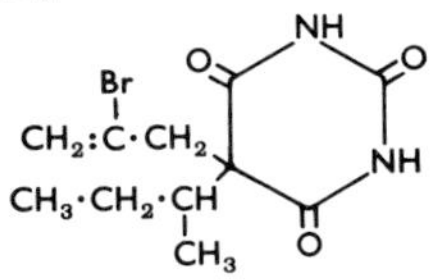

A fine white crystalline powder. M.p. 130° to 133°.
Solubility. Very slightly soluble in water; soluble in ethanol, ether, and aqueous solutions of alkalis.

Screening Tests. See under Barbiturates, p. 208.

Extraction. Butallylonal may be isolated in the A2 fraction (see p. 27).

Chromatography. THIN-LAYER: system T10—Rf 0·28 (location reagents: *fluorescein spray*, pink; *mercurous nitrate spray*, black; *potassium permanganate spray*, yellow-brown).

Colour Test. Zwikker's test—violet-blue.

Ultraviolet Absorption Spectrum. Butallylonal is a 5,5-derivative—see Screening Test 3 under Barbiturates, p. 208.

Quantitative Estimation. See under Barbiturates, p. 208.

Metabolism. Butallylonal is an intermediate-acting barbiturate—see under Barbiturates, p. 207. It has been found to be converted in man, by side-chain oxidation, to 5-(2-acetonyl)-5-(1-methylpropyl)barbituric acid, 5 to 17% of the dose appearing in the urine in this form with only traces of unchanged drug (Fretwurst *et al.*, 1930).

Dose. Usually 200 mg.

Toxicity. The minimum oral lethal dose in rabbits is 400 mg/kg.

BUTANILICAINE *Local Anaesthetic*

Synonym: Hostacain.

α-Butylamino-*N*-(6-chloro-2-methylphenyl)-acetamide
$C_{13}H_{19}ClN_2O = 254{\cdot}8$

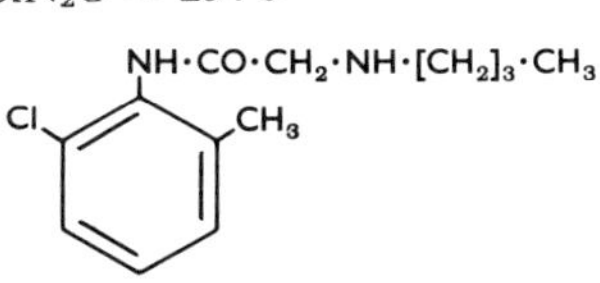

BUTANILICAINE PHOSPHATE
Butanilicaine phosphate melts at 126° to 127°.

Extraction. Butanilicaine is extracted by organic solvents from aqueous alkaline solutions.

Chromatography. PAPER: system P1—Rf 0·78 (location reagents: *iodoplatinate spray*, white; *bromocresol green spray*, weak reaction).
THIN-LAYER: system T1—Rf 0·70 (location reagent *acidified iodoplatinate spray*, positive reaction).
GAS: system G2/225—retention time 1·65 relative to diphenhydramine; system G4—retention time 0·47 relative to codeine.

Colour Test. MICRO: ammonium molybdate test—faint blue (*sensitivity:* 1·0 μg).

Crystal Tests. MICRO: *picric acid*—rosettes of rods (*sensitivity:* 1 in 1000); *platinic iodide solution*—masses of rods (*sensitivity:* 1 in 1000).

Ultraviolet Absorption Spectrum. Butanilicaine in 0·1N sulphuric acid, maxima at 267·5 mμ (E1%, 1cm 15) and 274·5 mμ (E1%, 1cm 12).

Infra-red Absorption Spectrum. Butanilicaine (base). Potassium bromide disk. The principal peaks are: A 1495 or 1694, B 1460, C 770 (p. 777).

BUTAPERAZINE *Tranquilliser*

Synonyms: Bayer 1362; Butyrylperazin; Riker 595.

2-Butyryl-10-[3-(4-methylpiperazin-1-yl)propyl]phenothiazine
$C_{24}H_{31}N_3OS = 409{\cdot}6$

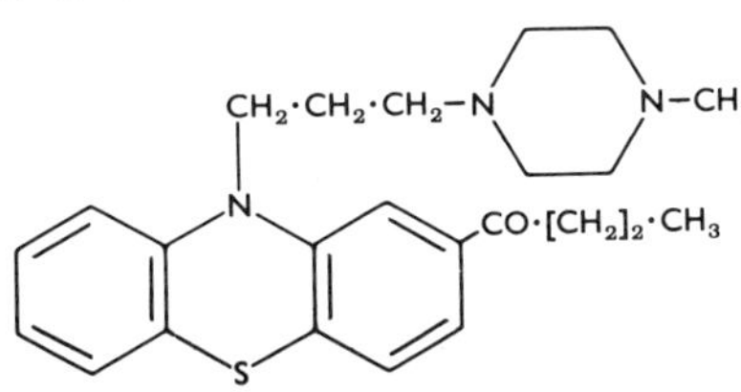

A yellow oil. B.p. 195° to 210°.

BUTAPERAZINE DIMALEATE
Proprietary Name: Randolectil (tablets).
A yellow crystalline powder. M.p. about 195°.
Solubility. Soluble in water; insoluble in ether and chloroform.

BUTAPERAZINE DIPHOSPHATE
Proprietary Name: Randolectil (injection).
A yellow crystalline powder. M.p. 161° to 162°.
Solubility. Soluble in water; insoluble in ether and chloroform.

Screening Test. See under Screening Tests, p. 10.

Extraction. Butaperazine is extracted by organic solvents from aqueous alkaline solutions.

Chromatography. PAPER: system P1—Rf 0·30 (location under ultraviolet light, yellow fluorescence; location reagents: *iodine vapour*, weak reaction; *potassium permanganate spray*, weak reaction).

THIN-LAYER: system T1—Rf 0·48 (location reagent *potassium permanganate spray*, positive reaction).

Colour Tests. MICRO: sulphuric acid–formaldehyde test—brown-purple (*sensitivity:* 0·1 μg); ammonium molybdate test—grey-purple (*sensitivity:* 0·1 μg); ammonium vanadate test—brown-purple (*sensitivity:* 0·5 μg); Vitali's test—pale yellow/pale yellow/pale yellow (*sensitivity:* 1·0 μg).

Crystal Tests. MICRO: *potassium chromate solution*—bunches of plates (*sensitivity:* 1 in 200); *zinc chloride solution*—small rosettes or fans of needles (*sensitivity:* 1 in 400).

Dose. Up to 200 mg daily.

BUTETHAMATE *Sympathomimetic*

Synonyms: Butetamate; Diphenamine.

2-Diethylaminoethyl α-phenylbutyrate

$C_{16}H_{25}NO_2$ = 263·4

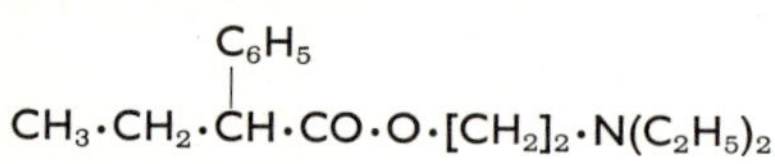

BUTETHAMATE CITRATE

Proprietary Names: Convenil. It is an ingredient of Hicoseen, Rybar Diabetic Cough Mixture, Rybrol, and Theophen.

Colourless crystals. M.p. 107°.

Solubility. Soluble 1 in 10 of water and 1 in 40 of ethanol.

Extraction. Butethamate is extracted by organic solvents from aqueous alkaline solutions.

Chromatography. PAPER: system P1—Rf 0·72 (location reagents: *iodoplatinate spray*, strong reaction; *bromocresol green spray*, weak reaction).

THIN-LAYER: system T1—Rf 0·63 (location reagent *acidified iodoplatinate spray*, positive reaction).

GAS: system G2/225—retention time 0·75 relative to diphenhydramine; system G4—retention time 0·58 relative to diphenhydramine.

Colour Test. MICRO: Vitali's test— –/–/deep purple (*sensitivity:* 0·1 μg).

Crystal Test. MICRO: *lead iodide solution*—fans of needles (*sensitivity:* 1 in 1000).

Ultraviolet Absorption Spectrum. Butethamate in 0·1N sulphuric acid, maxima at 247 mμ (E1%, 1 cm 3), 252·5 mμ (E1%, 1 cm 3), 258 mμ (E1%, 1 cm 4), and 264 mμ (E1%, 1 cm 3), and an inflexion at 267 mμ.

Infra-red Absorption Spectrum. Butethamate (base). Potassium bromide disk. The principal peaks are: A 1730, B 1158, C 1194 (p. 777).

Dose. Up to 30 mg.

BUTETHAMINE *Local Anaesthetic*

2-Isobutylaminoethyl *p*-aminobenzoate

$C_{13}H_{20}N_2O_2$ = 236·3

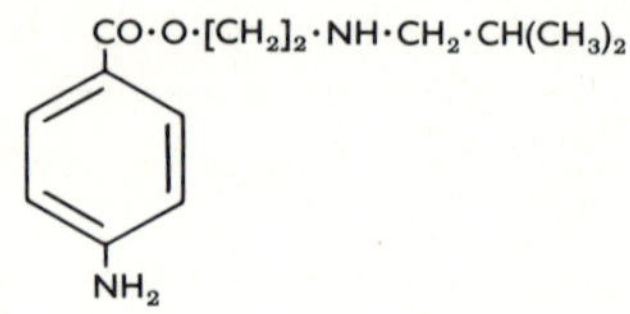

NOTE. Butethamine and Metabutethamine (p. 405) are isomers.

BUTETHAMINE FORMATE

Proprietary Name: Monocaine Formate.

White crystals or crystalline powder. M.p. 136° to 139°.

Solubility. Readily soluble in water and ethanol; slightly soluble in ether and chloroform.

BUTETHAMINE HYDROCHLORIDE

Proprietary Name: Monocaine Hydrochloride.

A white crystalline powder. M.p. 192° to 196°.

Solubility. Sparingly soluble in water; slightly soluble in ethanol and chloroform; practically insoluble in ether.

Extraction. Butethamine is extracted by organic solvents from aqueous alkaline solutions.

Chromatography. PAPER: system P1—Rf 0·51 (location under ultraviolet light, blue fluorescence; location reagents: *iodoplatinate spray*, strong reaction; *bromocresol green spray*, weak reaction); system RP1a—Rf 0·82 (location under ultraviolet light, absorption); system RP1b—Rf 0·24 (location as for RP1a).

THIN-LAYER: system T1—Rf 0·60 (location reagents: *acidified iodoplatinate spray*, positive reaction; p-*dimethylaminobenzaldehyde spray*, yellow).

GAS: system G2/225—retention time 1·8 relative to diphenhydramine.

Colour Tests. MICRO: diazotisation test—red; Vitali's test— –/yellow/yellow (*sensitivity:* 1·0 μg).

Crystal Tests. MICRO: *gold bromide–hydrochloric acid solution*—long needles (*sensitivity:* 1 in 1000); *picric acid*—rosettes of plates (*sensitivity:* 1 in 1000).

Ultraviolet Absorption Spectrum. Butethamine in water, maximum at 290 mμ (E1%, 1 cm 631); in 0·1N sulphuric acid, maxima at 228 mμ and 280 mμ, and inflexions at 275 mμ and 290 mμ.

Infra-red Absorption Spectrum. Butethamine (base). Potassium bromide disk. The principal peaks are: A 1272, B 1600, C 1702 (p. 777).

Metabolism. Butethamine is metabolised by hydrolysis to *p*-aminobenzoic acid.

Toxicity. Butethamine is used by injection as a 1 to 1·5% solution with adrenaline. It is one-third more potent and one-third more toxic than procaine hydrochloride; it is not recommended as a surface anaesthetic for mucous membranes. The maximum safe amount by

injection or topical application is 750 mg, or 75 ml of a 1% solution.
LD50 (intraperitoneal): in rats 183 mg/kg.

BUTOBARBITONE *Barbiturate*

Synonyms: Butethal; Butobarbital (distinguish from Butabarbital).
Proprietary Names: Monodorm; Soneryl.

5-Butyl-5-ethylbarbituric acid
$C_{10}H_{16}N_2O_3 = 212{\cdot}3$

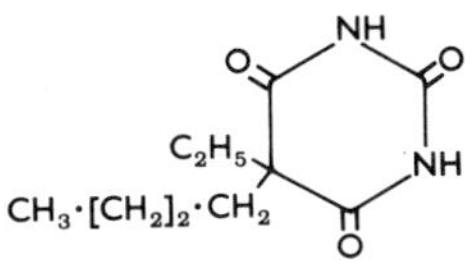

A fine white crystalline powder. M.p. 122° to 125°.

Solubility. Soluble 1 in 250 of water, 1 in 1 of ethanol, 1 in 10 of ether, 1 in 3 of chloroform, and in aqueous solutions of alkali hydroxides and carbonates.

Screening Tests. See under Barbiturates, p. 208.

Extraction. Butobarbitone may be isolated in the A2 fraction (see p. 27).

Chromatography. PAPER: system P2—Rf 0·52 relative to amylobarbitone (location under ultraviolet light, dark spot); system P3—Rf 0·24 (location reagent *silver nitrate spray*, white); system P4—Rf 0·35 (location as for P3); system RP1b—Rf 0·27 (location under ultraviolet light after exposure to ammonia; location reagent *potassium permanganate spray*, yellow on pink).

THIN-LAYER: system T10—Rf 0·33 (location reagents: *mercurous nitrate spray*, black; *Zwikker's reagent spray*, pink).

GAS: system G5—retention time 1·84 relative to barbitone; system G7—retention time 1·60 relative to barbitone.

Colour Test. Zwikker's test—violet-blue.

Ultraviolet Absorption Spectrum. Butobarbitone is a 5,5-derivative—see Screening Test 3 under Barbiturates, p. 208.

Infra-red Absorption Spectrum. Potassium bromide disk. The principal peaks are: A 1683 or 1712 or 1745 (p. 732).

Quantitative Estimation. See under Barbiturates, p. 208.

Metabolism. Butobarbitone is an intermediate-acting barbiturate—see under Barbiturates, p. 207. About 26% of the butobarbitone present in blood post mortem appears to be protein-bound (Turner, 1964b). About 10% of oral doses have been recovered from the urine of dogs as the hydroxy-derivative, 5-(3′-hydroxybutyl)-5-ethylbarbituric acid (Maynert, 1952).

Dose. Up to 200 mg; maximum in 24 hours 600 mg.

Toxicity. The minimum lethal oral dose in rabbits is 160 mg/kg.

BUTOXAMINE *Antidiabetic*

Synonym: BW 64–9.

(±)-*erythro*-1-(2,5-Dimethoxyphenyl)-2-t-butylaminopropan-1-ol
$C_{15}H_{25}NO_3 = 267{\cdot}4$

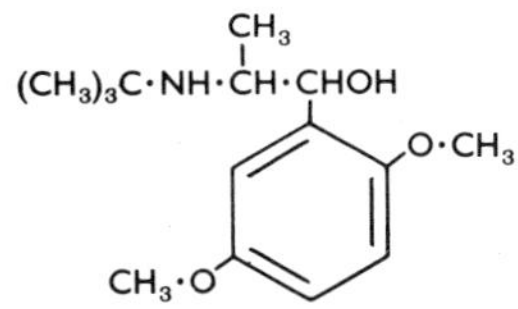

Extraction. Butoxamine is extracted by organic solvents from aqueous alkaline solutions.

Chromatography. PAPER: system P1—Rf 0·75 (location reagents: *bromocresol green spray*, strong reaction; *iodine vapour*, weak reaction; *Marquis reagent*, green).

THIN-LAYER: system T1—Rf 0·60 (location reagent *potassium permanganate spray*, positive reaction).

Colour Tests. MICRO: sulphuric acid–formaldehyde test—green (*sensitivity:* 0·1 μg); ammonium molybdate test—green (*sensitivity:* 0·1 μg); Vitali's test—yellow/yellow/yellow (*sensitivity:* 0·5 μg).

Crystal Tests. MICRO: *potassium chromate solution*—bunches of plates (*sensitivity:* 1 in 200); *sodium carbonate solution*—clusters of blades (*sensitivity:* 1 in 200).

Infra-red Absorption Spectrum. Potassium chloride disk. The principal peaks are: A 1485, B 1206, C 1263 (p. 777).

BUTRIPTYLINE *Antidepressant*

Synonym: AY 62014.

10,11-Dihydro-5-(3-dimethylamino-2-methylpropyl)-5*H*-dibenzo[*a,d*]cycloheptene
$C_{21}H_{27}N = 293{\cdot}4$

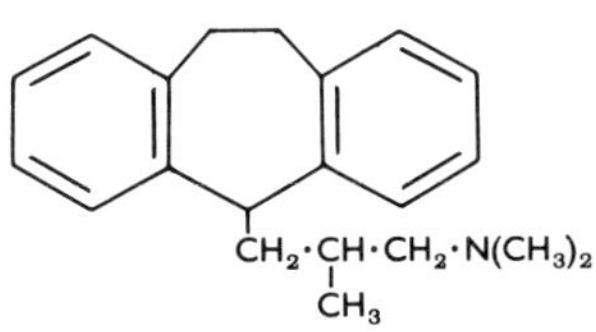

BUTRIPTYLINE HYDROCHLORIDE
A white crystalline powder.
Solubility. Soluble in water.

Extraction. Butriptyline is extracted by organic solvents from aqueous alkaline solutions.

Chromatography. PAPER: system P1—Rf 0·78 (location reagents: *iodoplatinate spray*, strong reaction; *bromocresol green spray*, weak reaction).
THIN-LAYER: system T1—Rf 0·61 (location reagent *acidified iodoplatinate spray*, positive reaction).
GAS: system G2/225—retention time 2·65 relative to diphenhydramine; retention time 0·56 relative to codeine; system G4—retention time 2·20 relative to diphenhydramine.

Colour Tests. MICRO: sulphuric acid–formaldehyde test—dull purple (*sensitivity:* 0·1 μg); ammonium molybdate test—blue-purple → green (*sensitivity:* 0·1 μg).

Crystal Tests. MICRO: *platinic bromide solution*—feathery crystals, forming overnight (*sensitivity:* 1 in 1000); *platinic chloride solution*—feathery rosettes (*sensitivity:* 1 in 1000).

Infra-red Absorption Spectrum. Butriptyline (base). Potassium chloride disk. The principal peaks are: A 757, B 1455, C 1033 (p. 777).

BUTYL AMINOBENZOATE

Local Anaesthetic

Synonyms: Butoforme; Scuroforme.
Proprietary Names: Butesin; Planoform.

Butyl *p*-aminobenzoate
$C_{11}H_{15}NO_2 = 193{\cdot}2$

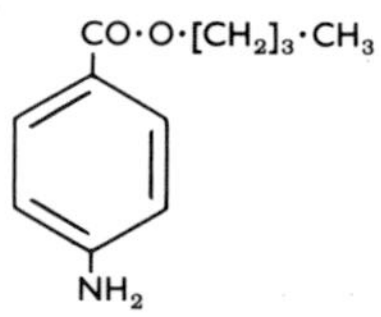

A white crystalline powder which is slowly hydrolysed when boiled with water. M.p. 57° to 59°. B.p. 174°.
Solubility. Soluble 1 in 7000 of water, 1 in 3 of ethanol, 1 in 2 of ether; soluble in chloroform and dilute mineral acids.

Extraction. Butyl aminobenzoate is extracted by organic solvents from aqueous alkaline solutions.

Chromatography. PAPER: system P1—Rf 0·91 (location under ultraviolet light, strong absorption; location reagents: *diazotised* p-*nitroaniline–sodium hydroxide spray*, red; p-*dimethylaminobenzaldehyde spray*, yellow); system RP1b—Rf 0·04 (location under ultraviolet light, absorption).

Colour Test. MICRO: diazotisation test—red.

Crystal Tests. MICRO: *gold bromide solution*—small blades in stars (*sensitivity:* 1 in 1000); *lead iodide solution*—long plates (*sensitivity:* 1 in 1000).

Ultraviolet Absorption Spectrum. Butyl aminobenzoate in ethanol, maximum at 294 mμ (E 1%, 1 cm 1080).

Infra-red Absorption Spectrum. Potassium bromide disk. The principal peaks are: A 1272, B 1164, C 1600 (p. 732).

Toxicity. Butyl aminobenzoate has been employed in concentrations from 1 to 6% as a dusting-powder or ointment. The maximum safe amount for topical use is stated to be 5 g.

BUTYLATED HYDROXYANISOLE

Antoxidant

Synonyms: 3-t-Butyl-4-hydroxyanisole; BHA.
Proprietary Names: Embanox; Nipantiox 1-F; Tenox BHA.

4-Methoxy-2-t-butylphenol
$C_{11}H_{16}O_2 = 180{\cdot}2$

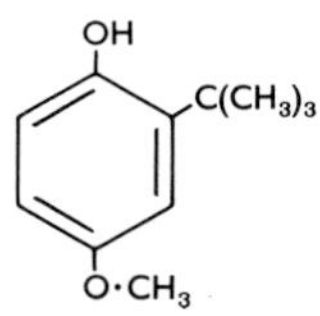

A white crystalline powder. M.p. 62° to 65°.
Solubility. Insoluble in water; soluble 1 in 4 of ethanol and in solutions of alkali hydroxides.

Extraction. Biological material must be dehydrated and extracted with ethanol (see p. 29).

Colour Tests. Dissolve 0·1 g of butylated hydroxyanisole in 10 ml of ethanol, add 2 ml of a 2% solution of borax and a few crystals of 2,6-dichloroquinonechloroimide—blue (compare blue colour produced by butylated hydroxytoluene). Dissolve a few crystals of butylated hydroxyanisole in 10 ml of ethanol and add 0·5 ml of a 0·2% solution of ferric ammonium sulphate in 1N sulphuric acid—greenish-blue.

Ultraviolet Absorption Spectrum. Butylated hydroxyanisole in ethanol:1N hydrochloric acid (49:1), maxima at 228 mμ (E 1%, 1 cm 340) and 292 mμ (E 1%, 1 cm 205); minimum at 253 mμ (E 1%, 1 cm 8).

Quantitative Estimation. Butylated hydroxyanisole may be estimated colorimetrically after reaction with 2,6-dichloroquinonechloroimide following reverse phase chromatography (Berger *et al.*, 1960).

Metabolism. Butylated hydroxyanisole is used as an antoxidant for oils and fats. It is absorbed from the gastro-intestinal tract and there is some evidence that when ingested in large amounts it accumulates in the depot fat. In the rabbit, butylated hydroxyanisole is excreted mainly as a conjugate with glucuronic acid or sulphuric acid; only a small amount is excreted unchanged. In the rat, it is excreted chiefly as a glucuronide. It does not seem to be oxidised prior to conjugation (FAO/WHO Expert Committee on Food Additives, Sixth Report, 1962).

Toxicity. The estimated acceptable daily intake for man is up to 0·5 mg/kg.
LD50 (oral): in mice 2 and in rats 2·2 to more than 5 g/kg.

BUTYLATED HYDROXYTOLUENE *Antoxidant*

Synonyms: BHT; DBPC.
Proprietary Names: Tenox BHT; Topanol BHT.

4-Methyl-2,6-di-t-butylphenol
$C_{15}H_{24}O = 220{\cdot}4$

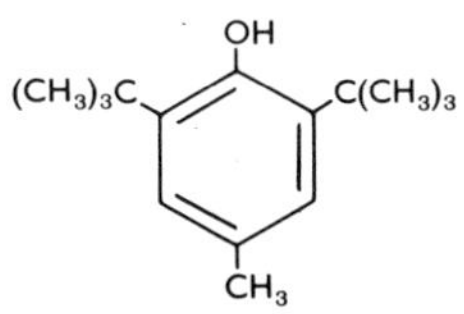

A white crystalline powder. M.p. not lower than 69°. B.p. 265°.
Solubility. Insoluble in water; soluble 1 in 4 of ethanol and 1 in 0·5 of ether.

Extraction. Biological material must be dehydrated and extracted with ethanol (see p. 29).

Colour Test. Dissolve 0·1 g of butylated hydroxytoluene in 10 ml of ethanol, add 2 ml of a 2% solution of borax and a few crystals of 2,6-dichloroquinonechloroimide — faint blue (compare blue colour produced by butylated hydroxyanisole).

Ultraviolet Absorption Spectrum. Butylated hydroxytoluene in ethanol, maximum at 278 mμ (E1%, 1 cm 85).

Quantitative Estimation. Butylated hydroxytoluene may be estimated spectrophotometrically in alkaline ethanolic solutions (Berger *et al.*, 1960).

Metabolism. Butylated hydroxytoluene is used as an antoxidant for oils and fats. It has been recommended, however, that it should not be used in food on account of its possible hazard to health (Food Standards Committee Report on Antioxidants in Food, 1963).
Butylated hydroxytoluene is readily absorbed. Following the ingestion of large doses by rats, some deposition in adipose tissue has been reported. The metabolism of butylated hydroxytoluene is complicated by the presence of the t-butyl groups on either side of the hydroxyl group. Two types of oxidation may occur: one of the butyl groups may be oxidised to a 2-hydroxy-2,2-dimethyl-2-ethyl group or the methyl group may be oxidised to yield 3,5-di-t-butyl-4-hydroxybenzoic acid. The former is excreted as a glucuronide conjugate while the latter may be excreted as a conjugate with glucuronic acid or glycine. Some of the oxidation products may be excreted unconjugated (FAO/WHO Expert Committee on Food Additives, Sixth Report, 1962).
Further studies in rats have shown that slow urinary excretion accounts for 32 to 35% of butylated hydroxytoluene and faecal excretion for 35 to 37%. The following metabolites have been detected in the bile: 3,5-di-t-butyl-4-hydroxybenzyl alcohol, 3,5-di-t-butyl-4-hydroxybenzaldehyde, 3,5-di-t-butyl-4-hydroxybenzoic acid, and smaller amounts of 1,2-bis(3,5-di-t-butyl-4-hydroxyphenyl)ethane. Three other metabolites appeared to be present in relatively large amounts (Ladomery, 1967).

Toxicity. LD50 (oral): in rats 1·7 to 1·97 g/kg.

BUTYLCHLORAL HYDRATE *Hypnotic*

Synonyms: Croton-Chloral Hydrate; Trichlorobutylidene Glycol.

2,2,3-Trichlorobutane-1,1-diol
$C_4H_7Cl_3O_2 = 193{\cdot}5$

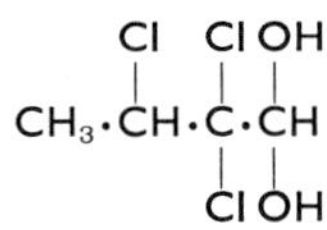

Pearly-white crystalline scales. M.p. about 78°.
Solubility. Soluble 1 in 40 of water, 5 in 3 of ethanol forming an ethanolate, 1 in 2 of ether, and 1 in 20 of chloroform.

Extraction. Butylchloral hydrate is extracted by organic solvents from aqueous acid or alkaline solutions.

Chromatography. GAS: system G5—retention time 0·14 relative to barbitone.

Infra-red Absorption Spectrum. Potassium bromide disk. The principal peaks are: A 830, B 1090, C 1051 (p. 733).

Metabolism. Butylchloral hydrate is probably metabolised to 2,2,3-trichlorobutanol since 2,2,3-trichlorobutyl glucuronide has been found in the urine of dogs.

Dose. Up to 1·2 g.

CADAVERINE *Putrefactive Base*

Pentamethylenediamine
$NH_2{\cdot}[CH_2]_5{\cdot}NH_2 = 102{\cdot}2$

A colourless syrupy basic liquid, which fumes and absorbs carbon dioxide on exposure to air. F.p. 9°. B.p. 178° to 180°.
Solubility. Soluble in water and ethanol; slightly soluble in ether.

Extraction. Cadaverine is extracted by organic solvents from aqueous alkaline solutions.

Chromatography. PAPER: system P1—Rf 0·00

(location under ultraviolet light, white fluorescence; location reagent *iodoplatinate spray*, weak reaction).
THIN-LAYER: system T1—Rf 0·02 (location reagent *acidified iodoplatinate spray*, positive reaction).

Crystal Tests. MICRO: *picric acid*—rods, forming overnight (*sensitivity:* 1 in 400); *platinic iodide solution*—small irregular blades (*sensitivity:* 1 in 3000).

Metabolism. Cadaverine is formed during putrefaction by bacterial decarboxylation of lysine in the gastro-intestinal tract. It may be deaminated to yield ammonia and an aldehyde and it may undergo cyclisation to piperidine. The piperidine normally excreted in the urine is formed from cadaverine.

CAFFEINE *Xanthine Derivative*

Synonyms: Guaranine; Methyltheobromine; Theine.

1,3,7-Trimethylxanthine

$C_8H_{10}N_4O_2 = 194{\cdot}2$

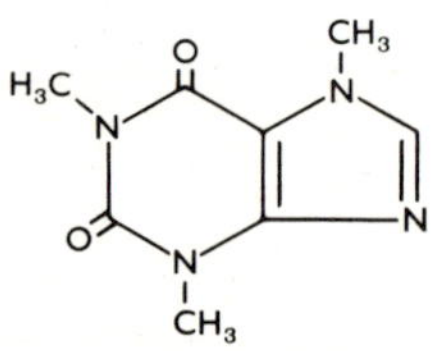

A white powder or white glistening needles, usually matted together. M.p. 235° to 237°. When crystallised from water, caffeine contains one molecule of water of crystallisation, but it is anhydrous when crystallised from ethanol, chloroform, or ether. It is decomposed by strong solutions of caustic alkalis.

Solubility. Soluble 1 in 60 of water, 1 in 2 of boiling water, 1 in 130 of ethanol, and 1 in 7 of chloroform; sparingly soluble in ether; more soluble in dilute acids.

CAFFEINE CITRATE

Synonym: Citrated Caffeine.

A white powder which is decomposed by water.

Solubility. Soluble 1 in 4 of hot water, dissociating on further dilution with the separation of caffeine which redissolves in 32 of water; soluble 1 in 25 of ethanol.

CAFFEINE HYDRATE

A white powder or white glistening needles usually matted together. It effloresces in dry air and sublimes at about 180°.

Solubility. Soluble 1 in 60 of water and 1 in 110 of ethanol; sparingly soluble in ether; readily soluble in chloroform, with the separation of water.

Extraction. Caffeine may be isolated in the D1 fraction (see p. 27). As caffeine is a weak base, a small amount may be extracted by organic solvents from aqueous acid solutions.

Chromatography. PAPER: system P1—Rf 0·65 (location under ultraviolet light, deep blue fluorescence; location by the Clarke-Kalayci test, reddish-purple); system RP1b—Rf 0·74 (location reagent *bromine–starch–potassium bromide*).
THIN-LAYER: system T1—Rf 0·63 (location reagents: *strongly acid iodoplatinate spray*, positve reaction; *iodine–carbon tetrachloride spray*, positive reaction). A system employing chloroform: ethanol (9:1) has been described for the separation of caffeine, theobromine, and theophylline (Szász *et al.*, 1965).
GAS: system G1/180—retention time 0·87 relative to diphenhydramine; system G3—retention time 1·90 relative to diphenhydramine; system G5—retention time 4·38 relative to barbitone; system G6—retention time 0·22 relative to codeine.

Colour Test. Amalic acid test—purple (see p. 127).

Crystal Tests. MICRO: *gold chloride solution*—small rods (*sensitivity:* 1 in 1500); *mercuric chloride solution*—long needles (*sensitivity:* 1 in 1500).

Ultraviolet Absorption Spectrum. Caffeine in ethanol, maximum at 273 mμ (E 1%, 1 cm 519); in 0·1N hydrochloric acid, maximum at 272 mμ (E 1%, 1 cm about 470).

Infra-red Absorption Spectrum. Caffeine (base). Potassium bromide disk. The principal peaks are: A 1658 or 1695, B 745 (p. 733).

Quantitative Estimation. Caffeine may be eluted from paper chromatograms and estimated spectrophotometrically (Moore, 1957).

Metabolism. Caffeine is rapidly absorbed in man, peak plasma levels being obtained about 1 hour after oral administration. It is metabolised at the rate of about 15% per hour, only about 0·5 to 1·5% of intravenous doses of 0·5 g being excreted unchanged in the urine. No apparent accumulation takes place in the body. Caffeine may undergo demethylation and oxidation in the 8-position to give uric acid derivatives. Within 48 hours of ingestion in man, 46% of the dose has been found to be excreted as 1-methyluric acid and 1-methylxanthine; in addition, 1,7-dimethylxanthine, 7-methylxanthine, and 1,3-dimethyluric acid may also be found.

Dose. Usually up to 300 mg.

Toxicity. The estimated lethal dose in man is probably about 10 g, but there is no recorded case of death. Doses of 1 g or over may produce toxic symptoms; recovery has occurred after the ingestion of 30 g of caffeine.
LD50 (oral): in rats 200 to 250 mg/kg.

NOTE. Caffeine has been used to stimulate the performance of racehorses.

CALCIFEROL *Vitamin*

Synonyms: Ergocalciferol; Irradiated Ergosterol; Viosterol; Vitamin D_2.

Proprietary Names: Fortodyl; Radiostol; Sterogyl-15 Oral; Vitavel-D.

24 - Methyl - 9,10 - secocholesta - 5,7,10(19),22-tetraen-3-ol

$C_{28}H_{44}O = 396{\cdot}7$

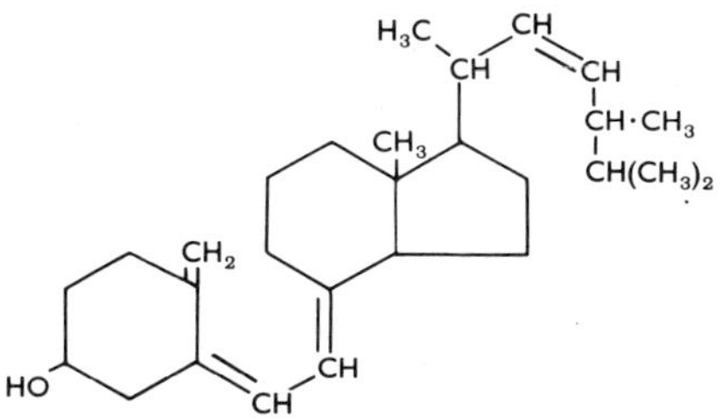

A white crystalline powder. M.p. 115° to 118°. Calciferol should be kept in a hermetically sealed glass container in which the air has been replaced by an inert gas, protected from light, and stored in a cool place.

Solubility. Insoluble in water; soluble 1 in 2 of ethanol, 1 in 2 of ether, 1 in 0·7 of chloroform, and 1 in 10 of acetone.

Chromatography. THIN-LAYER: system T21a—Rf 0·33 (location reagent *0·2M sulphuric acid spray*, positive reaction); system T21b—Rf 0·44 (location as for T21a); system T21c—Rf 0·15 (location as for T21a).

Colour Test. Lyness and Quackenbush (1955) describe a colour reaction for calciferol and cholecalciferol using an iodine-ethylene dichloride reagent which produces a strong yellow colour with both compounds but which does not react with cholesterol or with sitosterols.

Ultraviolet Absorption Spectrum. Calciferol in ethanol, maximum at 265 mμ (E1%, 1 cm about 460); in cyclohexane, maximum at 265 mμ (E1%, 1 cm not less than 460).

Quantitative Estimation. Barua and Rao (1964) describe a method of determination of calciferol and cholecalciferol in the presence of vitamin A involving column chromatographic separation followed by spectrophotometric estimation. Clements *et al.* (1967) describe a spectrophotometric determination of calciferol involving the formation of a stable yellow complex with trifluoroacetic acid.

Metabolism. Vitamin D is necessary for the absorption of calcium and phosphorus from the gastro-intestinal tract. The daily requirements of vitamin D in adults are small and need not be met directly in the diet.

Toxicity. Single doses of 25 mg (1 million units) or more have been given without untoward effects but prolonged administration of 2·5 to 3·75 mg (100,000 to 150,000 units) daily in adults is liable to give rise to toxic symptoms. Symptoms of overdosage include an increase in the calcium and phosphorus levels in serum and urine; calcium may be deposited in many tissues including the arteries and kidneys. The effects are reversible if the drug is withdrawn in time.

CAMPHOR *Carminative/Rubefacient*

Synonyms: Alcanfor; 2-Bornanone; 2-Camphanone; Camphre du Japon (natural); Camphre Droit (natural).

2-Oxo-1,7,7-trimethylbicyclo(2,2,1)heptane

$C_{10}H_{16}O = 152{\cdot}2$

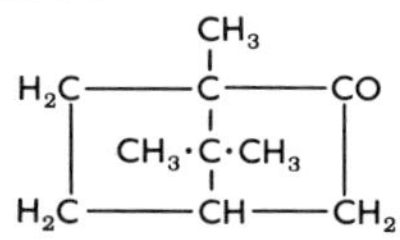

Camphor is obtained by distillation from the wood of *Cinnamomum camphora* (Lauraceae) and purified by sublimation, or it may be prepared synthetically.

Colourless transparent crystals, crystalline masses, blocks, or powdery masses known as 'flowers of camphor'. M.p. 174° to 179°.

Solubility. Soluble 1 in 700 of water, 1 in 1 of ethanol, 1 in 1 of ether, and 1 in 0·25 of chloroform.

Extraction. Camphor may be isolated by distillation from acid solutions followed by ether extraction of the distillate and final evaporation.

Chromatography. GAS: system G5—retention time 0·1 relative to barbitone.

Ultraviolet Absorption Spectrum. Camphor in ethanol, maximum at 289 mμ (E1%, 1 cm 2).

Metabolism. Camphor is metabolised by hydroxylation to yield mainly 5-hydroxycamphor with appreciable amounts of 3-hydroxycamphor. These 2 metabolites are excreted in the urine as glucuronide conjugates. Oxidation also occurs in the 7-position yielding a small amount of a carboxylic acid. It is of interest that the keto-group of camphor suffers no change during metabolism.

Dose. Up to 300 mg.

Toxicity. The fatal dose in a one-year-old child is approximately 1 g, although some children have survived as much as 5 g. Camphor stimulates the cerebral cortex and causes convulsions. LD50 (intraperitoneal): in rats 900 mg/kg.

CASE EXAMPLES. A 20-month-old child swallowed and aspirated camphorated oil. The resultant asphyxia was successfully treated by atropine 0·2 mg and subcutaneous oxygen (Laurie, 1950).

A 77-year-old man was admitted to hospital after the ingestion of about 12 g of camphorated oil. Within 4 hours lipid haemodialysis was instituted for 4½ hours and 6·56 g of camphor was found in the dialysate. The patient recovered rapidly (Ginn *et al.*, 1968).

CANNABIS *Narcotic*

Synonyms: Bhang; Cannabis Indica; Indian Hemp; Ganja; Guaza; Marihuana.

The dried flowering or fruiting tops of the pistillate plant of *Cannabis sativa* (Cannabinaceae).

The active principle of the drug is contained in the resin (charas; hashish) which contains at least 4 substances:
1. Cannabidiolic Acid. M.p. 43° to 47°.
2. Cannabidiol. M.p. 66° to 67°.
3. Cannabinol. M.p. 75° to 76°.
4. Tetrahydrocannabinol. An oily liquid from which 2 isomers may be crystallised. These have melting-points of 146° and 128°, respectively. The isomer which melts at 146° has ultraviolet absorption maxima at about 208 mμ, 273 mμ, and 283 mμ; the isomer which melts at 128° has ultraviolet maxima at 227 mμ and 266 mμ.
The euphoric activity of the drug is reported to be associated only with tetrahydrocannabinol.

Cannabis and cannabis resin may be identified by the following method. The material is extracted with 3 aliquots of benzene which are decanted through a short column of Florisil (60 to 100 mesh). The pooled extract is then evaporated to small bulk, about 2 drops, and submitted to either paper chromatography using Whatman SG 81 paper and a solvent consisting of carbon tetrachloride: benzene (1:1), or to thin-layer chromatography on plates coated with silica gel G, the solvent being benzene: chloroform (3:7). After development, the chromatograms are dried and sprayed with *Beam's reagent*. A purple spot at about Rf 0·80 (cannabidiol) indicates the presence of cannabis. Other location reagents which may be used include alkaline 0·1% fast blue B and *diazotised p-nitroaniline–sodium hydroxide spray*.
Further methods of identifying cannabis involving paper, thin-layer, and gas chromatographic analyses are described by Farmilo and Davis (1961); Davis *et al.* (1963); Caddy and Fish (1967); Heaysman *et al.* (1967); Caddy *et al.* (1967); Betts and Holloway (1967).

Use. Cannabis was formerly employed in mania and nervous disorders as a sedative or narcotic but it is now rarely used as a therapeutic agent since its action is very unreliable.

Toxicity. Toxic doses cause vertigo and collapse but serious poisoning is rare and fatalities unknown since the margin between the effective and the fatal dose is wide. Addiction does not give rise to serious physical consequences and, except in severe cases, withdrawal symptoms are insignificant.

CANTHARIDIN *Vesicant*

3,6 - Epoxy - 1,2 - dimethylcyclohexane - 1,2 - dicarboxylic anhydride
$C_{10}H_{12}O_4 = 196{\cdot}2$

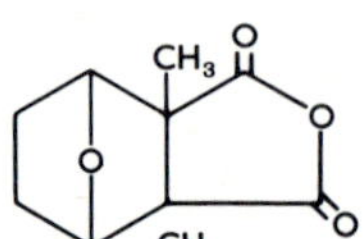

Cantharidin is found in cantharides, the dried beetle *Cantharis vesicatoria* (Meloidae), which may contain from 0·4 to 0·8%.
Colourless glistening crystals which sublime at about 120°. M.p. 216° to 218°.
Solubility. Very slightly soluble in water; soluble 1 in about 1100 of ethanol, 1 in 700 of ether, and 1 in 55 of chloroform.

Extraction and **Detection.** Cantharidin may be extracted from acidified stomach contents and other viscera with ether, or from an ethanolic or aqueous extract of viscera by chloroform. No simple characteristic chemical reactions have been found to identify cantharidin. A 'blistering technique' for its identification is described in *Taylor's Principles and Practice of Medical Jurisprudence*, 12th Edn, J. & A. Churchill Ltd., 1965, Vol. II, p. 577.

Quantitative Estimation. A very full account of the extraction and quantitative estimation of cantharidin in 2 fatal cases is given by Nickolls and Teare (1954).

Metabolism. Cantharidin is readily absorbed from the skin and mucous membranes. When taken orally it causes great pain as well as blistering and gross inflammation of the whole of the alimentary canal, the kidneys, and the bladder. It does not seem to be decomposed in the body.
Cantharidin was formerly employed as a counter-irritant and vesicant.

Toxicity. The lethal dose of cantharidin in man is less than 60 mg, and a minute crystal weighing not more than 0·5 mg lodging in the mucosa will produce a blister which could prove fatal.
CASE EXAMPLES. A 27-year-old woman died about 17 hours after she had eaten coconut ice into which a small quantity of cantharidin had been introduced by a fellow employee. The post-mortem findings revealed that between 65 and 130 mg of cantharidin was circulating in the organs. At the same time as the above incident a 19-year-old girl also ate a piece of the cantharidin-impregnated coconut ice. She died 26 hours later. The post-mortem level of cantharidin in the organs was somewhat less than in the former case (Nickolls and Teare, 1954).
Recovery of a 42-year-old man who developed haematuria after taking a teaspoonful of liquor epispasticus containing cantharidin (approximately 20 mg). When seen 9 hours after ingestion, he was treated with a high fluid intake of milk, a magnesium sulphate enema, analgesics, and sedation (Rosin, 1967).

CAPTODIAME *Tranquilliser*

p-Butylthiodiphenylmethyl 2-dimethylaminoethyl sulphide
$C_{21}H_{29}NS_2 = 359{\cdot}6$

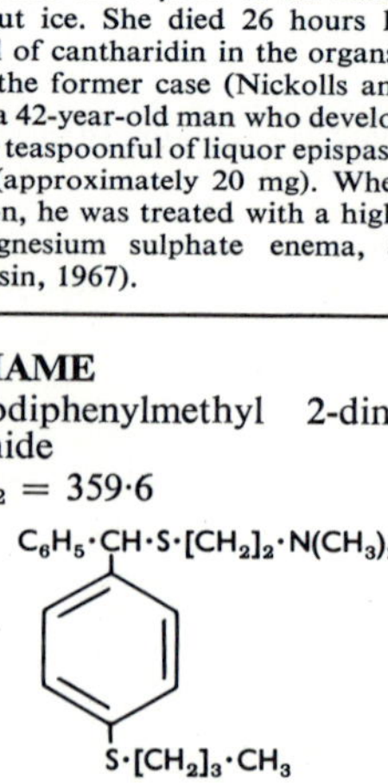

CAPTODIAME HYDROCHLORIDE
Synonym: Captodiamine Hydrochloride.
Proprietary Names: Covatin; Suvren.

Extraction. Captodiame is extracted by organic solvents from aqueous alkaline solutions.

Chromatography. PAPER: system P1—Rf 0·84 (location under ultraviolet light, strong absorption; location reagent *iodoplatinate spray*, weak reaction).

THIN-LAYER: system T1—Rf 0·66 (location reagent *acidified iodoplatinate spray*, positive reaction).

GAS: system G2/225—retention time 2·76 relative to codeine; system G4—retention time 2·66 relative to diphenhydramine.

Colour Tests. MICRO: sulphuric acid–formaldehyde test—bright purple; ammonium molybdate test—blue-purple; ammonium vanadate test—light purple.

Crystal Test. MICRO: *potassium bismuth iodide solution*—curved needles, forming overnight (*sensitivity:* 1 in 200).

Ultraviolet Absorption Spectrum. Captodiame in 0·1N sulphuric acid, maximum at 265 mμ (E1%, 1cm 372).

Infra-red Absorption Spectrum. Captodiame (base). Potassium bromide disk. The principal peaks are: A 1450, B 695, C 1485 (p. 777).

Dose. Up to 300 mg daily.

Toxicity. The estimated lethal dose in man is 25 to 250 mg/kg.

CARAMIPHEN *Parasympatholytic*

2-Diethylaminoethyl 1-phenylcyclopentane-1-carboxylate

$C_{18}H_{27}NO_2 = 289·4$

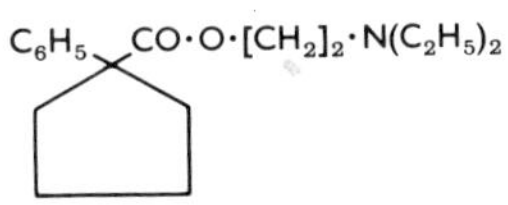

B.p. 110° to 115° at 20 mm Hg.

CARAMIPHEN EDISYLATE

Synonym: Caramiphen Ethanedisulphonate
Proprietary Name: Taoryl.

It occurs as crystals from acetone. M.p. 115° to 116°.
Solubility. Soluble in water and ethanol.

CARAMIPHEN HYDROCHLORIDE

Proprietary Names: Panparnit; Parpanit.

A white crystalline powder. M.p. 142° to 146°.
Solubility. Soluble 1 in 4 of water and 1 in 8 of ethanol; almost insoluble in ether.

Extraction. Caramiphen is extracted by organic solvents from aqueous alkaline solutions.

Chromatography. PAPER: system P1—Rf 0·72 (location reagents: *iodoplatinate spray*, strong reaction; *bromocresol green spray*, weak reaction); system RP1a—Rf 0·35 (location reagent *iodoplatinate spray*, positive reaction); system RP1b—Rf 0·00 (location as for RP1a).

THIN-LAYER: system T1—Rf 0·66 (location reagent *acidified iodoplatinate spray*, positive reaction).

GAS: system G2/225—retention time 1·4 relative to diphenhydramine; system G4—retention time 1·17 relative to diphenhydramine.

Colour Test. MICRO: sulphuric acid–formaldehyde test—yellow (*sensitivity:* 1·0 μg).

Crystal Tests. MICRO: *lead iodide solution*—rosettes of needles, forming overnight (*sensitivity:* 1 in 1000); *platinic chloride solution*—rhomboidal plates (*sensitivity:* 1 in 400).

Ultraviolet Absorption Spectrum. Caramiphen in 0·1N sulphuric acid, maxima at 252 mμ (E1%, 1cm 5), 258 mμ (E1%, 1cm 6), and 264·5 mμ (E1%, 1cm 4).

Infra-red Absorption Spectrum. Caramiphen (base). Potassium bromide disk. The principal peaks are: A 1718, B 1154, C 694 or 1173 (p. 778).

Metabolism. Caramiphen hydrochloride has parasympatholytic and antispasmodic properties. The maximum effect of therapeutic doses does not last longer than 2 or 3 hours. Caramiphen edisylate has been employed as an antitussive.

Dose. Daily doses of 50 mg, increasing gradually to 600 mg, have been given.

Toxicity. The lethal dose in man is probably between 10 and 100 mg/kg.

CARBACHOL *Parasympathomimetic*

Synonyms: Carbacholine; Carbamoylcholine Chloride; Choline Chloride Carbamate.

(2-Carbamoyloxyethyl)trimethylammonium chloride

$C_6H_{15}ClN_2O_2 = 182·7$

$$[NH_2·CO·O·[CH_2]_2·N(CH_3)_3]^+ \ Cl^-$$

A white hygroscopic crystalline powder. M.p. about 210°, with decomposition.
Solubility. Soluble 1 in 1 of water and 1 in 55 of ethanol; very slightly soluble in dehydrated ethanol but more readily so on boiling; almost insoluble in ether and chloroform.

Screening Test. See under Screening Tests (carbamates), p. 13.

Extraction. Carbachol is a quaternary ammonium compound (see p. 29).

Chromatography. PAPER: system P1—Rf 0·03 (location reagent *iodoplatinate spray*, strong reaction); system P7—Rf 0·82 (location reagent *furfural–hydrochloric acid spray*, positive reaction).

THIN-LAYER: system T1—Rf 0·01 (location reagent *acidified iodoplatinate spray*, positive reaction).

Crystal Tests. MICRO: *gold bromide–hydrochloric acid solution*—rectangular plates (*sensitivity:* 1 in 1000); *potassium bismuth–iodide solution*—small needles (*sensitivity:* 1 in 1000).

Actions. Carbachol has the muscarinic and nicotinic actions of acetylcholine but it is not rapidly inactivated by cholinesterase; its action is therefore more prolonged. It stimulates the parasympathetic nervous system and reduces intra-ocular pressure and is a powerful miotic.

Dose. Up to 0·5 mg subcutaneously; up to 4 mg by mouth.

Toxicity. Fatalities have occurred due to accidental overdosage.
LD50 (oral): in mice 15 and in rats 40 mg/kg.

CARBAMAZEPINE *Anticonvulsant*
Synonym: G 32883.
Proprietary Names: Tegretal; Tegretol.

5-Carbamoyl-5*H*-dibenz[*b*,*f*]azepine
$C_{15}H_{12}N_2O = 236{\cdot}3$

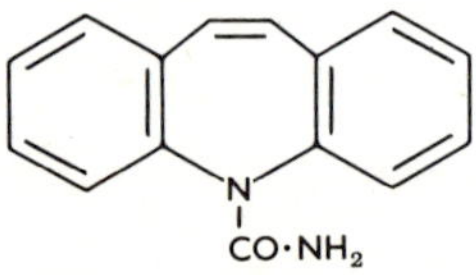

A white crystalline powder. M.p. 190° to 193°.
Solubility. Practically insoluble in water; soluble in ethanol, acetone, and propylene glycol.

Extraction. Carbamazepine is extracted by organic solvents from aqueous alkaline solutions.

Chromatography. PAPER: system P1—Rf 0·84 (location under ultraviolet light, blue fluorescence; location reagent *potassium permanganate spray*, strong reaction); system RP1a—Rf 0·29 (location under ultraviolet light, blue fluorescence); system RP1b—Rf 0·30 (location under ultraviolet light, blue fluorescence).
THIN-LAYER: system T1—Rf 0·73 (location reagent *potassium permanganate spray*, positive reaction).
GAS: system G2/225—retention time 0·81 relative to codeine; retention time 3·76 relative to diphenhydramine.

Colour Test. MICRO: ammonium molybdate test—faint blue (*sensitivity:* 1·0 μg).

Crystal Test. MICRO: *lead iodide solution*—needles.

Ultraviolet Absorption Spectrum. Carbamazepine in ethanol, maxima at 215 mμ and 285 mμ; minimum at about 257 mμ; in 0·1N sulphuric acid, maximum at 283 mμ (E1%, 1 cm 147) and an inflexion at about 255 mμ (E1%, 1 cm 274).

Infra-red Absorption Spectrum. Potassium bromide disk. The principal peaks are: A 1678, B 1388, C 1594 (p. 778).

Dose. Usually up to 200 mg daily, increasing if necessary up to 1·6 g.

Toxicity. LD50 (oral): in mice about 3·75 and in rats 4 g/kg.

CARBETAPENTANE *Antitussive*
Synonym: Pentoxyverine.

2-(2-Diethylaminoethoxy)ethyl 1-phenylcyclopentane-1-carboxylate
$C_{20}H_{31}NO_3 = 333{\cdot}5$

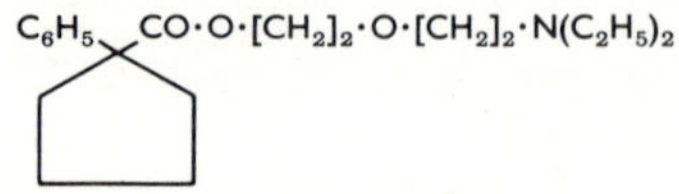

CARBETAPENTANE CITRATE
Proprietary Names: Toclase; Tuclase.

A white or almost white crystalline powder. M.p. 90° to 95°.
Solubility. Freely soluble in water and chloroform; slightly soluble in ethanol; almost insoluble in ether.

Extraction. Carbetapentane is extracted by organic solvents from aqueous alkaline solutions.

Chromatography. PAPER: system P1—Rf 0·76 (location reagents: *iodoplatinate spray*, strong reaction; *bromocresol green spray*, weak reaction); system RP1a—Rf 0·73 (location reagent *iodoplatinate spray*, positive reaction); system RP1b—Rf 0·08 (location as for RP1a).
THIN-LAYER: system T1—Rf 0·46 (location reagent *acidified iodoplatinate spray*, positive reaction).

Colour Tests. MICRO: sulphuric acid–formaldehyde test—orange, slowly (*sensitivity:* 1·0 μg); ammonium vanadate test—brown, slowly (*sensitivity:* 1·0 μg).

Crystal Test. MICRO: *lead iodide solution*—network of hairlike crystals (*sensitivity:* 1 in 200).

Ultraviolet Absorption Spectrum. Carbetapentane in methanol, maxima at 252 mμ (E1%, 1 cm 3·6), 258 mμ (E1%, 1 cm 4), and 265 mμ (E1%, 1 cm 3); in 0·1N sulphuric acid, maxima at 252 mμ (E1%, 1 cm 3), 258·5 mμ (E1%, 1 cm 3·6), and 264·5 mμ (E1%, 1 cm 3).

Infra-red Absorption Spectrum. Carbetapentane (base). Potassium bromide disk. The principal peaks are: A 1725, B 1120, C 1158 (p. 778).

Dose. Usually up to 120 mg daily.

Toxicity. Its toxicity is low and it is not narcotic.

CARBIMAZOLE *Antithyroid Agent*
Synonym: Ethyl 3-methyl-2-thioimidazoline-1-carboxylate.
Proprietary Name: Neo-Mercazole.

1-Ethoxycarbonyl-3-methyl-2-thio-4-imidazoline

$C_7H_{10}N_2O_2S$ = 186·2

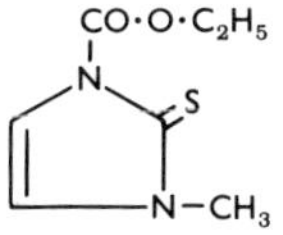

A white crystalline powder. M.p. 122° to 125°.

Solubility. Soluble 1 in 500 of water, 1 in 50 of ethanol, 1 in 330 of ether, and 1 in 3 of chloroform.

Extraction. Carbimazole is extracted by organic solvents from aqueous acid or alkaline solutions.

Chromatography. PAPER: system P1—Rf 0·90 (location under ultraviolet light, absorption; location reagents: *iodoplatinate spray*, yellow; *potassium permanganate spray*, weak reaction).

THIN-LAYER: system T1—Rf 0·72 (location reagent *acidified iodoplatinate spray*, positive reaction).

GAS: system G2/225—retention time 0·61 relative to diphenhydramine.

Colour Tests. To a small quantity add 1 drop of *iodobismuthous acid solution*—scarlet.

MICRO: ammonium molybdate test—faint blue (*sensitivity:* 1·0 μg).

Crystal Tests. MICRO: *mercuric chloride solution*—irregular rosettes (*sensitivity:* 1 in 1000); *potassium cadmium iodide solution*—bunches of very small plates (*sensitivity:* 1 in 400).

Ultraviolet Absorption Spectrum. Carbimazole in 0·1N hydrochloric acid:water (1:8), maximum at 291 mμ (E1%, 1 cm 557); in 0·1N sulphuric acid, maxima at 227 mμ and 291 mμ (E1%, 1 cm 557).

Infra-red Absorption Spectrum. Potassium bromide disk. The principal peaks are: A 1748 B 1278, C 1320 (p. 733).

Metabolism. Carbimazole is an antithyroid substance which depresses the formation of thyroid hormone and so lowers the basal metabolic rate. It reduces the uptake and concentration of inorganic iodine by the thyroid but its main effect is to reduce the formation of di-iodotyrosine and thyroxine, although, once formed, their action is not antagonised.

Carbimazole is absorbed rapidly from the intestinal tract and is widely distributed throughout the body. It slowly releases methimazole in the body to exert slow prolonged antithyroid action. It readily crosses the placental barrier; it also attains a high concentration in the milk of lactating women. Excretion in the urine is rapid, being almost complete within 24 hours.

Dose. Up to 60 mg daily.

Toxicity. Agranulocytosis, aplastic anaemia, and thrombocytopenic purpura have occasionally been reported following carbimazole therapy.

CARBINOXAMINE *Antihistamine*

2-(*p*-Chloro-α-pyrid-2-ylbenzyloxy)-*NN*-dimethylethylamine

$C_{16}H_{19}ClN_2O$ = 290·8

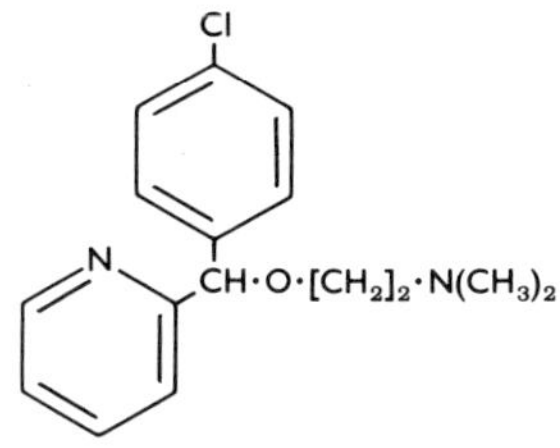

A liquid. B.p. 158° to 162° at 0·1 mm Hg.

CARBINOXAMINE MALEATE

Proprietary Names: Clistin Maleate. It is an ingredient of Davenol.

A white crystalline powder. M.p. 116° to 121°.

Solubility. Very soluble in water; freely soluble in ethanol and chloroform; very slightly soluble in ether.

Extraction. Carbinoxamine is extracted by organic solvents from aqueous alkaline solutions.

Chromatography. PAPER: system P1—Rf 0·46 (location under ultraviolet light, blue fluorescence; location reagents: *iodoplatinate spray*, strong reaction; *bromocresol green spray*, weak reaction); system RP1a—Rf 0·78 (location under ultraviolet light, absorption; location reagent *iodoplatinate spray*, positive reaction); system RP1b—Rf 0·10 (location as for RP1a).

THIN-LAYER: system T1—Rf 0·38 (location reagent *acidified iodoplatinate spray*, positive reaction); system T2—Rf 0·63 (location reagent *iodoplatinate spray*, positive reaction); system T3—Rf 0·33 (location as for T2).

GAS: system G2/225—retention time 2·1 relative to diphenydramine; retention time 0·45 relative to codeine.

Crystal Tests. MICRO: *gold chloride solution*—bunches of rods (*sensitivity:* 1 in 400); *lead iodide solution*—dense rosettes (*sensitivity:* 1 in 100).

Ultraviolet Absorption Spectrum. Carbinoxamine in methanol, maximum at about 260 mμ; in 0·1N sodium hydroxide, maximum at 260 mμ (E1%, 1 cm 208); in 0·1N sulphuric acid, maximum at 264 mμ (E1%, 1 cm 271) and an inflexion at about 270 mμ (E1%, 1 cm 226).

Infra-red Absorption Spectrum. Carbinoxamine (base). Potassium bromide disk. The principal peaks are: A 1084, B 1110, C 1462 or 1484 or 1584 (p. 778).

Dose. Up to 32 mg daily.

Toxicity. The estimated acute lethal dose in man is 25 to 250 mg/kg. The lethal dose in guinea-pigs is 411 mg/kg.

CARBON TETRACHLORIDE *Anthelmintic*

Synonym: Carbonei Tetrachloridum.

Tetrachloromethane

$CCl_4 = 153{\cdot}8$

A colourless volatile liquid which is slowly decomposed by light and by various metals, if moisture is present. B.p. 76° to 77·5°. Refractive index 1·4607.

Solubility. Soluble 1 in 2000 of water; miscible with ethanol, ether, and chloroform.

Extraction. Carbon tetrachloride is volatile and may be isolated by distillation (see p. 18).

Quantitative Estimation. Carbon tetrachloride may be estimated in blood by aeration of samples and subsequent infra-red spectrophotometry (Stewart *et al.*, 1960; Feldstein, 1965); it may be estimated similarly in expired air (Stewart *et al.*, 1961c).

Metabolism. Carbon tetrachloride is absorbed very readily from the lungs, gastro-intestinal tract, and skin. The rate of absorption is increased by concomitant ingestion of alcohol. The tissue distribution of carbon tetrachloride is probably dependent on absorption, concentration, and exposure time. Carbon tetrachloride injures almost all cells of the body, including those of the blood, central nervous system, liver, and kidney; the kidneys and liver of fatal cases often show marked fatty degeneration.

Carbon tetrachloride is eliminated rapidly from the body; none is detected in the blood after 48 hours, although complete excretion takes about 5 days. Expiration from the lungs appears to be the major route of excretion; between 50 and 90% of the absorbed carbon tetrachloride has been variously reported to be excreted in this way. About 20% of the absorbed carbon tetrachloride is metabolised to carbon dioxide which is exhaled. Carbon tetrachloride does not seem to be excreted unchanged in the urine; two metabolites have been detected in the urine, urea and one, as yet uncharacterised, which may be a conjugate.

Dose. Up to 4 ml, as a single dose, has been given.

Toxicity. The minimum lethal dose in man is between 3 and 5 ml but recoveries have occurred following ingestion of 30 to 40 ml. The estimated safe atmospheric concentration is 25 p.p.m. although this level cannot be detected by odour. Inhalation of concentrations of 1000 p.p.m., even for short periods, may cause acute toxic reactions. Continued exposure to concentrations of even less than 100 p.p.m. may give rise to chronic poisoning. When carbon tetrachloride is ingested together with or immediately after the ingestion of alcohol its toxicity is greatly increased, due probably to the fact that it dissolves readily in alcohol and so is freely absorbed from the gastro-intestinal tract. Alcohol is thought to increase the urinary excretion of carbon tetrachloride and it may contribute towards the nephrotoxic action which has been observed when carbon tetrachloride is taken together with alcohol.

LD50 (oral): in mice 13 and in rats 7·5 g/kg.

NOTE. Carbon tetrachloride is used as an anthelmintic in animals. It was formerly used for this purpose in man but has been superseded by less toxic anthelmintics. It is employed in industry as a solvent and degreaser and is a constituent of certain types of fire extinguisher. It was formerly widely used as an industrial and domestic dry cleaner but it has been largely replaced by less toxic cleaners. Thawpit, for example, which originally contained carbon tetrachloride, now contains trichloroethane (p. 581).

CASE EXAMPLE. A middle-aged alcoholic ingested about 30 ml of carbon tetrachloride under the impression that it was alcohol. He was seriously ill but recovered. On his admission to hospital the serum level of carbon tetrachloride was 2 mg%. The first 24-hour urine collection contained 0·8 mg% and the first peritoneal dialysate contained 0·1 mg% of carbon tetrachloride (Tompsett, 1967b).

For numerous reports on carbon tetrachloride poisoning by ingestion and inhalation and in alcoholics see Extra Pharmacopoeia (Martindale), 25th Edn, pp. 1114–5.

CARBROMAL *Hypnotic*

Synonyms: Bromadal; Bromodiethylacetylurea; Uradal.
Proprietary Names: Adalin. An ingredient of Carbrital.

N-(α-Bromo-α-ethylbutyryl)urea

$C_7H_{13}Br\,N_2O_2 = 237{\cdot}1$

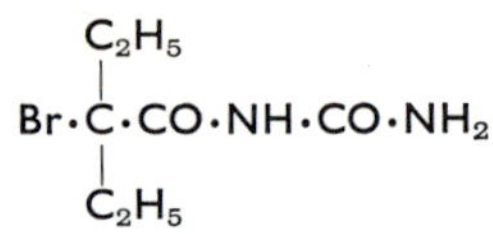

A white crystalline powder. M.p. 116° to 118°.

Solubility. Soluble 1 in 3000 of water, 1 in 18 of ethanol, 1 in 25 of ether, and 1 in 2 of chloroform.

Screening Tests. See under Screening Tests, p. 10.

Extraction. Carbromal is extracted by organic solvents from aqueous acid or alkaline solutions.

Chromatography. PAPER: system P1—Rf 0·93 (location under ultraviolet light, absorption; location reagent *bromine–starch–potassium iodide*, weak reaction); system RP1b—Rf 0·15 (location reagent *bromine–starch–potassium iodide*).

THIN-LAYER: system T10—Rf 0·50 (location reagents: *fluorescein spray*, pink; *potassium permanganate spray*, yellow-brown).

GAS: system G5—retention time 0·31 relative to barbitone.

Crystal Test. MICRO: *lead iodide solution*—bunches of needles.

Infra-red Absorption Spectrum. Potassium bromide disk. The principal peaks are: A 1692, B 1388, C 1600 (p. 733).

Quantitative Estimation. Carbromal may be

estimated spectrophotometrically in blood as free bromide (Street, 1960). Goldbaum and Domanski (1966) have described a procedure for extraction and quantitative estimation applicable to carbromal in biological fluids and tissues involving gas chromatography.

Metabolism. Carbromal is a weak hypnotic. In therapeutic doses, it induces sleep in about half an hour. The effect lasts for 4 to 5 hours. It is excreted partly as 2-ethyl-2-hydroxybutyric acid and appears in only very small quantities as the unchanged drug. It has been isolated as diethylacetylurea from the gastro-intestinal tract (Curry, 1960).
In the mouse, carbromal is rapidly metabolised by debromination to *N*-(α-ethylbutyryl) urea and by hydroxylation to *N*-(α-bromo-α-ethyl-3-hydroxybutyryl)urea. It is metabolised more slowly in the rat and a smaller proportion is converted to the hydroxy-derivative (Butler, 1964).

Dose. Usually up to 1 g.

Toxicity. Fatalities have occurred in adults following the ingestion of 10 to 25 g. Continued therapy with carbromal may lead to blood-levels of over 100 mg% of inorganic bromide and at this level psychiatric disturbances may occur.
LD50 (oral): in dogs 450 and in rabbits 500 to 700 mg/kg.

CASE EXAMPLES. Report of 2 deaths following the ingestion of 10 and 25 g of carbromal. In 2 chronic poisoning cases the serum bromide-level was 245 and 139 mg% and the level in the cerebrospinal fluid was 104 and 57 mg% (Magnussen, 1947).
Accidental death is reported in a 54-year-old woman who had taken Persomnia tablets (containing carbromal and bromvaletone) in large numbers for at least 10 years. Post-mortem levels of bromide: blood, 132 mg%; urine, 110 mg%; cerebrospinal fluid, 105 mg%. The stomach fluid contained about 125 mg% of bromide (Steel and Johnstone, 1959).

CARBUTAMIDE *Antidiabetic*

Synonyms: BZ 55; Glybutamide; U 6987.
Proprietary Names: Bucrol; Invenol; Nadisan.

N-p-Aminobenzenesulphonyl-*N'*-butylurea
$C_{11}H_{17}N_3O_3S = 271{\cdot}3$

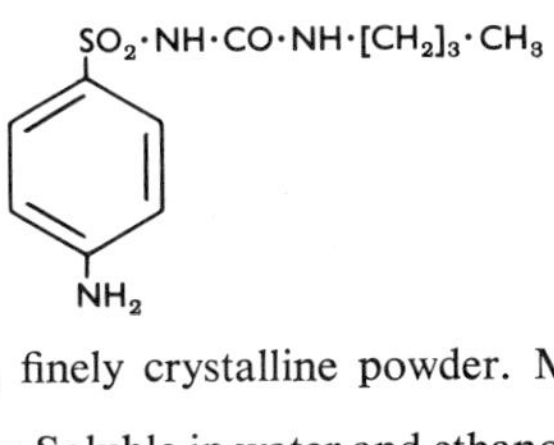

A white, finely crystalline powder. M.p. 144° to 145°.
Solubility. Soluble in water and ethanol; almost insoluble in ether and chloroform.

Chromatography. PAPER: system P1—Rf 0·95 (location reagents: diazotisation followed by *alkaline betanaphthol spray*, red; p-*dimethylaminobenzaldehyde spray*, yellow).
THIN-LAYER: system T1—Rf 0·78 (location reagent diazotisation followed by *alkaline betanaphthol spray*, positive reaction).

Crystal Tests. MICRO: *gold bromide solution*—sheaves of small needles (*sensitivity:* 1 in 400); *platinic iodide solution*—rods, best viewed under polarised light (*sensitivity:* 1 in 200).

Ultraviolet Absorption Spectrum. Carbutamide in ethanol, maximum at 269 mμ (E1%, 1 cm 756); in 0·1N hydrochloric acid, maxima at 266 mμ (E1%, 1 cm 151) and 272 mμ (E1%, 1 cm 143); in 0·1N sodium hydroxide, maximum at 255 mμ (E1%, 1 cm 598).

Infra-red Absorption Spectrum. Potassium bromide disk. The principal peaks are: A 1661, B 1147 or 1599, C 1089 or 1635 (p. 778).

Quantitative Estimation. Kern (1963) describes a method of extraction of carbutamide from blood followed by nitration of the phenyl moiety, diazotisation, coupling with *N*-1-naphthylethylenediamine, and final spectrophotometric determination.

Metabolism. In man, carbutamide appears in the urine mainly as the acetyl derivative which is soluble in water and biological fluids. In dogs, the metabolism of carbutamide may give rise to hepatotoxic intermediates (Levine and Berger, 1960).

Toxicity. Carbutamide is an antidiabetic drug which was administered orally in doses ranging from 1 to 4·5 g daily. It was later withdrawn from use on account of serious toxic effects including liver damage, blood dyscrasias, and exfoliative dermatitis.
LD50 (oral): in mice 11·5 g/kg.

CARISOPRODOL *Muscle Relaxant*

Synonyms: CB 8019; *N*-Isopropylmeprobamate.
Proprietary Names: Carisoma; Flexartal; Rela; Soma.

2-Carbamoyloxymethyl-2-isopropylcarbamoyloxymethylpentane
$C_{12}H_{24}N_2O_4 = 260{\cdot}3$

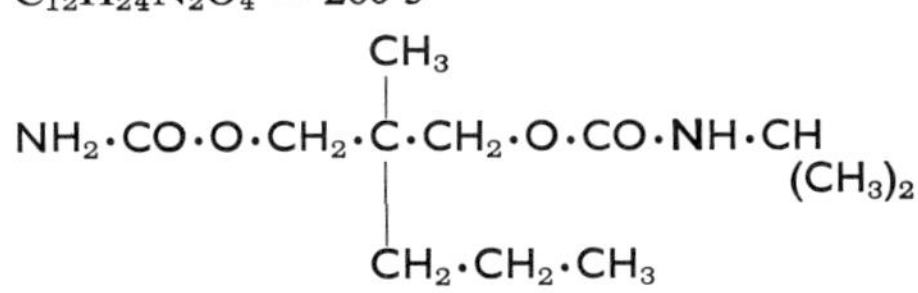

A white crystalline powder. M.p. 92° to 94°.
Solubility. Soluble 1 in 3300 of water; soluble in most common organic solvents.

Screening Test. See under Screening Tests (carbamates), p. 13.

Extraction. Carisoprodol is extracted by organic solvents from aqueous acid or alkaline solutions.

Chromatography. GAS: system G5—retention time 3·49 relative to barbitone.

Quantitative Estimation. Goldbaum and Domanski (1966) have described a procedure, involving gas chromatography, for extraction and quantitative determination applicable to carisoprodol in biological fluids and tissues.

Metabolism. In the dog, carisoprodol is largely excreted in the urine as hydroxycarisoprodol; small quantities of hydroxymeprobamate and meprobamate are also present and traces of carisoprodol itself. In the blood, after intravenous injection, the major circulating carbamate is the unchanged drug although hydroxycarisoprodol, hydroxymeprobamate, and meprobamate are also present (Douglas *et al.*, 1962).

Dose. Up to 1·4 g daily.

CARPHENAZINE *Tranquilliser*

Synonyms: Carfenazine; Wy 2445.

10-{3-[4-(2-Hydroxyethyl)piperazin-1-yl]propyl}-2-propionylphenothiazine

$C_{24}H_{31}N_3O_2S = 425{\cdot}6$

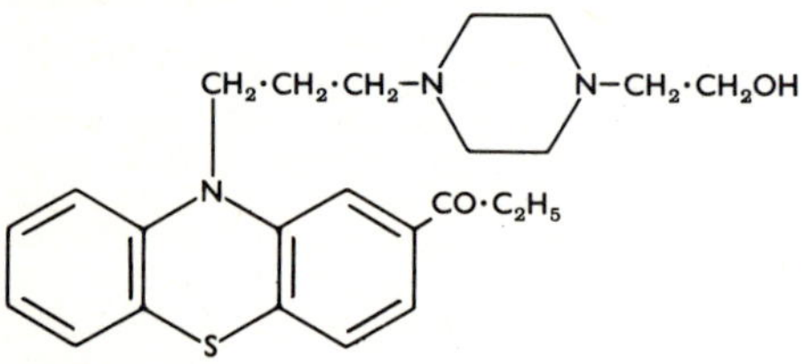

CARPHENAZINE MALEATE

Proprietary Name: Proketazine Maleate.

A finely divided yellow powder. M.p. 162° to 167°, with decomposition.

Solubility. Slightly soluble in water and ethanol; practically insoluble in ether.

Screening Test. *FPN reagent* with urine—red-violet (see p. 10).

Extraction. Carphenazine is extracted by organic solvents from aqueous alkaline solutions.

Chromatography. PAPER: system P1—Rf 0·26 (location under ultraviolet light, yellow fluorescence; location reagents: *iodoplatinate spray*, strong reaction; *potassium permanganate spray*, weak reaction).

THIN-LAYER: system T1—Rf 0·53 (location reagent *acidified iodoplatinate spray*, positive reaction); system T6—Rf 0·71 (the spot may be converted on the plate to the sulphoxide, Rf 0·16; location of both spots under ultraviolet light).

Colour Tests. MICRO: sulphuric acid–formaldehyde test—orange → red-purple (*sensitivity:* 0·1 μg); ammonium molybdate test—blue-purple (*sensitivity:* 0·1 μg); ammonium vanadate test—red-purple (*sensitivity:* 0·5 μg).

Crystal Tests. MICRO: *picric acid*—small irregular plates or needles (*sensitivity:* 1 in 1000); *potassium bismuth iodide solution*—bunches of curved needles, forming overnight (*sensitivity:* 1 in 1000).

Ultraviolet Absorption Spectrum. Carphenazine in ethanol, maxima at 243 mμ (E1%, 1cm 385) and 278 mμ (E1%, 1cm 328); carphenazine in 0·1N sulphuric acid, maxima at about 243 mμ (E1%, 1cm about 595) and about 277 mμ (E1%, 1cm about 441); minima at about 228 mμ and about 260 mμ.

Infra-red Absorption Spectrum. Carphenazine (base). Potassium bromide disk. The principal peaks are: A 1455, B 1408 or 1585, C 1557 (p. 778).

Dose. Usually up to 400 mg daily.

Toxicity. The acute lethal dose in man of phenothiazine tranquillisers appears to be in the range 15 to 150 mg/kg, although severe toxic symptoms have occurred with doses of less than 1 mg/kg.

CEPHAËLINE *Emetic and Expectorant*

Synonym: Desmethylemetine.

$C_{28}H_{38}N_2O_4 = 466{\cdot}6$

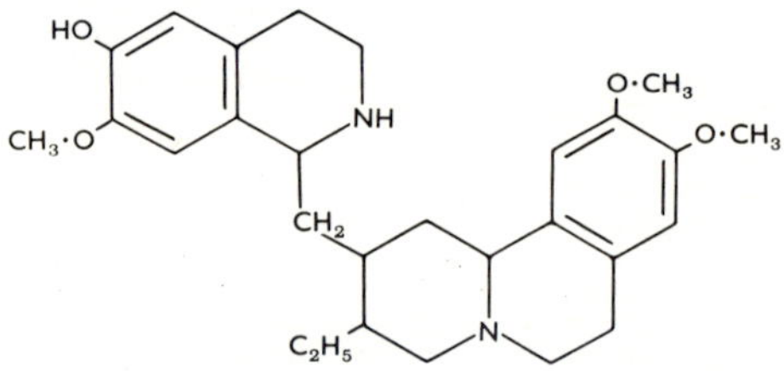

An alkaloid of ipecacuanha, the dried rhizome and root of *Cephaëlis ipecacuanha* (Rubiaceae). It forms needles. M.p. 115° to 116°.

Solubility. Insoluble in water; soluble in ethanol and chloroform; slightly soluble in ether.

CEPHAËLINE HYDROCHLORIDE

Proprietary Name: It is an ingredient of Sedatussin.

White crystals or crystalline powder. Sinters at 245°, slowly melts up to 270°. Solutions turn yellow.

Solubility. Soluble in water, ethanol, and chloroform.

Extraction. Cephaëline is extracted by organic solvents from aqueous alkaline solutions.

Chromatography. PAPER: system P1—Rf 0·11 (location under ultraviolet light, blue fluorescence; location reagent *iodoplatinate spray*, strong reaction).

THIN-LAYER: system T1—Rf 0·51 (location reagent *acidified iodoplatinate spray*, positive reaction).

Colour Tests. MICRO: ammonium molybdate test—deep grey → blue (*sensitivity:* 0·5 μg); Vitali's test—yellow/yellow/brown (*sensitivity:* 0·5 μg).

Toxicity. The lethal dose of emetine in man is estimated to be between 0·7 and 1 g; cephaëline is said to be more irritant and more toxic than emetine.

CEPHALORIDINE *Antibiotic*

Synonyms: Ceph. 87/4; Compound 40602.
Proprietary Names: Ceporan; Ceporin; Keflordin.

8-Oxo-3-(pyrid-1-ylmethyl)-7-(α-thien-2-ylacetamido)-5-thia-1-azabicyclo[4,2,0]oct-2-ene-2-carboxylic acid betaine

$C_{19}H_{17}N_3O_4S_2 = 415{\cdot}5$

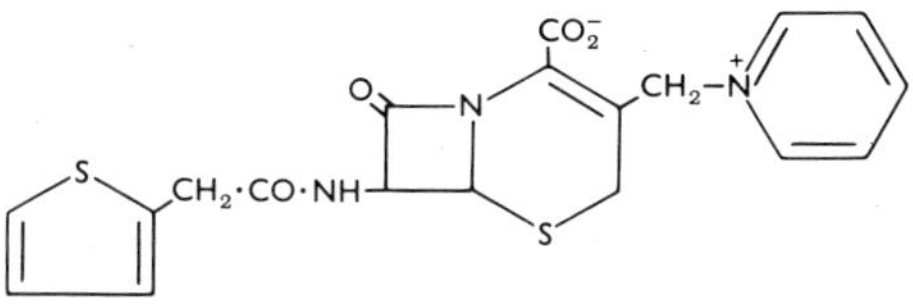

A white crystalline powder which discolours on exposure to light. Specific rotation of a 1% aqueous solution, +46° to +50°.

Solubility. Soluble 1 in 12 water; practically insoluble in ethanol, ether, and chloroform; moderately soluble in dimethylformamide, dimethylacetamide, and dimethyl sulphoxide.

Chromatography. PAPER: system P1—Rf 0·05 (location under ultraviolet light, absorption; location reagents: *iodoplatinate spray*, strong reaction; *potassium permanganate spray*, strong reaction).

THIN-LAYER: system T1—Rf 0·73 (location reagent *potassium permanganate spray*, positive reaction).

Colour Tests. Treat a 0·05% aqueous solution with 1 ml of chloramine solution and 2 ml of 0·1N sodium hydroxide—dull red, persisting for 1 minute. Stir a few milligrams of the solid with 80% v/v sulphuric acid : concentrated nitric acid (100:1)—deep bluish-green, immediately.

MICRO: sulphuric acid–formaldehyde test—red-purple; ammonium molybdate test—blue; ammonium vanadate test—dull purple.

Ultraviolet Absorption Spectrum. Cephaloridine in water, maximum at about 240 mμ (E1%, 1 cm about 390); minimum at about 220 mμ.

Metabolism. Cephaloridine is poorly absorbed from the gastro-intestinal tract; it must be administered parenterally. It is widely distributed in the body tissues, except the brain and cerebrospinal fluid. Serum levels of cephaloridine have been reported to range from 0·75 to 1·72 mg% following a dose of 500 mg. Cephaloridine is rapidly excreted, about 75% of an intravenous dose and 66% of an intramuscular dose being accounted for as active drug in the urine.

Dose. Up to 3 g daily, by intramuscular or deep subcutaneous injection.

Toxicity. LD50 (oral): in mice 15 and in rats 2·5 to 4 g/kg.

CETALKONIUM CHLORIDE *Bactericide*

Proprietary Name: Bacfor CC 100.

Benzylhexadecyldimethylammonium chloride

$C_{25}H_{46}ClN = 396{\cdot}1$

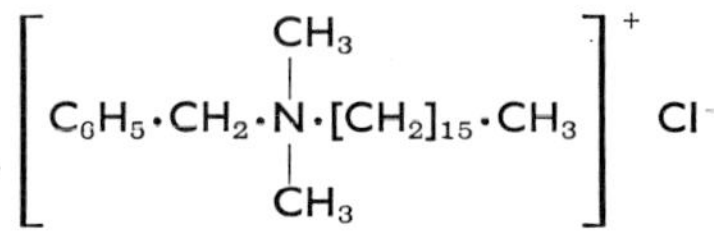

Colourless crystalline powder. M.p. 58° to 60°.

Solubility. Sparingly soluble in cold water, more soluble in hot water; soluble in ethanol.

Extraction. Cetalkonium chloride is a quaternary ammonium compound (see p. 29).

Chromatography. PAPER: system P1—Rf 0·92 (location reagents: *iodoplatinate spray*, strong reaction; *bromocresol green spray*, strong reaction).

THIN-LAYER: system T1—Rf 0·12, streaking (location reagent *acidified iodoplatinate spray*, positive reaction).

Crystal Tests. MICRO: *gold bromide solution*—oily plates, best viewed under polarised light (*sensitivity:* 1 in 1000); *potassium tri-iodide solution* (*I*)—small crystals, best viewed under polarised light (*sensitivity:* 1 in 1000).

Ultraviolet Absorption Spectrum. Cetalkonium chloride in 0·1N sulphuric acid, maxima at 258 mμ (E1%, 1 cm 8), 264 mμ (E1%, 1 cm 10), and 270 mμ (E1%, 1 cm 8), and an inflexion at 253 mμ.

Infra-red Absorption Spectrum. Potassium bromide disk. The principal peaks are: A 1450, B 722, C 698 (p. 778).

Toxicity. The lethal dose in man of cetalkonium chloride, which is closely related to benzalkonium chloride, is estimated to be 1 to 3 g.

CETOXIME *Antihistamine*

N-Benzylanilinoacetamidoxime

$C_{15}H_{17}N_3O = 255{\cdot}3$

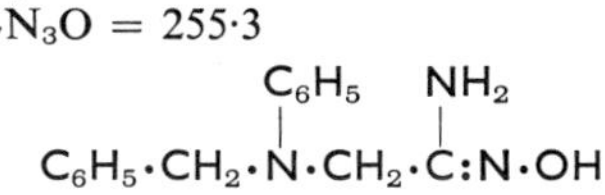

CETOXIME HYDROCHLORIDE

Proprietary Name: Febramine.

Cetoxime hydrochloride melts at about 160°.

Solubility. Soluble in water.

Chromatography. PAPER: system P1—Rf 0·75 (location under ultraviolet light, strong absorption; location reagents: *iodine vapour*, strong reaction; *potassium permanganate spray*, strong reaction); system RP1a—Rf 0·08 (location under ultraviolet light, absorption; location reagent *iodoplatinate spray*, positive reaction).

THIN-LAYER: system T1—Rf 0·75 (location reagent *potassium permanganate spray*, positive reaction).

Colour Tests. MICRO: ammonium vanadate test—red (*sensitivity:* 0·1 μg); Vitali's test—red/yellow/red-brown (*sensitivity:* 0·1 μg).

Crystal Tests. MICRO: *gold bromide solution*—leaflike plates (*sensitivity:* 1 in 400); *gold bromide–hydrochloric acid solution*—feathery plates (*sensitivity:* 1 in 400).

Ultraviolet Absorption Spectrum. Cetoxime in 0·1N sodium hydroxide, maxima at 249 mμ (E1%, 1cm 518) and 300 mμ (E1%, 1cm 83); in 0·1N sulphuric acid, maxima at 242 mμ (E1%, 1cm about 558) and 290 mμ (E1%, 1cm 71).

Dose. Up to 800 mg daily has been given.

Toxicity. LD50 (oral): in mice 300 mg/kg.

CETRIMIDE *Antiseptic Detergent*

Synonyms: CTAB; Cetrimonium Bromide.
Proprietary Names: Biocetab; Cetavlon; Morpan CHSA.

Cetrimide consists chiefly of tetradecyltrimethylammonium bromide, together with smaller amounts of dodecyl- and hexadecyltrimethylammonium bromides.

$$[CH_3\cdot[CH_2]_{13}\cdot N(CH_3)_3]^+ \, Br^-$$

Cetrimide occurs as a white powder.

Solubility. Soluble 1 in 2 of water; very soluble in ethanol; soluble in ether.

Extraction. Cetrimide is a quaternary ammonium compound (see p. 29).

Chromatography. PAPER: system P1—Rf 0·71 (location reagent *iodoplatinate spray*, strong reaction).

THIN-LAYER: system T1—Rf 0·02 (location reagent *acidified iodoplatinate spray*, positive reaction).

Crystal Tests. MICRO: *potassium tri-iodide solution* (*1*)—oily needles or plates, best viewed under polarised light (*sensitivity:* 1 in 200); *styphnic acid*—oily plates or needles, best viewed under polarised light (*sensitivity:* 1 in 1000).

Infra-red Absorption Spectrum. Potassium chloride disk. The principal peaks are: A 1480, B 1462, C 961 (p. 778).

CETYLPYRIDINIUM CHLORIDE *Antiseptic Detergent*

Proprietary Name: Ceepryn Chloride.

1-Hexadecylpyridinium chloride monohydrate

$C_{21}H_{38}ClN,H_2O = 358{\cdot}0$

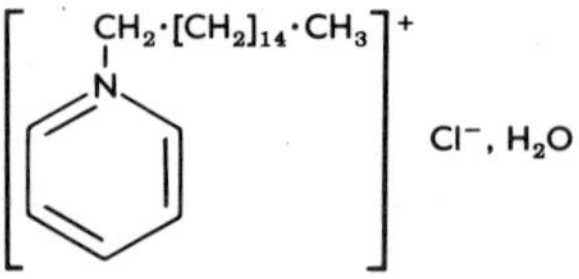

A white powder. M.p. 77° to 83°.

Solubility. Soluble 1 in 20 of water; soluble in ethanol and chloroform; slightly soluble in ether.

Extraction. Cetylpyridinium chloride is a quaternary ammonium compound (see p. 29).

Chromatography. PAPER: system P1—Rf 0·79 (location under ultraviolet light, absorption; location reagent *iodoplatinate spray*, strong reaction).

THIN-LAYER: system T1—Rf 0·20 (location reagent *acidified iodoplatinate spray*, positive reaction).

Crystal Tests. MICRO: *Potassium tri-iodide solution* (2)—plates, sometimes very small, best seen under polarised light; *styphnic acid*—branching needles or very small plates, best seen under polarised light.

Ultraviolet Absorption Spectrum. Cetylpyridinium chloride in water, maximum at 259 mμ (E1%, 1cm 124).

Toxicity. The estimated lethal dose in man is 1 to 3 g. Cetylpyridinium chloride is used as an aqueous solution in strengths from 1 in 10,000 to 1 in 100.

LD50 (oral): in rats 200 mg/kg.

CHLOPHEDIANOL *Antitussive*

Synonyms: Clofedanol; Bayer B186; SL 501.

1-*o*-Chlorophenyl-3-dimethylamino-1-phenylpropan-1-ol

$C_{17}H_{20}ClNO = 289{\cdot}8$

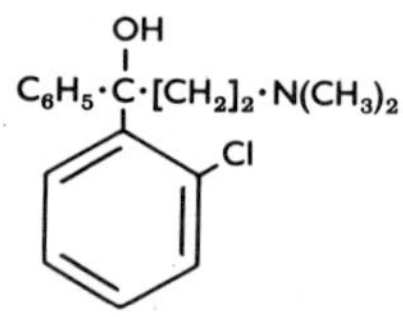

CHLOPHEDIANOL HYDROCHLORIDE

Proprietary Names: Detigon; Ulo.

Chlophedianol hydrochloride occurs as crystals.

Solubility. Soluble in water and ethanol; sparingly soluble in ether.

Extraction. Chlophedianol is extracted by organic solvents from aqueous alkaline solutions.

Chromatography. PAPER: system P1—Rf 0·63 (location under ultraviolet light, absorption; location reagents: *iodoplatinate spray*, strong reaction; *bromocresol green spray*, weak reaction); system RP1a—Rf 0·43 (location under ultraviolet light, absorption).

THIN-LAYER: system T1—Rf 0·54 (location reagent *acidified iodoplatinate spray*, positive reaction).

GAS: system G2/225—retention time 2·0 relative to diphenhydramine; system G4—retention time 2·92 relative to diphenhydramine.

Colour Tests. MICRO: sulphuric acid–formaldehyde test—red-purple → brown (*sensitivity:* 0·1 μg); ammonium molybdate test—yellow (*sensitivity:* 1·0 μg); ammonium vanadate test—greenish-blue (*sensitivity:* 1·0 μg).

Crystal Test. MICRO: *sodium carbonate solution*—rosettes of branching needles (*sensitivity:* 1 in 400).

Ultraviolet Absorption Spectrum. Chlophedianol in 0·1N sulphuric acid, maxima at about 253·5 mμ (E1%, 1cm 11), 259 mμ (E1%, 1cm 13), 265 mμ (E1%, 1cm 12), and an inflexion at about 273 mμ (E1%, 1cm 6).

Infra-red Absorption Spectrum. Chlophedianol (base). Potassium bromide disk. The principal peaks are: A 700 or 756, B 1035 or 1463 (p. 733).

Dose. Up to 150 mg daily.

Toxicity. LD50 (oral): in mice about 315 and in rats about 422 mg/kg.

CHLORAL HYDRATE *Hypnotic*

Synonym: Chloral.

2,2,2-Trichloroethane-1,1-diol

$C_2H_3Cl_3O_2$ = 165·4

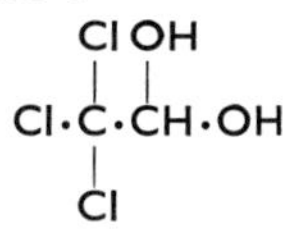

Colourless crystals which volatilise slowly on exposure to air and are decomposed by caustic alkalis, liberating chloroform. Chloral hydrate liquefies between 50° and 58° and boils at 98° with dissociation into water and trichloroacetaldehyde.

Solubility. Soluble 1 in 0·3 of water, 1 in 0·2 of ethanol, 1 in less than 1 of ether, and 1 in 3 of chloroform.

Screening Test. Fujiwara's test—red (see p. 15).

Extraction. Chloral hydrate is volatile and may be isolated by distillation; it may also be extracted by organic solvents from aqueous acid or alkaline solutions. Moss and Kenyon (1964) have described a method of extraction and detection of chloral hydrate and its metabolites in urine involving the Fujiwara reaction and gas chromatography.

Colour Test. Chloral hydrate may be distinguished from other trichloro- compounds by mixing an aqueous solution with a little resorcinol and making the mixture alkaline with 2N sodium hydroxide. The mixture gradually becomes pink and then red in the cold; after about 1 hour it exhibits a green fluorescence under ultraviolet light.

Ultraviolet Absorption Spectrum. Chloral hydrate does not absorb significantly between 200 and 400 mμ.

Infra-red Absorption Spectrum. Potassium bromide disk. The principal peaks are: A 838, B 1078, C 1750 (p. 733).

Quantitative Estimation. Chloral hydrate may be determined quantitatively by modifications of the Fujiwara reaction (Leibman and Hindman, 1964; Bonnichsen and Maehly, 1966) or by spectrophotometric estimation of the blue cyanine dye produced by reaction with quinaldine ethiodide (Archer and Haugas, 1960). Jain *et al.* (1967a) describe a specific and sensitive method for the determination of chloral hydrate and trichloroethanol in biological materials; this involves direct gas chromatographic analysis of the sample mixed with chlorbutol, which is used as the internal standard.

Metabolism. Chloral hydrate is rapidly absorbed from the stomach and begins to act within half an hour. It is metabolised in man to trichloroethanol, which is thought to be responsible for the effects of the drug, and to trichloroacetic acid; the latter appears to be formed both directly from chloral hydrate and later from trichloroethanol since it appears rapidly in the plasma following absorption.

Chloral hydrate is excreted in the urine as free trichloroethanol, trichloroethyl glucuronide (urochloralic acid), and trichloroacetic acid; the main urinary metabolite is trichloroacetic acid which is excreted relatively slowly; between 16 and 35% of the dose has been recovered in 24 hours as trichloroethanol and its glucuronide, about 5% of the dose being in the form of free trichloroethanol.

Chloral hydrate may be found unchanged in the liver, stomach contents, and upper gastro-intestinal tract shortly after death.

In the dog, almost twice as much trichloroethanol and trichloroethyl glucuronide are produced as in man and very little trichloroacetic acid is excreted.

Chloral hydrate taken shortly after alcoholic drinks may lead to marked alterations of the chloral hydrate metabolism; the blood trichloroethanol concentrations reach earlier and higher peak levels and remain elevated during the following 6 hours.

Dose. Usually up to 2 g.

Toxicity. The lethal dose in man averages about 10 g, but varies greatly. Fatalities have followed the ingestion of 1·25 and 3 g but recovery has occurred after the ingestion of 30 g.

LD50 (oral): in rats 200 to 500 mg/kg.

CASE EXAMPLES. Two fatal cases involving the ingestion of overdoses of chloral hydrate are described. In one case the following post-mortem levels were found: blood, 5·8 mg%; kidney, 2·5 mg%; liver, 0·9 mg%; stomach contents 80 mg%; urine, 3 mg%. In the second case: brain, 1·4 mg%; blood, 3·4 mg%. In a suicide case involving chloral hydrate the post-mortem levels were: kidney, 1·1 mg%; liver, 3·1 mg% (Bonnichsen and Maehly, 1966).

A 50-year-old woman was found dead 3 days after disappearing in a state of great intoxication. Nearby were 3 bottles of drugs, one containing chloral hydrate. A blood sample contained 0·9 mg% of trichloroethanol; no unchanged chloral hydrate or alcohol was found (Jain *et al.*, 1967b).

CHLORAMPHENICOL *Antibiotic*

Synonyms: Cloramfenicol; Laevomycetin.
Proprietary Names: Alficetyn; Chloromycetin; Kemicetine.

D-*threo*-2-Dichloroacetamido-1-*p*-nitrophenylpropane-1,3-diol
$C_{11}H_{12}Cl_2N_2O_5 = 323{\cdot}1$

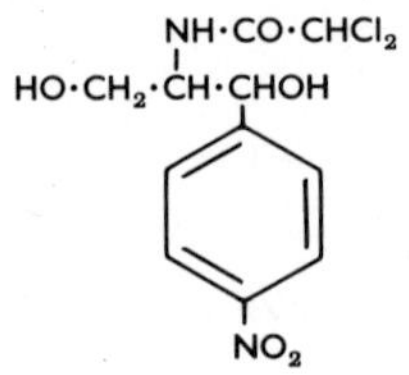

White crystals. M.p. 150° to 153°. Specific rotation of a 5% solution in ethanol, +18·5° to +21·5°. A solution in ethyl acetate is laevorotatory; a solution in ethanol is dextrorotatory.
Solubility. Soluble 1 in 400 of water and 1 in 2·5 of ethanol; slightly soluble in ether and chloroform.

CHLORAMPHENICOL CINNAMATE
A white crystalline powder. M.p. about 119°. Specific rotation of a 10% solution in ethyl acetate, +55° to +58°.
Solubility. Very slightly soluble in water; soluble 1 in 25 of ethanol, 1 in 500 of ether, and 1 in 50 of chloroform.

CHLORAMPHENICOL PALMITATE
A fine white unctuous crystalline powder. M.p. about 89°. Specific rotation of a 5% solution in ethanol, +22·5° to +25·5°.
Solubility. Insoluble in water; soluble 1 in 45 of ethanol, 1 in 14 of ether, and 1 in 6 of chloroform; soluble in acetone and ethyl acetate.

CHLORAMPHENICOL SODIUM SUCCINATE
A light yellow crystalline powder.
Solubility. Freely soluble in water and ethanol; almost insoluble in ether and chloroform.

Chromatography. PAPER: system P1—Rf 0·95 (location under ultraviolet light, strong absorption).

Colour Tests. When heated with 5% sodium hydroxide solution—orange-red (and ammonia vapour given off). Chloramphenicol gives a positive reaction to Fujiwara's test (see p. 128). MICRO: ammonium molybdate test—faint blue.

Ultraviolet Absorption Spectrum. Chloramphenicol in water, maximum at 278 mμ (E1%, 1 cm 298); in 0·1N sodium hydroxide, maximum at 276 mμ (E1%, 1 cm 200); in 0·1N sulphuric acid, maximum at 278 mμ (E1%, 1 cm 284); chloramphenicol cinnamate in ethanol, maximum at about 276 mμ (E1%, 1 cm 710); chloramphenicol palmitate in ethanol, maximum at about 271 mμ (E1%, 1 cm 176).

Infra-red Absorption Spectrum. Chloramphenicol. Potassium bromide disk. The principal peaks are: A 1682, B 1061, C 1351 or 1526 (p. 734).

Quantitative Estimation. Chloramphenicol may be determined by the spectrophotometric estimation of the yellow colour produced by heating it with isonicotinic acid and sodium hydroxide solution (Hughes and Diamond, 1964).

Metabolism. Chloramphenicol is rapidly absorbed from the gastro-intestinal tract. Following a single 1-g dose, maximum blood-levels of about 0·9 mg% are reached in 2 to 4 hours; a dose of 250 mg every 6 hours usually maintains blood-levels above 0·2 mg%; about 60% in the blood is bound to protein. The serum half-life of active chloramphenicol is 1·6 to 3·3 hours while that of the metabolites is 3·7 to 4·6 hours (Kunin *et al.*, 1959).
Chloramphenicol is widely distributed in body tissues and is excreted in the bile and urine. The portion in the bile, however, is resorbed from the alimentary tract so that little is excreted in the faeces. The greater proportion is excreted in the urine during the first 6 hours after ingestion; approximately 10% is excreted unchanged and about 80% is excreted as inactive conjugated metabolites. The 2 major metabolites are the 3-glucuronide of chloramphenicol and the deacylated form of chloramphenicol. In man, very little reduction of the nitro-group to form an aryl amine occurs.
Chloramphenicol cinnamate and palmitate are both inactive but they are each hydrolysed slowly to active chloramphenicol in the gastro-intestinal tract.

Dose. Usually up to 3 g daily.

Toxicity. Daily doses of 50 mg/kg or more lead to plasma chloramphenicol levels of 25 μg/ml which have been found to be associated with bone-marrow depression (Scott *et al.*, 1965).

CHLORBUTOL *Preservative and Sedative*

Synonyms: Acetone-Chloroform; Chlorbutanol; Chlorbutanol Hydrate; Chlorobutanol; Trichlorbutanol; Trichlorisobutyl Alcohol.
Proprietary Name: Chloretone.

2,2,2 - Trichloro -1,1 - dimethylethanol hemihydrate
$C_4H_7Cl_3O,\frac{1}{2}H_2O = 186{\cdot}5$

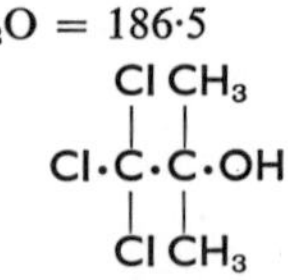

Colourless crystals which are volatile at ordinary temperatures. It is unstable in alkaline solution even at room temperatures; in acid solution it is more stable at room temperatures. M.p. not lower than 77°; anhydrous chlorbutol, about 95°. B.p. about 167°.
Solubility. Soluble 1 in 130 of water, 1 in 1 of ethanol, and 1 in 3 of chloroform; readily soluble in ether.

Screening Test. Fujiwara's test—red (see p. 15).

Extraction. Chlorbutol is volatile and may be isolated by distillation (see p. 18).

Moss and Kenyon (1964) have described a method of extraction and detection of chlorbutol in urine involving the Fujiwara reaction and gas chromatography.

Chromatography. GAS: system G5—retention time 0·16 relative to barbitone.

Colour Test. Iodoform test—positive reaction.

Infra-red Absorption Spectrum. Potassium bromide disk. The principal peaks are: A 802, B 845, C 1150 (p. 734).

Quantitative Estimation. Chlorbutol may be estimated by polarography (Birner, 1961) and by gas chromatography (Koshy *et al.*, 1967).

Metabolism. In man, chlorbutol is probably excreted mainly as a glucuronide conjugate. It has been detected unchanged in the urine of the dog and horse.

Dose. It has been given in doses of 0·3 to 1·2 g.

Toxicity. The minimum lethal oral dose in dogs is 238 mg/kg.
LD50 (oral): in rabbits 200 mg/kg.

CHLORCYCLIZINE *Antihistamine*

Synonym: Histachlorazine.

(±)-1-(*p*-Chlorodiphenylmethyl)-4-methylpiperazine
$C_{18}H_{21}ClN_2 = 300·8$

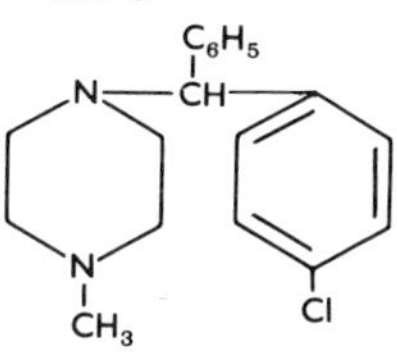

A liquid which boils between 137° and 145° at 0·1 mm Hg.

CHLORCYCLIZINE HYDROCHLORIDE
Proprietary Names: Di-Paralene; Histantin.

A white crystalline powder. M.p. about 225°, with decomposition.
Solubility. Soluble 1 in 2 of water, 1 in 11 of ethanol, and 1 in 4 of chloroform; almost insoluble in ether.

Extraction. Chlorcyclizine is extracted by organic solvents from aqueous alkaline solutions.

Chromatography. PAPER: system P1—Rf 0·74 (location under ultraviolet light, absorption; location reagents: *iodoplatinate spray*, strong reaction; *bromocresol green spray*, weak reaction); system RP1a—Rf 0·02 (location under ultraviolet light, absorption; location reagent *iodoplatinate spray*, positive reaction); system RP1b—Rf 0·00.

THIN-LAYER: system T1—Rf 0·57 (location reagent *acidified iodoplatinate spray*, positive reaction); system T2—Rf 0·49 (location reagent *iodoplatinate spray*, positive reaction); system T3—Rf 0·90 (location as for T2).

GAS: system G1/180—retention time 3·56 relative to diphenhydramine; system G1/250—retention time 0·72 relative to codeine; system G2/225—retention time 3·13 relative to diphenhydramine; retention time 0·67 relative to codeine; system G3—retention time 2·30 relative to diphenhydramine; system G4—retention time 3·2 relative to diphenhydramine.

Colour Test. To 10 mg of chlorcyclizine hydrochloride add 2 ml of sulphuric acid—bright yellow, disappearing when the solution is diluted with water.

Crystal Tests. MICRO: *platinic chloride solution*—small oily needles (*sensitivity:* 1 in 1000); *potassium bismuth iodide solution*—small needles and plates (*sensitivity:* 1 in 1000).

Ultraviolet Absorption Spectrum. Chlorcyclizine in ethanol, maximum at 230 mμ (E1%, 1 cm 495); in 0·1N sulphuric acid, maxima at 232 mμ (E1%, 1 cm 628), 258·5 mμ (E1%, 1 cm 23), 263·5 mμ (E1%, 1 cm 25), 270 mμ (E1%, 1 cm 20), and 276 mμ (E1%, 1 cm 8).

Infra-red Absorption Spectrum. Chlorcyclizine (base). Potassium bromide disk. The principal peaks are: A 1000, B 1135, C 752 or 1283 or 1478 (p. 779).

Metabolism. Chlorcyclizine has a prolonged antihistamine action of similar duration to that of promethazine but it is less potent. Studies in dogs and rats have shown that the major route of metabolism is demethylation to norchlorcyclizine. The highest levels of the drug and its metabolite were found in the kidneys, liver, lungs, and spleen (Kuntzman *et al.*, 1965).

Dose. Up to 200 mg daily.

Toxicity. The estimated lethal dose in man is between 25 and 250 mg/kg. Reports have suggested a possibility of human foetal abnormalities resulting from the administration of chlorcyclizine but a causal relationship has not been confirmed.
LD50 (oral): in mice 347 mg/kg.

CHLORDANE *Pesticide*

Synonyms: CD 68; Chlordan.
Proprietary Names: Octachlor; Octa-Klor; Toxichlor; Velsicol 1068.

Chlordane consists of a mixture of isomers of 1,2,4,5,6,7,8,8 - Octachloro - 3a,4,7,7a - tetrahydro-4,7(*endo*)-methanoindane
$C_{10}H_6Cl_8 = 409·8$

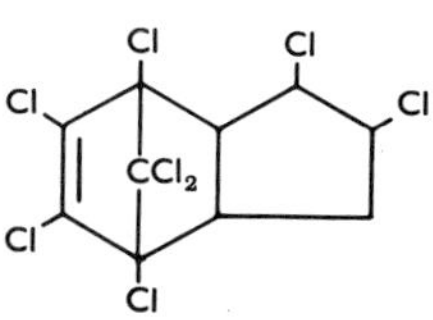

An amber viscous liquid which is decomposed by alkalis.

Solubility. Insoluble in water; soluble in ethanol, ether, and chloroform.

Extraction. Chlordane is extracted by organic solvents from acid or alkaline solutions.

Quantitative Estimation. Chlordane may be extracted from blood by acetone: ether (1 : 1) and quantitatively determined by gas chromatography (Jain *et al.*, 1965).

Metabolism. Chlordane is readily absorbed from the gastro-intestinal tract, the respiratory tract, and the skin. It is stored in the fat, the maximum level being attained 5 days after the beginning of daily doses. Some accumulation also occurs in glandular tissue. Chlordane is removed fairly rapidly from the fat, very little being detectable 20 days after cessation of exposure. The urinary excretion levels reach a maximum 2 to 3 days after a single dose and significant excretion continues for several days longer. About 12 to 24% of the dose is eliminated in the urine; several acidic urinary metabolites have been detected but they have not yet been identified.

Toxicity. Severe symptoms follow ingestion of or skin contamination with 15 to 50 mg/kg or 1 to 3 g of chlordane. Fatalities have occurred following ingestion of 2 to 6 g and contamination with 100 to 500 ml.

LD50 (oral): in rabbits 100 to 300, in rats about 335, and in sheep about 50 mg/kg.

CHLORDIAZEPOXIDE *Tranquilliser*

Synonyms: CMPB; Methaminodiazepoxide; Ro 5-0690.

7-Chloro-2-methylamino-5-phenyl-3*H*-1,4-benzodiazepine 4-oxide

$C_{16}H_{14}ClN_3O = 299{\cdot}8$

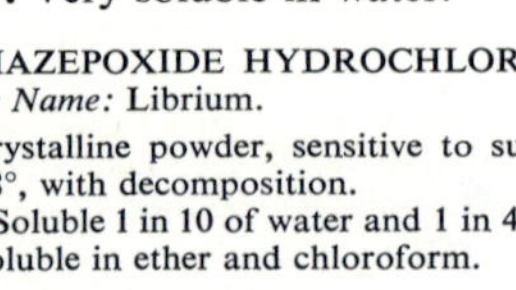

A colourless crystalline powder. M.p. 236°.

Solubility. Very soluble in water.

CHLORDIAZEPOXIDE HYDROCHLORIDE

Proprietary Name: Librium.

A white crystalline powder, sensitive to sunlight. M.p. 212° to 218°, with decomposition.

Solubility. Soluble 1 in 10 of water and 1 in 40 of ethanol; almost insoluble in ether and chloroform.

Screening Test. Acid hydrolysis followed by diazotisation and coupling with *N*-1-naphthylethylenediamine—mauve (see p. 10). A blank test should be carried out on the unhydrolysed material.

Extraction. Chlordiazepoxide is extracted by organic solvents from aqueous alkaline solutions. The lactam metabolite is extracted by ether from neutral and acidic solutions.

Chromatography. PAPER: system P1—Rf 0·82 (location under ultraviolet light, strong absorption; location reagents: *iodoplatinate spray*, strong reaction; *bromocresol green spray*, weak reaction).

THIN-LAYER: system T1—Rf 0·67 (location reagent *acidified iodoplatinate spray*, positive reaction); system T2—Rf 0·70 (location reagent *iodoplatinate spray*, positive reaction); system T3—Rf 0·10 (location as for T2).

GAS: system G1/250—retention time 0·89 relative to codeine; system G2/225—retention time 1·46 relative to codeine; system G3—retention time 4·80 relative to diphenhydramine; system G4—retention time 2·08 relative to codeine.

Colour Tests. MICRO: sulphuric acid–formaldehyde test—yellow (*sensitivity:* 1·0 μg); ammonium molybdate test—dull orange (*sensitivity:* 1·0 μg); Vitali's test— –/faint brown/faint yellow (*sensitivity:* 1·0 μg).

Crystal Tests. MICRO: *lead iodide solution*—dense rosettes (*sensitivity:* 1 in 200); *sodium carbonate solution*—dense rosettes (*sensitivity:* 1 in 400).

Ultraviolet Absorption Spectrum. Chlordiazepoxide in 0·1N sodium hydroxide, maxima at about 243 mμ (E1%, 1 cm 1000) and 260 mμ (E1%, 1 cm 1080); in 0·1N sulphuric acid, maxima at 245 mμ (E1%, 1 cm 1100) and 306 mμ (E1%, 1 cm 310); chlordiazepoxide hydrochloride in 0·1N hydrochloric acid, maxima at 246 mμ (E1%, 1 cm about 1020) and 308 mμ (E1%, 1 cm about 292).

Infra-red Absorption Spectrum. Chlordiazepoxide (base). Potassium bromide disk. The principal peaks are: A 1625, B 1458, C 760 (p. 779).

Quantitative Estimation. Chlordiazepoxide, diazepam, and the *N*-demethylated metabolite of diazepam, after preliminary separation and hydrolysis to their respective benzophenones, may be quantitatively estimated by gas chromatography (de Silva *et al.*, 1964); a sensitive and selective spectrofluorimetric method has been developed for the determination of chlordiazepoxide and, upon slight modification, its lactam metabolite in plasma (Koechlin and d'Arconte, 1963); and a combined spectrofluorimetric assay for chlordiazepoxide, its *N*-demethyl metabolite, and its lactam metabolite in plasma is described by Schwartz and Postma (1966).

Metabolism. Chlordiazepoxide is rapidly absorbed in man; following the oral or intramuscular administration of single 30-mg doses, maximum plasma levels of 0·1 to 0·2 mg% occurred within 2 to 4 hours (Koechlin and d'Arconte, 1963).

It has a plasma half-life in man of 22 to 24 hours and the major metabolic route involves a primary hydrolytic cleavage of the 2-methylamino substituent to yield a lactam derivative. This metabolite is excreted in the urine as well as being further cleaved to the corresponding amino-acid, an 'opened lactam', which is excreted as such or as alkali-labile conjugates. The metabolism of chlordiazepoxide in the dog is similar to that in man but in the rat a basic derivative has been found to be the major metabolite (Koechlin *et al.*, 1965).

The lactam metabolite has been found to be pharmacologically active but the corresponding amino-acid is inactive (Randall *et al.*, 1965).

The *N*-demethyl derivative of chlordiazepoxide, which is a logical intermediate in the formation of the lactam derivative, has been detected in human blood (Schwartz and Postma, 1966).

Evidence for the metabolic conversion of chlordiazepoxide to oxazepam in the dog in small but significant amounts has been obtained: after a single dose of 26 mg/kg of chlordiazepoxide, 1·1% of oxazepam was found in the urine and 1·3% in the faeces (Kimmel and Walkenstein, 1967).

Dose. Up to 100 mg daily, by mouth or intramuscularly.

Toxicity. Recoveries have occurred after ingestion of single doses of 2·25 g and serum levels of between 0·55 and 1·78 mg% have been found in non-fatal poisoning cases. A 500-mg overdose produced a plasma level of 2·5 mg% of chlordiazepoxide and in a fatal case in which the drug was found in the intestines the plasma level was 1·9 mg% (McBay, 1966).

CHLORHEXIDINE *Antiseptic*

Proprietary Name: Hibitane.

Hexamethylenebis[*N*-(*N'*-4-chlorophenylamidino)guanidine]

$C_{22}H_{30}Cl_2N_{10} = 505{\cdot}5$

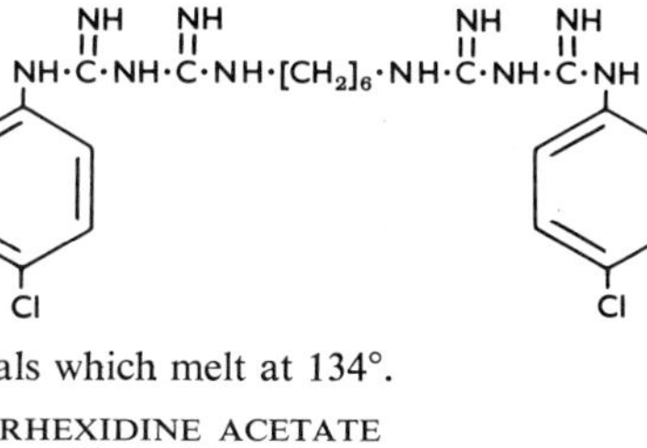

Crystals which melt at 134°.

CHLORHEXIDINE ACETATE

Synonym: Chlorhexidine Diacetate.

A white microcrystalline powder. M.p. 153° to 154°.

Solubility. Soluble 1 in 55 of water and 1 in 15 of ethanol.

CHLORHEXIDINE GLUCONATE SOLUTION

An almost colourless to straw-coloured liquid containing between 19 and 21% of chlorhexidine digluconate. It is affected by light.

Solubility. Miscible with water, with up to 5 parts of ethanol, and up to 3 parts of acetone.

CHLORHEXIDINE HYDROCHLORIDE

Synonym: Chlorhexidine Dihydrochloride.

A white crystalline powder, affected by light. M.p. about 255°, with decomposition.

Solubility. Soluble 1 in 1700 of water and 1 in 450 of ethanol.

Chromatography. PAPER: system P1—Rf 0·28 (location under ultraviolet light, strong absorption; location reagent *iodoplatinate spray* weak reaction).

THIN-LAYER: system T1—Rf 0·33 (location reagents: *strongly acid iodoplatinate spray*, positive reaction; *iodine–carbon tetrachloride spray*, positive reaction).

Colour Test. Stir a small quantity of chlorhexidine on a white tile with a drop of a saturated solution of bromine in water followed by a drop of 20% sodium hydroxide solution—red.

Crystal Tests. MICRO: *picrolonic acid*—very small crystals (*sensitivity:* 1 in 100); *sodium carbonate solution*—rosettes of blades (*sensitivity:* 1 in 100).

Ultraviolet Absorption Spectrum. Chlorhexidine in 0·1N sulphuric acid, maximum at about 254 mμ (E 1%, 1 cm 447).

Infra-red Absorption Spectrum. Chlorhexidine (base). Potassium bromide disk. The principal peaks are: A 1527, B 1628, C 1486 or 1575 (p. 779).

CHLORISONDAMINE CHLORIDE *Antihypertensive*

Synonym: SU 3088.

Propietary Name: Ecolid.

Ethylene-1-(4,5,6,7-tetrachloro-2-methylisoindolinium)-2-trimethylammonium dichloride

$C_{14}H_{20}Cl_6N_2 = 429{\cdot}0$

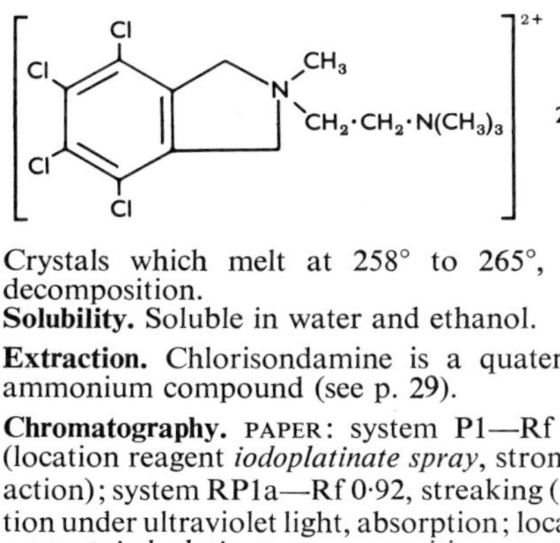

Crystals which melt at 258° to 265°, with decomposition.

Solubility. Soluble in water and ethanol.

Extraction. Chlorisondamine is a quaternary ammonium compound (see p. 29).

Chromatography. PAPER: system P1—Rf 0·06 (location reagent *iodoplatinate spray*, strong reaction); system RP1a—Rf 0·92, streaking (location under ultraviolet light, absorption; location reagent *iodoplatinate spray*, positive reaction).

THIN-LAYER: system T1—Rf 0·01 (location reagent *acidified iodoplatinate spray*, positive reaction).

Crystal Tests. MICRO: *potassium chromate solution*—small plates and needles (*sensitivity:* 1 in 1000); *zinc chloride solution*—masses of small irregular needles (*sensitivity:* 1 in 1000).

Ultraviolet Absorption Spectrum. Chlorisondamine chloride in 0·1N sulphuric acid, maxima at about 274 mμ (E 1%, 1 cm 6), 282 mμ (E 1%, 1 cm 8), and about 290 mμ (E 1%, 1 cm 6).

Infra-red Absorption Spectrum. Potassium bromide disk. The principal peaks are: A 1392, B 964 or 1480, C 1177 (p. 734).

Dose. Up to 200 mg daily.

CHLORMETHIAZOLE *Hypnotic*

Synonym: SCTZ; Wy 1485.

5-(2-Chloroethyl)-4-methylthiazole

$C_{12}H_{16}Cl_2N_2S_2 = 323{\cdot}3$

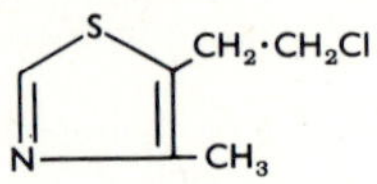

CHLORMETHIAZOLE EDISYLATE

Synonyms: Chlormethiazole Ethanedisulphonate; Clomethiazole Ethanedisulphonate.

Proprietary Name: Heminevrin.

A white crystalline solid. M.p. 126° to 129°.

Solubility. Freely soluble in water and ethanol; insoluble in ether.

Extraction. Chlormethiazole is extracted by organic solvents from aqueous alkaline solutions.

Chromatography. PAPER: system P1—Rf 0·93 (location under ultraviolet light, absorption; location reagent *iodoplatinate spray*, white).

THIN-LAYER: system T1—Rf 0·72 (location reagent *acidified iodoplatinate spray*, positive reaction).

Crystal Tests. MICRO: *picric acid*—rods or needles (*sensitivity:* 1 in 1500); *potassium bismuth iodide solution*—rods and plates (*sensitivity:* 1 in 400).

Ultraviolet Absorption Spectrum. Chlormethiazole in 0·1N sulphuric acid, maximum at 257 mμ (E1%, 1cm 122).

Infra-red Absorption Spectrum. Chlormethiazole (base). Potassium bromide disk. The principal peaks are: A 1409, B 650, C 1438 (p. 779).

Dose. Up to 2 g as a hypnotic; up to 5 g daily in the treatment of alcoholism and acute mania.

CHLORMEZANONE *Tranquilliser*

Synonym: Chlormethazanone.

Proprietary Name: Trancopal.

2-*p*-Chlorophenyltetrahydro-3-methyl-2*H*-1,3-thiazin-4-one 1,1-dioxide

$C_{11}H_{12}ClNO_3S = 273{\cdot}7$

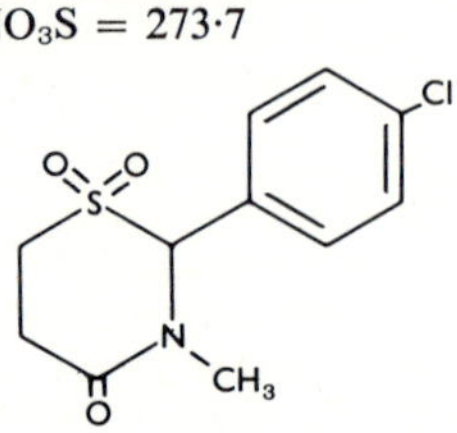

White crystals. M.p. about 117°.

Solubility. Soluble 1 in 400 of water and 1 in less than 100 of ethanol.

Extraction. Chlormezanone is extracted by organic solvents from aqueous acid or alkaline solutions.

Chromatography. GAS: system G2/225—retention times of the 2 major peaks: 0·35 and 2·91 relative to diphenhydramine; there are other intermediate peaks.

Ultraviolet Absorption Spectrum. Chlormezanone in 0·1N sulphuric acid, maxima at 258 mμ (E1%, 1cm 21) and 265 mμ (E1%, 1cm 23); a shoulder at about 270 mμ (E1%, 1cm 16); minima at 249 mμ and 261 mμ.

Infra-red Absorption Spectrum. Potassium bromide disk. The principal peaks are: A 1645, B 1128 or 1145, C 1336 (p. 734).

Metabolism. Studies in mice indicate that at least 2 metabolites are formed (Lockett and Patel, 1961).

Dose. Up to 800 mg daily.

Toxicity. The estimated lethal dose in man is 100 to 500 mg/kg; recovery has followed the ingestion of 10 g.

CHLOROFORM *General Anaesthetic*

Trichloromethane

$CHCl_3 = 119{\cdot}4$

A colourless volatile liquid. B.p. 60° to 62°. Refractive index 1·4464.

Solubility. Soluble 1 in 200 of water; miscible with dehydrated ethanol and ether.

Screening Test. Fujiwara's test—red (see p. 15).

Extraction. Chloroform is volatile and may be isolated by distillation (see p. 18).

Chromatography. GAS: system G8/160—retention time 1·45 relative to n-propanol.

Colour Tests. Heat a little chloroform with a small amount of resorcinol in 2N sodium hydroxide—red. If the resorcinol is replaced by either alpha- or beta-naphthol in this test—blue.

Quantitative Estimation. Chloroform may be quantitatively determined by infra-red spectrophotometry in blood (Feldstein, 1965), in expired air (Stewart *et al.*, 1965), and from steam distillates of fluids and tissues by a modification of the Fujiwara reaction (Bonnichsen and Maehly, 1966).

Metabolism. Chloroform is a more potent general anaesthetic than ether. It diffuses rapidly throughout the body and is rapidly eliminated from the blood. Between 30 and 50% may be exhaled unchanged in 15 to 20 minutes and 90% within an hour; small amounts may be detected in the blood up to 8 hours after the cessation of exposure. Chloroform is not metabolised to any appreciable extent in man; very slow dehalogenation may occur.

Case	Stomach contents	Blood	Liver	Kidney	Urine	Brain	Remarks
K 1	49	43	44	16	3	—	Homicide by forced inhalation of chloroform.
K 2	25	17	6	—	0	55	Homicide by forced inhalation of chloroform.
K 3	39	48	37	27	7	—	Suicide by inhalation of chloroform from plastic bag.
K 4	7	10	—	—	60	—	Overdose by 'sniffing' of chloroform. Died in hospital 12 hours later.
K 5	2	1	1	—	15	—	Exposure to chloroform. Overdose of meprobamate; probably suicide.
K 6	—	36	71	18	3	143	Suicide by inhalation of chloroform and ether. Ethanol present.

Reprinted from *Journal of Forensic Sciences*, 1966, **11**, 422, published by Callaghan & Company, 6141 North Cicero Avenue, Chicago, Illinois 60646, U.S.A.

Toxicity. A concentration of 2 to 3% of chloroform vapour is adequate for the induction of anaesthesia and 1 to 2% for its maintenance. In man, a blood-level of 7 mg% indicates a condition of light anaesthesia and a level of 15 to 25 mg% indicates a condition of fourth-plane anaesthesia. The lethal dose in man by ingestion is about 10 ml. Accumulated amounts of chloroform taken in repeated doses of preparations containing it, e.g. chlorodyne, may lead to liver damage.

LD50 (oral): in rats 2·2 g/kg.

CASE EXAMPLES. Bonnichsen and Maehly (1966) have reported the 6 cases of fatal poisoning due to chloroform presented in the table above. The post-mortem levels of chloroform are given in p.p.m.

CHLOROPROCAINE *Local Anaesthetic*

2-Diethylaminoethyl 4-amino-2-chlorobenzoate

$C_{13}H_{19}ClN_2O_2 = 270{\cdot}8$

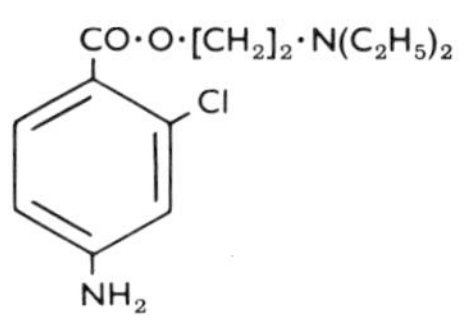

CHLOROPROCAINE HYDROCHLORIDE

Proprietary Name: Nesacaine Hydrochloride.

A white crystalline powder. M.p. 173° to 176°.

Solubility. Soluble 1 in about 20 of water and 1 in about 100 of ethanol; almost insoluble in ether; very slightly soluble in chloroform.

Extraction. Chloroprocaine is extracted by organic solvents from aqueous alkaline solutions.

Chromatography. PAPER: system P1—Rf 0·45 (location under ultraviolet light, strong absorption; location reagents: *iodoplatinate spray*, strong reaction; *bromocresol green spray*, weak reaction; *potassium permanganate spray*, weak reaction).

THIN-LAYER: system T1—Rf 0·60 (location reagents: *acidified iodoplatinate spray*, positive reaction; p-*dimethylaminobenzaldehyde spray*, yellow).

GAS: system G2/225—retention time 2·7 relative to diphenhydramine; retention time 0·58 relative to codeine.

Colour Test. MICRO: diazotisation test—red.

Crystal Tests. MICRO: *gold bromide–hydrochloric acid solution*—irregular needles, best viewed under polarised light (*sensitivity:* 1 in 1000); *styphnic acid*—feathery rosettes (*sensitivity:* 1 in 1000).

Ultraviolet Absorption Spectrum. Chloroprocaine in 0·1N sulphuric acid, maxima at 230 mμ (E1%, 1 cm 330) and 288 mμ (E1%, 1 cm 311): chloroprocaine hydrochloride in *phosphate buffer* (pH 4·5), maxima at 229 mμ (E1%, 1 cm 350) and 291 mμ (E1%, 1 cm 524); minima at about 221 mμ and 249 mμ.

Infra-red Absorption Spectrum. Chloroprocaine (base). Potassium bromide disk. The principal peaks are: A 1595, B 1240 or 1698, C 1625 (p. 779).

Metabolism. Chloroprocaine is a local anaesthetic similar to procaine but it has a more rapid onset of action and is about twice as potent. It is rapidly hydrolysed by plasma cholinesterase.

Dose. Up to 1 g as a 0·5 to 3% solution.

CHLOROPYRILENE *Antihistamine*

Synonyms: Chloromethapyrilene; Chloropyrilen; Chlorothen; Histachlorylene.

N - (5 - Chlorothen - 2 -yl) - *N'N'*- dimethyl - *N*-(pyrid-2-yl)ethylenediamine
$C_{14}H_{18}ClN_3S = 295{\cdot}8$

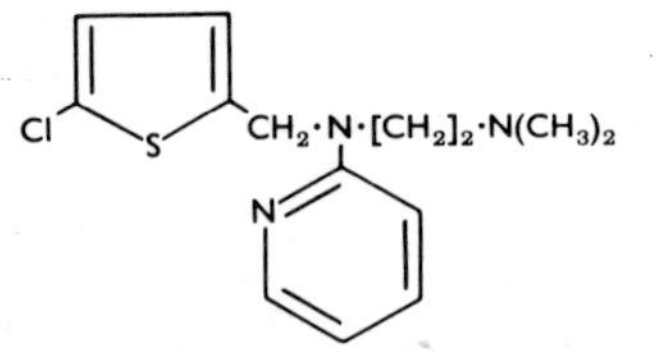

A liquid. B.p. 155° to 156° at 1 mm Hg.

CHLOROPYRILENE CITRATE
Proprietary Name: Tagathen.

A white crystalline powder. M.p. 112° to 116°, then it solidifies and remelts between 125° and 140°, with decomposition.
Solubility. Soluble 1 in about 35 of water; slightly soluble in ethanol; almost insoluble in ether and chloroform.

Extraction. Chloropyrilene is extracted by organic solvents from aqueous alkaline solutions.

Chromatography. PAPER: system P1—Rf 0·54 (location under ultraviolet light, bright blue fluorescence; location reagent *iodoplatinate spray*, strong reaction).
THIN-LAYER: system T1—Rf 0·53 (location reagent *acidified iodoplatinate spray*, positive reaction); system T2—Rf 0·66 (location reagent *iodoplatinate spray*, positive reaction); system T3—Rf 0·70 (location as for T2).
GAS: system G2/225—retention time 1·8 relative to diphenhydramine; system G4—retention time 2·95 relative to diphenhydramine.

Colour Tests. MICRO: sulphuric acid–formaldehyde test—purple (*sensitivity:* 0·1 μg); ammonium molybdate test—purple → green (*sensitivity:* 0·1 μg); ammonium vanadate test—purple → orange (*sensitivity:* 0·1 μg); Vitali's test— –/pale yellow/pale yellow (*sensitivity:* 1·0 μg).

Crystal Tests. MICRO: *gold bromide solution*—oily plates or rods, best viewed under polarised light (*sensitivity:* 1 in 1000); *gold chloride solution*—dense rosettes, forming overnight (*sensitivity:* 1 in 1000).

Ultraviolet Absorption Spectrum. Chloropyrilene in 0·1N sodium hydroxide, maxima at 243 mμ (E1%, 1 cm 676) and 308 mμ (E1%, 1 cm 148); in 0·1N sulphuric acid, maxima at 237·5 mμ (E1%, 1 cm 655) and 312 mμ (E1%, 1 cm 297).

Infra-red Absorption Spectrum. Chloropyrilene (base). Potassium bromide disk. The principal peaks are: A 1488 or 1595, B 1437, C 767 (p. 779).

Dose. Up to 100 mg daily.

Toxicity. The estimated lethal dose in man is 25 to 250 mg/kg.

CHLOROQUINE *Antimalarial*

Synonyms: RP 3377; SN 7618.

7 - Chloro - 4 - (4 - diethylamino - 1 - methylbutyl-amino)quinoline
$C_{18}H_{26}ClN_3 = 319{\cdot}9$

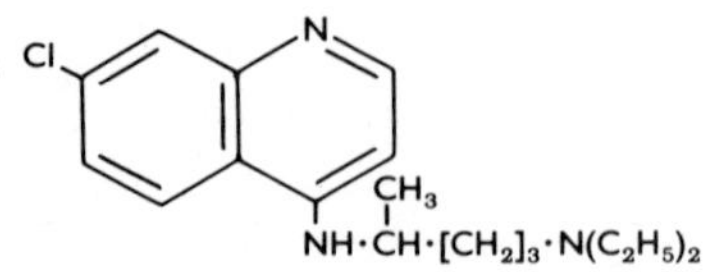

Chloroquine occurs as crystals. M.p. 87° to 88°. B.p. 212° to 214° at 0·2 mm Hg.

CHLOROQUINE PHOSPHATE
Synonym: Chloroquin Diphosphate.
Proprietary Names: Aralen; Avloclor; Bemaphate; Resochin.

A white crystalline powder. Chloroquine phosphate occurs in two forms, one of which melts at 193° to 195°, the other at 215° to 218°.
Solubility. Soluble 1 in 4 of water; very slightly soluble in ethanol; almost insoluble in ether and chloroform.

CHLOROQUINE SULPHATE
Proprietary Names: Bemasulph; Nivaquine.

A white crystalline powder.
Solubility. Soluble 1 in 3 of water; almost insoluble in ethanol; sparingly soluble in ether and chloroform.

Extraction. Chloroquine is extracted by organic solvents from aqueous alkaline solutions. Alternatively, the biological material may be homogenised, brought to pH 10 with ammonia, and then extracted with n-hexane. The extract is re-extracted into 0·1N sulphuric acid and then extracted back into hexane (Bonnichsen and Maehly, 1965).

Chromatography. PAPER: system P1—Rf 0·19 (location under ultraviolet light, blue fluorescence; location reagents: *iodoplatinate spray*, strong reaction; *bromocresol green spray*, strong reaction); system RP1a—Rf 0·70 (location under ultraviolet light, blue fluorescence; location reagent *iodoplatinate spray*, positive reaction); system RP1b—Rf 0·14 (location as for RP1a).
THIN-LAYER: system T1—Rf 0·31 (location reagent *acidified iodoplatinate spray*, positive reaction).
GAS: system G1/250—retention time 1·44 relative to codeine.

Crystal Tests. MICRO: *picric acid*—rosettes of plates (*sensitivity:* 1 in 1000); *styphnic acid*—rosettes of plates (*sensitivity:* 1 in 1000).

Ultraviolet Absorption Spectrum. Chloroquine in 0·1N sulphuric acid, maxima at 221·5 mμ (E1%, 1 cm 900), 236 mμ (E1%, 1 cm 515), 257·5 mμ (E1%, 1 cm 457), 329·5 mμ (E1%, 1 cm 461), and 343 mμ (E1%, 1 cm 496); chloroquine phosphate in 0·01N hydrochloric acid, maxima at 257 mμ (E1%, 1 cm 468), 329 mμ (E1%, 1 cm 516), and 343 mμ (E1%, 1 cm 596).

Infra-red Absorption Spectrum. Chloroquine (base). Potassium bromide disk. The principal peaks are: A 1573, B 1538, C 1372 or 1448 (p. 779).

Quantitative Estimation. Wilson and Edeson (1954) and Haskins (1958) have described methods of detection of chloroquine in urine. A quantitative method of determination of chloroquine in blood has been described by Waarst (1964), involving haemolysis with a 10% solution of saponin followed by extraction with alkaline chloroform and re-extraction into 0·1N hydrochloric acid and subsequent spectrophotometric measurement at 343 mμ.

Metabolism. Chloroquine is metabolised primarily by side-chain degradation to yield eventually a carboxylic acid. Conjugation with glucuronic acid seems to occur but the nature of the conjugates is not known. In 24 hours 4 patients, maintained on 155 mg daily of chloroquine, excreted in the urine between 50 and 70% as unchanged drug, between 25 and 50% as the mono-*N*-de-ethylated metabolite, and 3% as the di-*N*-de-ethylated metabolite (McChesney *et al.*, 1966).

Animal studies have demonstrated that chloroquine is preferentially deposited in melanin-containing cells, especially those of the eye. This leads to the occasional development of irreversible retinal damage. Visual disturbances do not ordinarily occur until a patient has taken the drug for a year or more.

Chloroquine is rapidly absorbed from the gastro-intestinal tract, maximum plasma levels are reached 1 to 2 hours after ingestion and they decline slowly. Ingestion of 500 mg of chloroquine phosphate has been found to lead to a blood-level after haemolysis of 0·07 mg% four hours later. About 55% of the drug is bound to plasma proteins and the rest is concentrated in the red blood-cells. High concentrations of chloroquine are attained in the kidneys, liver, lungs, and spleen; the drug is excreted very slowly so that it may be detected in the tissues for more than a week. The urinary excretion of unchanged chloroquine is influenced by the urinary pH; usually between 15 and 50% of the dose is excreted but, when the urine becomes unusually acid, 20 to 90% may be excreted.

Dose. Up to 1 g daily has been given.

Toxicity. The accepted minimum lethal dose in man is usually given as 20 mg/kg. Doses as low as 1 g have caused deaths in children and fatalities have occurred in adults after the ingestion of 3 to 44 g. A 2-year-old boy recovered after the ingestion of 2·5 g of chloroquine phosphate (Markowitz and McGinley, 1964).

CASE EXAMPLES. A 28-year-old man drank brandy and took 12 to 15 tablets, each containing 0·25 g of chloroquine phosphate. He was found dead the next morning. Post-mortem levels: blood, 0·3 mg%; liver, 15 mg%. No analysis was made for metabolites or for glucuronides (Bonnichsen and Maehly, 1965).

A 45-year-old woman was found dead after ingesting an unknown quantity of chloroquine sulphate. She had been dead for approximately 24 hours before she was found. Post-mortem levels: blood, 9·9 mg%; kidneys, 18·8 mg%; liver, 88·3 mg%; stomach contents, 10·1 mg (Hoole, 1966).

A report of thirteen cases of death due to chloroquine overdosage is given by Kiel (1964).

CHLOROTHIAZIDE *Diuretic*

Proprietary Names: Aquil; Chlorazide; Chlorfluvin; Chlotride; Diuril; Diurite; Flumen; Ipsodema; Minzil; Neo-Dema; Salisan; Saluren; Saluret; Saluric; Yadalan.

6-Chloro-7-sulphamoyl-2*H*-benzo-1,2,4-thiadiazine 1,1-dioxide

$C_7H_6ClN_3O_4S_2 = 295{\cdot}7$

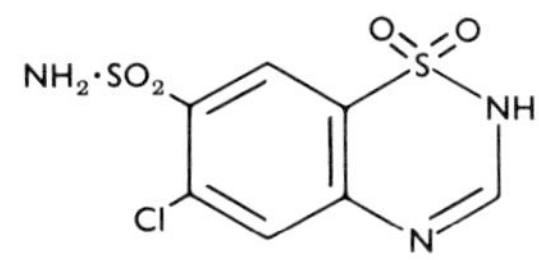

A white crystalline powder. Alkaline solutions undergo hydrolysis upon standing. M.p. 342° to 343°, with decomposition.

Solubility. Almost insoluble in water; soluble 1 in 650 of ethanol; insoluble in ether and chloroform; soluble 1 in 100 of acetone; soluble in solutions of alkali hydroxides.

CHLOROTHIAZIDE SODIUM

Synonym: Sodium Chlorothiazide.

Proprietary Names: Lyovac Diuril; Lyovac Saluric.

A crystalline solid.

Solubility. Soluble in water.

Extraction. Chlorothiazide may be isolated in the A1 fraction (see p. 27); it is distinguished from the salicylates by chromatography (see below), by the fact that it does not react with *ferric chloride solution*, and by the presence of additional ultraviolet maxima in the region 270 to 330 mμ.

Chromatography. PAPER: system P16—Rf 0·05 (location under ultraviolet light, absorption; location reagent *sodium naphthaquinone spray*, strong reaction); system RP1b—Rf 0·75 (location as for P16).

Ultraviolet Absorption Spectrum. Chlorothiazide in 0·1N sodium hydroxide, maxima at 228 mμ (E1%, 1 cm 700), 292 mμ (E1%, 1 cm 450), and a shoulder at 310 mμ (E1%, 1 cm 320).

Infra-red Absorption Spectrum. Chlorothiazide (base). Potassium bromide disk. The principal peaks are: A 1157, B 1305, C 1342 (p. 734).

Metabolism. Chlorothiazide is well absorbed from the gastro-intestinal tract and yields measurable plasma levels within a few minutes. The onset of diuresis after ingestion of 750 mg occurs in about 30 minutes and it may be maintained for 6 to 12 hours. Chlorothiazide is almost completely eliminated in the unchanged form by the kidneys within 12 hours (Kessler, 1962). The rate of glomerular filtration and the renal flow are not significantly altered.

Dose. Up to 2 g daily.

Toxicity. Doses as high as 8 g have been given without producing toxic effects.

LD50 (oral): in mice 8·5 and in rats more than 10 g/kg.

CASE EXAMPLE. A fatal case of agranulocytosis with thrombocytopenia occurred in a 70-year-old man following the administration of 25 g of chlorothiazide over a period of 13 days (Zuckerman and Chazan, 1958).

CHLOROTRIANISENE *Oestrogen*

Synonym: Tri-*p*-anisylchloroethylene.
Proprietary Name: TACE.

1 - Chloro - 1,2,2 - tri(*p* - methoxyphenyl) - ethylene

$C_{23}H_{21}ClO_3$ = 380·9

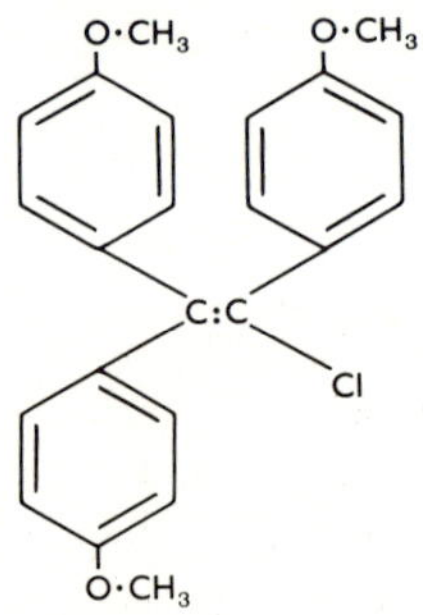

A white crystalline powder. M.p. about 118°.
Solubility. Soluble 1 in 4200 of water, 1 in 360 of ethanol, 1 in 28 of ether, and 1 in 1·5 of chloroform.

CAUTION. *Chlorotrianisene is a powerful oestrogen. Contact with the skin or inhalation of the dust should be avoided. Rubber gloves and a face mask should be worn when handling the powder.*

Extraction. Chlorotrianisene is extracted by organic solvents from aqueous acid solutions.

Colour Test. Dissolve 10 mg in 2 ml of sulphuric acid—very dark purple; addition of 5 ml of water—pink, becoming turbid.

Ultraviolet Absorption Spectrum. Chlorotrianisene in ethanol, maxima at 247 mμ (E1%, 1 cm 633) and 307 mμ (E1%, 1 cm 410).

Infra-red Absorption Spectrum. Potassium bromide disk. The principal peaks are: A 1246, B 1514, C 1165 or 1600 (p. 734).

Metabolism. Chlorotrianisene is stored in the body fat and is slowly converted, probably in the liver, to an oestrogenically active compound.

Dose. Up to 48 mg daily.

CHLOROXYLENOL *Antiseptic*

Synonyms: 4-Chloro-3,5-xylenol; *p*-Chloro-*m*-xylenol; PCMX; Parachlorometaxylenol.

4-Chloro-3,5-dimethylphenol

C_8H_9ClO = 156·6

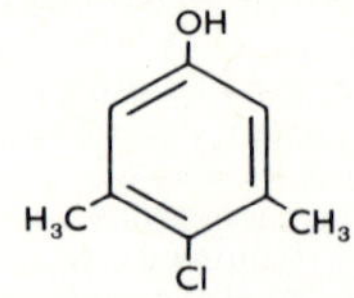

A white crystalline powder, which is volatile in steam. M.p. 114° to 116°. B.p. 246°.
Solubility. Soluble 1 in 3000 of water, 1 in 200 of boiling water, and 1 in 1 of ethanol; soluble in ether and in solutions of alkali hydroxides.

Extraction. Chloroxylenol is volatile and may be isolated by distillation (see p. 18).

Ultraviolet Absorption Spectrum. Chloroxylenol in ethanol, maximum at 282 mμ (E1%, 1 cm 108); in 0·1N hydrochloric acid, maximum at 279 mμ (E1%, 1 cm 83); in 0·1N sodium hydroxide, maximum at 296 mμ (E1%, 1 cm 161).

Metabolism. Chloroxylenol is a potent non-irritant bactericide of low toxicity which is usually employed in solution with terpineol as an antiseptic for the skin in surgery and obstetrics. Of a dose of 5 g injected into man, about 14% was found to be excreted in the urine as a glucuronide conjugate and 17% as a sulphate conjugate, only traces of the unchanged free phenol being found. Alkaline urine was found to contain as much as 8% in the free form.

CASE EXAMPLE. The death of a 28-year-old woman, 2½ months pregnant, was due to an air embolism alleged to have been caused by abortion with soap and antiseptic solutions. Post-mortem examination of steam distillates of heart, uterus, and vaginal fluids by gas chromatography revealed the presence of chloroxylenol and terpineol; control blood and the suspected antiseptic solution gave identical results (Wilson, 1965).

CHLORPHENIRAMINE *Antihistamine*

Synonym: Chlorprophenpyridamine.

(±)-3-*p*-Chlorophenyl-*NN*-dimethyl-3-pyrid-2′-ylpropylamine

$C_{16}H_{19}ClN_2$ = 274·8

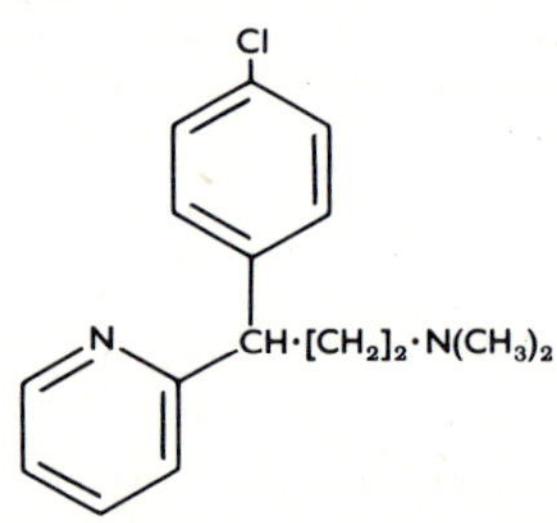

An oily liquid. B.p. 142° at 1 mm Hg.

NOTE. The chromatographic data and crystal tests of chlorpheniramine are similar to those of dexchlorpheniramine (p. 289) which is the (+)-isomer of chlorpheniramine—see also Microcrystal Tests, p. 140.

CHLORPHENIRAMINE MALEATE
Proprietary Names: Chlor-Trimeton; Piriton; Teldrin.

A white crystalline powder. M.p. 132° to 135°.
Solubility. Soluble 1 in 4 of water, 1 in 10 of ethanol, and 1 in 10 of chloroform; slightly soluble in ether.

Extraction. Chlorpheniramine is extracted by organic solvents from aqueous alkaline solutions.

Chromatography. PAPER: system P1—Rf 0·45 (location under ultraviolet light, blue fluorescence; location reagent *iodoplatinate spray*, strong reaction).
THIN-LAYER: system T1—Rf 0·38 (location reagent *acidified iodoplatinate spray*, positive reaction); system T2—Rf 0·52 (location as for T1); system T3—Rf 0·40 (location as for T1).
GAS: system G1/180—retention time 1·56 relative to diphenhydramine.

Crystal Tests. MICRO: *lead iodide solution*—dense rosettes (*sensitivity:* 1 in 1000); *platinic iodide solution*—long plates and needles (*sensitivity:* 1 in 1000).

Ultraviolet Absorption Spectrum. Chlorpheniramine in 0·1N sodium hydroxide, maximum at about 261·5 mμ (E1%, 1 cm 213), and a shoulder at 268 mμ (E1%, 1 cm 156); in 0·1N sulphuric acid, maximum at 265 mμ (E1%, 1 cm about 240) and a shoulder at about 271 mμ (E1%, 1 cm 194).

Infra-red Absorption Spectrum. Chlorpheniramine (base). Potassium bromide disk. The principal peaks are: A 1585, B 1465 or 1486, C 1430 (p. 779).

Quantitative Estimation. Chlorpheniramine may be estimated spectrophotometrically after reaction with sulphanilic acid and cyanogen bromide (Hudanick, 1964).

Dose. Usually up to 20 mg by mouth or by injection; max. in 24 hours 40 mg.

Toxicity. The estimated lethal dose in man is 5 to 10 mg/kg. It is one of the most potent of the antihistamines.

CHLORPHENOXAMINE *Parasympatholytic*
2-[1-(*p*-Chlorophenyl)-1-phenylethoxy]-*NN*-dimethylethylamine
$C_{18}H_{22}ClNO = 303{\cdot}8$

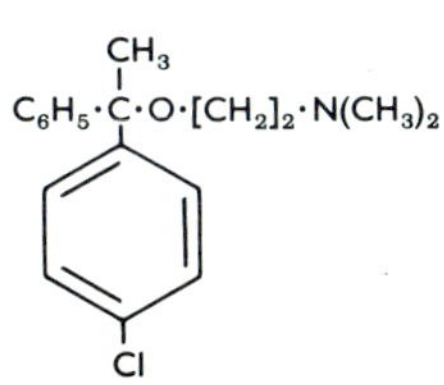

An oil. B.p. 150° to 155° at 0·05 mm Hg.

CHLORPHENOXAMINE HYDROCHLORIDE
Proprietary Name: Clorevan.

A white crystalline powder. M.p. 128°.
Solubility. Soluble in water.

Extraction. Chlorphenoxamine is extracted by organic solvents from aqueous alkaline solutions.

Chromatography. PAPER: system P1—Rf 0·75 (location reagents: *iodoplatinate spray*, strong reaction; *bromocresol green spray*, weak reaction).
THIN-LAYER: system T1—Rf 0·50 (location reagent *acidified iodoplatinate spray*, positive reaction).
GAS: system G2/225—retention time 1·9 relative to diphenhydramine; system G4—retention time 1·89 relative to diphenhydramine.

Colour Tests. MICRO: sulphuric acid–formaldehyde test—yellow → green (*sensitivity:* 0·5 μg); ammonium molybdate test—yellow (*sensitivity:* 0·5 μg); Vitali's test—light brown/light brown/light brown (*sensitivity:* 0·5 μg).

Crystal Test. MICRO: *zinc chloride solution*—bunches of plates or rods, forming overnight (*sensitivity:* 1 in 200).

Ultraviolet Absorption Spectrum. Chlorphenoxamine in 0·1N sulphuric acid, maxima at 253 mμ (E1%, 1 cm 14), 259 mμ (E1%, 1 cm 16), about 265 mμ (E1%, 1 cm 15), and about 275 mμ (E1%, 1 cm 7).

Infra-red Absorption Spectrum. Chlorphenoxamine hydrochloride. Potassium bromide disk. The principal peaks are: A 1088, B 1490, C 1010 or 1448 (p. 735).

Dose. Up to 400 mg daily.

Toxicity. The minimum lethal dose in man is probably between 10 and 100 mg/kg.
LD50 (oral): in mice 575 mg/kg.

CHLORPHENTERMINE *Anorectic*
Synonym: S 62.

p-Chloro-αα-dimethylphenethylamine
$C_{10}H_{14}ClN = 183{\cdot}7$

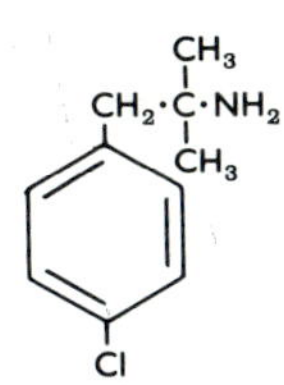

CHLORPHENTERMINE HYDROCHLORIDE
Proprietary Names: Lucofen; Pre-Sate.

A white crystalline powder. M.p. 232° to 234°.
Solubility. Soluble 1 in 5 of water; freely soluble in ethanol; almost insoluble in ether; sparingly soluble in chloroform.

Extraction. Chlorphentermine is extracted by

organic solvents from aqueous alkaline solutions; it may also be isolated by distillation. Chlorphentamine is very volatile; loss occurs if it is subjected to paper or thin-layer chromatography therefore it is advisable to convert it to the hydrochloride immediately after extraction.

Chromatography. PAPER: system P1—Rf 0·65 (location reagents: *iodoplatinate spray*, weak reaction; *bromocresol green spray*, strong reaction).

THIN-LAYER: system T1—Rf 0·54 (location reagent *acidified iodoplatinate spray*, positive reaction).

GAS: system G2/120—retention time 0·77 relative to ephedrine; system G2/225—retention time 0·24 relative to diphenhydramine; system G4—retention time 0·3 relative to diphenhydramine.

Crystal Tests. MICRO: *picric acid*—bunches of rods and needles (*sensitivity:* 1 in 1000); *picrolonic acid*—serrated blades or rods (*sensitivity:* 1 in 200).

Ultraviolet Absorption Spectrum. Chlorphentermine hydrochloride in ethanol, maxima at about 259 mμ, about 266 mμ, and about 275 mμ; minima at 240 mμ, 262 mμ, and 273 mμ; in 0·2N sulphuric acid or 0·1N hydrochloric acid, maxima at about 259 mμ, about 265 mμ, and about 274 mμ; minima at 239 mμ and 272 mμ.

Infra-red Absorption Spectrum. Chlorphentermine (base). Potassium bromide disk. The principal peaks are: A 1487, B 810, C 1084 (p. 780).

Quantitative Estimation. Chlorphentermine in blood and tissues may be determined by gas chromatography following steam distillation (Mason *et al.*, 1966).

Dose. Usually 75 mg daily.

Toxicity. LD50 (oral): in rats 180 mg/kg.

CHLORPROGUANIL *Antimalarial*

Synonym: M 5943.

N^1- (3,4 - Dichlorophenyl) - N^5 - isopropyldiguanide

$C_{11}H_{15}Cl_2N_5 = 288{\cdot}2$

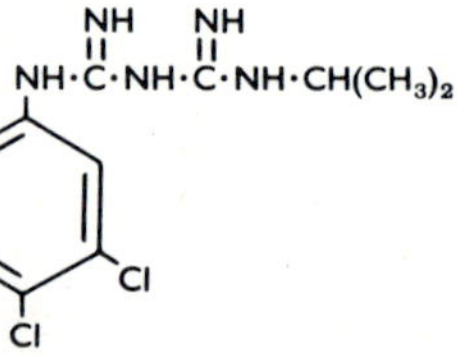

CHLORPROGUANIL HYDROCHLORIDE

Proprietary Name: Lapudrine. It is an ingredient of Lapaquin.

A white crystalline powder. M.p. 246° to 247°.

Solubility. Soluble 1 in 140 of water and 1 in 50 of ethanol; insoluble in ether and chloroform.

Extraction. Chlorproguanil is extracted by organic solvents from aqueous alkaline solutions.

Chromatography. PAPER: system P1—Rf 0·65 (location under ultraviolet light, strong absorption; location reagent *iodoplatinate spray*, weak reaction); system RP1a—Rf tailing (location under ultraviolet light, absorption); system RP1b—Rf 0·31 (location as for RP1a).

THIN-LAYER: system T1—Rf 0·58 (location reagent *potassium permanganate spray*, positive reaction).

Colour Tests. To 10 ml of a saturated solution of chlorproguanil hydrochloride add 1 drop of 10% copper sulphate solution and 2·5 ml of *dilute ammonia solution* and shake well; add 5 ml of toluene and shake again—toluene layer is purplish-red. Dissolve 5 mg in 5 ml of a warm 1% solution of cetrimide in water, add 1 ml of 20% sodium hydroxide solution and 1 ml of a saturated solution of bromine in water—deep red.

Crystal Tests. MICRO: *gold bromide–hydrochloric acid solution*—long plates, often serrated (*sensitivity:* 1 in 400); *platinic iodide solution*—rosettes of irregular rods or prisms (*sensitivity:* 1 in 400).

Ultraviolet Absorption Spectrum. Chlorproguanil in 0·1N sulphuric acid, maximum at 250 mμ (E 1%, 1 cm 347).

Infra-red Absorption Spectrum. Chlorproguanil (base). Potassium bromide disk. The principal peaks are: A 1525, B 1602 or 1614, C 1468 (p. 780).

Metabolism. Detailed metabolic studies have not been carried out but it has been shown that one of its metabolites is a triazine derivative and this is ten times more active than the corresponding metabolite of proguanil.

Dose. 20 mg weekly, as a single dose.

CHLORPROMAZINE *Tranquilliser*

2-Chloro-10-(3-dimethylaminopropyl)phenothiazine

$C_{17}H_{19}ClN_2S = 318{\cdot}9$

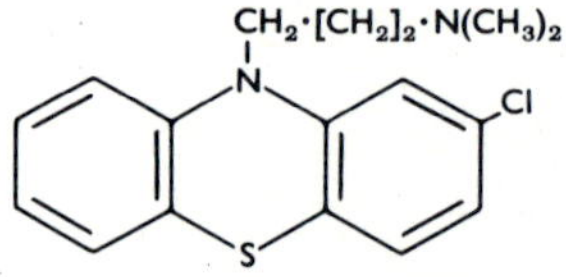

An oily liquid. B.p. 200° to 205° at 0·8 mm Hg.

CHLORPROMAZINE HYDROCHLORIDE

Synonym: Aminazin.

Proprietary Names: Hibernal; Largactil; Megaphen; Thorazine.

A white crystalline powder which darkens on exposure to light. M.p. 194° to 197°.

Solubility. Soluble 1 in 0·4 of water, 1 in 1·3 of ethanol, and 1 in 1 of chloroform; insoluble in ether.

Screening Test. *FPN reagent* with urine—red-purple (see p. 10).

Extraction. Chlorpromazine may be isolated in the D1 fraction; hydrolysis of biological material is required in order to improve the yield (see p. 27).

Chromatography. PAPER: system P1—Rf 0·68 (location under ultraviolet light, blue fluorescence; location reagents: *iodoplatinate spray*, strong reaction; *bromocresol green spray*, strong reaction; *FPN spray*, purple); system RP1a—Rf 0·20 (location reagent *iodoplatinate spray*, positive reaction); system RP1b—Rf 0·02 (location under ultraviolet light, turquoise fluorescence).

THIN-LAYER: system T1—Rf 0·49 (location reagent *acidified iodoplatinate spray*, positive reaction); system T3—Rf 0·94 (location reagents: *iodoplatinate spray*, positive reaction; *sulphuric acid–ethanol spray*, reddish-pink); system T6—Rf 0·62 (the spot may be converted on the plate to the sulphoxide, Rf 0·48; location of both spots under ultraviolet light).

GAS: system G1/250—retention time 1·22 relative to codeine; system G2/225—retention time 1·38 relative to codeine.

Colour Tests. MICRO: sulphuric acid–formaldehyde test—purple (*sensitivity:* 0·1 μg); ammonium molybdate test—blue-violet → purple (*sensitivity:* 0·25 μg); ammonium vanadate test —green → purple (*sensitivity:* 0·1 μg); Vitali's test—purple → yellow/yellow (*sensitivity:* 0·25 μg).

Crystal Tests. MICRO: *gold bromide–hydrochloric acid solution*—bundles of curved needles (*sensitivity:* 1 in 400); *gold chloride solution*—bunches of plates (*sensitivity:* 1 in 1000).

Ultraviolet Absorption Spectrum. Chlorpromazine in 0·1N sulphuric acid, maxima at 255 mμ (E1%, 1cm 1280) and 307 mμ (E1%, 1cm 175); chlorpromazine sulphoxide in 0·1N sulphuric acid, maxima at 239 mμ, 274 mμ, 300 mμ, and 341 mμ.

Infra-red Absorption Spectrum. Chlorpromazine (base). Potassium bromide disk. The principal peaks are: A 1455, B 747, C 1240 or 1402 or 1561 (p. 780).

Quantitative Estimation. Chlorpromazine in biological fluids and tissues may be estimated spectrophotometrically after conversion to its sulphoxide (Gothelf and Karczmar, 1963) and polarographically (Porter and Beresford, 1966). Johnson *et al.* (1963) describe an extraction procedure for separating the chlorpromazine metabolites occurring in urine; the separation may be followed by thin-layer or gas chromatography; a similar extraction procedure, which separates the two groups of metabolites, conjugated and unconjugated, and is followed by spectrophotometric determination, is described by Bolt *et al.* (1966). Driscoll *et al.* (1964) describe a gas chromatographic method for the quantitative determination of some urinary metabolites.

Metabolism. Over 20 metabolites of chlorpromazine have been found in the urine—see The Metabolism of Drugs, p. 163; 20% of the metabolites are non-conjugated sulphoxides and less than 1% is free chlorpromazine; the remaining 80% consists of hydroxy-derivatives and their conjugates, *N*-oxides, and unidentified metabolites (Forrest and Forrest, 1964). The 2 main metabolites are chlorpromazine sulphoxide and *N*-demethylchorpromazine sulphoxide (Cochin and Daly, 1963b).
Chlorpromazine is rapidly absorbed following oral or parenteral administration. Its action persists for 6 to 12 hours, it is rapidly distributed in all body tissues, and remains in the body for a long time; following the cessation of long-term therapy with chlorpromazine, the unchanged drug and its metabolites may continue to be excreted in the urine for 6 to 12 months.

Dose. The usual therapeutic dose is 75 to 500 mg daily, in divided doses, but larger doses are often given to psychotic patients.

Toxicity. The acute lethal dose of phenothiazine tranquillisers in man appears to be in the range 15 to 150 mg/kg, although severe toxic symptoms have occurred with doses of less than 1 mg/kg. Recoveries have occurred following prompt treatment involving gastric lavage in cases where 9 g and 4 g of chlorpromazine were ingested as single doses. A single dose of 1 g of chlorpromazine may be expected to lead to blood-levels of about 0·1 to 0·2 mg%.

LD50 (oral): in mice 580 mg/kg.

CASE EXAMPLES. An 11-month-old girl died about 20 hours after ingesting an unknown quantity of chloropromazine. Post-mortem levels: brain, about 20 mg%; liver, about 13·5 mg%; stomach contents, 21 mg%. There was no evidence to suggest the presence of sulphoxide metabolites (Jóhannesson and Lausen, 1961).
A 67-year-old woman was found dead about 5 months after beginning a course of treatment of 100 mg of chlorpromazine thrice daily. She may have ingested as many as one hundred 100-mg tablets in a single dose. Post-mortem levels: blood, 1·2 mg%; gastro-intestinal contents, 92 mg; liver, 45 mg%. No alkaloids, alcohol, salicylates, or barbiturates were found (Fatteh, 1964).
A 31-year-old man died suddenly. He had been undergoing intensive treatment with chlorpromazine and thioridazine for about 3½ years. By the time of his death, the doses had been reduced to 400 mg of chlorpromazine daily with 2 mg of biperiden hydrochloride. The post-mortem blood-level of chlorpromazine was 0·3 mg%. A strongly positive qualitative test for chlorpromazine was obtained from the urine (Hollister and Kosek, 1965).

CHLORPROPAMIDE *Antidiabetic*

Synonyms: Chlorglypropamide; P 607.
Proprietary Names: Catanil; Diabinese; Dialane; Mellinese; Upidiamin.

N-p-Chlorobenzenesulphonyl-*N'*-propylurea
$C_{10}H_{13}ClN_2O_3S = 276{\cdot}7$

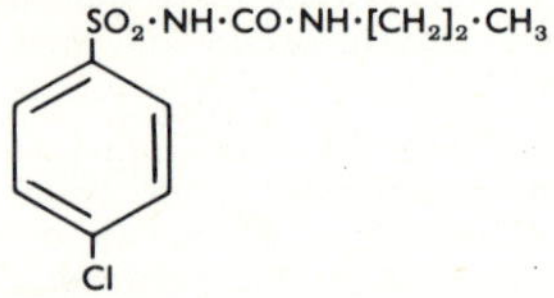

A white crystalline powder. M.p. 126° to 130°.

Solubility. Insoluble in water; soluble 1 in 12 of ethanol, 1 in 200 of ether, and 1 in 9 of chloroform.

Extraction. Chlorpropamide is extracted by organic solvents from aqueous acid or alkaline solutions.

Chromatography. PAPER: system P1—Rf 0·96 (location under ultraviolet light, absorption; location reagent *ninhydrin spray*, purple).

THIN-LAYER: system T1—Rf 0·72 (location reagent *potassium permanganate spray*, positive reaction).

GAS: system G2/225—retention time 0·77 relative to diphenhydramine; system G5—retention time 2·92 relative to barbitone.

Ultraviolet Absorption Spectrum. Chlorpropamide in 0·01N hydrochloric acid, maximum at 232 mμ (E1%, 1 cm 600).

Infra-red Absorption Spectrum. Potassium bromide disk. The principal peaks are: A 1661, B 1159, C 1553 (p. 735).

Quantitative Estimation. Kern (1963) describes a method of extraction of chlorpropamide from blood followed by nitration of the phenyl moiety, diazotisation, coupling with *N*-1-naphthylethylenediamine, and final spectrophotometric determination.

Metabolism. Chlorpropamide is an orally active hypoglycaemic agent which reduces the blood-sugar level without affecting glucose tolerance. It probably acts by stimulating insulin secretion. It is excreted slowly, primarily in the unchanged form, but a metabolite, *p*-chlorobenzene-sulphonamide, has been detected. Maximum blood-levels following a single dose are reached in 2 to 4 hours but the peak activity does not develop until approximately 10 hours after administration and persists for at least 24 hours.

Dose. Up to 500 mg daily.

Toxicity. Toxic effects appear quite soon if more than the maximum daily dose is given. The dose threshold varies according to the severity of the diabetes and the age of the patient. Fatal blood dyscrasias have been reported.

A 2-year-old child recovered after swallowing probably 18 chlorpropamide tablets equivalent to a dose of about 500 mg/kg (Youberg, 1960).

CASE EXAMPLES. A diabetic, aged 59, was treated with 250 mg of chlorpropamide daily for 7 days followed by 500 mg daily for 24 days. Although the drug was withdrawn and symptomatic treatment given, he died from agranulocytosis (Karlin, 1960).

For about 7 weeks a woman aged 63 had been taking 375 mg of chlorpropamide daily; she then developed fatal marrow aplasia (White, 1962).

Of 19 pregnancies in which women with mild diabetes were given 500 mg of chlorpropamide daily, there were 14 cases of foetal death (Campbell, 1963).

CHLORPROTHIXENE *Tranquilliser*

Synonyms: Chlorprothixan; N 714; Ro 4-0403.
Proprietary Names: Taractan; Tarasan; Truxal.

α-2-Chloro-9-(3-dimethylaminopropylidine)-thiaxanthen
$C_{18}H_{18}ClNS = 315{\cdot}9$

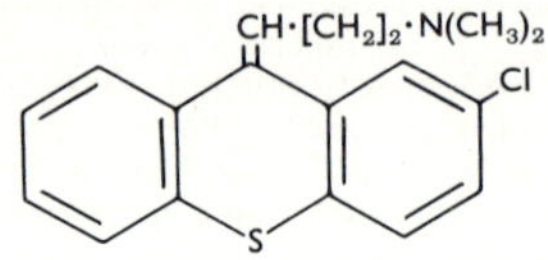

A pale yellow crystalline powder. M.p. 98°.

Solubility. Almost insoluble in water; soluble in ethanol, ether, and chloroform.

Extraction. Chlorprothixene is extracted by organic solvents from aqueous acid solutions.

Chromatography. PAPER: system P1—Rf 0·75 (location under ultraviolet light, dark blue fluorescence; location reagent *iodoplatinate spray*, strong reaction).

THIN-LAYER: system T1—Rf 0·55 (location reagent *acidified iodoplatinate spray*, positive reaction); system T3—Rf 0·80 (location reagents: *iodoplatinate spray*, positive reaction; *sulphuric acid–ethanol spray*, light orange); system T6—Rf 0·66 (the spot may be converted on the plate to the sulphoxide, Rf 0·45; location of both spots under ultraviolet light).

GAS: system G2/225—retention time 1·43 relative to codeine; system G4—retention time 0·81 relative to codeine.

Colour Tests. MICRO: sulphuric acid–formaldehyde test—red-orange (*sensitivity:* 0·1 μg); ammonium molybdate test—dull purple →red (*sensitivity:* 0·1 μg); ammonium vanadate test—red (*sensitivity:* 0·1 μg); Vitali's test—red/yellow/grey-green (*sensitivity:* 0·5 μg).

Crystal Tests. MICRO: *platinic chloride solution*—yellow smudge rosettes (*sensitivity:* 1 in 400); *potassium chromate solution*—branching needles (*sensitivity:* 1 in 400).

Infra-red Absorption Spectrum. Potassium bromide disk. The principal peaks are: A 776, B 1104, C 832 or 1446 or 1468 (p. 735).

Quantitative Estimation. Mellinger *et al.* (1964) describe a spectrofluorimetric method of determining chlorprothixene in urine which has been diluted with phosphoric acid. An ultraviolet spectrophotometric method of determining chlorprothixene and its principal sulphoxide metabolite in biological materials is presented by Wallace (1967).

Metabolism. Chlorprothixene is structurally similar to the phenothiazines and has similar properties. After a single oral dose of 50 mg, blood-levels of 0·004 mg% are found 8 hours after administration. After four oral doses of 100 mg given every 3 hours, levels of 0·006 to 0·03 mg% may be found. Chlorprothixene has a half-life in the blood of 17 to 24 hours. Approximately 6% of a dose is excreted in the urine within 24 hours as unchanged chlorprothixene and its sulphoxide derivative.

Dose. Up to 600 mg daily has been given.

Toxicity. Recoveries have occurred after the ingestion of 2 g and 5 g.

CHLORTETRACYCLINE *Antibiotic*

7-Chloro-4-dimethylamino-1,4,4a,5,5a,6,11,-12a-octahydro-3,6,10,12,12a-pentahydroxy-6-methyl-1,11-dioxonaphthacene-2-carboxyamide

$C_{22}H_{23}ClN_2O_8 = 478{\cdot}9$

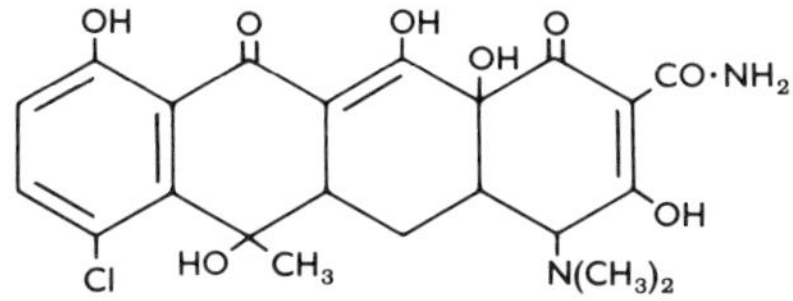

Golden-yellow crystals. M.p. 168° to 169°.
Solubility. Soluble 1 in 200 of water; slightly soluble in ethanol.

CHLORTETRACYCLINE CALCIUM
A white powder.
Solubility. Soluble in water.

CHLORTETRACYCLINE HYDROCHLORIDE
Proprietary Name: Aureomycin.

Yellow crystals. M.p. 210°, with decomposition.
Solubility. Soluble 1 in 110 of water and 1 in 250 of ethanol; practically insoluble in ether and chloroform; soluble in solutions of alkali hydroxides and carbonates.

Extraction. Chlortetracycline is extracted by organic solvents from aqueous alkaline solutions.

Chromatography. PAPER: system P1—Rf 0·37 (location under ultraviolet light, orange fluorescence; location reagents: *iodine vapour*, weak reaction; *potassium permanganate spray*, weak reaction).
A paper chromatographic method of separation of tetracycline derivatives in blood and urine is described by Addison and Clark (1963).
THIN-LAYER: system T1—Rf 0·05, streaking (location under ultraviolet light, orange fluorescence; location reagent *potassium permanganate spray*, positive reaction).
Ascione *et al.* (1967) describe a thin-layer method for the separation of tetracyclines and their derivatives.

Colour Tests. MICRO: sulphuric acid–formaldehyde test—yellow → dull green; ammonium molybdate test—purple-brown → yellow; ammonium vanadate test—purple-brown → yellow; sulphuric acid test—blue-black → brown → yellow; Vitali's test—faint yellow/yellow/red.

Ultraviolet Absorption Spectrum. Chlortetracycline in 0·1N hydrochloric acid, maxima at 228 mμ (E1%, 1 cm 344), 265 mμ (E1%, 1 cm 366), and 319 mμ (E1%, 1 cm 161); in 0·1N sodium hydroxide, maxima at 223 mμ (E1%, 1 cm 1184), 253 mμ (E1%, 1 cm 610), and 346 mμ (E1%, 1 cm 287).

Infra-red Absorption Spectrum. Chlortetracycline (base). Potassium bromide disk. The principal peaks are: A 1617, B 1573, C 1663 (p. 780).

Quantitative Estimation. Chlortetracycline may be estimated spectrophotometrically in biological materials as its thorium chelate (Sakaguchi and Taguchi, 1955) and spectrofluorimetrically in blood and urine (Saltzman, 1950).

Metabolism. The tetracyclines are incompletely absorbed from the gastro-intestinal tract. Absorption is diminished by calcium, magnesium, aluminium, and other alkaline metals. Following the administration of single oral doses of 500 mg of chlortetracycline, maximum serum levels of 0·15 mg% were obtained after 3 hours (Kunin and Finland, 1961).
The tetracyclines are bound in varying degrees to plasma protein, chlortetracycline showing the greatest extent of binding, and are slowly excreted in the bile and urine; 20 to 25% of an oral dose and 50% of an intravenous dose is excreted in the urine.
Studies in dogs and rats have detected the presence of unchanged chlortetracycline and 4-epichlortetracycline in the urine (Eisner and Wulf, 1963).
Chlortetracycline is inactivated to a certain extent in the body, possibly by conjugation or dealkylation.

Dose. Up to 3 g daily.

Toxicity. Chlortetracycline has caused fatal liver damage after large oral or intravenous doses. It is believed that blood-levels exceeding 1·6 mg% may contribute to the development of liver damage.
LD50 (intravenous): in rats 118 mg/kg.

CHLORTHALIDONE *Diuretic*

Synonyms: Chlortalidone; G 33182.
Proprietary Names: Hygroton; Igroton.

3-(4-Chloro-3-sulphamoylphenyl)-3-hydroxy-1-oxoisoindoline

$C_{14}H_{11}ClN_2O_4S = 338{\cdot}8$

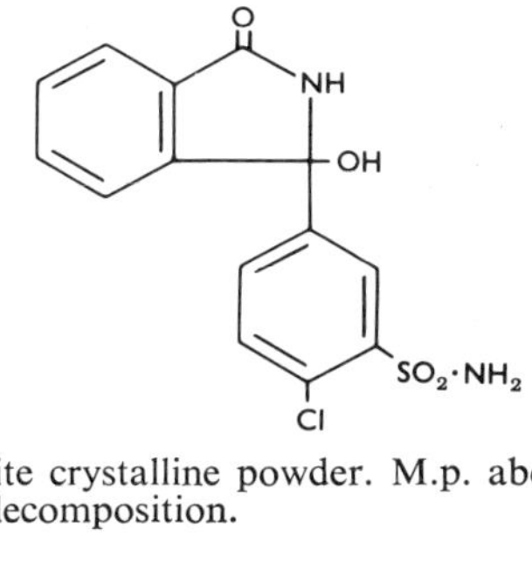

A white crystalline powder. M.p. about 220°, with decomposition.

Solubility. Very slightly soluble in water; soluble 1 in 150 of ethanol and 1 in 650 of chloroform; slightly soluble in ether.

Extraction. Chlorthalidone is extracted by organic solvents from aqueous acid or alkaline solutions.

Chromatography. PAPER: system P1—Rf 0·85 (location under ultraviolet light, absorption).

Colour Test. Dissolve 50 mg in 3 ml of sulphuric acid—yellow.
MICRO: sulphuric acid–formaldehyde test—yellow (*sensitivity:* 1·0 μg); ammonium molybdate test—yellow (*sensitivity:* 1·0 μg); Vitali's test—yellow (fading)/–/– (*sensitivity:* 1·0 μg).

Ultraviolet Absorption Spectrum. Chlorthalidone in ethanol, maxima at 275 mμ (E1%, 1 cm about 600) and 284 mμ (E1%, 1 cm about 450).

Infra-red Absorption Spectrum. Potassium bromide disk. The principal peaks are: A 1685, B 1036, C 1163 or 1345 (p. 780).

Metabolism. Chlorthalidone is a long-acting diuretic with actions similar to those of chlorothiazide. It is absorbed from the gastro-intestinal tract more slowly than chlorothiazide. It is excreted slowly in the urine, largely as unchanged drug. In therapeutic doses, it produces diuresis in about 2 hours, the maximum effect being reached within 6 hours and continuing for another 12 hours. The overall duration of effect is 48 to 72 hours.

Dose. Usually up to 200 mg on alternate days.

CHLORZOXAZONE *Muscle Relaxant*

Synonym: Chlorobenzoxazolinone.
Proprietary Name: Paraflex.

5-Chloro-2,3-dihydro-2-oxobenzoxazole
$C_7H_4ClNO_2 = 169{\cdot}6$

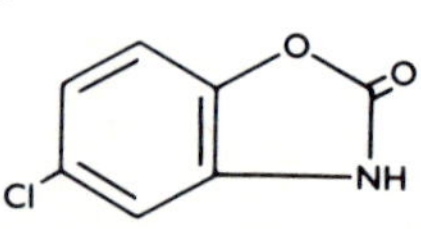

A white crystalline powder. M.p. 189° to 193°.
Solubility. Slightly soluble in water; soluble in ethanol; slightly soluble in dilute ammonia and alkalis.

Extraction. Chlorzoxazone is extracted with 1·5% isoamyl alcohol in light petroleum from alkaline solution (Poole and Gardocki, 1963).

Chromatography. PAPER: system P1—Rf 0·93 (location under ultraviolet light, absorption).
GAS: system G2/225—retention time 0·69 relative to diphenhydramine.

Colour Test. MICRO: Vitali's test— –/–/yellow (*sensitivity:* 1·0 μg).

Ultraviolet Absorption Spectrum. Chlorzoxazone in 0·1N sodium hydroxide, maxima at 243 mμ (E1%, 1 cm 600) and 287·5 mμ (E1%, 1 cm 420); in 0·1N sulphuric acid, a shoulder at 227 mμ (E1%, 1 cm 400) and a maximum at 279 mμ (E1%, 1 cm 300).

Infra-red Absorption Spectrum. Potassium bromide disk. The principal peaks are: A 1762, B 801, C 962 or 1480 (p. 735).

Quantitative Estimation. Chlorzoxazone may be estimated spectrophotometrically in alkaline solution following extraction from biological fluids and tissues with 1·5% isoamyl alcohol in light petroleum (Poole and Gardocki, 1963).

Metabolism. Studies have shown that chlorzoxazone is well absorbed in man and is rapidly metabolised to 6-hydroxychlorzoxazone which is excreted in the urine primarily as the glucuronide (Conney and Burns, 1960). Peak plasma levels of about 0·7 mg% were obtained in 2 subjects after 120 to 180 minutes following oral administration of 500 mg of chlorzoxazone. The biological half-life was about 170 minutes (Poole and Gardocki, 1963).

Dose. Up to 3 g daily.

Toxicity. The estimated minimum lethal dose in man is 100 to 500 mg/kg.

CHOLECALCIFEROL *Vitamin*

Synonyms: Activated 7-dehydrocholesterol; Colecalciferol; Vitamin D_3.

9,10-Secocholesta-5,7,10(19)-trien-3-ol
$C_{27}H_{44}O = 384{\cdot}7$

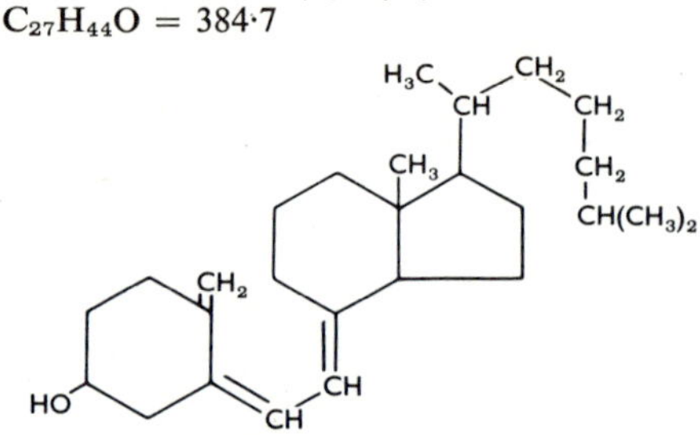

White crystals. M.p. 84° to 88°. Cholecalciferol is affected by air and light and should be stored under nitrogen in hermetically sealed containers. Specific rotation of a 0·5% solution in ethanol, +105° to +112°.
Solubility. Insoluble in water; soluble in ethanol, ether, chloroform, and fixed oils.

Chromatography. THIN-LAYER: system T21a—Rf 0·32 (location reagent *0·2M sulphuric acid spray*, positive reaction); system T21b—Rf 0·44 (location as for T21a); system T21c—Rf 0·15 (location as for T21a).

Colour Tests. To a 10% solution in chloroform, add 0·3 ml of acetic anhydride and 0·1 ml of sulphuric acid—bright red → violet → blue-green.
Lyness and Quackenbush (1955) describe a colour reaction for calciferol and cholecalciferol using an iodine–ethylene dichloride reagent which produces a strong yellow colour with

both compounds but which does not react with cholesterol or sitosterols.

Quantitative Estimation. Barua and Rao (1964) describe a method of determination of calciferol and cholecalciferol in the presence of vitamin A involving column chromatographic separation followed by spectrophotometric estimation.

Metabolism. As for Calciferol, p. 235. Cholecalciferol is the chief form of vitamin D in fish-liver oils.

Toxicity. As for Calciferol, p. 235.

CHOLESTEROL

Synonym: Cholesterin.
Proprietary Name: Dythol.

Cholest-5-en-3-ol

$C_{27}H_{46}O = 386{\cdot}7$

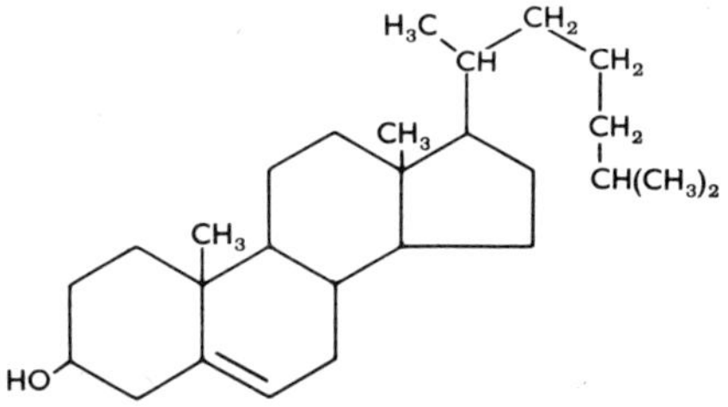

White pearly leaflets or granules which on prolonged exposure to light acquire a yellow to pale tan colour. M.p. 147° to 150°. Specific rotation of a 2% solution in dioxan, −34° to −38°.
Solubility. Insoluble in water; slowly soluble 1 in 100 of ethanol; soluble 1 in 50 of dehydrated ethanol; soluble in ether, acetone, dioxan, and light petroleum.

Extraction. Cholesterol is extracted by organic solvents from aqueous acid solutions.

Chromatography. THIN-LAYER: system T21a—Rf 0·30 (location reagent *0·2M sulphuric acid spray*, positive reaction); system T21b—Rf 0·41 (location as for T21a). Coleman and Parke (1963) have described a 2-dimensional thin-layer chromatographic system for the separation of cholesterol and enoxolone.

GAS: system G2/225—retention time 6·95 relative to codeine; system G4—retention time 3·0 relative to codeine.

Colour Tests. To a solution of 10 mg in 1 ml of chloroform add 1 ml of sulphuric acid; chloroform layer—blood-red, sulphuric acid layer—green fluorescence. Dissolve about 5 mg in 2 ml of chloroform, add 1 ml of acetic anhydride and 1 drop of sulphuric acid—pink → red → blue → brilliant green.

Quantitative Estimation. Total and free cholesterol in blood and other biological materials may be determined colorimetrically as the digitonide (Schoenheimer and Sperry, 1934). Methods of spectrophotometric determination of total and free cholesterol in blood have been described by Shin and Lee (1961), Momose *et al.* (1963), Huang *et al.* (1963), Glick *et al.* (1964).

Metabolism. Cholesterol is an unsaponifiable lipid which is found in all body tissues, particularly in the brain, the cerebrospinal cord, and the nerve tissues. It is relatively poorly absorbed in man. About 50% of the absorbed cholesterol is esterified, the major portion of the cholesterol in the plasma being in the form of fatty acid esters. The normal serum level is between 150 and 280 mg%.
Cholesterol is excreted to a greater extent in the faeces than in the urine and appears together with coprostanol, which arises from the action of the gastro-intestinal bacteria on cholesterol, and cholestanol which is the final product of the reduction of cholesterol in the tissues. The bile acids are quantitatively the most important end-products of cholesterol metabolism in higher animals although cholesterol also serves as a precursor of the steroid hormones.

CHOLINE

2-Hydroxyethyltrimethylammonium hydroxide

$C_5H_{15}NO_2 = 121{\cdot}2$

$$[HO{\cdot}[CH_2]_2{\cdot}N(CH_3)_3]^+\ OH^-$$

A colourless, hygroscopic, viscous, alkaline liquid.
Solubility. Very soluble in water and ethanol; insoluble in ether.

CHOLINE CHLORIDE
White, very hygroscopic crystals.
Solubility. Very soluble in water and ethanol; almost insoluble in ether and chloroform.

CHOLINE DIHYDROGEN CITRATE
Synonym: Choline Citrate.
Proprietary Names: Chothyn; Citrocholine; Lipocholine.
Colourless translucent crystals or a white granular to fine crystalline powder. M.p. 103° to 107·5°.
Solubility. Soluble 1 in 1 of water and 1 in 45 of ethanol; very slightly soluble in ether and chloroform.

Extraction. Choline is a quaternary ammonium compound (see p. 29).

Chromatography. PAPER: system P1—Rf 0·05 (location reagent *iodoplatinate spray*, strong reaction).

THIN-LAYER: system T1—Rf 0·02 (location reagents: *acidified iodoplatinate spray*, positive reaction; *potassium permanganate spray*, positive reaction).

Crystal Tests. MICRO: *gold bromide–hydrochloric acid solution*—small irregular crystals (*sensitivity:* 1 in 1000); *mercuric chloride solution*—small irregular crystals which may vanish (*sensitivity:* 1 in 3000).

Infra-red Absorption Spectrum. Choline chloride. Capillary film between potassium bromide windows. The principal peaks are: A 1636, B 1477, C 953 (p. 735).

Metabolism. Choline is an essential element in animal and human nutrition but it cannot strictly be classed as a vitamin. It acts as a methyl-group donor to tissue methionine and is capable of preventing or curing fatty infiltration of the liver. It is readily absorbed from the gastro-intestinal tract and as much as 20% of the administered dose may appear in the urine as trimethylamine. It is thought that trimethylamine is formed through the action of the gastro-intestinal bacteria on choline.

Dose. Usually up to 4 g daily. Doses of up to 32 g daily have been given.

Toxicity. LD50 (subcutaneous): in mice 700 and in rabbits 500 mg/kg.

CINCHOCAINE *Local Anaesthetic*

Synonyms: Cincain; Dibucaine.
Proprietary Name: Nupercaine.

2-Butoxy-*N*-(2-diethylaminoethyl)quinoline-4-carboxyamide

$C_{20}H_{29}N_3O_2 = 343{\cdot}5$

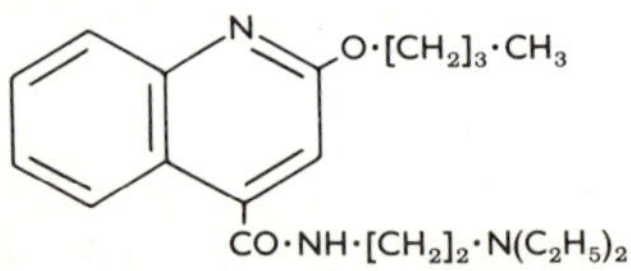

A white, somewhat hygroscopic powder. M.p. 63·5° to 65·5°.

Solubility. Very slightly soluble in water; soluble in ethanol, ether, and chloroform; dissolves in light petroleum and in hydrochloric acid on warming.

CINCHOCAINE HYDROCHLORIDE

Synonym: Sovcaine.
Proprietary Name: Nupercaine.

NOTE. This compound was originally marketed under the proprietary name Percaine, but accidents occurred owing to the confusion of this name with procaine.

Fine, white hygroscopic crystals. M.p. 96° to 100°.

Solubility. Soluble 1 in 0·5 of water; freely soluble in ethanol and chloroform; insoluble in ether.

Extraction. Cinchocaine is extracted by organic solvents from aqueous alkaline solutions.

Chromatography. PAPER: system P1—Rf 0·78 (location under ultraviolet light, blue fluorescence; location reagents: *iodoplatinate spray*, strong reaction; *bromocresol green spray*, weak reaction); system RP1a—Rf 0·30 (location reagent *iodoplatinate spray*, positive reaction); system RP1b—Rf 0·00 (location as for RP1a). THIN-LAYER: system T1—Rf 0·63 (location reagent *acidified iodoplatinate spray*, positive reaction).

GAS: system G1/250—retention time 1·72 relative to codeine; system G2/225—retention time 2·62 relative to codeine; system G6—retention time 2·12 relative to codeine.

Crystal Tests. MICRO: *gold bromide–hydrochloric acid solution*—irregular plates and needles (*sensitivity:* 1 in 3000); *lead iodide solution*—dense rosettes (*sensitivity:* 1 in 1000).

Ultraviolet Absorption Spectrum. Cinchocaine in 0·1N sulphuric acid, maxima at 247 mμ (E1%, 1 cm 856) and 318 mμ (E1%, 1 cm 222).

Infra-red Absorption Spectrum. Cinchocaine (base). Potassium bromide disk. The principal peaks are: A 1596, B 1543 or 1639, C 1337 or 1397 (p. 780).

Metabolism. Cinchocaine is not hydrolysed by tissue enzymes (Adriani, 1960).

Toxicity. Cinchocaine is more toxic than procaine by injection and more toxic than cocaine by local application but it is relatively safer in use because its local anaesthetic action is greater and it can therefore be used in lower concentrations than are normally employed with procaine and cocaine.

CINCHONIDINE *Antimalarial*

An alkaloid present in the bark of various species of *Cinchona* (Rubiaceae). Cinchonidine is the (−)-stereoisomer of cinchonine; quinine is its (−)-6′-methoxy-derivative.

$C_{19}H_{22}N_2O = 294{\cdot}4$

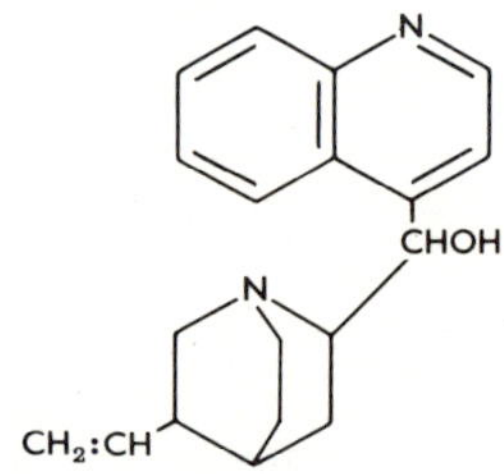

White prisms or powder. M.p. about 210°, with decomposition.

Solubility. Slightly soluble in water and ether; soluble in ethanol.

CINCHONIDINE SULPHATE

Colourless crystals.

Solubility. Soluble 1 in 100 of water and 1 in 60 of ethanol; almost insoluble in ether and chloroform.

Extraction. Cinchonidine is extracted by organic solvents from aqueous alkaline solutions.

Chromatography. PAPER: system P1—Rf 0·41 (location under ultraviolet light, blue fluorescence; location reagents: *iodoplatinate spray*, strong reaction; *bromocresol green spray*, weak reaction); system RP1a—Rf 0·70 (location under ultraviolet light, absorption; location reagent *iodoplatinate spray*, positive reaction); system RP1b—Rf 0·20 (location as for RP1a). THIN-LAYER: system T1—Rf 0·51 (location reagent *acidified iodoplatinate spray*, positive reaction).

GAS: system G1/250—retention time 1·55 relative to codeine; system G6—retention time 1·45 relative to codeine.

Crystal Tests. MICRO: *platinic chloride solution*—small rods (*sensitivity:* 1 in 3000); *sodium carbonate solution*—small rosettes (*sensitivity:* 1 in 1000).

Ultraviolet Absorption Spectrum. Cinchonidine in 0·1N sulphuric acid, maxima at 236 mμ (E1%, 1 cm 1874) and 316 mμ (E1%, 1 cm 320).

Infra-red Absorption Spectrum. Cinchonidine (base). Potassium bromide disk. The principal peaks are: A 754, B 899 or 1090, C 800 (p. 780).

Metabolism. In man, cinchonidine has been found to be oxidised first at the 2′-position of the quinoline nucleus and then at the 2-position of the quinuclidine nucleus; both 2′-hydroxycinchonidine and 2,2′-dihydroxycinchonidine have been detected in the urine.

Dose. Up to 600 mg has been given.

Toxicity. Large doses may cause convulsions. The fatal dose in man may be as low as 1 g.
LD50 (intraperitoneal): in rats 206 mg/kg.

CINCHONINE *Antimalarial*

An alkaloid present in the bark of various species of *Cinchona* (Rubiaceae). Cinchonine is the (+)-stereoisomer of cinchonidine; quinidine is its (+)-6′-methoxy-derivative.
$C_{19}H_{22}N_2O = 294{\cdot}4$

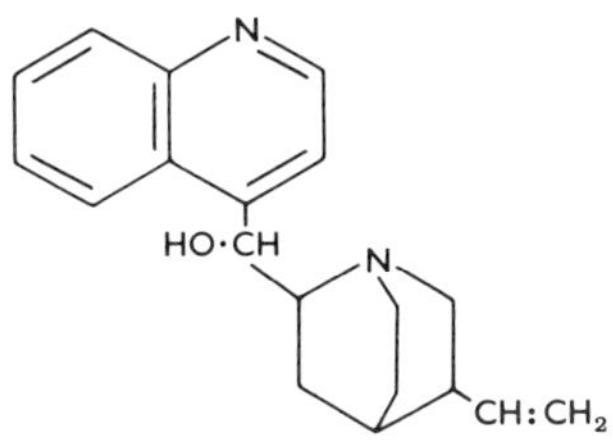

White shining prisms or needles. M.p. 264·3°, subliming at 220°.
Solubility. Practically insoluble in water; slightly soluble in ethanol, ether, and chloroform.

CINCHONINE HYDROCHLORIDE
White microcrystalline flakes or needles.
Solubility. Soluble 1 in 20 of water, 1 in 2 of ethanol, and 1 in 300 of ether.

Extraction. Cinchonine is extracted by organic solvents from aqueous alkaline solutions.

Chromatography. PAPER: system P1—Rf 0·47 (location under ultraviolet light, bright blue fluorescence; location reagents: *iodoplatinate spray*, strong reaction; *bromocresol green spray*, weak reaction); system RP1a—Rf 0·72 (location under ultraviolet light, absorption; location reagent *iodoplatinate spray*, positive reaction); system RP1b—Rf 0·10 (location as for RP1a).

THIN-LAYER: system T1—Rf 0·48 (location reagent *acidified iodoplatinate spray*, positive reaction).

GAS: system G1/250—retention time 1·55 relative to codeine; system G6—retention time 1·45 relative to codeine.

Crystal Tests. MICRO: *platinic iodide solution*—curved needles, forming overnight (*sensitivity:* 1 in 1500); *sodium carbonate solution*—rosettes (*sensitivity:* 1 in 3000).

Ultraviolet Absorption Spectrum. Cinchonine in ethanol, maxima at 227 mμ (E1%, 1 cm 1214), 282 mμ (E1%, 1 cm 176), 301 mμ (E1%, 1 cm 126), 314 mμ (E1%, 1 cm 111), and 332 mμ (E1%, 1 cm 68); in 0·1N sulphuric acid, maxima at 235 mμ (E1%, 1 cm 1134) and 315 mμ (E1%, 1 cm 217).

Infra-red Absorption Spectrum. Cinchonine (base). Potassium bromide disk. The principal peaks are: A 760, B 1110, C 1505 or 1590 (p. 780).

Metabolism. In man, cinchonine is rapidly and almost completely absorbed from the gastro-intestinal tract, maximum plasma levels being reached in 1 to 2 hours. It is concentrated in most of the tissues, especially the kidneys, liver, and lungs. Between 3·6 and 5% of a dose is excreted unchanged in the urine and 2 to 3% of a dose is recovered in the faeces.
Cinchonine is rapidly oxidised, first at the 2′-position of the quinoline nucleus and then at the 2-position of the quinuclidine nucleus; following single oral doses, 55% of the dose has been recovered as 2′-hydroxycinchonine (cinchonine carbostyril) and 22% as 2,2′-dihydroxycinchonine.

Dose. Up to 600 mg has been given.

Toxicity. The lethal dose in man may be as low as 1 g.
LD50 (intraperitoneal): in rats 152 mg/kg.

CINNARIZINE *Antihistamine*

Synonyms: MD516; R516; R1575; 1-Benzhydryl-4-cinnamylpiperazine.
Proprietary Names: Dimitron; Glanil; Mitronal.

1-*trans*-Cinnamyl-4-diphenylmethylpiperazine
$C_{26}H_{28}N_2 = 368{\cdot}5$

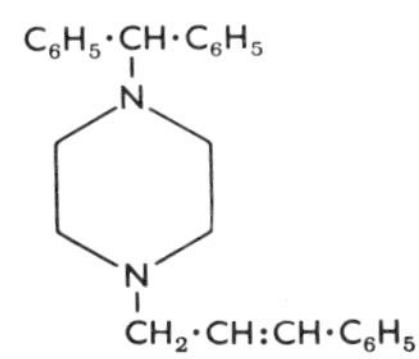

Solubility. Practically insoluble in water; soluble in dilute hydrochloric acid.

Extraction. Cinnarizine is extracted by organic solvents from aqueous alkaline solutions.

Chromatography. PAPER: system P1—Rf 0·90 (location reagents: *iodoplatinate spray*, weak reaction; *bromocresol green spray*, strong reaction).

THIN-LAYER: system T1—Rf 0·72 (location reagent *acidified iodoplatinate spray*, positive reaction).

GAS: system G2/225—retention time 6·90 relative to codeine.

Crystal Tests. MICRO: *potassium cyanide solution*—masses of plates and needles, forming overnight (*sensitivity:* 1 in 100); *sodium carbonate solution*—masses of plates and needles, forming overnight (*sensitivity:* 1 in 100).

Ultraviolet Absorption Spectrum. Cinnarizine in 0·1N sulphuric acid, maxima at 227·5 mμ (E1%, 1 cm 633), 254 mμ (E1%, 1 cm 800), and 291·5 mμ (E1%, 1 cm 31), and an inflexion at 281 mμ.

Infra-red Absorption Spectrum. Potassium bromide disk. The principal peaks are: A 702, B 691 or 1138, C 964 or 1452 (p. 736).

Dose. 45 mg daily; doses of up to 90 mg daily have been given.

Toxicity. The estimated lethal dose in man is 100 to 500 mg/kg.

LD50 (oral): in mice and rats, greater than 1 g/kg.

CITRONELLA OIL *Essential Oil*

Contains citronellal ($C_{10}H_{18}O$ = 154·3) and geraniol ($C_{10}H_{18}O$ = 154·3).

A pale to deep yellow oil, obtained by distillation from *Cymbopogon nardus* or *C. winterianus* (Gramineae).

Solubility. Soluble 1 in 4 of ethanol (80%), forming a clear or slightly opalescent solution.

Extraction. Citronella oil is volatile and may be isolated by distillation (see p. 18).

Metabolism. Citronellal has been shown to undergo a cyclisation reaction in rabbits under the influence of hydrochloric acid in the stomach, the product, *p*-menthane-3,8-diol, being excreted as a glucuronide conjugate. Geraniol has been found to undergo a double ω-oxidation and also reduction of the 2,3-double bond, 2 acids being produced.

CASE EXAMPLE. A case is described of a 21-month-old child who accidentally ingested 3 drachms (10·5 ml), at the most, of Antimate (active constituent citronella oil) and died 5½ hours later. The odour of citronella was apparent in the vomit and in all the body cavities post mortem; no measurable quantities, however, were extracted from the tissues (Mant, 1961).

CLAMOXYQUIN *Anti-amoebic*

5 - Chloro - 7 - [(3 - diethylaminopropyl)aminomethyl]-8-hydroxyquinoline

$C_{17}H_{24}ClN_3O$ = 321·9

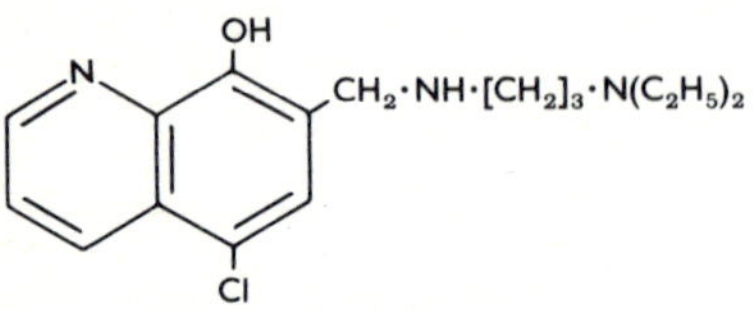

CLAMOXYQUIN HYDROCHLORIDE

Synonyms: CI 433; PAA 3854.

Extraction. Clamoxyquin is extracted by organic solvents from aqueous alkaline solutions.

Chromatography. PAPER: system P1—Rf 0·12 (location under ultraviolet light, pale yellow fluorescence; location reagents: *iodoplatinate spray*, strong reaction; *bromocresol green spray*, strong reaction).

THIN-LAYER: system T1—Rf 0·02 (location reagent *acidified iodoplatinate spray*, positive reaction).

Crystal Tests. MICRO: *platinic bromide solution*—feathery needles (*sensitivity:* 1 in 1000); *platinic chloride solution*—rosettes or fans of branching needles (*sensitivity:* 1 in 1000).

Infra-red Absorption Spectrum. Clamoxyquin (base). Potassium bromide disk. The principal peaks are: A 1387, B 1347, C 1444 (p. 781).

CLEMIZOLE *Antihistamine*

1 - *p* - Chlorbenzyl - 2 - pyrrolidin - 1′- ylmethylbenziminazole

$C_{19}H_{20}ClN_3$ = 325·8

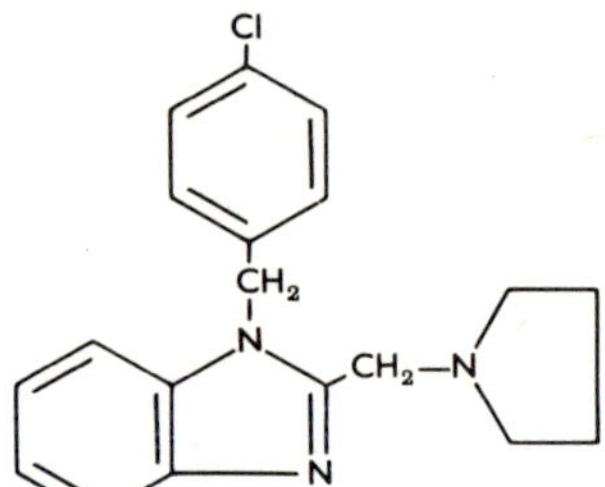

Crystals from dilute ethanol. M.p. 167°.

CLEMIZOLE HYDROCHLORIDE

Proprietary Names: Allercur; Reactrol.

White crystals or powder. M.p. 245° to 247°.

Solubility. Sparingly soluble in water; soluble in ethanol and chloroform; insoluble in ether.

Extraction. Clemizole is extracted by organic solvents from aqueous alkaline solutions.

Chromatography. PAPER: system P1—Rf 0·77 (location under ultraviolet light, dark blue fluorescence; location reagents: *iodoplatinate spray*, strong reaction; *bromocresol green spray*, strong reaction); system RP1a—Rf 0·04 (location under ultraviolet light, absorption; location reagent *iodoplatinate spray*, positive reaction); system RP1b—Rf 0·00.

THIN-LAYER: system T1—Rf 0·72 (location reagent *acidified iodoplatinate spray*, positive reaction).

GAS: system G2/225—retention time 2·25 relative to codeine.

Colour Test. MICRO: Vitali's test— –/yellow rim/yellow rim (*sensitivity:* 1·0 μg).

Crystal Tests. MICRO: *potassium cyanide solution*

—plates (*sensitivity:* 1 in 200); *zinc chloride solution*—rosettes or fans of needles (*sensitivity:* 1 in 1000).

Ultraviolet Absorption Spectrum. Clemizole in 0·1N sodium hydroxide, maxima at 253 mμ (E1%, 1 cm 253), 267 mμ (E1%, 1 cm 187), 274 mμ (E1%, 1 cm 209), and 282 mμ; in 0·1N sulphuric acid, maximum at 274 mμ (E1%, 1 cm 330).

Infra-red Absorption Spectrum. Clemizole (base). Potassium bromide disk. The principal peaks are: A 748, B 765 or 1400 or 1460 (p. 781).

Dose. Up to 100 mg daily, by mouth or by injection.

Toxicity. The estimated lethal dose in man is 25 to 250 mg/kg.

CLIDINIUM BROMIDE *Parasympatholytic*

Synonym: Ro 2-3773.
Proprietary Names: Quarzan Bromide. It is an ingredient of Libraxin.

3-Benziloyloxy-1-methylquinuclidinium bromide

$C_{22}H_{26}BrNO_3 = 432{\cdot}4$

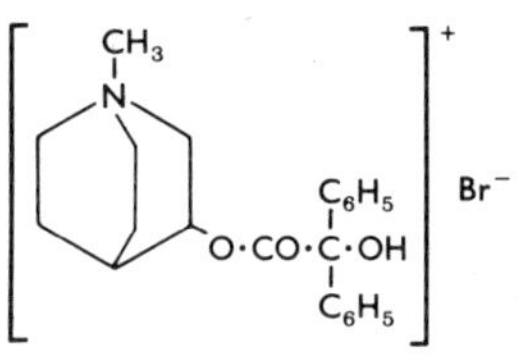

Extraction. Clidinium bromide is a quaternary ammonium compound (see p. 29).

Chromatography. PAPER: system P1—Rf 0·53 (location reagents: *iodoplatinate spray*, strong reaction; *bromocresol green spray*, weak reaction); system RP1a—Rf 0·86 (location reagent *iodoplatinate spray*, positive reaction); system RP1b—Rf 0·85 (location under ultraviolet light, absorption; location reagent *iodoplatinate spray*, positive reaction).

THIN-LAYER: system T1—Rf 0·02 (location reagent *acidified iodoplatinate spray*, positive reaction).

Colour Tests. MICRO: sulphuric acid–formaldehyde test—orange → blue (*sensitivity:* 0·5 μg); ammonium molybdate test—orange → green (*sensitivity:* 0·5 μg).

Crystal Tests. MICRO: *platinic iodide solution*—small oily needles, forming overnight (*sensitivity:* 1 in 200).

Ultraviolet Absorption Spectrum. Clidinium bromide in 0·1N sulphuric acid, maxima at 252 mμ (E1%, 1 cm 11), 258 mμ (E1%, 1 cm 12), about 263 mμ (E1%, 1 cm 10), and about 268 mμ (E1%, 1 cm 7).

Metabolism. Clidinium bromide has peripheral parasympatholytic properties similar to those of atropine. It cannot be detected in the blood following oral administration as it is taken up by tissues immediately after its absorption.

Dose. Up to 20 mg daily.

Toxicity. The lethal dose in man is probably in the range 10 to 100 mg/kg.

CLIOQUINOL *Anti-amoebic*

Synonyms: Chinoform; Chloroiodoquine; Iodochlorhydroxyquin; Iodochlorhydroxyquinoline.
Proprietary Names: Barquinol; Vioform; Viozol. It is an ingredient of Entero-Vioform.

5-Chloro-8-hydroxy-7-iodoquinoline

$C_9H_5ClINO = 305{\cdot}5$

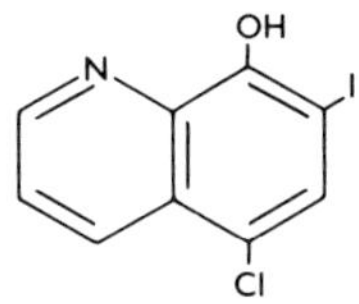

A yellowish-white powder, which darkens on exposure to light. M.p. about 180°, with decomposition.

Solubility. Practically insoluble in water and ethanol; soluble 1 in 45 of boiling ethanol and 1 in 130 of chloroform.

Chromatography. THIN-LAYER: Korzun *et al.* (1964) have described a thin-layer chromatographic system for the separation of clioquinol from its intermediates.

Ultraviolet Absorption Spectrum. Clioquinol in 3N hydrochloric acid, maximum at 267 mμ.

Quantitative Estimation. Clioquinol may be estimated colorimetrically (Vadodaria *et al.*, 1965) and by infra-red spectrophotometry (Urbanyi *et al.*, 1966).

Metabolism. Clioquinol is administered by mouth in the treatment of intestinal amoebiasis and bacillary dysentery. On repeated oral administration in man the peak blood-level appears to be reached not later than the seventh day. In rabbits, 78% of the ingested iodine was excreted, three-quarters of this amount in the urine and one-quarter in the faeces. The urine contained sulphuric acid and glucuronic acid conjugates.

Dose. Up to 1·5 g.

Toxicity. LD50 (oral): in cats 400 mg/kg.

CLOMIPHENE *Anterior Pituitary Activator*

Synonyms: Chloramiphene; Clomifene; MRL 41; NSC 35770.

2-[p-(β-Chloro-α-phenylstyryl)phenoxy]triethylamine
$C_{26}H_{28}ClNO = 406{\cdot}0$

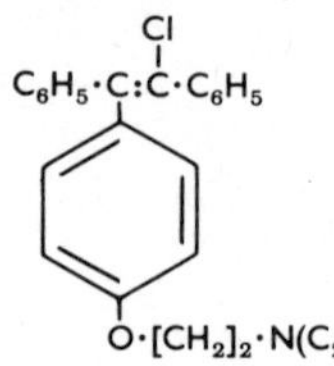

A white to pale yellow solid. M.p. 111° to 115°.
Solubility. Sparingly soluble in water and ethanol; slightly soluble in chloroform.

CLOMIPHENE CITRATE
Proprietary Name: Clomid.

Clomiphene citrate melts at 144° to 147°, with decomposition.

Extraction. Clomiphene is extracted by organic solvents from aqueous alkaline solutions.

Chromatography. PAPER: system P1—Rf 0·88 (location under ultraviolet light, absorption; location reagents: *iodoplatinate spray*, strong reaction; *Dragendorff spray*, strong reaction).
THIN-LAYER: system T1—Rf 0·59 (location reagent *acidified iodoplatinate spray*, positive reaction).

Colour Tests. MICRO: sulphuric acid–formaldehyde test—purple-brown (*sensitivity:* 0·1 μg); ammonium molybdate test—purple → brown (*sensitivity:* 0·25 μg); ammonium vanadate test—dull purple → orange-brown (*sensitivity:* 0·1 μg); Vitali's test—red/pale yellow/pale yellow (*sensitivity:* 0·1 μg).

Ultraviolet Absorption Spectrum. Clomiphene in 0·1N sulphuric acid, maxima at 233 mμ (E1%, 1cm 770) and 288 mμ (E1%, 1cm 226): clomiphene citrate in 0·1N hydrochloric acid, maxima at 235 mμ (E1%, 1cm 319) and 290 mμ (E1%, 1cm 175); minimum at about 265 mμ.

Infra-red Absorption Spectrum. Clomiphene (base). Potassium bromide disk. The principal peaks are: A 1590, B 1111, C 1245 or 1605 (p. 781).

Metabolism. Clomiphene stimulates pituitary gonadotrophic hormones, particularly the luteinising hormone. It is possible that the primary action is upon the enzyme systems concerned with the formation of ovarian hormones.

Dose. Up to 250 mg daily has been given.

Toxicity. LD50 (oral): in rats 5·75 g/kg.

CLONITAZENE *Narcotic*

Synonym: Clonitazine.

2-(p-Chlorobenzyl)-1-(2-diethylaminoethyl)-5-nitrobenzimidazole
$C_{20}H_{23}ClN_4O_2 = 386{\cdot}9$

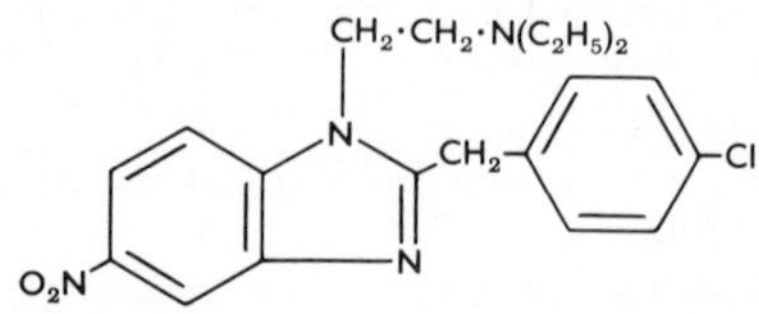

Chromatography. PAPER: system P1—Rf 0·68 (location under ultraviolet light, strong absorption; location reagent *iodoplatinate spray*, strong reaction).
THIN-LAYER: system T1—Rf 0·70 (location reagent *acidified iodoplatinate spray*, positive reaction).

Colour Tests. MICRO: ammonium molybdate test—faint grey-blue (*sensitivity:* 1·0 μg); Vitali's test—faint brown/faint brown/faint brown (*sensitivity:* 1·0 μg).

Crystal Tests. MICRO: *potassium tri-iodide solution (1)*—small plates or needles, forming overnight (*sensitivity:* 1 in 1000); *zinc chloride solution*—very small rosettes (*sensitivity:* 1 in 1000).

Ultraviolet Absorption Spectrum. Clonitazene in 0·1N sulphuric acid, maxima at 232 mμ (E1%, 1cm 571) and 285 mμ (E1%, 1cm 217).

CLOPENTHIXOL *Tranquilliser*

Synonyms: Cloperphenthixan; N 746.
Proprietary Name: Sordinol.

2-Chloro-9-{3-[4-(2-hydroxyethyl)piperazin-1-yl]propylidene}thiaxanthen
$C_{22}H_{25}ClN_2OS = 401{\cdot}0$

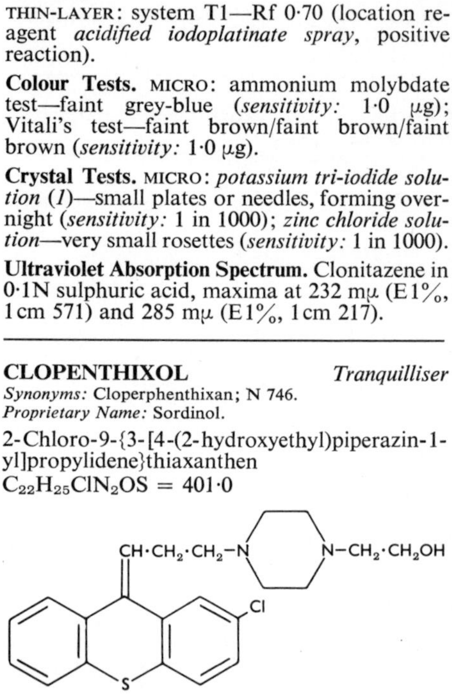

Chromatography. PAPER: system P1—Rf 0·34 (location under ultraviolet light, dark blue fluorescence; location reagents: *iodoplatinate spray*, strong reaction; *bromocresol green spray*, strong reaction).
THIN-LAYER: system T1—Rf 0·58 (location reagent *acidified iodoplatinate spray*, positive reaction).

Crystal Tests. MICRO: *platinic chloride solution*—gelatinous rosettes (*sensitivity:* 1 in 1000); *styphnic acid*—very small plates, best viewed under polarised light (*sensitivity:* 1 in 200).

Ultraviolet Absorption Spectrum. Clopenthixol in 0·1N sulphuric acid, maxima at 231 mμ (E1%, 1cm 956), 269 mμ (E1%, 1cm 317), and 325 mμ (E1%, 1cm 66).

Infra-red Absorption Spectrum. Potassium bromide disk. The principal peaks are: A 1451, B 1090 or 1150, C 757 (p. 781).

Dose. Up to 30 mg daily.

CLORPRENALINE *Sympathomimetic*

Synonym: Isoprophenamine.

1-*o*-Chlorophenyl-2-isopropylaminoethanol

$C_{11}H_{16}ClNO = 213{\cdot}7$

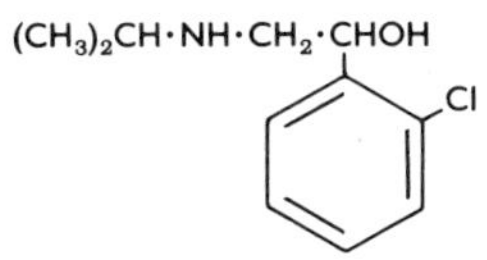

Solubility. Soluble in chloroform.

CLORPRENALINE HYDROCHLORIDE

Proprietary Name: It is an ingredient of Vortel.

White crystals. M.p. 161° to 162°.

Solubility. Soluble in water.

Extraction. Clorprenaline is extracted by organic solvents from aqueous alkaline solutions.

Chromatography. PAPER: system P1—Rf 0·67 (location reagent *bromocresol green spray*, positive reaction).

THIN-LAYER: system T1—Rf 0·63 (location reagent *potassium permanganate spray*, positive reaction).

Dose. Up to 80 mg daily.

Toxicity. LD50 (intravenous): in mice 61·8 mg/kg.

CLOTHIAPINE *Tranquilliser*

Synonyms: Clotiapine; HF 2159.

Proprietary Name: Etumine.

2-Chloro-11-(4-methylpiperazin-1-yl)dibenzo-[*b*,*f*][1,4]thiazepine

$C_{18}H_{18}ClN_3S = 343{\cdot}9$

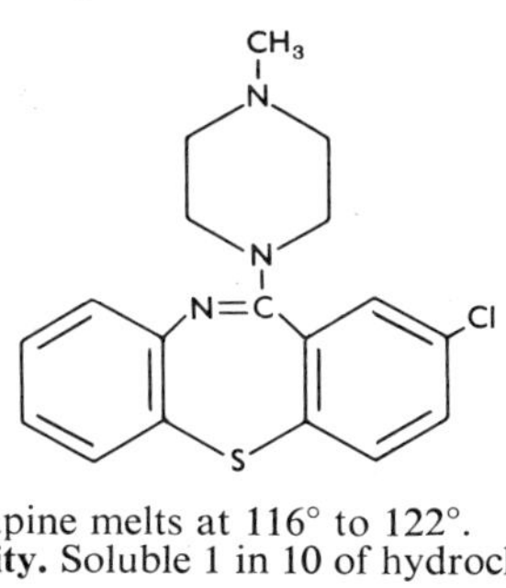

Clothiapine melts at 116° to 122°.

Solubility. Soluble 1 in 10 of hydrochloric acid.

Extraction. Clothiapine is extracted by organic solvents from aqueous alkaline solutions.

Chromatography. PAPER: system P1—Rf 0·71 (location under ultraviolet light, strong absorption; location reagents: *iodoplatinate spray*, strong reaction; *Dragendorff spray*, strong reaction).

THIN-LAYER: system T1—Rf 0·60 (location reagent *acidified iodoplatinate spray*, positive reaction).

Colour Tests. MICRO: ammonium molybdate test—faint blue (*sensitivity:* 1·0 μg); Vitali's test— –/yellow/yellow (*sensitivity:* 1·0 μg).

Crystal Tests. MICRO: *ammonium thiocyanate solution*—dense rosettes or rosettes of needles.

Ultraviolet Absorption Spectrum. Clothiapine in ethanol, maximum at about 212 mμ; weak inflexions at 235 to 240 mμ and 249 to 270 mμ; in 0·1N sulphuric acid, maximum at 220 mμ (E1%, 1 cm 1560) and an inflexion at about 288 mμ (E1%, 1 cm 224).

Infra-red Absorption Spectrum. Potassium bromide disk. The principal peaks are: A 1570 or 1596, B 1453, C 1295 or 1548 (p. 781).

COCAINE *Local Anaesthetic*

Synonym: Neurocaine.

Methyl benzoylecgonine

$C_{17}H_{21}NO_4 = 303{\cdot}4$

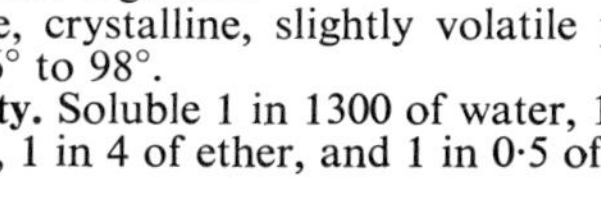

An alkaloid obtained from coca, the dried leaves of *Erythroxylum coca* and other species of *Erythroxylum* (Erythroxylaceae), or by synthesis from ecgonine.

A white, crystalline, slightly volatile powder. M.p. 96° to 98°.

Solubility. Soluble 1 in 1300 of water, 1 in 7 of ethanol, 1 in 4 of ether, and 1 in 0·5 of chloroform.

COCAINE HYDROCHLORIDE

A white crystalline hygroscopic powder. M.p. not lower than 197°. Specific rotation of a 2% solution, −70° to −72°.

Solubility. Soluble 1 in 0·5 of water, 1 in 4·5 of ethanol, and 1 in 18 of chloroform; almost insoluble in ether.

Extraction. Cocaine may be isolated in the D2 fraction (see p. 27).

Chromatography. PAPER: system P1—Rf 0·38 (location under ultraviolet light, strong absorption; location reagent *iodoplatinate spray*, strong reaction).

THIN-LAYER: system T1—Rf 0·60 (location reagent *acidified iodoplatinate spray*, positive reaction).

GAS: system G6—retention time 0·57 relative to codeine.

Crystal Tests. MICRO: *gold chloride solution*—serrated needles (*sensitivity:* 1 in 3000); *lead*

iodide solution—feathery rosettes (*sensitivity:* 1 in 3000).

Ultraviolet Absorption Spectrum. Cocaine in ethanol, maxima at 230 mμ, 274 mμ, and 281 mμ; minima at about 217 mμ, 260 mμ, and 279 mμ; in 0·1N sulphuric acid, maxima at 233 mμ (E1%, 1 cm 470) and 275 mμ (E1%, 1 cm 38), and an inflexion at 281 mμ. Cocaine hydrochloride in water, maxima at 233 mμ and 274 mμ; minima at 211 mμ and 261 mμ.

Infra-red Absorption Spectrum. Cocaine (base). Potassium bromide disk. The principal peaks are: A 1275, B 1700, C 1106 or 1728 (p. 736).

Quantitative Estimation. Cocaine may be quantitatively estimated in biological materials by spectrophotometry following reaction with bromocresol purple solution (Woods *et al.*, 1951) or with methyl orange solution (Gettler and Sunshine, 1951).

Metabolism. After absorption, cocaine is extensively metabolised in the liver. In rabbits, the metabolism is thought to proceed by hydrolysis of the 2 ester groups to yield benzoylecgonine and finally ecgonine and benzoic acid. However, ecgonine has not been detected in the urine; it is possibly further transformed.

Cocaine is excreted slowly, the amount of unchanged drug appearing in the urine being dependent on the pH. In man, between 1 and 12% of an injected dose is excreted in the first 24 hours, the excretion being most rapid in the first 5 to 6 hours. No cocaine is detected in the faeces.

Toxicity. Ingested cocaine is much less toxic than cocaine taken or administered by other routes; not more than 50 mg or 1 ml of a 5% solution should be used on mucous membranes. The course of acute poisoning is very rapid; the usual fatal dose is about 1·2 g but death has occurred from doses as low as 20 mg. Cocaine has marked addiction-producing properties and addicts may tolerate as much as 5 g daily.

LD50 (intravenous): in rabbits 17 and in rats 17·5 mg/kg.

CODEINE *Analgesic*

Synonyms: Methylmorphine; Morphine Methyl Ether.

7,8-Dehydro-4,5-epoxy-6-hydroxy-3-methoxy-*N*-methylmorphinan

$C_{18}H_{21}NO_3 = 299·4$

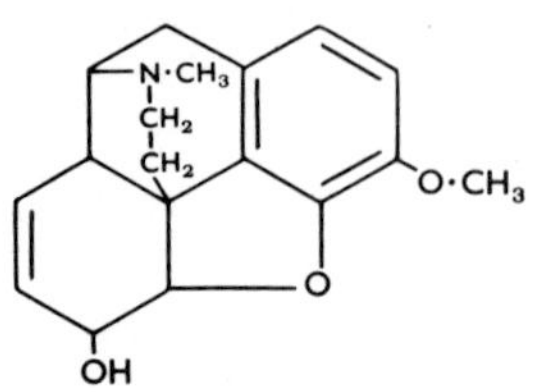

An alkaloid obtained from opium or prepared by methylation of morphine.

A white crystalline powder, which effloresces slowly in dry air and is affected by light. In acid or ethanol solution it is laevorotatory. M.p. of the anhydrous compound, 154° to 158°.

Solubility. Soluble 1 in 120 of water, 1 in 20 of boiling water, 1 in 2 of ethanol, 1 in 50 of ether, and 1 in 2 of chloroform.

CODEINE HYDROCHLORIDE

A white crystalline powder. M.p. about 280°, with decomposition.

Solubility. Soluble 1 in 30 of water, 1 in 100 of ethanol, and 1 in 800 of chloroform.

CODEINE PHOSPHATE

A white crystalline powder.

Solubility. Soluble 1 in 4 of water and 1 in 450 of ethanol; sparingly soluble in ether and chloroform.

CODEINE SULPHATE

A white crystalline powder.

Solubility. Soluble 1 in 30 of water and 1 in 1300 of ethanol; insoluble in ether and chloroform.

Screening Tests. See under Screening Tests, p. 11.

Extraction. Codeine is extracted by organic solvents from aqueous alkaline solutions.

Chromatography. PAPER: system P1—Rf 0·16 (location under ultraviolet light, strong absorption; location reagents: *iodoplatinate spray*, strong reaction; *bromocresol green spray*, weak reaction); system RP1a—Rf 0·89 (location under ultraviolet light, absorption; location reagent *iodoplatinate spray*, positive reaction); system RP1b—Rf 0·22 (location as for RP1a). THIN-LAYER: system T1—Rf 0·35 (location reagent *acidified iodoplatinate spray*, positive reaction); system T7—Rf 0·39 (location reagent *iodoplatinate spray*, positive reaction); system T8—Rf 0·29 (location as for T7). GAS: system G2/225—retention time 4·65 relative to diphenhydramine; system G4—retention time 9·6 relative to diphenhydramine.

Colour Tests. MICRO: sulphuric acid–formaldehyde test—purple (*sensitivity:* 0·05 μg); ammonium molybdate test—blue-green (*sensitivity:* 0·1 μg); ammonium vanadate test—green (*sensitivity:* 1·0 μg); Vitali's test—yellow/yellow/orange.

Crystal Tests. MICRO: *potassium cadmium iodide solution*—gelatinous rosettes, changing to aggregates of small tablets (*sensitivity:* 1 in 1500); *potassium tri-iodide solution* (*1*)—feathery rosettes, forming overnight (*sensitivity:* 1 in 1000).

Ultraviolet Absorption Spectrum. Codeine in ethanol, maximum at 286 mμ and minimum at 263 mμ; codeine phosphate in water, maximum at 284 mμ (E1%, 1 cm about 52·3).

Infra-red Absorption Spectrum. Codeine (base). Potassium bromide disk. The principal peaks are: A 1052, B 1268, C 1500 (p. 736).

Quantitative Estimation. Codeine may be estimated spectrophotometrically following the formation of a complex with methyl orange (Woods *et al.*, 1956; Takemori and Mannering, 1958).

Metabolism. Codeine is well absorbed after both oral and parenteral administration. Very little is known regarding the tissue distribution and levels of codeine in man. Codeine is metabolised mainly in the liver by 3 major routes: conjugation, possibly with glucuronic acid; *O*-demethylation to morphine and subsequent conjugation; *N*-demethylation to norcodeine and subsequent conjugation. Excretion is rapid, about two-thirds of the total material excreted being found in the urine within 6 hours of administration, and is virtually complete in 24 hours although trace amounts of the conjugated alkaloids may be detected for several days.

After normal therapeutic doses the major fraction of each alkaloid appears in the urine in the conjugated form, although after large doses measurable amounts of free morphine and free norcodeine have been demonstrated. After single oral doses of 22 mg, the 24-hour excretion of codeine and its metabolites ranged from 63 to 86% of the dose, a similar proportion being observed after 22-mg intravenous doses; but only 48% of the dose was recovered from the urine of a subject who received 70·5 mg every 4 hours for 12 hours (Adler *et al.*, 1955). In 24 hours following the oral administration of 4 mg/kg in divided doses, 4% of the dose was excreted in the urine as free norcodeine, 14% as conjugated norcodeine, 1% as free morphine, and 7% as conjugated morphine.

Very little is known regarding the part played by morphine in the pharmacological action of codeine; the amounts of morphine released during the period of drug action do not necessarily have any marked biological effects.

Dose. Up to 60 mg.

Toxicity. Codeine is much less toxic than morphine and even large overdoses do not produce the central depression characteristic of morphine; death directly attributable to codeine is very rare. Both tolerance and addiction to codeine can occur but, as it has only a feeble euphoric action when taken by mouth when compared with that of morphine, it is seldom used as a drug of addiction. The estimated lethal dose in man is 800 mg and more than 200 mg is dangerous, although addicts may tolerate much higher doses.

LD50 (subcutaneous): in mice 300 and in rabbits 32 mg/kg.

CODEINE *N*-OXIDE — *Narcotic*

Synonym: Genocodeine.

$C_{18}H_{21}NO_4$ = 315·4

Chromatography. PAPER: system P1—Rf 0·19 (location under ultraviolet light, strong absorption; location reagent *iodoplatinate spray*, strong reaction).

THIN-LAYER: system T1—Rf 0·23 (location reagent *acidified iodoplatinate spray*, positive reaction).

Colour Tests. MICRO: sulphuric acid–formaldehyde test—deep purple (*sensitivity:* 0·1 μg); ammonium molybdate test—green → blue (*sensitivity:* 0·1 μg); Vitali's test—yellow/faint orange/purple → chocolate-brown (*sensitivity:* 0·1 μg).

Crystal Tests. MICRO: *gold bromide–hydrochloric acid solution*—blades, forming overnight (*sensitivity:* 1 in 100); *potassium tri-iodide solution* (*I*)—bunches of blades (*sensitivity:* 1 in 200).

COLCHICINE — *Suppressant for Gout*

$C_{22}H_{25}NO_6$ = 399·4

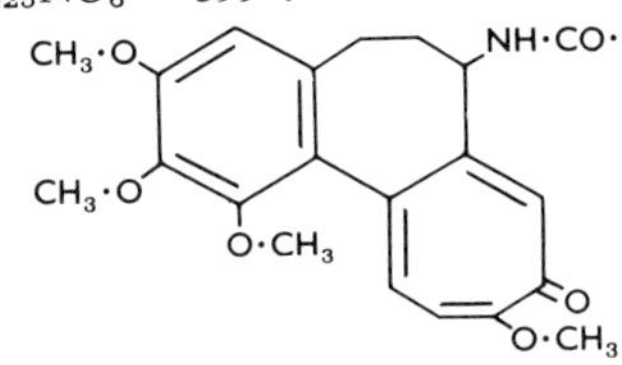

Colchicine is an alkaloid obtained from the corm and seeds of the meadow saffron, *Colchicum autumnale* (Liliaceae).

Pale yellow crystals or powder, darkening on exposure to light. M.p. 153° to 157°.

Solubility. Soluble 1 in 20 of water but moderately concentrated solutions may deposit crystals of the 6-hydrate, which is sparingly soluble in cold water. Freely soluble in ethanol and chloroform; soluble 1 in 160 of ether at 15·5°.

Extraction. Colchicine is extracted by chloroform from aqueous alkaline solutions.

Chromatography. PAPER: system P1—Rf 0·83 (location under ultraviolet light, yellow fluorescence).

THIN-LAYER: system T1—Rf 0·62 (location reagent p-*dimethylaminobenzaldehyde spray*, yellow).

GAS: system G6—retention time 1·15 relative to codeine.

Colour Tests. MICRO: sulphuric acid–formaldehyde test—yellow (*sensitivity:* 0·25 μg); ammonium molybdate test—yellow (*sensitivity:* 0·25 μg); ammonium vanadate test—green (*sensitivity:* 0·25 μg); Vitali's test—yellow → purple/brown/red-brown (*sensitivity:* 0·25 μg).

Ultraviolet Absorption Spectrum. Colchicine in ethanol, maxima at 243 mμ (E1%, 1 cm 730) and 350 mμ (E1%, 1 cm 420).

Infra-red Absorption Spectrum. Potassium bromide disk. The principal peaks are: A 1248, B 1566, C 1589 (p. 736).

Quantitative Estimation. King (1951) describes a spectrophotometric method of estimation of colchicine involving its conversion by acid hydrolysis to colchiceine and subsequent formation of a green complex with ferric chloride.

Metabolism. Little is known regarding the

absorption of colchicine from the gastro-intestinal tract. There is no evidence of any specific accumulation in the tissues or in tumours. About 50% of an injected dose has been recovered from the mouse within 16 hours. Excretion occurs rapidly, especially at high blood-levels, the bulk of the drug being excreted in the first 24 hours. Colchicine may be excreted in the bile and also directly into the gastro-intestinal tract; mice excrete between 2·5 and 14% of the dose in the faeces and rats between 10 and 25%.

Studies with ^{14}C-labelled colchicine have shown that the subjects without neoplastic or renal diseases excrete between 15·6 and 40·7% of a dose as unchanged colchicine in 48 hours and between 4·3 and 14% as a chloroform-soluble metabolite (Walaszek *et al.*, 1960, per Carr, 1965).

It is thought that colchicine is converted in the body to oxydicolchicine which is extremely irritating to all cells.

Toxicity. The total amount of colchicine required to relieve an acute attack of gout is usually between 3 and 6 mg; a total dose of 6 mg should not be exceeded during a single course of treatment and a total dose of 3 mg should not be exceeded in 24 hours.

Symptoms of poisoning may set in within 3 to 6 hours and death from exhaustion or from respiratory paralysis occurs in 7 to 36 hours. The lethal dose in man may be as low as 6 mg, although recovery has occurred after much larger doses.

CASE EXAMPLES. A youth swallowed 10 to 13 mg of colchicine in tablet form and 7 hours later became acutely ill, complaining of nausea, vomiting, diarrhoea, and severe abdominal pain. After 6 days, loss of hair was noted and within a further 2 weeks loss of over 90% of the scalp hair occurred (Thompson, 1964).

A gouty patient, aged 36 years, who also had renal failure, was given 47 mg of colchicine by mouth over 16 days, then 4 mg intravenously. He promptly developed classic signs of colchicine toxicity—fever, malaise, vomiting, diarrhoea, mental confusion, alopecia, and liver damage, as well as severe bone-marrow depression indicated by leucopenia, granulocytopenia, and thrombocytopenia (Carr, 1965).

CONIINE *Alkaloid*

Synonyms: Cicutine; Conicine; Conine.

2-Propylpiperidine

$C_8H_{17}N = 127{\cdot}2$

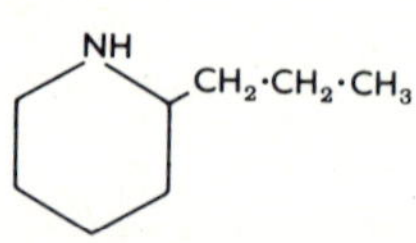

An alkaloid obtained mainly from the fruits and leaves of hemlock, *Conium maculatum* (Umbelliferae).

An almost colourless volatile liquid with a mouse-like odour. M.p. −2°. B.p. 166°.

Solubility. Soluble 1 in 100 of water and slightly soluble in chloroform; miscible with ethanol and ether.

CONIINE HYDROBROMIDE

Colourless prismatic crystals. M.p. about 211°.

Solubility. Soluble 1 in 2 of water and 1 in 3 of ethanol; soluble in ether and chloroform.

Extraction. Coniine is extracted by organic solvents from aqueous alkaline solutions; it may also be isolated by steam distillation from alkaline solutions (see p. 19).

Chromatography. PAPER: system P1—Rf 0·56 (location reagents: *iodoplatinate spray*, weak reaction; *bromocresol green spray*, weak reaction).

THIN-LAYER: system T1—Rf 0·26 (location reagent *acidified iodoplatinate spray*, positive reaction).

GAS: system G5—retention time 0·23 relative to barbitone.

Crystal Tests. MICRO: *platinic iodide solution*—plates (*sensitivity:* 1 in 400); *potassium bismuth iodide solution*—rhomboids (*sensitivity:* 1 in 3000).

Ultraviolet Absorption Spectrum. Coniine in 0·2N sulphuric acid, maximum at 266 to 270 mμ.

Toxicity. Coniine is very poisonous; death may occur within half an hour or may be delayed 3 to 12 hours. It resembles nicotine in its peripheral action but it produces more pronounced paralysis of the central nervous system and of the skeletal muscle nerve endings. It is well absorbed from the gastro-intestinal tract. The estimated lethal dose in man is 120 to 300 mg and toxic symptoms may occur after 60 mg.

Coniine has been responsible for numerous cases of poisoning in farm stock which have eaten hemlock.

The oral lethal dose in guinea-pigs is 150 and in rabbits 56 mg/kg.

CORTISONE *Corticosteroid*

Synonyms: Compound E; 17-Hydroxy-11-dehydrocorticosterone.

17α,21-Dihydroxypregn-4-ene-3,11,20-trione

$C_{21}H_{28}O_5 = 360{\cdot}5$

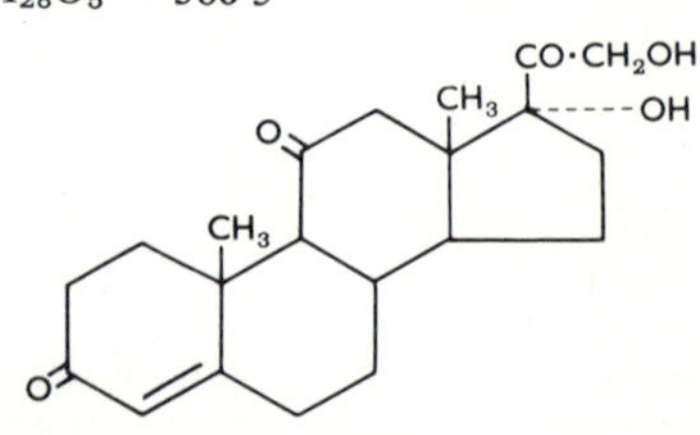

It occurs as crystals. M.p. 217° to 224°, with some decomposition.

Solubility. Very slightly soluble in water; soluble in ethanol; sparingly soluble in ether and chloroform.

CORTISONE ACETATE
21 - Acetoxy - 17α - hydroxypregn - 4 - ene - 3,11,20 - trione
Synonym: Cortisone 21-Acetate.
Proprietary Names: Adreson; Cortelan; Cortistab; Cortisyl.

A white crystalline powder. M.p. about 240°, with decomposition. Specific rotation of a 1% solution in dioxan, +208° to +219°.
Solubility. Almost insoluble in water; soluble 1 in 300 of ethanol and 1 in 4 of chloroform; soluble in ether.

Extraction. Cortisone is extracted from neutral solutions with freshly distilled ethyl acetate.

Chromatography. PAPER, for the cortisone: system P13—Rf 0·62 (location reagent *DPST solution*, violet on yellow); for cortisone acetate: system P14—Rf 0·80 (location as for P13).
THIN-LAYER, for cortisone acetate: system T19—Rf 1·88 (location reagent *DPST spray*).

Ultraviolet Absorption Spectrum. Cortisone acetate in ethanol, maximum at 240 mμ (E1%, 1 cm about 390).

Metabolism. Cortisone is a glucocorticoid secreted by the human adrenal cortex. It is used for replacement therapy in adrenal insufficiency, as an anti-inflammatory agent, and occasionally as an anti-allergic agent. It is metabolised mainly in the liver but also in the kidneys to a number of physiologically inactive compounds. The metabolites may be excreted in the faeces and urine, largely as conjugates of glucuronic acid or sulphuric acid.
Four main metabolic reactions may occur: reduction of the 4,5-double bond, reduction of the 3-carbonyl group, reduction of the 11-carbonyl group, and reduction of the 20-carbonyl group.

Dose. Up to 400 mg daily.

COTARNINE *Alkaloid*

8 - Methoxy - 2 - methyl - 6,7 - methylenedioxy-1,2,3,4-tetrahydroisoquinolin-1-ol
$C_{12}H_{15}NO_4 = 237{\cdot}3$

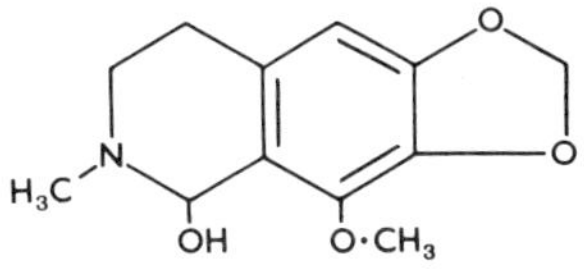

An alkaloid obtained by oxidising noscapine with nitric acid.
It occurs as small needles. M.p. 132° to 137°, with decomposition.
Solubility. Slightly soluble in water; soluble in ethanol, ether, and chloroform.

COTARNINE CHLORIDE
Synonyms: Cotarnine Hydrochloride; Stypticine.
Proprietary Name: Cotarnine phthalate is marketed under the name Styptol.

A pale yellow deliquescent powder or needles. M.p. 197°. When heated to decomposition, highly toxic fumes are evolved.
Solubility. Soluble in water, ethanol, and chloroform.

Extraction. Cotarnine is extracted by organic solvents from aqueous alkaline solutions.

Chromatography. PAPER: system P1—Rf 0·19 (location under ultraviolet light, green fluorescence; location reagent *iodoplatinate spray*, strong reaction); system RP1a—Rf 0·80 (location reagent *iodoplatinate spray*, positive reaction); system RP1b—Rf 0·90 (location as for RP1a).
THIN-LAYER: system T1—Rf 0·02 (location reagent *acidified iodoplatinate spray*, positive reaction).
GAS: system G6—retention time 0·23 relative to codeine.

Colour Tests. MICRO: ammonium molybdate test—pale purple → green (*sensitivity:* 0·25 μg); ammonium vanadate test—red-orange → brown (*sensitivity:* 0·05 μg); Vitali's test—yellow/yellow/brown (*sensitivity:* 1·0 μg).

Crystal Tests. MICRO: *platinic chloride solution*—rods (*sensitivity:* 1 in 3000); *potassium tri-iodide solution* (*3*)—small rods (*sensitivity:* 1 in 3000).

Ultraviolet Absorption Spectrum. Cotarnine in 0·1N sulphuric acid, maxima at 253 mμ (E1%, 1 cm 582) and 332 mμ (E1%, 1 cm 666).

Infra-red Absorption Spectrum. Cotarnine (base). Potassium bromide disk. The principal peaks are: A 1089, B 1478, C 1035 (p. 781).

Dose. Up to 100 mg has been given, by mouth or by injection.

CRESOL *Antiseptic and Preservative*

Synonyms: Cresyl Oil; Cresylic Acid.
Preparation: Cresol and Soap Solution (Lysol).

Cresol is a mixture of *o*-, *m*-, and *p*-cresols, $CH_3{\cdot}C_6H_4{\cdot}OH$, in which the *m*-isomer predominates, and of other phenols obtained from coal tar.

An almost colourless to pale brownish-yellow liquid which darkens with age or on exposure to light. B.p. 195° to 205°.
Solubility. Soluble 1 in 50 of water; freely soluble in ethanol, ether, and chloroform.

Extraction. Cresol is volatile and may be isolated by distillation (see p. 18).

Colour Test. Heat a little cresol with about an equal quantity of phthalic anhydride and a few drops of *sulphuric acid* until the mixture is orange-brown; cool the mixture with a few drops of water; make alkaline with sodium hydroxide solution—red with *o*-cresol and blue-violet with *m*-cresol.

Ultraviolet Absorption Spectrum. Cresol in ethanol, maxima at 275 mμ (E1%, 1 cm 163) and 279 mμ (E1%, 1 cm 145); in 0·1N sodium hydroxide, maxima at 239 mμ (E1%, 1 cm 949) and 290 mμ (E1%, 1 cm 251).

Metabolism. Cresol is similar to phenol (p. 487) in its action on the body; it has a corrosive action on the skin and mucous membranes. In rabbits, about 15% of ingested cresol is excreted as a sulphuric acid conjugate and 60 to 70% as a glucuronic acid conjugate; about 3% is found to be excreted as dihydroxytoluene. *p*-Cresol but not *o*-cresol or *m*-cresol is oxidised in both dogs and rabbits at the methyl group to yield *p*-hydroxybenzoic acid; in rabbits, up to 10% of an oral dose may be excreted as *p*-hydroxybenzoic acid, partly as the free acid and partly conjugated.

Toxicity. The maximum permissible concentration of cresol in air is stated to be 5 p.p.m. The fatal dose is about 2 g or 2 ml; the fatal dose of Cresol and Soap Solution (Lysol), the form in which cresol is most frequently used, is about 10 g or 10 ml.

CROPROPAMIDE *Respiratory Stimulant*

NN-Dimethyl-α-(*N*-propylcrotonamido)butyramide

$C_{13}H_{24}N_2O_2 = 240{\cdot}3$

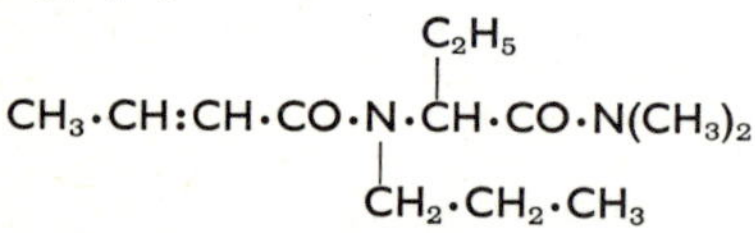

Cropropamide is an ingredient of **prethcamide** (Micoren) which is a mixture of equal parts by weight of cropropamide and crotethamide.

Chromatography. PAPER: system P1—Rf 0·93 (location under ultraviolet light, strong absorption; location reagent *potassium permanganate spray*, strong reaction); system RP1a—Rf 0·40 (location under ultraviolet light, absorption); system RP1b—Rf 0·30 (location as for RP1a).
THIN-LAYER: system T1—Rf 0·72 (location reagent *potassium permanganate spray*, positive reaction).

Crystal Test. MICRO: *gold bromide–hydrochloric acid solution*—bunches of prisms.

Infra-red Absorption Spectrum. Potassium bromide disk. The principal peaks are: A 1654, B 1617, C 1413 (p. 781).

Toxicity. LD50 (intravenous) of prethcamide (cropropamide with crotethamide): in rabbits 250 mg/kg.

CROTETHAMIDE *Respiratory Stimulant*

α-(*N*-Ethylcrotonamido)-*NN*-dimethylbutyramide

$C_{12}H_{22}N_2O_2 = 226{\cdot}3$

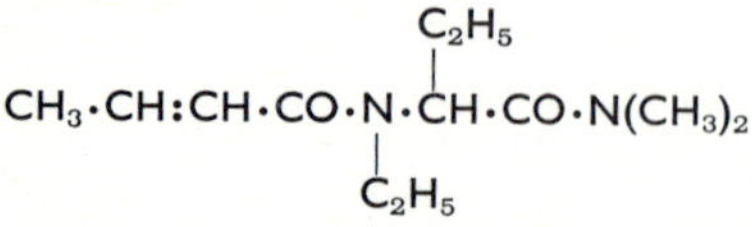

Crotethamide is an ingredient of **prethcamide** (Micoren) which is a mixture of equal parts by weight of cropropamide and crotethamide.

Chromatography. PAPER: system P1—Rf 0·93 (location under ultraviolet light, strong absorption; location reagent *potassium permanganate spray*, strong reaction); system RP1a—Rf 0·90 (location under ultraviolet light, absorption; location reagent *iodoplatinate spray*, positive reaction); system RP1b—Rf 0·50 (location under ultraviolet light, absorption).
THIN-LAYER: system T1—Rf 0·73 (location reagent *potassium permanganate spray*, positive reaction).

Ultraviolet Absorption Spectrum. Crotethamide in 0·1N sulphuric acid, maximum at 210 mμ (E1%, 1 cm 1358) and an inflexion at about 243 mμ (E1%, 1 cm 538).

Infra-red Absorption Spectrum. Potassium bromide disk. The principal peaks are: A 1655, B 1617, C 1417 (p. 781).

Toxicity. See under Cropropamide.

CYANOCOBALAMIN *Haemopoietic Agent*

Synonyms: Cobamin; Cycobemin; Vitamin B_{12}.
Proprietary Names: Bitevan; Cobalin; Cobastab; Cytacon; Fermin.

α-(5,6-Dimethylbenzimidazolyl)cobamide cyanide

$C_{63}H_{88}CoN_{14}O_{14}P = 1355{\cdot}4$

Dark red crystals or crystalline powder; very hygroscopic when anhydrous.

Solubility. Soluble 1 in 80 of water and 1 in 180 of ethanol; insoluble in ether and chloroform.

Extraction. Biological material must be dehydrated and extracted with ethanol (see p. 29); Hall and Allen (1964) describe 2 methods for the extraction of cyanocobalamin from serum; one involves papain digestion in an acidified sodium cyanide solution, the second involves heat treatment of a sodium cyanide solution of the serum. A bioassay is also described.

Ultraviolet Absorption Spectrum. Cyanocobalamin in water, maxima at 278 mμ (E1%, 1 cm 119), 361 mμ (E1%, 1 cm 207), and 550 mμ (E1%, 1 cm 63).

Metabolism. Cyanocobalamin is the most important member of a group of similar compounds which influence erythropoiesis. It is present in liver, kidneys, milk, eggs, and muscle tissue, and is produced by bacterial synthesis in the colon. Cyanocobalamin is involved together with folic acid in the formation and metabolism of purines and pyrimidines, and hence in the synthesis of nucleoproteins and in the maintenance of normal haemopoiesis.
Absorption of cyanocobalamin from the gastro-intestinal tract is irregular and unpredictable and it is therefore usually administered by injection. Following absorption from the

intestine, little if any cyanocobalamin is found in urine but, after administration by injection, it circulates in the blood in an unbound form for about 8 hours during which time it is rapidly excreted in the urine; subsequently, that remaining in the blood is present in a bound form and very little urinary excretion occurs. It is probable that cyanocobalamin is slowly converted to hydroxocobalamin in human tissues (Reizenstein, 1967).

Dose. In megaloblastic anaemia, up to 2 mg weekly, intramuscularly, in divided doses.

CYCLAMIC ACID *Sweetening Agent*

Proprietary Name: Hexamic Acid.

N-Cyclohexylsulphamic acid

$C_6H_{13}NO_3S = 179{\cdot}2$

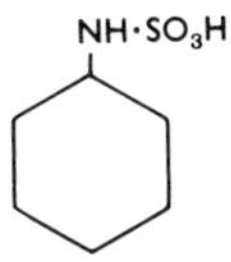

A white crystalline powder. M.p. 175°.
Solubility. Soluble 1 in 7·5 of water, 1 in 3 of ethanol, 1 in 250 of chloroform, and 1 in 4 of propylene glycol.

CALCIUM CYCLAMATE
Synonym: Calcium Cyclohexanesulphamate.
Proprietary Name: Sucaryl Calcium.

White crystals or crystalline powder.
Solubility. Soluble 1 in 4 of water and 1 in 50 of ethanol; almost insoluble in ether and chloroform.

SODIUM CYCLAMATE
Synonym: Sodium Cyclohexanesulphamate.
Proprietary Name: Sucaryl Sodium.

White crystals or crystalline powder.
Solubility. Soluble 1 in 5 of water and 1 in 250 of ethanol; almost insoluble in ether and chloroform.

Extraction. Richardson (1967) has reviewed many methods for the extraction and determination of cyclamates, including paper, thin-layer, and gas chromatographic systems.

Metabolism. When administered as the sodium or calcium salt in man, cyclamic acid has been found to be largely excreted unchanged, mainly in the urine and to a lesser extent in the faeces; however, there is some evidence that a very small proportion may be converted to cyclohexylamine, which is reported to be toxic.

Toxicity. Single 1-g doses of sodium and calcium cyclamate have been administered intravenously without ill effect and up to 12 g of calcium cyclamate has been administered orally, the only side-effect being the production of soft stools.
LD50 (oral): sodium cyclamate in rats, 6 to 12 g/kg.

CYCLIZINE *Antihistamine/Anti-emetic*

1-Diphenylmethyl-4-methylpiperazine

$C_{18}H_{22}N_2 = 266{\cdot}4$

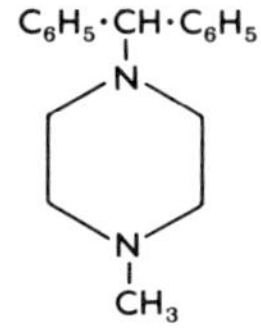

Cyclizine occurs as crystals from light petroleum. M.p. 107° to 108°.
Solubility. Slightly soluble in water; freely soluble in ethanol and ether.

CYCLIZINE HYDROCHLORIDE
Proprietary Names: Marezine Hydrochloride; Marzine; Sereen; Valoid (tablets and suppositories).

A white crystalline powder. M.p. about 285°, with decomposition.
Solubility. Soluble 1 in 125 of water, 1 in 120 of ethanol, and 1 in 75 of chloroform; insoluble in ether.

CYCLIZINE LACTATE
Proprietary Names: Marezine Lactate; Valoid (injection).
Solubility. Freely soluble in water.

Extraction. Cyclizine is extracted by organic solvents from aqueous alkaline solutions.

Chromatography. PAPER: system P1—Rf 0·55 (location under ultraviolet light, absorption; location reagents: *iodoplatinate spray*, strong reaction; *bromocresol green spray*, strong reaction); system RP1a—Rf 0·47 (location under ultraviolet light, absorption; location reagent *iodoplatinate spray*, positive reaction); system RP1b—Rf 0·00.
THIN-LAYER: system T1—Rf 0·24, streaking (location reagent *acidified iodoplatinate spray*, positive reaction).
GAS: system G2/225—retention time 1·77 relative to diphenhydramine; system G4—retention time 1·6 relative to diphenhydramine.

Colour Tests. MICRO: sulphuric acid–formaldehyde test—faint yellow; ammonium molybdate test—faint yellow.

Crystal Tests. MICRO: *potassium bismuth iodide solution*—bunches of small irregular needles (*sensitivity:* 1 in 400); *sodium carbonate solution*—plates (*sensitivity:* 1 in 200).

Ultraviolet Absorption Spectrum. Cyclizine in methanol, maximum at 259·5 mμ (E 1%, 1 cm 16); in 0·1N sulphuric acid, maxima at 225 mμ (E 1%, 1 cm 455), 257 mμ (E 1%, 1 cm 27), 262·5 mμ (E 1%, 1 cm 28), and 269 mμ; cyclizine hydrochloride in 0·1N hydrochloric acid, maxima at 225 mμ (E 1%, 1 cm 394), 257 mμ (E 1%, 1 cm 24), 262 mμ (E 1%, 1 cm 25), and 268 mμ (E 1%, 1 cm 19); minima at 244·5 mμ, 260 mμ, and 266 mμ.

Infra-red Absorption Spectrum. Cyclizine (base). Potassium bromide disk. The principal peaks are: A 708, B 1150 or 1447, C 745 or 759 or 1285 (p. 782).

Metabolism. Cyclizine is an antihistamine that is used mainly for its anti-emetic action which is potent and begins within a few minutes of administration. Studies in dogs and rats show that the major route of metabolism is demethylation to norcyclizine which must be further metabolised since no accumulation occurs (Kuntzman *et al.*, 1965); cyclizine and norcyclizine are found to be distributed throughout the tissues of the rat, the highest levels occurring in the kidneys, liver, lungs and spleen. Cyclizine is metabolised more rapidly than chlorcyclizine.

Dose. Up to 150 mg daily by mouth; up to 300 mg daily by suppository.

Toxicity. There have been reports which suggest a possibility of human foetal abnormalities resulting from the administration of cyclizine but a causal relationship has not been confirmed. The estimated lethal dose in man is in the range 25 to 250 mg/kg.
LD50 (oral): in mice 147 mg/kg.

CYCLOBARBITONE *Barbiturate*

Synonyms: Cyclobarbital; Ethylhexabital; Hexemalum.
Proprietary Name: Phanodorm.

5-Cyclohex-1′-enyl-5-ethylbarbituric acid
$C_{12}H_{16}N_2O_3 = 236{\cdot}3$

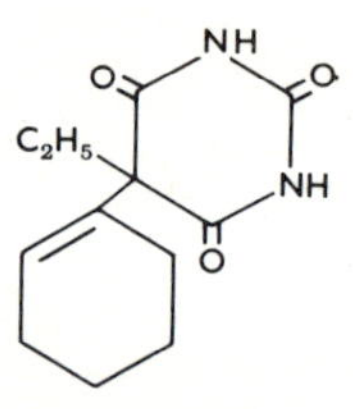

A white crystalline powder, which gradually decomposes on storage. M.p. 171° to 174°.
Solubility. Soluble 1 in 800 of water, 1 in 4 of ethanol, 1 in 15 of ether, and 1 in 20 of chloroform; soluble in solutions of alkali hydroxides and carbonates.

CYCLOBARBITONE CALCIUM

Synonym: Hexemalcalcium.
Proprietary Names: Phanodorm; Phanodorn; Rapidal.
A white powder.
Solubility. Soluble 1 in 100 of water; almost insoluble in ethanol, ether, and chloroform.

Screening Tests. See under Barbiturates, p. 208.

Extraction. Cyclobarbitone may be isolated in the A2 fraction (see p. 27).

Chromatography. PAPER: system P2—Rf 0·24 relative to amylobarbitone (location under ultraviolet light, dark spot); system P4—Rf 0·23 (location reagent *silver nitrate spray*, white); system RP1b—Rf 0·20 (location under ultraviolet light after exposure to ammonia; location reagent *potassium permanganate spray*, yellow on pink).

THIN-LAYER: system T10—Rf 0·32 (location reagents: *mercurous nitrate spray*, black; *potassium permanganate spray*, yellow-brown on purple; *Zwikker's reagent spray*, pink); system T11—Rf 0·55 (location reagents: *mercurous nitrate spray*, white on grey; *potassium permanganate spray*, yellow on purple).

GAS: system G5—retention time 7·2 relative to barbitone; system G7—retention time 5·0 relative to barbitone.

Colour Test. Zwikker's test—violet-blue.

Ultraviolet Absorption Spectrum. Cyclobarbitone is a 5,5-derivative—see Screening Test 3 under Barbiturates, p. 208.

Infra-red Absorption Spectrum. Cyclobarbitone. Potassium bromide disk. The principal peaks are: A 1693, B 1725, C 1430 (p. 736).

Quantitative Estimation. See under Barbiturates, p. 208.

Metabolism. Cyclobarbitone is a short-acting barbiturate—see under Barbiturates, p. 207. In man, it is oxidised in the cyclohexenyl ring in a position adjacent to the double bond to yield 5 - (3′ - oxo - 1′,2′ - cyclohexenyl) - 5 - ethylbarbituric acid; between 18 and 22% of this metabolite is excreted in the urine while 2 to 7% of the original drug is excreted unchanged (Mark, 1963). The metabolite has been detected up to 5 to 6 days after a single dose. A 3′-hydroxy-derivative may also be formed.

Dose. Up to 400 mg.

Toxicity. The estimated minimum lethal dose in man is about 2 g; the blood-level associated with severe poisoning is 1 to 3 mg%.
The oral lethal dose in cats is 120 to 200, in dogs 200 to 300, and in rabbits 450 mg/kg.

CYCLOGUANIL *Antimalarial*

Synonym: CI 501.

4,6-Diamino-1-*p*-chlorophenyl-1,2-dihydro-2,2-dimethyl-1,3,5-triazine
$C_{11}H_{14}ClN_5 = 251{\cdot}7$

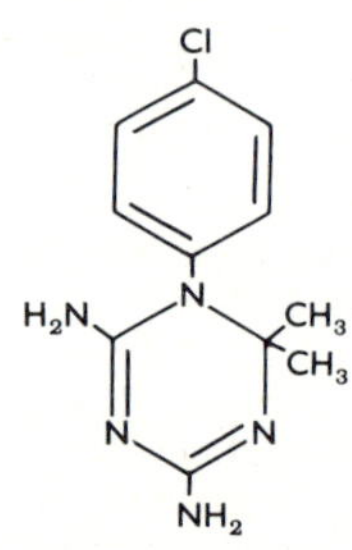

CYCLOGUANIL EMBONATE

Synonym: Cycloguanil Pamoate.
Proprietary Name: Camolar.
Solubility. Very slightly soluble in water.

Extraction. Cycloguanil is extracted by organic solvents from aqueous alkaline solutions.

Chromatography. PAPER: system P1—Rf 0·25 (location under ultraviolet light, weak absorption).

Crystal Tests. MICRO: *picric acid*—fans of needles (*sensitivity:* 1 in 1000); *platinic iodide solution*—curved needles (*sensitivity:* 1 in 1000).

Ultraviolet Absorption Spectrum. Cycloguanil in 0·1N sulphuric acid, inflexions at 220 mμ (E1%, 1cm 358) and 238 mμ (E1%, 1cm 176).

Infra-red Absorption Spectrum. Cycloguanil (base). Potassium bromide disk. The principal peaks are: A 1393 or 1452 or 1515 or 1673 (p. 782).

Metabolism. Cycloguanil is the active metabolite of proguanil (p. 516). Because of its low solubility in water, it is absorbed very slowly from the depot at the injection site, resulting in very low but persisting concentrations of the drug in body fluids and tissues.

Dose. 5 mg/kg, intramuscularly.

Toxicity. LD50 (oral): in rats 331 mg/kg.

CYCLOMETHYCAINE *Local Anaesthetic*

3-(2-Methylpiperidino)propyl *p*-cyclohexyloxybenzoate

$C_{22}H_{33}NO_3 = 359·5$

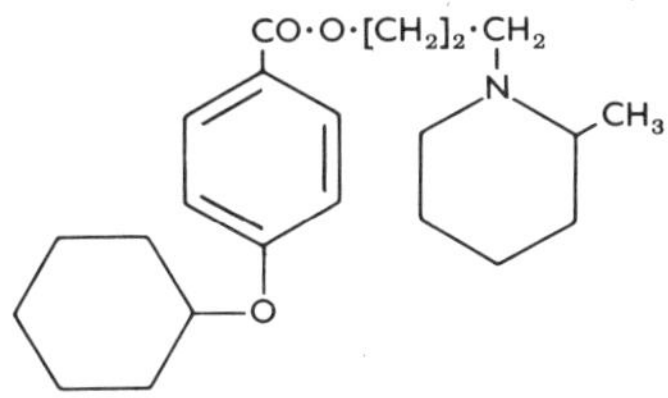

A white crystalline powder.

Solubility. Sparingly soluble in water, ethanol, and ether; very slightly soluble in chloroform.

CYCLOMETHYCAINE SULPHATE

Proprietary Names: Surfacaine; Surfathesin.

A white crystalline powder. M.p. 162·5° to 165·5°.

Solubility. Soluble 1 in 50 of water, 1 in 50 of ethanol, and 1 in 227 of chloroform.

Extraction. Cyclomethycaine is extracted by organic solvents from aqueous alkaline solutions.

Chromatography. PAPER: system P1—Rf 0·87 (location under ultraviolet light, blue fluorescence; location reagents: *iodoplatinate spray*, strong reaction; *bromocresol green spray*, weak reaction).

THIN-LAYER: system T1—Rf 0·53 (location reagent *acidified iodoplatinate spray*, positive reaction).

Colour Tests. MICRO: ammonium vanadate test —green → pale brown (*sensitivity:* 1·0 μg); Vitali's test— -/-/faint yellow (*sensitivity:* 1·0 μg).

Crystal Tests. MICRO: *potassium iodide solution* —sheaves of blades (*sensitivity:* 1 in 400); *potassium tri-iodide solution* (2)—sheaves of needles (*sensitivity:* 1 in 100).

Ultraviolet Absorption Spectrum. Cyclomethycaine in 0·1N sulphuric acid, maximum at 261 mμ (E1%, 1cm 535).

Infra-red Absorption Spectrum. Cyclomethycaine (base). Potassium bromide disk. The principal peaks are: A 1247, B 1696, C 1600 (p. 736).

Toxicity. Cyclomethycaine sulphate is used only for local application; it is applied in the form of ointments, creams, and sprays, containing 0·25 to 1%. The maximum safe amount for surface use is stated to be 500 mg or 25 ml of a 2% solution.

CYCLOPENTAMINE *Sympathomimetic*

Synonym: Cyclopentadrin.

1-Cyclopentylmethyl-*N*-methylethylamine

$C_9H_{19}N = 141·3$

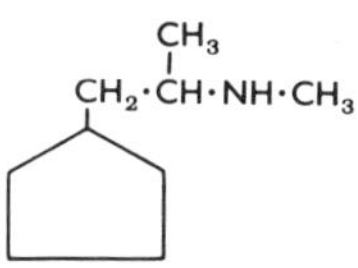

CYCLOPENTAMINE HYDROCHLORIDE

Proprietary Name: Clopane Hydrochloride.

A white crystalline powder. M.p. 113° to 116°.

Solubility. Soluble 1 in 1 of water, 1 in 2 of ethanol, and 1 in 1·5 of chloroform; slightly soluble in ether.

Extraction. Cyclopentamine is extracted by organic solvents from aqueous alkaline solutions.

Chromatography. PAPER: system P1—Rf 0·64 (location reagents: *iodoplatinate spray*, weak reaction; *bromocresol green spray*, weak reaction).

THIN-LAYER: system T1—Rf 0·18, streaking (location reagent *potassium permanganate spray*, positive reaction).

GAS: system G2/120—retention time 0·21 relative to ephedrine.

Crystal Tests. MICRO: *picrolonic acid*—small stout rods or prisms (*sensitivity:* 1 in 200); *trinitrobenzoic acid solution*—irregular rods and prisms, best viewed under polarised light (*sensitivity:* 1 in 200).

Dose. Up to 10 mg intravenously; 25 mg intramuscularly. A 0·5 to 1% solution is used as a nasal decongestant.

CYCLOPENTHIAZIDE *Diuretic*

Synonym: SU 8341.
Proprietary Names: Navidrex; Navidrix.

6-Chloro-3-cyclopentylmethyl-3,4-dihydro-7-sulphamoyl-2*H*-benzo-1,2,4-thiadiazine 1,1-dioxide

$C_{13}H_{18}ClN_3O_4S_2$ = 379·9

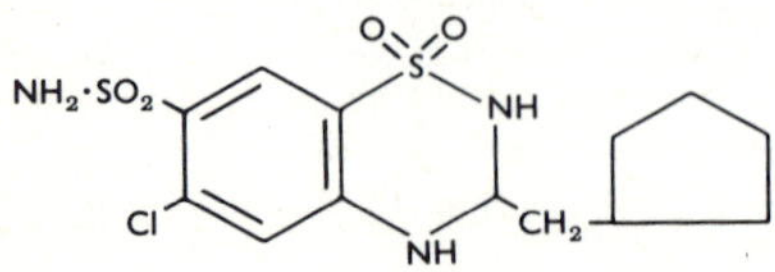

A white crystalline solid. M.p. 235°, with decomposition.
Solubility. Soluble 1 in 12,000 of water, 1 in 125 of ethanol, and 1 in 600 of chloroform.

Extraction. Cyclopenthiazide may be isolated in the A2 fraction (see p. 27). It may be distinguished from the barbiturates by chromatography (see below) and by the presence of additional ultraviolet maxima in the region 270 to 330 mμ.

Chromatography. PAPER: system P16—Rf 0·80 (location under ultraviolet light, absorption; location reagent *sodium naphthaquinone spray*, weak reaction); system RP1b—Rf 0·06 (location as for P16).

Ultraviolet Absorption Spectrum. Cyclopenthiazide in distilled water make alkaline to pH 10 with 2N ammonium hydroxide solution, maxima at 273 mμ (E1%, 1 cm 375) and 320 mμ (E1%, 1 cm 40); cyclopenthiazide in the above solution made acid to pH 2 with sulphuric acid, maxima at 272 mμ (E1%, 1 cm 470) and 315 mμ (E1%, 1 cm 45).

Infra-red Absorption Spectrum. Potassium bromide disk. The principal peaks are: A 1158 or 1598, B 1343 (p. 737).

Quantitative Estimation. Cyclopenthiazide in urine may be determined by extraction with ethyl acetate followed by either direct complexing with chromotropic acid or by alkaline hydrolysis, diazotisation and coupling with *N*-(1-naphthyl)ethylenediamine (Sheppard *et al.*, 1960).

Metabolism. Cyclopenthiazide is a diuretic with similar actions and uses to chlorothiazide (p. 253). Sodium and chloride ions are excreted in approximately equal quantities but there is little loss of bicarbonate. Diuresis is induced in 1 to 2 hours, reaches its maximum after 4 to 8 hours, and lasts about 12 hours. It exerts its diuretic effect by inhibiting reabsorption of sodium in the renal tubules.

Dose. Up to 2 mg daily.

Toxicity. LD50 (intravenous): in mice 232 and in rats 142 mg/kg.

CYCLOPENTOLATE *Parasympatholytic*

2-Dimethylaminoethyl-α-(1-hydroxycyclopentyl)-α-phenylacetate

$C_{17}H_{25}NO_3$ = 291·4

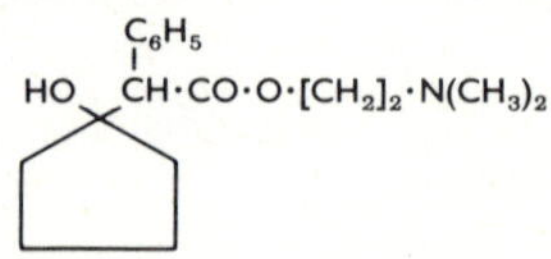

CYCLOPENTOLATE HYDROCHLORIDE

Proprietary Names: Cyclogyl; Mydrilate.

A white crystalline powder. M.p. 137° to 141°.
Solubility. Very soluble in water; soluble 1 in 5 of ethanol; insoluble in ether.

Extraction. Cyclopentolate is extracted by organic solvents from aqueous alkaline solutions.

Chromatography. PAPER: system P1—Rf 0·60 (location reagent *iodoplatinate spray*, strong reaction).

GAS: system G2/225—retention time 1·66 relative to diphenhydramine.

Colour Tests. MICRO: ammonium vanadate test—brown (*sensitivity:* 0·5 μg); Vitali's test—-/-/purple (*sensitivity:* 0·05 μg).

Crystal Tests. MICRO: *gold bromide–hydrochloric acid solution*—stars (*sensitivity:* 1 in 1500); *platinic chloride solution*—plates and prisms (*sensitivity:* 1 in 200).

Metabolism. Cyclopentolate has mydriatic and cycloplegic properties. The maximum effect is produced in 30 to 60 minutes after instillation into the eye and lasts for up to 24 hours. Slight systemic absorption may occur.

Application. Topically, 0·1 ml of a 0·5 to 1% solution to the conjuctiva, up to 6 times daily.

Toxicity. The lethal dose in man is probably in the range 10 to 100 mg/kg.
LD50 (intravenous): in mice 84 mg/kg.

CYCLOSERINE *Antibiotic/Tuberculostatic*

Synonym: D-Cycloserine.
Proprietary Names: Oxamycin; Seromycin.

D-4-Aminoisoxazolid-3-one

$C_3H_6N_2O_2$ = 102·1

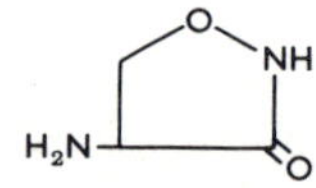

A white or pale yellow, hygroscopic, crystalline powder. Cycloserine is unstable in neutral or acid solutions; it should be protected from moisture and stored at a temperature not exceeding 25°. M.p. 153° to 155°. Specific rotation of a 5% solution in 2N sodium hydroxide, +110° to +114°.
Solubility. Soluble 1 in 10 of water and 1 in 50 of ethanol; slightly soluble in ether and chloroform.

Chromatography. PAPER: system P1—Rf 0·02 (location under ultraviolet light, absorption; location reagents: *iodoplatinate spray*, white; *bromocresol green spray*, weak reaction; *ninhydrin spray*, purple; *potassium permanganate spray*, strong reaction).
THIN-LAYER: system T1—Rf 0·15, streaking (location reagent *acidified iodoplatinate spray*, positive reaction).

Ultraviolet Absorption Spectrum. Cycloserine in 0·1N sulphuric acid, maximum at 220 mμ (E 1%, 1 cm 421).

Infra-red Absorption Spectrum. Potassium bromide disk. The principal peaks are: A 1577, B 1399 or 1526 or 1550 (p. 782).

Quantitative Estimation. Cycloserine may be estimated spectrophotometrically as the blue complex formed when it is treated with sodium nitroprusside pentacyanoferroate (Jones, 1956).

Metabolism. Cycloserine is rapidly absorbed when given orally, absorption taking place from both the stomach and the gastro-intestinal tract. Peak blood-levels occur about 4 hours after an oral dose and accumulation occurs for the first 3 to 4 days. It is widely distributed throughout the body fluids and tissues. In man, 64% of an oral dose is excreted unchanged in the urine in 72 hours, 40 to 50% in the first 12 to 24 hours. The fate of the remaining 36% is not known (Atkins *et al.*, 1965).

Dose. Usually up to 750 mg daily; maximum in 24 hours 1 g.

Toxicity. Experience has shown that toxic effects may be minimised if blood-levels do not exceed 25 to 30 μg/ml.

LD50 (oral): in guinea-pigs more than 2, in mice 5·3, and in rats more than 5 g/kg.

CASE EXAMPLE. A 25-year-old woman was admitted semi-conscious to hospital 11 hours after taking 3 g of cycloserine. Prior to admission she had been on long-term therapy with cycloserine, taking 250 mg on alternate days. On admission the cycloserine plasma level was 9·1 mg%. After 20 hours of peritoneal dialysis the plasma level had fallen to 2·5 mg%, and a total of 520 mg of cycloserine was recovered from the dialysate. The patient recovered (Atkins *et al.*, 1965).

CYCLOTHIAZIDE *Diuretic*

Synonym: MDi 193.
Proprietary Name: Anhydron.

3-(Bicyclo[2,2,1]hept-5-en-2-yl)-6-chloro-3,4-dihydro-7-sulphamoyl-2*H*-benzo-1,2,4-thiadiazine 1,1-dioxide

$C_{14}H_{16}ClN_3O_4S_2 = 389·9$

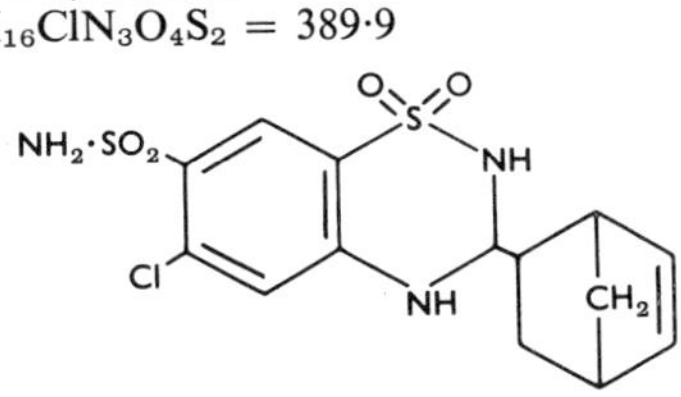

A white crystalline solid. M.p. about 220°.

Solubility. Soluble in hot ethanol; insoluble in ether and chloroform.

Extraction. Cyclothiazide may be isolated in the A2 fraction (see p. 27). It may be distinguished from the barbiturates by chromatography (see below), and by the presence of additional ultraviolet maxima in the region 270 to 330 mμ.

Chromatography. PAPER: system P1—Rf 0·92 (location under ultraviolet light, absorption; location reagent *potassium permanganate spray*, weak reaction); system RP1a—Rf 0·10 (location under ultraviolet light, absorption).
THIN-LAYER: system T1—Rf 0·77 (location reagent *potassium permanganate spray*, positive reaction).

Colour Test. MICRO: ammonium molybdate test—pale grey-blue → faint brown, slowly (*sensitivity:* 1·0 μg).

Ultraviolet Absorption Spectrum. Cyclothiazide in 0·1N sulphuric acid, maxima at 226 mμ (E 1%, 1 cm 228) and 272 mμ (E 1%, 1 cm 130).

Infra-red Absorption Spectrum. Potassium bromide disk. The principal peaks are: A 1596, B 1153 or 1168, C 1337 (p. 782).

Dose. Usually up to 2 mg daily; doses of up to 8 mg daily have been given.

Cyclothiazide is a much more potent diuretic than chlorothiazide (p. 253).

CYCRIMINE *Parasympatholytic*

1-Cyclopentyl-1-phenyl-3-piperidinopropan-1-ol

$C_{19}H_{29}NO = 287·4$

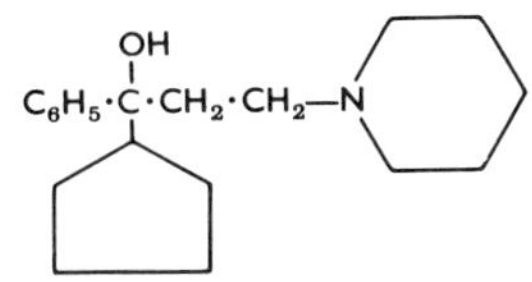

Cycrimine melts at 90° to 96°.

CYCRIMINE HYDROCHLORIDE
Proprietary Name: Pagitane Hydrochloride.

A white solid. M.p. 241° to 244°, with decomposition.
Solubility. Soluble 1 in 175 of water, 1 in 50 of ethanol, and 1 in 35 of chloroform; almost insoluble in ether.

Extraction. Cycrimine is extracted by organic solvents from aqueous alkaline solutions.

Chromatography. PAPER: system P1—Rf 0·83 (location reagents: *iodoplatinate spray*, strong reaction; *bromocresol green spray*, weak reaction); system RP1a—Rf 0·38 (location reagent *iodoplatinate spray*, positive reaction).
THIN-LAYER: system T1—Rf 0·65 (location reagent *acidified iodoplatinate spray*, positive reaction).

Colour Tests. MICRO: sulphuric acid–formaldehyde test—orange → dull red (*sensitivity:* 1·0

μg); ammonium molybdate test—brown (*sensitivity:* 0·5 μg); ammonium vanadate test—red-brown (*sensitivity:* 0·25 μg); Vitali's test— –/brown/brown (*sensitivity:* 1·0 μg).

Crystal Tests. MICRO: *potassium iodide solution*—rosettes of rods (*sensitivity:* 1 in 100); *sodium carbonate solution*—masses of rods (*sensitivity:* 1 in 200).

Ultraviolet Absorption Spectrum. Cycrimine in 0·1N sulphuric acid, maxima at 246·5 mμ (E1%, 1 cm 4), 251 mμ (E1%, 1 cm 5), 256·5 mμ (E1%, 1 cm 6), and 263 mμ (E1%, 1 cm 5): cycrimine hydrochloride in water, maxima at about 251 mμ (E1%, 1 cm about 5·4), about 257 mμ (E1%, 1 cm about 6·2), and about 263 mμ (E1%, 1 cm about 5·0); minima at about 230 mμ, 254 mμ, and 261 mμ.

Infra-red Absorption Spectrum. Cycrimine (base). Potassium bromide disk. The principal peaks are: A 696, B 1117 or 1438, C 755 or 1468 (p. 782).

Dose. Up to 45 mg daily.

Toxicity. The estimated lethal dose in man is in the range 10 to 100 mg/kg.

CYPRENORPHINE *Narcotic Antagonist*

Synonyms: N-Cyclopropylmethyl-19-methylnororvinol; M 285.

N-Cyclopropylmethyl-7,8-dihydro-7α-(1-hydroxy-1-methylethyl)-O^6-methyl-6,14-*endo*-ethenonormorphine

$C_{26}H_{33}NO_4 = 423·6$

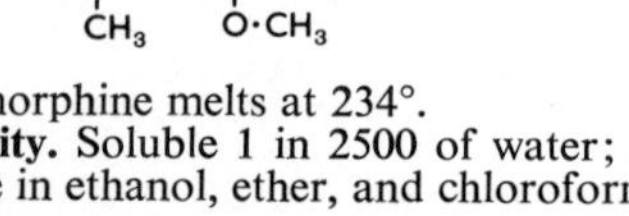

Cyprenorphine melts at 234°.
Solubility. Soluble 1 in 2500 of water; readily soluble in ethanol, ether, and chloroform.

CYPRENORPHINE HYDROCHLORIDE

A white crystalline powder. M.p. 254° to 255°.
Solubility. Soluble 1 in 30 of water and 1 in 16 of ethanol.

Extraction. Cyprenorphine is extracted by organic solvents from aqueous alkaline solutions.

Chromatography. PAPER: system P1—Rf 0·63 (location under ultraviolet light, absorption; location reagents: *iodoplatinate spray*, weak reaction; *Marquis reagent*, blue-grey).
THIN-LAYER: system T1—Rf 0·75 (location reagents: *acidified iodoplatinate spray*, positive reaction; *Marquis reagent*, grey).

Colour Tests. MICRO: sulphuric acid–formaldehyde test—bluish-grey → yellow-brown (*sensitivity:* 0·1 μg); ammonium molybdate test—bluish-purple → blue → dull green (*sensitivity:* 0·1 μg); Vitali's test— –/–/faint orange (*sensitivity:* 1·0 μg).

Crystal Tests. MICRO: *gold cyanide solution*—bunches of rods or prisms (*sensitivity:* 1 in 400).

Ultraviolet Absorption Spectrum. Cyprenorphine in 0·1N hydrochloric acid, maximum at 287 mμ (E1%, 1 cm 36); in 0·1N sodium hydroxide, maximum at 301 mμ (E1%, 1 cm 65).

NOTE. Cyprenorphine is a highly potent narcotic antagonist with actions similar to those of nalorphine. It has been used to antagonise the effects of acetorphine and etorphine.

CYPROHEPTADINE *Antihistamine*

4-(5*H*-Dibenzo[*a,d*]cyclohepten-5-ylidene)-1-methylpiperidine

$C_{21}H_{21}N = 287·4$

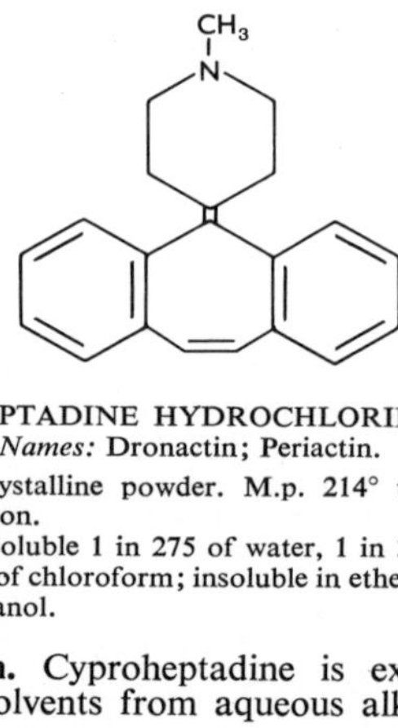

CYPROHEPTADINE HYDROCHLORIDE

Proprietary Names: Dronactin; Periactin.

A white crystalline powder. M.p. 214° to 216°, with decomposition.
Solubility. Soluble 1 in 275 of water, 1 in 35 of ethanol, and 1 in 16 of chloroform; insoluble in ether; soluble 1 in 1·5 of methanol.

Extraction. Cyproheptadine is extracted by organic solvents from aqueous alkaline solutions.

Chromatography. PAPER: system P1—Rf 0·77 (location under ultraviolet light, blue fluorescence; location reagents: *iodoplatinate spray*, weak reaction; *bromocresol green spray*, weak reaction); system RP1a—Rf 0·20 (location under ultraviolet light, absorption; location reagent *iodoplatinate spray*, positive reaction); system RP1b—Rf 0·00.
THIN-LAYER: system T1—Rf 0·50 (location reagent *acidified iodoplatinate spray*, positive reaction).
GAS: system G2/225—retention time 0·94 relative to codeine.

Colour Tests. MICRO: sulphuric acid–formaldehyde test—grey-green (*sensitivity:* 0·5 μg); ammonium molybdate test—green-blue → green (*sensitivity:* 0·1 μg); ammonium vanadate test—purple-brown (*sensitivity:* 0·5 μg).

Crystal Tests. MICRO: *ammonium thiocyanate solution*—branching needles (*sensitivity:* 1 in 1000); *potassium iodide solution*—dense rosettes or fans of rods (*sensitivity:* 1 in 1000).

Ultraviolet Absorption Spectrum. Cyproheptadine in 0·1N sulphuric acid, maxima at 224 mμ (E1%, 1cm 1656) and 285 mμ (E1%, 1cm 355), and an inflexion at 240 mμ.

Infra-red Absorption Spectrum. Cyproheptadine (base). Potassium bromide disk. The principal peaks are: A 749 or 797, B 765, C 776 (p. 782).

Quantitative Estimation. Cyproheptadine may be estimated colorimetrically as the green complex formed with bromocresol green (Adamski, 1965).

Dose. Up to 20 mg daily.

Toxicity. The estimated lethal dose in man is 25 to 250 mg/kg.

NOTE. Cyproheptadine is one of the most potent of the antihistamines and it is effective in smaller doses than promethazine hydrochloride although the effect is of shorter duration.

CYTISINE *Alkaloid*

Synonyms: Baptitoxine; Cytiton; Laburnine; Sophorine; Ulexine.

$C_{11}H_{14}N_2O = 190{\cdot}2$

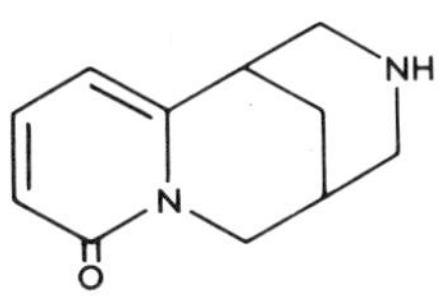

An alkaloid found in all parts of the laburnum, *Laburnum anagyroides* (Leguminosae), particularly in the pods and seeds, and in some other leguminous plants.
Cytisine melts at 152° to 153°.
Solubility. Soluble 1 in 1·3 of water, 1 in 3·5 of ethanol, and 1 in 2 of chloroform.

Extraction. Cytisine is extracted by organic solvents from aqueous alkaline solutions.

Chromatography. PAPER: system P1—Rf 0·03 (location under ultraviolet light, blue fluorescence; location reagent *iodoplatinate spray*, strong reaction).
THIN-LAYER: system T1—Rf 0·32 (location reagent *acidified iodoplatinate spray*, positive reaction).

Crystal Tests. MICRO: *potassium mercuric iodide solution*—fans of needles (*sensitivity:* 1 in 100); *potassium tri-iodide solution* (*1*)—short rods (*sensitivity:* 1 in 3000).

Ultraviolet Absorption Spectrum. Cytisine in methanol, maxima at 235 mμ (E1%, 1cm 263) and 308 mμ (E1%, 1cm 331).

Dose. It has been used similarly to lobeline as a respiratory stimulant in doses up to a maximum of 3 mg daily.

Toxicity. Cytisine is a highly toxic alkaloid which resembles nicotine in its actions. In the horse, the oral lethal dose of laburnum seeds is about 0·5 g/kg and in the dog it is about 6 g/kg. The lethal dose of the pure alkaloid in dogs and cats is 3 to 4 mg/kg.
Numerous cases of poisoning in farm stock have been recorded.

CASE EXAMPLES. Mitchell (1951) has reported 10 cases of laburnum poisoning in children.

DEBRISOQUINE *Antihypertensive*

Synonyms: Isocaramidine; Ro 5-3307/1.

2-Amidino-1,2,3,4-tetrahydroisoquinoline
$C_{10}H_{13}N_3 = 175{\cdot}2$

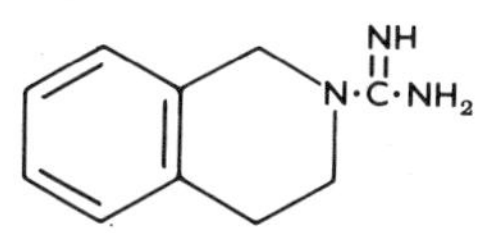

DEBRISOQUINE SULPHATE
Proprietary Name: Declinax.
A white crystalline powder. M.p. 278° to 280°.
Solubility. Soluble in water.

Extraction. Debrisoquine is extracted by organic solvents from aqueous alkaline solutions.

Chromatography. PAPER: system P1—Rf 0·43 (location reagents: *iodoplatinate spray*, strong reaction; *potassium permanganate spray*, weak reaction).
THIN-LAYER: system T1—Rf 0·20, streaking (location reagent *acidified iodoplatinate spray*, positive reaction).

Colour Tests. MICRO: sulphuric acid–formaldehyde test—red-brown (*sensitivity:* 1·0 μg); ammonium molybdate test—(faintly blue) blue (*sensitivity:* 0·5 μg); ammonium vanadate test—(green) faint green (*sensitivity:* 1·0 μg); Vitali's test— -/-/yellow, fading (*sensitivity:* 1·0 μg).

Crystal Tests. MICRO: *picrolonic acid*—small rosettes (*sensitivity:* 1 in 1000); *potassium mercuric iodide solution*—segmented blades, best viewed under polarised light (*sensitivity:* 1 in 1000).

Ultraviolet Absorption Spectrum. Debrisoquine in 0·1N sulphuric acid, maxima at 262 mμ (E1%, 1cm 13) and 270 mμ (E1%, 1cm 10); minima at 235 mμ and 268 mμ.

Infra-red Absorption Spectrum. Debrisoquine (base). Potassium bromide disk. The principal peaks are: A 1615, B 1647, C 1439 or 1451 (p. 782).

Metabolism. Debrisoquine is a hypotensive agent whose action is similar to that of guanethidine sulphate although its effect is of shorter duration. Following oral administration in man, approximately 75% of the dose is excreted in the first 24 hours in the urine; eventually between 80 and 90% of the dose is excreted by this route; about 12 to 15% is excreted in the first 48 hours in the faeces. Debrisoquine is rapidly metabolised; 3 metabolites have been found in the urine, each containing an intact guanidine moiety. The tissue distribution of debrisoquine has been studied in rats, the highest levels being found in the kidneys and liver.

Dose. Usually up to 20 mg daily, increasing very gradually up to a maximum of 150 mg daily.

Toxicity. LD50 (oral): in mice 235 mg/kg and in rats 1·6 g/kg.

DECAMETHONIUM IODIDE

Muscle Relaxant

Synonym: C 10.
Proprietary Names: Eulissin; Syncurine.

Decamethylenebis(trimethylammonium iodide)
$C_{16}H_{38}I_2N_2$ = 512·3

$$[(CH_3)_3N \cdot [CH_2]_{10} \cdot N(CH_3)_3]^{2+} \ 2I^-$$

A white crystalline powder. M.p. 244° to 246°.

Solubility. Soluble 1 in 10 of water and 1 in 50 of ethanol; almost insoluble in ether and chloroform.

Extraction. Decamethonium iodide is a quaternary ammonium compound (see p. 29).

Chromatography. PAPER: system P1—Rf 0·04 (location reagent *iodoplatinate spray*, strong reaction); system RP1a—Rf 0·99 (location reagent *iodoplatinate spray*, positive reaction); system RP1b—Rf 0·96 (location as for RP1a). THIN-LAYER: system T1—Rf 0·00 (location reagent *acidified iodoplatinate spray*, positive reaction).

Crystal Tests. MICRO: *lead iodide solution*—sheaves of oily needles (*sensitivity:* 1 in 1000); *styphnic acid*—bunches of curving blades (*sensitivity:* 1 in 1000).

Ultraviolet Absorption Spectrum. Decamethonium iodide in 0·1N sulphuric acid, maximum at 227 mμ (E1%, 1 cm 584).

Infra-red Absorption Spectrum. Potassium bromide disk. The principal peaks are: A 910 or 1479 or 1627, B 965 (p. 782).

Metabolism. Decamethonium iodide is a depolarising muscle relaxant which has been used to obtain muscular relaxation during surgical operations. It is very poorly absorbed from the gastro-intestinal tract, hence it is administered by intravenous injection. Since it is highly ionised it would be expected to be excreted unchanged but studies in rabbits have disclosed traces of a suspected metabolite appearing more than 2 hours after administration (Christensen, 1966a).
Following the intravenous administration of 90 μg/kg of decamethonium to rabbits, more than 80% of the dose was excreted unchanged in the urine within 24 hours. A varying amount was bound to an unidentified component of urine from which it was liberated by extraction with acid alcohol. Paper chromatographic studies of the urine and of extracts of liver and muscle tissue gave no support to the assumption that decamethonium is metabolised (Christensen, 1967).

Dose. Usually up to 5 mg by slow intravenous injection.

Toxicity. LD50 (oral): in mice, greater than 125 mg/kg.

DEHYDROEMETINE

Anti-amoebic

Synonyms: DHE; Ro 1-9934.

3-Ethyl-1,6,7,11b-tetrahydro-9,10-dimethoxy-2-(1,2,3,4-tetrahydro-6,7-dimethoxyisoquinol-1-ylmethyl)-4*H*-benzo[*a*]quinolizine
$C_{29}H_{38}N_2O_4$ = 478·6

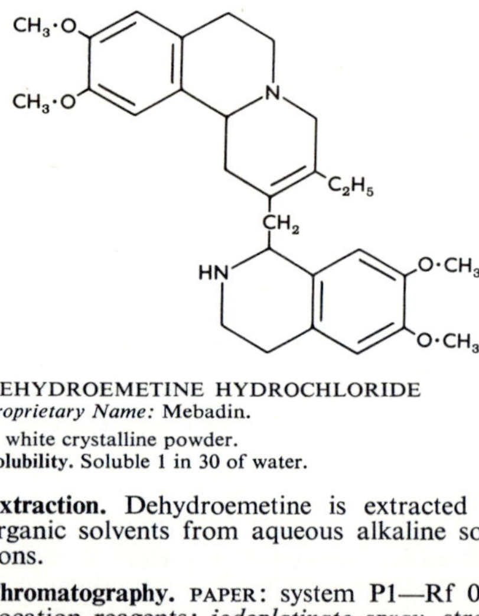

DEHYDROEMETINE HYDROCHLORIDE
Proprietary Name: Mebadin.

A white crystalline powder.
Solubility. Soluble 1 in 30 of water.

Extraction. Dehydroemetine is extracted by organic solvents from aqueous alkaline solutions.

Chromatography. PAPER: system P1—Rf 0·11 (location reagents: *iodoplatinate spray*, strong reaction; *potassium permanganate spray*, weak reaction).
THIN-LAYER: system T1—Rf 0·36 (location reagent *acidified iodoplatinate spray*, positive reaction).

Colour Tests. MICRO: sulphuric acid–formaldehyde test—faint orange (*sensitivity:* 1·0 μg); ammonium molybdate test—dull green → blue (*sensitivity:* 0·1 μg); Vitali's test—pale yellow/brown/brown (*sensitivity:* 0·5 μg).

Crystal Test. MICRO: *gold cyanide solution*—dense rosettes and rosettes of needles (*sensitivity:* 1 in 1000).

Ultraviolet Absorption Spectrum. Dehydroemetine in ethanol, maxima at 232 mμ (E1%, 1 cm 316) and 284 mμ (E1%, 1 cm 151).

Metabolism. Dehydroemetine is a potent amoebicide which is used similarly to emetine hydrochloride in the treatment of amoebiasis. It is quickly eliminated from the body, thus reducing the risk of cumulative toxicity which is a hazard of emetine therapy.

Dose. Up to 2 mg/kg daily.

DEMECOLCINE *Antimitotic*

Synonyms: Colchamine; Desacetylmethylcolchicine; Omaine.
Proprietary Name: Colcemid.

Deacetylmethylcolchicine
$C_{21}H_{25}NO_5 = 371{\cdot}4$

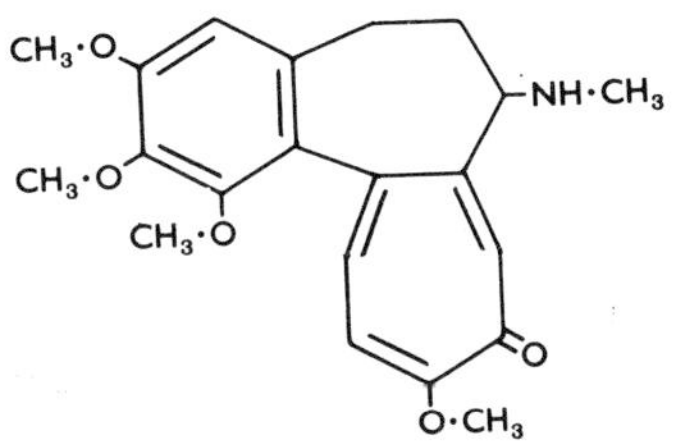

Demecolcine is an alkaloid isolated from the corms of the meadow saffron, *Colchicum autumnale* (Liliaceae).

Pale yellow crystals. M.p. 186°.
Solubility. Soluble 1 in 50 of water; soluble in ethanol, ether, and chloroform.

Extraction. Demecolcine is extracted by organic solvents from aqueous alkaline solutions.

Chromatography. PAPER: system P1—Rf 0·29 (location under ultraviolet light, pale yellow fluorescence).
THIN-LAYER: system T1—Rf 0·56 (location reagent p-*dimethylaminobenzaldehyde spray*, positive reaction).

Colour Tests. MICRO: ammonium molybdate test—green → yellow (*sensitivity:* 0·05 μg); ammonium vanadate test—brown-purple → yellow (*sensitivity:* 0·025 μg); Vitali's test—yellow → purple/brown/red-violet (*sensitivity:* 0·05 μg).

Crystal Tests. MICRO: *gold chloride solution*—feathery rosettes (*sensitivity:* 1 in 1000); *platinic chloride solution*—dense rosettes (*sensitivity:* 1 in 200).

Infra-red Absorption Spectrum. Potassium bromide disk. The principal peaks are: A 1241 or 1562, B 1582, C 1090 (p. 737).

Dose. Up to 10 mg daily.

DEMETHYLCHLORTETRACYCLINE *Antibiotic*

Synonym: DMCT.

7-Chloro-4-dimethylamino-1,4,4a,5,5a,6,11,12a-octahydro-3,6,10,12,12a-pentahydroxy-1,11-dioxonaphthacene-2-carboxyamide
$C_{21}H_{21}ClN_2O_8 = 464{\cdot}9$

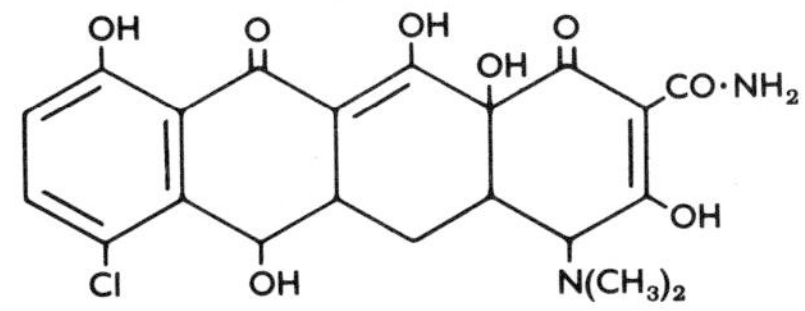

DEMETHYLCHLORTETRACYCLINE HYDROCHLORIDE
Proprietary Names: Declomycin; Ledermycin.

A yellow crystalline amphoteric powder.
Solubility. Soluble 1 in 30 of water, 1 in 45 of ethanol, and 1 in 1000 of chloroform; almost insoluble in ether; soluble 1 in 1200 of acetone.

Extraction. Demethylchlortetracycline is extracted by organic solvents from aqueous alkaline solutions.

Chromatography. PAPER: system P1—Rf 0·32 (location under ultraviolet light, orange fluorescence; location reagents: *Dragendorff spray*, weak reaction; *potassium permanganate spray*, weak reaction).
A paper chromatographic method of separation of tetracycline derivatives in blood and urine is described by Addison and Clark (1963).
THIN-LAYER: system T1—Rf 0·05, streaking (location under ultraviolet light, orange fluorescence; location reagent *potassium permanganate spray*, positive reaction).
Ascione *et al.* (1967) describe a thin-layer method for the separation of tetracyclines and their derivatives.

Colour Tests. MICRO: sulphuric acid–formaldehyde test—(faint yellow) yellow → dull green (*sensitivity:* 1·0 μg); ammonium molybdate test—(faint yellow) purple-brown → yellow (*sensitivity:* 1·0 μg); ammonium vanadate test —(faint yellow) purple-brown → yellow (*sensitivity:* 1·0 μg); sulphuric acid test—purple → yellow; Vitali's test—(faint yellow) faint yellow/yellow/red (*sensitivity:* 1·0 μg).

Ultraviolet Absorption Spectrum. Demethylchlortetracycline in water, maximum at 385 mμ (E1%, 1 cm about 369); in 0·1N sulphuric acid, maxima at 227 mμ (E1%, 1 cm 517), 268 mμ (E1%, 1 cm 517), and 368 mμ (E1%, 1 cm 348).

Infra-red Absorption Spectrum. Demethylchlortetracycline (base). Potassium bromide disk. The principal peaks are: A 1616, B 1573, C 1660 (p. 783).

Metabolism. Demethylchlortetracycline is incompletely and irregularly absorbed from the gastro-intestinal tract. Maximum serum levels are attained within 3 to 6 hours of oral administration; following a dose of 150 mg, peak serum levels have been reported to range from 0·025 to 0·175 mg/ml. Demethylchlortetracycline is excreted in the urine more slowly than

the other tetracyclines; it is concentrated in the liver and some is excreted in the bile. Six hours after dogs were given 5 consecutive doses of 15 mg/kg of demethylchlortetracycline by stomach tube the following drug levels were found: heart, 0·33 mg%; kidney, 1·17 mg%; liver, 0·77 mg%; lung, 0·24 mg%; muscle, 0·24 to 0·29 mg%; serum, 0·22 mg% (von Wittenau and Delahunt, 1966).
Demethylchlortetracycline may cause photosensitisation of parts of the skin exposed to strong sunlight.

Dose. Up to 1·8 g daily.

Toxicity. Liver damage may develop where serum levels exceed 1·6 mg%.

DEMETON-O *Pesticide*

Other Name: Mercaptofos.
A mixture of demeton-O and demeton-S is known by the common name demeton and by the proprietary name Systox.

Diethyl 2-ethylthioethyl phosphorothionate
$C_8H_{19}O_3PS_2 = 258{\cdot}3$

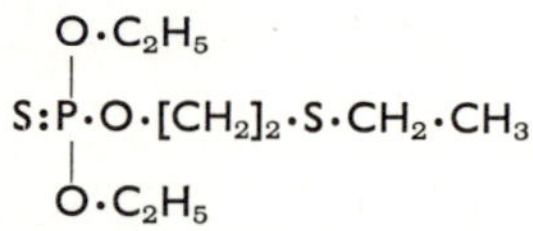

An oily liquid. B.p. 128° at 1·2 mm Hg.

DEMETON-O-METHYL
Other Names: SPOC Compound; Thionate.
A mixture of demeton-O-methyl and demeton-S-methyl is known by the common name demeton-methyl and by the proprietary name Metasystox.
A yellowish-brown oil. B.p. 74° at 0·15 mm Hg. Refractive index 1·5063.
Solubility. Soluble 1 in about 3000 of water. In solution or upon storage, 30% of demeton-O-methyl is transformed into demeton-S-methyl.

Extraction. Demeton-O and demeton-O-methyl are extracted by organic solvents from aqueous acid or alkaline solutions.

Chromatography. THIN-LAYER, for demeton-O: system T16—Rf 0·60 (location reagent *bromophenol blue spray* followed by *5% aqueous acetic acid spray*, mauve).

Quantitative Estimation. Laws and Webley (1959) have described a method of estimation of demeton-methyl in plant material involving column chromatography followed by spectrophotometric determination of the phosphorus in the form of the molybdenum blue complex.

Metabolism. Demeton-O and demeton-O-methyl are very readily absorbed by all routes; they have a particularly high percutaneous toxicity. They exert a direct inhibitory action on cholinesterase and are rapidly hydrolysed in the tissues.

Toxicity. The estimated acute lethal dose in man is 5 g but exposure to as little as 300 mg daily may be dangerous.

DEMETON-S *Pesticide*

Other Names: Disystox; Isosystox; Mercaptofos teolovy; Thiolosystox.
A mixture of demeton-S and demeton-O is known by the common name demeton and by the proprietary name Systox.

Diethyl *S*-2-ethylthioethyl phosphorothiolate
$C_8H_{19}O_3PS_2 = 258{\cdot}3$

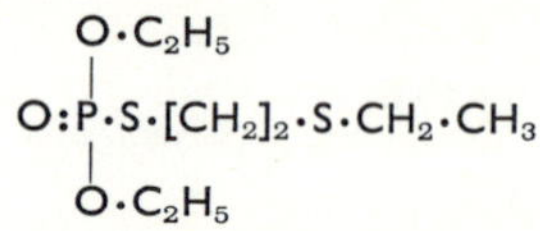

Demeton-S boils at 132° to 134° at 2 mm Hg.

DEMETON-S-METHYL.
Other Names: Metaisosystox; OPSC Compound; Thiolate.
A mixture of demeton-S-methyl and demeton-O-methyl is known by the common name demeton-methyl and by the proprietary name Metasystox.
A yellow oil of low viscosity with an unpleasant odour. B.p. 89° at 0·15 mm Hg. Refractive index 1·5065.
Solubility. Soluble 1 in 300 of water. In solution or upon storage demeton-S-methyl is oxidised to the sulphoxide and the sulphone.

Extraction. Demeton-S is extracted by organic solvents from aqueous acid or alkaline solutions.

Chromatography. THIN-LAYER, for demeton-S: system T16—Rf 0·19 (location reagent *bromophenol blue spray* followed by *5% aqueous acetic acid spray*, blue).

Quantitative Estimation. See under Demeton-O.

Metabolism. Demeton-S and demeton-S-methyl are very readily absorbed by all routes; they have a particularly high percutaneous toxicity. They exert a direct inhibitory action on cholinesterase and are rapidly hydrolysed in the tissues. They are metabolised to the corresponding sulphoxide and sulphone.

Toxicity. The estimated acute lethal dose in man is 5 g but exposure to as little as 300 mg daily may be dangerous.

DENATONIUM BENZOATE *Denaturant for Alcohol*

Proprietary Name: Bitrex.

Benzyldiethyl(2,6-xylylcarbamoylmethyl)ammonium benzoate
$C_{28}H_{34}N_2O_3 = 446{\cdot}6$

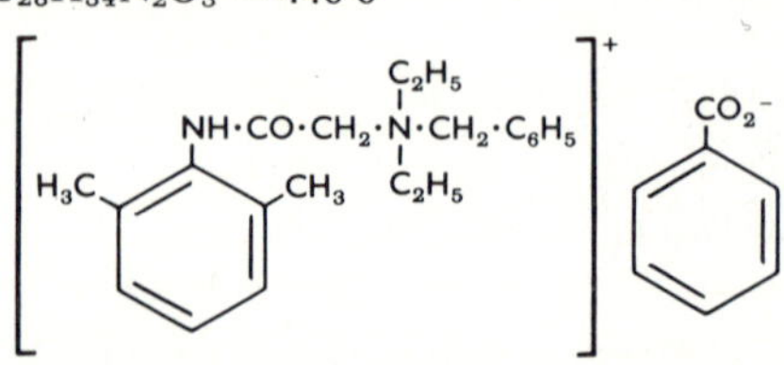

A white crystalline powder.
Solubility. Soluble 1 in 4 of water and 1 in 2 of ethanol.

Extraction. Denatonium benzoate is a quaternary ammonium compound (see p. 29).

Chromatography. PAPER: system P1—Rf 0·70 (location reagents: *iodoplatinate spray*, weak reaction; *Dragendorff spray*, weak reaction); system RP1a—Rf 0·84 (location reagent *iodoplatinate spray*, positive reaction); system RP1b—Rf 0·00.

THIN-LAYER: system T1—Rf 0·10 (location reagent *acidified iodoplatinate spray*, positive reaction).

Colour Test. MICRO: ammonium vanadate test —purple, fading (*sensitivity:* 0·5 µg).

Crystal Tests. MICRO: *gold cyanide solution*—long prisms (*sensitivity:* 1 in 1000); *lead iodide solution*—burrs (*sensitivity:* 1 in 1000).

Ultraviolet Absorption Spectrum. Denatonium benzoate in ethanol, maxima at 263·5 mµ (E1%, 1cm 44) and 269 mµ (E1%, 1cm 40).

Infra-red Absorption Spectrum. Potassium bromide disk. The principal peaks are: A 1550, B 1596, C 1370 or 1407 or 1680 (p. 783).

DEOXYCORTONE — *Corticosteroid*

Synonyms: Decortone; Deoxycorticosterone; Desoxycorticosterone; Desoxycortone; 21-Hydroxyprogesterone.

21-Hydroxypregn-4-ene-3,20-dione

$C_{21}H_{30}O_3$ = 330·5

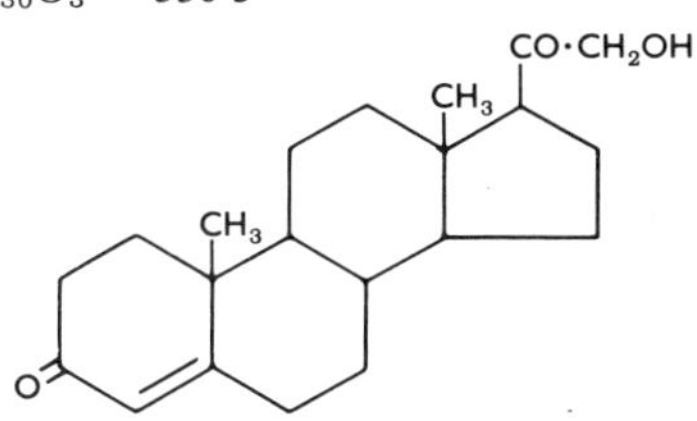

DEOXYCORTONE ACETATE

Proprietary Names: DOCA; Decortacete; Percorten; Syncortyl.

Colourless crystals, or a white crystalline powder. M.p. 158° to 161°. Specific rotation of a 1% solution in ethanol, +179° to +184°.

Solubility. Almost insoluble in water; soluble 1 in 50 of ethanol, 1 in 170 of ether, 1 in 1·5 of chloroform, and 1 in 30 of acetone.

DEOXYCORTONE PIVALATE

Synonym: Deoxycortone Trimethylacetate.

Proprietary Name: Percorten M Crystules.

A white crystalline powder. M.p. 198° to 204°. Specific rotation of a 1% solution in dioxan, +153° to +161°.

Solubility. Almost insoluble in water; soluble 1 in 350 of ethanol and 1 in 160 of methanol; slightly soluble in ether.

Extraction. Deoxycortone is extracted from neutral solutions with freshly distilled ethyl acetate.

Chromatography. THIN-LAYER, for deoxycortone acetate: system T18—Rf 1·92 (location reagent *DPST spray*); for deoxycortone pivalate: system T18—Rf 2·22 (location reagent *DPST spray*).

Ultraviolet Absorption Spectrum. Deoxycortone acetate in ethanol, maximum at about 240 mµ (E1%, 1cm 440). Deoxycortone pivalate in ethanol, maximum at about 240 mµ (E1%, 1cm 405).

Metabolism. Deoxycortone is a mineralocorticoid secreted in small amounts by the adrenal cortex. It has a pronounced effect on electrolyte balance but no significant glucocorticoid action. It is readily absorbed after parenteral administration or when applied to mucous membranes. It is excreted in the urine partly as pregnane-3α,20α-diol. There is no increase in urinary 17-ketosteroids when small therapeutic doses are administered but large doses are converted to 17-ketosteroids.

Toxicity. The usual therapeutic dose is 2 to 10 mg daily, or 100 to 400 mg as a total implantation dose every 4 to 5 months. The therapeutic and toxic doses are often closely akin.

DEPTROPINE — *Antihistamine*

Synonyms: BS 6987; Dibenzheptropine.

3-(10,11-Dihydro-5*H*-dibenzo[*a,d*]cyclohepten-5-yloxy)tropane

$C_{23}H_{27}NO$ = 333·5

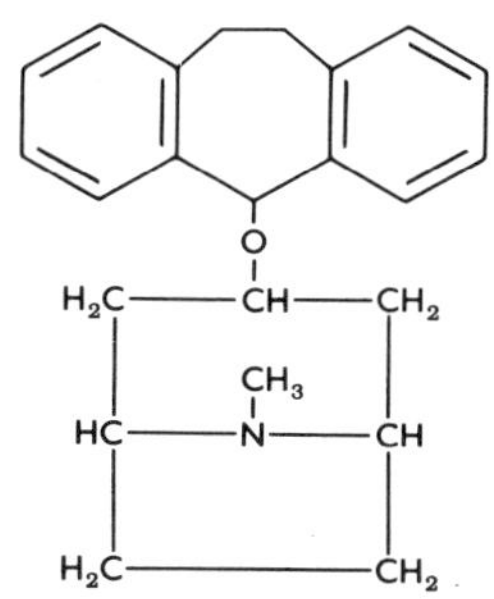

DEPTROPINE CITRATE

Proprietary Names: Brontina; Brontine.

A white to colourless microcrystalline powder.

Solubility. Very slightly soluble in water and ethanol; insoluble in ether and chloroform.

Extraction. Deptropine is extracted by organic solvents from aqueous alkaline solutions.

Chromatography. THIN-LAYER: system T1—Rf 0·69 (location reagent *potassium permanganate spray*, positive reaction).

GAS: system G2/225—retention time 1·93 relative to codeine.

Colour Tests. MICRO: sulphuric acid–formaldehyde test—yellow (*sensitivity:* 0·1 µg); ammonium molybdate test—yellow (*sensitivity:* 0·1 µg); ammonium vanadate test—(green) yellow (*sensitivity:* 0·1 µg).

Crystal Tests. MICRO: *platinic iodide solution*—small rods which vanish (*sensitivity:* 1 in 200); *potassium bismuth iodide solution*—clusters of stout rods (*sensitivity:* 1 in 200).

Metabolism. Deptropine is well absorbed after oral administration and appears to reach the tissues in active form.

Dose. Up to 4 mg.

Toxicity. Deptropine is a much more potent antihistamine than promethazine (p. 518). It has marked anticholinergic and antiserotonin properties.

LD50 (oral): in mice 300, in rats 445, and in dogs 75 mg/kg.

DEQUALINIUM CHLORIDE *Antibacterial*

Proprietary Name: Dequadin.

Decamethylenebis(4-aminoquinaldinium chloride)

$C_{30}H_{40}Cl_2N_4 = 527{\cdot}6$

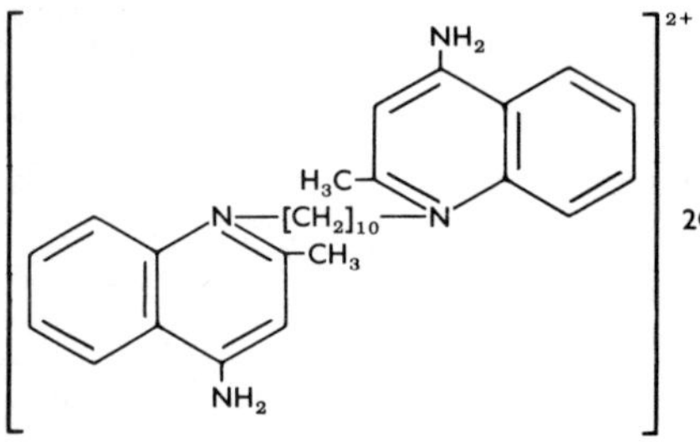

A creamy-white powder. M.p. about 315°, with decomposition.

Solubility. Slightly soluble in water but soluble 1 in 30 of boiling water; soluble 1 in 60 of methanol and 1 in 200 of propylene glycol.

DEQUALINIUM ACETATE

A white, slightly hygroscopic powder. M.p. about 280°, with decomposition.

Solubility. Soluble 1 in 2 of water and 1 in 12 of ethanol.

Extraction. The dequalinium salts are quaternary ammonium compounds (see p. 29).

Chromatography. PAPER: system P1—Rf 0·27 (location under ultraviolet light, bright blue fluorescence; location reagents: *iodoplatinate spray*, weak reaction; *bromocresol green spray*, weak reaction).

THIN-LAYER: system T1—Rf 0·03 (location reagent *acidified iodoplatinate spray*, positive reaction).

Colour Test. MICRO: Vitali's test—pale yellow/ pale yellow/ pale yellow (*sensitivity:* 1·0 μg).

Crystal Tests. MICRO: *picric acid*—small oily needles (*sensitivity:* 1 in 100); *potassium bismuth iodide solution*—oily branching needles (*sensitivity:* 1 in 100).

Ultraviolet Absorption Spectrum. Dequalinium salts in water, maxima at 240 mμ (E1%, 1 cm 890), 326 mμ (E1%, 1 cm 510), and 335 mμ (E1%, 1 cm 425).

Infra-red Absorption Spectrum. Potassium bromide disk. The principal peaks are: A 1605, B 1652, C 764 (p. 737).

Toxicity. The lethal dose in man is estimated to be between 1 and 3 mg. Prolonged or frequently repeated application of dermatological preparations containing dequalinium may on rare occasions lead to the development of necrotic lesions.

DESERPIDINE *Antihypertensive*

Synonyms: Canescine; 11-Demethoxyreserpine.
Proprietary Name: Harmonyl.

Methyl 11-demethoxy-18-(3,4,5-trimethoxybenzoyl)reserpate

$C_{32}H_{38}N_2O_8 = 578{\cdot}7$

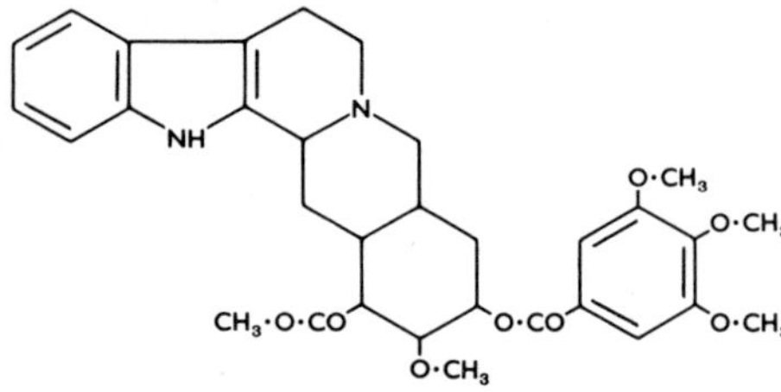

An ester alkaloid isolated from *Rauwolfia canescens* (Apocynaceae).

It occurs as needles or prisms. M.p. 230° to 234°, with decomposition.

Solubility. Insoluble in water; soluble in hot ethanol and chloroform.

Extraction. Deserpidine is extracted by organic solvents from aqueous alkaline solutions.

Chromatography. PAPER: system P1—Rf 0·72 (location under ultraviolet light, pale blue fluorescence; location reagents: *iodoplatinate spray*, weak reaction; *bromocresol green spray*, weak reaction).

THIN-LAYER: system T1—Rf 0·75 (location reagent *acidified iodoplatinate spray*, positive reaction).

Colour Tests. MICRO: sulphuric acid–formaldehyde test—grey-green (*sensitivity:* 0·5 μg); ammonium molybdate test—blue (*sensitivity:* 0·5 μg); ammonium vanadate test—blue → green; Vitali's test—brown/brown/purple-brown (*sensitivity:* 1·0 μg).

Crystal Tests. MICRO: *potassium chromate solution*—irregular smudge rosettes (*sensitivity:* 1 in 400); *zinc chloride solution*—bunches of irregular plates (*sensitivity:* 1 in 400).

Ultraviolet Absorption Spectrum. Deserpidine in ethanol, maxima at 220 mμ (E1%, 1 cm 990) and 272 mμ (E1%, 1 cm 300); minimum at 243 mμ; in methanol, maxima at 216 mμ, 271 mμ, and 289 mμ.

Infra-red Absorption Spectrum. Potassium bromide disk. The principal peaks are: A 1121 or 1220, B 1330 (p. 737).

Dose. Up to 3 mg daily has been given.

Toxicity. LD50 (oral): in mice about 500 mg/kg.

DESFERRIOXAMINE *Chelating Agent*

Synonyms: Ba-33112; DFM; DFOM; Deferoxamine.

30 - Amino - 3,14,25 - trihydroxy - 3,9,14,20,25- penta - azatriacontane - 2,10,13,21,24 - pentaone

$C_{25}H_{48}N_6O_8 = 560{\cdot}7$

DESFERRIOXAMINE MESYLATE

Synonyms: Desferrioxamine B Mesylate; Desferrioxamine Methanesulphonate.

Proprietary Name: Desferal.

A white crystalline powder.

Solubility. Soluble 1 in 4 of water.

Chromatography. PAPER: system P1—Rf 0·29 (location reagents: *iodine vapour*, weak reaction; *potassium permanganate spray*, strong reaction).

THIN-LAYER: system T1—Rf 0·08, streaking (location reagent *potassium permanganate spray*, positive reaction).

Colour Tests. MICRO: ammonium molybdate test—orange (*sensitivity:* 1·0 μg); ammonium vanadate test—(grey) blue → faint purple (*sensitivity:* 0·1 μg).

Crystal Tests. MICRO: *gold bromide solution*—tablets, forming overnight (*sensitivity:* 1 in 1000); *picrolonic acid*—oily crystals, forming overnight, best viewed under polarised light (*sensitivity:* 1 in 1000).

Ultraviolet Absorption Spectrum. Desferrioxamine in 0·1N sulphuric acid, maximum at 208·5 mμ (E1%, 1cm 313).

Infra-red Absorption Spectrum. Desferrioxamine (base). Potassium bromide disk. The principal peaks are: A 1628, B 1195, C 1455 or 1562 (p. 783).

Metabolism. Desferrioxamine is an iron chelating agent which is used in the treatment of acute iron poisoning and in conditions associated with excessive iron storage in the tissues. It is poorly absorbed from the gastro-intestinal tract and is therefore usually given by injection. It specifically chelates any ferric iron present in the gastro-intestinal tract, blood, and tissues to form an octahedral complex, ferrioxamine, which is readily excreted by the kidneys. Theoretically, 100 mg of desferrioxamine can chelate approximately 8·5 mg of iron; thus 5 g can chelate the iron contained in about 10 tablets of ferrous sulphate or ferrous gluconate.

Dose. In acute iron poisoning desferrioxamine is administered in doses of 5 g orally or by stomach tube, 2 g intramuscularly, and 15 mg/kg by slow intravenous infusion.

Toxicity. LD50 (oral): in mice greater than 3 and in rats greater than 1 g/kg.

DESIPRAMINE *Antidepressant*

Synonyms: Desmethylimipramine; DMI; GMI; G 35020; JB 8181.

10,11-Dihydro-5-(3-methylaminopropyl)-5*H*-dibenz[*b*,*f*]azepine

$C_{18}H_{22}N_2 = 266{\cdot}4$

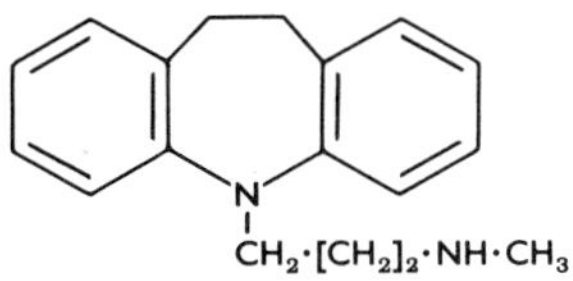

DESIPRAMINE HYDROCHLORIDE

Proprietary Names: Norpramin; Pertofran.

A white crystalline powder. M.p. 214° to 218°.

Solubility. Soluble 1 in 20 of water, 1 in 20 of ethanol, and 1 in 4 of chloroform; very slightly soluble in ether.

Screening Test. See Screening Tests, p. 13.

Extraction. Desipramine may be isolated in the D2 fraction (see p. 27).

Chromatography. PAPER: system P1—Rf 0·65 (location under ultraviolet light, dark blue fluorescence; location reagents: *iodoplatinate spray*, strong reaction; *bromocresol green spray*, weak reaction); system RP1a—Rf 0·70 (location under ultraviolet light, absorption); system RP1b—Rf 0·06 (location under ultraviolet light, absorption; location reagent *iodoplatinate spray*, positive reaction).

THIN-LAYER: system T1—Rf 0·24 (location reagent *acidified iodoplatinate spray*, positive reaction).

GAS: system G2/225—retention time 0·68 relative to codeine.

Colour Tests. MICRO: ammonium molybdate test—blue (*sensitivity:* 0·25 μg); ammonium vanadate test—yellow (blue rim) → blue (*sensitivity:* 0·1 μg); Vitali's test—dark green/light brown/light brown (*sensitivity:* 0·1 μg).

Crystal Tests. MICRO: *gold cyanide solution*—feathery crystals (*sensitivity:* 1 in 1000); *potassium chromate solution*—serrated blades (*sensitivity:* 1 in 1000).

Ultraviolet Absorption Spectrum. Desipramine in 0·1N sulphuric acid, maxima at 251 mμ (E1%, 1cm 363) and about 275 mμ (E1%, 1cm 294).

Infra-red Absorption Spectrum. Desipramine (base). Potassium chloride disk. The principal peaks are: A 1482, B 747, C 757 or 1228 (p. 783).

Metabolism. Desipramine is a primary active metabolite of imipramine and possesses similar but more rapid antidepressant properties. Desipramine does not inhibit monoamine oxidase activity in the brain. In a group of patients whose dosage was gradually increased to 150 mg per day for 3 weeks, the range of plasma levels found during this period was 0·59 to 1·38 μg/ml, the levels in each patient remaining fairly constant (Yates *et al.*, 1963).

Dose. Up to 200 mg daily.

Toxicity. The death of a two-year-old child after swallowing about 50 mg of desipramine has been reported but adults have survived the ingestion of 1·15 g and 2·5 g.

CASE EXAMPLE. In a fatal case involving the ingestion of desipramine (amount not stated) the following post-mortem drug-levels were found: blood, 0·3 mg%; kidney, 3·5 mg%; liver, 2·7 mg%; stomach contents, a total of 9·6 mg. Ethchlorvynol was also thought to have been involved but it was not detected (Wilson, 1966).

DESLANOSIDE *Cardiac Glycoside*

Synonyms: Desacetyl-lanatoside C; Deacetyl-lanatoside C.

Proprietary Name: Cedilanid.

NOTE. The name Cedilanid is applied also to preparations of lanatoside C (p. 388).

3-Glucosyltridigitoxoside of digoxigenin

$C_{47}H_{74}O_{19} = 943{\cdot}1$

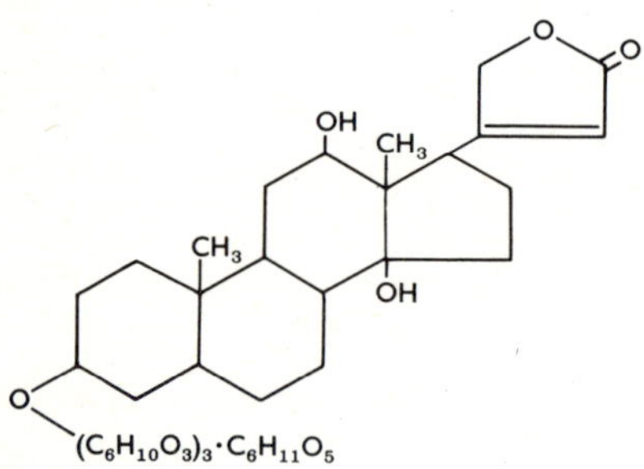

White hygroscopic crystals or crystalline powder. It melts indistinctly between 220° and 235°. It is more stable in solution than lanatoside C.

Solubility. Very slightly soluble in water and chloroform; soluble 1 in 300 of ethanol and 1 in 200 of methanol.

Extraction. Deslanoside may be isolated by continuous extraction under reduced pressure with ethanol (see p. 29).

Chromatography. THIN-LAYER: system T14—Rf 0·27 (location reagents: *perchloric acid spray*, followed by examination under ultraviolet light, blue fluorescence; p-*anisaldehyde spray*, blue).

Colour Test. Dissolve 2 to 3 mg in 5 ml of a solution containing 0·5 ml of 9% ferric chloride solution and 100 ml of glacial acetic acid; underlay with 5 ml of sulphuric acid—intense blue in the glacial acetic acid layer and a brown ring free from red at the junction of the two liquids (see also lanatoside C, p. 388).

Ultraviolet Absorption Spectrum. Deslanoside in *sulphuric acid*, maxima at 235 mμ (E1%, 1 cm 215), 325 mμ (E1%, 1 cm 120), 390 mμ (E1%, 1 cm 260), and 480 mμ (E1%, 1 cm 180); minima at 265 mμ, 340 mμ, and 440 mμ.

Dose. Deslanoside is more stable in solution than lanatoside C (p. 388) and is the form of the glycoside generally administered intravenously, the initial dose being 1·2 to 1·6 mg and the maintenance dose 0·2 to 0·6 mg.

DESOMORPHINE *Narcotic Analgesic*

Synonym: Dihydrodesoxymorphine.

4,5-Epoxy-3-hydroxy-*N*-methylmorphinan

$C_{17}H_{21}NO_2 = 271{\cdot}4$

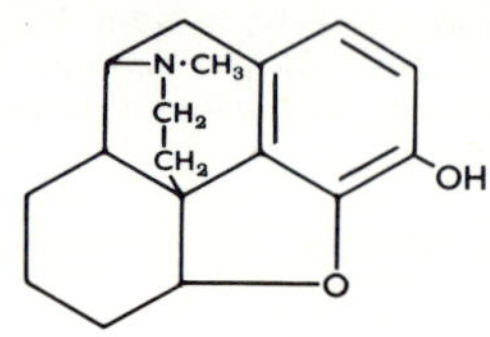

Desomorphine forms rectangular plates from an acetone:water mixture. The anhydrous base melts at 189°.

Solubility. Soluble in acetone and ethyl acetate.

DESOMORPHINE HYDROBROMIDE

Proprietary Name: Permonid.

Extraction. Desomorphine may be isolated in the D3 fraction (see p. 27).

Chromatography. PAPER: system P1—Rf 0·35 (location under ultraviolet light, absorption; location reagents: *iodoplatinate spray*, strong reaction; *bromocresol green spray*, weak reaction); system RP1a—Rf 0·87 (location reagent *iodoplatinate spray*, positive reaction); system RP1b—Rf 0·22 (location as for RP1a).

THIN-LAYER: system T1—Rf 0·29 (location reagent *acidified iodoplatinate spray*, positive reaction).

GAS: system G2/225—retention time 0·78 relative to codeine; system G4—retention time 0·66 relative to codeine.

Colour Tests. MICRO: sulphuric acid–formaldehyde test—purple (*sensitivity:* 0·1 μg); ammonium molybdate test—deep purple → blue → green → yellow (*sensitivity:* 0·1 μg); ammonium vanadate test—grey-purple (*sensitivity:* 1·0 μg); Vitali's test—yellow/yellow/orange.

Crystal Test. MICRO: *mercuric chloride solution*—plates, best viewed under polarised light (*sensitivity:* 1 in 200).

Ultraviolet Absorption Spectrum. Desomorphine in 0·1N sulphuric acid, maximum at 277 mμ (E1%, 1 cm 50·5), and inflexions at about 225 mμ and about 282 mμ.

Toxicity. The estimated minimum lethal dose in man is in the region of 200 mg. Desomorphine has been reported to have greater addiction-producing properties than morphine.

DEXAMETHASONE *Corticosteroid*

Synonym: 9α-Fluoro-16α-methylprednisolone.
Proprietary Names: Decadron; DexaCortisyl; Oradexon.

9α-Fluoro-11β,17α,21-trihydroxy-16α-methylpregna-1,4-diene-3,20-dione

$C_{22}H_{29}FO_5 = 392{\cdot}5$

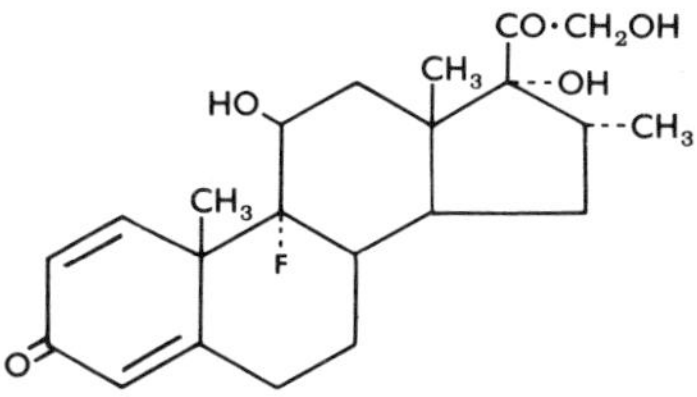

White to light tan crystals or crystalline powder. M.p. about 255°, with decomposition. Specific rotation of a 1% solution in dioxan, +75° to +80°.

Solubility. Almost insoluble in water; soluble 1 in 42 of ethanol and 1 in 165 of chloroform; very slightly soluble in ether; soluble in acetone.

DEXAMETHASONE ACETATE
21 - Acetoxy - 9α - fluoro - 11β,17α - dihydroxy - 16α - methylpregna-1,4-diene-3,20-dione
Synonym: Dexamethasone 21-Acetate.

A white powder. M.p. about 225°, with decomposition. Specific rotation of a 1% solution in dioxan, +82° to +88°.

Solubility. Almost insoluble in water; soluble 1 in 40 of ethanol, 1 in 25 of dehydrated ethanol, 1 in 1000 of ether, and 1 in 33 of chloroform.

DEXAMETHASONE BUTYLACETATE
Synonyms: Dexamethasone TBA; Dexamethasone Tertiary Butyl Acetate.
Proprietary Name: Decadron TBA.

Solubility. Sparingly soluble in water; soluble in ethanol and acetone.

DEXAMETHASONE SODIUM PHOSPHATE
Synonyms: Dexamethasone Phosphate Sodium; Dexamethasone 21-(Disodium Phosphate); Sodium Dexamethasone Phosphate; Sodium 9α-fluoro-16α-methylprednisolone-21-phosphate.
Proprietary Names: Decadron Phosphate Injection; Oradexon Injection.

A white or slightly yellow, crystalline, very hygroscopic powder. Specific rotation of 1% solution, +74° to +82°.
Solubility. Soluble 1 in 2 of water; slightly soluble in ethanol; insoluble in ether and chloroform.

Extraction. Dexamethasone is extracted from neutral solutions with freshly distilled ethyl acetate.

Chromatography. PAPER, for dexamethasone: system P13—Rf 0·21 (location reagent *DPST solution*, violet on yellow); for dexamethasone acetate: system P14—Rf 0·60 (location reagent *DPST solution*, violet on yellow).

THIN-LAYER, for dexamethasone: system T19—Rf 1·00 (location reagent *DPST spray*); for dexamethasone acetate: system T18—Rf 0·79 (location reagent *DPST spray*).

Ultraviolet Absorption Spectrum. Dexamethasone in methanol, maxima at 240 mμ (E1%, 1 cm 355) and about 263 mμ (E1%, 1 cm 422 to 455). Dexamethasone acetate in ethanol, maxima at about 240 mμ (E1%, 1 cm 340 to 370) and 263 mμ (E1%, 1 cm 375 to 408).

Infra-red Absorption Spectrum. Dexamethasone. Potassium bromide disk. The principal peaks are: A 1655, B 1616, C 892 (p. 737).

Metabolism. Dexamethasone is a synthetic glucocorticoid and is an isomer of betamethasone.

Dose. The usual therapeutic dose of dexamethasone and dexamethasone acetate is up to 10 mg daily orally. Dexamethasone sodium phosphate is administered by injection in doses of up to 20 mg and is also applied topically usually in concentrations of 0·05 to 0·1%; the total daily dose of dexamethasone sodium phoshate should not exceed 80 mg.

DEXAMPHETAMINE *Central Stimulant*

Synonyms: Dextroamphetamine; (+)-Phenylisopropylamine.

(+)-α-Methylphenethylamine

$C_9H_{13}N = 135{\cdot}2$

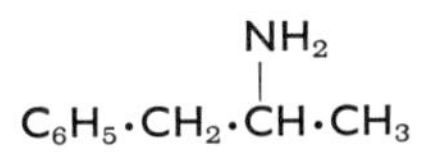

NOTE. It is extremely difficult to distinguish dexamphetamine from amphetamine. It may, however, be accomplished by examination, under polarised light, of the crystals formed with platinic bromide solution. Those of dexamphetamine are strongly birefringent, those of the (±)-form only weakly so. For a microcrystalline method of differentiation of dexamphetamine from levamphetamine see Microcrystal Tests, p. 140.

DEXAMPHETAMINE PHOSPHATE
A white crystalline powder.
Solubility. Soluble 1 in 20 of water; slightly soluble in ethanol; practically insoluble in ether and chloroform.

DEXAMPHETAMINE SULPHATE
Proprietary Names: Dephadren; Dexamed; Dexedrine; Dexten. It is an ingredient of Amphetone, Anxine, Appetrol, Barbidex, Daprisal, Dexobarb, Dexytal, Drinamyl, Durophet, Mylodex-A, Steladex, Thyrodex, and Thyrophem.

A white crystalline powder. M.p. above 300°.
Solubility. Soluble 1 in 9 of water and 1 in 800 of ethanol; insoluble in ether.

Screening Test. See under Screening Tests, p. 7.

Extraction. Dexamphetamine may be isolated in the D2 fraction (see p. 27); it is volatile and may be isolated by distillation from alkaline solutions (see p. 18).

Chromatography. PAPER: system P1—Rf 0·51 (location reagents: *iodoplatinate spray*, white; *bromocresol green spray*, strong reaction).

THIN-LAYER: system T1—Rf 0·48 (location reagent *potassium permanganate spray*, positive reaction).

Colour Test. MICRO: sulphuric acid–formaldehyde test—orange → brown (*sensitivity:* 0·5 μg).

Crystal Tests. MICRO: *platinic bromide solution*—long rhomboidal plates and prisms, strongly birefringent (*sensitivity:* 1 in 200); *platinic iodide solution*—plates, mostly hexagonal (*sensitivity:* 1 in 400).

Ultraviolet Absorption Spectrum. Dexamphetamine in 0·1N sulphuric acid, maxima at 252 mμ (E1%, 1cm 15), 257·5 mμ (E1%, 1cm 19), and 265 mμ (E1%, 1cm 14).

Infra-red Absorption Spectrum. Dexamphetamine sulphate. Potassium bromide disk. The principal peaks are: A 1118, B 1495, C 1582 (p. 737).

Metabolism. Dexamphetamine has actions qualitatively similar to those of amphetamine but it is approximately twice as potent. It is well absorbed from the gastro-intestinal tract. In man, the major portion of a single dose is excreted unchanged in the urine; the actual amount of unchanged dexamphetamine excreted is influenced by the urinary pH, being as much as 54% at pH 5 and as low as 2·9% at pH 8 (Beckett *et al.*, 1965b). In 3 human subjects, 37·6% of a 10-mg dose of dexamphetamine was recovered in the urine in 24 hours (Keller and Ellenbogen, 1952). In dogs and rats hydroxylation to yield hydroxyamphetamine (p. 373) appears to be an important metabolic pathway; over a period of 48 hours, 31% of a 5-mg/kg dose of dexamphetamine given to dogs was excreted unchanged in the urine and 20% was recovered as hydroxyamphetamine (Axelrod, 1954). Hydroxylation was also observed in rats given a similar dose, the respective percentages being 13 and 31.

Dose. Up to 30 mg daily.
Continued use of dexamphetamine may cause addiction, and ingestion of up to 10 times the usual therapeutic dose is common among addicts.

Toxicity. The estimated minimum lethal dose in children is 20 mg; that for adults may be 10 times as great; however, fatalities are rare. One common and alarming result of acute amphetamine poisoning may be the development of an acute psychosis; severe cases often present as acute mental disturbances.

LD50 (oral): in rats 36 mg/kg.

CASE EXAMPLES. A 32-year-old woman, who was admitted to hospital 12 hours after swallowing 200 mg of dexamphetamine sulphate, recovered within 3 days. The urine passed in hospital contained 54·7 mg of amphetamine sulphate which would correspond to an oral dose of between 109 and 187 mg of dexamphetamine sulphate (Greenwood and Peachey, 1957).

A 36-year-old man died within 14 hours of swallowing a large number of sustained-release tablets, each of which contained 32 mg of phenobarbitone in an inner core and between 10 and 15 mg of dexamphetamine in an outer shell. Post-mortem amphetamine-levels: blood, 0·2 mg%; kidney, 1·5 mg%; liver, 0·9 mg%; spleen, 1·4 mg%; urine, 2·7 mg%; gastric contents, a total of 103 mg. Phenobarbitone was found only in the gastric contents, a total of 71 mg, and in the spleen, 1·5 mg%. The gastric contents contained 103 partially digested tablets. The inner cores of the tablets were still intact and the apparent disparity between the 2 drug levels was probably due to this (Finkle, 1967b).

DEXBROMPHENIRAMINE *Antihistamine*

(+)-3-*p*-Bromophenyl-*NN*-dimethyl-3-pyrid-2′-ylpropylamine

$C_{16}H_{19}BrN_2 = 319{\cdot}3$

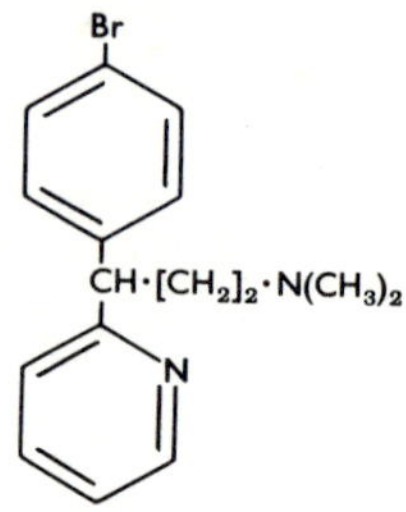

NOTE. The chromatographic data and crystal tests of dexbrompheniramine are similar to those of brompheniramine which is the racemic mixture—see also Microcrystal Tests, p. 140.

DEXBROMPHENIRAMINE MALEATE
Proprietary Name: Disomer.

Extraction. Dexbrompheniramine is extracted by organic solvents from aqueous alkaline solutions.

Chromatography. PAPER: system P1—Rf 0·45 (location under ultraviolet light, strong absorption; location reagents: *iodoplatinate spray*, strong reaction; *bromocresol green spray*, weak reaction).

THIN-LAYER: system T1—Rf 0·33 (location reagent *acidified iodoplatinate spray*, positive reaction).

GAS: system G2/225—retention time 2·0 relative to diphenydramine; system G4—retention time 2·5 relative to diphenhydramine.

Crystal Test. MICRO: *lead iodide solution*—feathery rosettes and sheaves, strong birefringent (*sensitivity:* 1 in 1000).

Ultraviolet Absorption Spectrum. Dexbrompheniramine in 0·1N sulphuric acid, maximum at 265 mμ (E1%, 1cm 223); minimum at 245 mμ.

Infra-red Absorption Spectrum. Dexbrompheniramine maleate. Potassium bromide disk. The principal peaks are: A 1590, B 1470 or 1485, C 1395 (p. 783).

Dose. Up to 16 mg daily has been given.

Toxicity. Dexbrompheniramine is about twice as potent as brompheniramine.

DEXCHLORPHENIRAMINE *Antihistamine*

(+)-3-*p*-Chlorophenyl-*NN*-dimethyl-3-pyrid-2′-ylpropylamine

$C_{16}H_{19}ClN_2 = 274{\cdot}8$

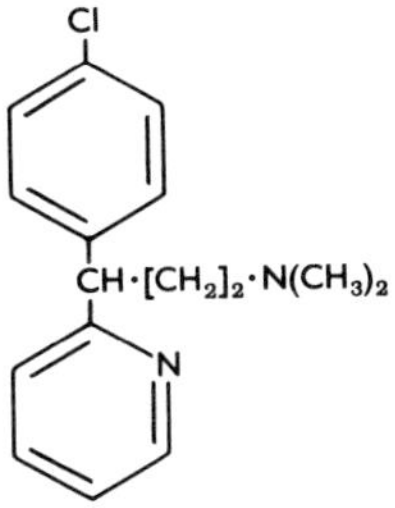

Solubility. Soluble in chloroform.

NOTE. The chromatographic data and crystal tests of dexchlorpheniramine are similar to those of chlorpheniramine which is the racemic mixture—see also Microcrystal Tests, p. 140.

DEXCHLORPHENIRAMINE MALEATE

Proprietary Name: Polaramine Maleate.

A white crystalline powder. M.p. 110° to 115°.

Solubility. Soluble 1 in 4 of water; soluble in ethanol and chloroform; slightly soluble in ether.

Extraction. Dexchlorpheniramine is extracted by organic solvents from aqueous alkaline solutions.

Chromatography. PAPER: system P1—Rf 0·45 (location under ultraviolet light, blue fluorescence; location reagents: *iodoplatinate spray*, strong reaction; *bromocresol green spray*, strong reaction).

THIN-LAYER: system T1—0·32 (location reagent *acidified iodoplatinate spray*, positive reaction).

GAS: system G2/225—retention time 1·53 relative to diphenhydramine; system G4—retention time 2·0 relative to diphenhydramine.

Crystal Tests. MICRO: *lead iodide solution*—feathery rosettes and sheaves, strongly birefringent (*sensitivity:* 1 in 1000); *platinic iodide solution*—long plates and needles (*sensitivity:* 1 in 1000).

Ultraviolet Absorption Spectrum. Dexchlorpheniramine in 0·1N sulphuric acid, maximum at 265 mμ (E1%, 1 cm 236); dexchlorpheniramine maleate in water, maximum at about 261 mμ.

Quantitative Estimation. Dexchlorpheniramine may be estimated spectrophotometrically after reaction with sulphanilic acid and cyanogen bromide (Hudanick, 1964).

Dose. Usually up to 8 mg daily.

Toxicity. Dexchlorpheniramine is about twice as potent as chlorpheniramine.

DEXTROMETHORPHAN *Antitussive*

(+)-3-Methoxy-*N*-methylmorphinan

$C_{18}H_{25}NO = 271{\cdot}4$

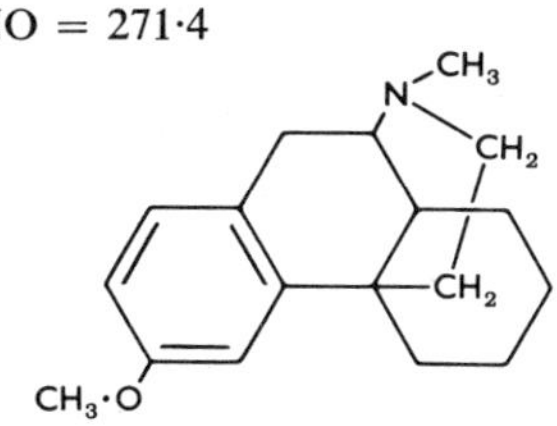

NOTE. Dextromethorphan is not subject to international control but its (−)-isomer, levomethorphan, and the (±)-form, racemethorphan, are. For a microcrystalline method of differentiation of dextromethorphan from levomethorphan and racemethorphan see Microcrystal Tests, p. 140.

Specific rotation of dextromethorphan determined on a chloroform extract of the hydrobromide, +64·3° to +66·3°.

DEXTROMETHORPHAN HYDROBROMIDE

Proprietary Name: Romilar.

A white crystalline powder. M.p. about 125°, with decomposition.

Solubility. Soluble 1 in 60 of water and 1 in 10 of ethanol; insoluble in ether; freely soluble in chloroform with the separation of water.

Extraction. Dextromethorphan may be isolated in the D2 fraction (see p. 27).

Chromatography. PAPER: system P1—Rf 0·60 (location reagents: *iodoplatinate spray*, strong reaction; *bromocresol green spray*, weak reaction); system RP1a—Rf 0·77 (location reagent *iodoplatinate spray*, positive reaction); system RP1b—Rf 0·04 (location as for RP1a).

THIN-LAYER: system T1—Rf 0·24 (location reagent *acidified iodoplatinate spray*, positive reaction).

GAS: system G2/225—retention time 0·50 relative to codeine; system G4—retention time 0·22 relative to codeine.

Colour Test. MICRO: ammonium molybdate test —blue → green (*sensitivity:* 0·25 μg).

Crystal Tests. MICRO: *lead iodide solution*—bunches of serrated plates (*sensitivity:* 1 in 400); *platinic chloride solution*—feathery rosettes (*sensitivity:* 1 in 400).

Ultraviolet Absorption Spectrum. Dextromethorphan in water, maximum at 278 mμ (E1%, 1 cm 69); in 0·1N sulphuric acid, maximum at 278 mμ (E1%, 1 cm 62·5) and an inflexion at about 283 mμ.

Metabolism. Dextromethorphan possesses antitussive activity approximately equivalent to that of codeine but it has no significant analgesic or narcotic action. Following oral administration in man, unchanged dextromethorphan and two demethylated metabolites, dextrorphan and (+)-3-hydroxymorphinan, may be recovered from 24-hour urine samples. (+)-3-Methoxymorphinan, a third theoretically possible metabolite, has not been identified

(Willner, 1963). Conjugation of these compounds with glucuronic acid may take place.

Dose. Up to 120 mg daily.

Toxicity. The estimated minimum lethal dose in man is 500 mg.

DEXTROMORAMIDE *Narcotic Analgesic*

Synonyms: Dextrodiphenopyrine; Jetrium; MCP 875; D-Moramid; Pyrrolamidol; R875; SKF 5137.

(+)-1-(3-Methyl-4-morpholino-2,2-diphenylbutyryl)pyrrolidine

$C_{25}H_{32}N_2O_2 = 392{\cdot}5$

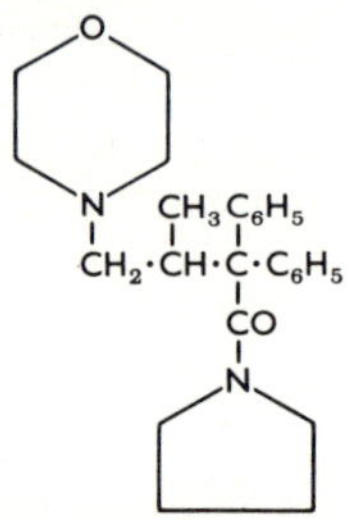

A white amorphous or microcrystalline powder. M.p. 183·5° to 184·5°.

Solubility. Insoluble in water; soluble 1 in 50 of ethanol and 1 in 3 of chloroform; slightly soluble in ether; soluble 1 in 5 of benzene.

NOTE. For a microcrystalline method of differentiation of dextromoramide from levomoramide and racemoramide see Microcrystal Tests, p. 140.

DEXTROMORAMIDE TARTRATE

Synonym: Dextromoramide Acid Tartrate.

Proprietary Names: Dimorlin Tartrate; Palfium.

A white amorphous or crystalline powder. M.p. 187° to 189°, with slight decomposition. Specific rotation of a 5% aqueous solution, +25·5°.

Solubility. Soluble 1 in 25 of water and 1 in 85 of ethanol; slightly soluble in ether; insoluble in chloroform.

Extraction. Dextromoramide may be isolated in the D2 fraction (see p. 27).

Chromatography. PAPER: system P1—Rf 0·61 (location reagent *iodoplatinate spray*, weak reaction); system RP1a—Rf 0·67 (location under ultraviolet light, blue fluorescence); system RP1b—Rf 0·06 (location under ultraviolet light, pale blue fluorescence).

THIN-LAYER: system T1—Rf 0·70 (location reagent *acidified iodoplatinate spray*, positive reaction).

GAS: system G2/225—retention time 4·86 relative to codeine.

Crystal Tests. MICRO: *gold chloride solution*—oily needles, some serrated, forming overnight (*sensitivity:* 1 in 1000); *picrolonic acid*—dense rosettes or rosettes of rods (*sensitivity:* 1 in 200).

Ultraviolet Absorption Spectrum. Dextromoramide in 0·01N hydrochloric acid, maxima at 256 mμ (E1%, 1 cm 355), 261 mμ (E1%, 1 cm 385), and 267 mμ (E1%, 1 cm 305); minima at 253 mμ, 258·5 mμ, and 266 mμ.

Dose. Usually 5 mg, increasing if necessary up to 20 mg.
Dextromoramide may cause addiction; cases have been reported of addicts taking up to 50 mg daily. Doses of up to 400 mg daily have been given to cancer patients.

Toxicity. The estimated minimum lethal dose in man is 500 mg.
LD50 (oral): in mice 220 mg/kg.

DEXTROPROPOXYPHENE *Narcotic Analgesic*

Synonym: Propoxyphene.

(+)-α-4-Dimethylamino-3-methyl-1,2-diphenylbut-2-yl propionate

$C_{22}H_{29}NO_2 = 339{\cdot}5$

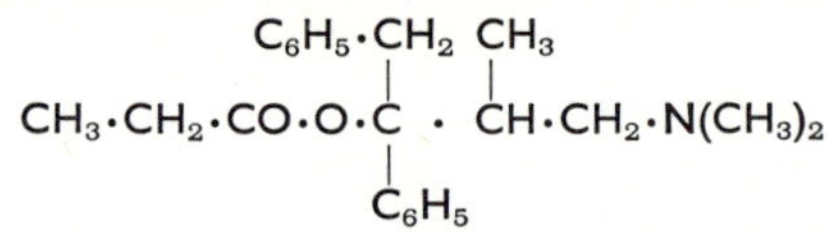

Solubility. Soluble 1 in 10,000 of water.

NOTE. For a microcrystalline method of differentiation of dextropropoxyphene from levopropoxyphene see Microcrystal Tests, p. 140.

DEXTROPROPOXYPHENE HYDROCHLORIDE

Proprietary Names: Darvon; Doloxene.

A white crystalline powder. M.p. 162·5° to 168·5°. Specific rotation of a 10% solution, +36° to +40°.

Solubility. Soluble 1 in 0·3 of water, 1 in 1·5 of ethanol, and 1 in 0·6 of chloroform; insoluble in ether.

DEXTROPROPOXYPHENE NAPSYLATE

Synonym: Dextropropoxyphene Naphthalene-2-sulphonate.

Proprietary Names: Napsalgesic. It is an ingredient of Doloxene Compound-65.

A white powder. M.p. about 160°.

Solubility. Slightly soluble in water; soluble 1 in 13 of ethanol and 1 in 3 of chloroform.

Extraction. Dextropropoxyphene may be isolated in the D1 fraction (see p. 27).

Chromatography. PAPER: system P1—Rf 0·75 (location reagent *iodoplatinate spray*, strong reaction); system RP1a—Rf 0·25 (location reagent *iodoplatinate spray*, positive reaction).

THIN-LAYER: system T1—Rf 0·66 (location reagent *acidified iodoplatinate spray*, positive reaction); system T7—Rf 0·97 (location reagent *iodoplatinate spray*, positive reaction); system T8—Rf 0·68 (location as for T7).

GAS: system G1/180—retention time 3·17 relative to diphenhydramine; system G2/225—retention time 0·63 (1·27), (2·71) relative to diphenhydramine; system G3—retention time 0·92 relative to diphenhydramine; system G4—retention time 0·60 relative to diphenhydramine.

Colour Tests. MICRO: sulphuric acid–formaldehyde test—black-purple → dull green (*sensitivity:* 0·5 μg); ammonium molybdate test—

black → green (*sensitivity:* 0·5 μg); ammonium vanadate test—grey-brown (*sensitivity:* 0·5 μg).

Crystal Tests. MICRO: *gold bromide–hydrochloric acid solution*—curving blades, forming overnight (*sensitivity:* 1 in 400); *potassium tri-iodide solution* (*1*)—small plates in fernlike patterns, best viewed under polarised light (*sensitivity:* 1 in 400).

Ultraviolet Absorption Spectrum. Dextropropoxyphene in 0·1N sodium hydroxide, maxima at 252 mμ and 264 mμ; minima at 238 mμ and 254 mμ: in 0·1N sulphuric acid, maxima at 251·5 mμ (E1%, 1 cm 10), at 257 mμ (E1%, 1 cm 12), and 263 mμ (E1%, 1 cm 9); minima at 232 mμ, 254 mμ, and 262 mμ.

Quantitative Estimation. Dextropropoxyphene in blood and urine may be estimated spectrophotometrically following extraction into alkaline ether, re-extraction into hydrochloric acid, refluxing, and final steam distillation of the conjugated product (Wallace *et al.*, 1965).

Metabolism. Dextropropoxyphene is a narcotic analgesic which is readily absorbed after oral administration. It appears to undergo *N*-demethylation in the liver; only a small fraction of the unaltered compound is excreted in the urine; the remainder is excreted as *N*-demethyldextropropoxyphene.

Dextropropoxyphene disappears from the blood within 5 minutes after the oral or parenteral administration of large doses. It has been shown to concentrate quickly in the brain, lungs, liver, and kidneys of animals (Qureshi, 1964). Approximately 25% of a 65-mg dose was recovered within 48 hours as a mixture of unchanged drug and the *N*-demethylated metabolite. The unchanged drug was excreted mainly in the first 6 hours after ingestion and the metabolite from 6 to 48 hours after ingestion (Amundson *et al.*, 1965). Approximately 3% of a 130-mg dose appeared unchanged in the urine within 24 hours and about 5% in 72 hours; very little was demonstrated thereafter. No dextropropoxyphene was demonstrated in the blood up to 6 hours after ingestion (Wallace *et al.*, 1965).

Dose. Up to 260 mg (hydrochloride) daily.

Toxicity. The estimated minimum lethal dose of dextropropoxyphene in man is 500 mg but recovery has followed the ingestion of 960 mg and of 3·2 g, and children have recovered after swallowing up to 260 mg. Dextropropoxyphene has low addiction-producing properties but a case has been reported of a 28-year-old man who appeared to be taking about 1 g daily and in hospital he tolerated 780 mg daily with no deleterious effects (Elson and Domino, 1963).

LD50 (oral): in mice 425 and in rats about 185 mg/kg.

CASE EXAMPLES. In a fatal poisoning attributed to dextropropoxyphene, 5·7 mg% was found in the blood and 10 mg% in the liver. Following oral doses of 130 mg no drug could be detected in the blood (McBay, 1966).

A 65-year-old woman died 9 days after ingesting about 2·3 g of dextropropoxyphene, despite repeated administration of nalorphine and peritoneal dialysis. On admission to hospital, about 1 hour after taking the drug, the dextropropoxyphene levels were 0·097 mg% in the serum and 0·92 mg% in the urine. At post-mortem examination there was no trace of dextropropoxyphene in the liver (Karliner, 1967).

After taking about 2 g of dextropropoxyphene, a 22-year-old woman died. Post-mortem levels: bile, 14·8 mg%; blood, 2·1 mg%; kidney, 2·1 mg%; liver, 3·6 mg%; spleen, 3·1 mg%; urine, 0·9 mg%. The stomach contents contained a total of 0·5 mg (Finkle, 1967a).

DEXTRORPHAN *Antitussive*

(+)-3-Hydroxy-*N*-methylmorphinan

$C_{17}H_{23}NO = 257{\cdot}4$

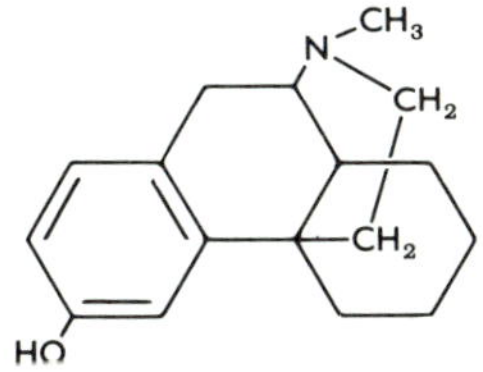

NOTE. Dextrorphan is not subject to international control buts its (−)-isomer, levorphanol, and the (±)-form, racemorphan, are.

For a microcrystalline method of differentiation of dextrorphan from levorphanol and racemorphan see Microcrystal Tests, p. 140.

Dextrorphan melts at 198° to 199°.

Extraction. Dextrorphan may be isolated in the D3 fraction (see p. 27).

Chromatography. PAPER: system P1—Rf 0·60 (location reagents: *iodoplatinate spray*, strong reaction; *bromocresol green spray*, weak reaction); system RP1a—Rf 0·78 (location reagent *iodoplatinate spray*, positive reaction).

THIN-LAYER: system T1—Rf 0·24 (location reagent *acidified iodoplatinate spray*, positive reaction); system T7—Rf 0·80 (location reagent *iodoplatinate spray*, positive reaction); system T8—Rf 0·47 (location as for T7).

Colour Tests. MICRO: ammonium molybdate test—blue → green (*sensitivity:* 0·25 μg); Vitali's test—yellow/yellow/orange (*sensitivity:* 0·25 μg).

Crystal Tests. MICRO: *platinic bromide solution*—bunches of small irregular plates (*sensitivity:* 1 in 400); *platinic chloride solution*—masses of small irregular crystals (*sensitivity:* 1 in 400).

Ultraviolet Absorption Spectrum. Dextrorphan in 0·1N sulphuric acid, maximum at 279 mμ (E1%, 1 cm 91·7) and an inflexion at about 285 mμ.

Metabolism. Dextrorphan has antitussive activity but it does not have the marked analgesic properties of its isomer levorphanol. Dextrorphan and levorphanol appear to be metabolised *in vivo* in a similar manner. Studies in dogs have shown that both are excreted chiefly in the urine as conjugates of glucuronic acid, only insignificant amounts being excreted in the faeces in either the free or bound form. In certain species, both compounds may be *N*-demethylated to some extent.

Dextrorphan has been found to be the major metabolite of dextromethorphan in man, but it is less potent as an antitussive than dextromethorphan.

DIAMORPHINE *Narcotic Analgesic*

Synonyms: Acetomorphine; Diacetylmorphine; Heroin.

3,6 - Diacetoxy - 7,8 - dehydro - 4,5 - epoxy - *N*-methylmorphinan

$C_{21}H_{23}NO_5 = 369{\cdot}4$

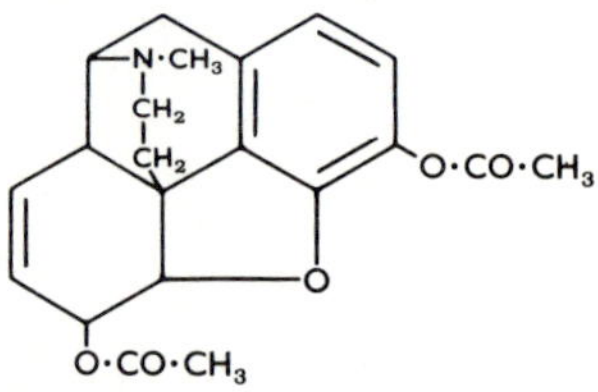

White crystals. M.p. about 170°. It is rapidly hydrolysed by alkalis.

Solubility. Soluble 1 in 1700 of water, 1 in 31 of ethanol, 1 in 100 of ether, and 1 in 1·5 of chloroform.

DIAMORPHINE HYDROCHLORIDE

A white crystalline powder. M.p. 229° to 233°.

Solubility. Soluble 1 in 1·6 of water, 1 in 12 of ethanol, and 1 in 1·6 of chloroform; insoluble in ether.

Extraction. Diamorphine may be isolated in the D1 fraction (see p. 27) but it is usually found as morphine in biological material. Shaffer (1953) describes a schematic separation of complex diamorphine mixtures sold illicitly.

Chromatography. PAPER: system P1—Rf 0·33 (location under ultraviolet light, absorption; location reagent *iodoplatinate spray*, strong reaction); system RP1a—Rf 0·84 (location reagent *iodoplatinate spray*, positive reaction); system RP1b—Rf 0·12 (location as for RP1a). THIN-LAYER: system T1—Rf 0·45 (location reagent *acidified iodoplatinate spray*, positive reaction); system T7—Rf 0·76 (location reagent *iodoplatinate spray*, positive reaction); system T8—Rf 0·35 (location as for T7).

GAS: system G1/250—retention time 1·67 relative to codeine; system G2/225—retention time 2·08 relative to codeine; system G6—retention time 1·39 relative to codeine.

For the metabolite, 6-monoacetylmorphine (see under Metabolism): system G2/225—retention time 1·45 relative to codeine.

Colour Tests. MICRO: sulphuric acid–formaldehyde test—purple (*sensitivity:* 0·05 μg); ammonium molybdate test—red-purple → blue → light green (*sensitivity:* 0·05 μg); ammonium vanadate test—faint blue-grey (*sensitivity:* 1·0 μg); Vitali's test—faint yellow/faint yellow/orange (*sensitivity:* 1·0 μg).

Crystal Tests. MICRO: *mercuric chloride solution*—fine dendrites (*sensitivity:* 1 in 1000).

Ultraviolet Absorption Spectrum. Diamorphine in ethanol, maximum at 281 mμ; minimum at 255 mμ; in 0·1N hydrochloric acid, maximum at 278 mμ (E1%, 1 cm 39); in 0·5N sodium hydroxide, maximum at 298 mμ and minimum at 278 mμ; in 0·1N sulphuric acid, maximum at 279 mμ (E1%, 1 cm 52) and an inflexion at about 275 mμ.

Metabolism. Diamorphine is a short-acting narcotic analgesic with an effect lasting only about 2 hours. It is rapidly hydrolysed in the body to 6-monoacetylmorphine, which is further hydrolysed to morphine but much more slowly. The amount of diamorphine detected in the urine as morphine after a single intramuscular injection of 5 mg is about one-third that detected after a single intramuscular injection of 15 mg of morphine. Diamorphine is excreted in the urine chiefly as morphine glucuronide and morphine (Parker *et al.*, 1966).

NOTE. In forensic investigations, where diamorphine ingestion is suspected, the blood should be tested for the presence of 6-monoacetylmorphine. However, the blood must be collected within 30 minutes of administration (Nakamura and Ukita, 1967).

Dose. The usual therapeutic dose of diamorphine is 5 to 10 mg by mouth or by injection; the maximum safe dose in 24 hours is stated to be 15 mg. Addicts, however, have been found to tolerate 75 mg to 900 mg in 24 hours; for an account of 30 diamorphine addicts see Cameron (1964).

Toxicity. Diamorphine is 2 to 3 times as potent as morphine; the estimated minimum lethal dose in man is 200 mg but fatalities have occurred after 10-mg doses; in addicts the lethal dose may be up to 10 times as high.

CASE EXAMPLE. About 1·3 g of diamorphine was found post mortem in the body of a 28-year-old addict. One doctor had been prescribing 420 mg daily and another, unaware of the first doctor's treatment, was prescribing a similar amount. It is probable that the man had ingested 2 days' dosage in a single dose, that is, about 1·6 g (per *Pharm. J.*, i/1955, 298).

DIAMPROMIDE *Narcotic*

N - [2 - (Methylphenethylamino)propyl]propionanilide

$C_{21}H_{28}N_2O = 324{\cdot}5$

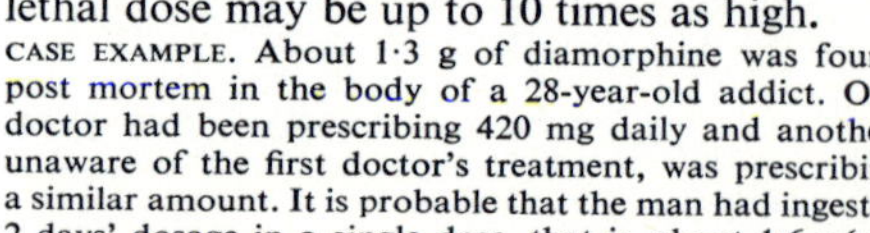

Extraction. Diampromide is extracted by organic solvents from aqueous alkaline solutions.

Chromatography. PAPER: system P1—Rf 0·76

(location reagent *iodoplatinate spray*, weak reaction); system RP1a—Rf 0·19 (location reagent *iodoplatinate spray*, positive reaction).

THIN-LAYER: system T1—Rf 0·42 (location reagent *acidified iodoplatinate spray*, positive reaction).

Colour Test. MICRO: sulphuric acid–formaldehyde test—orange (*sensitivity:* 1·0 μg).

Crystal Test. MICRO: *lead iodide solution*—dense rosettes, forming overnight (*sensitivity:* 1 in 100).

Ultraviolet Absorption Spectrum. Diampromide in 0·1N sulphuric acid, maxima at about 225 mμ (E1%, 1cm 201), 257 mμ (E1%, 1cm 28), and about 263 mμ (E1%, 1cm 22).

DIAMTHAZOLE *Antimycotic*

Synonyms: Amycazol; Ro 2-2453.

6-(2-Diethylaminoethoxy)-2-dimethylaminobenzothiazole

$C_{15}H_{23}N_3OS = 293·4$

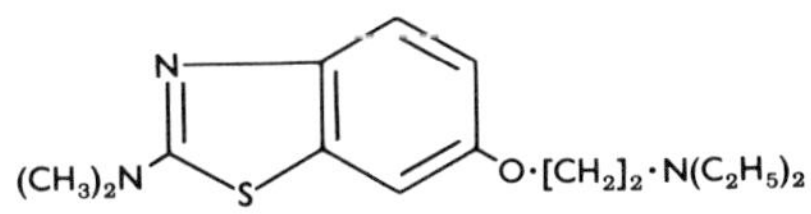

DIAMTHAZOLE HYDROCHLORIDE

Synonym: Diamthazole Dihydrochloride.

Proprietary Name: Asterol.

A white crystalline powder.

Solubility. Freely soluble in water; soluble in ethanol.

Extraction. Diamthazole is extracted by organic solvents from aqueous alkaline solutions.

Chromatography. PAPER: system P1—Rf 0·28 (location under ultraviolet light, absorption; location reagent *iodoplatinate spray*, weak reaction).

THIN-LAYER: system T1—Rf 0·50 (location reagent *acidified iodoplatinate spray*, positive reaction).

Colour Test. MICRO: ammonium molybdate test—blue, fading (*sensitivity:* 1·0 μg).

Crystal Tests. MICRO: *gold chloride solution*—bunches of serrated blades (*sensitivity:* 1 in 100); *picrolonic acid*—rosettes of fine needles (*sensitivity:* 1 in 100).

Infra-red Absorption Spectrum. Diamthazole (base). Potassium bromide disk. The principal peaks are: A 1015, B 667, C 1460 or 1548 or 1602 (p. 783).

Toxicity. Ataxia, tremors, convulsions, hallucinations, and changes in behaviour have been reported in infants and young children due to sucking fingers or clothing contaminated with diamthazole.

LD50 (oral): in mice 500 mg/kg.

NOTE. Diamthazole is applied as an ointment, dusting-powder, and tincture, the usual concentration being 5%. It should be applied cautiously to mucous membranes.

DIAVERIDINE *Coccidiostatic (Veterinary)*

Proprietary Name: It is an ingredient of Darvisul.

2,4-Diamino-5-(3,4-dimethoxybenzyl)pyrimidine

$C_{13}H_{16}H_4O_2 = 260·3$

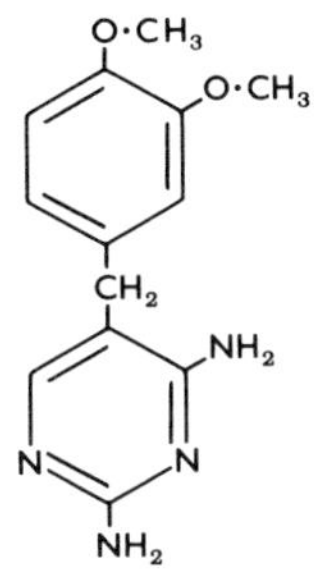

A white crystalline powder. M.p. about 233°.

Solubility. Very slightly soluble in water and ethanol; soluble 1 in 600 of chloroform.

Extraction. Diaveridine is extracted by organic solvents from aqueous alkaline solutions.

Chromatography. PAPER: system P1—Rf 0·21 (location under ultraviolet light, white fluorescence; location reagents: *iodoplatinate spray*, weak reaction; *bromocresol green spray*, weak reaction).

THIN-LAYER: system T1—Rf 0·58 (location reagent *acidified iodoplatinate spray*, positive reaction).

Colour Tests. MICRO: sulphuric acid–formaldehyde test—grey → purple-brown (*sensitivity:* 0·5 μg); ammonium molybdate test—blue (*sensitivity:* 0·25 μg); ammonium vanadate test—olive (*sensitivity:* 0·5 μg); Vitali's test—pale yellow/pale yellow/orange (*sensitivity:* 0·5 μg).

Crystal Tests. MICRO: *picrolonic acid*—small needles in bunches (*sensitivity:* 1 in 3000); *potassium tri-iodide solution* (3)—burrs (*sensitivity:* 1 in 1000).

Ultraviolet Absorption Spectrum. Diaveridine in 0·1N sulphuric acid, maximum at 276 mμ (E1%, 1cm 337).

Infra-red Absorption Spectrum. Potassium bromide disk. The principal peaks are: A 1460, B 1630, C 1252 or 1598 or 1645 (p. 783).

Metabolism. Diaveridine is used in veterinary medicine for the prevention of coccidiosis in poultry. It is administered in conjunction with sulphaquinoxaline with which it acts synergistically. This synergism results from each drug influencing a different phase of one metabolic pathway of the parasite, the diaveridine interfering with folic acid metabolism and the sulphaquinoxaline with *p*-aminobenzoic acid metabolism.

DIAZEPAM *Tranquilliser*

Synonyms: LA 111; Ro 5-2807; Wy 3467.
Proprietary Name: Valium.

7-Chloro-1,2-dihydro-1-methyl-2-oxo-5-phenyl-3*H*-1,4-benzodiazepine

$C_{16}H_{13}ClN_2O = 284{\cdot}7$

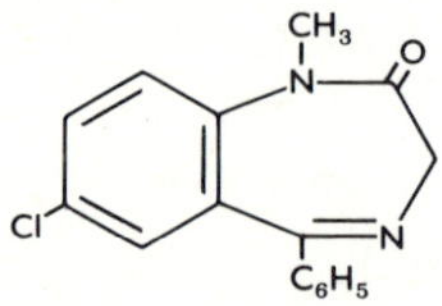

A white crystalline powder. M.p. 131·5° to 134·5°.

Solubility. Insoluble in water; freely soluble in chloroform.

Screening Tests. See under Screening Tests, p. 11.

Extraction. Diazepam is extracted by organic solvents from aqueous acid or alkaline solutions.

Chromatography. PAPER: system P1—Rf 0·89 (location reagents: *iodoplatinate spray*, weak, reaction; *bromocresol green spray*, weak reaction); system RP1a—Rf 0·26 (location under ultraviolet light, absorption; location reagent *iodoplatinate spray*, positive reaction).
THIN-LAYER: system T1—Rf 0·75 (location reagent *Dragendorff spray*, positive reaction).
GAS: system G2/225—retention time 1·16 relative to codeine; system G4—retention time 1·77 relative to codeine.

Crystal Tests. MICRO: *potassium cadmium iodide solution*—bunches of prisms, forming overnight (*sensitivity:* 1 in 400); *potassium mercuric iodide solution*—irregular rosettes, forming overnight (*sensitivity:* 1 in 400).

Ultraviolet Absorption Spectrum. Diazepam in 2N hydrochloric acid, maxima at about 242 mμ and about 287 mμ; minimum at about 262 mμ; in 0·1N sulphuric acid, maxima at 241 mμ (E1%, 1 cm 1402), 284 mμ (E1%, 1 cm 700), and 359 mμ (E1%, 1 cm 170).

Infra-red Absorption Spectrum. Potassium bromide disk. The principal peaks are: A 1681, B 1484, C 1313 (p. 738).

Quantitative Estimation. Diazepam, its *N*-demethylated metabolite, and chlordiazepoxide in blood and urine, after preliminary separation and hydrolysis to their respective benzophenones, may be quantitatively estimated by gas chromatography (de Silva *et al.*, 1964); diazepam in blood may be estimated spectrophotometrically following extraction into ether (de Silva *et al.*, 1966); diazepam in biological materials may be estimated polarographically, an advantage of this method being that the estimation may be carried out in the presence of the acid hydrolysis product (Oelschlaeger *et al.*, 1964).

Metabolism. Diazepam is rapidly absorbed from the gastro-intestinal tract. It is metabolised principally through *N*-demethylation and this metabolite is then hydroxylated at position 3 to give oxazepam. There is also evidence for a 3-hydroxylation before *N*-demethylation, again yielding oxazepam; diazepam and these 3 metabolites may be separated by thin-layer chromatography with acetone: chloroform (1 : 9) as the solvent (de Silva *et al.*, 1966).
The hydroxylated compounds are excreted as glucuronides, whereas the main *N*-demethylated metabolite seems to be excreted both in the conjugated and unconjugated forms. Oxazepam glucuronide is the major urinary metabolite of diazepam in man. Both the *N*-demethylated metabolite and oxazepam have been shown to have a diminished pharmacological activity as compared with diazepam itself whereas the 3-hydroxylated metabolite shows no loss of activity (Randall *et al.*, 1965).
Following the administration of single 10-mg doses orally, peak blood-levels of 0·016 to 0·2 mg% were seen 1 hour after dosage; in another study, following the administration of 20-mg to 25-mg oral doses daily for up to 5 days, blood-levels ranging from 0·016 to 0·04 mg% were observed; after 2 days the blood-levels of diazepam and its *N*-demethylated metabolite were the same, indicating a rapid turnover and equilibration of the drug (de Silva *et al.*, 1964). The levels of the metabolite in the blood remained appreciable for up to 7 days after medication ceased, whereas the level of diazepam decreased more rapidly.
Following the oral ingestion of 10-mg doses, 71% of the drug was excreted in the urine and 10% in the faeces; the urine contained about 33% of the dose in the form of oxazepam glucuronide, 10% as the conjugated *N*-demethylated metabolite, and 10% as the conjugated 3-hydroxylated metabolite (Schwartz *et al.*, 1965).

Dose. Up to 40 mg daily.

Toxicity. The estimated minimum lethal dose in man is between 100 and 500 mg/kg. Recoveries have occurred in children who ingested 20 and 150 mg, and in a young adult who ingested 125 mg (Picchioni, 1965).
LD50 (oral): in dogs 1, in mice 0·7, and in rats 1·2 g/kg.

CASE EXAMPLE. A driver was involved in 3 hit-and-run accidents in the space of several hours. Afterwards he claimed he had taken ten 5-mg tablets of diazepam on each of the 2 previous days and twenty-four to twenty-seven 5-mg tablets earlier on the day in question, with the intention of committing suicide. His blood diazepam level was 0·25 mg% (Turner, 1966).

DIAZINON *Pesticide*

Other Names: Basudin; DBD; Diazitol; Dimpylate; G 24480; Neocidal; Nucidol.

Diethyl 2-isopropyl-6-methylpyrimidin-4-yl phosphorothionate
$C_{12}H_{21}N_2O_3PS = 304{\cdot}4$

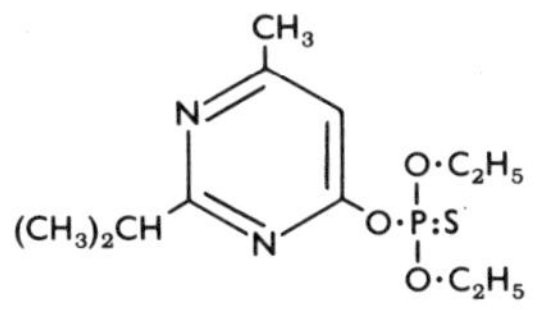

The pure compound is a colourless liquid; the technical grade is a pale to dark brown liquid. It is stable in alkaline solutions but is slowly hydrolysed in water and dilute acids. B.p. 83° to 84° at 0·002 mm Hg.
Solubility. Slightly soluble in water; soluble in petroleum oils.

Screening Test. Fisk *et al.* (1965) have described a rapid qualitative screening test involving extraction into n-heptane and subsequent spectrophotometric determination.

Extraction. Diazinon is extracted by organic solvents from aqueous acid or alkaline solutions.

Chromatography. PAPER: system P11—Rf 0·56 (location reagent *bromine vapour* followed by *congo red spray*, clear blue against red background).
THIN-LAYER: system T15—Rf 0·50 (location reagent *palladium chloride spray*, positive reaction); system T16—Rf 0·38 (location reagent *bromophenol blue spray* followed by *5% aqueous acetic acid spray*, mauve).

Metabolism. Diazinon is rapidly absorbed from the lungs and through the skin. Very little accumulation appears to take place.

Toxicity. The lethal dose in man is stated to be 25 g.
LD50 (oral): in guinea-pigs 240 to 320, in mice 80 to 135, and in rats 76 to 150 mg/kg.

DIBENZEPIN *Antidepressant*

Synonym: HF 1927.

10-(2-Dimethylaminoethyl)-10,11-dihydro-5-methyl-11-oxo-5*H*-dibenzo[*b*,*e*][1,4]-diazepine
$C_{18}H_{21}N_3O = 295{\cdot}4$

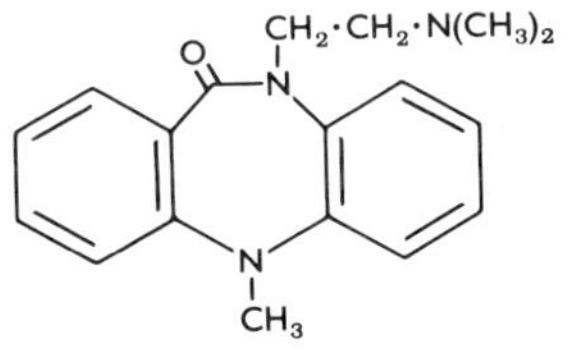

Dibenzepin melts at 116° to 117° and boils at 185° at 0·01 mm Hg.

DIBENZEPIN HYDROCHLORIDE
Proprietary Name: Noveril.

A white crystalline powder. M.p. 234° to 240°.

Solubility. Soluble 1 in 16 of water; soluble in ethanol and chloroform.

Extraction. Dibenzepin is extracted by organic solvents from aqueous alkaline solutions.

Chromatography. PAPER: system P1—Rf 0·47 (location under ultraviolet light, pale yellow fluorescence; location reagents: *iodoplatinate spray*, strong reaction; *bromocresol green spray*, weak reaction).
THIN-LAYER: system T1—Rf 0·52 (location reagent *acidified iodoplatinate spray*, positive reaction).
GAS: system G2/225—retention time 1·28 relative to codeine; system G4—retention time 1·34 relative to codeine.

Colour Tests. MICRO: ammonium vanadate test—(pale green) green → olive (*sensitivity:* 0·5 μg); Vitali's test—yellow/yellow/dull purple (*sensitivity:* 0·1 μg).

Crystal Tests. MICRO: *platinic bromide solution*—smudge rosettes or rosettes of needles (*sensitivity:* 1 in 1000); *platinic chloride solution*—very small rosettes.

Ultraviolet Absorption Spectrum. Dibenzepin in 0·1N sulphuric acid, maximum at 221 mμ (E1%, 1 cm 925) and an inflexion at about 280 mμ; dibenzepin hydrochloride in methanol, maximum at about 226 mμ and plateau between 210 and 217 mμ.

Dose. Usually about 200 to 240 mg daily, but doses of up to 600 mg have been given.

DIBROMOPROPAMIDINE *Antiseptic*

1,3-Di(4-amidino-2-bromophenoxy)propane
$C_{17}H_{18}Br_2N_4O_2 = 470{\cdot}2$

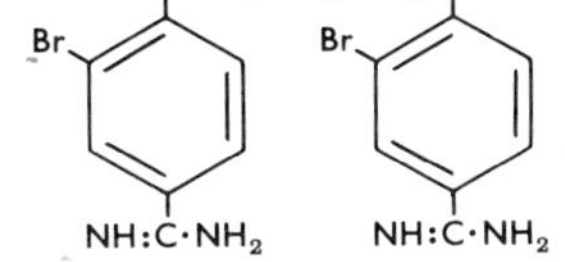

DIBROMOPROPAMIDINE EMBONATE
Synonym: Dibromopropamidine Pamoate.
Proprietary Name: it is an ingredient of Planidets.

DIBROMOPROPAMIDINE ISETHIONATE
Proprietary Names: Brolene; Brulidine.

A white crystalline powder.
Solubility. Soluble 1 in 2 of water and 1 in 60 of ethanol; insoluble in ether and chloroform.

Extraction. Dibromopropamidine is extracted by organic solvents from aqueous alkaline solutions.

Chromatography. PAPER: system P1—Rf 0·13 (location under ultraviolet light, strong absorption; location reagents: *iodoplatinate spray*, strong reaction; *bromocresol green spray*, weak reaction).

THIN-LAYER: system T1—Rf 0·01 (location reagent *acidified iodoplatinate spray*, positive reaction).

Colour Test. MICRO: Vitali's test— –/–/pale orange (*sensitivity:* 1·0 μg).

Crystal Tests. MICRO: *ammonium thiocyanate solution*—small needles, best viewed under polarised light (*sensitivity:* 1 in 1000); *potassium permanganate solution*—bunches of fine needles (*sensitivity:* 1 in 1000).

Ultraviolet Absorption Spectrum. Dibromopropamidine in 0·1N sulphuric acid, maximum at 261 mμ (E1%, 1 cm 413).

Infra-red Absorption Spectrum. Dibromopropamidine (base). Potassium bromide disk. The principal peaks are: A 1589, B 1485, C 1470 or 1569 (p. 783).

NOTE. Dibromopropamidine has bacteriostatic, bactericidal, and fungistatic properties which are not inhibited by blood, pus, or *p*-aminobenzoic acid. It is employed in creams and ointments (0·15%) and in throat lozenges.

DIBUTOLINE SULPHATE

Parasympatholytic

Proprietary Name: Dibuline Sulphate.

(2 - Dibutylcarbamoyloxyethyl)ethyldimethylammonium sulphate

$(C_{15}H_{33}N_2O_2)_2, SO_4 = 642{\cdot}9$

An extremely hygroscopic powder. Aqueous solutions decompose on heating at 100°.

Solubility. Soluble in water and benzene.

Extraction. Dibutoline is a quaternary ammonium compound (see p. 29).

Chromatography. PAPER: system P1—Rf 0·58 (location reagent *iodoplatinate spray*, strong reaction).

THIN-LAYER: system T1—Rf 0·02 (location reagent *acidified iodoplatinate spray*, positive reaction).

Colour Tests. MICRO: sulphuric acid–formaldehyde test—red (*sensitivity:* 1·0 μg); ammonium molybdate test—faint blue-grey (*sensitivity:* 1·0 μg); Vitali's test— –/–/faint yellow (*sensitivity:* 1·0 μg).

Crystal Tests. MICRO: *gold bromide solution*—masses of small plates, best viewed under polarised light (*sensitivity:* 1 in 200); *mercuric chloride solution*—small plates, forming overnight (*sensitivity:* 1 in 3000).

Dose. Up to 100 mg daily, intramuscularly or subcutaneously.

Toxicity. The lethal dose in man is probably between 10 and 100 mg/kg. Its effect is weaker and of shorter duration than that of atropine. It is poorly absorbed from the gastro-intestinal tract.

DIBUTYL PHTHALATE

Insect Repellent

Synonyms: Butyl Phthalate; DBP.

Butyl benzene-*o*-dicarboxylate

$C_{16}H_{22}O_4 = 278{\cdot}4$

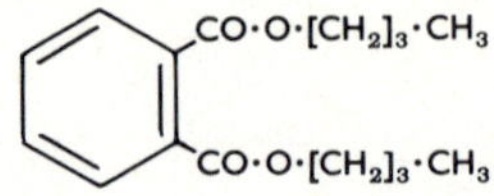

A clear, colourless or faintly coloured, somewhat viscous liquid. B.p. about 330°. Refractive index 1·492 to 1·495.

Solubility. Soluble 1 in 2500 of water; miscible with ethanol, ether, and most organic solvents.

Extraction. Dibutyl phthalate is extracted by organic solvents from aqueous acid solutions.

Ultraviolet Absorption Spectrum. Dibutyl phthalate in ethanol, maxima at 221·5 mμ, 230 mμ, 234 mμ, 240 mμ, 274 mμ, and 281 mμ.

Metabolism. Dibutyl phthalate is probably hydrolysed *in vivo* to phthalic acid. Phthalic acid is a strong acid and is excreted almost entirely unchanged by animals.

Toxicity. The estimated lethal dose in man is 50 g.

LD50 (intraperitoneal): in mice 4 g/kg.

NOTE. Dibutyl phthalate is slightly less effective than dimethyl phthalate as an insect repellent. It is less volatile and less easily removed by washing than dimethyl phthalate, and its chief use is for the impregnation of clothing.

DICHLORALPHENAZONE

Hypnotic

Proprietary Names: Bonadorm; Dormwell; Welldorm.

A molecular complex of chloral hydrate and phenazone.

$C_{15}H_{18}Cl_6N_2O_5 = 519{\cdot}0$

A white microcrystalline powder, decomposed by dilute alkalis. M.p. 64° to 67°.

Solubility. Soluble 1 in 7 of water, 1 in 1 of ethanol, 1 in 2 of chloroform, and in dilute acids.

NOTE. Dichloralphenazone is decomposed in aqueous and ethanolic solutions to chloral hydrate and phenazone. It appears that on administration dichloralphenazone acts simply as a mixture of chloral hydrate (p. 245) and phenazone (p. 480).

Infra-red Absorption Spectrum. Potassium bromide disk. The principal peaks are: A 1656, B 767, C 1484 (p. 738).

Dose. Up to 2 g.

Toxicity. Symptoms of poisoning similar to those of chloral hydrate may occur.

LD50 (oral): in mice 1·5 to 2 g/kg.

CASE EXAMPLES. A 65-year-old man died in under 3 hours following the ingestion of between 39 and 65 g of dichloralphenazone (between 60 and 100 Welldorm tablets). A post-mortem examination revealed marked oedema of the lungs and intense congestion of the stomach mucosa (Curry, 1962).

Following the ingestion of one 650-mg tablet of dichloralphenazone a 60-year-old woman experienced symptoms typical of phenazone toxicity including vomiting, diarrhoea, erythematous rash, and pyrexia. Although she recovered within a few days, skin patch-tests revealed positive sensitivity reactions to dichloralphenazone and phenazone but none to chloral hydrate (Gomersall *et al.*, 1966).

DICHLOROPHEN *Taenicide*

Synonyms: Di-phenthane-70; G 4.
Proprietary Names: Anthiphen; Antiphene; Dicestal; Teniathane; Teniatol.

Di(5-chloro-2-hydroxyphenyl)methane
$C_{13}H_{10}Cl_2O_2 = 269{\cdot}1$

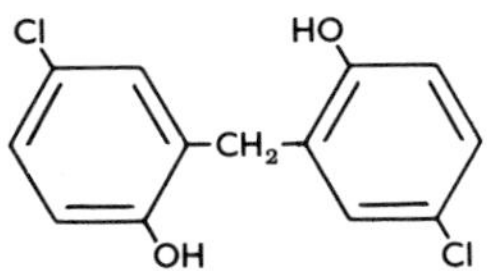

A white powder. M.p. 174° to 178°.
Solubility. Almost insoluble in water; soluble 1 in 1 of ethanol and 1 in less than 1 of ether.

Extraction. Dichlorophen is extracted by organic solvents from aqueous acid or alkaline solutions.

Ultraviolet Absorption Spectrum. Dichlorophen in ethanol, maxima at 228 mμ (E1%, 1 cm 540) and 287 mμ (E1%, 1 cm 165); in 0·1N sodium hydroxide, maxima at 246 mμ (E1%, 1 cm 667) and 305 mμ (E1%, 1 cm 274).

Infra-red Absorption Spectrum. Potassium bromide disk. The principal peaks are: A 1226, B 817, C 1111 or 1487 (p. 738).

Quantitative Estimation. Ashton (1960) has described a spectrophotometric method of estimating dichlorophen involving reaction with 4-aminoantipyrine in the presence of potassium periodate as oxidising agent.

Metabolism. Dichlorophen is a taenicide with a direct lethal action on the tapeworm. It is employed both in human and in veterinary medicine.

Dose. In man, 6 g on each of two successive days; in dogs and cats, 200 mg/kg.

DICHLOROPHENOXYACETIC ACID *Herbicide*

Synonym: 2,4-D.
Proprietary Names: Herbatox; Herbitox.

2,4-Dichlorophenoxyacetic acid
$C_8H_6Cl_2O_3 = 221{\cdot}0$

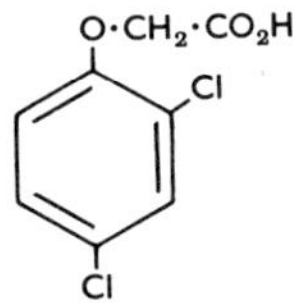

A white crystalline powder. M.p. 138°. B.p. 160° at 0·4 mm Hg.

Solubility. Almost insoluble in water; soluble in ethanol.

Extraction and **Quantitative Estimation.** Nielsen *et al.* (1965) have described a procedure involving extraction with ether and chloroform and transference to a slightly alkaline aqueous phase which is made strongly acid and re-extracted with chloroform, the final extraction being made with water at pH 10·6; the aqueous extract is measured spectrophotometrically at 282 mμ.

Colour Test. Add a few crystals of chromotropic acid to the dry material then add 2 ml of *sulphuric acid* and heat in a glycerin bath for 2 minutes—pink → purple → deep wine-purple.

Ultraviolet Absorption Spectrum. Dichlorophenoxyacetic acid in both acid and alkaline solution, maximum at 282 mμ and an inflexion at 290 mμ.

Toxicity. Dichlorophenoxyacetic acid is a plant hormone which stimulates growth at a concentration of 10 p.p.m. Higher strengths stimulate abnormal growth and the plant becomes distorted and dies. Strengths of 100 to 1000 p.p.m. are widely used as selective herbicides, being particularly effective for broad-leaved plants. Dichlorophenoxyacetic acid is very irritating to the eyes, nose, and throat, but inhalation has been shown to be relatively harmless. It should be used with caution in the vicinity of food and water supplies.

LD50 (oral): in dogs 0·1, in guinea-pigs 1, in mice 0·375, and in rabbits 0·8 g/kg.

CASE EXAMPLES. Absorption of dichlorophenoxyacetic acid through the skin of the arms and legs caused pain, paraesthesia, and paralysis in 3 cases. Recovery was not complete for several years (Goldstein *et al.*, 1959).

A 23-year-old man died following ingestion of dichlorophenoxyacetic acid. Post-mortem levels were: blood, 66·9 mg%; brain, 1·25 mg%; fatty tissue, 12·9 mg%; kidney, 6·3 mg%; liver, 1·83 mg%; muscles, 7 mg%; spleen, 1·34 mg%; urine, 26·4 to 27·0 mg%. In the stomach contents (75 ml), 583 mg was found. In all, at least 6 g was found in the body. Acute congestion had occurred in most organs and, in the brain, degenerating ganglion-cell changes with shrunken degranulated nuclei were seen (Nielsen *et al.*, 1965).

DICOPHANE *Pesticide*

Synonyms: Chlorophenothane; Chlorphenan; DDT; Dichlorodiphenyltrichloroethane; Parachlorocide; Penticide.

Not less than 70% consists of 1,1,1-trichloro-2,2-di(*p*-chlorophenyl)ethane.
$C_{14}H_9Cl_5 = 354{\cdot}5$

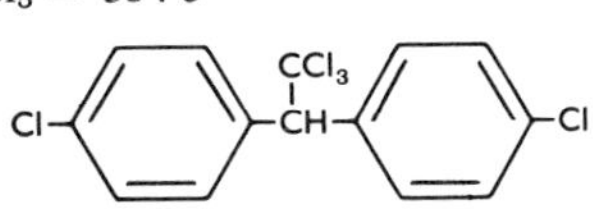

White crystals or powder affected by high storage temperatures and slowly by light. M.p. 108·5° to 109°.
Solubility. Almost insoluble in water; soluble 1

in 50 of ethanol, 1 in about 6 of boiling ethanol, 1 in about 4 of ether, and 1 in 3·5 of chloroform; readily soluble in benzene and carbon tetrachloride; soluble 1 in 2·5 of acetone.

Chromatography. GAS: system G1/180—retention time 6·0 relative to diphenhydramine; system G2/225—retention time 0·82 relative to codeine.

Extraction. Dicophane is extracted by organic solvents from aqueous acid solutions.

Colour Test. Heat a small quantity with a 0·5% solution of hydroquinone in *sulphuric acid*—wine-red.

NOTE. Dicophane does not react to Fujiwara's test.

Ultraviolet Absorption Spectrum. Dicophane in 0·1N sulphuric acid, maxima at 236 mμ, 266 mμ, and 276 mμ; minimum at 225 mμ.

Quantitative Estimation. Pollard *et al.* (1955) describe a quantitative infra-red spectrophotometric method of determination of dicophane and dieldrin when present in mixtures; a method of extraction, nitration, and colour-test microdetermination of dicophane is described by Irudayasamy and Natarajan (1961); a method of extraction and thin-layer chromatographic estimation is described by Luckens (1966).
Hamence *et al.* (1965) describe a method of extraction involving column chromatographic purification followed by differential gas chromatography of the untreated extract and of the extract after treatment with alcoholic potassium hydroxide solution, and Maunder *et al.* (1964a and b) discuss various extraction, clean-up, and gas chromatographic procedures for the determination of chlorinated insecticides.

Metabolism. Dicophane is an insecticide and larvicide. It is a stomach and contact poison, active whether ingested by the insect or absorbed through the cuticle and, because of its low volatility, it retains its activity for long periods under a variety of conditions. In man, the dry powder is poorly absorbed from the gastro-intestinal tract and not at all through the skin; however, cutaneous absorption is rapid when dicophane is dissolved in lipid solvents such as ethanol, kerosene, dimethyl phthalate, and oils; solutions in oils are also readily absorbed from the gastro-intestinal tract. Dicophane accumulates in the body fat both in the unchanged form and in the form of its primary degradation product, DDE[1,1-dichloro-2,2-di-(*p*-chlorophenyl)ethylene]; it may also be stored in the liver.
Analysis of fat samples from 130 subjects indicated that the general population of the U.S.A. had a mean storage level of 0·4 mg% of dicophane and 0·78 mg% of DDE (Quinby *et al.*, 1965).
Following the cessation of ingestion of dicophane occurring in food, the level in the fat gradually decreases to zero over a period of 6 months. Human urine has been found to contain no unchanged dicophane; only metabolites, DDE, TDE [1,1-dichloro-2,2-di(*p*-chlorophenyl)ethane], and DDA[2,2-di(*p*-chlorophenyl)acetic acid] have been detected, although unchanged dicophane has been found to be excreted in the milk. After the administration of 200 mg/kg of dicophane in olive oil by stomach tube to 3 rats, between 0·6 and 0·7 mg% of unchanged dicophane was detected in the blood after 4 hours and 0·7 mg% of the *o,p*-isomer, but 5 mg% of DDE was detected (Jain *et al.*, 1965).

Toxicity. A single oral dose of 10 mg/kg in man will cause toxic symptoms; the estimated lethal dose in man is 30 g (about 400 mg/kg).
The toxicity of some of the organic solvents, such as kerosene, used in the application of dicophane may be as great as that of the pesticide; 150 mg/kg of dicophane in kerosene is considered to be a toxic dose in man.

DICOUMAROL *Anticoagulant*

Synonyms: Bishydroxycoumarin; Dicoumarin; Melitoxin

3,3′-Methylenebis-4-hydroxycoumarin

$C_{19}H_{12}O_6 = 336{\cdot}3$

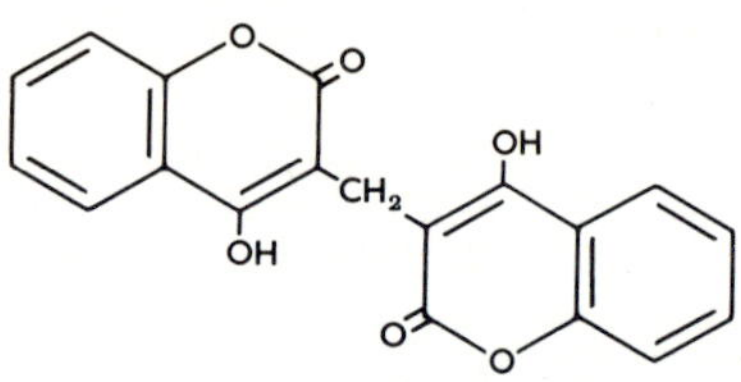

A white crystalline powder. M.p. 287° to 293°.
Solubility. Practically insoluble in water, ethanol, and ether; slightly soluble in chloroform; readily soluble in alkali hydroxides.

Extraction. Dicoumarol is extracted by organic solvents from aqueous acid or alkaline solutions. Christensen (1964) has described a method of extraction from acidified biological fluids and tissue homogenates using ethylene dichloride followed by centrifugation, neutralisation, and final extraction into chloroform.

Chromatography. PAPER: system P8—Rf 0·76 (location under ultraviolet light, weak yellow-green fluorescence; location reagents: *diazotised o-dianisidine spray*, purple; *diazotised sulphanilic acid spray*, orange); system P9—Rf 0·31 (location as for P8); system P10—Rf 0·96 (location as for P8).

Ultraviolet Absorption Spectrum. Dicoumarol in 0·1N sodium hydroxide, maximum at 312 mμ (E1%, 1 cm 850) and an inflexion at about 238 mμ.

Quantitative Estimation. Dicoumarol may be estimated by infra-red spectrophotometry (Stubbs *et al.*, 1962) or spectrophotometrically following paper chromatography and coupling with diazotised sulphanilic acid

(Christensen, 1964). Nagashima *et al.* (1968) have described a spectrophotometric method of estimation of dicoumarol in plasma after its extraction into heptane at a strictly controlled pH of 3.

Metabolism. Dicoumarol is an anticoagulant which is effective when given orally. It acts by inhibiting prothrombin formation by the liver. In man it is very slowly metabolised and, after a single dose, may persist for a week or more. The dicoumarol serum concentration rises to a peak between 6 and 28 hours after ingestion, then slowly declines over a period of a week (Stubbs, 1962).
Very little dicoumarol is excreted in the urine unchanged. Studies in rats have demonstrated the presence of several metabolites in the faeces, tissues, and urine; the most abundant has been shown to have the coumarin ring systems intact (Christensen, 1964 and 1966b).
Dicoumarol has been reported to inhibit the metabolism of phenytoin, phenobarbitone, and tolbutamide (Hansen *et al.*, 1966).

Dose. Up to 300 mg daily, depending on the prothrombin activity of the blood.

Toxicity. Fatalities have been recorded after doses of 100 mg daily, the usual fatal toxic effect being severe haemorrhage. Dicoumarol readily passes through the placenta.
LD50 (oral): in mice about 230 and in rats about 540 mg/kg.

CASE EXAMPLES. Report on 21 deaths due to haemorrhage attributed to dicoumarol during anticoagulant therapy. No analyses presented (Duff and Shull, 1949).
Review of 32 deaths due to haemorrhage resulting from treatment, in many cases overdoses, with dicoumarol (Wright and Rothman, 1951).

DICYCLOMINE *Parasympatholytic*

Synonym: Dicycloverine.

2-Diethylaminoethyl bi(cyclohexyl)-1-carboxylate

$C_{19}H_{35}NO_2 = 309{\cdot}5$

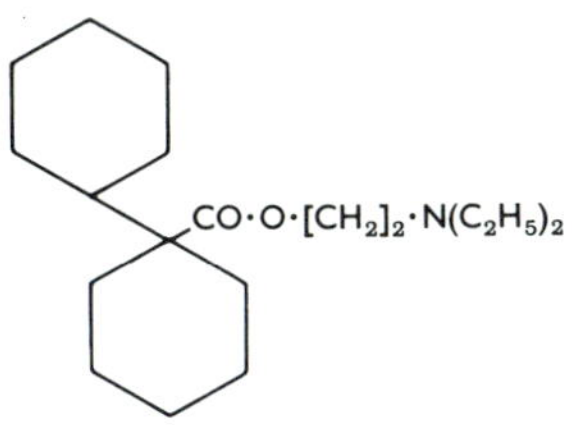

DICYCLOMINE HYDROCHLORIDE

Proprietary Names: Bentyl; Merbentyl; Wyovin.

A white crystalline powder. M.p. 172° to 174°.
Solubility. Soluble 1 in 20 of water, 1 in 5 of ethanol, and 1 in 2 of chloroform; insoluble in ether.

Extraction. Dicyclomine may be isolated in the D1 fraction (see p. 27).

Chromatography. PAPER: system P1—Rf 0·84 (location reagents: *iodoplatinate spray*, strong reaction; *bromocresol green spray*, strong reaction); system RP1a—Rf 0·07 (location reagent *iodoplatinate spray*, positive reaction).
THIN-LAYER: system T1—Rf 0·66 (location reagent *acidified iodoplatinate spray*, positive reaction).
GAS: system G2/225—retention time 0·65 relative to diphenhydramine; system G4—retention time 0·93 relative to diphenhydramine.

Crystal Tests. MICRO: *potassium iodide solution*—branching needles (*sensitivity:* 1 in 200); *trinitrobenzoic acid solution*—rosettes of plates (*sensitivity:* 1 in 200).

Ultraviolet Absorption Spectrum. Dicyclomine in 0·1N sulphuric acid, maximum at 215 mμ.

Infra-red Absorption Spectrum. Dicyclomine (base). Potassium bromide disk. The principal peaks are: A 1122 or 1128, B 1724, C 1154 or 1188 (p. 784).

Dose. Up to 100 mg daily has been given.

Toxicity. The lethal dose in man is probably in the range 10 to 100 mg/kg.

NOTE. Dicyclomine has antispasmodic actions weaker than those of atropine; it also has a local anaesthetic action.

DIELDRIN *Pesticide*

Synonym: Compound 497.

Proprietary Names: It is an ingredient of Dieldrex, Dilstan EC-15, Kypodrin, Murdiel, Octalox, and Superdiel.

Dieldrin contains about 85% w/w HEOD [1,2,3,4,10,10-hexachloro-6,7-epoxy-1,4,4a,5,6,7,8,8a-octahydro-1,4(*exo*):5,8(*endo*)-dimethanonaphthalene] and 15% w/w of active isomeric compounds.

$C_{12}H_8Cl_6O = 380{\cdot}9$

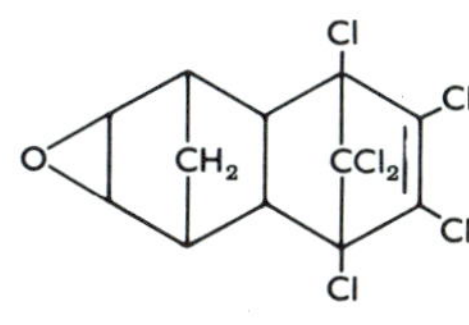

The technical product occurs as a light tan flaky crystalline solid or cream-coloured powder, with a setting-point of 115° to 120° (determined by the method of the *B.P.* 1968 for the setting-point of dicophane, but heating the sample to 125° to 130° in an oil-bath and immersing in a water-bath at 80° during cooling).
Dieldrin is stable in the presence of alkalis, weak acids, and light.
Solubility. Insoluble in water; soluble 1 in 4 of ethanol, 1 in 1 of methanol, and 1 in 40 of carbon tetrachloride; moderately soluble in chloroform.

Extraction. Dieldrin is extracted by organic solvents from aqueous acid or alkaline solutions.

Chromatography. PAPER: Mitchell (1956) has described 4 systems for the separation of chlorinated insecticides, including dieldrin.

GAS: system G2/225—retention time 0·56 relative to codeine.

Colour Tests. Johnson (1956) has described a specific colour test for dieldrin. To 0·1 ml of a 1% solution in xylene add 2 ml of a mixture consisting of 30% fuming sulphuric acid:concentrated sulphuric acid (1:4)—intense red immediately (*sensitivity:* 0·05 mg). Aldrin and endrin produce less intense red colours gradually upon shaking.

Ultraviolet Absorption Spectrum. Dieldrin in ethanol, maximum at 329 mμ (E1%, 1cm 2).

Quantitative Estimation. Garhart *et al.* (1952) describe a method of quantitative estimation of dieldrin involving extraction with acetone, evaporation, and infra-red spectrophotometric measurement in carbon disulphide; Pollard *et al.* (1955) describe a quantitative infra-red spectrophotometric method of determination of dieldrin and dicophane when present in mixtures; Baker and Skerrett (1960) describe a method of estimation of dieldrin involving its conversion to the 2,4-dinitrophenylhydrazone derivative of an isomeric ketone. Hamence *et al.* (1965) describe a method of estimation from biological tissues by gas chromatography.

Metabolism. Dieldrin is a contact and stomach poison which has been widely used in insecticidal dips, sprays, and dusting-powders in agriculture and horticulture. It is readily absorbed through the gastro-intestinal tract, the respiratory tract, and the skin. In contrast to dicophane, dieldrin powder is absorbed through intact skin almost as readily as when in solution. Dieldrin is selectively stored in human body fat, levels of 0·21 p.p.m. of HEOD having been found at 131 post-mortem examinations (Hunter *et al.*, 1963). In cattle, pigs, rats, and sheep, dieldrin is stored unchanged, and it persists for several weeks after the cessation of ingestion.

Toxicity. The estimated lethal dose in man is 5 g. Symptoms of intoxication have occurred after oral doses of 10 mg/kg, and the dermal application of 100 ml of a 25% solution may be dangerous.

LD50 (oral): in rats about 65, in cattle, sheep, and horses 25 mg/kg (estimated).

CASE EXAMPLES. A 9-month-old girl died 20 hours after being found with her face covered with dieldrin powder. She had probably ingested the powder which was loose on paper on the floor. She lost consciousness and developed severe convulsions some 6 hours after taking the powder (Committee on Toxicology, 1960).

A 31-year-old woman administered Ellman's Dieldrin 15 Solution intravenously to herself and died shortly afterwards. Post-mortem examination revealed a dieldrin blood-level of 5 mg% but none could be detected in the kidneys, liver, stomach contents, or urine. It was observed that the hydrocarbon solvent of the preparation is as toxic as the dieldrin (Schwär, 1965).

From a young woman who handled dressed seed, two gallstones were removed and found to contain 0·045 mg% of dieldrin (Simmons and Tattan, 1966).

DIENOESTROL *Oestrogen*

Synonyms: Dehydrostilbestrol; Dienestrol; Oestrodienolum.

Proprietary Names: Hormofemin; Restrol; Synestrol.

3,4-Di(4-hydroxyphenyl)hexa-2,4-diene

$C_{18}H_{18}O_2 = 266·3$

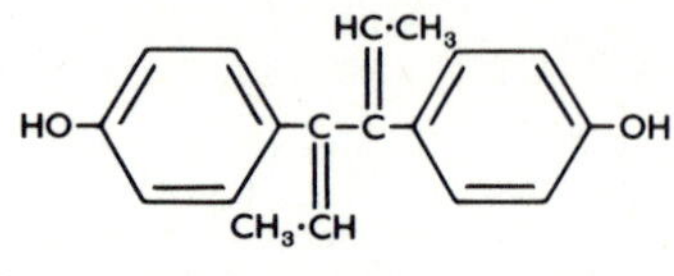

A white crystalline powder. M.p. 230° to 235°.

Solubility. Almost insoluble in water; soluble 1 in 8 of ethanol, 1 in 15 of ether, and 1 in 5 of acetone; slightly soluble in chloroform.

Extraction. Dienoestrol is extracted from neutral solutions with freshly distilled ethyl acetate.

Chromatography. PAPER: system P15—Rf 0·85 (location reagents: *diazotised* p-*nitroaniline spray*, brown; *Pauly's reagent*, purple).

Colour Test. Dissolve about 0·5 mg in 0·2 ml of glacial acetic acid, add 1 ml of phosphoric acid, and heat on a water-bath for 3 minutes—magenta, becoming slightly more blue on dilution with 3 ml of glacial acetic acid. (This test distinguishes dienoestrol from stilboestrol, which produces a yellow colour.)

Ultraviolet Absorption Spectrum. Dienoestrol in ethanol, maxima at 228 mμ (E1%, 1cm 1200) and 276 mμ (E1%, 1cm 160).

Infra-red Absorption Spectrum. Potassium bromide disk. The principal peaks are: A 1199, B 1513, C 828 or 1241 or 1330 (p. 738).

Metabolism. Dienoestrol is a synthetic oestrogen similar to stilboestrol. It is readily absorbed from the gastro-intestinal tract and a high proportion is excreted as a glucuronide conjugate.

Dose. Dienoestrol is administered in doses of up to 45 mg daily.

DIETHAZINE *Parasympatholytic*

Synonyms: Eazamine; RP 2987.

10-(2-Diethylaminoethyl)phenothiazine

$C_{18}H_{22}N_2S = 298·5$

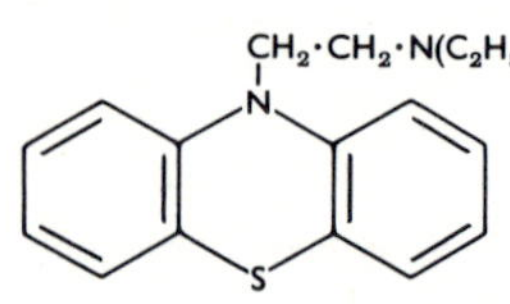

An oily liquid. B.p. 195° to 208° at 0·4 to 0·5 mm Hg.

DIETHAZINE HYDROCHLORIDE

Proprietary Names: Casantin; Diparcol; Latibon.

A white crystalline powder. M.p. 185° to 188°.

Solubility. Soluble 1 in 2·5 of water, 1 in 5 of ethanol, and 1 in 2 of chloroform; insoluble in ether.

Screening Test. *FPN reagent* with urine (see p. 10).

Extraction. Diethazine may be isolated in the D1 fraction (see p. 27); hydrolysis of biological material is required in order to improve the yield.

Chromatography. PAPER: system P1—Rf 0·75 (location under ultraviolet light, yellow fluorescence; location reagents: *iodoplatinate spray*, strong reaction; *bromocresol green spray*, strong reaction); system RP1a—Rf 0·23 (location reagent *iodoplatinate spray*, positive reaction); system RP1b—Rf 0·04 (location as for RP1a).

THIN-LAYER: system T1—Rf 0·61 (location reagent *acidified iodoplatinate spray*, positive reaction); system T6—Rf 0·69 (the spot may be converted on the plate to the sulphoxide, Rf 0·44; location of both spots under ultraviolet light).

GAS: system G2/225—retention time 1·04 relative to codeine; system G4—retention time 0·60 relative to codeine.

Colour Tests. MICRO: sulphuric acid–formaldehyde test—purple-brown (*sensitivity:* 1·0 μg); ammonium molybdate test—green → purple (*sensitivity:* 0·1 μg); ammonium vanadate test—green → purple (excess reagent) (*sensitivity:* 0·1 μg); Vitali's test—purple → yellow/yellow rim/yellow (*sensitivity:* 1·0 μg).

Crystal Tests. MICRO: *platinic bromide solution*—small wedges (*sensitivity:* 1 in 400); *platinic chloride solution*—small serrated needles (*sensitivity:* 1 in 1000).

Ultraviolet Absorption Spectrum. Diethazine in water or 0·1N sulphuric acid, maxima at 250 mμ (E1%, 1 cm 1200) and 298 mμ (E1%, 1 cm 125).

Infra-red Absorption Spectrum. Diethazine (base). Potassium bromide disk. The principal peaks are: A 1456, B 748, C 1245 (p. 784).

Toxicity. The lethal dose in man is probably in the range 15 to 150 mg/kg. Fatalities have been reported.

DIETHYLCARBAMAZINE *Antifilarial*

1-Diethylcarbamoyl-4-methylpiperazine

$C_{10}H_{21}N_3O = 199·3$

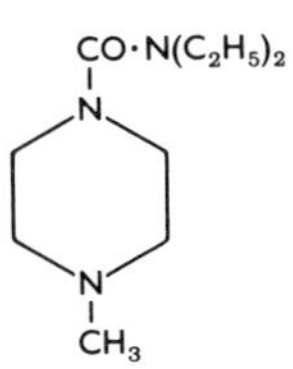

A crystalline powder. M.p. 49°.

Solubility. Soluble in water, ethanol, ether, and chloroform.

DIETHYLCARBAMAZINE CITRATE

Synonym: Diethylcarbamazine Acid Citrate.

Proprietary Names: Banocide; Carbilazine; Ethodryl; Franocide; Hetrazan; Notézine; Spatonin.

A white, slightly hygroscopic, crystalline powder. M.p. 136° to 138°.

Solubility. Very soluble in water; soluble 1 in 35 of ethanol; insoluble in ether and chloroform.

Extraction. Diethylcarbamazine is extracted by organic solvents from aqueous alkaline solutions.

Chromatography. PAPER: system P1—Rf 0·28 (location reagent *iodoplatinate spray*, weak reaction).

THIN-LAYER: system T1—Rf 0·48 (location reagent *Dragendorff spray*, positive reaction).

Colour Test. MICRO: ammonium molybdate test—faint blue (*sensitivity:* 1·0 μg).

Crystal Tests. MICRO: *gold bromide solution*—long plates (*sensitivity:* 1 in 1000); *potassium tri-iodide solution* (*1*)—rods (*sensitivity:* 1 in 1000).

Ultraviolet Absorption Spectrum. Diethylcarbamazine in 0·1N sulphuric acid, maximum at 211 mμ (E1%, 1 cm 581).

Metabolism. Diethylcarbamazine is rapidly absorbed in man and after a single oral dose a peak blood-level is reached in 3 hours. In studies in rats and monkeys with ^{14}C-labelled diethylcarbamazine, about 70% was excreted in 24 hours. The drug was distributed throughout all organs, tissues, and body fluids (Brown, 1960).

Dose. Usually up to 500 mg daily; doses of up to 30 mg/kg have been used.

Toxicity. LD50 (oral): in mice 550 and in rats 395 mg/kg.

DIETHYLPROPION *Anorectic*

Synonym: Amfépramone.

α-Diethylaminopropiophenone

$C_{13}H_{19}NO = 205·3$

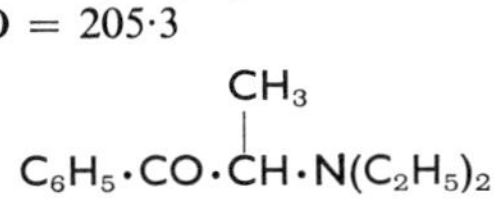

DIETHYLPROPION HYDROCHLORIDE

Proprietary Names: Apisate; Dobesin; Regenon; Tenuate; Tepanil.

Diethylpropion hydrochloride occurs as crystals which melt at 168°.

Solubility. Soluble in water.

Extraction. Diethylpropion may be isolated in the D2 fraction (see p. 27).

Chromatography. PAPER: system P1—Rf 0·58 (location under ultraviolet light, strong absorption; location reagents: *iodoplatinate spray*, weak reaction; *bromocresol green spray*, weak reaction); system RP1a—Rf 0·52 (location under ultraviolet light, absorption); system RP1b—Rf 0·00.

THIN-LAYER: system T1—Rf 0·71 (location reagent *acidified iodoplatinate spray*, positive reaction).

GAS: system G2/120—retention time 1·6 relative to ephedrine.

Crystal Tests. MICRO: *gold bromide solution*—curved serrated needles (*sensitivity:* 1 in 400); *gold chloride solution*—plates, some serrated (*sensitivity:* 1 in 400).

Ultraviolet Absorption Spectrum. Diethylpropion in 0·1N sodium hydroxide, maximum at 246 mμ (E1%, 1 cm 460); in 0·1N sulphuric acid, maximum at 253 mμ (E1%, 1 cm 580). Diethylpropion hydrochloride in 0·1N hydrochloric acid, maxima at 245 mμ (E1%, 1 cm 574), 252 mμ, and 260 mμ.

Infra-red Absorption Spectrum. Diethylpropion (base). Potassium choride disk. The principal peaks are: A 1682, B 1220, C 689 or 1378 or 1445 (p. 784).

Metabolism. Twenty-one metabolites were identified in the urine of subjects who had been given ^{14}C-labelled diethylpropion. Hippuric acid was present in the greatest quantity and represented about 27% of the radioactivity excreted in the urine between 8 and 12 hours after the ingestion of the diethylpropion. Two major basic metabolites remained unidentified (Schreiber *et al.*, 1968).

Dose. Up to 100 mg daily.

Toxicity. The administration of 30 mg/kg to a child has caused cardiac arrest.

LD50 (intravenous): in mice 50 mg/kg.

NOTE. Diethylpropion is related to amphetamine and is used to suppress appetite in obesity. It can lead to addiction.

DIETHYLTHIAMBUTENE

Narcotic Analgesic (Veterinary)

3-Diethylamino-1,1-dithien-2′-ylbut-1-ene

$C_{16}H_{21}NS_2 = 291·5$

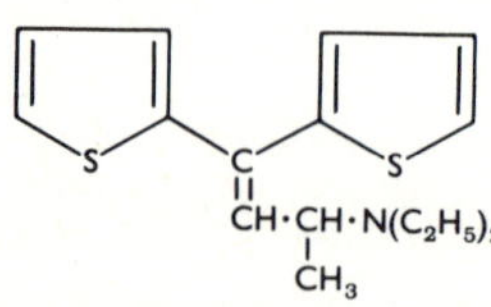

DIETHYLTHIAMBUTENE HYDROCHLORIDE

Proprietary Name: Themalon.

A white crystalline powder. M.p. 151° to 154°.

Solubility. Soluble 1 in 2 of water and 1 in 1 of ethanol; insoluble in ether.

Extraction. Diethylthiambutene is extracted by organic solvents from aqueous alkaline solutions.

Chromatography. PAPER: system P1—Rf 0·67 (location under ultraviolet light, strong absorption; location reagents: *iodoplatinate spray*, strong reaction; *bromocresol green spray*, weak reaction; system RP1a—Rf 0·22 (location under ultraviolet light, absorption); system RP1b—Rf 0·06 (location as for RP1a).

THIN-LAYER: system T1—Rf 0·63 (location reagent *acidified iodoplatinate spray*, positive reaction).

GAS: system G2/225—retention time 1·6 relative to diphenhydramine; system G4—retention time 0·75 relative to diphenhydramine.

Colour Tests. MICRO: sulphuric acid–formaldehyde test—purple (*sensitivity:* 0·1 μg); ammonium vanadate test—green → greenish-blue (*sensitivity:* 0·1 μg); Vitali's test—red → green/brown/brown (*sensitivity:* 0·5 μg).

Crystal Tests. MICRO: *picric acid*—irregular blades, forming overnight, best viewed under polarised light (*sensitivity:* 1 in 400); *potassium iodide solution*—rosettes of plates (*sensitivity:* 1 in 200).

Ultraviolet Absorption Spectrum. Diethylthiambutene in 0·1N sulphuric acid, maxima at 225 mμ (E1%, 1 cm 212), 268 mμ (E1%, 1 cm 327), and 287·5 mμ (E1%, 1 cm 346).

Dose. In dogs, up to 4 mg intravenously, up to 10 mg intramuscularly, and up to 20 mg subcutaneously.

Toxicity. Occasional fatalities and toxic effects have been reported from its use (Owen, 1955).

DIGITOXIN

Cardiac Glycoside

Synonyms: Digitaline Cristallisée; Digitoxoside.

Proprietary Names: Crystodigin; Digimerck; Nativelle's Digitaline; Purpurid.

$C_{41}H_{64}O_{13} = 765·0$

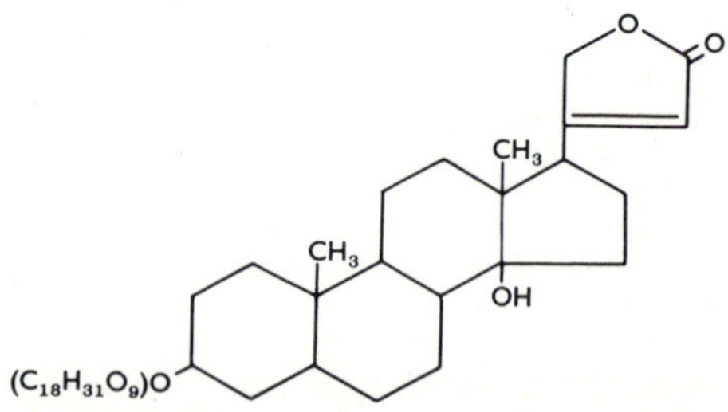

A white crystalline powder, obtained from suitable species of *Digitalis* (Scrophulariaceae). M.p. 256°.

Solubility. Insoluble in water; soluble 1 in 150 of ethanol and 1 in 40 of chloroform; slightly soluble in ether.

Extraction. Digitoxin may be isolated by continuous extraction under reduced pressure with ethanol (see p. 29).

Chromatography. THIN-LAYER: system T14—Rf 0·72 (location reagents: *perchloric acid* *spray*, followed by ultraviolet light, red fluorescence; p-*anisaldehyde spray*, blue). Two thin-layer chromatographic systems which separate digitoxin and digoxin are given in *Pharm. J.*, ii/1965, 80.

Colour Test. Digitoxin and digoxin in solutions of ethanol:chloroform (1:1) are spotted on Whatman No. 7 paper in varying amounts and a 10% solution of *antimony pentachloride in chloroform* is sprayed on the paper—yellow → purple; after warming the sprayed paper in hot air for 5 to 10 minutes—black. After heating, the test is sensitive to 1 to 5 μg.

Ultraviolet Absorption Spectrum. Digitoxin in *sulphuric acid*, maxima at 235 mμ (E1%, 1cm 270), 340 mμ (E1%, 1cm 240), 420 mμ (E1%, 1cm 240), and 485 mμ (E1%, 1cm 230); minima at 265 mμ, 375 mμ, and 440 mμ.

Quantitative Estimation. The simultaneous determination of digitoxin and digoxin in the same sample may be carried out by spectrofluorimetry (Jakovljevic, 1963). A double isotope dilution derivative assay of digitoxin in the plasma, urine, and faeces is described by Lukas and Peterson (1966).

Metabolism. Digitoxin is rapidly and completely absorbed following oral ingestion and its full effect appears as rapidly as by intravenous injection. The liver is the main site of detoxification of the drug, metabolism occurring very rapidly. One metabolite has been identified as digoxigenin di-digitoxoside, produced by hydroxylation and the loss of one molecule of digitoxose. The unchanged drug and metabolites are passed into the gastro-intestinal tract and reabsorbed; they are finally excreted very slowly in the urine. Following the administration of maintenance doses of 0·1 to 0·3 mg daily, 10% of the dose is excreted unchanged. The plasma of patients with chronic cardiac disease treated with the drug contains 1 to 5·6 μg%. Patients on a daily dose of 0·1 mg excrete 8 to 30 μg in the urine during 24 hours and 9 μg to 19 μg in the faeces. Ten days after an injection, half of the dose is still present in the body and some still remains after 20 days.

Dose. Up to 0·2 mg daily; for rapid digitalisation, an initial dosage of up to 1·5 mg, in divided doses over 24 to 48 hours, may be given.

Toxicity. 2 mg may prove fatal. Patients manifesting toxic effects after large doses have been found to have plasma concentrations of 4·3 to 6·7 μg%, these levels being more than twice those in patients taking 0·1 mg daily (Lukas and Peterson, 1966).

CASE EXAMPLES. Report of deaths following ingestion of 0·2 mg daily for a month (17-month-old child), and 8·9 mg (26-year-old woman) (McNamara *et al.*, 1964).

DIGOXIN *Cardiac Glycoside*

Proprietary Names: Lanicor; Lanoxin.

3β-Tridigitoxoside of digoxigenin

$C_{41}H_{64}O_{14} = 781{\cdot}0$

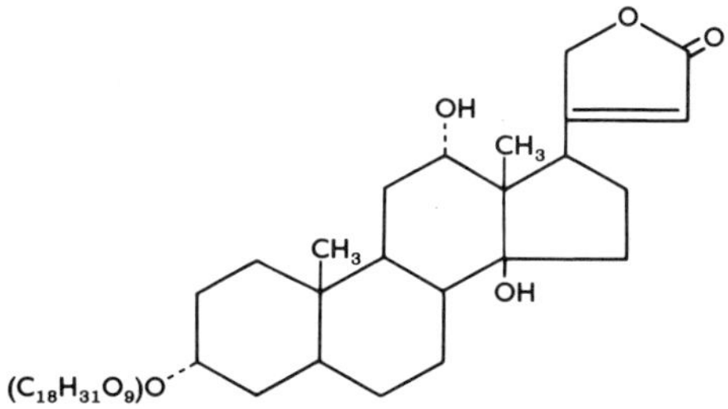

A white crystalline powder, obtained from the leaves of the woolly foxglove, *Digitalis lanata* (Scrophulariaceae). M.p. about 240°, with decomposition.

Solubility. Almost insoluble in water, ethanol, ether, and chloroform; soluble 1 in 122 of 80% ethanol and 1 in 4 of pyridine.

Extraction. Digoxin may be isolated by continuous extraction under reduced pressure with ethanol (see p. 29).

Chromatography. THIN-LAYER: system T14—Rf 0·62 (location reagents: *perchloric acid spray* followed by ultraviolet light, blue fluorescence; p-*anisaldehyde spray*, blue). Two thin-layer chromatographic systems which separate digitoxin and digoxin are given in *Pharm. J.*, ii/1965, 80.

Colour Test. See under Digitoxin, above.

Ultraviolet Absorption Spectrum. Digoxin in *sulphuric acid*, maxima at 230 mμ (E1%, 1cm 260), 320 mμ (E1%, 1cm 225), 390 mμ (E1%, 1cm 305), and 490 mμ (E1%, 1cm 210); minima at 265 mμ, 340 mμ, and 430 mμ.

Infra-red Absorption Spectrum. Potassium bromide disk. The principal peaks are: A 1075, B 1709, C 1020 or 1055 (p. 738).

Quantitative Estimation. The simultaneous determination of digitoxin and digoxin may be carried out by spectrofluorimetry (Jakovljevic, 1963).

Metabolism. Digoxin is rapidly absorbed and distributed in the tissues. It is largely excreted unchanged in the urine and more rapidly so than digitoxin. Following intravenous injections of 1 mg in normal subjects, 26·8% of the dose appeared in the urine in the first 24 hours, 93·9% in the form of digoxin; 14·8% of the dose appeared in the faeces, mainly as metabolites (Marcus *et al.*, 1964). One metabolite of digoxin has been identified as digoxigenin di-digitoxoside which is obtained by the loss of one sugar residue (Wright, 1962).

Dose. Up to 0·75 mg daily; for rapid digitilisation, an initial dose of up to 1·5 mg may be given.

Toxicity. Digoxin is more rapidly excreted than digitoxin so that it is less likely to give rise to cumulative toxic effects.

LD50 (intravenous): in guinea-pigs 0·355 mg/kg.

CASE EXAMPLES. A girl aged 19 months died 82 hours after swallowing about 10 mg of digoxin just before a meal (*J. Pediat.*, 1964, **64**, 188).
Death of a 2-year-old girl after taking about 30 digoxin tablets (0·25 mg each) (*Pharm. J.*, ii/1967, 143).

DIHYDRALLAZINE *Antihypertensive*

Synonyms: C 7441; Dihydralazine.

1,4-Dihydrazinophthalazine
$C_8H_{10}N_6 = 190{\cdot}2$

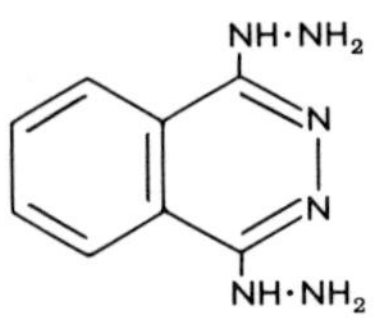

DIHYDRALLAZINE SULPHATE
Proprietary Names: Nepresol; Népressol. It is an ingredient of Adelphane, Desencin, and Ipharon.

Yellowish crystalline needles. M.p. 245°.
Solubility. Soluble 1 in about 300 of water.

Extraction. Dihydrallazine is extracted by organic solvents from aqueous alkaline solutions.

Chromatography. PAPER: system P1—Rf 0·36 (location under ultraviolet light, blue fluorescent streak; location reagent *iodoplatinate spray*, weak reaction).

Colour Tests. MICRO: ammonium molybdate test—(red-brown) red-brown (*sensitivity:* 1·0 µg); ammonium vanadate test—(dull green) yellow (*sensitivity:* 1·0 µg); Vitali's test— -/-/ brown, fading (*sensitivity:* 0·1 µg).

Crystal Tests. MICRO: *gold bromide–hydrochloric acid solution*—needles, often hairlike, which vanish (*sensitivity:* 1 in 400); *platinic iodide solution*—dense rosettes or bunches of needles (*sensitivity:* 1 in 1000).

Ultraviolet Absorption Spectrum. Dihydrallazine in 0·1N sulphuric acid, maxima at 219 mµ (E1%, 1cm 1466), about 240 mµ (E1%, 1cm 388), 274 mµ (E1%, 1cm 207), and 308 mµ (E1%, 1cm 213).

Infra-red Absorption Spectrum. Dihydrallazine (base). Potassium bromide disk. The principal peaks are: A 1608, B 1575 or 1633, C 1375 or 1458 or 1537 (p. 784).

DIHYDROCODEINE *Narcotic Analgesic*

Synonym: Morphine 3-Methyl Ether.

4,5 - Epoxy - 6 - hydroxy - 3 - methoxy - *N* - methylmorphinan
$C_{18}H_{23}NO_3 = 301{\cdot}4$

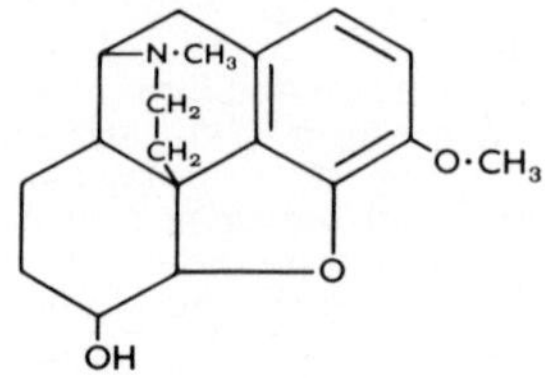

Crystals which melt at 112° to 113°. B.p. 248°.

DIHYDROCODEINE ACID TARTRATE
Synonyms: Dihydrocodeine Bitartrate; Hydrocodeine Bitartrate.
Proprietary Names: DF 118; Didrate; Paracodin.

A white crystalline powder. M.p. 190° to 194°.
Solubility. Soluble 1 in 4·5 of water; slightly soluble in ethanol; almost insoluble in ether.

DIHYDROCODEINE PHOSPHATE
Synonym: Hydrocodeine Phosphate.

A white powder.
Solubility. Soluble 1 in 3 of water; almost insoluble in ethanol.

Extraction. Dihydrocodeine is extracted by organic solvents from aqueous alkaline solutions; hydrolysis of biological material is required in order to improve the yield.

Chromatography. PAPER: system P1—Rf 0·20 (location under ultraviolet light, strong absorption; location reagents: *iodoplatinate spray*, strong reaction; *bromocresol green spray*, weak reaction); system RP1a—Rf 0·89 (location reagent *iodoplatinate spray*, positive reaction); system RP1b—Rf 0·35 (location as for RP1a).
THIN-LAYER: system T1—Rf 0·25 (location reagent *acidified iodoplatinate spray*, positive reaction).
GAS: system G2/225—retention time 1·0 relative to codeine; system G4—retention time 0·95 relative to codeine.

Colour Tests. MICRO: sulphuric acid–formaldehyde test—purple (*sensitivity:* 0·1 µg); ammonium molybdate test—green → blue (*sensitivity:* 0·1 µg); ammonium vanadate test—faint grey-green (*sensitivity:* 1·0 µg); Vitali's test—faint yellow/faint yellow/orange (*sensitivity:* 1·0 µg).

Crystal Test. MICRO: *potassium bismuth iodide solution*—bunches of plates (*sensitivity:* 1 in 6000).

Ultraviolet Absorption Spectrum. Dihydrocodeine in ethanol, maximum at 284 to 285 mµ; in 0·1N sulphuric acid, maximum at 282·5 mµ (E1%, 1cm 41·7) and inflexion at 277 mµ.

Metabolism. Following administration in man, between 7 and 18% is excreted in the conjugated form and 13 to 22% as unchanged drug.

Dose. Up to 60 mg.

Toxicity. The estimated minimum lethal dose

in man is 800 mg but it may be 10 times as high in addicts.

CASE EXAMPLE. Examination of a man, found dead after ingesting a few barbiturate tablets and some 22 tablets containing in all about 660 mg of dihydrocodeine, showed the stomach contents to contain 6 mg and the liver 2 mg% of dihydrocodeine (Kimber, 1966).

DIHYDROERGOTAMINE *Ergot Alkaloid*

$C_{33}H_{37}N_5O_5$ = 583·7

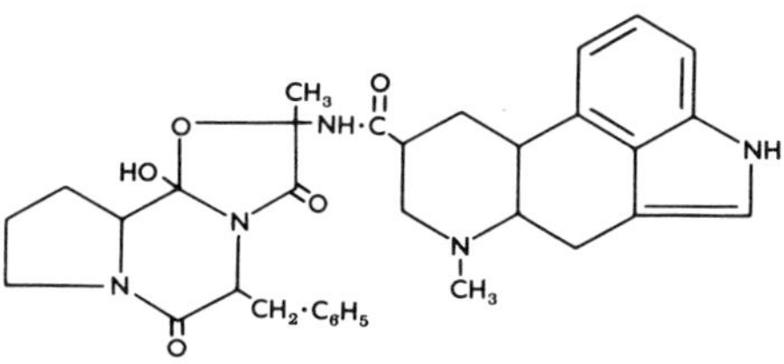

White crystals. M.p. 239°.

Solubility. Insoluble in water; slightly soluble in ethanol and chloroform.

DIHYDROERGOTAMINE MESYLATE

Synonyms: DHE 45; Dihydroergotamine Methanesulphonate.

A white microcrystalline powder which should be protected from light in an atmosphere of nitrogen in sealed containers, in a cool place.

Solubility. Moderately soluble in water and ethanol.

DIHYDROERGOTAMINE TARTRATE

A white powder.

Solubility. Soluble in water and pyridine.

Extraction. Dihydroergotamine is extracted by organic solvents from aqueous alkaline solutions.

Chromatography. PAPER: system P1—Rf 0·63 (location under ultraviolet light, pale green fluorescence; location reagent p-*dimethylaminobenzaldehyde spray*, blue).

THIN-LAYER: system T1—Rf 0·63 (location reagent p-*dimethylaminobenzaldehyde spray*, blue); system T9—Rf 0·35 (location under ultraviolet light, green fluorescence; location reagent p-*dimethylaminobenzaldehyde spray*, blue).

Colour Tests. MICRO: sulphuric acid–formaldehyde test—grey-brown (*sensitivity:* 1·0 μg); ammonium molybdate test—blue → brown (*sensitivity:* 0·5 μg); ammonium vanadate test—purple-brown (*sensitivity:* 1·0 μg); Vitali's test—dull orange/dull orange/brown (*sensitivity:* 1·0 μg).

Dose. Up to 3 mg.

Toxicity. LD50 (intravenous): in mice 118, in rabbits 25, and in rats 110 mg/kg.

DIHYDROERGOTOXINE MESYLATE *Ergot Alkaloid*

Synonym: Dihydroergotoxine Methanesulphonate.

Proprietary Name: Hydergine.

A mixture of the methanesulphonates of dihydroergocornine, dihydroergocristine, and dihydroergocryptine, the hydrogenated derivatives of the 3 alkaloids of ergotoxine.

Extraction. Dihydroergotoxine is extracted by organic solvents from aqueous alkaline solutions.

Chromatography. PAPER: system P1—Rf 0·80 (location under ultraviolet light, green fluorescence; location reagents: p-*dimethylaminobenzaldehyde spray*, blue; *potassium permanganate spray*, strong reaction).

THIN-LAYER: system T1—0·71 (location reagent p-*dimethylaminobenzaldehyde spray*, blue).

Dose. Up to 2 mg daily.

DIHYDROMORPHINE *Narcotic Analgesic*

4,5 - Epoxy - 3,6 - dihydroxy - *N* - methylmorphinan

$C_{17}H_{21}NO_3$ = 287·4

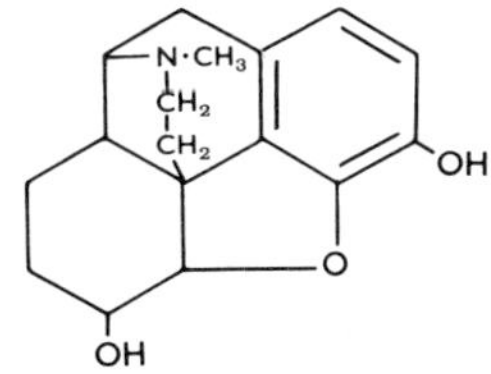

White crystals. M.p. of the hydrated compound, 157°, with decomposition.

Solubility. Insoluble in water; soluble in ethanol and chloroform.

DIHYDROMORPHINE HYDROCHLORIDE

Solubility. Very soluble in water; slightly soluble in ethanol.

Extraction. Dihydromorphine may be extracted by organic solvents from aqueous ammoniacal solutions; hydrolysis of biological material is required in order to increase the yield.

Chromatography. PAPER: system P1—Rf 0·16 (location under ultraviolet light, strong absorption; location reagents: *iodoplatinate spray*, strong reaction; *bromocresol green spray*, weak reaction); system RP1a—Rf 0·90 (location reagent *iodoplatinate spray*, positive reaction); system RP1b—Rf 0·88 (location as for RP1a).

THIN-LAYER: system T1—Rf 0·23 (location reagent *acidified iodoplatinate spray*, positive reaction); system T7—Rf 0·10 (location reagent *iodoplatinate spray*, positive reaction); system T8—Rf 0·21 (location as for T7).

GAS: system G2/225—retention time 1·2 relative to codeine.

Colour Tests. MICRO: sulphuric acid–formaldehyde test—red-purple (*sensitivity:* 0·025 μg); ammonium molybdate test—blue-purple (*sensitivity:* 0·025 μg); ammonium vanadate test—grey (*sensitivity:* 1·0 μg); Vitali's test—yellow/yellow/orange (*sensitivity:* 0·5 μg).

Crystal Tests. MICRO: *platinic iodide solution*—smudge rosettes (*sensitivity:* 1 in 3000); *potassium mercuric iodide solution*—sheaves of fine needles (*sensitivity:* 1 in 1000).

Ultraviolet Absorption Spectrum. Dihydromorphine in ethanol, maximum at 286 mμ; minimum at 258 mμ; in 0·1N sulphuric acid, maximum at 283 mμ (E1%, 1cm 42) and an inflexion at 278 mμ.

Metabolism. When injected subcutaneously into rats, tritium-labelled dihydromorphine was metabolised primarily by conjugation. A very small amount of the drug underwent *N*-demethylation; a total of 85% of the administered dose was excreted in the urine and faeces, partly in the conjugated form and partly in the free form (Hug and Mellett, 1965).

Toxicity. LD50 (subcutaneous): in mice 133 and in rabbits 160 mg/kg.

DIHYDROSTREPTOMYCIN

Antibiotic/Tuberculostatic

2,4 - Diguanidino - 3,5,6 - trihydroxycyclohexyl 5 - deoxy - 2 - *O* - (2 - deoxy - 2 - methylamino - α - L - glucopyranosyl) - 3 - hydroxymethyl - β - L - *lyxo*pentanofuranoside

$C_{21}H_{41}N_7O_{12}$ = 583·6

DIHYDROSTREPTOMYCIN SULPHATE

Proprietary Name: Didromycine.

A white solid.

Solubility. Very soluble in water; almost insoluble in ethanol, ether, and chloroform.

Chromatography. PAPER: system P1—Rf 0·00 (location reagents: *bromine–starch–potassium iodide*, weak reaction; *iodine vapour*, weak reaction).

THIN-LAYER: system T1—Rf 0·01 (location reagent *potassium permanganate spray*, positive reaction).

Colour Test. MICRO: ammonium molybdate test—faint blue.

Metabolism. Dihydrostreptomycin is readily absorbed and excreted in man, following intramuscular administration. About 50 to 75% is excreted in the urine within 24 hours, peak serum concentrations occurring after one hour. Practically no absorption takes place after oral administration.

Dose. Up to 1 g daily, intramuscularly.

Toxicity. Toxic effects following administration of dihydrostreptomycin may not become apparent until several weeks after treatment has ceased.

LD50 (oral): in mice 9 g/kg.

DI-IODOHYDROXYQUINOLINE

Anti-amoebic

Synonyms: Diiodohydroxyquin; Diodoxyquinoline.

Proprietary Names: Diodoquin; Embequin; Ioquin; Savorquin.

8-Hydroxy-5,7-diiodoquinoline

$C_9H_5I_2NO$ = 397·0

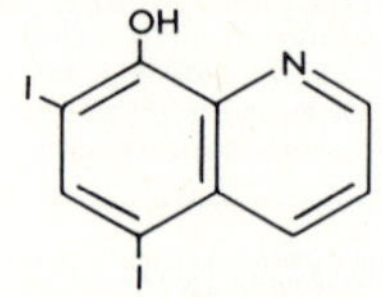

A yellowish microcrystalline powder. M.p. 200° to 215°, with decomposition.

Solubility. Almost insoluble in water; sparingly soluble in ethanol, ether, and acetone.

Extraction. Di-iodohydroxyquinoline is extracted by organic solvents from aqueous alkaline solutions.

Colour Test. Heat a few crystals with 1 ml of sulphuric acid—violet iodine vapour.

Ultraviolet Absorption Spectrum. Di-iodohydroxyquinoline in ethanol, maximum at 258 mμ (E1%, 1cm 1060).

Infra-red Absorption Spectrum. Potassium bromide disk. The principal peaks are: A 1330 or 1390, B 1484 (p. 738).

Metabolism. Di-iodohydroxyquinoline is irregularly absorbed from the small intestine and because of its low solubility much of the dose reaches the large intestine where it is thought to act upon the amoebae living in the lumen or upon the bacteria on which they feed. Di-iodohydroxyquinoline slowly releases iodine which has been found in appreciable amounts in the thyroid gland, the spleen, the lungs, and muscle. Excretion of di-iodohydroxyquinoline seems to be dependent upon the mode of administration; rabbits, after oral doses, excrete in the urine 39% of the iodine administered and 61% in the faeces whereas, after intravenous doses, only 39% of the iodine is excreted, nearly all of it in the urine. The drug is excreted mostly in the form of glucuronide and sulphate conjugates.

Dose. Up to 2·4 g daily.

DIMEFLINE

Analeptic

Synonyms: DW 62; Rec 7-0267.

8 - Dimethylaminomethyl - 7 - methoxy - 3 - methyl-2-phenyl-4*H*-chromen-4-one

$C_{20}H_{21}NO_3$ = 323·4

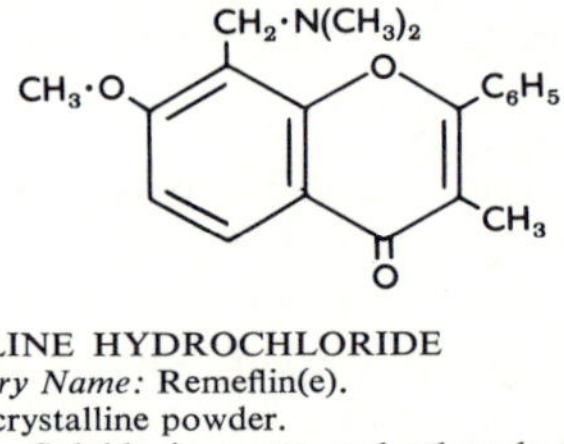

DIMEFLINE HYDROCHLORIDE

Proprietary Name: Remeflin(e).

A white crystalline powder.

Solubility. Soluble in water and ethanol; insoluble in ether and chloroform.

Extraction. Dimefline is extracted by organic solvents from aqueous alkaline solutions.

Chromatography. PAPER: system P1—Rf 0·53 (location under ultraviolet light, dark blue fluorescence; location reagents: *iodoplatinate spray*, strong reaction; *bromocresol green spray*, weak reaction).

THIN-LAYER: system T1—Rf 0·56 (location reagent *acidified iodoplatinate spray*, positive reaction).

Crystal Tests. MICRO: *gold cyanide solution*—blades or plates, best viewed under polarised light (*sensitivity:* 1 in 1000); *lead iodide solution*—irregular rosettes (*sensitivity:* 1 in 1000).

Ultraviolet Absorption Spectrum. Dimefline in 0·1N sulphuric acid, maxima at 245 mμ (E1%, 1 cm 785) and 309 mμ (E1%, 1 cm 950).

Infra-red Absorption Spectrum. Dimefline (base). Potassium bromide disk. The principal peaks are: A 1637, B 1278 or 1389, C 1081 or 1428 or 1602 (p. 784).

Quantitative Estimation. De Fina and Setnikar (1966) have described a method for the extraction and spectrophotometric determination of dimefline from rat tissue.

Dose. Up to 45 mg by mouth; up to 24 mg by injection.

Toxicity. LD50 (intraperitoneal): in mice 6·2 mg/kg.

DIMENOXADOLE *Narcotic*

2-Dimethylaminoethyl α-ethoxy-α,α-diphenylacetate

$C_{20}H_{25}NO_3$ = 327·4

$$CH_3\cdot CH_2\cdot O\cdot C(C_6H_5)_2\cdot CO\cdot O\cdot [CH_2]_2\cdot N(CH_3)_2$$

Dimenoxadole melts at 170° to 172°.

Chromatography. PAPER: system P1—Rf 0·62 (location under ultraviolet light, absorption; location reagents: *iodoplatinate spray*, strong reaction; *bromocresol green spray*, weak reaction).

THIN-LAYER: system T1—Rf 0·60 (location reagent *acidified iodoplatinate spray*, positive reaction).

Colour Tests. MICRO: sulphuric acid–formaldehyde test—orange → greenish-blue (*sensitivity:* 0·1 μg); ammonium molybdate test—orange → dull purple (*sensitivity:* 0·1 μg); ammonium vanadate test—orange → dull purple (*sensitivity:* 0·1 μg).

Crystal Tests. MICRO: *platinic bromide solution*—rosettes of branching rods (*sensitivity:* 1 in 3000); *styphnic acid*—bunches of plates (*sensitivity:* 1 in 3000).

Toxicity. LD50 (oral): in mice 700 to 800 mg/kg.

DIMERCAPROL

Synonyms: BAL; British Anti-Lewisite; Dimercaptopropanol.

2,3-Dimercaptopropan-1-ol

$C_3H_8OS_2$ = 124·2

$$HS\cdot CH_2\cdot CH(SH)\cdot CH_2OH$$

A clear colourless liquid. It should be kept in a small, well-filled, well-closed container in a cool place. B.p. 80° at 1·9 mm Hg. Refractive index 1·570 to 1·575.

Solubility. Soluble 1 in 20 of water; miscible with ethanol.

Ultraviolet Absorption Spectrum. Dimercaprol in water, maximum at 197·5 mμ.

Infra-red Absorption Spectrum. Liquid film. The principal peaks are: A 1022, B 1050, C 990 or 1418 (p. 739).

Metabolism. Dimercaprol combines in the body with arsenic, mercury, and other heavy metals. It is used in the treatment of acute poisoning by antimony, arsenic, bismuth, gold and mercury. It combines with these metals through its two sulphydryl groups and the resulting compounds are stable and rapidly excreted by the kidneys. Following intramuscular injection, the maximum concentration in the blood is reached in about 2 hours. Dimercaprol is entirely excreted or metabolised within 6 to 24 hours.

Dose. Usually up to 800 mg daily, intramuscularly; max. in 24 hours 1·5 g.

Toxicity. Doses of dimercaprol at a rate of 4 to 5 mg/kg produce transitory side-effects, including nausea, vomiting, lachrymation and salivation, muscle pains, and muscle spasm, in about 50% of patients. Dimercaprol is intensely irritating when applied to the skin and mucous membranes.

LD50 (intramuscular): in rats 105 mg/kg.

DIMETHINDENE *Antihistamine*

Synonyms: Dimethpyrindene; SU 6518.

2 - {1 - [2 - (2 - Dimethylaminoethyl)inden - 3 - yl]ethyl}pyridine

$C_{20}H_{24}N_2$ = 292·4

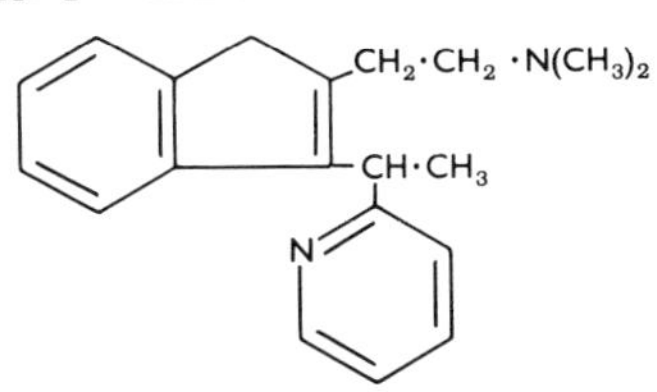

DIMETHINDENE MALEATE

Proprietary Names: Fenostil; Forhistal.

A white crystalline powder.

Solubility. Soluble in water.

Extraction. Dimethindene is extracted by

organic solvents from aqueous alkaline solutions.

Chromatography. PAPER: system P1—Rf 0·38 (location under ultraviolet light, white fluorescence; location reagents: *iodoplatinate spray*, strong reaction; *bromocresol green spray*, weak reaction); system RP1a—Rf 0·12 (location reagent *iodoplatinate spray*, positive reaction); system RP1b—Rf 0·04 (location as for RP1a).
THIN-LAYER: system T1—Rf 0·36 (location reagent *acidified iodoplatinate spray*, positive reaction).
GAS: system G2/225—retention time 0·75 relative to codeine; system G4—retention time 0·47 relative to codeine.

Colour Tests. MICRO: sulphuric acid–formaldehyde test—purple → deep blue (*sensitivity:* 0·1 μg); ammonium molybdate test—green → blue (*sensitivity:* 0·1 μg); ammonium vanadate test—green (*sensitivity:* 0·25 μg); Vitali's test—yellow/faint orange/deep green (*sensitivity:* 0·25 μg).

Crystal Tests. MICRO: *gold cyanide solution*—rosettes of long plates (*sensitivity:* 1 in 1000); *platinic chloride solution*—irregular rosettes of plates (*sensitivity:* 1 in 1000).

Dose. Usually 3 mg daily.

Toxicity. The estimated acute lethal dose in man is in the range 25 to 250 mg/kg.
LD50 (oral): in guinea-pigs 888 mg/kg.

DIMETHISOQUIN *Local Anaesthetic*

Synonyms: Chinisocaine; Quinisocaine; SKF 538A.

3 - Butyl - 1 - (2 - dimethylaminoethoxy)isoquinoline
$C_{17}H_{24}N_2O = 272{\cdot}4$

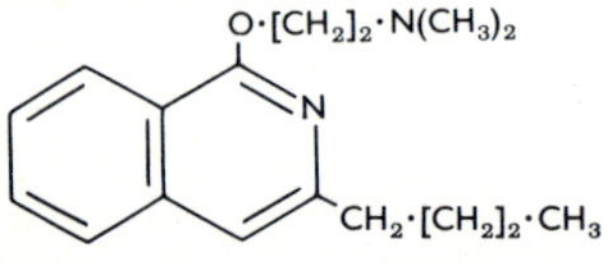

Dimethisoquin occurs as a liquid. B.p. about 156°.

DIMETHISOQUIN HYDROCHLORIDE
Proprietary Names: Pruralgin; Quotane.

A white crystalline powder. M.p. 144° to 148°.
Solubility. Soluble 1 in 8 of water, 1 in 3 of ethanol, and 1 in 2 of chloroform; very slightly soluble in ether.

Extraction. Dimethisoquin is extracted by organic solvents from aqueous alkaline solutions.

Chromatography. PAPER: system P1—Rf 0·70 (location under ultraviolet light, bright blue fluorescence; location reagents: *iodoplatinate spray*, strong reaction; *bromocresol green spray*, weak reaction); system RP1a—Rf 0·99 (location reagent *iodoplatinate spray*, positive reaction); system RP1b—Rf 0·00 (location as for RP1a).
THIN-LAYER: system T1—Rf 0·56 (location reagent *acidified iodoplatinate spray*, positive reaction).

Crystal Tests. MICRO: *potassium iodide solution*—bunches of serrated blades (*sensitivity:* 1 in 1500); *trinitrobenzoic acid solution*—masses of needles (*sensitivity:* 1 in 1500).

Ultraviolet Absorption Spectrum. Dimethisoquin in ethanol, an inflexion at 265 mμ and maxima at 274 mμ (E1%, 1cm 240), 283 mμ (E1%, 1cm 210), 316 mμ (E1%, 1cm 110), and 328 mμ (E1%, 1cm 100); in 0·1N sulphuric acid, maxima at 227 mμ (E1%, 1cm 1254), 261 mμ (E1%, 1cm 153), 269 mμ (E1%, 1cm 158), 331 mμ (E1%, 1cm 151), and 343 mμ (E1%, 1cm 126); dimethisoquin hydrochloride in isopropanol (0·00005% solution), maxima at about 285 mμ, about 316 mμ, and about 328 mμ.

Toxicity. Dimethisoquin is usually employed as a lotion or ointment in a concentration of 0·5%. The maximum amount considered safe for surface analgesia is 100 mg or 10 ml of a 1% solution.
LD50 (intraperitoneal): in rats 50 mg/kg.

DIMETHISTERONE *Progestational Steroid*

Synonyms: 6α,21-Dimethylethisterone; P 5048.
Proprietary Name: Secrosteron. It is an ingredient of Secrodyl.

17β - Hydroxy - 6α,21 - dimethyl - 17α - pregn - 4-en-20-yn-3-one monohydrate
$C_{23}H_{32}O_2,H_2O = 358{\cdot}5$

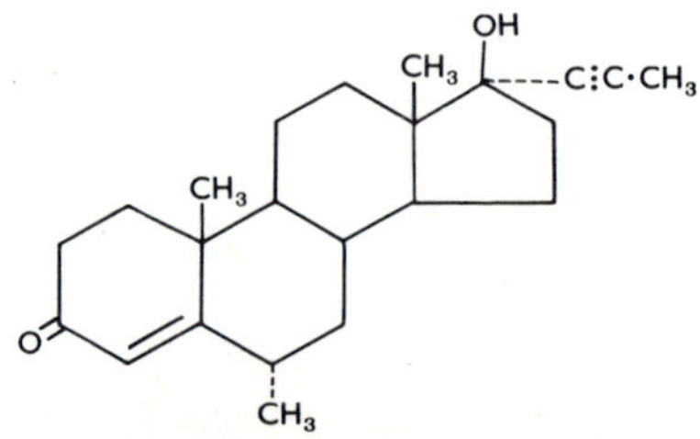

A white crystalline powder. M.p. about 100°, with decomposition. Specific rotation of a 2% solution in chloroform, +16° to +21·5°.
Solubility. Insoluble in water; soluble 1 in 3 of ethanol, 1 in 0·7 of chloroform, and 1 in 1 of pyridine.

Extraction. Dimethisterone is extracted from neutral solutions with freshly distilled ethyl acetate.

Ultraviolet Absorption Spectrum. Dimethisterone in ethanol, maximum at about 240 mμ (E1%, 1cm 467).

Infra-red Absorption Spectrum. Potassium bromide disk. The principal peaks are: A 1650, B 1269, C 1600 (p. 739).

Metabolism. Dimethisterone is a progestational agent which also possesses slight oestrogenic activity. It is frequently administered in conjunction with ethinyloestradiol in oral contraceptive preparations.

Dose. Up to 40 mg daily.

DIMETHOATE *Pesticide*

Synonyms: Am. Cyanamid 12880; L 395; Rogor.
Proprietary Names: Boots Systemic Insecticide Concentrate; Cygon Dimethoate; Perfekthion.

Dimethyl *S*-methylcarbamoylmethyl phosphorothiolothionate

$C_5H_{12}NO_3PS_2 = 229{\cdot}3$

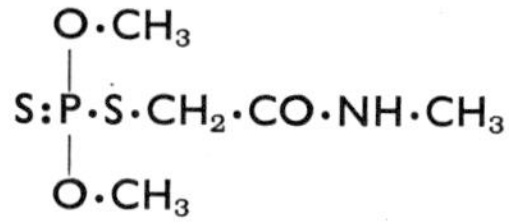

A white solid. M.p. 51° to 52°.

Solubility. Moderately soluble in water; soluble in most organic solvents except hydrocarbons.

Extraction. Dimethoate is extracted by organic solvents from aqueous acid solutions.

Chromatography. THIN-LAYER: system T16—Rf 0·03 (location reagent *bromophenol blue spray* followed by 5% *aqueous acetic acid spray*, blue).

Metabolism. Dimethoate is used as a systemic insecticide in cattle. Studies in cows have shown dimethoate to be rapidly metabolised and excreted; 12 days after treatment it was present in the tissues in only trace amounts. Hydrolysis of dimethoate occurred initially at the methyl-phosphate, phosphate-sulphur, sulphur-carbon, and particularly at the carbonyl-nitrogen bonds (Dauterman *et al.*, 1959).

Toxicity. Dimethoate can be harmful to animals, birds, bees, and fish. The minimum lethal dose in calves is 80 mg/kg.

LD50 (oral): in cats 150, in mice 250, and in rats 300 mg/kg.

NOTE. The maximum acceptable daily intake in man is 0·004 mg/kg (FAO/WHO Expert Committee on Pesticide Residues, 1967). Following studies of the response of adult volunteers to the daily ingestion of dimethoate, Edson *et al.* (1967) have concluded that this maximum figure might safely be raised to 0·02 mg/kg.

DIMETHOTHIAZINE *Antihistamine*

Synonyms: Dimethitazine; Dimetotiazine; RP 8599.
Proprietary Name: Migristène.

10 - (2 - Dimethylaminopropyl) - *NN* - dimethylphenothiazine-2-sulphonamide

$C_{19}H_{25}N_3O_2S_2 = 391{\cdot}6$

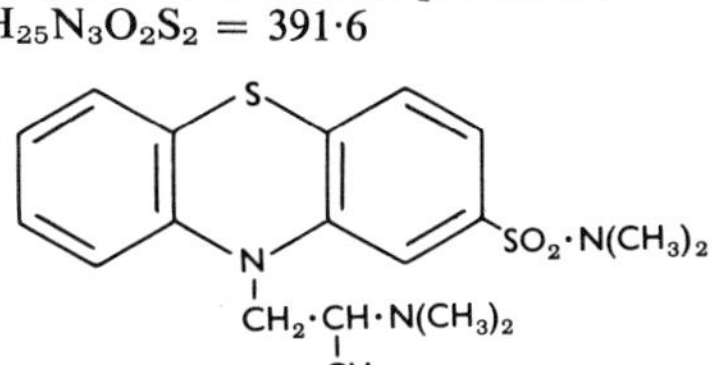

Extraction. Dimethothiazine is extracted by organic solvents from aqueous alkaline solutions; hydrolysis of biological material is required in order to improve the yield.

Chromatography. PAPER: system P1—Rf 0·63 (location under ultraviolet light, pale green fluorescence; location reagents: *iodoplatinate spray*, weak reaction; *bromocresol green spray*, weak reaction; *potassium permanganate spray*, weak reaction).

THIN-LAYER: system T1—Rf 0·54 (location reagent *acidified iodoplatinate spray*, positive reaction).

Colour Tests. MICRO: sulphuric acid–formaldehyde test—red (*sensitivity:* 0·1 µg); ammonium molybdate test—purple (*sensitivity:* 0·1 µg); ammonium vanadate test—red-purple (*sensitivity:* 0·25 µg).

Crystal Tests. MICRO: *gold bromide solution*—tablets, forming overnight (*sensitivity:* 1 in 1000); *gold bromide–hydrochloric acid solution*—branching needles, forming overnight (*sensitivity:* 1 in 100).

Ultraviolet Absorption Spectrum. Dimethothiazine in 0·1N sulphuric acid, maxima at 235 mµ (E1%, 1 cm 525), 261 mµ (E1%, 1 cm 666), and 306 mµ (E1%, 1 cm 85).

Dose. Up to 80 mg daily.

DIMETHOXANATE *Antitussive*

2-(2-Dimethylaminoethoxy)ethyl phenothiazine-10-carboxylate

$C_{19}H_{22}N_2O_3S = 358{\cdot}5$

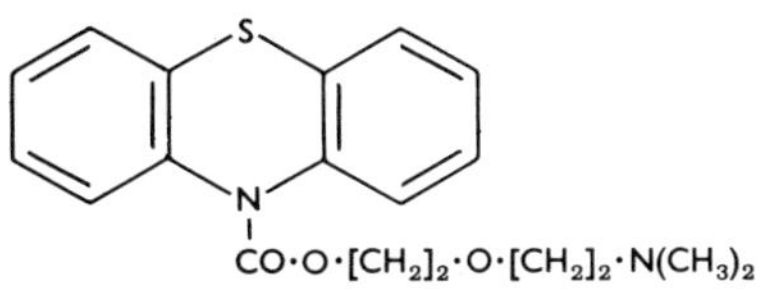

DIMETHOXANATE HYDROCHLORIDE
Proprietary Names: Cothera; Cotrane.

Dimethoxanate hydrochloride melts at 161° to 163°, with decomposition.

Extraction. Dimethoxanate is extracted by organic solvents from aqueous alkaline solutions.

Chromatography. PAPER: system P1—Rf 0·54 (location under ultraviolet light, yellow-green fluorescence; location reagent *iodoplatinate spray*, strong reaction); system RP1a—Rf 0·61 (location under ultraviolet light, green fluorescence; location reagent *iodoplatinate spray*, positive reaction); system RP1b—Rf 0·04 (location reagent *iodoplatinate spray*, positive reaction).

THIN-LAYER: system T1—Rf 0·36 (location reagent *acidified iodoplatinate spray*, positive reaction); system T6—Rf 0·56 (the spot may be converted on the plate to the sulphoxide, Rf 0·41; location of both spots under ultraviolet light).

Colour Tests. MICRO: sulphuric acid–formaldehyde test—faint purple (*sensitivity:* 1·0 μg); ammonium molybdate test—dull purple → brown (*sensitivity:* 1·0 μg); ammonium vanadate test—green → brown (*sensitivity:* 1·0 μg).

Crystal Tests. MICRO: *mercuric chloride solution*—feathery rosettes, forming overnight (*sensitivity:* 1 in 400); *sodium carbonate solution*—small threadlike crystals (*sensitivity:* 1 in 400).

Ultraviolet Absorption Spectrum. Dimethoxanate in 0·1N sulphuric acid, maxima at 226 mμ (E1%, 1cm 93) and 254 mμ (E1%, 1cm 24).

Infra-red Absorption Spectrum. Dimethoxanate (base). Potassium bromide disk. The principal peaks are: A 1718, B 1317, C 1217 or 1460 (p. 784).

Dose. Up to 200 mg daily.

Toxicity. The estimated lethal dose in man is in the range 100 to 500 mg/kg.

DIMETHYL PHTHALATE *Insect Repellent*

Synonyms: DMP; Methyl Phthalate.

Methyl benzene-*o*-dicarboxylate

$C_{10}H_{10}O_4$ = 194·2

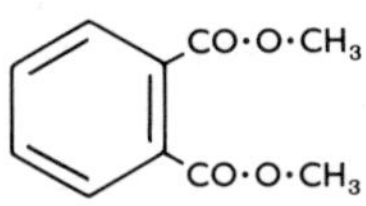

A colourless liquid. B.p. about 280°, with decomposition. Refractive index 1·515 to 1·517.

Solubility. Soluble 1 in 250 of water; miscible with ethanol, ether, and most organic solvents.

Extraction. Dimethyl phthalate is extracted by organic solvents from acid or alkaline solutions.

Ultraviolet Absorption Spectrum. Dimethyl phthalate in ethanol, maximum at 275 mμ (E1%, 1cm 75).

Metabolism. Dimethyl phthalate is probably hydrolysed *in vivo* to phthalic acid and methanol.

Toxicity. The estimated lethal dose in man is 50 g.

LD50 (intraperitoneal): in mice 1·58 g/kg.

DIMETHYL SULPHOXIDE *Industrial Solvent*

Synonyms: DMSO; SQ 9453.
Proprietary Names: Dolicur; Dromisol; Hyadur; Infiltrina.

Methyl sulphoxide

$(CH_3)_2S{:}O$ = 78·13

A colourless hygroscopic liquid. M.p. 18·4°. B.p. 189°. Refractive index 1·4783.

Solubility. Soluble in water, ethanol, ether, and chloroform; miscible with acetaldehyde, acetone, benzene, dioxan, formic acid, glycerol, and methanol.

Extraction. After preliminary extraction with heptane, which is discarded, urine is saturated with sodium chloride and the dimethyl sulphoxide (and dimethylsulphone) extracted with chloroform.

Colour Test. Dimethyl sulphoxide decolorises a 1% potassium permanganate solution.

Quantitative Estimation. Hucker *et al.* (1967) describe the determination of dimethyl sulphoxide by gas chromatography.

Metabolism. Dimethyl sulphoxide is a highly polar substance which has exceptional solvent properties for both organic and inorganic chemicals. It is rapidly absorbed when applied to the skin.

Following the daily administration of 21 g of dimethyl sulphoxide in man, 3% of the dose was excreted in the urine as dimethylsulphone (Hucker *et al.*, 1966).

Toxicity. Dimethyl sulphoxide seems to have a relatively low systemic toxicity in mammals but, when it is injected intravenously, local toxic effects, including tissue destruction, have been reported.

LD50 (oral): in mice 21·4 and in rats 28·3 g/kg.

DIMETHYLTHIAMBUTENE *Narcotic*

Synonyms: Aminobutene; Cobatone; Dimethibutin.

*NN*1 - Trimethyl - 3,3 - di(thien - 2′ - yl) allylamine

$C_{14}H_{17}NS_2$ = 263·4

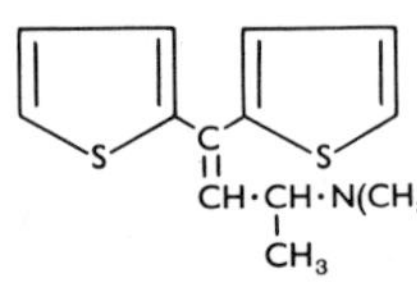

A viscous oil. B.p. 123° to 125° at 0·5 mm Hg.

Solubility. Soluble in ether and chloroform.

DIMETHYLTHIAMBUTENE HYDROCHLORIDE
Dimethylthiambutene hydrochloride melts at 168° to 169°.
Solubility. Soluble in water and chloroform.

Extraction. Dimethylthiambutene is extracted by organic solvents from aqueous alkaline solutions.

Chromatography. PAPER: system P1—Rf 0·60 (location under ultraviolet light, strong absorption; location reagent *iodoplatinate spray*, weak reaction); system RP1a—Rf 0·40 (location under ultraviolet light, absorption); system RP1b—Rf 0·08 (location as for RP1a).

THIN-LAYER: system T1—Rf 0·55 (location reagent *acidified iodoplatinate spray*, positive reaction).

GAS: system G2/225—retention time 1·1 relative to diphenhydramine; system G4—retention time 0·74 relative to diphenhydramine.

Colour Tests. MICRO: sulphuric acid–formaldehyde test—purple → brown (*sensitivity:* 0·1 μg); ammonium molybdate test—orange-brown → pale green (*sensitivity:* 0·1 μg); ammonium vanadate test—brown → blue-green (*sensitivity:* 0·1 μg); Vitali's test—red → green/brown/dark brown (*sensitivity:* 0·5 μg).

Crystal Tests. MICRO: *lead iodide solution*—dense rosettes or rosettes of branching rods (*sensitivity:* 1 in 1000); *potassium mercuric iodide solution*—long plates, forming overnight (*sensitivity:* 1 in 1000).

Ultraviolet Absorption Spectrum. Dimethylthiambutene in 0·1N sulphuric acid, maxima at 227 mμ (E 1%, 1 cm 254), 267·5 mμ (E 1%, 1 cm 351), and 286 mμ (E 1%, 1 cm 360).

Toxicity. LD50 (oral): in mice 199 mg/kg.

DIMETHYLTRYPTAMINE *Hallucinogen*

3-(2-Dimethylaminoethyl)indole

$C_{12}H_{16}N_2 = 188{\cdot}3$

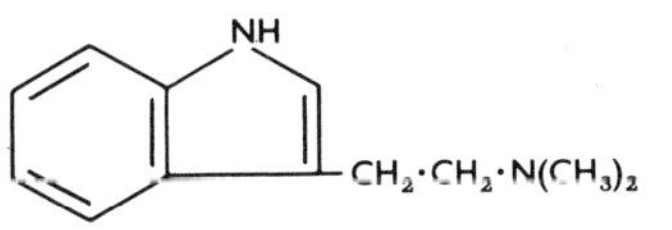

Dimethyltryptamine is an active principle obtained from the seeds and leaves of *Piptadenia peregrina* (Mimosaceae).

DIMETHYLTRYPTAMINE HYDROCHLORIDE

A white crystalline powder. M.p. 165° to 167·5°.

Solubility. Soluble in water.

Extraction. Dimethyltryptamine is extracted by organic solvents from aqueous alkaline solutions.

Chromatography. PAPER: system P1—Rf 0·38 (location under ultraviolet light, blue fluorescence; location reagents: *iodoplatinate spray*, strong reaction; *bromocresol green spray*, weak reaction; *Marquis reagent*, brown, slowly; *potassium permanganate spray*, strong reaction).

THIN-LAYER: system T1—Rf 0·34 (location reagents: *acidified iodoplatinate spray*, positive reaction; p-*dimethylaminobenzaldehyde spray*, blue).

GAS: system G2/225—retention time 0·74 relative to diphenhydramine; system G4—retention time 2·0 relative to diphenhydramine.

Colour Tests. MICRO: sulphuric acid–formaldehyde test—dull orange (*sensitivity:* 1·0 μg); ammonium molybdate test—blue → green → yellow (*sensitivity:* 0·1 μg).

Crystal Tests. MICRO: *gold cyanide solution*—rectangular plates, best viewed under polarised light (*sensitivity:* 1 in 200); *lead iodide solution*—fans and sheaves of needles (*sensitivity:* 1 in 200).

Ultraviolet Absorption Spectrum. Dimethyltryptamine hydrochloride in water, maximum at 282 mμ (E 1%, 1 cm 333).

Metabolism. Dimethyltryptamine produces effects on the mental state which are similar in some respects to those produced by lysergide (p. 395). It is excreted mainly unchanged but 6- and 7-hydroxydimethyltryptamine are also excreted, chiefly as glucuronides.

DIMETHYLTUBOCURARINE BROMIDE

Muscle Relaxant

Proprietary Name: Diamethine.

Dimethyl ether of (+)-tubocurarine bromide

$C_{40}H_{48}Br_2N_2O_6 = 812{\cdot}7$

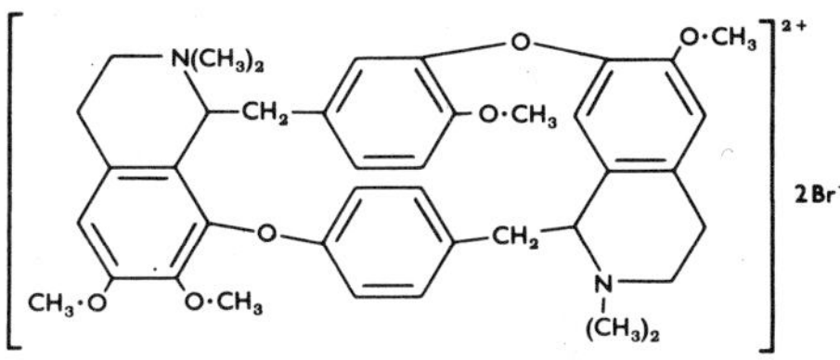

Solubility. Soluble 1 in 50 of water; soluble in methanol.

DIMETHYLTUBOCURARINE CHLORIDE

Proprietary Name: Mecostrin Chloride.

A white crystalline powder. When heated to 236°, it decomposes with the evolution of gas.

Solubility. Soluble in water; sparingly soluble in ethanol; almost insoluble in ether; very slightly soluble in chloroform.

DIMETHYLTUBOCURARINE IODIDE

Proprietary Name: Metubine Iodide.

A white crystalline powder. When heated to 257°, it decomposes with the evolution of gas. Specific rotation of a 0·4% aqueous solution, +148° to +158°.

Solubility. Slightly soluble in water; very slightly soluble in ethanol; practically insoluble in ether and chloroform; slightly soluble in dilute hydrochloride acid and dilute sodium hydroxide solution.

Extraction. The dimethyltubocurarine salts are quaternary ammonium compounds (see p. 29).

Chromatography. PAPER: system P1—Rf 0·07 (location under ultraviolet light, strong absorption; location reagents: *iodoplatinate spray*, strong reaction; *bromocresol green spray*, weak reaction).

THIN-LAYER: system T1—Rf 0·00 (location reagent *acidified iodoplatinate spray*, positive reaction).

Colour Test. MICRO: ammonium molybdate test—blue → green (*sensitivity:* 0·05 μg).

Crystal Tests. MICRO: *potassium chromate solution*—bunches of irregular plates, best viewed under polarised light (*sensitivity:* 1 in 3000); *potassium iodide solution*—plates (*sensitivity:* 1 in 1000).

Ultraviolet Absorption Spectrum. Dimethyltubocurarine in ethanol, maxima at 275 mμ (E 1%, 1 cm 70) and 281 mμ (E 1%, 1 cm 72).

Metabolism. When dimethyltubocurarine is injected intravenously in man, the plasma level decreases to two-thirds of the initial level in less than 10 minutes; 55% of the administered dose is excreted unchanged in the urine within 2 hours.

Dose. Up to 8 mg intravenously.

Toxicity. Dimethyltubocurarine is more potent than tubocurarine (p. 591), but, in therapeutic doses, it has a shorter duration of action.

DIMINAZENE *Antiprotozoal*

pp'-Diamidinodiazoaminobenzene

$C_{14}H_{15}N_7 = 281{\cdot}3$

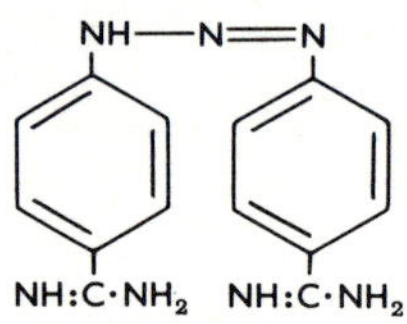

DIMINAZENE ACETURATE

Proprietary Name: It is an ingredient of Berenil.

A yellow powder. M.p. 217°, with decomposition.

Solubility. Soluble 1 in 14 of water; slightly soluble in ethanol; very slightly soluble in ether and chloroform.

Extraction. Diminazene is extracted by organic solvents from aqueous alkaline solutions.

Chromatography. PAPER: system P1—Rf 0·02 (location under ultraviolet light, orange fluorescence; location reagents: *iodoplatinate spray*, weak reaction; *potassium permanganate spray*, weak reaction).

THIN-LAYER: system T1—Rf 0·04 (location reagent *acidified iodoplatinate spray*, positive reaction).

Crystal Tests. MICRO: *potassium cadmium iodide solution*—masses of small needles (*sensitivity:* 1 in 1000); *sodium phosphate solution*—fans and sheaves of needles (*sensitivity:* 1 in 1000).

Ultraviolet Absorption Spectrum. Diminazene in 0·1N sulphuric acid, maximum at 258 mμ (E1%, 1 cm 935); diminazene aceturate in water, maximum at 370 mμ (E1%, 1 cm 650).

Toxicity. Diminazene is used mainly in animals. Doses in excess of 10 mg/kg have caused death in cattle but up to 6 times the normal dose (up to 4 g) has been given without causing toxic effects.

In man, trial doses of 2 mg/kg have been well tolerated.

DINITRO-ORTHOCRESOL *Pesticide/Herbicide*

Synonyms: DN; DNC; DNOC; Dinitrocresol; Dinitrol; Dinitrosol; Ditrosol; KIII; KIV.

Proprietary Names: Capsine; Dekrysil; Effusan; Prokarbol; Sinox (DNOC-sodium).

2-Methyl-4,6-dinitrophenol

$C_7H_6N_2O_5 = 198{\cdot}1$

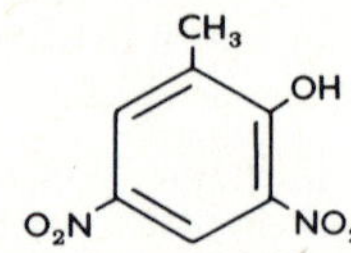

Dinitro-orthocresol melts at 85·8°.

Solubility. Almost insoluble in water; soluble in most organic solvents, acetic acid, and lipids.

Extraction. Dinitro-orthocresol may be extracted by shaking 5 ml of methyl ethyl ketone with 1 ml of blood to which 1 g of a solid mixture of sodium chloride and sodium carbonate (9 : 1) has been added (Fenwick and Parker, 1955).

Chromatography. GAS: system G5—retention time 2·30 relative to barbitone.

Ultraviolet Absorption Spectrum. Dinitro-orthocresol in 0·1N hydrochloric acid, maximum at 268 mμ (E1%, 1 cm 631); in 0·1N sodium hydroxide, maxima at 265 mμ (E1%, 1 cm 251), 370 mμ (E1%, 1 cm 646), and 409 mμ (E1%, 1 cm 501).

Quantitative Estimation. Dinitro-orthocresol may be estimated spectrophotometrically (Fenwick and Parker, 1955), and by the method of Edson (1954).

Metabolism. Dinitro-orthocresol may be absorbed through the skin or by inhalation or accidental ingestion. It acts as a cumulative poison causing an increase in the metabolic rate and it is eliminated slowly over a period of weeks. In man, following daily doses of 75 mg for 5 or 7 days, only 1 to 2% was excreted in the urine (Harvey *et al.*, 1951). In the rabbit, the main metabolite and detoxication product has been found to be conjugated 6-acetamido-2-methyl-4-nitrophenol which accounts for 12% of the dose; small amounts of 3-amino-5-nitrosalicylic acid and conjugates of 4-amino-2-methyl-6-nitrophenol are also excreted (Smith *et al.*, 1953).

Toxicity. Yellow discoloration of the sclera indicates absorption of significant amounts, and toxic effects in man appear at blood-levels of about 3 to 4 mg%. Levels of above 7·5 mg% will probably be fatal. Further contact with the preparation must be avoided if the quantity present in the blood exceeds 2 mg% eight hours after the last exposure. The acute toxic dose in man is stated to be about 200 mg.

LD50 (oral): in rats 40 to 65 mg/kg for the sodium salt.

CASE EXAMPLES. Fatal poisoning cases have been described by Steer (1951), Bidstrup and Payne (1951), and Edson (1955). Reviews on poisoning by dinitro-orthocresol have been published by Hunter (1950) and Bidstrup *et al.* (1952).

DIOXAPHETYL BUTYRATE

Narcotic Analgesic

Ethyl γ-morpholino-αα-diphenylbutyrate
$C_{22}H_{27}NO_3 = 353{\cdot}5$

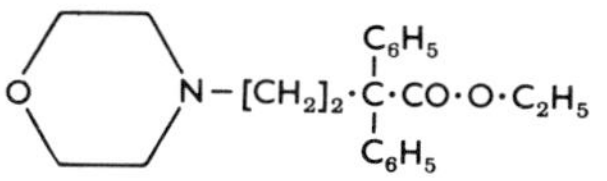

Dioxaphetyl butyrate melts at 68·5° to 70° and boils at 170° to 180°.

DIOXAPHETYL BUTYRATE HYDROCHLORIDE
Synonym: Amidalgon.
Proprietary Name: Spasmoxale.
Dioxaphetyl butyrate hydrochloride melts at 167·5° to 168·5°.

Extraction. Dioxaphetyl butyrate is extracted by organic solvents from aqueous alkaline solutions.

Chromatography. PAPER: system P1—Rf 0·75 (location under ultraviolet light, absorption; location reagent *iodoplatinate spray*, weak reaction).
THIN-LAYER: system T1—Rf 0·72 (location reagent *acidified iodoplatinate spray*, positive reaction).

Crystal Tests. MICRO: *ammonium thiocyanate solution*—fine dendrites (*sensitivity:* 1 in 400); *potassium chromate solution*—fans of fine needles (*sensitivity:* 1 in 200).

DIOXATHION

Pesticide

Other Names: Bercotox; Delnav; Hercules AC 528; Kavadel; Navadel; Polythion.

Dioxathion is mainly a mixture of the *cis* and *trans* isomers of *SS'*-1,4-dioxane-2,3-diylbis-(*OO*-diethyl phosphorothiolothionate)
$C_{12}H_{26}O_6P_2S_4 = 456{\cdot}5$

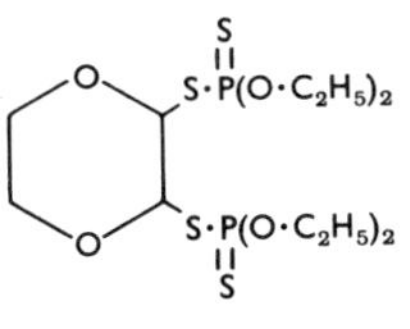

A dark amber-coloured liquid which should be stored in well-closed containers in a cool place.
Solubility. Immiscible with water; miscible with ethanol, acetone, benzene, and xylene.

Extraction. Dioxathion is extracted by organic solvents from aqueous acid solutions.

Metabolism. Dioxathion is an organophosphorus insecticide used chiefly for the control of cattle ticks. It depresses cholinesterase activity in mammals but, when applied externally in the recommended concentrations, it has a good margin of safety. When dioxathion is absorbed, it is rapidly metabolised and leaves insignificant residues in tissues.

Toxicity. Very toxic when inhaled, swallowed, or spilled on the skin. The recommended strength of washes for weekly dipping or spraying of infested cattle is 0·05%.

DIOXYLINE

Antispasmodic

Synonym: Dimoxyline.

1-(4-Ethoxy-3-methoxybenzyl)-6,7-dimethoxy-3-methylisoquinoline
$C_{22}H_{25}NO_4 = 367{\cdot}4$

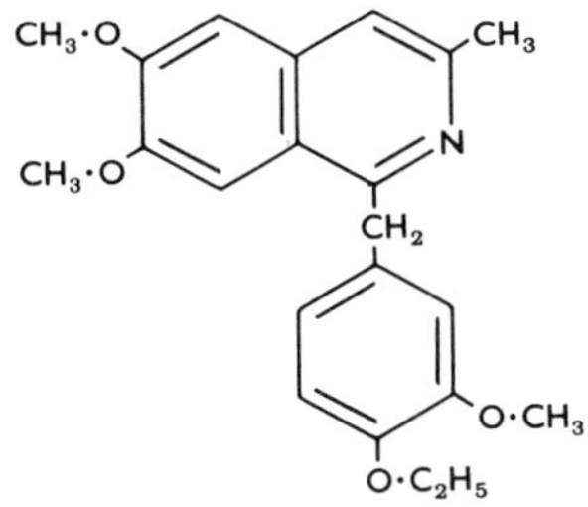

Dioxyline occurs as crystals. M.p. 124° to 125°.

DIOXYLINE PHOSPHATE
Proprietary Name: Paveril.
Crystals which melt at 197° to 199°.
Solubility. Soluble in water.

Extraction. Dioxyline is extracted by organic solvents from aqueous alkaline solutions.

Chromatography. PAPER: system P1—Rf 0·65 (location under ultraviolet light, yellow fluorescence; location reagent *iodoplatinate spray*, weak reaction); system RP1a—Rf 0·07 (location under ultraviolet light, yellow fluorescence); system RP1b—Rf 0·02 (location as for RP1a).
THIN-LAYER: system T1—Rf 0·69 (location reagent *acidified iodoplatinate spray*, positive reaction).

Colour Tests. MICRO: sulphuric acid–formaldehyde test—brown (*sensitivity:* 0·5 μg); ammonium molybdate test—blue (*sensitivity:* 0·5 μg); ammonium vanadate test—green (*sensitivity:* 0·5 μg); Vitali's test—yellow/yellow/brown (*sensitivity:* 1·0 μg).

Crystal Tests. MICRO: *potassium cadmium iodide solution*—rosettes of small irregular plates (*sensitivity:* 1 in 1000); *potassium iodide solution*—bunches of blades (*sensitivity:* 1 in 400).

Ultraviolet Absorption Spectrum. Dioxyline in 0·1N sulphuric acid, maxima at 285 mμ (E1%, 1 cm 120), 309 mμ (E1%, 1 cm 179), and 335 mμ (E1%, 1 cm 136), and an inflexion at about 348 mμ.

Infra-red Absorption Spectrum. Dioxyline (base). Potassium chloride disk. The principal peaks are: A 1504, B 1247, C 1145 or 1208 (p. 784).

Metabolism. Dioxyline is rapidly and almost

completely metabolised in the dog, and excreted as unknown metabolites (Root and Comer, 1953).

Dose. Usually up to 600 mg daily; max. in 24 hours 2 g.

Toxicity. LD50 (intravenous): in mice about 112 mg/kg.

DIPERODON *Local Anaesthetic*

Synonym: Diperocaine.

1,2 - Diphenylcarbamoyloxy - 3 - piperidinopropane

$C_{22}H_{27}N_3O_4 = 397{\cdot}5$

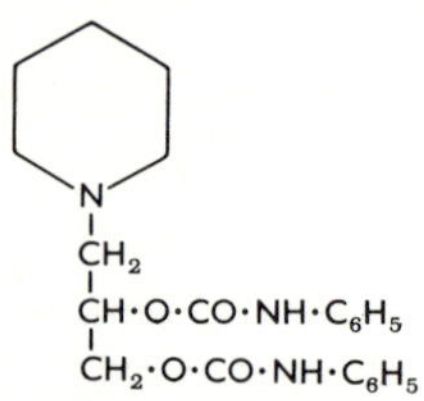

DIPERODON HYDROCHLORIDE

Proprietary Name: Diothane Hydrochloride.

A white crystalline powder. M.p. 195° to 200°.

Solubility. Soluble 1 in 100 of water; soluble in ethanol; insoluble in ether; slightly soluble in ethyl acetate.

Extraction. Diperodon is extracted by organic solvents from aqueous alkaline solutions.

Chromatography. PAPER: system P1—Rf 0·85 (location under ultraviolet light, strong absorption; location reagent *iodoplatinate spray*, strong reaction); system RP1a—Rf 0·16 (location under ultraviolet light, absorption); system RP1b—Rf 0·00 (location as for RP1a).

THIN-LAYER: system T1—Rf 0·72 (location reagent *acidified iodoplatinate spray*, positive reaction).

Colour Test. MICRO: ammonium vanadate test—red → green (*sensitivity:* 0·025 μg).

Crystal Tests. MICRO: *potassium cyanide solution*—rosettes of rods (*sensitivity:* 1 in 400); *trinitrobenzoic acid solution*—rosettes of rods or plates (*sensitivity:* 1 in 200).

Ultraviolet Absorption Spectrum. Diperodon in 0·1N sulphuric acid, maxima at 231 mμ (E1%, 1 cm 1322), 264 mμ (E1%, 1 cm 47), about 270 mμ (E1%, 1 cm 46), and about 277 mμ (E1%, 1 cm 32).

Infra-red Absorption Spectrum. Diperodon (base). Potassium bromide disk. The principal peaks are: A 1210 or 1705, B 1530, C 1442 or 1600 (p. 784).

Toxicity. Solutions for infiltration anaesthesia stronger than 0·5% may cause tissue damage. The maximum amount considered safe for surface use is 10 ml of a 1% solution.

DIPHEMANIL METHYLSULPHATE *Parasympatholytic*

Synonym: Diphenmethanil Methylsulfate.

Proprietary Names: Demotil; Diphenatil; Prantal.

4-Diphenylmethylene-1,1-dimethylpiperidinium methyl sulphate

$C_{20}H_{24}N,CH_3SO_4 = 389{\cdot}5$

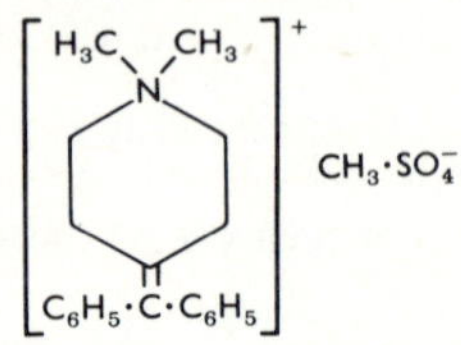

A white hygroscopic crystalline powder. M.p. 194° to 195°.

Solubility. Soluble 1 in 33 of water, 1 in 33 of ethanol, and 1 in 33 of chloroform; very slightly soluble in ether.

Extraction. Diphemanil methylsulphate is a quaternary ammonium compound (see p. 29).

Chromatography. PAPER: system P1—Rf 0·60 (location under ultraviolet light, strong absorption; location reagents: *iodoplatinate spray*, weak reaction; *bromocresol green spray*, weak reaction); system RP1a—Rf 0·82 (location under ultraviolet light, absorption); system RP1b—Rf 0·74 (location under ultraviolet light, absorption; location reagent *iodoplatinate spray*, positive reaction).

THIN-LAYER: system T1—Rf 0·02 (location reagent *acidified iodoplatinate spray*, positive reaction).

Colour Tests. MICRO: sulphuric acid–formaldehyde test—orange-red (*sensitivity:* 0·1 μg); ammonium molybdate test—yellow → green → blue (*sensitivity:* 0·25 μg); ammonium vanadate test—brown (*sensitivity:* 0·25 μg); Vitali's test—-/-/black-purple (*sensitivity:* 0·1 μg).

Crystal Tests. MICRO: *mercuric chloride solution*—rhomboidal plates, best viewed under polarised light (*sensitivity:* 1 in 1000); *zinc chloride solution*—masses of rods (*sensitivity:* 1 in 1000).

Ultraviolet Absorption Spectrum. Diphemanil methylsulphate in 0·1N sulphuric acid, maximum at 232 mμ (E1%, 1 cm 342).

Quantitative Estimation. Diphemanil methylsulphate may be estimated colorimetrically (Perlman *et al.*, 1953a).

Metabolism. Diphemanil methylsulphate is not very readily absorbed from the gastro-intestinal tract. In dogs, whatever the route of administration, about 50% of the diphemanil dose is eliminated as the original cation; more than half of this is eliminated in the urine and the remainder in the faeces. The fate of the other 50% is not known but it does not appear to be stored (Perlman *et al.*, 1953a).

Toxicity. The estimated lethal dose in man is probably between 10 and 100 mg/kg.

DIPHENADIONE *Anticoagulant*

Proprietary Name: Dipaxin.

2-Diphenylacetylindane-1,3-dione

$C_{23}H_{16}O_3 = 340{\cdot}4$

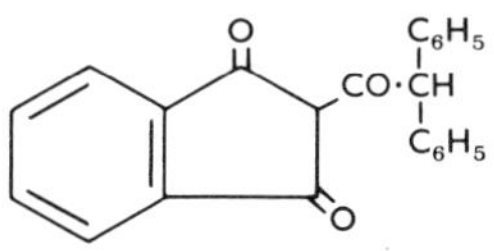

Yellow crystals or a yellow crystalline powder. M.p. 144° to 150°.

Solubility. Practically insoluble in water; slightly soluble in ethanol; soluble in ether, benzene, and glacial acetic acid.

Extraction. Diphenadione is extracted by organic solvents from aqueous acid or alkaline solutions.

Ultraviolet Absorption Spectrum. Diphenadione in ethanol:0·1N sodium hydroxide (19:1), maxima at 246 mμ (E1%, 1cm 500), 275 mμ (E1%, 1cm 700), 284 mμ (E1%, 1cm 1220), 312 mμ (E1%, 1cm 560), and 323 mμ (E1%, 1cm 580); in ethanol:0·1N sulphuric acid (19:1), maxima at 238 mμ (E1%, 1cm 1800), 277 mμ (E1%, 1cm 1600), 288 mμ (E1%, 1cm 2050), 306 mμ (E1%, 1cm 950), and 314 mμ (E1%, 1cm 950).

Dose. Up to 30 mg daily.

DIPHENHYDRAMINE *Antihistamine*

Synonym: Benzhydraminum.

2-Diphenylmethoxy-*NN*-dimethylethylamine

$C_{17}H_{21}NO = 255{\cdot}4$

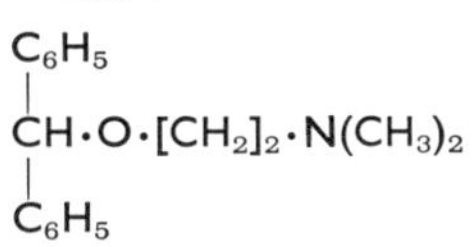

NOTE. Diphenhydramine is an isomer of phenyltoloxamine (p. 495).

DIPHENHYDRAMINE HYDROCHLORIDE

Synonym: Dimedrol.

Proprietary Names: Benadryl; Benodine; Benylin; Paranausine.

A white crystalline powder. M.p. 168° to 172°.

Solubility. Soluble 1 in 1 of water, 1 in 2 of ethanol, and 1 in 2 of chloroform; sparingly soluble in ether.

DIPHENHYDRAMINE METHYLSULPHOMETHYLATE

Proprietary Name: Allerga.

DIPHENHYDRAMINE THEOCLATE

Synonyms: Anautin(e); Chloranautine; Dimenhydrinate; Diphenhydramine 8-Chlorotheophyllinate.

Proprietary Names: Dramamine; Gravol; Nautamine.

A white crystalline powder. M.p. 102° to 107°.

Solubility. Soluble 1 in 95 of water, 1 in 2 of ethanol, and 1 in 2 of chloroform; sparingly soluble in ether.

Extraction. Diphenhydramine is extracted by organic solvents from aqueous alkaline solutions.

Chromatography. PAPER: system P1—Rf 0·62 (location under ultraviolet light, absorption; location reagents: *iodoplatinate spray*, strong reaction; *bromocresol green spray*, weak reaction); system RP1a—Rf 0·70 (location reagent *iodoplatinate spray*, positive reaction); system RP1b—Rf 0·00.

THIN-LAYER: system T1—Rf 0·51 (location reagent *acidified iodoplatinate spray*, positive reaction); system T2—Rf 0·53 (location reagent *iodoplatinate spray*, positive reaction); system T3—Rf 0·91 (location as for T2).

GAS: system G2/225—retention time 0·21 relative to codeine; system G4—retention time 0·1 relative to codeine.

Colour Tests. MICRO: sulphuric acid–formaldehyde test—bright yellow (*sensitivity:* 0·1 μg); ammonium molybdate test—bright yellow (*sensitivity:* 0·1 μg); ammonium vanadate test—bright yellow (*sensitivity:* 0·1 μg).

Crystal Tests. MICRO: *gold bromide–hydrochloric acid solution*—blades or needles, some curved (*sensitivity:* 1 in 1000); *potassium tri-iodide solution (1)* plates or prisms (*sensitivity:* 1 in 1000).

Ultraviolet Absorption Spectrum. Diphenhydramine in 0·1N sulphuric acid, maxima at 252 mμ (E1%, 1cm 16) and 257 mμ (E1%, 1cm 18) and minimum at about 244 mμ; diphenhydramine theoclate in 0·1N sulphuric acid, maximum at 276 mμ (E1%, 1cm 275) and minimum at about 245 mμ.

Infra-red Absorption Spectrum. Diphenhydramine theoclate. Potassium bromide disk. The principal peaks are: A 699, B 1100, C 1448 (p. 785).

Quantitative Estimation. Diphenhydramine may be estimated colorimetrically as the complex formed with cobalt thiocyanate and sulphuric acid (Sekules and Guadagnini, 1964).

Metabolism. Diphenhydramine is rapidly absorbed from the gastro-intestinal tract, peak concentrations being attained in the tissues in about half an hour. The highest concentrations are found in the lungs, spleen, kidneys, liver, brain, and muscle. In 6 hours the drug can no longer be detected in the tissues; within 24 hours most of it is excreted in the urine. Only a small amount is excreted unchanged, most of it being hydrolysed to benzhydrol which is then conjugated with glucuronic acid.

Dose. Usually up to 300 mg daily.

Toxicity. An acute lethal dose in man of 40 mg/kg of the hydrochloride has been recorded and the estimated lethal dose of the theoclate in man is reported to be between 25 and 250 mg/kg.

CASE EXAMPLE. A 16-year-old girl experienced a toxic psychosis which included schizophrenic-like behaviour and features of an acute brain syndrome about 2 hours after the ingestion of 500 mg of diphenhydramine hydrochloride. She became co-operative and rational 29 hours after ingestion (Nigro, 1968).

DIPHENIDOL *Anti-emetic*

Proprietary Names: Nometic; Vontrol.

1,1-Diphenyl-4-piperidinobutanol

$C_{21}H_{27}NO = 309{\cdot}5$

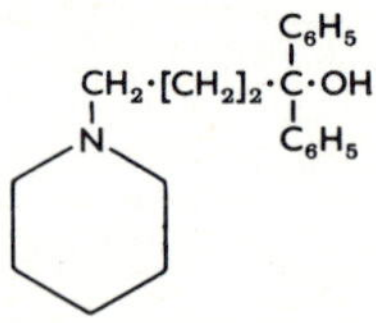

Diphenidol melts at 103° to 104°.

Extraction. Diphenidol is extracted by organic solvents from aqueous alkaline solutions.

Chromatography. PAPER: system P1—Rf 0·77 (location reagents: *iodoplatinate spray*, strong reaction; *bromocresol green spray*, weak reaction).

THIN-LAYER: system T1—Rf 0·58 (location reagent *acidified iodoplatinate spray*, positive reaction).

Colour Tests. MICRO: sulphuric acid–formaldehyde test—yellow (*sensitivity:* 0·1 μg); ammonium molybdate test—yellow (*sensitivity:* 0·1 μg); ammonium vanadate test—yellow (*sensitivity:* 0·5 μg); Vitali's test—yellow flash/–/– (*sensitivity:* 1·0 μg).

Crystal Tests. MICRO: *potassium iodide solution*—masses of hairlike needles (*sensitivity:* 1 in 1000); *potassium permanganate solution*—feathery rosettes (*sensitivity:* 1 in 1000).

Ultraviolet Absorption Spectrum. Diphenidol in 0·1N sulphuric acid, maxima at about 248 mμ (E1%, 1cm 52), 251·5 mμ (E1%, 1cm 54), and 259 mμ (E1%, 1cm 53).

Infra-red Absorption Spectrum. Potassium bromide disk. The principal peaks are: A 697 or 701, B 1447, C 749 or 773 (p. 785).

DIPHENOXYLATE *Narcotic*

Synonym: R 1132.

Ethyl 1-(3-cyano-3,3-diphenylpropyl)-4-phenylpiperidine-4-carboxylate

$C_{30}H_{32}N_2O_2 = 452{\cdot}6$

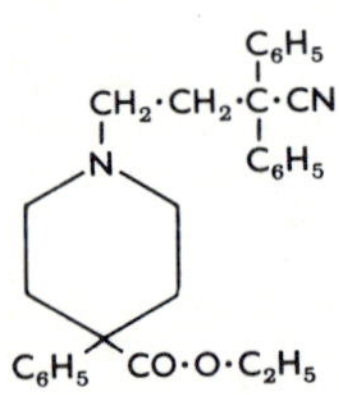

DIPHENOXYLATE HYDROCHLORIDE

Proprietary Names: Reasec. It is an ingredient of Lomotil and Retardin.

Solubility. Almost insoluble in water; soluble in propylene glycol; almost insoluble in most organic solvents.

Extraction. Diphenoxylate is extracted by organic solvents from aqueous alkaline solutions.

Chromatography. PAPER: system P1—Rf 0·90 (location reagents: *iodoplatinate spray*, weak reaction; *bromocresol green spray*, weak reaction); system RP1a—Rf 0·00 (location reagent *iodoplatinate spray*, positive reaction); system RP1b—Rf 0·00 (location under ultraviolet light, absorption).

THIN-LAYER: system T1—Rf 0·79 (location reagent *acidified iodoplatinate spray*, positive reaction).

Crystal Tests. MICRO: *potassium iodide solution*—smudge rosettes (*sensitivity:* 1 in 400); *potassium tri-iodide solution* (*2*)—bunches of plates (*sensitivity:* 1 in 400).

Dose. Up to 20 mg daily, in the treatment of diarrhoea.

Toxicity. The minimum lethal dose in man is 200 mg/kg. Diphenoxylate has addiction-producing properties; a dose of 40 to 60 mg is followed by euphoria.

DIPHENYL *Fungistatic*

Synonym: Biphenyl.

Phenylbenzene

$C_{12}H_{10} = 154{\cdot}2$

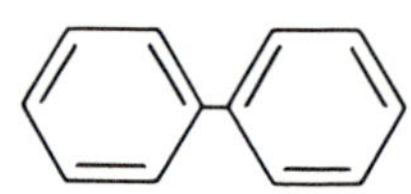

A white crystalline powder. M.p. 69° to 71°. B.p. 254° to 255°.

Solubility. Insoluble in water; soluble in ethanol and ether.

Extraction. Diphenyl is extracted by organic solvents from aqueous acid or alkaline solutions.

Quantitative Estimation. Several methods have been reported for the determination of diphenyl with particular reference to its occurrence in citrus fruits and juices: gas chromatographically (Thomas, 1960), colorimetrically (Rajzman, 1960 and 1963), and spectrophotometrically (Gunther *et al.*, 1963).

Metabolism. In rats and rabbits diphenyl is metabolised to various phenolic compounds, mainly 4-hydroxydiphenyl which is excreted in the urine in the free form and as the ethereal sulphate and glucuronide conjugates.

Toxicity. The estimated acceptable daily intake for man is up to 0·05 mg/kg.

LD50 (oral): in rabbits 2·4 and in rats 3·5 to 5 g/kg.

NOTE. Diphenyl is a fungistatic agent which inhibits the growth of the species of *Penicillium* which cause the decay of citrus fruits and it is employed for impregnating the material used for wrapping such fruits.

DIPHENYLPYRALINE *Antihistamine*

Synonyms: Diphenylpyrilene; P 253.

4-Diphenylmethoxy-1-methylpiperidine

$C_{19}H_{23}NO = 281{\cdot}4$

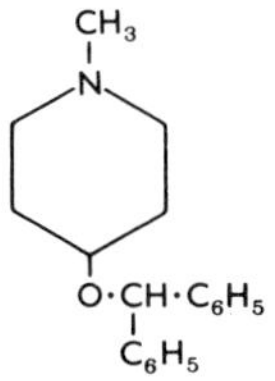

DIPHENYLPYRALINE HYDROCHLORIDE

Proprietary Names: Diafen; Hispril; Histryl.

A white crystalline powder. M.p. 206°.

Solubility. Soluble in water and ethanol; insoluble in ether.

Extraction. Diphenylpyraline is extracted by organic solvents from aqueous alkaline solutions.

Chromatography. PAPER: system P1—Rf 0·46 (location under ultraviolet light, absorption; location reagents: *iodoplatinate spray*, strong reaction; *bromocresol green spray*, weak reaction); system RP1a—Rf 0·50 (location under ultraviolet light, absorption; location reagent *iodoplatinate spray*, positive reaction); system RP1b—Rf 0·04 (location as for RP1a).

THIN-LAYER: system T1—Rf 0·41 (location reagent *acidified iodoplatinate spray*, positive reaction).

GAS: system G2/225—retention time 2·05 relative to diphenhydramine; system G4—retention time 2·1 relative to diphenhydramine.

Colour Tests. MICRO: sulphuric acid–formaldehyde test—yellow (*sensitivity:* 0·1 μg); ammonium molybdate test—yellow (*sensitivity:* 0·1 μg); ammonium vanadate test—yellow (*sensitivity:* 0·1 μg).

Crystal Tests. MICRO: *platinic chloride solution*—rosettes of oily blades (*sensitivity:* 1 in 200); *styphnic acid*—feathery rosettes (*sensitivity:* 1 in 400).

Ultraviolet Absorption Spectrum. Diphenylpyraline in 0·1N sulphuric acid, maximum at 258 mμ (E1%, 1 cm 20), and inflexions at about 251 mμ and about 264 mμ.

Dose. Up to 10 mg daily.

Toxicity. The estimated acute lethal dose in man is 5 to 10 mg/kg.

DIPIPANONE *Narcotic Analgesic*

Synonyms: Fenpidon; Hoechst 10805; Pamedone; Phenylpiperone; Piperidyl Methadone; Piperidylamidone.

(±)-4,4-Diphenyl-6-piperidinoheptan-3-one

$C_{24}H_{31}NO = 349{\cdot}5$

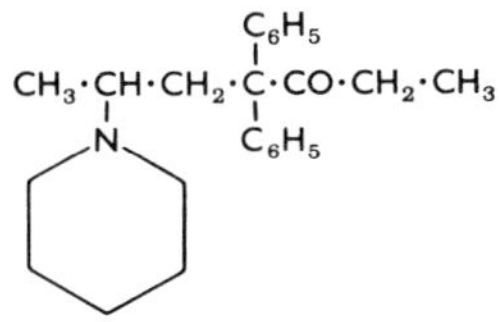

DIPIPANONE HYDROCHLORIDE

Proprietary Name: Pipadone.

A white crystalline powder. M.p. 124° to 127°.

Solubility. Soluble 1 in 40 of water and 1 in 1·5 of ethanol; insoluble in ether.

Extraction. Dipipanone is extracted by organic solvents from aqueous alkaline solutions.

Chromatography. PAPER: system P1—Rf 0·85 (location under ultraviolet light, absorption; location reagent *iodoplatinate spray*, strong reaction); system RP1a—Rf 0·16 (location under ultraviolet light, absorption; location reagent *iodoplatinate spray*, positive reaction); system RP1b—Rf 0·00 (location as for RP1a).

THIN-LAYER: system T1—Rf 0·60, streaking (location reagent *acidified iodoplatinate spray*, positive reaction).

GAS: system G2/225—retention time 1·35 relative to codeine; system G4—retention time 0·55 relative to codeine.

Colour Test. MICRO: ammonium vanadate test—green → blue (*sensitivity:* 0·25 μg).

Crystal Tests. MICRO: *platinic bromide solution*—curving blades, mostly serrated (*sensitivity:* 1 in 400); *platinic chloride solution*—bunches of serrated blades (*sensitivity:* 1 in 1000).

Ultraviolet Absorption Spectrum. Dipipanone in 0·1N sodium hydroxide, maxima at about 259 mμ (E1%, 1 cm 25) and 292 mμ (E1%, 1 cm 16); in 0·1N sulphuric acid, maxima at 252·5 mμ (E1%, 1 cm 14·6), 259 mμ (E1%, 1 cm 15·5), 265 mμ (E1%, 1 cm 14·8), and 293 mμ (E1%, 1 cm 16·3).

Metabolism. Dipipanone is a narcotic analgesic with a rapid onset of action. Like methadone it is metabolised in the liver and excreted in the faeces and urine.

Toxicity. The toxicity of dipipanone is of the same order as that of methadone (p. 408); it has addiction-producing properties.

LD50 (oral): in mice 124 mg/kg.

CASE EXAMPLE. A 51-year-old man took an unknown quantity of dipipanone with suicidal intent. Analysis of the urine by the Straub test is described (Taylor, 1965).

DIPROPHYLLINE *Xanthine Derivative*

Synonyms: Dihydroxypropyltheophyllinum; Dyphylline; Glyphyllin; Hyphylline.

Proprietary Names: Isophylline; Neothylline; Neutraphylline; Silbephylline.

7-(2,3-Dihydroxypropyl)-1,3-dimethylxanthine
$C_{10}H_{14}N_4O_4$ = 254·2

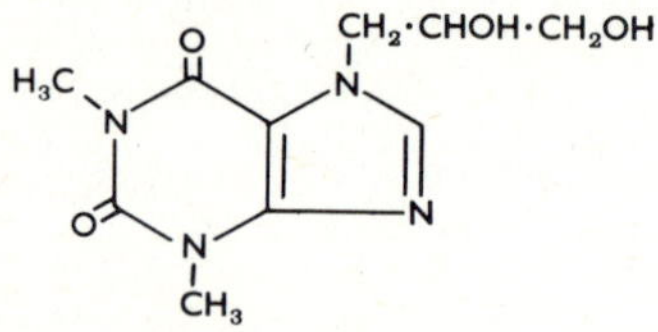

A white powder. M.p. 158°.

Solubility. Soluble 1 in 10 of water, 1 in 150 of ethanol, and 1 in 600 of chloroform; almost insoluble in ether.

Extraction. Diprophylline is extracted by organic solvents from aqueous alkaline solutions.

Chromatography. PAPER: system P1—Rf 0·47 (location under ultraviolet light, dark blue fluorescence; location by the Clarke–Kalayci test, purple).

THIN-LAYER: system T1—Rf 0·61 (location reagent *potassium permanganate spray*, positive reaction).

Colour Test. Amalic acid test—purple (see p. 127).

Crystal Test. MICRO: *gold bromide–hydrochloric acid solution*—fans of needles (*sensitivity:* 1 in 200).

Infra-red Absorption Spectrum. Potassium bromide disk. The principal peaks are: A 1660 or 1700, B 1039, C 747 (p. 785).

Dose. Usually up to 600 mg daily; max. in 24 hours 1·5 g.

Toxicity. Studies in mice show diprophylline to be much less toxic than aminophylline (see under Theophylline, p. 567); this difference has not been shown in man except that diprophylline produces less gastric irritation.

DIPYRIDAMOLE *Coronary Vasodilator*

Synonym: RA 8.
Proprietary Name: Persantin.

2,6-Di[di(2-hydroxyethyl)amino]-4,8-dipiperidinopyrimido[5,4-*d*]pyrimidine
$C_{24}H_{40}N_8O_4$ = 504·6

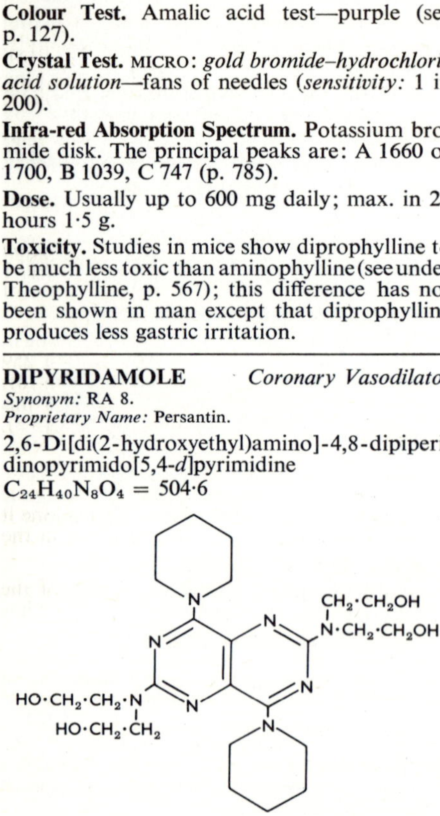

A yellow crystalline powder. M.p. 163°.

Solubility. Slightly soluble in water; very soluble in ethanol; almost insoluble in ether; soluble in chloroform.

Extraction. Dipyridamole is extracted by organic solvents from aqueous alkaline solutions.

Chromatography. PAPER: system P1—Rf 0·74 (location under ultraviolet light, bright yellow fluorescence; location reagent *iodoplatinate spray*, weak reaction); system RP1a—Rf 0·13 (location under ultraviolet light, yellow fluorescence); system RP1b—Rf 0·07 (location as for RP1a).

THIN-LAYER: system T1—Rf 0·72 (location reagent *acidified iodoplatinate spray*, positive reaction).

Colour Tests. MICRO: sulphuric acid–formaldehyde test—(yellow) orange (*sensitivity:* 0·25 μg); ammonium molybdate test—(yellow) orange (*sensitivity:* 1·0 μg); ammonium vanadate test—(yellow) dull purple (*sensitivity:* 0·1 μg); Vitali's test—(yellow) deep purple/pale yellow/pale yellow (*sensitivity:* 0·1 μg).

Crystal Tests. MICRO: *lead iodide solution*—small needles (*sensitivity:* 1 in 1000); *styphnic acid*—bunches of curved needles (*sensitivity:* 1 in 1000).

Ultraviolet Absorption Spectrum. Dipyridamole in 0·1N sulphuric acid, maxima at 236 mμ (E1%, 1 cm 520), 283 mμ (E1%, 1 cm 533), and 398 mμ (E1%, 1 cm 123).

Dose. Up to 150 mg daily.

DIPYRONE *Analgesic*

Synonyms: Analgin; Metamizole; Methampyrone; Noramidazophen; Sodium Noramidopyrine Methanesulphonate; Sulpyrin(e).
Proprietary Names: Barone; Novaldin; Novalgin; Novapyrine; Pydirone.

Sodium[*N*-(1,5-dimethyl-3-oxo-2-phenylpyrazolin-4-yl)-*N*-methylamino]methanesulphonate monohydrate
$C_{13}H_{16}N_3NaO_4S, H_2O$ = 351·4

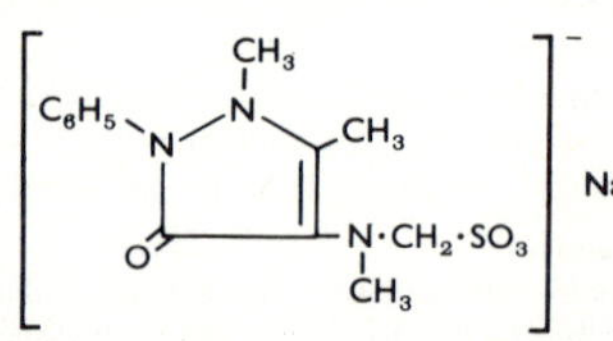

A white crystalline powder. M.p. 172°.

Solubility. Soluble 1 in 1·5 of water and 1 in 30 of ethanol; almost insoluble in ether and chloroform.

Chromatography. PAPER: system P1—Rf 0·32 (location under ultraviolet light, absorption; location reagent *potassium permanganate spray*, strong reaction).

THIN-LAYER: system T1—Rf 0·60 (location reagent *acidified iodoplatinate spray*, white).

Colour Tests. MICRO: ammonium molybdate test—very pale purple ring (*sensitivity:* 1·0 μg); ammonium vanadate test—brown (*sensitivity:* 1·0 μg); ferric chloride test—blue → purple; Vitali's test— –/light brown/orange (*sensitivity:* 1·0 μg).

Crystal Tests. MICRO: *gold bromide–hydrochloric acid solution*—very small plates or rosettes (*sensitivity:* 1 in 200); *potassium tri-iodide solution (1)*—rods or prisms (*sensitivity:* 1 in 200).

Dose. Up to 3 g by mouth, or 6 ml of a 50% solution by injection.

Toxicity. The acute fatal dose is 5 to 30 g but fatalities from acute poisoning have been rare.

DIQUAT *Herbicide*

Synonym: 1,1′-Ethylene-2,2′-bipyridylium dibromide.
Proprietary Preparation: Reglone.

9,10 - Dihydro - 8a,10a - diazoniaphenanthrene dibromide
$C_{12}H_{12}N_2Br_2$ = 344·1

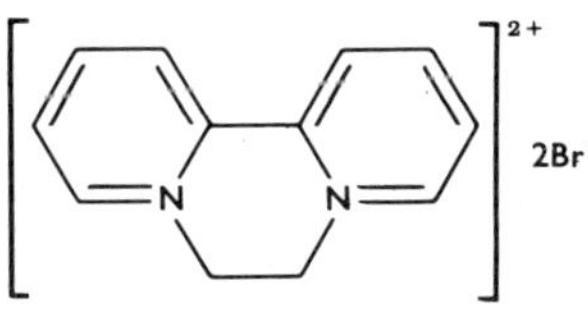

Yellow crystals. M.p. about 335°.
Solubility. Soluble in water.

Extraction. Diquat is a quaternary ammonium compound (see p. 29).

Chromatography. PAPER: system P1—Rf 0·01 (location under ultraviolet light, pale green fluorescence with an absorbing centre; location reagents: *iodoplatinate spray*, strong reaction; *bromocresol green spray*, weak reaction).
THIN-LAYER: system T1—Rf 0·00 (location reagent *acidified iodoplatinate spray*, positive reaction).

Colour Test. MICRO: Vitali's test— –/–/yellow-brown (*sensitivity:* 1·0 μg).

A rapid test for the detection of diquat in gastric aspirate/lavage and urine has been devised by S. L. Tompsett and may be carried out as follows. To 5 ml of fluid add 100 mg of sodium bicarbonate and 100 mg of sodium dithionite and mix. Diquat gives a yellowish-green colour; 2 to 5 mg% can be detected without difficulty. Urine may require dilution, and gastric aspirate/lavage may require filtration and dilution before application of the test. Paraquat gives a blue colour with this test (Kerr *et al.*, 1968).

Crystal Tests. MICRO: *styphnic acid*—needles, mostly curved (*sensitivity:* 1 in 1000); *picric acid*—irregular blades (*sensitivity:* 1 in 1000).

Ultraviolet Absorption Spectrum. Diquat in 0·1N sulphuric acid, maximum at 310 mμ (E 1%, 1 cm 518), inflexions at 258 mμ and 318 mμ, and minor inflexions at about 245 mμ and about 267 mμ.

Toxicity. The estimated lethal dose in man is 20 g.
LD50 (oral): in rats 400 mg/kg.

DISTIGMINE BROMIDE *Anticholinesterase*

Synonyms: BC 51; Bis-pyridostigmine.
Proprietary Name: Ubretid.

N,N′-Hexamethylenebis[1 - methyl - 3 - (methylcarbamoyloxy)pyridinium bromide]
$C_{22}H_{32}Br_2N_4O_4$ = 576·3

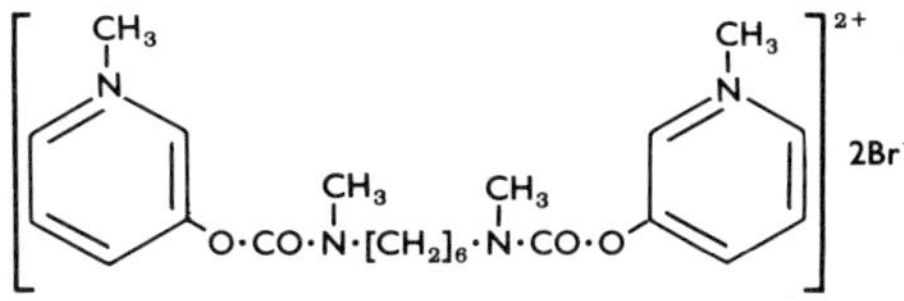

Extraction. Distigmine bromide is a quaternary ammonium compound (see p. 29).

Chromatography. PAPER: system P1—Rf 0·03 (location under ultraviolet light, strong absorption; location reagents: *iodoplatinate spray*, weak reaction; *bromocresol green spray*, strong reaction); system RP1a—Rf 1·00 (location under ultraviolet light, absorption; location reagent *iodoplatinate spray*, positive reaction); system RP1b—Rf 0·96 (location as for RP1a).
THIN-LAYER: system T1—Rf 0·00 (location reagent *acidified iodoplatinate spray*, positive reaction).

Crystal Tests. MICRO: *platinic chloride solution*—dense rosettes (*sensitivity:* 1 in 100); *styphnic acid*—dense rosettes or rosettes of plates (*sensitivity:* 1 in 1000).

Ultraviolet Absorption Spectrum. Distigmine bromide in 0·1N sulphuric acid, maximum at 270 mμ (E 1%, 1 cm 111).

Dose. Usually 5 mg daily; up to 15 mg daily has been given.

DISULFIRAM *Alcohol Deterrent*

Synonyms: Ethyldithiourame; TTD.
Proprietary Names: Antabuse; Cronetal.

Tetraethylthiuram disulphide
$C_{10}H_{20}N_2S_4$ = 296·5

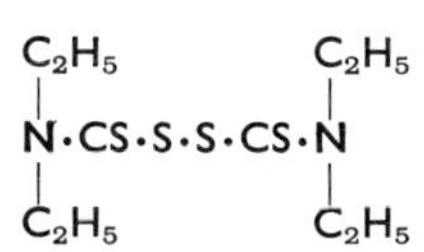

An almost white powder. F.p. 69·5° to 70·5°.
Solubility. Insoluble in water; soluble in ethanol, ether, and chloroform.

Extraction. Disulfiram is extracted with carbon tetrachloride from urine at pH 8.

Colour Test. Dissolve 0·05 g in 5 ml of ethanol

and add 1 ml of a 10% potassium cyanide solution—yellow → green → bluish-green.

A test for the presence in urine of the metabolite of disulfiram, diethyldithiocarbamic acid, may be carried out as follows. To 10 ml of urine add the following in order, mixing thoroughly after each addition: 1 ml of 10% sodium citrate solution, 1 ml of dilute ammonia solution, 1 ml of 5% copper sulphate solution, and 5 ml of amyl alcohol. After adding the amyl alcohol shake vigorously for 2 minutes and centrifuge. The presence of diethyldithiocarbamic acid is indicated by the amyl alcohol layer (top layer) assuming a yellow colour (per *Br. med. J.*, 1967, **2**, 687).

Quantitative Estimation. Disulfiram and diethyldithiocarbamic acid in blood and urine may be estimated colorimetrically after reaction with cuprous iodide (Tompsett, 1964).

Metabolism. Disulfiram is used in the treatment of chronic alcoholism. It produces hypersensitivity to alcohol since it interferes with the metabolism of alcohol, allowing acetaldehyde to accumulate. The concentrations of acetaldehyde in the blood and in the expired air are increased by 5 to 10 times.

Disulfiram is only slowly excreted so that up to 20% of an ingested dose may still remain in the body after 7 days. It may be found in the blood and urine within 24 hours unchanged, but mainly in a reduced form, diethyldithiocarbamic acid.

Dose. Up to 2 g daily.

Toxicity. Severe toxic reactions may occur at blood acetaldehyde levels greater than 0·5 mg% and fatalities may occur at blood alcohol levels of 100 mg% after as little as 0·5 to 1 g of disulfiram has been ingested. A single dose of 30 g of disulfiram is likely to produce serious toxic effects. Cases of serious phenytoin intoxication have occurred when disulfiram and phenytoin have been simultaneously administered; it is suggested that disulfiram inhibits the *p*-hydroxylation of phenytoin.

LD50 (oral): in rats 8·6 g/kg.

CASE EXAMPLES. A 29-year-old man died following ingestion of about 30 ml of rum after taking disulfiram (Jones, 1949).

A 49-year-old man died after taking a 'test drink' of about 30 ml of whisky while receiving disulfiram for chronic alcoholism (Becker and Sugarman, 1952).

DISULPHAMIDE *Diuretic*

Proprietary Name: Disamide.

5-Chlorotoluene-2,4-disulphonamide

$C_7H_9ClN_2O_4S_2 = 284{\cdot}7$

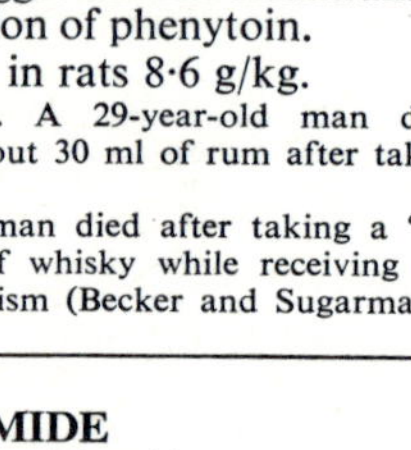

A white crystalline powder. M.p. about 260°.

Solubility. Soluble 1 in 500 of cold water, 1 in 50 of boiling water, 1 in 50 of ethanol, and 1 in 1000 of ether; slightly soluble in chloroform.

Extraction. Disulphamide is extracted by organic solvents from aqueous acid or alkaline solutions. A method of direct isolation from urine is described by Boggiano *et al.* (1960).

Ultraviolet Absorption Spectrum. Disulphamide in ethanol, maxima at 210 mμ, 235 mμ, 276 mμ, and 285 mμ.

Infra-red Absorption Spectrum. Potassium bromide disk. The principal peaks are: A 1172 or 1320, B 1552 (p. 739).

Metabolism. Disulphamide is a non-mercurial diuretic which has actions similar to those of chlorothiazide but which also inhibits the action of carbonic anhydrase. The onset of diuresis is rapid and the maximum response develops within 2 hours. In rats given disulphamide orally, 15% of the dose was excreted unchanged in the urine in 24 hours following doses of 300 mg/kg and 20 to 50% was excreted in 5 hours following 10 mg/kg. In rabbits given 10 mg/kg orally, peak levels in the serum were reached 1 to 2 hours after administration (Boggiano *et al.*, 1960).

Dose. Usually up to 200 mg daily; up to 500 mg daily has been given.

Toxicity. LD50 (oral): in mice 13 g/kg.

DITHIAZANINE IODIDE *Anthelmintic*

Synonym: 3,3′-Diethylthiadicarbocyanine Iodide.

Proprietary Names: Delvex; Telmid.

3 - Ethyl - 2 - [5 - (3 - ethylbenzothiazolidin - 2-ylidene)penta - 1,3 - dienyl]benzothiazolium iodide

$C_{23}H_{23}IN_2S_2 = 518{\cdot}5$

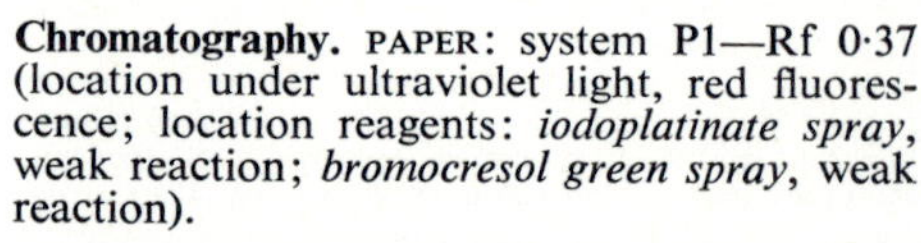

A dark greenish crystalline powder. M.p. 248°, with decomposition.

Solubility. Almost insoluble in water; very slightly soluble in ethanol; insoluble in ether.

Chromatography. PAPER: system P1—Rf 0·37 (location under ultraviolet light, red fluorescence; location reagents: *iodoplatinate spray*, weak reaction; *bromocresol green spray*, weak reaction).

Ultraviolet Absorption Spectrum. Dithiazanine iodide in ethanol, maxima at 276 mμ (E1%, 1 cm 22) and 327 mμ (E1%, 1 cm 34), and inflexions at about 255 mμ (E1%, 1 cm 24) and about 364 mμ (E1%, 1 cm 12); in methanol, maximum at 652 mμ (E1%, 1 cm 637).

Metabolism. Dithiazanine iodide is not readily absorbed from the gastro-intestinal tract and thus an effective concentration level of the dye may be attained in the faeces which it stains a bluish-green colour.

Dose. Up to 600 mg daily.

Toxicity. Dithiazanine is very toxic when absorbed from the gastro-intestinal tract and its use should be discontinued if the skin or sclera becomes blue.

LD50 (oral): in dogs 200, in mice 4 to 16, and in rats 165 to 192 mg/kg.

CASE EXAMPLES. A 3-year-old girl, given 150 mg of dithiazanine daily for 5 days, died on the sixth day. Dithiazanine was shown spectrophotometrically to be present in the liver in a concentration of 0·1 mg% but none was demonstrated in the blood. The intestinal mucosa and contents, and the surface of the kidney, were green and the heart and liver showed some green discoloration (Abadie and Samuels, 1965).

DODECYL GALLATE *Antoxidant*

Synonym: Lauryl Gallate.
Proprietary Name: Progallin LA.

Dodecyl 3,4,5-trihydroxybenzoate

$C_{19}H_{30}O_5 = 338{\cdot}4$

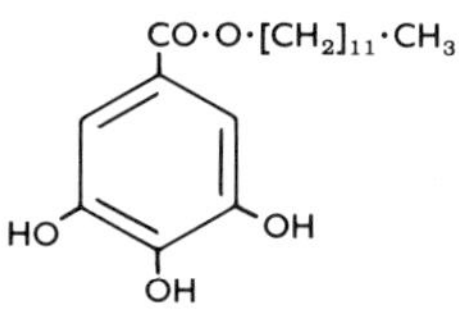

A white powder. M.p. 96° to 97·5°.

Solubility. Insoluble in water; soluble 1 in 3·5 of ethanol, 1 in 4 of ether, and 1 in 60 of chloroform.

Extraction. Dodecyl gallate is extracted by organic solvents from aqueous acid or alkaline solutions.

Colour Tests. Dissolve 10 mg in a mixture of 2·5 ml of acetone and 2·5 ml of water, and add 5 ml of dilute ammonia solution—deep pink, changing to orange-brown on standing; the pink colour is restored on shaking. Dissolve 5 mg in a mixture of 25 ml of acetone and 25 ml of water, and add 0·05 ml of ferric chloride solution—purplish-blue, rapidly changing to bluish-black.

Quantitative Estimation. Dodecyl gallate may be estimated colorimetrically after reaction with ferrous tartrate following reversed phase chromatography (Berger *et al.*, 1960).

Toxicity. The estimated acceptable daily intake for man is up to 0·2 mg/kg.

LD50 (oral): in rats 6·5 g/kg.

DOMIPHEN BROMIDE *Antiseptic Detergent*

Synonym: Phenododecinium Bromide.
Proprietary Names: Bradosol; Domittol.

Consists chiefly of dodecyldimethyl-2-phenoxyethylammonium bromide

$C_{22}H_{40}BrNO = 414{\cdot}5$

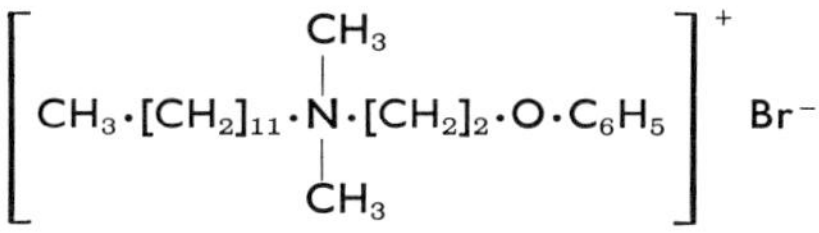

Colourless crystalline flakes. M.p. about 108°.

Solubility. Soluble 1 in less than 2 of water and of ethanol.

Extraction. Domiphen bromide is a quaternary ammonium compound (see p. 29).

Chromatography. PAPER: system P1—Rf 0·80 (location under ultraviolet light, absorption; location reagents: *iodoplatinate spray*, strong reaction; *bromocresol green spray*, weak reaction); system RP1a—Rf 0·32 (location reagent *iodoplatinate spray*, positive reaction); system RP1b—Rf 0·15 (location as for RP1a). THIN-LAYER: system T1—Rf 0·05 (location reagent *acidified iodoplatinate spray*, positive reaction).

Colour Test. Dissolve 10 mg in 10 ml of water, add 0·1 ml of a 0·5% aqueous eosin solution and 100 ml of water—intense pink.

Crystal Test. MICRO: *styphnic acid*—leaflike plates, best viewed under polarised light.

Ultraviolet Absorption Spectrum. Domiphen bromide in water, maxima at 268 mμ (E1%, 1 cm about 300) and 274 mμ (E1%, 1 cm about 250).

Infra-red Absorption Spectrum. Potassium bromide disk. The principal peaks are: A 1228, B 752, C 1500 (p. 739).

Toxicity. Domiphen bromide is used as 0·02 and 0·05% aqueous solutions, as a 0·5% solution in 70% ethanol, and as lozenges containing 0·5 mg. It is non-toxic in concentrations considerably higher than those normally used.

DOPAMINE

Synonym: 3-Hydroxytyramine.

3,4-Dihydroxyphenylethylamine

$C_8H_{11}NO_2 = 153{\cdot}2$

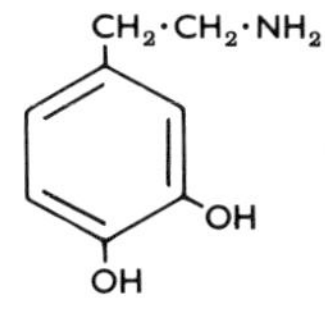

DOPAMINE HYDROCHLORIDE
A white crystalline powder.
Solubility. Soluble in water.

Extraction. Dopamine may be extracted into acidified butanol (Brownlee and Spriggs, 1965).

Chromatography. PAPER: system P1—Rf 0·12

(location under ultraviolet light, strong absorption; location reagents: *bromocresol green spray*, weak reaction; *potassium permanganate spray*, strong reaction).
THIN-LAYER: system T1—Rf 0·18, streaking (location reagent *potassium permanganate spray*, positive reaction).
GAS: system G2/225—retention time 0·56 relative to codeine (a poor peak, with tailing).

Colour Tests. MICRO: sulphuric acid–formaldehyde test—brown-purple (*sensitivity:* 0·5 µg); ammonium molybdate test—(yellow) blue (*sensitivity:* 1·0 µg); Vitali's test—yellow/yellow/brown (*sensitivity:* 1·0 µg).

Crystal Tests. MICRO: *gold bromide–hydrochloric acid solution*—very small plates (*sensitivity:* 1 in 100); *gold chloride solution*—very small plates (*sensitivity:* 1 in 100).

Ultraviolet Absorption Spectrum. Dopamine in 0·1N sulphuric acid, maximum at 279·5 mµ (E1%, 1 cm 133).

Quantitative Estimation. Choulis (1967) describes a method of separation of dopamine from adrenaline and noradrenaline involving thin-layer chromatography and its subsequent determination by spectrophotometry.

Metabolism. Dopamine is a naturally occurring catecholamine which is considered to be the immediate precursor of noradrenaline in the body. It is formed by decarboxylation of 3,4-dihydroxyphenylalanine; the latter may arise by oxidation of tyrosine. The decarboxylation can take place through bacterial action in the gastro-intestinal tract and also through enzymes present in the liver, kidney, and brain.

Use. Dopamine has been administered by injection in the treatment of congestive heart failure.

DOXAPRAM *Analeptic*

Synonym: AHR-619.

1-Ethyl-4-(2-morpholinoethyl)-2-oxo-3,3-diphenylpyrrolidine
$C_{24}H_{30}N_2O_2$ = 378·5

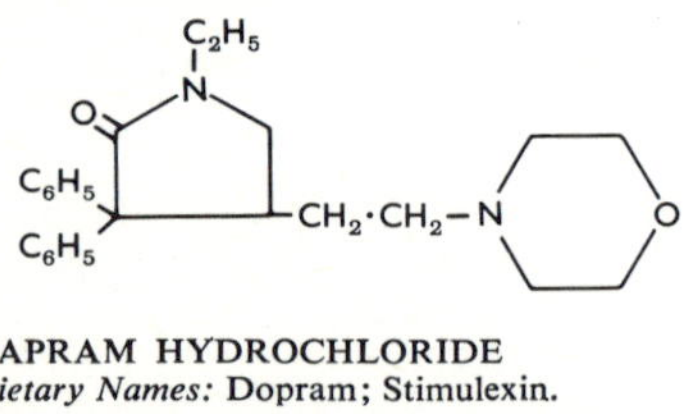

DOXAPRAM HYDROCHLORIDE
Proprietary Names: Dopram; Stimulexin.

A white crystalline powder. M.p. 217° to 221°.
Solubility. Sparingly soluble in water and ethanol; almost insoluble in ether; soluble in chloroform.

Extraction. Doxapram is extracted by organic solvents from aqueous alkaline solutions.

Chromatography. PAPER: system P1—Rf 0·60 (location reagents: *iodoplatinate spray*, strong reaction; *bromocresol green spray*, strong reaction); system RP1a—Rf 0·25 (location reagent *iodoplatinate spray*, positive reaction); system RP1b—Rf 0·00 (location as for RP1a).
THIN-LAYER: system T1—Rf 0·68 (location reagent *acidified iodoplatinate spray*, positive reaction).
GAS: system G2/225—retention time 4·20 relative to codeine; system G4—retention time 5·80 relative to codeine.

Colour Test. MICRO: ammonium vanadate test—faint blue (*sensitivity:* 1·0 µg).

Crystal Tests. MICRO: *potassium mercuric iodide solution*—feathery crystals (*sensitivity:* 1 in 1000); *potassium permanganate solution*—irregular blades (*sensitivity:* 1 in 1000).

Ultraviolet Absorption Spectrum. Doxapram in 0·1N sulphuric acid, maxima at about 248 mµ (E1%, 1 cm 8), 252·5 mµ (E1%, 1 cm 12), 258·5 mµ (E1%, 1 cm 14), 264 mµ (E1%, 1 cm 12), and about 268·5 mµ (E1%, 1 cm 8); doxapram hydrochloride in water, maxima at about 252 mµ, 258 mµ, and 264 mµ; minima at 244 mµ, 254 mµ, and 262 mµ.

Infra-red Absorption Spectrum. Doxapram (base). Potassium bromide disk. The principal peaks are: A 1685, B 1114, C 696 (p. 785).

Metabolism. Following intravenous injection into the dog, doxapram hydrochloride was rapidly metabolised in the liver, no unchanged drug being found in any biological material analysed. Large concentrations of the metabolites were found in the bile and high levels occurred in the fat and liver. Excretion of the metabolites took place rapidly in the urine during the first 24 hours. A large number of metabolites were formed, of which 2 were identified as 1-ethyl-4-(2-hydroxyethylaminoethyl)-2-oxo-3,3-diphenylpyrrolidine and 1-ethyl-4-(2-aminoethyl)-2-oxo-3,3-diphenylpyrrolidine (Bruce *et al.*, 1965).

Dose. Up to 400 mg by slow intravenous infusion.

DOXYLAMINE *Antihistamine*

Synonym: Histadoxylamine.

NN-Dimethyl-2-[1-phenyl-1-(pyrid-2-yl)-ethoxy]ethylamine
$C_{17}H_{22}N_2O$ = 270·4

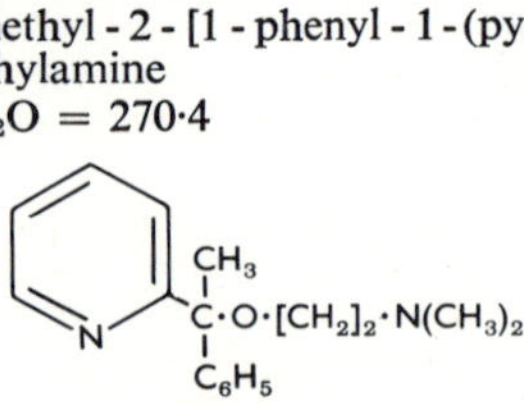

A liquid which boils at about 140°.

DOXYLAMINE SUCCINATE
Proprietary Name: Decapryn Succinate.

A white powder. M.p. 100° to 104°.
Solubility. Soluble 1 in 1 of water, 1 in 2 of ethanol, and 1 in 2 of chloroform; very slightly soluble in ether.

Extraction. Doxylamine is extracted by organic solvents from aqueous alkaline solutions.

Chromatography. PAPER: system P1—Rf 0·30 (location under ultraviolet light, blue fluorescence; location reagents: *iodoplatinate spray*, strong reaction; *bromocresol green spray*, weak reaction); system RP1a—Rf 0·77 (location reagent *iodoplatinate spray*, positive reaction); system RP1b—Rf 0·17 (location as for RP1a).
THIN-LAYER: system T1—Rf 0·43 (location reagent *acidified iodoplatinate spray*, positive reaction); system T2—Rf 0·60 (location reagent *iodoplatinate spray*, positive reaction); system T3—Rf 0·52 (location as for T2).
GAS: system G2/225—retention time 1·1 relative to diphenhydramine; system G4—retention time 1·4 relative to diphenhydramine.

Colour Test. MICRO: sulphuric acid–formaldehyde test—dull purple (*sensitivity:* 0·25 µg).

Crystal Tests. MICRO: *lead iodide solution*—irregular crystals or dense rosettes (*sensitivity:* 1 in 1000); *potassium cadmium iodide solution*—serrated needles (*sensitivity:* 1 in 1000).

Ultraviolet Absorption Spectrum. Doxylamine in 0·1N sodium hydroxide, maxima at 260 mµ (E1%, 1 cm 144) and 268 mµ (E1%, 1 cm 108); in 0·1N sulphuric acid, maximum at 261 mµ (E1%, 1 cm 421) and an inflexion at about 265 mµ (E1%, 1 cm 409).

Infra-red Absorption Spectrum. Doxylamine (base). Potassium bromide disk. The principal peaks are: A 700, B 1431 or 1470 or 1590 (p. 785).

Metabolism. Studies in rats and dogs have demonstrated that only 10 to 30% of a dose is excreted, the bulk appearing to be destroyed in the body (Snyder *et al.*, 1948).

Dose. Up to 100 mg daily.

Toxicity. The estimated lethal dose in man is between 25 and 250 mg/kg.

DROPERIDOL *Tranquilliser*

Synonyms: Dehydrobenzperidol; R 4749.
Proprietary Names: Inapsin. It is an ingredient of Innovar and Thalamonal.

1-{1,2,3,6-Tetrahydro-1-[4-(*p*-fluorophenyl)-4-oxobutyl]pyrid-4-yl}-2-oxobenzimidazoline
$C_{22}H_{22}FN_3O_2 = 379·4$

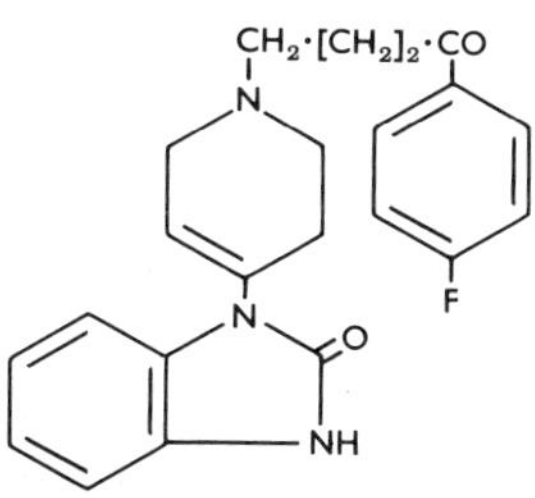

A yellowish to orange-brown amorphous powder which slowly darkens on exposure to light. M.p. 142° to 146°.

Solubility. Sparingly soluble in water; slightly soluble in ethanol and ether; freely soluble in chloroform.

Extraction. Droperidol is extracted by organic solvents from aqueous alkaline solutions.

Chromatography. PAPER: system P1—Rf 0·59 (location under ultraviolet light, strong absorption; location reagents: *iodoplatinate spray*, strong reaction; *bromocresol green spray*, strong reaction; *potassium permanganate spray*, weak reaction).
THIN-LAYER: system T1—Rf 0·50, streaking (location reagent *acidified iodoplatinate spray*, positive reaction).

Colour Tests. MICRO: ammonium molybdate test—pale blue-grey (*sensitivity:* 1·0 µg); ammonium vanadate test—dark blue → dull green (*sensitivity:* 0·1 µg); Vitali's test— –/faint brown/bright yellow (*sensitivity:* 0·25 µg).

Crystal Tests. MICRO: *ammonium thiocyanate solution*—dendrites, best viewed under polarised light (*sensitivity:* 1 in 1000); *platinic chloride solution*—small needles, sometimes in sheaves or bunches (*sensitivity:* 1 in 1000).

Infra-red Absorption Spectrum. Potassium bromide disk. The principal peaks are: A 1688, B 1591, C 1227 (p. 739).

Dose. Up to 20 mg.

Toxicity. LD50 (intravenous): in mice 43 and in rats 30 mg/kg.

DYCLONINE *Local Anaesthetic*

p-Butoxy-β-piperidinopropiophenone
$C_{18}H_{27}NO_2 = 289·4$

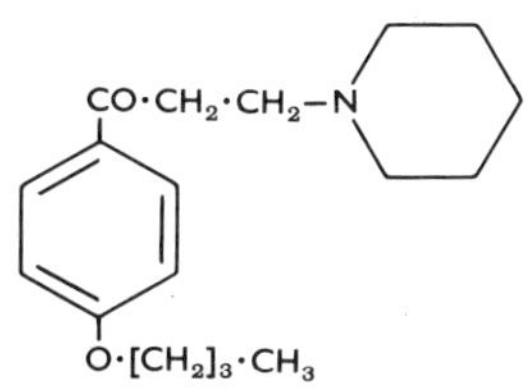

DYCLONINE HYDROCHLORIDE
Proprietary Name: Dyclone Hydrochloride.

A white crystalline powder. M.p. 175° to 176°.
Solubility. Soluble 1 in 50 of water; soluble in ethanol and acetone.

Extraction. Dyclonine is extracted by organic solvents from aqueous alkaline solutions.

Chromatography. PAPER: system P1—Rf 0·78 (location under ultraviolet light, absorption; location reagents: *iodoplatinate spray*, strong reaction; *bromocresol green spray*, weak reaction).
THIN-LAYER: system T1—Rf 0·57 (location reagent *acidified iodoplatinate spray*, positive reaction).

Colour Test. MICRO: Vitali's test— –/–/faint orange (*sensitivity:* 1·0 µg).

Crystal Tests. MICRO: *gold cyanide solution*—

oily rods (*sensitivity:* 1 in 1000); *trinitrobenzoic acid solution*—small rosettes or bunches of needles (*sensitivity:* 1 in 1000).

Ultraviolet Absorption Spectrum. Dyclonine in water, maximum at 282 mμ (E1%, 1 cm 492); in 0·1N sulphuric acid, maxima at 221 mμ (E1%, 1 cm 322) and 282 mμ (E1%, 1 cm 380).

Toxicity. Dyclonine is employed as a 1% vanishing cream or a 0·5% aqueous lotion. The maximum amount considered safe for surface use is 100 mg or 20 ml of a 0·5% solution.

ECGONINE *Alkaloid*

Synonym: Laevo-ecgonine.

3-Hydroxy-2-tropanecarboxylic acid

$C_9H_{15}NO_3$ = 185·2

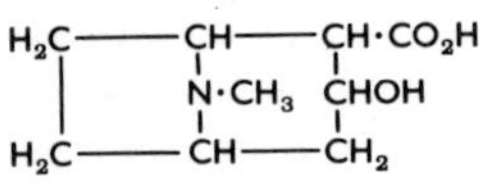

Ecgonine is a hydrolysis product of cocaine; it melts at 198°, with decomposition; the dry substance melts at 205°.

Solubility. Soluble in water; slightly soluble in ethanol; insoluble in ether.

Chromatography. PAPER: system P1—Rf 0·03 (location reagent *iodoplatinate spray*, strong reaction).

THIN-LAYER: system T1—Rf 0·17 (location reagent *acidified iodoplatinate spray*, positive reaction).

Crystal Tests. MICRO: *platinic iodide solution*—small rectangular plates (*sensitivity:* 1 in 400); *potassium bismuth iodide solution*—hexagons (*sensitivity:* 1 in 1000).

Ultraviolet Absorption Spectrum. Ecgonine in ethanol, maximum at about 275 mμ; minimum at about 250 mμ.

Metabolism. Ecgonine is the product of complete hydrolysis of cocaine; however, it does not seem to have been detected in the urine of animals dosed with cocaine. Ecgonine could be further metabolised but nothing seems to have been recorded.

EDROPHONIUM CHLORIDE *Anticholinesterase*

Proprietary Name: Tensilon.

Ethyl(3-hydroxyphenyl)dimethylammonium chloride

$C_{10}H_{16}ClNO$ = 201·7

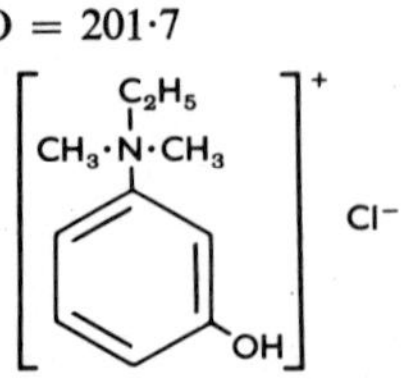

A white crystalline powder. M.p. about 168°, with decomposition.

Solubility. Soluble 1 in 0·5 of water; soluble 1 in 5 of ethanol; insoluble in ether and chloroform.

Extraction. Edrophonium chloride is a quaternary ammonium compound (see p. 29).

Chromatography. PAPER: system P1—Rf 0·25 (location under ultraviolet light, absorption; location reagents: *iodoplatinate spray*, strong reaction; *bromocresol green spray*, weak reaction); system RP1a—Rf 0·93 (location under ultraviolet light, absorption); system RP1b—Rf 0·94 (location under ultraviolet light, absorption; location reagent *iodoplatinate spray*, positive reaction).

THIN-LAYER: system T1—Rf 0·07 (location reagent *acidified iodoplatinate spray*, positive reaction).

Colour Tests. MICRO: ammonium vanadate test—blue-green (*sensitivity:* 0·5 μg); Vitali's test—–/yellow/yellow (*sensitivity:* 0·5 μg).

Crystal Tests. MICRO: *gold bromide–hydrochloric acid solution*—plates, often cruciform (*sensitivity:* 1 in 400); *lead iodide solution*—long plates or needles (*sensitivity:* 1 in 400).

Ultraviolet Absorption Spectrum. Edrophonium chloride in 0·1N hydrochloric acid, maximum at 273 mμ (E1%, 1 cm about 110); in 0·1N sodium hydroxide, maxima at 240 mμ (E1%, 1 cm about 550) and 294 mμ (E1%, 1 cm about 170).

Infra-red Absorption Spectrum. Potassium bromide disk. The principal peaks are: A 1479 or 1609, B 690 or 1217 or 1495 (p. 785).

Dose. Up to 10 mg intravenously, in the diagnosis of myasthenia gravis.

Toxicity. The estimated minimum lethal dose in man is 100 mg.

EMBRAMINE *Antihistamine*

Synonym: Mebrophenhydramine.

2-(1-*p*-Bromophenyl-1-phenylethoxy)-*NN*-dimethylethylamine

$C_{18}H_{22}BrNO$ = 348·3

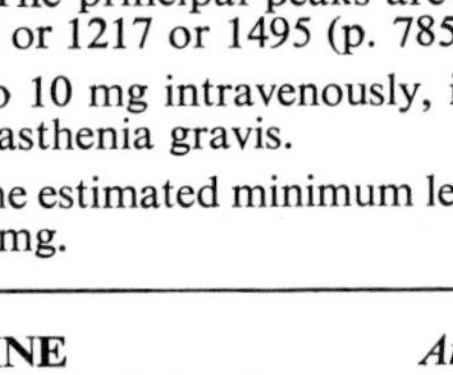

EMBRAMINE HYDROCHLORIDE

Proprietary Names: Bromadryl; Mebryl.

White crystals. M.p. 155°.

Solubility. Soluble in water.

Extraction. Embramine is extracted by organic solvents from aqueous alkaline solutions.

Chromatography. PAPER: system P1—Rf 0·79 (location under ultraviolet light, absorption; location reagent *iodoplatinate spray*, strong

reaction); system RP1a—Rf 0·32 (location reagent *iodoplatinate spray*, positive reaction); system RP1b—Rf 0·00 (location as for RP1a).
THIN-LAYER: system T1—Rf 0·54 (location reagent *acidified iodoplatinate spray*, positive reaction).
GAS: system G2/225—retention time 0·57 relative to codeine; system G4—retention time 0·27 relative to codeine.

Colour Tests. MICRO: sulphuric acid–formaldehyde test—orange (*sensitivity:* 0·1 μg); ammonium molybdate test—yellow → green → blue (*sensitivity:* 0·1 μg); ammonium vanadate test—orange-brown (*sensitivity:* 0·25 μg); Vitali's test—dull orange/dull orange/dull orange (*sensitivity:* 0·25 μg).

Crystal Tests. MICRO: *platinic bromide solution*—oily branching needles or smudge rosettes (*sensitivity:* 1 in 1000); *platinic chloride solution*—smudge rosettes or oily needles (*sensitivity:* 1 in 1000).

Ultraviolet Absorption Spectrum. Embramine in 0·1N sulphuric acid, maxima at 226 mμ (E1%, 1cm 400) and 258 mμ (E1%, 1cm 18).

Infra-red Absorption Spectrum. Embramine (base). Potassium bromide disk. The principal peaks are: A 1009, B 1095, C 699 (p. 785).

Metabolism. Embramine is rapidly absorbed from the intestinal tract. Six hours after a large dose, high levels of the drug were found in the liver, lungs, and spleen, and low levels in the brain and heart.

Dose. Up to 120 mg daily.

Toxicity. Long-term administration of large doses to dogs and cats have shown it to have negligible toxicity.
LD50 (oral): in mice 330 mg/kg.

EMBUTRAMIDE

Proprietary Name: It is an ingredient of T61, a preparation used for veterinary euthanasia.

N-[*β*-Ethyl-*β*-(*m*-methoxyphenyl)butyl]-*γ*-hydroxybutyramide
$C_{17}H_{27}NO_3 = 293{\cdot}4$

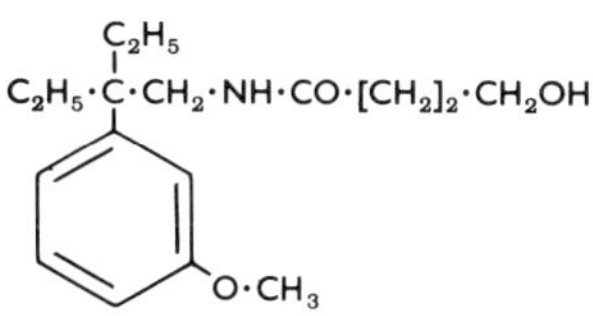

Extraction. Embutramide is extracted by organic solvents from aqueous acid or alkaline solutions.

Chromatography. THIN-LAYER: system T1—Rf 0·72 (location reagent *potassium permanganate spray*, positive reaction).

Colour Tests. MICRO: sulphuric acid–formaldehyde test—dull blue (*sensitivity:* 0·5 μg); ammonium molybdate test—faint blue (*sensitivity:* 1·0 μg); ammonium vanadate test—faint brown (*sensitivity:* 1·0 μg).

Ultraviolet Absorption Spectrum. Embutramide in 0·1N sulphuric acid, maxima at 271 mμ (E1%, 1cm 50) and 276·5 mμ (E1%, 1cm 45).

Infra-red Absorption Spectrum. Potassium bromide disk. The principal peaks are: A 1652, B 1248, C 1037 (p. 785).

EMETINE *Anti-amoebic*

Synonyms: Ipecine; Methylcephaëline.

Cephaëline-*O*-methyl ether
$C_{29}H_{40}N_2O_4 = 480{\cdot}7$

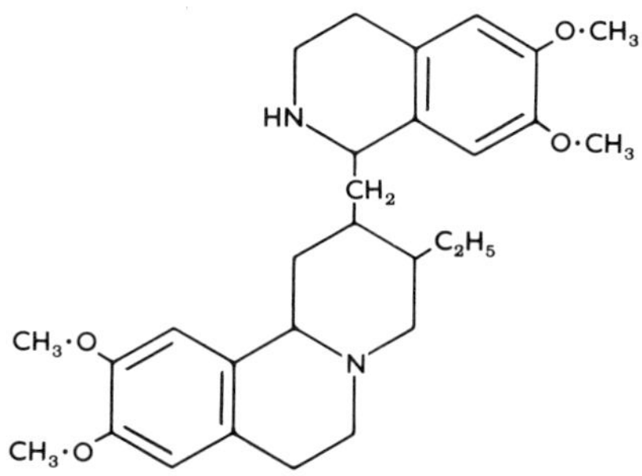

An alkaloid obtained from ipecacuanha, the dried rhizome and root of *Cephaëlis ipecacuanha* (Rubiaceae), or prepared by methylation of cephaëline.
A white amorphous powder. M.p. 74°.
Solubility. Slightly soluble in water; soluble in ethanol, ether, and chloroform.

EMETINE HYDROCHLORIDE
Synonym: Emetine Dihydrochloride.
A white crystalline powder.
Solubility. Soluble 1 in 8 of water, 1 in 12 of ethanol, and 1 in 4 of chloroform; insoluble in ether.

Extraction. Emetine is extracted by organic solvents from aqueous alkaline solutions.

Chromatography. PAPER: system P1—Rf 0·19 (location reagents: *iodoplatinate spray*, strong reaction; *bromocresol green spray*, strong reaction); system RP1b—Rf 0·07 (location reagent *iodoplatinate spray*, positive reaction).
THIN-LAYER: system T1—Rf 0·52 (location reagent *acidified iodoplatinate spray*, positive reaction).
GAS: system G6—retention time 1·21 relative to codeine.

Colour Tests. MICRO: ammonium molybdate test—green (*sensitivity:* 0·1 μg); Vitali's test—pale yellow/pale brown/yellow (*sensitivity:* 1·0 μg).

Ultraviolet Absorption Spectrum. Emetine in 0·1N sulphuric acid, maximum at 281·5 mμ (E1%, 1cm 227) and an inflexion at about 285 mμ (E1%, 1cm 208).

Infra-red Absorption Spectrum. Emetine (base). Potassium bromide disk. The principal peaks are: A 1514, B 1256, C 1228 or 1463 (p. 786).

Quantitative Estimation. Davis *et al.* (1962) describe a method of spectrofluorimetric determination of emetine in biological fluids and tissues.

Metabolism. Emetine is rapidly absorbed from the gastro-intestinal tract and also following injection. It is distributed rapidly throughout the body, the liver and spleen having the highest concentrations. In most organs, the maximum concentration of the drug occurs within 24 hours of injection. Emetine is only slowly excreted, mainly in the urine although some may be excreted back into the stomach. Urinary excretion of unchanged emetine has been reported to begin within 20 minutes after injection and to continue for as long as 2 months. This very slow excretion means that continuous use leads to cumulative action.

Toxicity. Death has occurred following a dose of 150 mg of emetine hydrochloride but about 700 mg is usually considered to be the fatal dose. Emetine is a protoplasmic poison acting on all tissues; large doses, or prolonged administration of therapeutic doses, may produce degenerative changes in the heart, liver, kidneys, intestinal tract, and skeletal muscle. It is also very irritant to mucous membranes.
LD50 (oral): in mice 30 mg/kg.

EMYLCAMATE *Tranquilliser*

Synonyms: KABI 925; MK 250; 1-Ethyl-1-methylpropyl Carbamate.
Proprietary Names: Nuncital; Striatran.

2-Ethylbut-2-yl carbamate
$C_7H_{15}NO_2 = 145{\cdot}2$

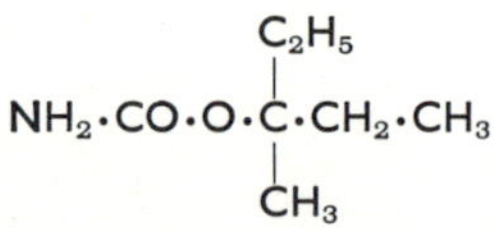

A white crystalline powder. M.p. 56° to 58°.
Solubility. Soluble 1 in 250 of water; very soluble in ethanol and ether.

Extraction. Emylcamate is extracted by organic solvents from aqueous acid or alkaline solutions.

Chromatography. Moss and Jackson (1961) have described 2 paper chromatographic systems, P6 and P7, which separate carbamate drugs and which therefore should be applicable to emylcamate.

Crystal Test. MICRO: *gold chloride solution*—smudge rosettes (*sensitivity:* 1 in 200).

Infra-red Absorption Spectrum. Potassium chloride disk. The principal peaks are: A 1690, B 1392, C 1610 (p. 739).

Metabolism. Emylcamate is structurally and pharmacologically similar to meprobamate (p. 403). It is rapidly absorbed from the gastro-intestinal tract, peak blood-levels being attained in 1 to 2 hours. It is metabolised in the liver and excreted in the urine.

Dose. Up to 800 mg daily.

Toxicity. The lethal dose in man is estimated to be between 100 and 500 mg/kg.

ENDRIN *Pesticide*

Other Names: CPA One-shot Dust; Compound 269; Endrex 20; Lacco Dust Endri Tox; Woodbury Brand End Borer.

1,2,3,4,10,10-Hexachloro-6,7-epoxy-1,4,4a,5,6,-7,8,8a-octahydro-1,4(*exo*):5,8(*exo*)-dimethanonaphthalene
$C_{12}H_8Cl_6O = 380{\cdot}9$

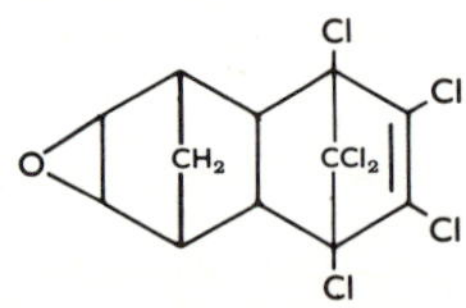

A white crystalline solid, which is stable to acids and alkalis. M.p. over 200°.
Solubility. Insoluble in water; sparingly soluble in ethanol.

Extraction. Endrin is extracted by organic solvents from aqueous acid or alkaline solutions.

Colour Test. Johnson (1956) describes a colour test which detects endrin in the presence of dieldrin and aldrin; a further test is described which is specific for dieldrin and endrin.

Ultraviolet Absorption Spectrum. Endrin in ethanol, maximum at 224 mμ (E1%, 1 cm 148).

Quantitative Estimation. Skerrett and Baker (1960) describe a method of estimation of endrin involving its conversion to the 2,4-dinitrophenylhydrazone derivative of an isomeric ketone, and it may be determined by gas chromatography (Jain *et al.*, 1965; Hamence *et al.*, 1965).

Metabolism. Endrin may be absorbed through the respiratory and gastro-intestinal tracts and through the skin; whatever the route, the absorption is facilitated if the endrin is dissolved in oils or other lipids.
Endrin has been found to accumulate in the body fat of cows and to be excreted in small amounts in their milk.

Toxicity. Endrin is said to have a greater mammalian toxicity than dieldrin but its percutaneous toxicity is said to be lower.
LD50 (oral): in rats 10 to 12 mg/kg.

CASE EXAMPLES. A case is reported of fatal intoxication with endrin which had been used as a pesticide in the cultivation of rice and remained as a residue in the rice (Charro Arias *et al.*, 1966).

Three people experienced sudden convulsions shortly after eating bread which had been made from flour contaminated with about 20 mg% of endrin. Recoveries were spontaneous and symptoms were minimal. Traces of endrin were detected in the serum and urine in all 3 cases. Several other people also ate the bread but experienced no ill effects (Coble *et al.*, 1967).

ENOXOLONE *Anti-inflammatory Agent*

Synonyms: Glycyrrhetic Acid; Glycyrrhetinic Acid.
Proprietary Name: Biosone.

3β-Hydroxy-11-oxo-olean-12-en-30-oic acid; there is evidence of the existence of at least 2 isomers.

$C_{30}H_{46}O_4 = 470{\cdot}7$

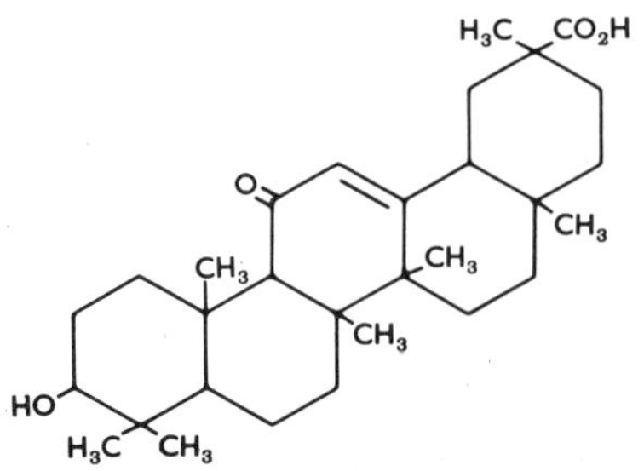

A white powder. M.p. 296°.

Solubility. Very sparingly soluble in water; soluble in ethanol and ether; freely soluble in chloroform.

Extraction and **Chromatography.** A method of extraction of enoxolone from biological fluids and tissues and consequent purification by 2-dimensional thin-layer chromatography is described by Coleman and Parke (1963).

Ultraviolet Absorption Spectrum. Enoxolone in ethanol, maxima at 204 mμ and 248 mμ.

Quantitative Estimation. Enoxolone may be estimated spectrophotometrically following purification by 2-dimensional thin-layer chromatography (Parke *et al.*, 1963).

Metabolism. The isomeric forms of enoxolone have different biological acitivity, but the most active have an anti-inflammatory action. Metabolic studies with tritium-labelled enoxolone in the rat have shown that it is excreted mainly via the bile in the form of three as yet unidentified metabolites. Less than 2% of the activity is found in the urine (Parke *et al.*, 1963).

EPHEDRINE *Sympathomimetic*

(−)-2-Methylamino-1-phenylpropan-1-ol hemihydrate

$C_{10}H_{15}NO,\frac{1}{2}H_2O = 174{\cdot}2$

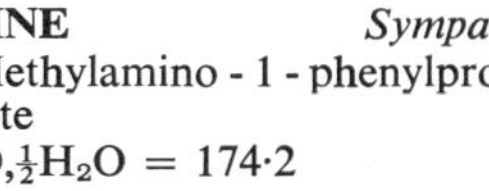

An alkaloid obtained from species of *Ephedra* (Ephedraceae), or prepared synthetically.

Colourless hexagonal prismatic crystals. M.p. 40° to 41°.

Solubility. Soluble 1 in 36 of water and 1 in less than 1 of ethanol; soluble in ether and chloroform but the solutions are turbid due to the separation of water.

NOTE. For racemic ephedrine, (±)-ephedrine, see Racephedrine, p. 535.

ANHYDROUS EPHEDRINE

An unctuous, almost colourless, very deliquescent solid which tends to crystallise in needles and rapidly absorbs carbon dioxide. M.p. 33° to 37·5°.

Solubility. Soluble 1 in 20 of water; soluble in ether and chloroform; readily soluble in ethanol.

EPHEDRINE HYDROCHLORIDE

A white crystalline powder. M.p. 217° to 220°.

Solubility. Soluble 1 in 4 of water and 1 in 17 of ethanol; insoluble in ether; almost insoluble in chloroform.

EPHEDRINE SULPHATE

Fine white crystals which darken on exposure to light. M.p. 258°, with decomposition.

Solubility. Soluble 1 in 2 of water and 1 in 60 of ethanol.

Extraction. Ephedrine is extracted by organic solvents from aqueous alkaline solutions; it is volatile and may also be isolated by distillation from alkaline solutions (see p. 18).

Chromatography. PAPER: system P1—Rf 0·45 (location under ultraviolet light, absorption; location reagents: *iodoplatinate spray*, weak reaction; *bromocresol green spray*, weak reaction).

THIN-LAYER: system T1—Rf 0·28 (location reagent *potassium permanganate spray*, positive reaction).

GAS: system G2/120—retention time 3·5 relative to amphetamine; system G2/225—retention time 0·25 relative to diphenhydramine.

Colour Test. Chen's test—purple.

Crystal Tests. MICRO: *platinic iodide solution*—plates, forming overnight (*sensitivity:* 1 in 100); *potassium bismuth iodide solution*—long jagged plates (*sensitivity:* 1 in 100).

Ultraviolet Absorption Spectrum. Ephedrine in 0·1N sulphuric acid, maxima at 251 mμ (E1%, 1 cm 9), 256·5 mμ (E1%, 1 cm 11·6), and 262·5 mμ (E1%, 1 cm 9); minima at 228 mμ, 253 mμ, and 260 mμ.

Infra-red Absorption Spectrum. Ephedrine (base). Potassium bromide disk. The principal peaks are: A 703, B 1455, C 745 (p. 740).

Quantitative Estimation. Karawya *et al.* (1967) describe two colorimetric methods for the quantitative estimation of ephedrine, one involving oxidation by hydrogen peroxide in alkali to give a red colour, the other involving reaction with carbon disulphide and ammoniacal copper sulphate solution to give copper dithiocarbamate which is brown. Tompsett (1967a) describes a spectrophotometric method of determination of ephedrine in biological materials. Beckett and Wilkinson (1965) have described a method of gas chromatographic analysis from urine.

Metabolism. Ephedrine is readily absorbed from the gastro-intestinal tract and after injection; it accumulates in tissues such as the liver, lung, kidney, brain, and spleen. In man, about 80% of the dose is excreted unchanged in the urine in 24 hours; only 4·3% of the dose has been found as the *N*-demethylated metabolite, phenylpropanolamine (Beckett and Wilkinson, 1965).
In the dog and the rabbit, demethylation is the major initial metabolic reaction; this is followed by hydroxylation but further transformation appears to take place.

Dose. Usually up to 300 mg.

Toxicity. The estimated minimum lethal dose in children up to 2 years of age is 200 mg and for adults 2 g. Single doses of as much as 400 mg have been given without causing serious toxic effects.

ERGOMETRINE *Ergot Alkaloid*

Synonyms: Ergobasine; Ergonovine.

(+)-*N*-(2-Hydroxy-1-methylethyl)lysergamide
$C_9H_{23}N_3O_2$ = 325·4

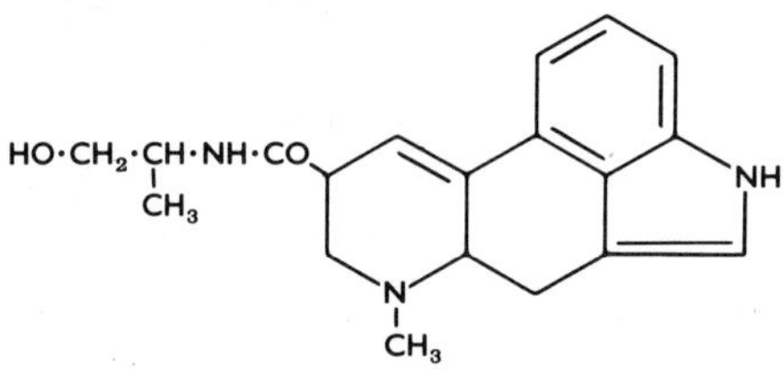

Colourless crystals. M.p. 162°.
Solubility. Slightly soluble in water, producing a solution with a blue fluorescence; more soluble in ethanol; sparingly soluble in chloroform.

ERGOMETRINE MALEATE
Synonym: Ergometrine Bimaleate.
Proprietary Names: Ergotrate. It is an ingredient of Syntometrine.
A white or faintly yellow, slightly hygroscopic, microcrystalline powder which darkens with age and exposure to light. M.p. 167°, with decomposition.
Solubility. Soluble 1 in 36 of water and 1 in 100 of ethanol; insoluble in ether and chloroform.

ERGOMETRINE TARTRATE
Proprietary Name: it is an ingredient of Neo-Femergin.
White, very light, matted masses of acicular crystals.
Solubility. Soluble in water and ethanol; slightly soluble in ether and chloroform.

Extraction. Ergometrine is extracted by organic solvents from aqueous alkaline solutions.

Chromatography. PAPER: system P1—Rf 0·25 (location under ultraviolet light, bright blue fluorescence; location reagents: *iodoplatinate spray*, weak reaction; p-*dimethylaminobenzaldehyde spray*, blue; *potassium permanganate spray*, strong reaction).
THIN-LAYER: system T1—Rf 0·67 (location reagent p-*dimethylaminobenzaldehyde spray*, blue); system T9—Rf 0·19 (location under ultraviolet light, blue fluorescence; location reagent p-*dimethylaminobenzaldehyde spray*, blue).
McLaughlin *et al.* (1964) have described 2 thin-layer systems which separate ergometrine, ergotamine, and other ergot alkaloids.

Colour Tests. MICRO: sulphuric acid–formaldehyde test—brown (*sensitivity:* 0·05 μg); ammonium molybdate test—deep green → red → grey → blue (*sensitivity:* 0·25 μg); Vitali's test—dull orange/yellow/dull purple (*sensitivity:* 0·25 μg).

Crystal Tests. MICRO: *trinitrobenzoic acid solution*—dendrites (*sensitivity:* 1 in 200); *picric acid*—clumps or fans of rods (*sensitivity:* 1 in 200).

Ultraviolet Absorption Spectrum. Ergometrine in 0·1N sulphuric acid, maximum at 312 mμ (E1%, 1 cm 250).

Quantitative Estimation. Curry (1959) describes an extraction and determination procedure for ergometrine in buttock tissue, liver, and urine.

Metabolism. Ergometrine is more rapidly absorbed from the gastro-intestinal tract than ergotamine. It has been detected unchanged in the urine up to 8½ hours after an injection, the maximum concentration generally occurring 2 to 3 hours after an injection (Curry, 1959).

Dose. Usually up to 1 mg.

Toxicity. Ergometrine is less toxic than ergotamine.
LD50 (intravenous): in mice 144 mg/kg.
CASE EXAMPLE. Following the intravenous injection of 0·2 mg of ergometrine maleate given with the birth of her baby, a 17-year-old girl developed nausea, a severe headache, increased blood-pressure, and coma. Death was caused 7 days later by excessive cerebral haemorrhage (Ringrose, 1962).

ERGOTAMINE *Ergot Alkaloid*

$C_{33}H_{35}N_5O_5$ = 581·7

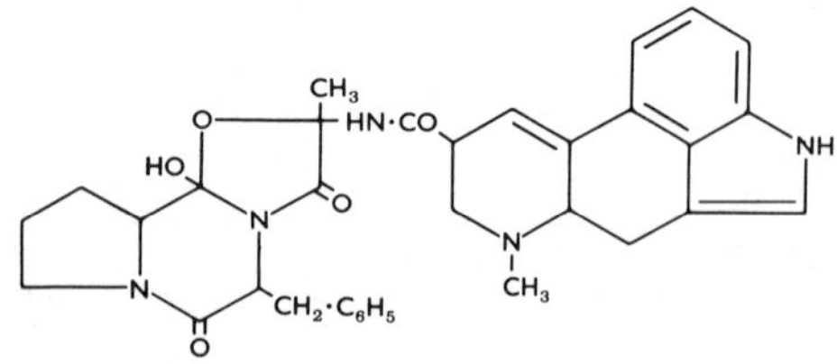

Ergotamine occurs as hygroscopic crystals which darken and decompose on exposure to air, heat, and light. M.p. 212° to 214°, with decomposition.
Solubility. Almost insoluble in water; slightly soluble in ethanol; freely soluble in chloroform.

ERGOTAMINE TARTRATE
Proprietary Names: Femergin; Gynergen; Lingraine; Lingräne. It is an ingredient of many proprietary prepara-

tions—see Extra Pharmacopoeia (Martindale) 25th Edn, p. 590.

A white crystalline powder, which softens at about 187° and decomposes at about 192° without melting. It should be stored in an atmosphere of nitrogen in a sealed tube, protected from light.
Solubility. Soluble 1 in 500 of water and 1 in 500 of ethanol; almost insoluble in ether and chloroform.

Extraction. Ergotamine is extracted by organic solvents from aqueous alkaline solutions.

Chromatography. PAPER: system P1—Rf 0·65 (location under ultraviolet light, blue fluorescence; location reagents: p-*dimethylaminobenzaldehyde spray*, blue; *potassium permanganate spray*, strong reaction).
THIN-LAYER: system T1—Rf 0·68 (location reagent p-*dimethylaminobenzaldehyde spray*, blue); system T9—Rf 0·51 (location under ultraviolet light, absorption; location reagent p-*dimethylaminobenzaldehyde spray*, blue).
McLaughlin *et al.* (1964) have described 2 thin-layer systems which separate ergometrine, ergotamine, and other ergot alkaloids.

Colour Tests. MICRO: sulphuric acid–formaldehyde test—faint brown (*sensitivity:* 1·0 μg); ammonium molybdate test—grey-blue (*sensitivity:* 1·0 μg); ammonium vanadate test—purple-brown (*sensitivity:* 1·0 μg); Vitali's test—dull orange/dull orange/purple-brown (*sensitivity:* 0·5 μg).

Ultraviolet Absorption Spectrum. Ergotamine in 0·1N sulphuric acid, maximum at 315 mμ (E1%, 1 cm 135); ergotamine tartrate in a 1% tartaric acid solution, maxima at 239 mμ (E1%, 1 cm 292) and 317·5 mμ (E1%, 1 cm 113); minimum at 270 mμ.

Metabolism. Ergotamine is poorly absorbed from the gastro-intestinal tract; it appears to be rapidly detoxified in the body, probably by the liver, and insignificant amounts of unchanged drug are excreted in the urine. Not more than 5% of an intravenous dose has been accounted for, even by analyses as early as 5 minutes after injection.

Dose. Up to 6 mg in 24 hours; not more than 12 mg in one week.

Toxicity. Ergotamine is highly toxic; in large repeated doses it can produce all the symptoms of ergot poisoning. Fatal poisoning has occurred after the oral administration of 26 mg of ergotamine over a period of several days, and also following single injections of only 0·5 to 1·5 mg.

LD50 (intravenous): in mice 52 and in rats 62 mg/kg.

CASE EXAMPLE. A 13-month-old girl ingested about 50 Bellergal tablets (20 mg phenobarbitone, 0·3 mg ergotamine tartrate, 0·1 mg belladonna per tablet). The estimated amount of ergotamine tartrate ingested was 15 mg. On admission to hospital a blood-level of more than 5 mg% of barbiturate was found. Peritoneal dialysis was performed and the first 200 ml of the dialysate contained 17·1 mg of phenobarbitone and 90 μg of ergotamine (present as ergotaminine). A substance appeared on the chromatogram which was probably a metabolite of ergotamine. The child recovered (Jones and Williams, 1966).

ERGOTOXINE *Ergot Alkaloid*

Synonym: Ecboline.

Ergotoxine has been shown to be a mixture of the three isomorphous alkaloids ergocornine, ergocristine, and ergocryptine.

$C_{31}H_{39}N_5O_5 = 561{\cdot}7$

It occurs as crystals. M.p. 190°, with decomposition.
Solubility. Almost insoluble in water; soluble in ethanol; slightly soluble in ether; very soluble in chloroform.

ERGOTOXINE ESYLATE

Synonym: Ergotoxine Ethanesulphonate.

Colourless acicular crystals which decompose at 209°.
Solubility. Sparingly soluble in water; more soluble in ethanol.

Extraction. Ergotoxine is extracted by organic solvents from aqueous alkaline solutions.

Chromatography. PAPER: system P1—Rf 0·82 (location under ultraviolet light, blue fluorescence; location reagents: p-*dimethylaminobenzaldehyde spray*, blue; *potassium permanganate spray*, strong reaction).
THIN-LAYER: system T1—Rf 0·73 (location as for system P1).
McLaughlin *et al.* (1964) have described 2 thin-layer systems which separate the constituents of ergotoxine from ergometrine, ergotamine, and other ergot alkaloids.

Ultraviolet Absorption Spectrum. Ergotoxine esylate in isopropanol, maximum at 320 mμ (E1%, 1 cm 123).

Dose. Up to 1 mg, subcutaneously or intramuscularly.

ERYTHRITYL TETRANITRATE *Coronary Vasodilator*

Synonyms: Erithritol Tetranitrate; Erythrol Nitrate or Tetranitrate; Erythrotetranitral; Nitro-Erythrite; Nitro-erythrol; Tetranitrol.
Proprietary Names: Cardilate. It is an ingredient of Dolorin and Erythin.

$C_4H_6(O{\cdot}NO_2)_4 = 302{\cdot}1$

$NO_3{\cdot}CH{\cdot}CH_2{\cdot}NO_3$
|
$NO_3{\cdot}CH{\cdot}CH_2{\cdot}NO_3$

Colourless crystals which are explosive unless mixed with an inert substance. M.p. about 61°.
Solubility. Almost insoluble in water; soluble in ethanol, ether, and glycerin.

Extraction. Erythrityl tetranitrate is extracted by organic solvents from aqueous acid or alkaline solutions.

Quantitative Estimation. A spectrophotometric method of assaying for nitrate and nitrite ions in blood is described by Lorenzetti *et al.* (1966).

Metabolism. Erythrityl tetranitrate is a vasodilator which acts more slowly than glyceryl trinitrate or amyl nitrite but has a much longer duration of action. Following oral administration, the maximum effect is attained in 20 to 30 minutes and lasts 3 to 4 hours. Erythrityl tetranitrate releases nitrite ions into the bloodstream but the amount does not appear to be sufficient to account for the pharmacological effect of the drug.

Dose. Up to 60 mg.

Toxicity. Prolonged use may result in methaemoglobinaemia.

ERYTHROMYCIN *Antibiotic*

Proprietary Names: Erycin; Erythrocin; Erythrogran; Ilotycin.

$C_{37}H_{67}NO_{13} = 733{\cdot}9$

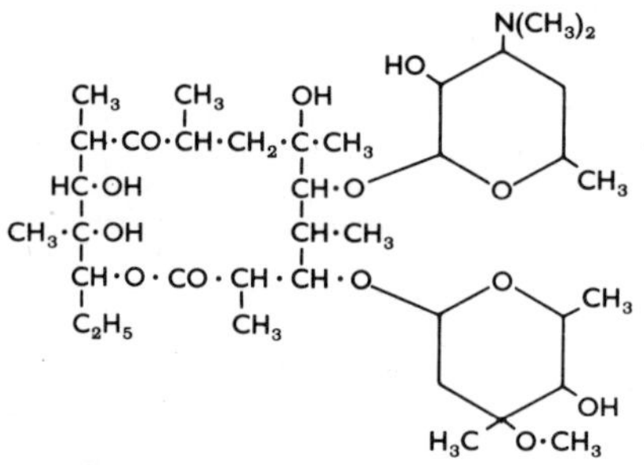

White hygroscopic crystals which should be protected from light. M.p. about 135°.
Solubility. Soluble 1 in 1000 of water; less soluble at higher temperatures; soluble 1 in 5 of ethanol, 1 in 5 of ether, 1 in 6 of chloroform, and 1 in 4 of acetone.

ERYTHROMYCIN ESTOLATE
Synonyms: Erythromycin Propionate Lauryl Sulphate; Propionyl Erythromycin Lauryl Sulphate.
Proprietary Name: Ilosone Lauryl Sulfate.

A white crystalline powder. M.p. 135° to 138°.
Solubility. Almost insoluble in water; soluble 1 in 2 of ethanol and in acetone; freely soluble in chloroform.

ERYTHROMYCIN ETHYL CARBONATE
Proprietary Name: Ilotycin Paediatric.

A white crystalline powder.
Solubility. Slightly soluble in water; soluble 1 in 10 of ethanol, 1 in 35 of ether, and 1 in 8 of chloroform.

ERYTHROMYCIN ETHYL SUCCINATE
Proprietary Names: Erythrocin I.M.; Erythroped.

Solubility. Insoluble in water; soluble in liquid macrogols.

ERYTHROMYCIN GLUCEPTATE
Synonym: Erythromycin Glucoheptonate.
Proprietary Name: Ilotycin Gluceptate Intravenous.

A white, slightly hygroscopic powder.
Solubility. Freely soluble in water and ethanol; practically insoluble in ether; slightly soluble in chloroform.

ERYTHROMYCIN LACTOBIONATE
Proprietary Names: Erythrocin I.V. (Lactobionate); Erythrocin Ophthalmic Ointment.

White crystals or powder.
Solubility. Freely soluble in water and ethanol; practically insoluble in ether; slightly soluble in chloroform.

ERYTHROMYCIN STEARATE
Proprietary Name: Erythrocin.

White crystals or powder.
Solubility. Practically insoluble in water; partly soluble in ethanol, ether, and chloroform; soluble in methanol.

Extraction. Erythromycin is extracted by organic solvents from aqueous alkaline solutions.

Chromatography. PAPER: system P1—Rf 0·90 (location reagent *iodoplatinate spray*, white).

Colour Tests. MICRO: sulphuric acid–formaldehyde test—brown (*sensitivity:* 1·0 μg); ammonium molybdate test—grey-blue → brown (*sensitivity:* 1·0 μg); Vitali's test—faint grey-purple/faint brown/faint brown (*sensitivity:* 1·0 μg).

Quantitative Estimation. A bioassay is described for the determination of erythromycin in serum and other body fluids (Zeigler and McGuire, 1953).

Metabolism. Erythromycin is readily absorbed from the gastro-intestinal tract and rapidly distributed in most of the body tissues and fluids. Following a single oral dose of 250 mg, a maximum blood-level of about 0·02 mg% is attained in about 1 hour and, after 1 g, a maximum level of about 0·12 mg% is attained in about 2 hours. Therapeutically effective amounts are present in the blood for about 6 hours. It is excreted mainly in the bile in which it attains a high concentration and, to a lesser extent, in the urine which contains 3 to 5% of the dose.

Dose. Up to 2 g (base) daily.

Toxicity. Toxic effects, including sensitisation reactions, are rare and usually mild.

ETAFEDRINE *Sympathomimetic*

Synonym: Ethylephedrine.

(−)-2-(Ethylmethylamino)-1-phenylpropan-1-ol

$C_{12}H_{19}NO = 193{\cdot}3$

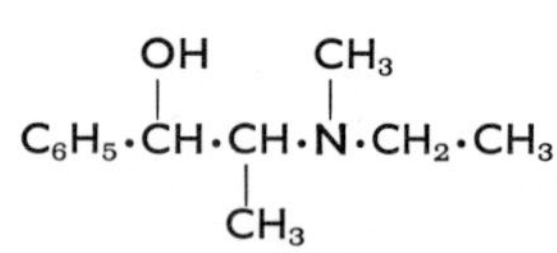

ETAFEDRINE HYDROCHLORIDE
Proprietary Names: Nethamine Hydrochloride. It is an ingredient of Nethaprin Dospan.
Solubility. Soluble 1 in 1·5 of water and 1 in 8 of ethanol.

Extraction. Etafedrine is extracted by organic solvents from aqueous alkaline solutions.

Chromatography. PAPER: system P1—Rf 0·56 (location reagents: *iodoplatinate spray*, strong reaction; *bromocresol green spray*, weak reaction).
THIN-LAYER: system T1—Rf 0·38 (location re-

agent *potassium permanganate spray*, positive reaction).

GAS: system G2/120—retention time 1·50 relative to ephedrine; system G2/225—retention time 0·33 relative to diphenhydramine.

Crystal Tests. MICRO: *gold bromide solution*—needles in combs or crosses (*sensitivity:* 1 in 1000); *gold bromide–hydrochloric acid solution*—segmented plates (*sensitivity:* 1 in 1000).

Ultraviolet Absorption Spectrum. Etafedrine in 0·1N sulphuric acid, maxima at about 247 mμ (E 1%, 1 cm 5), 251 mμ (E 1%, 1 cm 7), 257 mμ (E 1%, 1 cm 8), and 263 mμ (E 1%, 1 cm 6·5).

Infra-red Absorption Spectrum. Etafedrine (base). Potassium bromide disk. The principal peaks are: A 697, B 1448, C 1057 or 1375 (p. 786).

Dose. Up to 200 mg daily.

ETAMIPHYLLINE *Xanthine Derivative*

Synonyms: Diethamiphylline; Paraphylline.

7-(2-Diethylaminoethyl)-1,3-dimethylxanthine

$C_{13}H_{21}N_5O_2 = 279{\cdot}3$

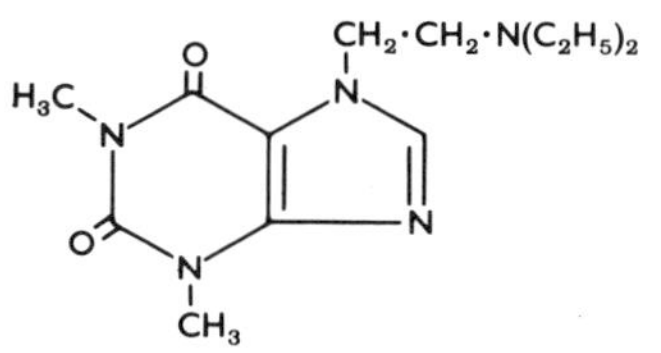

ETAMIPHYLLINE CAMSYLATE

Synonym: Etamiphylline Camphorsulphonate.

Proprietary Names: Camphophyline; Canfofillina; Millophyline.

A white crystalline powder.

Solubility. Soluble 1 in 2 of water.

Extraction. Etamiphylline is extracted by organic solvents from aqueous alkaline solutions.

Chromatography. PAPER: system P1—Rf 0·14 (location under ultraviolet light, absorption; location reagent *iodoplatinate spray*, positive reaction).

THIN-LAYER: system T1—Rf 0·49 (location reagent *acidified iodoplatinate spray*, positive reaction).

Colour Test. Amalic acid test—purple (see p. 127).

Crystal Tests. MICRO: *potassium bismuth iodide solution*—small crystals, often in clusters (*sensitivity:* 1 in 1000); *potassium tri-iodide solution (1)*—small irregular crystals (*sensitivity:* 1 in 1000).

Dose. Up to 600 mg by mouth; up to 1·4 g intramuscularly.

Toxicity. LD50 (subcutaneous): in mice 600 mg/kg.

ETHACRIDINE *Antiseptic*

Synonym: Acrinol.

6,9-Diamino-2-ethoxyacridine

$C_{15}H_{15}N_3O = 253{\cdot}3$

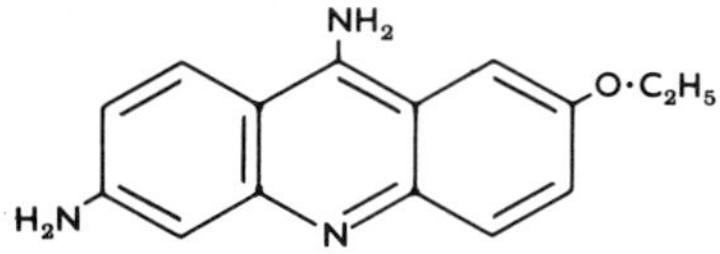

Orange crystals. M.p. 226°.

ETHACRIDINE LACTATE

Synonym: Lactoacridine.

Proprietary Names: Acrolactine; Ethodine; Rivanol; Vucine.

A yellow crystalline powder.

Solubility. Soluble 1 in 15 of cold water, 1 in 9 of boiling water, and 1 in 150 of ethanol.

Extraction. Ethacridine is extracted by organic solvents from aqueous alkaline solutions.

Chromatography. PAPER: system P1—Rf 0·48 (location under ultraviolet light, pale green fluorescence; location reagent *iodoplatinate spray*, weak reaction); system RP1a—Rf 0·11 (location under ultraviolet light, yellow fluorescence); system RP1b—Rf 0·13 (location as for RP1a).

THIN-LAYER: system T1—Rf 0·60 (location reagents: diazotisation followed by *alkaline beta-naphthol spray*, red-brown; *p-dimethylaminobenzaldehyde spray*, yellow).

Colour Tests. MICRO: sulphuric acid–formaldehyde test—(yellow) orange (*sensitivity:* 0·5 μg); diazotisation test—red-brown; Vitali's test—(yellow) purple/brown/brown (*sensitivity:* 1·0 μg).

Crystal Tests. MICRO: *potassium cadmium iodide solution*—bunches of small needles, often curved, forming overnight (*sensitivity:* 1 in 1000); *trinitrobenzoic acid solution*—fans of needles (*sensitivity:* 1 in 1000).

Ultraviolet Absorption Spectrum. Ethacridine in 0·1N sulphuric acid, maxima at 269·5 mμ (E 1%, 1 cm 1874), 364 mμ (E 1%, 1 cm 296) and 410 mμ (E 1%, 1 cm 171), and an inflexion at about 430 mμ (E 1%, 1 cm 151).

ETHACRYNIC ACID *Diuretic*

Synonyms: Etacrynic Acid; Methylenebutyrylphenoxyacetic Acid; MK 595.

Proprietary Name: Edecrin.

[2,3 - Dichloro - 4 - (α - ethylacryloyl)phenoxy]-acetic acid

$C_{13}H_{12}Cl_2O_4 = 303{\cdot}1$

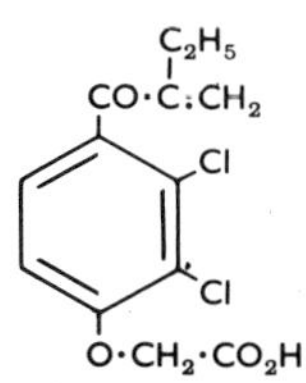

A white crystalline powder. M.p. about 122°.

Solubility. Sparingly soluble in water; soluble in ethanol, ether, and chloroform.

Ultraviolet Absorption Spectrum. Ethacrynic acid in 0·1N sodium hydroxide, maxima at 227 mμ (E1%, 1cm about 470) and 280 mμ (E1%, 1cm about 150).

Metabolism. Ethacrynic acid is well absorbed when administered orally and its action is extremely rapid in onset when it is given intravenously or orally. It is excreted in the bile and urine unchanged and as metabolites, including the cysteine conjugate.

Dose. Up to 400 mg daily.

Toxicity. Anorexia, dysphagia, nausea and vomiting, and diarrhoea have frequently occurred, particularly with large doses. Liver damage and fatal agranulocytosis have been reported.

CASE EXAMPLE. A 25-year-old patient with rheumatic heart disease and gross congestive cardiac failure was given ethacrynic acid as well as other appropriate treatment. Although the ethacrynic acid proved a better diuretic than others for the patient, he developed jaundice each period it was given and eventually died. Examination post mortem showed chronic venous congestion of the liver with necrosis around the dilated central veins; other necrotic areas resembled those produced experimentally in animals by carbon tetrachloride (Datey *et al.*, 1967).

ETHAMBUTOL *Tuberculostatic*

Synonym: EMB.

(+) - *NN′* - Di(1-hydroxymethylpropyl)ethylenediamine

$C_{10}H_{24}N_2O_2 = 204·3$

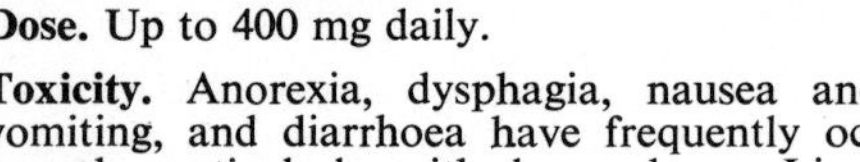

ETHAMBUTOL HYDROCHLORIDE

Proprietary Name: Myambutol Hydrochloride.

A white crystalline powder. M.p. about 202°.
Solubility. Very soluble in water.

Chromatography. PAPER: system P1—Rf 0·05 (location reagent *bromocresol green spray*, strong reaction).

THIN-LAYER: system T1—Rf 0·20 (location reagent *potassium permanganate spray*, positive reaction).

Crystal Tests. MICRO: *platinic iodide solution*—rectangular plates (*sensitivity:* 1 in 400); *potassium bismuth iodide solution*—small irregular crosses (*sensitivity:* 1 in 400).

Metabolism. Following the oral administration of 25 mg/kg daily of ethambutol in man the drug was absorbed rapidly, resulting in peak plasma levels of 0·5 mg% after 4 hours. Six days after administration, between 72 and 94% of an oral dose and 82% of an intravenous dose had been recovered in the urine; accumulation of the drug was not observed. In 24 hours, between 8 and 15% of a dose appeared in the urine as metabolites. Ethambutol appears to undergo oxidation first to an aldehyde and then to the acid, 2,2′-(ethylenedi-imino)dibutyric acid, both of which have been identified in the urine (Peets *et al.*, 1965).

Dose. Up to 50 mg/kg daily.

Toxicity. Prolonged treatment with ethambutol may cause visual impairment.

ETHANOL *Central Depressant*

Synonyms: Alcohol; Ethyl Alcohol.

$CH_3{\cdot}CH_2OH = 46·07$

The standard alcohol of the *British Pharmacopoeia* is Alcohol (95%). The *B.P.* also includes Dehydrated Alcohol (Absolute Alcohol) which contains 99·4 to 100% v/v of ethanol. Rectified Spirit is Alcohol (90%).

A clear, colourless, mobile, volatile, readily inflammable, hygroscopic liquid. Alcohol (95%) boils at about 78°; refractive index 1·3637 to 1·3639.

Solubility. Miscible with water, ether, and chloroform.

INDUSTRIAL METHYLATED SPIRIT (*B.P.*).
A mixture of 19 volumes of alcohol (95%) with 1 volume of approved wood naphtha. It complies with the description and solubility given above.

NOTE. Four other varieties of methylated spirits are recognised in Great Britain: mineralised methylated spirits, industrial methylated spirits (pyridinised), industrial methylated spirits (Q grade), and power methylated spirits. Mineralised methylated spirits is alcohol mixed with wood naphtha 9·5% and crude pyridine 0·5% and to every 100 gal of this mixture is added 3/8 gal of mineral naphtha (petroleum oil) and not less than 1/40 oz of methyl violet. Industrial methylated spirits (pyridinised) is alcohol mixed with wood naphtha 5% and to every 100 parts of this mixture is added ½ part of crude pyridine. Industrial methylated spirits (Q grade), which is used in the manufacture of perfumes, is alcohol mixed with pure methyl alcohol 5% and to every gal of this mixture is added 175 minims of standardised quassin solution. Power methylated spirits is a mixture of alcohol 100 parts with wood naphtha 2½ parts, crude pyridine ½ part, and petrol or benzol not less than 5 parts, and to this mixture is added ¼ oz of 'Spirit Red III' dye to every 1000 gal.

Screening Tests. See under Screening Tests, p. 6.

Extraction. Ethanol is volatile and may be isolated by distillation (see p. 18).

Chromatography. GAS: system G8/100—retention time 0·28 relative to n-propanol; system G8/160—retention time 0·44 relative to n-propanol.

Colour Tests. *Acidified potassium dichromate solution*—green, on warming; iodoform test—positive reaction.

Quantitative Estimation. Nickolls (1960) has described a modified Cavett diffusion procedure for the determination of ethanol in blood and urine which has a precision equal to that of the original method (Cavett, 1938) and a better reproducibility than the steam distillation method of Kozelka and Hine (1941). The diffusion chamber is a wide-mouthed, screw-capped bottle, with the top of the neck ground plane to effect closure with a circular glass plate inside the cap. The chamber contains 10 ml of 0·1N potassium dichromate in 18N sulphuric acid. A 2-ml sample of blood or urine is placed in a 2-inch Petri dish which is supported on a glass tripod inside the chamber. After diffusion has proceeded for 8 hours at 37°, the reaction fluid is diluted to 12 fluid ounces with distilled water, 2 g of solid potassium iodide is added, and the fluid is titrated with 0·1N sodium thiosulphate, a few millilitres of a 1% solution of soluble starch being used as indicator.

Brink *et al.* (1954) have described a method of estimation of ethanol by way of its oxidation to acetaldehyde in the presence of alcohol dehydrogenase and nicotinamide adenine dinucleotide; the reduced form of the latter is measured spectrophotometrically at the completion of the reaction.

Lundquist and Wolthers (1958) have used a modification of the alcohol dehydrogenase method to determine very low concentrations of ethanol in serum.

Kirk *et al.* (1958) have described an enzymic method of determination which also involves diffusion.

Machata (1961) has suggested ways in which maximum accuracy may be attained with the alcohol dehydrogenase method.

Metabolism. Ethanol is rapidly absorbed when ingested, 10 to 15 ml being metabolised per hour. The kidneys, liver, lungs, and muscles are all able to metabolise ethanol rapidly. Ethanol is rapidly oxidised to acetaldehyde and then to acetic acid. Acetic acid enters the metabolic pool of 2-carbon compounds and is eventually converted to carbon dioxide. Both unchanged ethanol and acetaldehyde may be excreted in the breath and small amounts of ethanol and a glucuronide conjugate may be found in the urine.

Toxicity. Ethanol may act as an acute or chronic poison. Death is rare in acute intoxication but deep coma persisting for over 12 hours is dangerous. Most people will have some disability or impairment of faculties if the concentration of ethanol in the blood is 150 mg% and above. A blood-level of 400 mg% may produce unconsciousness or may even be fatal.

In Great Britain (1969) it is an offence to have a blood alcohol concentration in excess of 80 mg% (or a urine concentration in excess of 107 mg%) whilst in charge of a motor vehicle.

ETHCHLORVYNOL *Hypnotic*

Synonym: β-Chlorovinyl Ethyl Ethynyl Carbinol.
Proprietary Names: Arvynol; Placidyl; Serenesil.

1-Chloro-3-ethylpent-1-en-4-yn-3-ol
$C_7H_9ClO = 144·6$

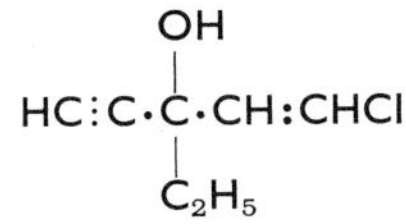

A colourless to yellow liquid which darkens on exposure to air and light. Refractive index, 1·4765 to 1·4800.

Solubility. Immiscible with water; miscible with most organic solvents.

Screening Tests. See under Screening Tests, p. 12.

Extraction. Ethchlorvynol is extracted by organic solvents from aqueous acid or alkaline solutions.

Chromatography. THIN-LAYER: system T11—Rf 0·32 (location reagents: *mercurous nitrate spray*, white on grey; *potassium permanganate spray*, yellow on purple); system T12—Rf 0·95 (location as for T11); system T13—Rf 0·95 (location as for T11).

Infra-red Absorption Spectrum. Capillary film between potassium bromide windows. The principal peaks are: A 935, B 950, C 830 (p. 740).

Quantitative Estimation. Ethchlorvynol may be estimated spectrophotometrically following conversion to its semicarbazone (Wallace *et al.*, 1964b).

Metabolism. Following ingestion of 500 mg of ethchlorvynol, concentrations were determined in venous blood, the highest concentrations occurring within 1 to 3 hours after ingestion and in the range 0·39 to 0·44 mg%. Approximately 10% of the ethchlorvynol was excreted unchanged in the urine within the first 24 hours. Subsequently, the amount of unaltered drug in the urine diminished rapidly (Wallace *et al.*, 1964b).

Toxicity. The usual hypnotic dose is up to 1 g but death has been reported in an alcoholic after daily doses of 500 mg (Ross and Gordon, 1964). The estimated lethal dose in man is 15 g and, in 2 fatal cases, the blood contained about 14 mg% (McBay, 1966). Cases of addiction to ethchlorvynol have been reported (Blumenthal and Reinhart, 1964; Aycrigg, 1964).

CASE EXAMPLES. A 27-year-old woman died 90 hours after the ingestion of about 12·5 g of ethchlorvynol and 200 mg of chlordiazepoxide. The ante-mortem blood-level of ethchlorvynol was 6·0 mg% and the post-mortem levels were: blood, 1·7 mg%; brain, 5·7 mg%; liver, 8·3 mg%. Chlordiazepoxide was detected in the liver only at a level of 0·2 mg% (*Pharm. J.*, ii/1965, 194).

A 29-year-old woman took 500 mg of ethchlorvynol each night for 6 years and then took 1 to 2 g nightly for the next 5 months. Three days after the last dose the serum ethchlorvynol level was 3·7 mg%, falling to 1·5 mg% over the next 2 days. Two weeks later the level was zero (Millhouse *et al.*, 1966).

A 37-year-old woman, 20 hours after ingesting 15 to 25 g

of ethchlorvynol, was admitted to hospital comatose and with a blood-level of 21·6 mg%. Haemodialysis over 10 hours removed 5·49 g of the drug; the post-dialysis blood-level was 9·05 mg%. Only 600 mg was recovered in the urine over the same period. Although dialysis removed significant amounts of the drug and sustained life, the patient remained comatose for 5 days then underwent withdrawal symptoms and seizures (Ogilvie *et al.*, 1966). Two patients recovered after taking overdoses of ethchlorvynol, 11 g and 10 g respectively. Both went into coma and had initial serum drug levels of 7·2 and 7·8 mg%. Totals of 2·45 and 3·52 g respectively were removed by haemodialysis. The amount of unchanged ethchlorvynol found in the urine was very small (Westervelt, 1966).

ETHER *General Anaesthetic*

Synonyms: Ethyl Ether; Ethyl Oxide.

Diethyl ether
$(C_2H_5)_2O = 74{\cdot}12$

A colourless transparent volatile liquid. B.p. 34° to 35°.

Solubility. Soluble 1 in 10 of water; miscible with ethanol and chloroform.

ANAESTHETIC ETHER (*B.P.*) is highly purified ether containing not more than 0·002% w/v of a stabiliser such as propyl gallate or hydroquinone.

SOLVENT ETHER (*B.P.*) is not so highly purified and is without a stabiliser.

CAUTION. *Ether is very volatile and inflammable and mixtures of its vapour with oxygen, nitrous oxide, or air at certain concentrations are explosive. It should not be used in the presence of an open flame or any electrical apparatus liable to produce a spark.*

Extraction. Ether is extracted by aeration.

Chromatography. GAS: system G8/100—retention time 1·03 relative to n-propanol; system G8/160—retention time 0·98 relative to n-propanol.

Quantitative Estimation. Ether may be estimated in blood by aeration of samples and subsequent infra-red spectrophotometry (Feldstein, 1965).

Metabolism. Ether is not metabolised in the body, approximately 90% of the amount absorbed during inhalation anaesthesia being recovered in the expired air after administration has ceased; elimination is very rapid for the first few minutes then it slows progressively. Ether may also be excreted unchanged in the urine. It is more soluble in brain tissue than in the blood and is much less soluble in muscle tissue.

Toxicity. Acute ether overdosage is characterised by respiratory failure followed by cardiac arrest.

The estimated minimum lethal oral dose in man is about 30 ml and the estimated maximum safe concentration in inhaled air is 400 p.p.m. The lethal dose (subcutaneous) in frogs is 1·68 g/kg.

CASE EXAMPLES. In 4 elderly persons who died after being given ether with other medication, the ether levels immediately after operation were: (a) blood, 60 mg%; brain, 70 mg%; liver, 40 mg%; lungs, 20 mg%; (b) blood, 375 mg%; brain, 61 mg%; liver, 128 mg%; lungs, 158 mg%; urine, 34 mg%: (c) blood, 288 mg%; brain, 272 mg%; liver, 26 mg%; lungs, 21 mg%; (d) blood, 19 mg%; brain, 31 mg%; liver, 23 mg%; mesentery, 23 mg%. In a child, who died in similar circumstances, the ether levels were: brain, 130 mg%; liver, 170 mg%; lungs, 220 mg% (Campbell, 1960).

ETHINAMATE *Hypnotic*

Proprietary Names: Valamin; Valmid; Valmidate.

1-Ethynylcyclohexyl carbamate
$C_9H_{13}NO_2 = 167{\cdot}2$

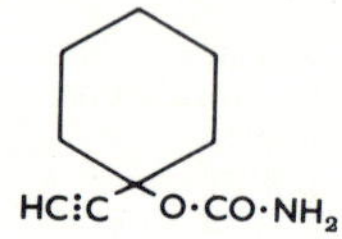

A white powder. M.p. 95° to 98°.

Solubility. Soluble 1 in 500 of water; freely soluble in ethanol, ether, and chloroform.

Screening Test. See under Screening Tests (carbamates), p. 13.

Extraction. Ethinamate is extracted by organic solvents from aqueous acid or alkaline solutions. Kum-Tatt (1961) has described a method of isolation of ethinamate and a metabolite from brain, liver, kidney, and stomach; the formation of derivatives and colour reactions are also described.

Chromatography. PAPER: system P1—Rf 0·93 (location reagents: *iodoplatinate spray*, white, forming overnight; *iodine vapour*, weak reaction); system P6—Rf 0·93 (location reagent *furfural–hydrochloric acid spray*, positive reaction); system P7—Rf 0·51 (location as for P6); system RP1b—Rf 0·26 (location as for P6).

THIN-LAYER: system T1—Rf 0·76 (location reagents: *furfural–hydrochloric acid spray*, positive reaction; *potassium permanganate spray*, positive reaction); system T11—Rf 0·65 (location reagents: *mercurous nitrate spray*, white on grey; *potassium permanganate spray*, yellow on purple).

GAS: system G5—retention time 0·49 relative to barbitone.

Crystal Tests. MICRO: *platinic iodide solution*—blades, sometimes in rosettes, forming overnight (*sensitivity:* 1 in 200); *potassium bismuth iodide solution*—blades, sometimes serrated (*sensitivity:* 1 in 1000).

Ultraviolet Absorption Spectrum. Ethinamate in 0·1N sulphuric acid, maximum at 265 mμ (E1%, 1cm 2·4).

Infra-red Absorption Spectrum. Potassium bromide disk. The principal peaks are: A 1713, B 1041, C 1370 (p. 740).

Quantitative Estimation. Ethinamate may be quantitatively determined by gas chromatography (Goldbaum and Domanski, 1966).

Metabolism. Following a dose of 500 mg, only a small amount of unchanged drug was excreted in the urine but a large amount of hydroxyethinamate was found (Cochin and Daly, 1963a).

Kum-Tatt (1961) isolated another metabolite of ethinamate from brain tissue but it did not appear to contain the carbamate group.

Dose. Up to 2 g.

Toxicity. Recovery has occurred after the ingestion of about 15 g (Siang, 1960). Two cases of habituation have been reported by Ellinwood *et al.* (1962).

ETHINYLOESTRADIOL *Oestrogen*

Synonym: Aethinyloestradiol.
Proprietary Names: Estigyn; Estinyl; Lynoral; Primogyn C.

19 - Nor - 17α - pregna - 1,3,5(10) - trien - 20 - yne-3,17-diol

$C_{20}H_{24}O_2 = 296{\cdot}4$

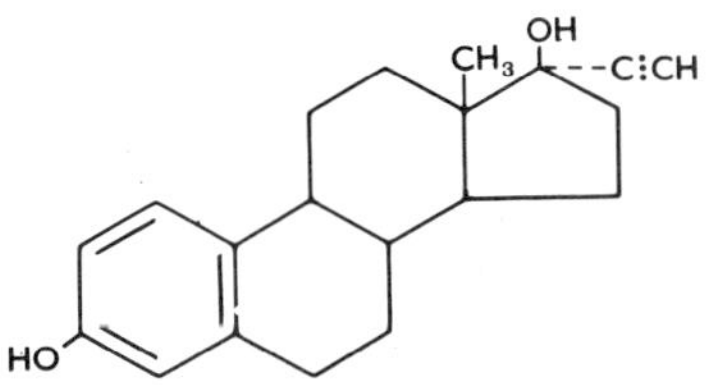

A fine white crystalline powder. M.p. 182° to 184° but it may occur in a form which melts at 141° to 146°.

Solubility. Almost insoluble in water; soluble 1 in 6 of ethanol, 1 in 4 of ether, and 1 in 20 of chloroform.

Extraction. Ethinyloestradiol is extracted from neutral solutions with freshly distilled ethyl acetate.

Chromatography. PAPER: a paper chromatographic method is described for the separation and identification of ethinyloestradiol and other oestrogens (Axelrod, 1953b).

THIN-LAYER: thin-layer chromatography on starch-bound silica gel layers involving several solvent systems is described for the separation of ethinyloestradiol and other steroids by Smith and Foell (1962).

Colour Test. Dissolve 2 mg in 2 ml of *sulphuric acid*—orange-red solution with yellowish-green fluorescence.

Ultraviolet Absorption Spectrum. Ethinyloestradiol in ethanol, maximum at about 280 mμ (E1%, 1cm 71); in 1N methanolic hydrochloric acid, maximum at 281 mμ; in 1N methanolic potassium hydroxide, maximum at 298 mμ (E1%, 1cm 88).

Infra-red Absorption Spectrum. Potassium bromide disk. The principal peaks are: A 1252 or 1505, B 1285 or 1298 (p. 740).

Quantitative Estimation. A quantitative gas chromatographic method of estimation of ethinyloestradiol involving prior separation from dimethisterone is described by Boughton *et al.* (1966). For the determination of ethinyloestradiol in pharmaceutical preparations a spectrofluorimetric method is described by Khoury and Cali (1967). Keay (1968) has devised an analytical scheme involving thin-layer chromatography and ultraviolet and infra-red absorption spectrophotometry which enables ethinyloestradiol to be identified and assayed, particularly when present in an oral contraceptive preparation.

Uses. Ethinyloestradiol is a synthetic oestrogen which is readily absorbed from the gastro-intestinal tract. It is at least twenty times more potent than stilboestrol. It is employed in conjunction with a progestational agent such as dimethisterone, megesterol acetate, or norethisterone acetate as an oral contraceptive, and for disorders of menstruation and fertility.

Dose. The usual therapeutic dose is up to 3 mg daily.

Toxicity. No symptoms of acute toxicity other than occasional vomiting have been reported following the accidental ingestion of overdoses of oral contraceptive preparations (Picchioni, 1965).

ETHIONAMIDE *Tuberculostatic*

Synonyms: Ethioniamide; TH 1314.
Proprietary Names: Trecator; Trescatyl.

2-Ethylpyridine-4-carbothionamide

$C_8H_{10}N_2S = 166{\cdot}2$

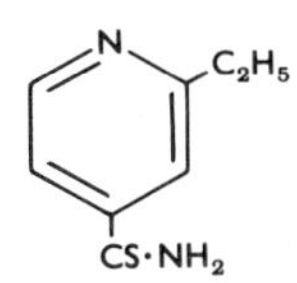

Yellow crystals. M.p. 161° to 165°, with decomposition.

Solubility. Almost insoluble in water; soluble 1 in 30 of ethanol, 1 in 350 of chloroform, and 1 in 600 of ether; soluble in dilute acetic acid.

Extraction. Ethionamide is extracted by organic solvents from aqueous alkaline solutions.

Chromatography. PAPER: system P1—Rf 0·72 (location under ultraviolet light, absorption; location reagent *iodoplatinate spray*, white); system RP1a—Rf 0·43 (location under ultraviolet light, absorption; location reagent *iodoplatinate spray*, positive reaction); system RP1b—Rf 0·39 (location as for RP1a).

THIN-LAYER: system T1—Rf 0·67 (location reagent *acidified iodoplatinate spray*, positive reaction).

Crystal Tests. MICRO: *lead iodide solution*—elongated plates, forming overnight (*sensitivity:* 1 in 100); *potassium tri-iodide solution (1)*—branching needles (*sensitivity:* 1 in 400).

Ultraviolet Absorption Spectrum. Ethionamide in ethanol, maximum at 290 mμ (E1%, 1cm 415); in 0·1N sulphuric acid, maxima at 229·5 mμ (E1%, 1cm 638), 276 mμ (E1%, 1cm 410), and about 317 mμ (E1%, 1cm 212).

Infra-red Absorption Spectrum. Potassium bromide disk. The principal peaks are: A 1418, B 808 or 865 or 1396 or 1588 (p. 740).

Quantitative Estimation. Pütter (1964) describes a spectrophotometric method of determination of ethionamide following its conversion to the sulphoxide.

Metabolism. Twenty-four hours after single oral doses of 500 mg or 1 g, ethionamide could no longer be detected in the serum and only minimal amounts of unchanged drug were excreted in the urine (Pütter, 1964).
Johnston *et al.* (1967) have shown, through studies in man, rats, mice, and dogs, that there is an extensive interconversion *in vivo* between ethionamide and ethionamide sulphoxide, both compounds appearing in the blood within 15 minutes of dosing, irrespective of which compound was administered. In man, 4 metabolites were detected in the urine, 2-ethylisonicotinamide, 2-ethylisonicotinic acid, and 2 unidentified metabolites; a paper chromatographic separation is described.

Dose. Up to 1 g daily.

Toxicity. Gastro-intestinal upset occurs in about 30% of patients receiving more than 500 mg daily.
LD50 (oral): in mice 1 g/kg.

ETHISTERONE *Progestational Steroid*

Synonyms: Aethisterone; Anhydrohydroxyprogesterone; Ethinyltestosterone; Praegnin; Pregneninolone.
Proprietary Names: Gestone-Oral; Lutocyclin (Linguets); Pranone; Progestoral; Trosinone. It is an ingredient of many proprietary preparations—see Extra Pharmacopoeia (Martindale), 25th Edn, p. 1285.

17-Hydroxy-17α-pregn-4-en-20-yn-3-one
$C_{21}H_{28}O_2$ = 312·6

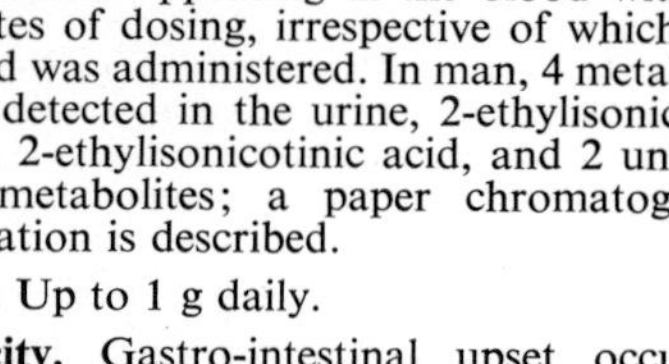

A white crystalline powder. M.p. 272° to 276°, with some decomposition. Specific rotation of a 1% solution in pyridine, +29° to +33°.
Solubility. Insoluble in water; soluble 1 in 1000 of ethanol, 1 in 3000 of ether, and 1 in 110 of chloroform.

Extraction. Ethisterone is extracted from neutral solutions with freshly distilled ethyl acetate.

Chromatography. THIN-LAYER: thin-layer chromatography on starch-bound silica gel layers involving several solvent systems is described for the separation of ethisterone and other steroids by Smith and Foell (1962).

Ultraviolet Absorption Spectrum. Ethisterone in ethanol, maximum at 240 mμ (E1%, 1 cm 520).

Dose. Up to 100 mg daily.
Structurally, ethisterone resembles both progesterone and testosterone; it possesses progestational and oestrogenic properties. It is better absorbed sublingually than from the gastro-intestinal tract. It is frequently administered in conjunction with ethinyloestradiol.

ETHOHEPTAZINE *Analgesic*

Synonyms: Heptacyclazine; Wy 401.

Ethyl 1 - methyl - 4 - phenyl - 1 - azacycloheptane-4-carboxylate
$C_{16}H_{23}NO_2$ = 261·4

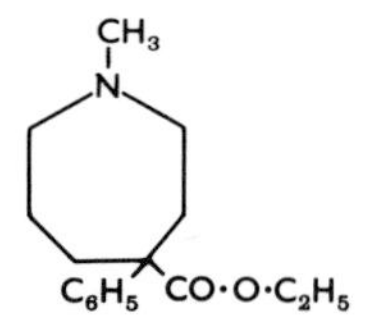

A liquid. B.p. 133° to 134° at 1 mm Hg.

ETHOHEPTAZINE CITRATE
Proprietary Names: Zactane. It is an ingredient of Equagesic, Zactipar, and Zactirin.
A white powder. M.p. about 140°.
Solubility. Sparingly soluble in water; very slightly soluble in ethanol; insoluble in ether.

Extraction. Ethoheptazine is extracted by organic solvents from aqueous alkaline solutions.

Chromatography. PAPER: system P1—Rf 0·52 (location reagent *iodoplatinate spray*, strong reaction); system RP1a—Rf 0·84 (location reagent *iodoplatinate spray*, positive reaction); system RP1b—Rf 0·17 (location as for RP1a).
THIN-LAYER: system T1—Rf 0·25 (location reagent *potassium permanganate spray*, positive reaction).
GAS: system G2/225—retention time 1·0 relative to diphenhydramine; system G4—retention time 1·07 relative to diphenhydramine.

Colour Test. MICRO: sulphuric acid–formaldehyde test—orange (*sensitivity:* 0·5 μg).

Crystal Tests. MICRO: *picric acid*—bunches of irregular rods, forming overnight (*sensitivity:* 1 in 200); *styphnic acid*—dense rosettes, forming overnight (*sensitivity:* 1 in 400).

Ultraviolet Absorption Spectrum. Ethoheptazine citrate in 0·1N hydrochloric acid, maxima at 251 mμ, 257 mμ, and 263 mμ; minima at 248 mμ, 254 mμ, and 261 mμ; in 0·1N sulphuric acid, maxima at 246 mμ (E1%, 1 cm 6·3), 251·5 mμ (E1%, 1 cm 7), 257·5 mμ (E1%, 1 cm 8), and 263·5 mμ (E1%, 1 cm 6).

Metabolism. Studies in animals (Walkenstein *et al.*, 1958) have shown ethoheptazine to be

rapidly absorbed, peak blood-levels being reached within 1 hour of ingestion. The highest concentrations of the drug are found after 30 minutes in the liver and kidneys.
Ethoheptazine appears to be extensively metabolised; the pathways include hydrolysis to the corresponding acid, oxidation to a hydroxy-derivative which may further undergo hydrolysis, and possibly *N*-demethylation to the corresponding nor-derivative which may be subsequently hydrolysed.
Very little ethoheptazine is excreted unchanged; in the dog, less than 4% of a dose was excreted unchanged within 24 hours and nearly 9% was excreted as a hydroxy-derivative.

Dose. Up to 600 mg daily.

Toxicity. The estimated minimum lethal dose for an adult is 1 g.

ETHOMOXANE *Tranquilliser*
2-Butylaminoethyl-8-ethoxy-1,4-benzodioxan
$C_{15}H_{23}NO_3 = 265{\cdot}4$

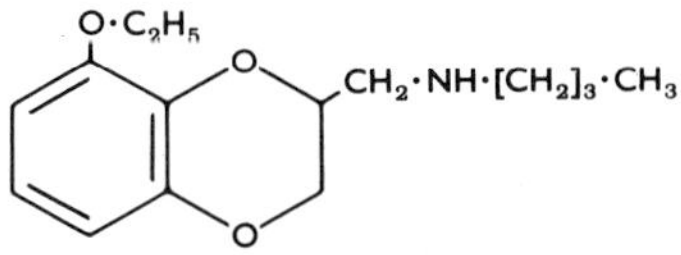

ETHOMOXANE HYDROCHLORIDE
Proprietary Name: It is an ingredient of Vortel.

Extraction. Ethomoxane is extracted by organic solvents from aqueous alkaline solutions.

Chromatography. PAPER: system P1—Rf 0·79 (location reagents: *iodoplatinate spray*, strong reaction; *bromocresol green spray*, weak reaction); system RP1a—Rf 0·64 (location reagent *iodoplatinate spray*, positive reaction); system RP1b—Rf 0·00.
THIN-LAYER: system T1—Rf 0·65 (location reagent *acidified iodoplatinate spray*, positive reaction).
GAS: system G2/225—retention time 1·5 relative to diphenhydramine; system G4—retention time 1·8 relative to diphenhydramine.

Colour Tests. MICRO: sulphuric acid–formaldehyde test—red-purple (*sensitivity:* 0·25 μg); ammonium molybdate test—green → yellow (*sensitivity:* 0·5 μg); ammonium vanadate test—red-brown (*sensitivity:* 0·5 μg).

Crystal Tests. MICRO: *gold cyanide solution*—bunches of blades or branching needles (*sensitivity:* 1 in 400); *platinic chloride solution*—rosettes of blades (*sensitivity:* 1 in 200).

Ultraviolet Absorption Spectrum. Ethomoxane in 0·1N sulphuric acid, maximum at 267 mμ (E1%, 1cm 23·2).

ETHOPROPAZINE *Parasympatholytic*
Synonyms: RP 3356; Isothazine; Phenopropazine; Profenamine; Prophenamine.
N-(2-Diethylaminopropyl)phenothiazine
$C_{19}H_{24}N_2S = 312{\cdot}5$

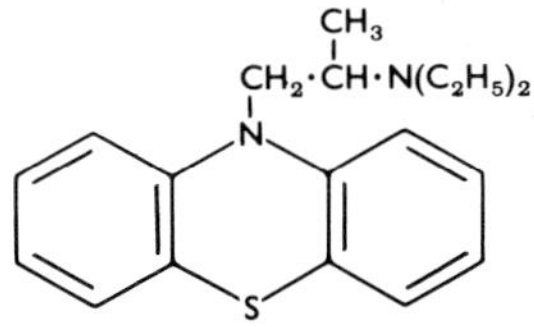

ETHOPROPAZINE HYDROCHLORIDE
Proprietary Names: Dibutil; Lysivane; Parfezin; Parsidol; Rodipal.

A white crystalline powder which darkens on exposure to light. M.p. about 225°, with decomposition.
Solubility. Soluble 1 in 225 of water, 1 in 35 of ethanol, and 1 in 7 of chloroform; insoluble in ether.

Screening Test. *FPN reagent* with urine—red (see p. 10).

Extraction. Ethopropazine is extracted by organic solvents from aqueous alkaline solutions; hydrolysis of biological material is required in order to improve the yield.

Chromatography. PAPER: system P1—Rf 0·72 (location under ultraviolet light, yellow fluorescence; location reagents: *iodoplatinate spray*, strong reaction; *FPN reagent*, red); system RP1a—Rf 0·14 (location under ultraviolet light, orange fluorescence; location reagent *iodoplatinate spray*, positive reaction); system RP1b—Rf 0·05 (location reagent *iodoplatinate spray*, positive reaction).
THIN-LAYER: system T1—Rf 0·63 (location reagent *acidified iodoplatinate spray*, positive reaction); system T6—Rf 0·70 (the spot may be converted on the plate to the sulphoxide, Rf 0·47; location of both spots under ultraviolet light).
GAS: system G2/225—retention time 1·0 relative to codeine; system G4—retention time 0·72 relative to codeine.

Colour Tests. MICRO: sulphuric acid–formaldehyde test—purple (*sensitivity:* 0·25 μg); ammonium molybdate test—blue-violet → purple (*sensitivity:* 0·1 μg); ammonium vanadate test—green → purple (*sensitivity:* 0·1 μg); Vitali's test — purple → yellow/brown/yellow-brown (*sensitivity:* 1·0 μg).

Crystal Tests. MICRO: *ammonium thiocyanate solution*—bunches of plates (*sensitivity:* 1 in 1000); *mercuric chloride solution*—curved needles (*sensitivity:* 1 in 1000).

Ultraviolet Absorption Spectrum. Ethopropazine in 0·1N sulphuric acid, maxima at 249 mμ (E1%, 1cm 2780), 299 mμ (E1%, 1cm 152), and 362 mμ (E1%, 1cm 46).

Dose. Up to 1·5 g daily has been given.

Toxicity. The acute lethal dose in man is in the range 15 to 150 mg/kg. Studies in animals show that there is only a slight difference between the acute and chronic toxicity figures,

indicating that there is little accumulation of the compound in the body.
LD50 (oral): in mice 720 mg/kg.

ETHOSUXIMIDE *Anticonvulsant*

Synonyms: Ethosuccimide; H 940; PM 671.
Proprietary Names: Emeside; Simatin; Zarontin.

α-Ethyl-α-methylsuccinimide
$C_7H_{11}NO_2 = 141{\cdot}2$

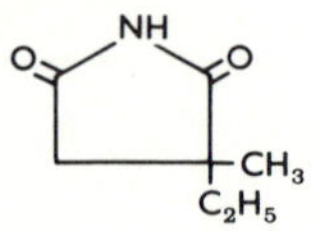

A white powder or waxy solid. M.p. about 46°. Refractive index at 50°, 1·4715 to 1·4745.
Solubility. Soluble 1 in 4·5 of water and 1 in less than 1 of ethanol, of ether, and of chloroform.

Extraction. Ethosuximide is extracted by organic solvents from aqueous acid or alkaline solutions.

Chromatography. PAPER: system P1—Rf 0·93 (location reagent *bromine–starch–potassium iodide*, weak reaction).
THIN-LAYER: system T1—Rf 0·70 (location reagent *iodine vapour*, positive reaction).
GAS: system G5—retention time 0·28 relative to barbitone.

Ultraviolet Absorption Spectrum. Ethosuximide in ethanol, maximum at 248 mμ (E1%, 1 cm about 8·5); in alkaline solution (pH 12) a strong maximum occurs at 218 mμ but in acid solution the absorption at 218 mμ is negligible and any significant alteration in the absorption at 248 mμ indicates the presence of barbiturates (Hansen, 1963).

Quantitative Estimation. Ethosuximide in serum may be determined spectrophotometrically following extraction into chloroform; this method also indicates the presence of barbiturates (Hansen, 1963).

Metabolism. Large daily doses of ethosuximide produce peak blood-levels 4 days after the beginning of treatment; these levels are maintained until treatment is discontinued. Elimination from the blood occurs approximately 2 days after treatment has ceased. A large single dose produces a peak blood concentration in 2 to 4 hours and this is maintained for about 24 hours.

Dose. 500 mg daily, increasing to a maximum of 2 g.

Toxicity. The estimated minimum lethal dose in man is 5 g.
LD50 (oral): in mice about 1·5 g/kg.

ETHOTOIN *Anticonvulsant*

Proprietary Name: Peganone.

3-Ethyl-5-phenylhydantoin
$C_{11}H_{12}N_2O_2 = 204{\cdot}2$

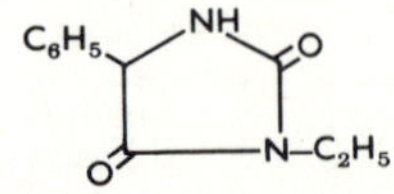

A white crystalline powder. M.p. about 90°.
Solubility. Insoluble in water; soluble 1 in 4 of dehydrated ethanol, 1 in 25 of ether, and 1 in 1·5 of chloroform.

Extraction. Ethotoin is extracted by organic solvents from aqueous acid or alkaline solutions.

Ultraviolet Absorption Spectrum. Ethotoin in ethanol, maxima at 259 mμ (E1%, 1 cm about 11) and 265 mμ (E1%, 1 cm about 8·2).

Infra-red Absorption Spectrum. Potassium bromide disk. The principal peaks are: A 1716, B 1455, C 700 (p. 740).

Metabolism. Ethotoin is readily absorbed from the gastro-intestinal tract.

Dose. 1 g daily, increasing to a maximum of 3 g. It is frequently administered in conjunction with other anticonvulsants such as phenobarbitone or phenytoin in the treatment of grand mal epilepsy.

Toxicity. The estimated minimum lethal dose in man is 5 g.
LD50 (oral): in mice 1·75 and in rats 1·5 g/kg.

ETHYL BISCOUMACETATE *Anticoagulant*

Synonyms: Aethyldicumarin; BOEA; Ethyldicoumarol; Neodicumarin.
Proprietary Names: Dicumacyl; Pelentan; Tromexan.

Ethyl di(4-hydroxycoumarin-3-yl)acetate
$C_{22}H_{16}O_8 = 408{\cdot}4$

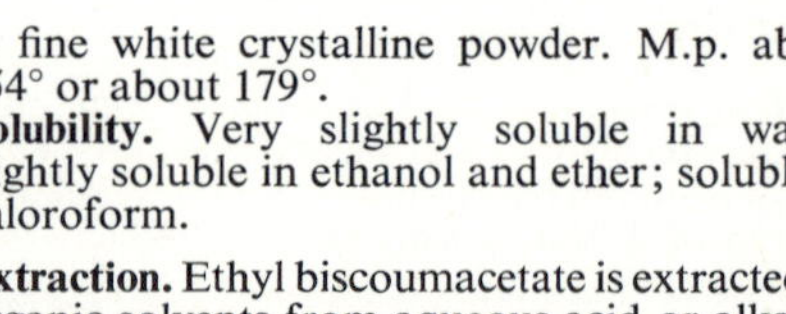

A fine white crystalline powder. M.p. about 154° or about 179°.
Solubility. Very slightly soluble in water; slightly soluble in ethanol and ether; soluble in chloroform.

Extraction. Ethyl biscoumacetate is extracted by organic solvents from aqueous acid or alkaline solutions.

Chromatography. PAPER: system P8—Rf 0·75 (location under ultraviolet light, weak yellow-green fluorescence; location reagents: *diazotised* o-*dianisidine spray*, red; *diazotised sulphanilic* *acid spray*, orange); system P9—Rf 0·23 (location as for P8); system P10—Rf 0·96 (location as for P8).

Colour Test. Add 0·15 ml of *sulphuric acid* to 0·1 g of ethyl biscoumacetate—orange-yellow.

Metabolism. Ethyl biscoumacetate is more rapidly absorbed and excreted than dicoumarol (p. 298). In man, following oral administration, peak blood-levels occur after 4½ to 8½ hours; after 24 hours it is no longer detectable in the blood. In man, ethyl biscoumacetate is metabolised very rapidly by hydroxylation in the liver to hydroxyethyl biscoumacetate which has been recovered from the urine in an amount equivalent to 5 to 15% of the administered dose. In contrast, in the rabbit, de-esterification to biscoumacetic acid occurs rapidly.

Dose. Up to 1·2 g daily, depending on the prothrombin activity of the blood.

Toxicity. Fatalities have occurred after 600 mg daily.

LD50 (oral): in mice 880 mg/kg.

CASE EXAMPLES. Report of one death and 2 nearly fatal haemorrhages following the use of ethyl biscoumacetate (Gripe, 1951).

ETHYLENE GLYCOL

Synonyms: Ethylene Alcohol; Glycol.

Ethane-1,2-diol

$HOCH_2{\cdot}CH_2OH = 62{\cdot}07$

A colourless hygroscopic syrupy liquid. F.p. about −13°. B.p. about 197°.

Solubility. Miscible with water and ethanol; slightly soluble in ether.

Extraction. Ethylene glycol is volatile and may be isolated by distillation (see p. 18).

Chromatography. THIN-LAYER: Conacher and Rees (1966) have described a method of detection and estimation of ethylene glycol involving thin-layer chromatography.

Quantitative Estimation. Ethylene glycol may be estimated by oxidation with periodic acid, treatment of the formaldehyde formed with Schiff's reagent, and subsequent colorimetric determination (Harger and Forney, 1959). Raekallio *et al.* (1967) have described a microscopic technique for the demonstration of calcium oxalate crystals in kidney sections.

Metabolism. Ethylene glycol itself is not lethally toxic but it is largely metabolised in the body to oxalic acid which is then converted to insoluble calcium oxalate. The calcium oxalate crystals are deposited in the renal tubules, often causing oliguria or anuria and necrosis. In many fatal cases ethylene glycol and calcium oxalate cannot be chemically determined in the urine (Raekallio *et al.*, 1967). Calcium oxalate crystals may also be found in the brain and spinal cord at post-mortem examination.

Toxicity. In adults, about 100 ml (3 to 4 ounces) of ethylene glycol is usually fatal but survival has been reported after the ingestion of 8 ounces.

LD50 (oral): in rats 5·8 ml/kg.

CASE EXAMPLES. Analysis of the blood, liver, stomach contents, and urine of 6 persons who died after drinking beverages containing ethylene glycol gave the following results: (1) blood, 423 mg%; liver, 812 mg%; stomach contents, 569 mg%: (2) traces only: (3) blood, 384 mg%; brain, 390 mg%; kidneys, 583 mg%; liver, 704 mg%; stomach contents, 616 mg%; urine, 1080 mg%: (4) blood, 24 mg%: (5) stomach, 412 mg%; tissue composite, 244 mg%: (6) stomach contents, 311 mg% (Harger and Forney, 1959).

Recovery reported in 2 cases in which the urine was heavily loaded with calcium oxalate crystals after the ingestion of 1 litre and about 250 ml respectively of an antifreeze mixture. Treatment: diuretics, dialysis, and intravenous ethanol (Wacker *et al.*, 1965).

Immediate post-mortem examination of an inebriated man who died in hospital revealed the following levels of ethylene glycol: kidney 1134 mg%; liver 1512 mg%. In another case in a 30-year-old woman the levels were: kidney 93 mg%; liver 310 mg% (Klenshoj and Rejent, 1966).

A 15-year-old youth drank 'blue vodka' at a party and died some 7 hours later. Analysis of the brain showed the presence of 196 mg% ethylene glycol (Klendshoj and Rejent, 1966).

Detailed cases of 4 American youths, 2 of whom died, poisoned by ingestion of ethylene glycol (Friedman *et al.*, 1962).

Numerous cases of poisoning in domestic animals have been recorded.

NOTE. Ethylene glycol is a constituent of some antifreeze solutions.

ETHYLMETHYLTHIAMBUTENE *Narcotic*

N-Ethyl-*N*, 1-dimethyl-3,3-di(thien-2′-yl)-allylamine

$C_{15}H_{19}NS_2 = 277{\cdot}5$

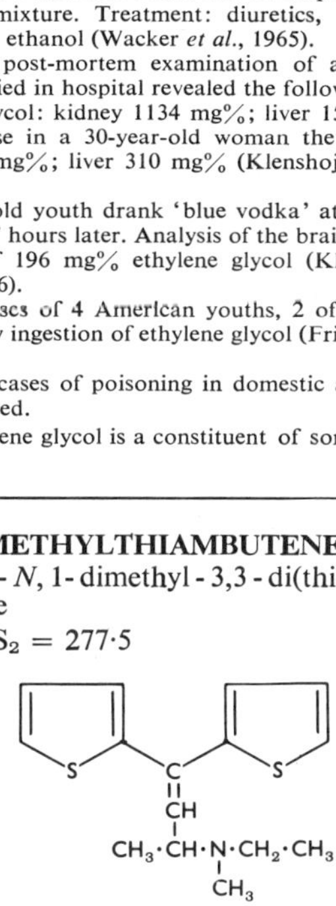

Extraction. Ethylmethylthiambutene is extracted by organic solvents from aqueous alkaline solutions.

Chromatography. PAPER: system P1—Rf 0·71 (location under ultraviolet light, absorption; location reagent *iodoplatinate spray*, weak reaction); system RP1a—Rf 0·28 (location under ultraviolet light, absorption); system RP1b—Rf 0·08 (location under ultraviolet light, absorption; location reagent *iodoplatinate spray*, positive reaction).

THIN-LAYER: system T1—Rf 0·58 (location reagent *acidified iodoplatinate spray*, positive reaction).

GAS: system G2/225—retention time 1·3 relative to diphenhydramine; system G4—retention time 0·8 relative to diphenhydramine.

Colour Tests. MICRO: sulphuric acid–formaldehyde test—purple-brown (*sensitivity:* 0·1 μg); ammonium molybdate test—orange-brown → pale green (*sensitivity:* 0·1 μg); ammonium vanadate test—green → greenish-blue (*sensitivity:* 0·1 μg); Vitali's test—red → green/brown/brown.

Crystal Tests. MICRO: *potassium chromate solution*—tablets, usually hexagonal (*sensitivity:* 1 in 200); *styphnic acid*—serrated needles (*sensitivity:* 1 in 400).

Ultraviolet Absorption Spectrum. Ethylmethylthiambutene in 0·1N sulphuric acid, maxima at 226 mμ (E1%, 1cm 270), 268 mμ (E1%, 1cm 400), and 285 mμ (E1%, 1cm 394).

ETHYLMORPHINE *Narcotic Analgesic*

Synonym: Morphine 3-Ethyl Ether.

7,8 - Dehydro - 4,5 - epoxy - 3 - ethoxy - 6 - hydroxy-*N*-methylmorphinan

$C_{19}H_{23}NO_3$ = 313·4

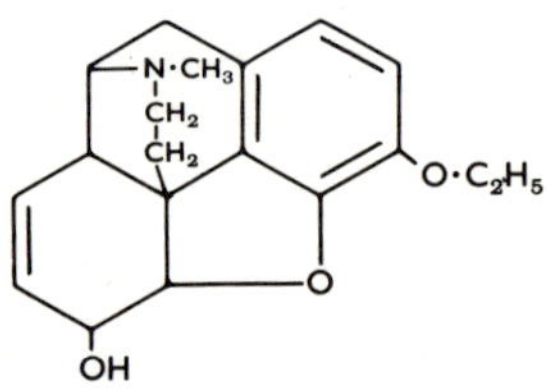

ETHYLMORPHINE HYDROCHLORIDE

Synonym: Chlorhydrate de Codethyline.

Proprietary Name: Dionin.

A white, minutely crystalline powder. M.p. about 123°, with decomposition.

Solubility. Soluble 1 in 12 of water, 1 in 25 of ethanol, and 1 in 1 of warm ethanol; almost insoluble in ether and chloroform.

Extraction. Ethylmorphine is extracted by organic solvents from aqueous alkaline solutions; hydrolysis of biological material is required in order to improve the yield.

Chromatography. PAPER: system P1—Rf 0·35 (location under ultraviolet light, dark blue fluorescence; location reagent *iodoplatinate spray*, strong reaction); system RP1a—Rf 0·88 (location reagent *iodoplatinate spray*, positive reaction); system RP1b—Rf 0·12 (location under ultraviolet light, purple fluorescence; location reagent *iodoplatinate spray*, positive reaction).

THIN-LAYER: system T1—Rf 0·36 (location reagent *acidified iodoplatinate spray*, positive reaction); system T7—Rf 0·46 (location reagent *iodoplatinate spray*, positive reaction); system T8—Rf 0·25 (location as for T7).

GAS: system G1/250—retention time 1·11 relative to codeine; system G2/225—retention time 1·1 relative to codeine; system G4—retention time 1·0 relative to codeine; system G6—retention time 1·21 relative to codeine.

Colour Tests. MICRO: sulphuric acid–formaldehyde test—yellow → purple → black (*sensitivity:* 0·1 μg); ammonium molybdate test—green → blue (*sensitivity:* 0·25 μg); Vitali's test—faint yellow/–/orange (*sensitivity:* 1·0 μg).

Crystal Tests. MICRO: *potassium mercuric iodide solution*—smudge rosettes (*sensitivity:* 1 in 200); *potassium tri-iodide solution* (*3*)—bunches of feathery needles (*sensitivity:* 1 in 1500).

Ultraviolet Absorption Spectrum. Ethylmorphine in 0·2N sulphuric acid, maximum at 285 mμ (E1%, 1cm 49) and inflexion at 277 mμ.

Dose. Usually up to 30 mg.

Toxicity. The minimum lethal dose in man is 500 mg.

ETHYLNORADRENALINE *Sympathomimetic*

Synonym: Ethylnorepinephrine.

Proprietary Names: Bronkephrine; Butanefrine.

2-Amino-1-(3,4-dihydroxyphenyl)butan-1-ol

$C_{10}H_{15}NO_3$ = 197·2

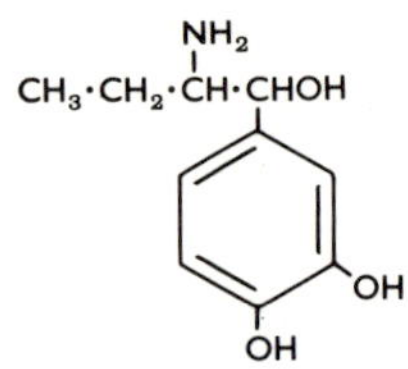

ETHYLNORADRENALINE HYDROCHLORIDE

A crystalline solid.

Solubility. Soluble in water.

Chromatography. PAPER: system P1—Rf 0·18 (location under ultraviolet light, absorption; location reagent *bromocresol green spray*, weak reaction).

THIN-LAYER: system T1—Rf 0·48, streaking (location reagent *potassium permanganate spray*, positive reaction).

Colour Tests. Chen's test—grey-green.

MICRO: sulphuric acid–formaldehyde test—pale orange → pale brown (*sensitivity:* 1·0 μg); ammonium molybdate test—(brown) dark grey → green (*sensitivity:* 1·0 μg); ammonium vanadate test—(grey) orange (*sensitivity:* 1·0 μg); Vitali's test — yellow/brown/brown (*sensitivity:* 1·0 μg).

Crystal Tests. MICRO: *gold bromide solution*—small plates or rosettes (*sensitivity:* 1 in 200); *gold chloride solution*—very small plates (*sensitivity:* 1 in 200).

Ultraviolet Absorption Spectrum. Ethylnoradrenaline in 0·1N sulphuric acid, maxima at 220 mμ (E1%, 1cm 332) and 278 mμ (E1% 1cm 154).

Infra-red Absorption Spectrum. Ethylnoradrenaline (base). Potassium bromide disk. The principal peaks are: A 1280 or 1500 or 1529, B 1331 or 1456 (p. 786).

Dose. Usually 2 mg subcutaneously.

ETONITAZENE *Narcotic Analgesic*

1 - (2 - Diethylaminoethyl) - 2 - *p* - ethoxybenzyl-5-nitrobenzimidazole

$C_{22}H_{28}N_4O_3$ = 396·5

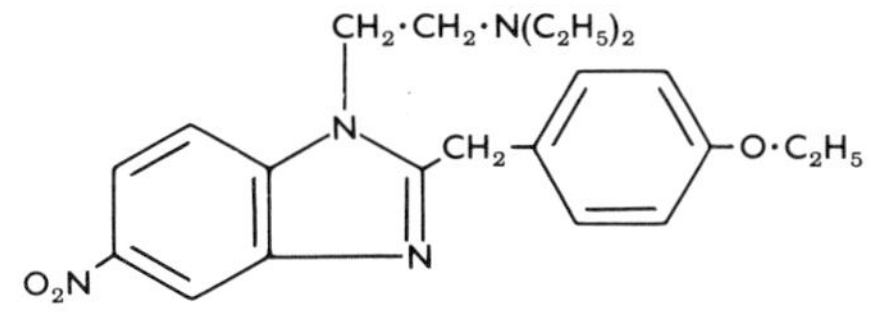

A white crystalline powder.

Solubility. Soluble in dilute hydrochloric acid.

Extraction. Etonitazene is extracted by organic solvents from aqueous alkaline solutions.

Chromatography. PAPER: system P1—Rf 0·72 (location under ultraviolet light, absorption; location reagents: *iodoplatinate spray*, weak reaction; *bromocresol green spray*, weak reaction).

THIN-LAYER: system T1—Rf 0·70 (location reagent *acidified iodoplatinate spray*, positive reaction).

Crystal Tests. MICRO: *picrolonic acid*—bunches of small rods and prisms (*sensitivity:* 1 in 400); *potassium chromate solution*—rosettes of plates and blades (*sensitivity:* 1 in 1000).

Ultraviolet Absorption Spectrum. Etonitazene in 0·1N sulphuric acid, maxima at 230 mμ (E1%, 1 cm 226) and 282 mμ (E1%, 1 cm 82).

ETORPHINE *Narcotic Analgesic*

Synonyms: M 99; 19-Propylorvinol.

7,8 - Dihydro - 7α - [1(*R*) - hydroxy - 1 - methyl-butyl]-O^6-methyl-6,14-*endo*ethenomorphine

$C_{25}H_{33}NO_4$ = 411·5

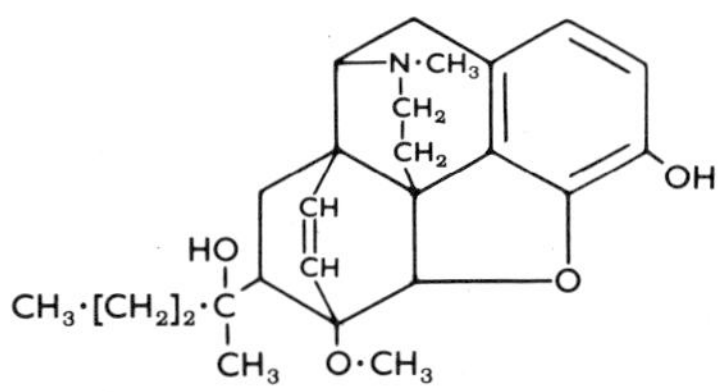

Etorphine melts at 214° to 215°.

CAUTION. *It is dangerous to smell or taste this material.*

Solubility. Soluble 1 in 30,000 of water; readily soluble in ethanol, ether, and chloroform.

ETORPHINE HYDROCHLORIDE

A white crystalline powder. M.p. 266° to 267°.

Solubility. Soluble 1 in 40 of water and 1 in 30 of ethanol.

Extraction. Etorphine is extracted by organic solvents from aqueous ammoniacal solutions.

Chromatography. PAPER: system P1—Rf 0·63 (location under ultraviolet light, absorption; location reagents: *iodoplatinate spray*, weak reaction; *potassium permanganate spray*, weak reaction).

THIN-LAYER: system T1—Rf 0·72 (location reagents: *acidified iodoplatinate spray*, positive reaction; *Marquis reagent*, grey; *potassium permanganate spray*, positive reaction).

Colour Tests. MICRO: sulphuric acid–formaldehyde test—bluish-grey → yellow-brown (*sensitivity:* 0·25 μg); ammonium molybdate test—bluish-purple → blue → dull green (*sensitivity:* 0·1 μg); Vitali's test— –/–/orange (*sensitivity:* 0·5 μg).

Crystal Test. MICRO: *picrolonic acid*—small rosettes of needles (*sensitivity:* 1 in 400).

Ultraviolet Absorption Spectrum. Etorphine in 0·1N hydrochloric acid, maximum at 287 mμ (E1%, 1 cm 36); in 0·1N sodium hydroxide, maximum at 301 mμ (E1%, 1 cm 63).

NOTE. Etorphine is a highly potent analgesic and narcotic which has been tried as a sedative to assist in the control of large animals. Its effects may be antagonised by cyprenorphine or nalorphine.

ETOXERIDINE *Narcotic*

Synonyms: Aténorax; Atenos; Carbetidine; UC 2073; UCB 2073; Wy 2039.

Ethyl 1 - [2 - (2 - hydroxyethoxy)ethyl] - 4 - phenylpiperidine-4-carboxylate

$C_{18}H_{27}NO_4$ = 321·4

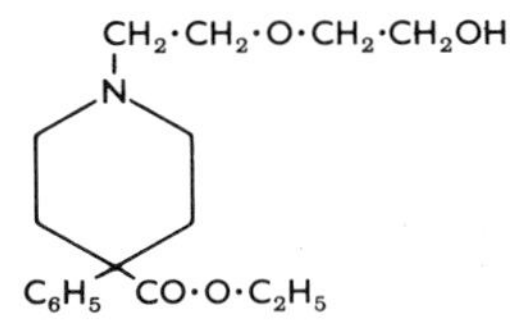

A white crystalline powder.

Solubility. Soluble in dilute hydrochloric acid.

Extraction. Etoxeridine is extracted by organic solvents from aqueous alkaline solutions.

Chromatography. PAPER: system P1—Rf 0·54 (location under ultraviolet light, absorption; location reagents: *iodoplatinate spray*, strong reaction; *bromocresol green spray*, weak reaction); system RP1a—Rf 0·90 (location reagent *iodoplatinate spray*, positive reaction); system RP1b—Rf 0·06 (location as for RP1a).

THIN-LAYER: system T1—Rf 0·64 (location reagent *acidified iodoplatinate spray*, positive reaction).

GAS: system G2/225—retention time 0·85 relative to codeine; system G4—retention time 1·05 relative to codeine.

Colour Test. MICRO: sulphuric acid–formaldehyde test—dull orange (*sensitivity:* 1·0 μg).

Crystal Tests. MICRO: *lead iodide solution*—bunches of fine needles (*sensitivity:* 1 in 100); *platinic iodide solution*—plates, forming overnight (*sensitivity:* 1 in 100).

Ultraviolet Absorption Spectrum. Etoxeridine in 0·1N sulphuric acid, maxima at 252 mμ (E1%, 1 cm 5), 258 mμ (E1%, 1 cm 6), and 264 mμ (E1%, 1 cm 4·8).

ETYMIDE *Analgesic*

Synonym: Carbiphene; Etomide; SQ 10269.

2 - Ethoxy - *N* - methyl - *N* - [2 - (*N* - methylphenethylamino)ethyl] - 2,2 - diphenylacetamide

$C_{28}H_{34}N_2O_2$ = 430·6

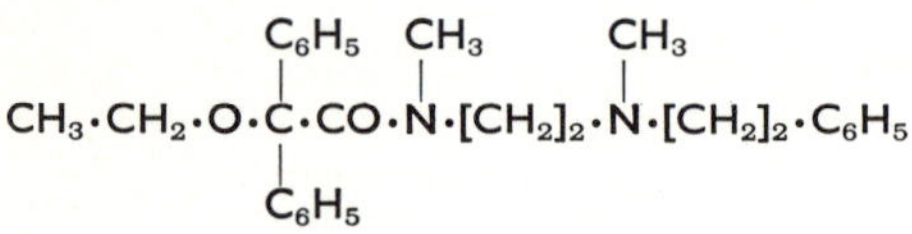

ETYMIDE HYDROCHLORIDE

Proprietary Name: Bandol.

Extraction. Etymide is extracted by organic solvents from aqueous alkaline solutions.

Chromatography. PAPER: system P1—Rf 0·90 (location reagent *iodoplatinate spray*, strong reaction).

THIN-LAYER: system T1—Rf 0·72 (location reagent *acidified iodoplatinate spray*, positive reaction).

Colour Test. MICRO: ammonium molybdate test—orange → blue (*sensitivity:* 0·1 μg).

Ultraviolet Absorption Spectrum. Etymide in 0·1N sulphuric acid, maxima at 258 mμ (E1%, 1 cm 15·7) and 263 mμ (E1%, 1 cm 13·2), and an inflexion at about 270 mμ (E1%, 1 cm 7·0).

Dose. Up to 450 mg daily has been given.

EUCALYPTOL *Essential Oil*

Synonyms: Cajuputol; Cineole.

Anhydromenthane-1,8-diol

$C_{10}H_{18}O$ = 154·3

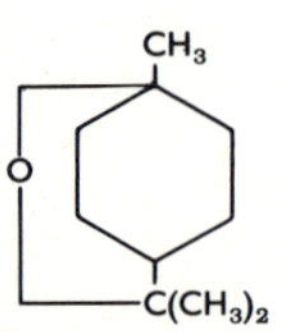

A colourless liquid, obtained from eucalyptus, cajuput, and other oils. F.p. not lower than 0°. Refractive index at 20°, 1·456 to 1·460.

Solubility. Insoluble in water; soluble 1 in 2 of ethanol (70%); miscible with ether, chloroform, fixed and volatile oils, and with most organic solvents.

Extraction. Eucalyptol is volatile and may be isolated by distillation (see p. 18).

Metabolism. Eucalyptol is metabolised by hydroxylation at the 2- or 3-positions and the hydroxy-derivative is excreted as a glucuronide conjugate.

Dose. Up to 0·2 ml.

Toxicity. In man, ingestion of 3 to 30 ml of eucalyptus oil has proved fatal. The oral lethal dose in rats is about 1·7 g/kg.

EUCATROPINE *Parasympatholytic*

Proprietary Name: Euphthalmine.

4-Mandeloyloxy-1,2,2,6-tetramethylpiperidine

$C_{17}H_{25}NO_3$ = 291·4

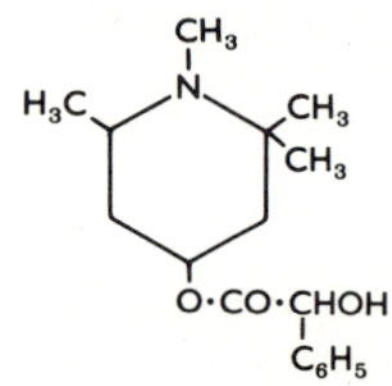

EUCATROPINE HYDROCHLORIDE

A white granular powder. M.p. 183° to 186°.

Solubility. Very soluble in water; freely soluble in ethanol and chloroform; insoluble in ether.

Extraction. Eucatropine is extracted by organic solvents from aqueous alkaline solutions.

Chromatography. PAPER: system P1—Rf 0·45 (location under ultraviolet light, absorption; location reagents: *iodoplatinate spray*, weak reaction; *bromocresol green spray*, weak reaction).

THIN-LAYER: system T1—Rf 0·45 (location reagent *acidified iodoplatinate spray*, positive reaction).

GAS: system G2/225—retention time 1·7 relative to diphenhydramine; retention time 0·37 relative to codeine; system G4—retention time 0·27 relative to codeine.

Crystal Tests. MICRO: *gold bromide solution*—bunches of curved plates (*sensitivity:* 1 in 3000); *potassium tri-iodide solution* (*3*)—elongated plates (*sensitivity:* 1 in 400).

Ultraviolet Absorption Spectrum. Eucatropine in 0·1N sulphuric acid, maxima at 252 mμ (E1%, 1 cm 5·5), 258 mμ (E1%, 1 cm 6·8), 264 mμ (E1%, 1 cm 5·8), and about 268 mμ (E1%, 1 cm 3·6).

Toxicity. The lethal dose is probably in the range 10 to 100 mg/kg.

NOTE. Eucatropine is used only as a mydriatic.

EUGENOL *Essential Oil*

Synonyms: Caryophyllic Acid; Eugenic Acid.

4-Allyl-2-methoxyphenol
$C_{10}H_{12}O_2 = 164{\cdot}2$

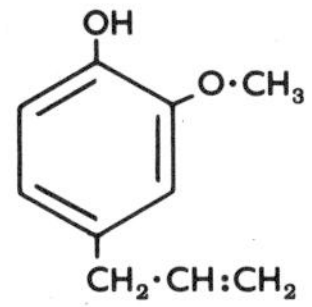

Eugenol is the principal constituent of clove oil.
A colourless or pale yellow liquid which darkens and thickens with age or on exposure to air. B.p. about 254°. Refractive index at 20°, 1·540 to 1·542.
Solubility. Almost insoluble in water; miscible 1 in 2 of ethanol (70%); miscible with ether, chloroform, and fixed oils.

Extraction. Eugenol is extracted by organic solvents from aqueous acid solutions.

Ultraviolet Absorption Spectrum. Eugenol in ethanol, maxima at 231·5 mμ (E1%, 1cm 406) and 282 mμ (E1%, 1cm 193); in 0·1N sodium hydroxide, maxima at 246 mμ (E1%, 1cm 552) and 296 mμ (E1%, 1cm 262).

Dose. Up to 0·2 ml.

Toxicity. LD50 (oral): in rats 2 g/kg.

FENCAMFAMIN *Central Stimulant*

Synonyms: H 610; W 1206.

2-Ethylamino-3-phenylnorbornane
$C_{15}H_{21}N = 215{\cdot}3$

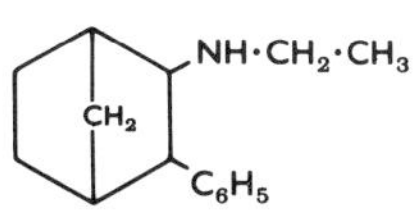

Solubility. Insoluble in water; soluble in chloroform.

FENCAMFAMIN HYDROCHLORIDE
Proprietary Name: Euvitol.

A white crystalline solid.
Solubility. Soluble in water.

Extraction. Fencamfamin is extracted by organic solvents from aqueous alkaline solutions.

Chromatography. PAPER: system P1—Rf 0·79 (location reagents: *iodoplatinate spray*, strong reaction; *bromocresol green spray*, strong reaction); system RP1a—Rf 0·80 (location reagent *iodoplatinate spray*, positive reaction); system RP1b—Rf 0·00.
THIN-LAYER: system T1—Rf 0·60 (location reagent *acidified iodoplatinate spray*, positive reaction).
GAS: system G2/120—retention time 3·7 relative to ephedrine.

Colour Test. MICRO: sulphuric acid–formaldehyde test—orange (*sensitivity:* 0·5 μg).

Crystal Tests. MICRO: *gold chloride solution*—plates, some serrated, best viewed under polarised light (*sensitivity:* 1 in 1500); *trinitrobenzoic acid solution*—irregular crystals (*sensitivity:* 1 in 400).

Ultraviolet Absorption Spectrum. Fencamfamin in 0·1N sulphuric acid, maxima at about 248 mμ (E1%, 1cm 6·6), 253 mμ (E1%, 1cm 8·7), 258·5 mμ (E1%, 1cm 10·5), 264·5 mμ (E1%, 1cm 8·1), and 268 mμ (E1%, 1cm 6·7).

Infra-red Absorption Spectrum. Fencamfamin (base). Potassium bromide disk. The principal peaks are: A 698, B 1449, C 1102 or 1130 (p. 786).

Dose. Up to 40 mg daily.

FENETHYLLINE *Xanthine Derivative*

Synonyms: Amfetyline; R 720-11.

7 - {2 - [(α - Methylphenethyl)amino]ethyl} - 1, 3-dimethylxanthine
$C_{18}H_{23}N_5O_2 = 341{\cdot}4$

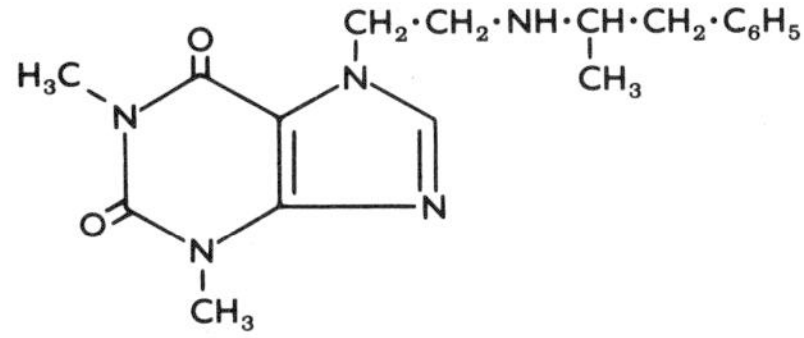

Solubility. Insoluble in water; soluble in chloroform.

FENETHYLLINE HYDROCHLORIDE
Proprietary Name: Captagon.

A white crystalline powder.
Solubility. Soluble in water.

Extraction. Fenethylline is extracted by organic solvents from aqueous alkaline solutions.

Chromatography. PAPER: system P1—Rf 0·53 (location under ultraviolet light, strong absorption; location reagents: *iodoplatinate spray*, strong reaction; *bromocresol green spray*, strong reaction).
THIN-LAYER: system T1—Rf 0·56 (location reagent *acidified iodoplatinate spray*, positive reaction).

Colour Tests. MICRO: sulphuric acid–formaldehyde test—dull orange (*sensitivity:* 0·5 μg); ammonium molybdate test—faint blue (*sensitivity:* 1·0 μg).

Crystal Tests. MICRO: *gold bromide–hydrochloric acid solution*—rosettes of blades (*sensitivity:* 1 in 1000); *styphnic acid*—rosettes of branching needles (*sensitivity:* 1 in 1000).

Ultraviolet Absorption Spectrum. Fenethylline 0·1N sulphuric acid, maximum at 274·5 mμ (E1%, 1cm 202).

Infra-red Absorption Spectrum. Fenethylline (base). Potassium bromide disk. The principal peaks are: A 1664, B 1705, C 1546 or 1600 (p. 786).

FENFLURAMINE *Anorectic*

Synonym: S 768.

N - Ethyl - α - methyl - 3 - trifluoromethylphenethylamine

$C_{12}H_{16}F_3N = 231{\cdot}3$

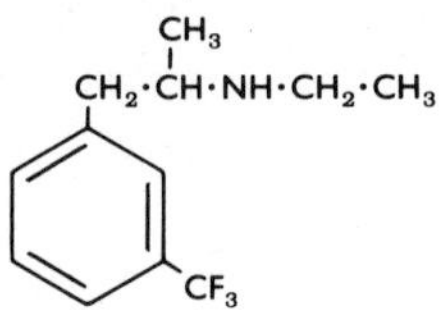

Solubility. Insoluble in water; soluble in chloroform.

FENFLURAMINE HYDROCHLORIDE

Proprietary Names: Pondéral; Ponderax.

A white crystalline powder.

Solubility. Soluble in water.

Extraction. Fenfluramine is extracted by organic solvents from aqueous alkaline solutions.

Chromatography. PAPER: system P1—Rf 0·82 (location under ultraviolet light, absorption; location reagents: *iodoplatinate spray*, strong reaction; *bromocresol green spray*, strong reaction).

THIN-LAYER: system T1—Rf 0·50 (location reagent *acidified iodoplatinate spray*, positive reaction).

GAS: system G2/120—retention time 0·46 relative to ephedrine.

Crystal Tests. MICRO: *picric acid*—rosettes of needles (*sensitivity:* 1 in 400); *platinic iodide solution*—bunches of plates (*sensitivity:* 1 in 1000).

Ultraviolet Absorption Spectrum. Fenfluramine in 0·1N sulphuric acid, maxima at about 259 mμ (E1%, 1cm 15·9), 263·5 mμ (E1%, 1cm 21·8), and 270·5 mμ (E1%, 1cm 19·5).

Infra-red Absorption Spectrum. Fenfluramine (base). Potassium bromide disk. The principal peaks are: A 1119, B 1160, C 1069 or 1330 (p. 786).

Metabolism. Following oral doses of 180 mg of fenfluramine hydrochloride, blood-levels of 0·008 and 0·016 mg% were obtained after one hour and two hours respectively; norfenfluramine, the *N*-de-ethylated derivative, has been detected in the blood (White *et al.*, 1967).

The urinary excretion of fenfluramine and its main metabolite, norfenfluramine, has been found to depend on the urinary pH, the excretion being greater when the urine is acid. Following a single oral dose of 20 mg of fenfluramine, about 20% is excreted in 48 hours as fenfluramine and 20% as norfenfluramine in acidic urine (Beckett and Brookes, 1967).

Dose. Up to 60 mg daily.

Toxicity. Recoveries have occurred following the ingestion of 1·6 to 1·8 g.

LD50 (oral): in mice 470 mg/kg.

CASE EXAMPLE. A 13-year-old girl recovered after taking 300 mg of fenfluramine hydrochloride. On admission to hospital, one and a half hours after ingestion, a blood sample was found to contain 0·024 mg% of fenfluramine and 0·004 mg% of norfenfluramine. The stomach washout contained approximately 3 mg of fenfluramine hydrochloride (White *et al.*, 1967).

FENIMIDE *Tranquilliser*

Synonyms: CI 419; Fenetimide.

α-Ethyl-α′-methyl-α′-phenylsuccinimide

$C_{13}H_{15}NO_2 = 217{\cdot}3$

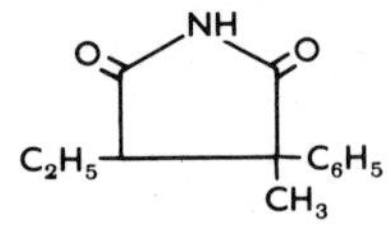

A white crystalline powder.

Solubility. Insoluble in water; soluble in ethanol and chloroform.

Extraction. Fenimide is extracted by organic solvents from aqueous acid or alkaline solutions.

Chromatography. PAPER: system P1—Rf 0·97 (location reagent *bromine–starch–potassium iodide*, weak reaction).

THIN-LAYER: system T1—Rf 0·75 (location reagents: *strongly acid iodoplatinate spray*, positive reaction; *iodine–carbon tetrachloride spray*, positive reaction).

Ultraviolet Absorption Spectrum. Fenimide in ethanol, maxima at 248 mμ (E1%, 1cm 13), 252·5 mμ (E1%, 1cm 15), 258·5 mμ (E1%, 1cm 15), and 265 mμ (E1%, 1cm 10).

FENPIPRAMIDE *Parasympatholytic*

Synonym: Hö 9980.

2, 2-Diphenyl-4-piperidinobutyramide

$C_{21}H_{26}N_2O = 322{\cdot}5$

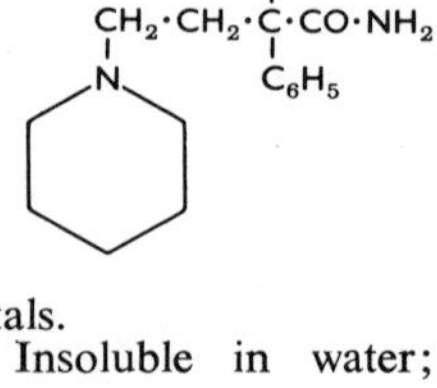

White crystals.

Solubility. Insoluble in water; soluble in chloroform.

FENPIPRAMIDE HYDROCHLORIDE

Proprietary Name: It is an ingredient of Efosin.

A white crystalline powder.

Solubility. Soluble in water.

FENPIPRAMIDE METHOBROMIDE
Proprietary Name: Resantin.

Extraction. Fenpipramide is extracted by organic solvents from aqueous alkaline solutions; fenpipramide methobromide is, however, a quaternary ammonium compound (see p. 29).

Chromatography. PAPER: system P1—Rf 0·68 (location reagents: *iodoplatinate spray*, strong reaction; *bromocresol green spray*, strong reaction).
THIN-LAYER: system T1—Rf 0·56 (location reagent *acidified iodoplatinate spray*, positive reaction).

Ultraviolet Absorption Spectrum. Fenpipramide in 0·1N sulphuric acid, maxima at 253 mμ (E1%, 1cm 10·4), 259 mμ (E1%, 1cm 11·8) and 265 mμ (E1%, 1cm 9·3).

FENPIPRANE *Parasympatholytic*

Synonym: Hö 10116.

1-(3,3-Diphenylpropyl)piperidine
$C_{20}H_{25}N = 279·4$

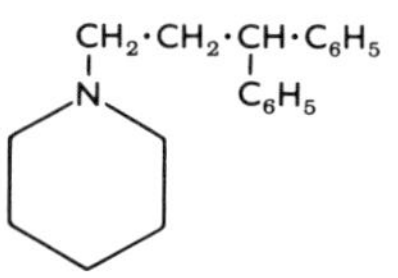

Solubility. Insoluble in water; soluble in chloroform.

FENPIPRANE HYDROCHLORIDE
Proprietary Name: It is an ingredient of Efosin.

A white crystalline powder.
Solubility. Soluble in water.

Extraction. Fenpiprane is extracted by organic solvents from aqueous alkaline solutions.

Chromatography. PAPER: system P1—Rf 0·82 (location under ultraviolet light, absorption; location reagents: *iodoplatinate spray*, strong reaction; *bromocresol green spray*, strong reaction).
THIN-LAYER: system T1—Rf 0·61 (location reagent *acidified iodoplatinate spray*, positive reaction).

Colour Tests. MICRO: sulphuric acid–formaldehyde test—red (*sensitivity:* 0·5 μg); Vitali's test— -/-/purple-brown (*sensitivity:* 0·1 μg).

Crystal Tests. MICRO: *ammonium thiocyanate solution*—long needles (*sensitivity:* 1 in 1000); *trinitrobenzoic acid solution*—bunches of rods or prisms (*sensitivity:* 1 in 1000).

Ultraviolet Absorption Spectrum. Fenpiprane in 0·1N sulphuric acid, maxima at about 254 mμ (E1%, 1cm 13·2), 259 mμ (E1%, 1cm 15), and 268·5 mμ (E1%, 1cm 9·9), and an inflexion at 249 mμ and a minor inflexion at about 265 mμ.

Infra-red Absorption Spectrum. Fenpiprane (base). Potassium bromide disk. The principal peaks are: A 1492, B 698 or 1092 or 1631 (p. 786).

FENTANYL *Narcotic Analgesic*

Synonym: Phentanyl; R 4263.

N-(1-Phenethylpiperid-4-yl)propionanilide
$C_{22}H_{28}N_2O = 336·5$

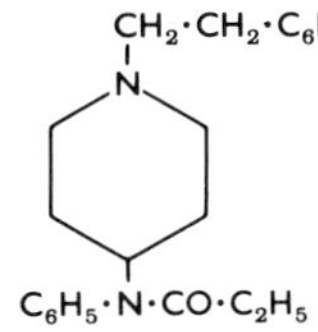

Fentanyl melts at 83° to 84°.
Solubility. Sparingly soluble in water.

FENTANYL CITRATE
Proprietary Name: Sublimaze. It is an ingredient of Innovar and Thalamonal.

A white crystalline powder. M.p. 149° to 151°.
Solubility. Soluble 1 in about 40 of water; sparingly soluble in ethanol, ether, and chloroform.

Extraction. Fentanyl is extracted by organic solvents from aqueous alkaline solutions.

Chromatography. PAPER: system P1—Rf 0·86 (location reagents: *iodoplatinate spray*, weak reaction; *bromocresol green spray*, weak reaction); system RP1a—Rf 0·27 (location reagent *iodoplatinate spray*, positive reaction); system RP1b—Rf 0·00 (location as for RP1a).
THIN-LAYER: system T1—Rf 0·71 (location reagent *acidified iodoplatinate spray*, positive reaction).
GAS: system G2/225—retention time 2·65 relative to codeine.

Colour Tests. MICRO: sulphuric acid–formaldehyde test—faint orange (*sensitivity:* 1·0 μg); ammonium molybdate test—faint grey (*sensitivity:* 1·0 μg).

Crystal Tests. MICRO: *picric acid*—small oily plates and needles (*sensitivity:* 1 in 1000); *potassium tri-iodide solution*(*1*)—branching needles and very small rods (*sensitivity:* 1 in 1000).

Ultraviolet Absorption Spectrum. Fentanyl in 0·1N sulphuric acid, maxima at 251 mμ (E1%, 1cm 12·4), 257·5 mμ (E1%, 1cm 13·7), and 263 mμ (E1%, 1cm 11·2).

Quantitative Estimation. Fentanyl in biological tissues may be determined spectrophotometrically following the formation of a complex with methyl orange (Gettler and Sunshine, 1951).

Dose. Up to 0·6 mg, intravenously.

Toxicity. LD50 (intravenous): in mice 11·2 mg/kg.

NOTE. Fentanyl citrate is a potent narcotic analgesic with similar actions to morphine. It is said to be 1000 times more potent than pethidine.

FLUANISONE *Tranquilliser*

Synonyms: Haloanisone; MD 2028.
Proprietary Names: Anti-Pica; Sédalande.

p-Fluoro-γ-(4-*o*-methoxyphenylpiperazin-1-yl)butyrophenone
$C_{21}H_{25}FN_2O_2 = 356{\cdot}4$

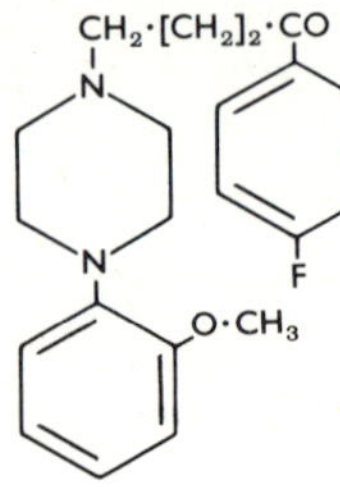

A white crystalline powder. M.p. about 68°.
Solubility. Practically insoluble in water; moderately soluble in ethanol; slightly soluble in ether; soluble in chloroform.

Extraction. Fluanisone is extracted by organic solvents from aqueous alkaline solutions.

Chromatography. PAPER: system P1—Rf 0·80 (location under ultraviolet light, strong absorption; location reagents: *iodoplatinate spray*, weak reaction; *potassium permanganate spray*, weak reaction).
THIN-LAYER: system T1—Rf 0·73 (location reagent *potassium permanganate spray*, positive reaction).

Colour Tests. MICRO: ammonium molybdate test—pale blue (*sensitivity:* 0·5 μg); ammonium vanadate test—pale brown (*sensitivity:* 0·5 μg); Vitali's test—yellow/yellow/yellow (*sensitivity:* 0·5 μg).

Crystal Tests. MICRO: *platinic iodide solution*—small rods and prisms (*sensitivity:* 1 in 1000); *zinc chloride solution*—rosettes of long plates (*sensitivity:* 1 in 1000).

Ultraviolet Absorption Spectrum. Fluanisone in 0·1N sulphuric acid, maxima at 247·5 mμ (E1%, 1 cm 845), 275 mμ (E1%, 1 cm 171), 305 mμ (E1%, 1 cm 14), and 360 mμ (E1%, 1 cm 12).

Infra-red Absorption Spectrum. Potassium bromide disk. The principal peaks are: A 1238 or 1690, B 1499, C 1599 (p. 786).

Dose. Up to 120 mg daily.

FLUDROCORTISONE *Corticosteroid*

Synonym: 9α-Fluorohydrocortisone.

9α-Fluoro-11β,17α,21-trihydroxypregn-4-ene-3,20-dione
$C_{21}H_{29}FO_5 = 380{\cdot}5$

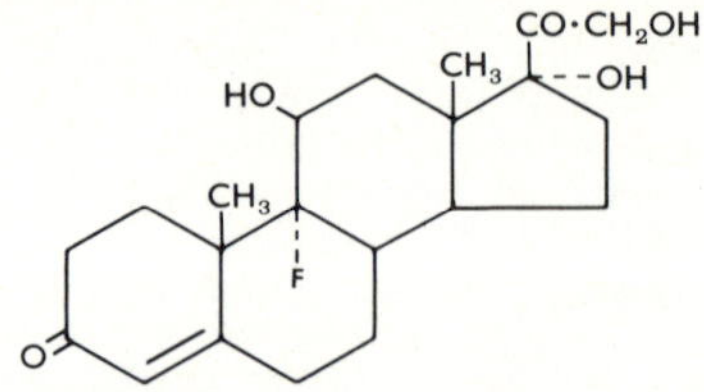

Fludrocortisone occurs as crystals which decompose between 260° and 262°.
Solubility. Very soluble in water.

FLUDROCORTISONE ACETATE
21-Acetoxy-9α-fluoro-11β,17α-dihydroxypregn-4-ene-3,20-dione.
Proprietary Names: Alfa-Fluorone; Alflorone Acetate; F-Cortef Acetate; Florinef Acetate; Scherofluron.
White hygroscopic crystals or crystalline powder. M.p. about 225°; it may also occur in a form which melts at about 209°. Specific rotation of a 1% solution in dioxan, +148° to +156°.
Solubility. Insoluble in water; soluble 1 in 50 of ethanol, 1 in 250 of ether, and 1 in 50 of chloroform.

Extraction. Fludrocortisone is extracted from neutral solutions with freshly distilled ethyl acetate.

Chromatography. PAPER, for fludrocortisone acetate: system P14—Rf 0·45 (location reagent *DPST solution*, violet).
THIN-LAYER, for fludrocortisone acetate: system T18—Rf 0·87 (location reagent *DPST spray*).

Ultraviolet Absorption Spectrum. Fludrocortisone acetate in ethanol, maximum at 240 mμ (E1%, 1 cm 405).

Metabolism. In doses of 2 to 3 mg daily, fludrocortisone effectively inhibits corticotrophin secretion.

Dose. Up to 2 mg initially; 0·2 mg daily as maintenance.

FLUOCINOLONE ACETONIDE *Corticosteroid*

Synonyms: 6α,9α-Difluoro-16α-hydroxyprednisolone-16,17-acetonide; RS 1401AT.
Proprietary Names: Jellin; Synalar; Synandone.

6α,9α-Difluoro-11β,21-dihydroxy-16α,17α-isopropylidenedioxypregna-1,4-diene-3,20-dione
$C_{24}H_{30}F_2O_6 = 452{\cdot}5$

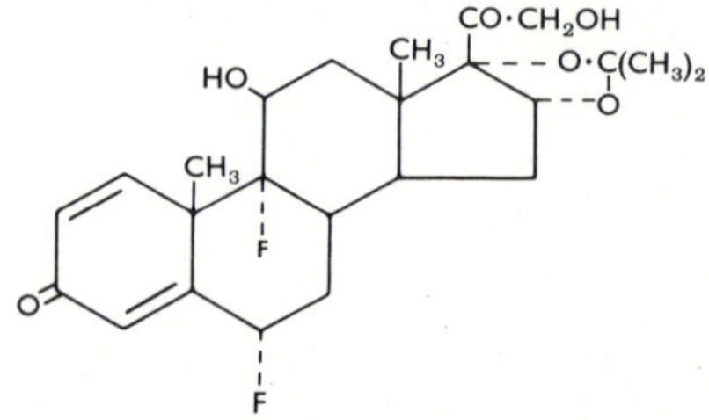

A white crystalline powder. M.p. about 275°,

with decomposition. Specific rotation of a 1% solution in dioxan, +92° to +96°.
Solubility. Insoluble in water; soluble 1 in 26 of dehydrated ethanol and 1 in 15 of chloroform.

Extraction. Fluocinolone acetonide is extracted from neutral solutions with freshly distilled ethyl acetate.

Chromatography. PAPER: system P14—Rf 0·40 (location reagent *DPST solution*, violet on yellow).
THIN-LAYER: system T18—Rf 0·53 (location reagent *DPST spray*); system T19—Rf 1·40 (location as for T18).

Ultraviolet Absorption Spectrum. Fluocinolone acetonide in ethanol, maximum at 240 mμ (E1%, 1cm 360).

NOTE. Fluocinolone acetonide is a synthetic glucocorticoid which is used topically to treat various skin disorders.

FLUOPROMAZINE *Tranquilliser*

Synonym: Triflupromazine.

10 - (3 - Dimethylaminopropyl) - 2 - trifluoromethylphenothiazine
$C_{18}H_{19}F_3N_2S$ = 352·4

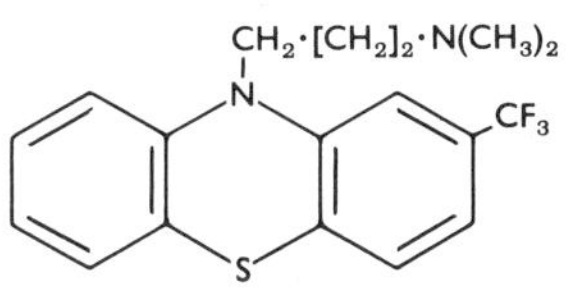

A liquid which boils at 176°.

FLUOPROMAZINE HYDROCHLORIDE
Proprietary Names: Adazine; Fluorofen; Nivoman; Psyquil; Siquil; Vespral; Vesprin.

A white powder. M.p. 173° to 174°.
Solubility. Soluble 1 in less than 10 of water; soluble in ethanol; insoluble in ether.

Screening Test. *FPN reagent* with urine—orange-yellow (see p. 10).

Extraction. Fluopromazine is extracted by organic solvents from aqueous alkaline solutions; hydrolysis of biological material is required in order to improve the yield.

Chromatography. PAPER: system P1—Rf 0·72 (location under ultraviolet light, yellow fluorescence; location reagents: *iodoplatinate spray*, strong reaction; *bromocresol green spray*, weak reaction); system RP1a—Rf 0·12 (location under ultraviolet light, green fluorescence; location reagent *iodoplatinate spray*, positive reaction); system RP1b—Rf 0·07 (location as for RP1a).
THIN-LAYER: system T1—Rf 0·53 (location reagent *acidified iodoplatinate spray*, positive reaction); system T3—Rf 0·95 (location reagents: *iodoplatinate spray*, positive reaction; *sulphuric acid–ethanol spray*, orange); system T4—Rf 0·79 (location as for T3); system T6—Rf 0·69 (the spot may be converted on the plate to the sulphoxide, Rf 0·50; location of both spots under ultraviolet light).
GAS: system G2/225—retention time 0·61 relative to codeine; system G4—retention time 0·44 relative to codeine.

Colour Tests. MICRO: sulphuric acid–formaldehyde test—red-purple (*sensitivity:* 0·5 μg); ammonium molybdate test—red-brown (*sensitivity:* 0·5 μg); ammonium vanadate test—red-brown (*sensitivity:* 0·5 μg); Vitali's test—purple → yellow/yellow (*sensitivity:* 1·0 μg).

Crystal Test. MICRO: *gold chloride solution*—small curved needles, best viewed under polarised light (*sensitivity:* 1 in 100).

Ultraviolet Absorption Spectrum. Fluopromazine in 0·1N sulphuric acid, maxima at 256 mμ (E1%, 1cm 1245) and 304 mμ (E1%, 1cm 139).

Infra-red Absorption Spectrum. Fluopromazine (base). Potassium bromide disk. The principal peaks are: A 1117, B 1319 or 1417, C 1159 or 1237 or 1459 (p. 787).

Dose. Up to 150 mg daily.

Toxicity. The acute lethal dose in man of phenothiazine tranquillisers appears to be in the range 15 to 150 mg/kg, although severe toxic symptoms have occurred with doses of less than 1 mg/kg.
LD50 (oral): in mice 330 mg/kg.

FLUOROACETAMIDE *Rodenticide*

$F{\cdot}CH_2{\cdot}CO{\cdot}NH_2$ = 77·06

A fine fluffy white powder which decomposes if heated appreciably above 100°.
Solubility. Very soluble in water; relatively insoluble in ether and other organic solvents.

Quantitative Estimation. Following hydrolysis to fluoroacetate, fluoroacetamide may be extracted with ether and separated from inorganic fluoride by column chromatography with silica gel (Ramsey and Clifford, 1949); the inorganic fluoride remains on the column and the organic fluoride which is eluted may be estimated spectrophotometrically or by gas chromatography (Sawyer *et al.*, 1967).

Metabolism. Fluoroacetamide is rapidly absorbed from the gastro-intestinal tract and can be readily absorbed through cuts and abrasions. Fluoroacetamide, like the fluoroacetates, is converted *in vivo* to fluoroacetic acid and then to fluorocitric acid which inhibits the citric acid cycle. The lethal action of fluoroacetamide is not so rapid as that of fluoroacetate; this may be because the hydrolysis takes place more slowly and a high level of fluorocitrate is not allowed to accumulate.

Toxicity. Fluoroacetamide is extremely toxic to animals and man. It is a highly effective rodenticide. Owing to the light consistency of the dry powder, masks should be worn when it is handled; gloves of rubber or p.v.c. should be worn when the rat-bait is handled.

In Great Britain, the use of fluoroacetamide is restricted to the destruction of rats in ships and in sewers.

CASE EXAMPLES. In a child who had consumed 23 mg/kg of fluoroacetamide, a level of 108 mg/kg of citric acid was found in the heart tissue and 23 mg/kg in the kidney tissue. Both organs contained 6·3 mg/kg of organic fluoride (dried weight). Lambs poisoned experimentally with 20 mg/kg of fluoroacetate died in 7 hours. Blood lactic acid levels and tissue citric acid levels were 3 times the normal. This may be of diagnostic value (Egyed and Brisk, 1965).

FLUOROACETIC ACID *Rodenticide*

Synonyms: Fluoroethanoic Acid; Gifblaar Poison; Monofluoroacetic Acid.

$F{\cdot}CH_2{\cdot}CO_2H = 78{\cdot}04$

Fluoroacetic acid is the toxic principle of the South African plant gifblaar, *Chailletia cymosa* (= *Dichapetalum cymosum*) (Chailletiaceae). It occurs as crystals which melt at 33° to 35°. B.p. 165° to 168°.

Solubility. Soluble in water and ethanol.

SODIUM FLUOROACETATE

Synonym: Sodium Monofluoroacetate.

A white powder.

Solubility. Very soluble in water; relatively insoluble in organic solvents.

Quantitative Estimation. Fluoroacetic acid and its salts may be extracted from biological material, water, and soils with ether; they are separated from inorganic fluoride by column chromatography on silica gel (Ramsey and Clifford, 1949); the inorganic fluoride remains on the column and the organic fluoride which is eluted may be estimated spectrophotometrically or by gas chromatography (Sawyer *et al.*, 1967).

Metabolism. Fluoroacetic acid and sodium fluoroacetate are absorbed rapidly through cuts and abrasions but not so rapidly through intact skin. Fluoroacetate is converted *in vivo* to fluoroacetic acid and then to fluorocitric acid which inhibits the citric acid cycle and leads to the accumulation of citrate.

Toxicity. Fluoroacetic acid and sodium fluoroacetate are extremely toxic to animals and man. Sodium fluoroacetate is a highly effective rodenticide but it must be used with great caution because of its toxicity. There is a latent period of ½ to 2 hours or more between administration of the rodenticide and the effects of poisoning. The lethal effects are related mainly to the myocardium and to the central nervous system. Survival for more than 24 hours gives a favourable prognosis. The lethal dose in man is estimated to be between 50 and 100 mg.

Several outbreaks of wholesale poisoning in domestic animals have been reported (Papworth, 1965).

In Great Britain, the use of sodium fluoroacetate is restricted to the destruction of rats in ships and in sewers.

FLUPHENAZINE *Tranquilliser*

10 - {3 - [4 - (2 - Hydroxyethyl)piperazin - 1 - yl]propyl} - 2 - trifluoromethylphenothiazine

$C_{22}H_{26}F_3N_3OS = 437{\cdot}5$

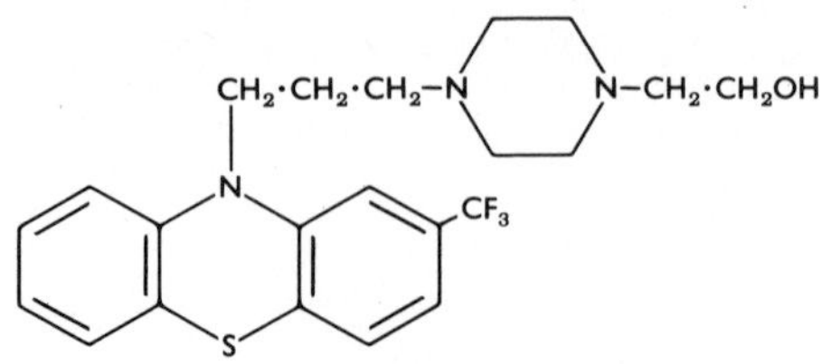

FLUPHENAZINE ENANTHATE

Synonym: Fluphenazine Heptanoate.

Proprietary Name: Moditen Enanthate.

FLUPHENAZINE HYDROCHLORIDE

Proprietary Names: Anatensol; Moditen; Omca; Permitil; Prolixin; Sevinol; Trancin.

A white powder. M.p. 184° to 185°.

Solubility. Soluble in water and ethanol.

Screening Test. *FPN reagent* with urine—orange (see p. 10).

Extraction. Fluphenazine is extracted by organic solvents from aqueous alkaline solutions; hydrolysis of biological material is required in order to improve the yield.

Chromatography. PAPER: system P1—Rf 0·36 (location under ultraviolet light, yellow fluorescence; location reagent *iodoplatinate spray*, strong reaction); system RP1a—Rf 0·13 (location under ultraviolet light, yellow fluorescence; location reagent *iodoplatinate spray*, positive reaction); system RP1b—Rf 0·07 (location as for RP1a).

THIN-LAYER: system T1—Rf 0·59 (location reagent *acidified iodoplatinate spray*, positive reaction); system T3—Rf 0·34 (location reagents: *iodoplatinate spray*, positive reaction; *sulphuric acid–ethanol spray*, orange); system T4—Rf 0·58 (location as for T3); system T6—Rf 0·75 (the spot may be converted on the plate to the sulphoxide, Rf 0·59; location of both spots under ultraviolet light).

Colour Tests. MICRO: sulphuric acid–formaldehyde test—red (*sensitivity:* 0·1 μg); ammonium molybdate test—brown→red (*sensitivity:* 0·1 μg); ammonium vanadate test—brown (*sensitivity:* 0·1 μg) Vitali's test—red → yellow/yellow/yellow-orange (*sensitivity:* 0·5 μg).

Crystal Tests. MICRO: *gold cyanide solution*—irregular bunches of needles (*sensitivity:* 1 in 1000); *platinic chloride solution*—smudge rosettes (*sensitivity:* 1 in 100).

Ultraviolet Absorption Spectrum. Fluphenazine in 0·01N sulphuric acid, maxima at 265 mμ and 306 mμ.

Infra-red Absorption Spectrum. Fluphenazine (base). Potassium bromide disk. The principal peaks are: A 1115 or 1425, B 1325, C 1142 or 1161 (p. 787).

Metabolism. Studies in rats (Ebert and Hess, 1965) with ^{14}C-labelled fluphenazine enanthate injected subcutaneously have shown it to be widely distributed, the major portion being found in the carcass and the least amount in the brain. Over a 3-week period, 46% of the injected radioactivity was recovered in the faeces but only 13% in the urine; both faeces and urine were found to contain fluphenazine, fluphenazine enanthate, and fluphenazine sulphoxide. The hydrolysis in the brain of fluphenazine enanthate to fluphenazine was demonstrated.

Toxicity. The usual therapeutic dose is up to 5 mg daily but toxic effects, e.g. blood dyscrasias, convulsions, and liver damage, begin to appear at or above this dosage. The acute lethal dose in man of phenothiazine tranquillisers appears to be in the range 15 to 150 mg/kg.

FOLIC ACID *Haemopoietic Vitamin*

Synonyms: Folacin; Folinsyre; Pteroylglutamic Acid.
Proprietary Name: Folvite.

4 - (2 - Amino - 4 - hydroxy - 6 - pteridinyl) methylaminobenzoyl - L - glutamic acid

$C_{19}H_{19}N_7O_6 = 441{\cdot}4$

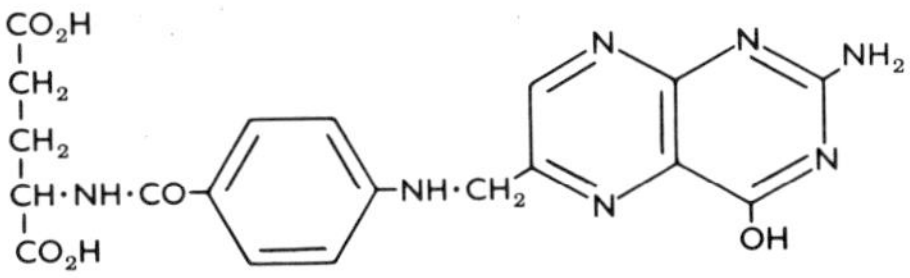

An orange-yellow microcrystalline powder.
Solubility. Insoluble in cold water; soluble 1 in 5000 of boiling water; insoluble in ethanol, ether, and chloroform. Solutions are inactivated by ultraviolet light, alkaline solutions are sensitive to oxidation, and acid solutions are sensitive to heat.

Ultraviolet Absorption Spectrum. Folic acid in 0·1N sodium hydroxide, maxima at 256 mμ (E1%, 1 cm about 546), 283 mμ (E1%, 1 cm about 533), and 365 mμ (E1%, 1 cm about 186).

Infra-red Absorption Spectrum. Potassium bromide disk. The principal peaks are: A 1688, B 1601, C 1484 or 1640 (p. 741).

Quantitative Estimation. Folic acid may be estimated by chromatography followed by spectrofluorimetry (Spinelli and Ciuffi, 1966).

Metabolism. Folic acid is a member of the vitamin-B group. It is present in many foods, partly as free folic acid but chiefly conjugated with several glutamic acid residues.
Folic acid is a growth factor; without it, normal cellular division cannot take place, mitosis being halted at the metaphase. It produces a haemopoietic response in many forms of anaemia. It is converted in the body to leucovorin, the active form, and the latter is then metabolised in the liver to inactive products, one of which is *p*-aminobenzoylglutamic acid.

Human Requirements. The normal human requirement is thought to be about 50 μg daily.

Dose. Up to 20 mg daily.

FORMALDEHYDE *Disinfectant*

Synonyms: Formic Aldehyde; Methanal; Methylene Oxide; Oxomethane.

$H{\cdot}CHO = 30{\cdot}03$

A colourless inflammable gas.
Solubility. Very soluble in water; slightly soluble in ethanol and ether.

FORMALDEHYDE SOLUTION
Synonyms: Formalin (this is a trade-mark in some countries); Formol.
A colourless liquid containing 34 to 38% w/w of formaldehyde. It should be stored in a moderately warm place (above 15°); a slight white deposit may form on keeping.
Solubility. Miscible with water and ethanol.

Extraction. Formaldehyde is volatile and may be isolated by distillation (see p. 18).

Chromatography. Sandler and Strom (1960) have described a method of determination of formaldehyde by gas chromatography.

Colour Tests. Add a few drops of a solution containing formaldehyde to a dilute solution of chromotropic acid in *sulphuric acid*—red.
Shake a little resorcinol with a solution containing formaldehyde and run some *sulphuric acid* down the inside of the tube to form a layer under the mixed solution—reddish-violet ring at the junction of the 2 layers.

Quantitative Estimation. Following microdiffusion from blood, urine, and tissue homogenates, formaldehyde may be determined spectrophotometrically (Klendshoj and Feldstein, 1955).

Metabolism. Formaldehyde is metabolised to formic acid (q.v.) and methanol; the formic acid may then be converted to methyl formate. Formaldehyde is also a metabolite of methanol. It combines rapidly with the amino-groups of proteins and amino-acids.

Toxicity. Formaldehyde is very irritant to mucous membranes and inhalation of the vapour causes intense irritation of the respiratory tract which may lead to bronchitis and pneumonia. Few fatalities have been recorded but 30 ml of formaldehyde solution may be fatal to an adult. The maximum allowable concentration in a factory atmosphere is 5 p.p.m.
LD50 (oral): in rats 800 mg/kg.

FORMIC ACID

$H{\cdot}CO_2H = 46{\cdot}03$

A colourless liquid with a pungent odour. M.p. 8·4°. B.p. 100·5°.
Solubility. Miscible with water, ethanol, and ether.

Extraction. Formic acid is extracted by organic solvents from aqueous acid solutions.

Colour Test. When warmed with *sulphuric acid* in a tube, formic acid evolves carbon monoxide vapour; the gas can be ignited at the mouth of the tube and burns with a blue flame.

Metabolism. Formic acid is an intermediate in normal metabolism and when administered it probably takes part in the metabolism of 1-carbon compounds to produce methyl groups; it is eventually oxidised to carbon dioxide. Together with formaldehyde, it is a metabolite of methanol and the two are thought to be responsible for the effect of methanol on vision.

Toxicity. The estimated lethal dose in man is about 30 ml. Formic acid is dangerously caustic on the skin.

CASE EXAMPLE. A 2-year-old child swallowed an unknown quantity of Kilrock-K, a kettle descaler, which contains 60% of formic acid, 39·7% of water, and 0·3% of an inhibitor (an aliphatic nitrogen compound). The most serious complication was severe laryngeal stridor which became steadily worse and a tracheostomy had to be performed about 18 hours after the poisoning. For at least 3 months the child could not take solid foods (Harvey, 1968).

NOTE. Formic acid is the principal ingredient (about 60%) of several proprietary preparations used for descaling kettles.

FRAMYCETIN *Antibiotic*

An antibiotic produced by the growth of *Streptomyces decaris*. It consists of neomycin B together with a small amount of neomycin C (cf. Neomycin, p. 437). Framycetin is heat-labile.

Solubility. Soluble in water.

FRAMYCETIN SULPHATE

Proprietary Names: Framygen; Soframycin.

A white hygroscopic powder.

Solubility. Soluble 1 in 1 of water; insoluble in ethanol, ether, and chloroform.

Extraction. Framycetin is soluble in water; special extraction methods are required (see p. 28).

Chromatography. PAPER: system P1—Rf 0·00 (location reagents: *bromine–starch–potassium iodide*, strong reaction; *ninhydrin spray*, purple).

THIN-LAYER: system T1—Rf 0·00 (location reagent *potassium permanganate spray*, positive reaction).

Ultraviolet Absorption Spectrum. Framycetin in 0·1N sulphuric acid, maxima at 249 mμ (E1%, 1cm 3), 305 mμ (E1%, 1cm 1), and 362 mμ (E1%, 1cm 1).

Metabolism. Framycetin is an antibiotic with a range of antimicrobial activity similar to that of neomycin (p. 437). It is poorly absorbed from the gastro-intestinal tract but readily absorbed and highly toxic when given by injection. Following the subcutaneous injection of 250 mg in man, serum levels of 0·23 to 2 mg% were obtained after 1 hour and 0·1 to 0·97 mg% after 4 hours.

Dose. Up to 1·5 g daily.

FRUSEMIDE *Diuretic*

Synonyms: Furosemid(e); Fursemide; Salu 058.

Proprietary Name: Lasix.

4 - Chloro - 2 - furfurylamino - 5 - sulphamoyl-benzoic acid

$C_{12}H_{11}ClN_2O_5S = 330{\cdot}7$

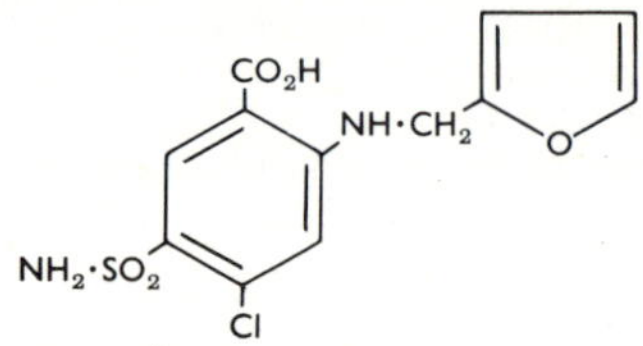

A white crystalline powder. M.p. about 208°, with decomposition.

Solubility. Very slightly soluble in water and chloroform; soluble 1 in 75 of ethanol and 1 in 850 of ether.

Extraction. Frusemide may be isolated in the A1 fraction (see p. 27); it is distinguished from the salicylates by chromatography (see below), also by the fact that it does not react with *ferric chloride solution*, and by the presence of additional ultraviolet maxima in the region 270 to 330 mμ.

Chromatography. PAPER: system P16—Rf 0·75 (location under ultraviolet light, green fluorescence; location reagent *sodium naphthaquinone spray*, strong reaction); system RP1b—Rf 0·17 (location as for P16).

Ultraviolet Absorption Spectrum. Frusemide in 0·01N sodium hydroxide, maxima at 229 mμ (E1%, 1cm 1088), 272 mμ (E1%, 1cm 600), and 335 mμ (E1%, 1cm 144); minima at 250 mμ and 300 mμ.

Infra-red Absorption Spectrum. Potassium bromide disk. The principal peaks are: A 1143, B 1668, C 1565 (p. 741).

Quantitative Estimation. Frusemide may be determined spectrophotometrically following acid hydrolysis and diazotisation (per *Drugs of Today*, 1965, **1**, 8). Häussler and Hajdú (1964) describe a spectrofluorimetric method of estimation.

Metabolism. Frusemide is a rapidly acting diuretic which is structurally similar to the thiazides. It has a short duration of action, the effect of a therapeutic dose lasting for about 4 hours.

Frusemide labelled with radioactive sulphur was given intramuscularly and orally to adults; peak plasma levels were found at 30 minutes and 60 minutes respectively after administration of single doses (Calesnick *et al.*, 1966). Approximately 80% of the dose is recovered in the urine 24 hours after intravenous or intramuscular injection of a single dose. The main metabolite found in the urine of man and dog has been shown to be the defurfurylated derivative, 2-amino-4-chloro-5-sulphamoylbenzoic acid (Häussler and Hajdú, 1964); other urinary metabolites have also been detected (Häussler and Wicha, 1965).

Dose. Up to 120 mg daily; doses of up to 500 mg daily have been employed under careful laboratory control.

Toxicity. Reversible leucopenia and thrombocytopenia have been reported following frusemide therapy.

LD50 (oral): in dogs 2, in rabbits 0·8, and in rats 4·6 g/kg.

FURALTADONE *Antibacterial*

Synonym: Furmethonol.
Proprietary Name: Altafur.

(±) - 5 - Morpholinomethyl - 3 - (5 - nitrofurfurylideneamino) - 2 - oxo - oxazolidine

$C_{13}H_{16}N_4O_6 = 324·3$

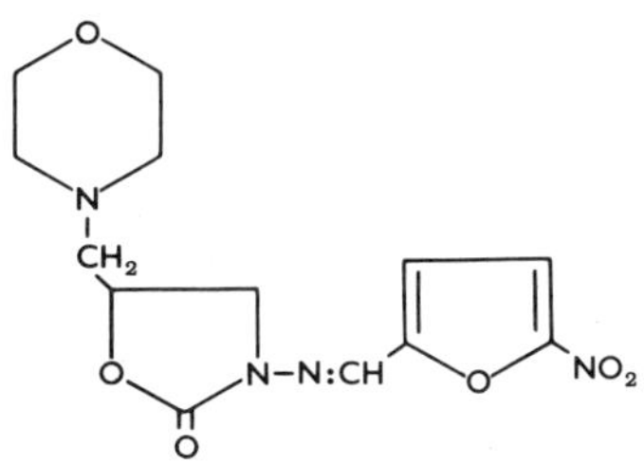

Furaltadone melts at 206°, with decomposition.

Chromatography. PAPER: system P1—Rf 0·08 (location under ultraviolet light, green fluorescence; location reagents: *iodoplatinate spray*, strong reaction; *bromocresol green spray*, weak reaction).

THIN-LAYER: system T1—Rf 0·46 (location reagent *acidified iodoplatinate spray*, positive reaction).

Colour Tests. MICRO: sulphuric acid–formaldehyde test—(yellow) yellow; ammonium molybdate test—(yellow) dull greenish-blue (*sensitivity:* 0·1 μg); Vitali's test—(yellow) yellow/yellow/deep brown (*sensitivity:* 1·0 μg).

Crystal Tests. MICRO: *gold chloride solution*—feathery rosettes (*sensitivity:* 1 in 200); *platinic iodide solution*—dense rosettes or burrs (*sensitivity:* 1 in 400).

Ultraviolet Absorption Spectrum. Furaltadone in 0·1N sulphuric acid, maxima at 255 mμ (E1%, 1cm 680) and 362 mμ (E1%, 1cm 847).

Infra-red Absorption Spectrum. Potassium bromide disk. The principal peaks are: A 1755, B 1352, C 1226 (p. 741).

Metabolism. The blood-level of furaltadone in 9 patients 5 hours after an initial dose of 500 mg averaged 0·31 mg% (Burn and Coleman, 1961).

Toxicity. Furaltadone was formerly administered by mouth as an antibacterial agent but was later withdrawn because of its toxicity.

FURAZOLIDONE *Antibacterial*

Proprietary Name: Furoxone.

3 - (5 - Nitrofurfurylideneamino) - 2 - oxo - oxazolidine

$C_8H_7N_3O_5 = 225·2$

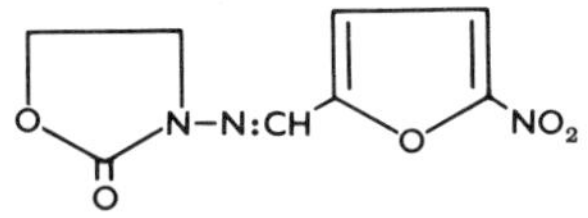

A yellow crystalline powder. M.p. about 259°, with decomposition.

Solubility. Almost insoluble in water and ethanol; insoluble in ether; slightly soluble in chloroform.

Extraction. Furazolidone is extracted by organic solvents from aqueous acid or alkaline solutions.

Colour Test. Dissolve 1 mg in 1 ml of dimethylformamide with 0·05 ml of 1N ethanolic potassium hydroxide—deep blue.

Ultraviolet Absorption Spectrum. Furazolidone in a solution prepared by dissolving 1 mg in 1 ml of dimethylformamide and diluting to 100 ml with a solution containing 3·5% of sodium acetate and 0·2% of glacial acetic acid in water, maximum at about 259 mμ (E1%, 1cm 746); minimum at about 302 mμ.

Infra-red Absorption Spectrum. Potassium bromide disk. The principal peaks are: A 1226 or 1345 or 1738 (p. 741).

Quantitative Estimation. Furazolidone may be estimated spectrophotometrically following its conversion to the phenylhydrazone derivative (Herrett and Buzard, 1960).

Metabolism. When administered by mouth, furazolidone is partly absorbed and excreted in the urine and partly retained in the bowel and excreted in the faeces. Much of the dose given cannot be recovered and is presumably destroyed either in the alimentary tract or in the tissues.

Dose. Up to 400 mg daily.

FURETHIDINE *Narcotic*

Synonym: TA 48.

Ethyl 4-phenyl-1-(2-tetrahydrofurfuryloxyethyl)piperidine-4-carboxylate
$C_{21}H_{31}NO_4 = 361{\cdot}5$

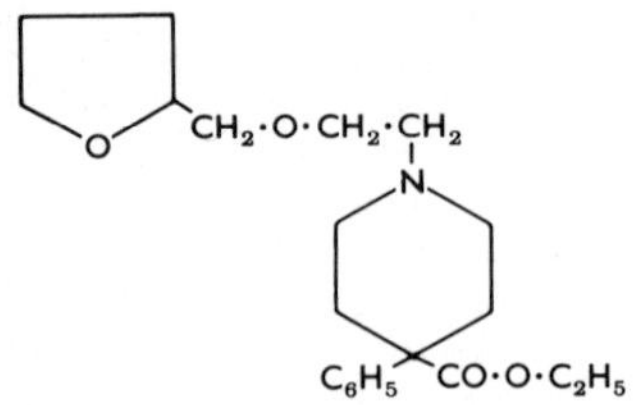

Furethidine is a yellow oil.

Solubility. Soluble in dilute hydrochloric acid.

Extraction. Furethidine is extracted by organic solvents from aqueous alkaline solutions.

Chromatography. PAPER: system P1—Rf 0·70 (location reagents: *iodoplatinate spray*, strong reaction; *bromocresol green spray*, strong reaction).

THIN-LAYER: system T1—Rf 0·66 (location reagent *acidified iodoplatinate spray*, positive reaction).

Colour Test. MICRO: sulphuric acid–formaldehyde test—orange (*sensitivity:* 0·5 μg).

GALLAMINE — *Muscle Relaxant*

Synonym: Bencurine.

1,2,3-Tri(2-diethylaminoethoxy)benzene
$C_{24}H_{45}N_3O_3 = 423{\cdot}6$

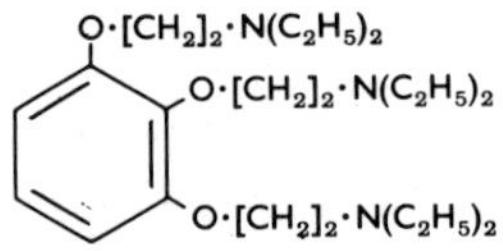

GALLAMINE TRIETHIODIDE
Proprietary Names: Flaxedil; Relaxan; Syntubin; Tricuran.

A white amorphous hygroscopic powder. M.p. about 235°, with decomposition.
Solubility. Soluble 1 in 0·6 of water, 1 in 115 of ethanol, and 1 in 1500 of chloroform; insoluble in ether.

Chromatography. PAPER: system P1—Rf 0·00 (location reagent *iodoplatinate spray*, weak reaction); system RP1a—tailing (location reagent *iodoplatinate spray*, positive reaction); system RP1b—tailing (location as for RP1a).

THIN-LAYER: system T1—Rf 0·00 (location reagent *acidified iodoplatinate spray*, positive reaction).

GAS: system G2/225—retention time 2·66 relative to codeine—there is also an early component running with the solvent peak.

Crystal Test. MICRO: *picric acid*—needles in fans (*sensitivity:* 1 in 1000).

Ultraviolet Absorption Spectrum. Gallamine in 0·1N sulphuric acid, maximum at 226 mμ (E1%, 1 cm 526).

Metabolism. Gallamine is absorbed slowly and incompletely from the gastro-intestinal tract. Absorption seems to be more rapid after sublingual administration. Following administration, the plasma concentration falls rapidly at first and then considerably more slowly for several hours. Gallamine is excreted unchanged, primarily by the kidneys (Foldes, 1960).

Toxicity. The average dose for a normal adult under anaesthesia is up to 120 mg intravenously; if a second dose is necessary it should not exceed 50% of the first dose. Tachycardia sometimes develops within 1 minute after injection. Overdosage may produce respiratory paralysis and circulatory collapse.

GAMMA BENZENE HEXACHLORIDE — *Pesticide*

Synonyms: 666; Gamma-BHC; Gamma-HCH; Hexachlorocyclohexane; Hexicide; Lindane.
Proprietary Names: Abol Gamma Seed Dressing; Gamma-Col; Gammalin; Gammexane; Gexane; Kwell; Lorexane.

γ-Isomer of 1,2,3,4,5,6-hexachlorocyclohexane
$C_6H_6Cl_6 = 290{\cdot}8$

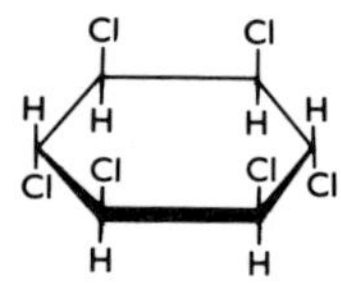

A white crystalline powder which crystallises at not lower than 112°.

Solubility. Insoluble in water; soluble 1 in 19 of dehydrated ethanol, 1 in 5·5 of ether, and 1 in 4 of chloroform.

Extraction. Gamma benzene hexachloride is extracted by organic solvents from aqueous acid or alkaline solutions.

Chromatography. PAPER: Mitchell (1956) has described 4 systems of paper chromatography which separate gamma benzene hexachloride from other chlorinated pesticides; Bridges *et al.* (1956) describe a method of separating the isomers of benzene hexachloride on paper impregnated with paraffin, and Cohen (1957) describes a method for distinguishing gamma benzene hexachloride from the other isomers of benzene hexachloride.

Quantitative Estimation. Wood (1960) describes a spectrophotometric method of determination of gamma benzene hexachloride following its dechlorination to benzene, nitration, and final complex formation with ethyl methyl ketone.
Gamma benzene hexachloride may be extracted from animal fat samples and certain dairy products by a dimethylformamide partition method and determined by gas chromatography (Maunder *et al.*, 1964a and b); it may be extracted from biological tissues by acetone

followed by hexane and determined by gas chromatography (Taylor *et al.*, 1964); it may be extracted from blood by acetone:ether (1:1) and determined by gas chromatography (Jain *et al.*, 1965).

Metabolism. Gamma benzene hexachloride is stored in the body fat and in the adrenal glands and is slowly eliminated through metabolism or by excretion in the urine, faeces, or milk.
It is an insecticide, larvicide, and acaricide. It has a more rapid action than dicophane and is effective in lower concentrations but as it is more volatile it has much less residual action.

Toxicity. Gamma benzene hexachloride is not highly toxic to man or the higher animals when applied externally in the concentrations usually employed (0·1 to 1%) but when ingested it may cause convulsions; dusts may irritate the nose and throat when used in a confined space. The estimated acute oral lethal dose in man is 200 mg/kg. Toxic doses or long-term exposure may cause liver necrosis in man and animals.
LD50 (oral): in rats 150 mg/kg.

CASE EXAMPLES. Stur and Zweymüller (1961) describe the treatment and course of 3 cases of gamma benzene hexachloride poisoning which occurred through oral ingestion in 3 young children. All 3 recovered.
An 8-year-old girl exposed to fumes from a gamma benzene hexachloride vaporiser for about 2 hours daily for 2 years and a 52-year-old man exposed for 8 to 15 hours weekly for about 3 months developed aplastic anaemia. Both died despite treatment with blood transfusions, prednisone, and methyltestosterone (Loge, 1965).

GELSEMINE — *Depressant*

$C_{20}H_{22}N_2O_2$ = 322·4

An alkaloid present in gelsemium, the dried rhizome and roots of *Gelsemium sempervirens* (Loganiaceae).
It occurs as crystals which melt at 178°.
Solubility. Slightly soluble in water; soluble in ethanol, ether, and chloroform.

Extraction. Gelsemine is extracted by organic solvents from aqueous alkaline solutions.

Chromatography. PAPER: system P1—Rf 0·40 (location under ultraviolet light, strong absorption; location reagents: *iodoplatinate spray*, strong reaction; *bromocresol green spray*, strong reaction).
THIN-LAYER: system T1—Rf 0·49 (location reagent *acidified iodoplatinate spray*, positive reaction).
GAS: system G6—retention time 2·81 relative to codeine.

Colour Tests. MICRO: ammonium vanadate test —red → green (*sensitivity:* 0·1 μg); Vitali's test — -/-/bright yellow (*sensitivity:* 0·25 μg).

Crystal Test. MICRO: *potassium iodide solution*—dense rosettes, or rosettes of plates, forming overnight (*sensitivity:* 1 in 100).

Ultraviolet Absorption Spectrum. Gelsemine in ethanol, maxima at 210 mμ (E1%, 1 cm 982) and 252 mμ (E1%, 1 cm 225), and an inflexion at 280 mμ (E1%, 1 cm 43).

Dose. Gelsemine has been used in the treatment of trigeminal neuralgia in doses of 0·5 to 2 mg.

Toxicity. Death has been caused by the ingestion of 3·6 ml of gelsemium fluid extract (1:1). Gelsemium poisoning has occurred in farm stock.
LD50 (intravenous): in mice 4 mg/kg.

GENTAMICIN — *Antibiotic*

A basic pseudo-oligosaccharide antibiotic which is a mixture of 2 isomeric components, C_1 and C_2, with the empirical formula $C_{17-18}H_{34-36}N_4O_7$, produced by *Micromonospora purpurea*.

GENTAMICIN SULPHATE
Proprietary Names: Cidomycin; Garamycin; Genticin; Refobacin.

A white powder. Solutions in water are stable to heat.
Solubility. Freely soluble in water; very slightly soluble in ethanol; practically insoluble in ether and chloroform.

Crystal Test. MICRO: *potassium bismuth iodide solution*—fans or bunches of needles (*sensitivity:* 1 in 1000).

Metabolism. Gentamicin is poorly absorbed from the gastro-intestinal tract but rapidly absorbed after intramuscular injection. Following a dose of about 0·5 mg/kg, peak concentrations in the blood of 0·2 to 0·3 mg% are reached in half to one hour. After 3 intramuscular injections of 30 mg of gentamicin daily for 4½ to 8 days, 30 to 96% of the total daily dose was excreted in the urine in 24 hours, the level of gentamicin ranging from 1·32 to 0·62 mg% (Bulger, 1963).

Dose. Up to 0·8 mg/kg, intramuscularly, every 8 hours.

Toxicity. Ototoxic changes have been reported and nephrotoxicity in experimental animals.
LD50 (oral): in mice 9·0 g/kg (base).

GLUTETHIMIDE — *Hypnotic*

Proprietary Name: Doriden.

α-Ethyl-α-phenylglutarimide
$C_{13}H_{15}NO_2$ = 217·3

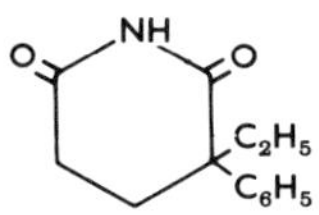

Colourless crystals which melt at 85° to 88°. Glutethimide is hydrolysed by alkalis.
Solubility. Insoluble in water; soluble 1 in 5 of ethanol, 1 in 12 of ether, and 1 in less than 1 of chloroform.

Screening Tests. See under Screening Tests, p. 12; for 2 tests which may be used to detect glutethimide—see Screening Tests 1 and 2 under Barbiturates, p. 208.

Extraction. Glutethimide is extracted by organic solvents from aqueous acid solutions.

Chromatography. PAPER: system P1—Rf 0·93 (location reagent *bromine–starch–potassium iodide*, weak reaction); system RP1a—Rf 0·13 (location under ultraviolet light, absorption); system RP1b—Rf 0·13 (location as for RP1a).
THIN-LAYER: system T1—Rf 0·75 (location reagent *strongly acid iodoplatinate spray* positive reaction); system T10—Rf 0·52 (location reagent *mercurous nitrate spray*, black); system T11—Rf 0·54 (location reagent *mercurous nitrate spray*, white on grey).
GAS: system G1/180—retention time 1·0 relative to diphenhydramine; system G3—retention time 3·30 relative to diphenhydramine; system G5—retention time 4·50 relative to barbitone.

Colour Test. *Liebermann's reagent*—orange.

Ultraviolet Absorption Spectrum. Glutethimide in ethanol, maxima at 251·5 mμ (E1%, 1 cm 17·2), 257·5 mμ (E1%, 1 cm 18·4), and 263·5 mμ (E1%, 1 cm 14·4). When the spectrum of glutethimide is observed in alkaline solution, i.e. ethanolic potassium hydroxide or 0·5N sodium hydroxide, a maximum appears at 235 mμ (E1%, 1 cm about 880) and a minimum at 223 to 225 mμ. However, measurement of the peak must be made within 90 seconds since it decreases rapidly due to hydrolysis of the piperidine ring (Goldbaum and Williams, 1960; Curry, 1963b).

Infra-red Absorption Spectrum. Potassium bromide disk. The principal peaks are: A 1686, B 1710, C 1200 (p. 741).

Quantitative Estimation. Glutethimide may be estimated spectrophotometrically in blood and urine (Goldbaum *et al.*, 1960) and in tissues (Goldbaum *et al.*, 1962) by utilising the gradual rate of hydrolysis of the piperidine ring in alkali. It may be estimated spectrophotometrically in vomitus (Phang *et al.*, 1961).
The main metabolite of glutethimide, α-phenylglutarimide, may be estimated colorimetrically following the formation of a hydroxamic acid derivative which then forms a purple complex with ferric ions (Sheppard *et al.*, 1956).
Goldbaum and Domanski (1966) have described a procedure, involving gas chromatography, for extraction and quantitative determination applicable to glutethimide in biological fluids and tissues.

Metabolism. Glutethimide is hydroxylated and the metabolites formed are excreted as conjugates; α-phenylglutarimide may also be formed—see The Metabolism of Drugs, p. 158.
Following the ingestion of 1 g of glutethimide, blood-levels of 0·28 mg% after 1 hour, 0·62 mg% after 2 hours, 0·5 mg% after 12 hours, 0·26 mg% after 24 hours, and 0·13 mg% after 48 hours were obtained (Algeri *et al.*, 1960).
Glutethimide may be found in the fat in high concentrations; it rapidly enters the kidneys and liver from the plasma (Goldbaum *et al.*, 1962).

Dose. Up to 1 g daily has been given.

Toxicity. The estimated minimum lethal dose of glutethimide is 5 g, although recoveries have occurred after the ingestion of up to 10 g. Blood-levels of about 3 mg% and over are indicative of serious poisoning.
CASE EXAMPLES. (1) A 56-year-old man died less than 24 hours after the ingestion of 15 g of glutethimide; the urine contained 34·2 mg% of the metabolite, α-phenylglutarimide. (2) A 23-year-old man died about 32 hours after the ingestion of about 12 g of glutethimide; the urine contained 24·2 mg% of the metabolite, α-phenylglutarimide. (3) A 40-year-old woman was found dead after the ingestion of up to 50 g of glutethimide; the urine contained 42 mg% of the metabolite, α-phenylglutarimide. (4) A 24-year-old woman recovered following the ingestion of 8·5 g of glutethimide; thirty-four hours later the urine contained 15 mg% of the metabolite, α-phenylglutarimide (McBay and Katsas, 1957).
(1) After the fatal ingestion of 15 g of glutethimide, the following post-mortem levels were obtained: blood, 4 mg%; liver, 12·2 mg%. (2) After the fatal ingestion of 12 g of glutethimide, the following post-mortem levels were obtained: blood, 7 mg%; liver, 18 mg%. (3) After the fatal ingestion of 50 g of glutethimide, the following post-mortem levels were obtained: blood, 1·1 mg%; liver, 18·8 mg% (Algeri *et al.*, 1960).
On admission to hospital 12 hours after the ingestion of 10 g of glutethimide, a patient was found to have a glutethimide plasma-level of 4·5 mg%. Twelve hours later the level had dropped to 3·15 mg%, 39 hours later to 1 mg%, and after 59 hours to only 0·35 mg% (Goldbaum *et al.*, 1960).

GLYCERYL TRINITRATE

Coronary Vasodilator

Synonyms: Glonoin; Nitroglycerin; Nitroglycerol; Trinitrin; Trinitroglycerin.

Proprietary Names: Angised; Antipressan; Cardamist; Nitrocine; Nitroglyn; Sustac.

$C_3H_5N_3O_9$ = 227·1

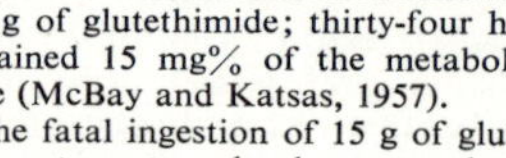

Dense, opaque, slightly volatile, oily liquid, appearing white but transparent when dehydrated. It explodes on rapid heating or on percussion.

Solubility. Soluble 1 in 800 of water and 1 in 4 of ethanol; miscible with ether and chloroform.

CAUTION. ***In ethanolic solution it is unstable and should be handled with the utmost caution.***

Extraction. Glyceryl trinitrate is extracted from blood and urine with n-hexane (Williams *et al.*, 1966).

Quantitative Estimation. Glyceryl trinitrate may be quantitatively determined in blood and urine by gas chromatography (Williams *et al.*, 1966). Blood-levels of nitrate ions and nitrite ions may be determined spectrophotometrically by the method of Lorenzetti *et al.* (1966). Lloyd (1967) has described the detection of microgram quantities of glyceryl trinitrate.

Metabolism. Glyceryl trinitrate has been shown to release both nitrate and nitrite ions into the blood-stream. It has been suggested that nitrate esters may be reduced to nitrite esters before hydrolysis, leading to the release of nitrite ions. Both glyceryl 1,2- and 1,3-dinitrate have been detected in the urine after the administration of glyceryl trinitrate (Needleman and Krantz, 1965).
Following oral administration in rabbits, nitrate and nitrite blood-concentrations reached peak levels within 90 to 120 minutes, then slowly returned to control levels; 60 minutes after either oral or intravenous administration of glyceryl trinitrate, blood-nitrate levels were almost twice the blood-nitrite levels (Lorenzetti *et al.*, 1966).

Dose. Up to 1 mg.

Toxicity. Ingestion of 2 g has been reported to have proved fatal. Chronic glyceryl trinitrate poisoning may occur in industry but tolerance develops when it is regularly handled. The maximum permissible concentration of glyceryl trinitrate in a factory atmosphere is 0·5 p.p.m. The oral minimum lethal dose in rats is 80 to 100 mg/kg.

GLYCOPYRRONIUM BROMIDE

Parasympatholytic

Synonyms: AHR 504; Glycopyrrolate.
Proprietary Names: Nodapton; Robinul; Tarodyn.

3-(α-Cyclopentyl-α-phenylglycolloyloxy)-1,1-dimethylpyrrolidinium bromide
$C_{18}H_{25}NO_3,CH_3Br = 398{\cdot}3$

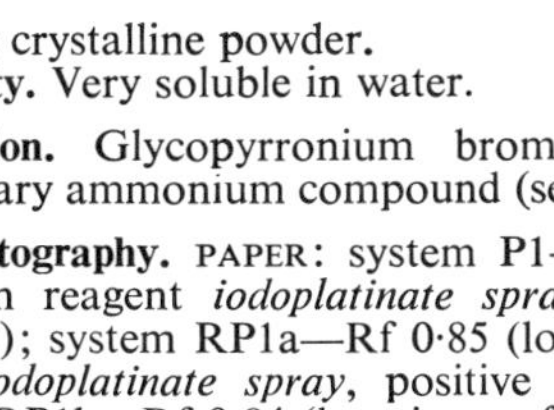

A white crystalline powder.
Solubility. Very soluble in water.

Extraction. Glycopyrronium bromide is a quaternary ammonium compound (see p. 29).

Chromatography. PAPER: system P1—Rf 0·50 (location reagent *iodoplatinate spray*, strong reaction); system RP1a—Rf 0·85 (location reagent *iodoplatinate spray*, positive reaction); system RP1b—Rf 0·84 (location as for RP1a). THIN-LAYER: system T1—Rf 0·03 (location reagent *acidified iodoplatinate spray*, positive reaction).

Crystal Tests. MICRO: *gold bromide solution*—leaflike plates, best viewed under polarised light (*sensitivity:* 1 in 1000); *gold chloride solution*—irregular plates, best viewed under polarised light (*sensitivity:* 1 in 1000).

Ultraviolet Absorption Spectrum. Glycopyrronium bromide in 0·1N sulphuric acid, maxima at 251 mμ (E1%, 1cm 7·4), 257·5 mμ (E1%, 1cm 7·8) and 263 mμ (E1%, 1cm 6·4).

Dose. Up to 6 mg daily has been given.

Toxicity. The lethal dose in man is probably between 10 and 100 mg/kg.

GRISEOFULVIN

Antibiotic/Antifungal

Synonym: Curling Factor.
Proprietary Names: Fulcin; Fulvicin; Grifulvin; Grisactin; Grisovin; Lamoryl.

7-Chloro-4,6,2′-trimethoxy-6′-methylspiro[benzofuran-2(3*H*),1′-cyclohex-2′-ene]-3,4′-dione
$C_{17}H_{17}ClO_6 = 352{\cdot}8$

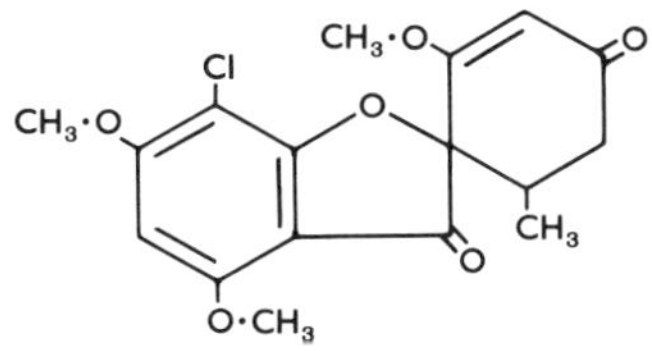

A colourless to white powder which occurs as griseofulvin (coarse particle) with particles mostly about 30 μ in diameter and as griseofulvin (fine particle) with particles mostly less than 5 μ in diameter. M.p. 218° to 224°. Specific rotation of a 1% solution in dimethylformamide, +354° to +364°.
Solubility. Soluble 1 in 1000 of water, 1 in 300 of dehydrated ethanol, and 1 in 25 of chloroform.

Extraction. Griseofulvin is extracted by organic solvents from aqueous acid or alkaline solutions.

Colour Test. Dissolve 5 mg in 1 ml of *sulphuric acid* and add 5 mg of powdered potassium dichromate—wine-red.

Ultraviolet Absorption Spectrum. Griseofulvin in ethanol, maximum at about 291 mμ (E1%, 1cm 686).

Quantitative Estimation. Griseofulvin may be quantitatively determined in blood by spectrofluorimetry (Bedford *et al.*, 1959; Duncan *et al.*, 1962; Kraml *et al.*, 1965).

Metabolism. Several metabolites of griseofulvin have been detected in the liver and urine of rats. The 2 major ones have been identified as 6- and 4-demethylgriseofulvin; both were present in the free and conjugated forms, more of the 4-demethyl derivative being conjugated.
In man, griseofulvin is absorbed from the gastro-intestinal tract following oral administration and is deposited in the deeper layers of the skin and the keratin of the nails and hair. Following single oral doses of 1 g, peak serum-levels were attained after 4 hours and traces of the drug were still present after 72 hours. Four hours after doses of 0·25 to 3 g, serum levels

have been reported to range from 0·03 to 0·17 mg%. Small amounts are excreted unchanged in the urine and faeces and some is excreted in the sweat.

Dose. Up to 1 g daily of the fine particle variety.

GUANETHIDINE *Antihypertensive*

Synonym: SU 5864.

1-(2-Guanidinoethyl)octahydroazocine

$C_{10}H_{22}N_4$ = 198·3

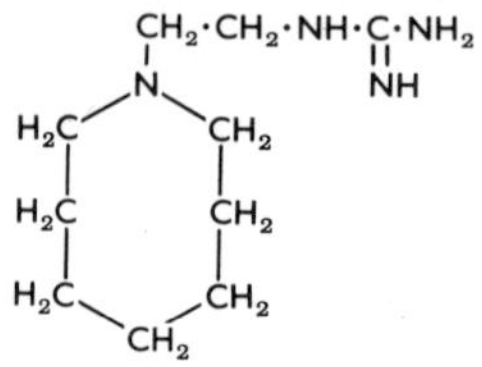

GUANETHIDINE SULPHATE

Proprietary Name: Ismelin.

A colourless crystalline powder. M.p. 251° to 256°.
Solubility. Soluble 1 in 1·5 of water; slightly soluble in ethanol; insoluble in ether and chloroform.

Extraction. Guanethidine is very soluble in water—for a discussion on the method of extraction see under Extraction Methods, Water-soluble Compounds, p. 28.

Chromatography. PAPER: system P1—Rf 0·03 (location reagents: *iodoplatinate spray*, strong reaction; *bromocresol green spray*, weak reaction); system RP1a—Rf 0·83 (location reagent *iodoplatinate spray*, positive reaction); system RP1b—Rf 0·82 (location as for RP1a).
THIN-LAYER: system T1—Rf 0·05 (location reagent *acidified iodoplatinate spray*, positive reaction).

Crystal Tests. MICRO: *picric acid*—branching rods or blades (*sensitivity:* 1 in 400); *platinic chloride solution*—small plates (*sensitivity:* 1 in 400).

Ultraviolet Absorption Spectrum. Guanethidine in 0·1N sulphuric acid, inflexions at 235 mμ (E1%, 1 cm 0·4), and 241 mμ (E1%, 1 cm 0·36), and a maximum at 306 mμ (E1%, 1 cm 0·12).

Quantitative Estimation. Tompsett *et al.* (1961) and Tompsett (1962) describe a method of extraction from serum and urine and subsequent quantitative determination—see under Extraction Methods, Water-soluble Compounds, p. 28. Bose and Vijayvargiya (1964) describe a spectrophotometric method for the estimation of guanethidine.

Metabolism. The amount of guanethidine excreted unchanged in the urine following oral ingestion appears to be quite small; after the administration of 200 mg orally, 38 mg was found in the urine within 24 hours, representing a recovery of 19%. After the administration of 30 mg, 4 mg (13·3%) was recovered in the urine (Tompsett *et al.*, 1961).

Guanethidine is administered orally but its effect may not be apparent for 2 or 3 days and may persist for several days after withdrawal of the drug.

Dose. Up to 10 mg initially, gradually increasing, as necessary, to a maximum of 300 mg.

GUANOCLOR *Antihypertensive*

Synonym: Compound 1029.

N-[2-(2,6-Dichlorophenoxy)ethylamino]guanidine

$C_9H_{12}Cl_2N_4O$ = 263·1

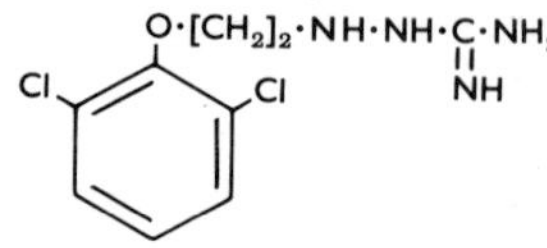

GUANOCLOR SULPHATE

Proprietary Name: Vatensol.

A white crystalline powder. M.p. 207° to 209°.
Solubility. Soluble 1 in 400 of water.

Extraction. Guanoclor is extracted by organic solvents from aqueous alkaline solutions.

Chromatography. PAPER: system P1—Rf 0·56 (location reagents: *iodoplatinate spray*, white; *bromocresol green spray*, weak reaction).
THIN-LAYER: system T1—Rf 0·48, streaking (location reagent *acidified iodoplatinate spray*, positive reaction).

Colour Tests. MICRO: ammonium vanadate test —(green) bright purple → orange-brown → yellow (*sensitivity:* 0·25 μg); Vitali's test— –/–/faint yellow (*sensitivity:* 1·0 μg).

Crystal Tests. MICRO: *platinic iodide solution*—masses of blades (*sensitivity:* 1 in 1000); *potassium mercuric iodide solution*—large plates, often twinned (*sensitivity:* 1 in 1000).

Ultraviolet Absorption Spectrum. Guanoclor in 0·1N sulphuric acid, maxima at 271 mμ (E1%, 1 cm 9·2) and about 277 mμ (E1%, 1 cm 8·1).

Dose. Adjusted according to the patient's needs; up to 200 mg daily has been given.

GUANOXAN *Antihypertensive*

2-Guanidinomethyl-1,4-benzodioxan

$C_{10}H_{13}N_3O_2$ = 207·2

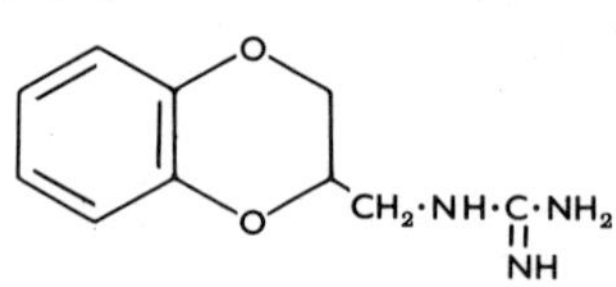

GUANOXAN SULPHATE

Proprietary Name: Envacar.

A white crystalline powder. M.p. 204° to 208°.
Solubility. Soluble 1 in 50 of water.

Extraction. Guanoxan is extracted by organic solvents from aqueous alkaline solutions.

Chromatography. PAPER: system P1—Rf 0·38 (location under ultraviolet light, absorption; location reagents: *bromocresol green spray*, weak reaction; *potassium permanganate spray*, weak reaction).
THIN-LAYER: system T1—Rf 0·43, streaking (location reagent *potassium permanganate spray*, positive reaction).

Colour Tests. MICRO: sulphuric acid–formaldehyde test—deep purple (*sensitivity:* 0·1 μg); ammonium molybdate test—dull blue → green (*sensitivity:* 0·1 μg); ammonium vanadate test—green, sometimes purple, depending on the relative proportions of test material and reagent (*sensitivity:* 0·25 μg).

Crystal Tests. MICRO: *platinic iodide solution*—bunches of blades (*sensitivity:* 1 in 1000); *styphnic acid*—dense rosettes (*sensitivity:* 1 in 1000).

Ultraviolet Absorption Spectrum. Guanoxan in 0·1N sulphuric acid, maximum at 275 mμ (E1%, 1 cm 92) and inflexion at about 280 mμ.

Dose. Adjusted according to the patient's needs; up to 120 mg daily has been given.

HALOPERIDOL *Tranquilliser*

Synonyms: Haloperiodole; R 1625.
Proprietary Names: Haldol; Serenace.

γ-[4-(*p*-Chlorophenyl)-4-hydroxypiperidino]-*p*-fluorobutyrophenone
$C_{21}H_{23}ClFNO_2$ = 375·9

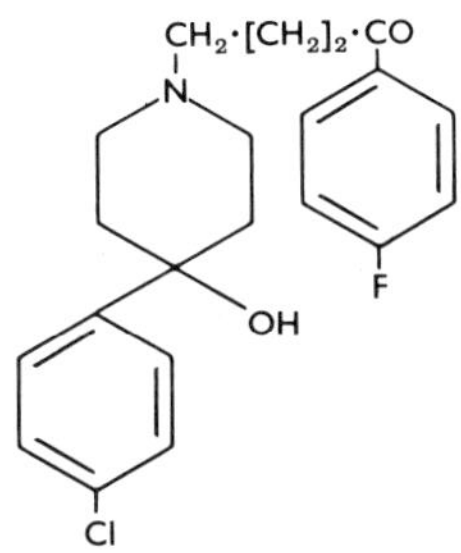

A white microcrystalline powder. M.p. 147° to 149°.
Solubility. Almost insoluble in water; soluble 1 in 55 of ethanol, 1 in 200 of ether, and 1 in 15 of chloroform.

Extraction. Haloperidol is extracted by organic solvents from aqueous alkaline solutions.

Chromatography. PAPER: system P1—Rf 0·84 (location under ultraviolet light, strong absorption; location reagents: *iodoplatinate spray*, strong reaction; *bromocresol green spray*, weak reaction); system RP1a—Rf 0·61 (location under ultraviolet light, absorption; location reagent *iodoplatinate spray*, positive reaction); system RP1b—Rf 0·00 (location reagent *iodoplatinate spray*, positive reaction).
THIN-LAYER: system T1—Rf 0·69 (location reagent *acidified iodoplatinate spray*, positive reaction).

Colour Test. MICRO: ammonium molybdate test—faint grey-blue (*sensitivity:* 1·0 μg).

Crystal Tests. MICRO: *mercuric chloride solution*—bundles of rods (*sensitivity:* 1 in 200); *potassium tri-iodide solution* (*1*)—small plates and needles, best viewed under polarised light (*sensitivity:* 1 in 400).

Ultraviolet Absorption Spectrum. Haloperidol in 0·1N hydrochloric acid:isopropanol (1:9), maxima at 220 mμ and 244 mμ; minimum at about 231 mμ: in 0·1N sulphuric acid, maxima at 220·5 mμ (E1%, 1 cm 393) and 248 mμ (E1%, 1 cm 346).

Infra-red Absorption Spectrum. Potassium bromide disk. The principal peaks are: A 832, B 1151, C 1217 or 1673 (p. 741).

Metabolism. Studies in rats (Soudijn *et al.*, 1967) have shown that oxidative *N*-dealkylation appears to be a major metabolic pathway giving rise to β-(*p*-fluorobenzoyl)propionic acid, which is rapidly metabolised to *p*-fluorophenylacetic acid and its glycine conjugate, *p*-fluorophenaceturic acid. When tritium-labelled haloperidol was injected subcutaneously, 20 to 30% of the excreted radioactivity in the urine was in the form of *p*-fluorophenylacetic acid while 60 to 70% was in the form of the glycine conjugate. Following oral administration of tritium-labelled haloperidol in rats (Braun *et al.*, 1967), the drug was rapidly absorbed; about 50% of the radioactivity was excreted in the urine and the other 50% in the faeces; in 24 hours about 33% of the dose was excreted in the urine. After 3 hours most of the radioactivity was concentrated in the liver.

Dose. Usually up to 10 mg daily.

HALOPYRAMINE *Antihistamine*

Synonyms: Chloropyramine; Chlorotripelennamine.

N-*p*-Chlorobenzyl-*N′N′*-dimethyl-*N*-pyrid-2-yl-ethylenediamine
$C_{16}H_{20}ClN_3$ = 289·8

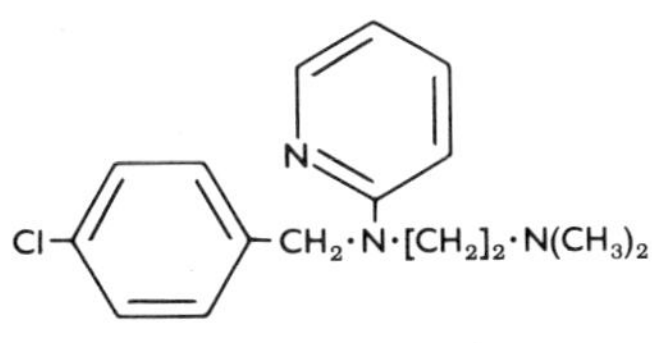

A yellow oil.

HALOPYRAMINE HYDROCHLORIDE
Proprietary Names: Synopen; Synpen.

A white powder. M.p. 172°.
Solubility. Readily soluble in water.

Extraction. Halopyramine is extracted by organic solvents from aqueous alkaline solutions.

Chromatography. PAPER: system P1—Rf 0·45 (location under ultraviolet light, blue fluorescence; location reagents: *iodoplatinate spray*, strong reaction; *bromocresol green spray*, weak reaction); system RP1a—Rf 0·58 (location under ultraviolet light, blue fluorescence; location reagent *iodoplatinate spray*, positive reaction); system RP1b—Rf 0·04 (location as for RP1a).
THIN-LAYER: system T1—Rf 0·48 (location reagent *acidified iodoplatinate spray*, positive reaction).

Crystal Tests. MICRO: *gold bromide–hydrochloric acid solution*—irregular rosettes and rods (*sensitivity:* 1 in 1000); *lead iodide solution*—rosettes of needles (*sensitivity:* 1 in 1000).

Ultraviolet Absorption Spectrum. Halopyramine in 0·1N sulphuric acid, maxima at 221·5 mμ (E1%, 1cm 409), 238·5 mμ (E1%, 1cm 517), and 314 mμ (E1%, 1cm 282).

Infra-red Absorption Spectrum. Halopyramine (base). Potassium bromide disk. The principal peaks are: A 1494, B 1598, C 1442 (p. 787).

Dose. Up to 150 mg daily.

HALOTHANE *General Anaesthetic*

Proprietary Name: Fluothane.

2-Bromo-2-chloro-1,1,1-trifluoroethane
$C_2HBrClF_3 = 197{\cdot}4$

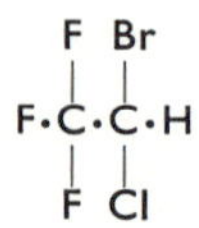

A colourless, mobile, non-inflammable, heavy liquid. B.p. 49° to 51°. Refractive index, at 20°, 1·3695 to 1·3705.
Solubility. Soluble 1 in 400 of water; miscible with ethanol, ether, and chloroform.

Extraction. Halothane is extracted by organic solvents from aqueous acid or alkaline solutions; it is volatile and may also be isolated by distillation (see p. 18).

Chromatography. GAS: system G8/160—retention time 1·62 relative to n-propanol.

Quantitative Estimation. Halothane in the blood and tissues may be determined spectrophotometrically (Duncan, 1959; Burns and Snow, 1961). It may also be determined by gas chromatography (Butler and Hill, 1961; Butler and Freeman, 1962).

Metabolism. Following the inhalation of halothane, the concentration in the arterial blood increases rapidly and is maintained for about 6 hours. There is a rapid accumulation of halothane in the adipose tissue. Little if any metabolism occurs; halothane is excreted in the expired air.

Use. Concentrations of up to 3% in oxygen or oxygen-nitrous oxide are commonly used for anaesthesia.

Toxicity. Ingestion of 10 ml has proved fatal. A contaminant of halothane, dichlorohexafluorobutene, is liable to be dangerous in animal anaesthesia since the species lethal range is very close to the clinical concentrations used (Cohen *et al.*, 1965).

HARMALINE *Hallucinogen*

3,4-Dihydroharmine
$C_{13}H_{14}N_2O = 214{\cdot}3$

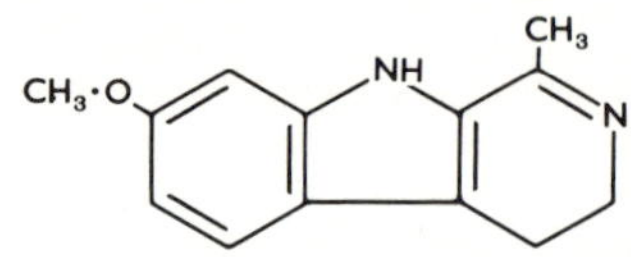

An alkaloid present in plants of the family Malpighiaceae and in the seeds of *Peganum harmala* (Rutaceae). It is found together with harmine in the South American narcotic drink 'caapi'. It melts at 249° to 250°, with decomposition.
Solubility. Slightly soluble in water, ethanol, and ether.

Extraction. Harmaline is extracted by organic solvents from aqueous alkaline solutions.

Chromatography. PAPER: system P1—Rf 0·39 (location under ultraviolet light, green fluorescence; location reagent *iodoplatinate spray*, strong reaction).
THIN-LAYER: system T1—Rf 0·38 (location reagent *acidified iodoplatinate spray*, positive reaction).

Colour Tests. MICRO: sulphuric acid–formaldehyde test—(yellow) brownish-green (*sensitivity:* 1·0 μg); ammonium molybdate test—(yellow) green (*sensitivity:* 0·5 μg); ammonium vanadate test—(yellow) olive-brown (*sensitivity:* 1·0 μg); Vitali's test— -/yellow/brown (*sensitivity:* 0·5 μg).

Crystal Tests. MICRO: *platinic chloride solution*—small fern-like crystals (*sensitivity:* 1 in 1000); *potassium chromate solution*—clusters of prisms (*sensitivity:* 1 in 1000).

Ultraviolet Absorption Spectrum. Harmaline in methanol, maxima at 218 mμ (E1%, 1cm 676), 260 mμ (E1%, 1cm 288), 344 mμ (E1%, 1cm 468), and 376 mμ (E1%, 1cm 380).

Toxicity. LD50 (subcutaneous): in rats 120 mg/kg.

HARMAN

Synonyms: Aribine; Harmane; Loturine; 1-Methyl-β-carboline; 1-Methylnorharman.

1-Methyl-9-pyrid[3,4-*b*]indole
$C_{12}H_{10}N_2 = 182{\cdot}2$

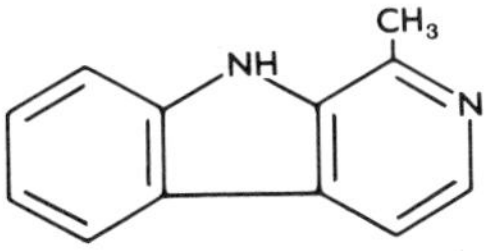

Harman occurs as crystals which melt at about 238°.

Solubility. Sparingly soluble in hot water; soluble in ethanol, ether, and chloroform.

Extraction. Harman is extracted by organic solvents from aqueous alkaline solutions.

Chromatography. PAPER: system P1—Rf 0·42 (location under ultraviolet light, blue fluorescence; location reagent *iodoplatinate spray*, strong reaction); system RP1a—Rf 0·50 (location under ultraviolet light, blue fluorescence; location reagent *iodoplatinate spray*, positive reaction); system RP1b—Rf 0·09 (location as for RP1a).

THIN-LAYER: system T1—Rf 0·70 (location reagent *acidified iodoplatinate spray*, positive reaction).

Colour Tests. MICRO: sulphuric acid–formaldehyde test—green (*sensitivity:* 0·5 μg); ammonium vanadate test—green (*sensitivity:* 0·5 μg); Vitali's test— –/–/orange-red (*sensitivity:* 0·5 μg).

Crystal Tests. MICRO: *gold bromide solution*—small needles (*sensitivity:* 1 in 400); *mercuric chloride solution*—bunches of needles (*sensitivity:* 1 in 400).

Ultraviolet Absorption Spectrum. Harman in 0·1N sulphuric acid, maxima at 245 mμ, 300 mμ, and about 358 mμ.

NOTE. Harman occurs naturally in some plants and it may be found in tobacco smoke and in home-made wine. It may also be found as a putrefactive base, particularly in cases where embalming has taken place. It is a condensation product of tryptophan and acetaldehyde.

HARMINE *Hallucinogen*

7-Methoxy-1-methyl-9-pyrid[3,4-*b*]indole
$C_{13}H_{12}N_2O = 212{\cdot}3$

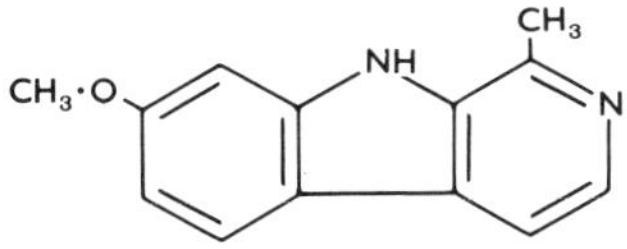

An alkaloid present in plants of the family Malpighiaceae and in the seeds of *Peganum harmala* (Rutaceae). It is found together with harmaline in the South American narcotic drink 'caapi'. It melts at 261°, with decomposition or sublimation.

Solubility. Slightly soluble in water, ethanol, ether, and chloroform.

Extraction. Harmine is extracted by organic solvents from aqueous alkaline solutions.

Chromatography. PAPER: system P1—Rf 0·37 (location under ultraviolet light, bright blue fluorescence; location reagent *iodoplatinate spray*, strong reaction).

THIN-LAYER: system T1—Rf 0·68 (location reagent *acidified iodoplatinate spray*, positive reaction).

GAS: system G2/225—retention time 0·67 relative to codeine.

Colour Tests. MICRO: sulphuric acid–formaldehyde test—orange (*sensitivity:* 0·025 μg); ammonium molybdate test—green (*sensitivity:* 0·1 μg); ammonium vanadate test—blue → green (*sensitivity:* 0·1 μg); Vitali's test—pale green/green/red (*sensitivity:* 0·1 μg).

Crystal Tests. MICRO: *gold chloride solution*—rods (*sensitivity:* 1 in 3000); *potassium iodide solution*—needles (*sensitivity:* 1 in 3000).

Ultraviolet Absorption Spectrum. Harmine in 0·1N sulphuric acid, maxima at 246·5 mμ (E1%, 1 cm 1942), 319 mμ (E1%, 1 cm 988), and 366 mμ (E1%, 1 cm 303).

Toxicity. By injection, 150 to 200 mg in man can produce hallucinations; by mouth, 300 to 400 mg will produce psychotic symptoms. The minimum lethal dose by subcutaneous injection in rats is 200 mg/kg.

HEPTABARBITONE *Barbiturate*

Synonyms: Heptabarb; Heptabarbital.
Proprietary Name: Medomin.

5-Cyclohept-1′-enyl-5-ethylbarbituric acid
$C_{13}H_{18}N_2O_3 = 250{\cdot}3$

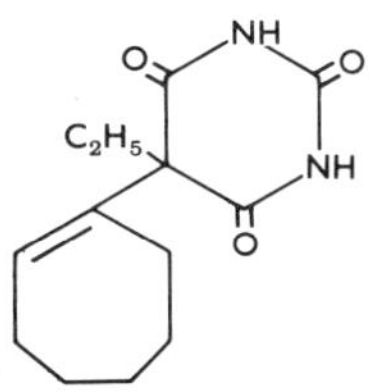

A white crystalline powder. M.p. 172°.

Solubility. Very sparingly soluble in water; soluble 1 in 30 of ethanol and 1 in 75 of chloroform; soluble in ether.

Screening Tests. See under Barbiturates, p. 208.

Extraction. Heptabarbitone may be isolated in the A2 fraction (see p. 27).

Chromatography. PAPER: system P2—Rf 0·58 relative to amylobarbitone (location under ultraviolet light, dark spot); system RP1b—Rf 0·18 (location under ultraviolet light after exposure to ammonia; location reagent *potassium permanganate spray*, yellow on pink).

THIN-LAYER: system T10—Rf 0·31 (location

reagents: *mercurous nitrate spray*, black; *potassium permanganate spray*, yellow-brown; *Zwikker's reagent spray*, pink).

GAS: system G5—retention time 10·5 relative to barbitone.

Ultraviolet Absorption Spectrum. Heptabarbitone is a 5,5-derivative—see Screening Test 3 under Barbiturates, p. 208.

Quantitative Estimation. See under Barbiturates, p. 208.

Metabolism. Heptabarbitone is a short-acting barbiturate—see under Barbiturates, p. 207. It may be oxidised in man to a cycloheptenone, 5-(3-oxo-1,2-cycloheptenyl)-5-ethylbarbituric acid, the oxygen atom probably being located on the carbon atom adjacent to the double bond (Pulver, 1943). Although the unchanged drug does not appear in the urine, the production of this metabolite may not represent a major metabolic pathway because it accounts for only 1% of the dose in man (Mark, 1963).

Dose. Up to 600 mg has been given.

Toxicity. The estimated minimum lethal dose in man is 2 g.

HEPTACHLOR *Pesticide*

Other Names: Ceresol; Master Brand Ant Killer; Heptasan; Velsicol 104.

1,4,5,6,7,8,8-Heptachloro-3a,4,7,7a-tetrahydro-4,7(*endo*)-methanoindene

$C_{10}H_5Cl_7 = 373·3$

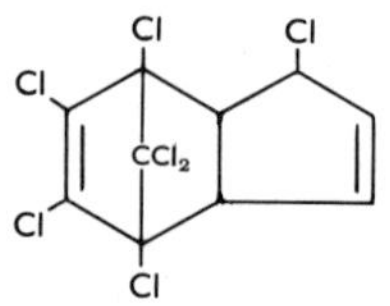

The pure substance is a white crystalline solid and the technical grade is a soft waxy solid which contains 72% of heptachlor and 28% of related compounds. Heptachlor may be found as an impurity in chlordane (p. 247). M.p. 95° to 96°.

Solubility. Almost insoluble in water; soluble 1 in 22 of ethanol and 1 in 5·3 of kerosene.

Extraction. Heptachlor is extracted by organic solvents from aqueous acid or alkaline solutions.

Quantitative Estimation. Heptachlor and heptachlor epoxide may be determined by gas chromatography (Jain *et al.*, 1965; Hamence *et al.*, 1965).

Metabolism. Heptachlor accumulates mainly in the fat as the metabolite, heptachlor epoxide (m.p. 157° to 159·5°).

HETERONIUM BROMIDE *Parasympatholytic*

Proprietary Name: Hetrum Bromide.

1,1-Dimethyl-3-[α-phenyl-α-(thien-2-yl)glycolloyloxy]pyrrolidinium bromide

$C_{18}H_{22}BrNO_3S = 412·4$

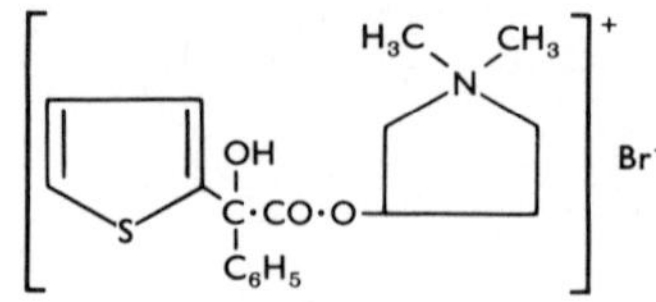

A white crystalline powder. M.p. 182° to 184°.

Solubility. Very soluble in water and ethanol.

Extraction. Heteronium bromide is a quaternary ammonium compound (see p. 29).

Chromatography. PAPER: system P1—Rf 0·44 (location under ultraviolet light, strong absorption; location reagent *iodoplatinate spray*, strong reaction).

THIN-LAYER: system T1—Rf 0·03 (location reagent *acidified iodoplatinate spray*, positive reaction).

Crystal Tests. MICRO: *lead iodide solution*—dense rosettes (*sensitivity:* 1 in 1000); *platinic chloride solution*—dense rosettes or bunches of prisms (*sensitivity:* 1 in 400).

Ultraviolet Absorption Spectrum. Heteronium bromide in 0·1N sulphuric acid, maximum at 234 mμ (E1%, 1 cm 235).

Infra-red Absorption Spectrum. Potassium bromide disk. The principal peaks are: A 1735, B 1219, C 1085 (p. 787).

HEXACHLOROPHANE *Antiseptic*

Synonyms: G 11; K 34; Hexachlorophene.

2,2′-Methylenebis(3,4,6-trichlorophenol)

$C_{13}H_6Cl_6O_2 = 406·9$

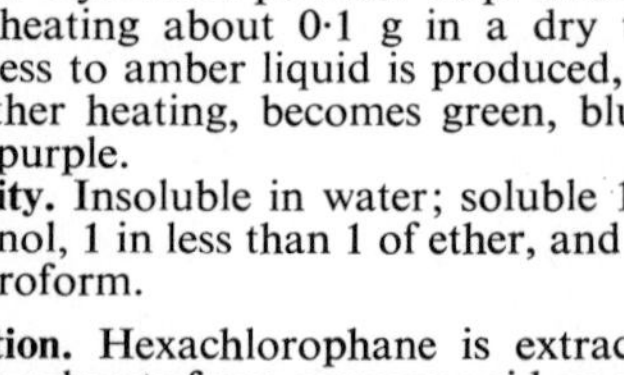

A white crystalline powder. M.p. about 164°. Upon heating about 0·1 g in a dry tube, a colourless to amber liquid is produced, which, on further heating, becomes green, blue, and finally purple.

Solubility. Insoluble in water; soluble 1 in 3·5 of ethanol, 1 in less than 1 of ether, and 1 in 25 of chloroform.

Extraction. Hexachlorophane is extracted by organic solvents from aqueous acid or alkaline solutions.

Chromatography. GAS: system G2/225—retention time 3·24 relative to codeine.

Colour Tests. Add 0·5 ml of *ferric chloride solution* to an ethanolic solution—transient purple colour is immediately produced. Dissolve 0·1 g in 0·5 ml of acetone, add *titanous chloride solution* and shake—yellowish-orange oil separates which is soluble in benzene, chloroform, and ether.

Ultraviolet Absorption Spectrum. Hexachlorophane in ethanol, maxima at 293 mμ (E1%, 1 cm 140) and 300 mμ (E1%, 1 cm 152); in 0·1N sodium hydroxide, maxima at 249 mμ (E1%, 1 cm 402) and 320 mμ (E1%, 1 cm 303).

Infra-red Absorption Spectrum. Potassium bromide disk. The principal peaks are: A 1442, B 1182 or 1276 (p. 742).

Quantitative Estimation. Johnston and Porcaro (1964) describe a method for the separation and spectrophotometric determination of hexachlorophane from biological material.

Use. It is chiefly used as an antiseptic in soaps and creams in a concentration of 1 to 3%.

Dose. Up to 20 mg/kg has been given in the treatment of clonorchiasis.

Toxicity. Side-effects have frequently followed the oral administration of therapeutic doses of 20 mg/kg. Recoveries have occurred following the accidental ingestion of up to 90 ml of a preparation containing 3% of hexachlorophane; the fatal dose in man is estimated to be between 2 and 10 g of hexachlorophane (Wear *et al.*, 1962).

HEXAMETHONIUM BROMIDE

Antihypertensive

Synonyms: Hexamethone Bromide; Hexonium Bromide.
Proprietary Names: Bistrium Bromide; Vegolysen.

Hexamethylenebis(trimethylammonium bromide)

$C_{12}H_{30}Br_2N_2 = 362{\cdot}2$

$$[(CH_3)_3N \cdot [CH_2]_6 \cdot N(CH_3)_3]^{2+}\ 2Br^-$$

A white hygroscopic powder. M.p. about 280°, with decomposition.
Solubility. Soluble 1 in less than 1 of water and 1 in 60 of ethanol; insoluble in ether and chloroform.

HEXAMETHONIUM TARTRATE

Synonyms: Hexamethonium Acid Tartrate; Hexamethonium Bitartrate.
Proprietary Name: Vegolysen T.

A white hygroscopic powder. M.p. about 186°, with decomposition.
Solubility. Soluble 1 in 0·7 of water and 1 in 500 of ethanol.

Extraction. The hexamethonium salts are quaternary ammonium compounds—for a discussion on the method of extraction see under Extraction Methods, Water-soluble Compounds, p. 28.

Chromatography. PAPER: system P1—Rf 0·00 (location reagent *iodoplatinate spray*, strong reaction); system RP1a—Rf 1·00 (location reagent *iodoplatinate spray*, positive reaction); system RP1b—Rf 1·00 (location as for RP1a). THIN-LAYER: system T1—Rf 0·00 (location reagent *acidified iodoplatinate spray*, positive reaction).

Crystal Tests. MICRO: *potassium chromate solution*—bunches of branching rods (*sensitivity:* 1 in 400); *potassium permanganate solution*—masses of blades or elongated plates (*sensitivity:* 1 in 1000).

Infra-red Absorption Spectrum. Hexamethonium bromide. Potassium bromide disk. The principal peaks are: A 913, B 1481, C 945 or 970 or 1630 (p. 787).

Quantitative Estimation. Hexamethonium salts in biological fluids may be determined spectrophotometrically following the formation of the reineckate salt (Harington, 1953) or following the formation of a complex with bromothymol blue (Ballard *et al.*, 1954). Tompsett *et al.* (1961) and Tompsett (1962) describe a method of extraction from serum and urine and subsequent quantitative determination—see under Extraction Methods, Water-soluble Compounds, p. 28.

Metabolism. Hexamethonium salts undergo little if any metabolism in the body. Harington (1953) found that the larger part of an oral dose in man was poorly absorbed from the gastro-intestinal tract and excreted unchanged mainly in the faeces; in 24 hours the total amount recovered from the urine did not exceed 10% of the dose. After parenteral administration, about 90% of a single dose could be recovered in the urine within 24 hours; excretion was more rapid after intravenous than after intramuscular or subcutaneous injection, 25 to 30% of the dose appearing in the first hour.

Dose. Hexamethonium bromide is usually given subcutaneously or intramuscularly in an initial dose of 5 to 15 mg gradually increasing, as necessary, up to a maximum of 500 mg daily; when it is given by mouth some patients may need a dose of 1 to 3 g; 14 mg of hexamethonium tartrate is approximately equivalent to 10 mg of hexamethonium bromide.

Toxicity. Hexamethonium exaggerates the blood-sugar-reducing action of insulin and, in the anaesthetised diabetic patient, it can mask many of the signs of severe hypoglycaemia induced by insulin. Continued ingestion of hexamethonium bromide may lead to bromism.

HEXETIDINE

Antimicrobial

Proprietary Names: Sterisil; Sterisol.

5 - Amino - 1,3 - di(2 - ethylhexyl)hexahydro - 5 - methylpyrimidine
$C_{21}H_{45}N_3$ = 339·6

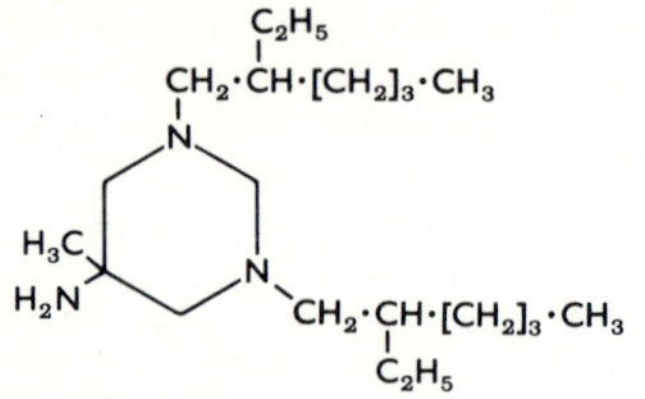

A viscous oil. B.p. 160° at 0·4 mm Hg. Refractive index 1·466.
Solubility. Soluble 1 in 10,000 of water; miscible with ethanol; soluble in ether, methanol, and benzene.

Extraction. Hexetidine is extracted by organic solvents from aqueous alkaline solutions.

Chromatography. PAPER: system P1—Rf 0·90 (location reagents: *iodoplatinate spray*, strong reaction, white; *bromocresol green spray*, strong reaction; *potassium permanganate spray*, weak reaction).

THIN-LAYER: system T1—Rf 0·70 (location reagent *acidified iodoplatinate spray*, positive reaction).

Ultraviolet Absorption Spectrum. Hexetidine in 0·1N sulphuric acid, maximum at 225 mμ (E1%, 1cm 11·1).

Infra-red Absorption Spectrum. Capillary film between potassium bromide windows. The principal peaks are: A 1455 or 1468, B 1093, C 1375 (p. 787).

Use. It has been applied intravaginally, usually as a 0·1% gel, in the treatment of vaginal infections.

HEXOBARBITONE *Barbiturate*

Synonyms: Enhexymalum; Enimal; Hexobarbital; Methexenyl; Methyl-cyclohexenyl-methyl-barbituric Acid; Methylhexabarbital; Narcosanum.
Proprietary Names: Cyclonal; Evipal; Evipan; Sombulex; Somnalert.

5-Cyclohex-1′-enyl-1,5-dimethylbarbituric acid
$C_{12}H_{16}N_2O_3$ = 236·3

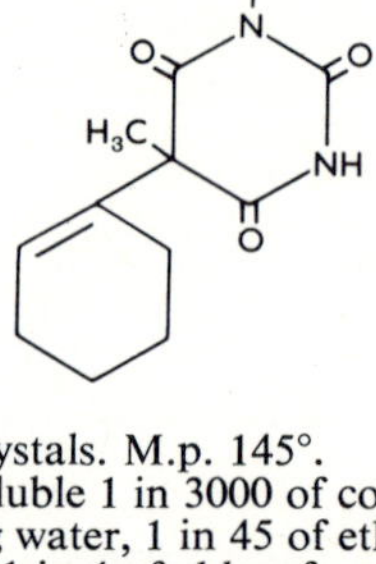

Colourless crystals. M.p. 145°.
Solubility. Soluble 1 in 3000 of cold water, 1 in 250 of boiling water, 1 in 45 of ethanol, 1 in 80 of ether, and 1 in 4 of chloroform.

HEXOBARBITONE SODIUM
Synonyms: Enhexymalnatrium; Enimalnatrium; Hexenalum; Soluble Hexobarbitone.
Proprietary Name: Cyclonal Sodium.

A white crystalline hygroscopic powder. It becames discoloured on exposure to air and solutions decompose on standing.
Solubility. Very soluble in water; soluble in ethanol and chloroform; very slightly soluble in ether.

Screening Tests. See under Barbiturates, p. 208.

Extraction. Hexobarbitone may be isolated in the A2 fraction (see p. 27).

Chromatography. PAPER: system P2—Rf 2·40 relative to amylobarbitone (location under ultraviolet light, dark spot); system P3—Rf 0·77 (location reagent *silver nitrate spray*, white); system P4—Rf 0·85 (location as for P3); system P5—Rf 2·35 relative to quinalbarbitone (location under ultraviolet light after exposure to ammonia, absorption); system RP1b—Rf 0·14 (location under ultraviolet light after exposure to ammonia; location reagent *potassium permanganate spray*, yellow on pink).

THIN-LAYER: system T10—Rf 0·50 (location reagents: *mercurous nitrate spray*, black; *potassium permanganate spray*, yellow-brown on purple); system T11—Rf 0·49 (location reagents: *mercurous nitrate spray*, white on grey; *potassium permanganate spray*, yellow on purple); system T12—Rf 0·58 (location as for T11); system T13—Rf 0·77 (location as for T11).

GAS: system G5—retention time 4·05 relative to barbitone; system G7—retention time 2·9 relative to barbitone.

Ultraviolet Absorption Spectrum. Hexobarbitone is a 1,5,5-derivative—see Screening Test 3 under Barbiturates, p. 208.

Infra-red Absorption Spectrum. Hexobarbitone. Potassium bromide disk. The principal peaks are: A 1660 or 1712, B 1358 or 1390 (p. 742).

Quantitative Estimation. See under Barbiturates, p. 208.

Metabolism. Hexobarbitone is a short-acting barbiturate—see under Barbiturates, p. 207. Its metabolism is discussed under The Metabolism of Drugs, p. 156.
By analogy with cyclobarbitone, oxidation of hexobarbitone in the cyclohexene ring to a ketone should be anticipated. Ketohexobarbitone has been demonstrated in human urine; the product is actually a mixture of 2 isomers, 5-(3′-oxo-cyclohex-1′-enyl)-1,5-dimethylbarbituric acid and presumably 5-(6′-oxo-cyclohex-1′-enyl)-1,5-dimethylbarbituric acid. *N*-Demethylation may take place; norhexobarbitone and 3′-ketohexobarbitone have also been detected (Frey *et al.*, 1959).

Dose. Hexobarbitone, up to 500 mg by mouth; hexobarbitone sodium, up to 1 g intravenously.

Toxicity. The estimated minimum lethal dose in man is 2 g of hexobarbitone sodium.

HEXOCYCLIUM METHYLSULPHATE

Parasympatholytic

Proprietary Name: Tral.

4-(β-Cyclohexyl-β-hydroxyphenethyl)-1,1-dimethylpiperazinium methylsulphate
$C_{20}H_{33}N_2O,CH_3SO_4$ = 428·6

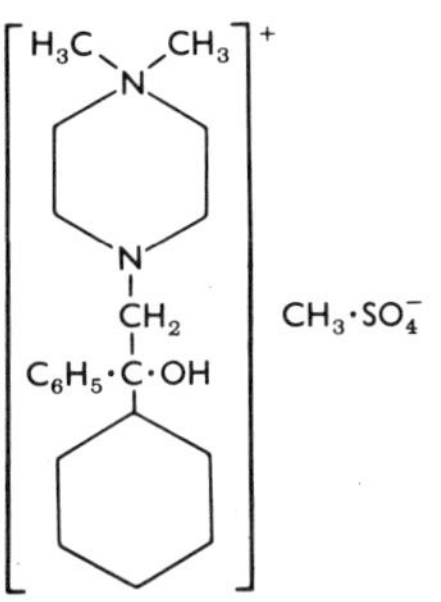

A white powder. M.p. 200° to 210°.

Solubility. Soluble 1 in 2 of water; insoluble in ether; slightly soluble in chloroform.

Extraction. Hexocyclium methylsulphate is a quaternary ammonium compound (see p. 29).

Chromatography. PAPER: system P1—Rf 0·38 (location reagents: *iodoplatinate spray*, strong reaction; *bromocresol green spray*, weak reaction); system RP1a—Rf 0·79 (location under ultraviolet light, absorption; location reagent *iodoplatinate spray*, positive reaction); system RP1b—Rf 0·76 (location as for RP1a).
THIN-LAYER: system T1—Rf 0·02 (location reagent *acidified iodoplatinate spray*, positive reaction).

Colour Tests. MICRO: sulphuric acid–formaldehyde test—dull purple (*sensitivity:* 1·0 μg); ammonium molybdate test—blue-grey (*sensitivity:* 0·25 μg); ammonium vanadate test—blue-purple (*sensitivity:* 1·0 μg).

Crystal Tests. MICRO: *ammonium thiocyanate solution*—bunches of rods (*sensitivity:* 1 in 100); *platinic chloride solution*—snowflake rosettes (*sensitivity:* 1 in 1000).

Ultraviolet Absorption Spectrum. Hexocyclium methylsulphate in 0·1N sulphuric acid, maxima at about 248 mμ (E1%, 1cm 2·5), 252 mμ (E1%, 1cm 3·5), 258 mμ (E1%, 1cm 4·2), 264 mμ (E1%, 1cm 3·2), and about 268 mμ (E1%, 1cm 1·7).

Infra-red Absorption Spectrum. Potassium bromide disk. The principal peaks are: A 1224, B 1005, C 748 (p. 742).

Metabolism. Hexocyclium methylsulphate is excreted mainly unchanged in the urine and the bile. Some unabsorbed drug may appear in the faeces, although it is readily absorbed from the gastro-intestinal tract.

Dose. Up to 100 mg daily.

Toxicity. The lethal dose in man is probably in the range 10 to 100 mg/kg.

HEXOESTROL

Oestrogen

Synonyms: Dihydrostilboestrol; Hexanoestrol; Hexestrol; Hexoestryl; Synoestrol.
Proprietary Names: Cycloestrol; Folliplex; Synthrogène.

(±)-3,4-Di(*p*-hydroxyphenyl)hexane
$C_{18}H_{22}O_2$ = 270·4

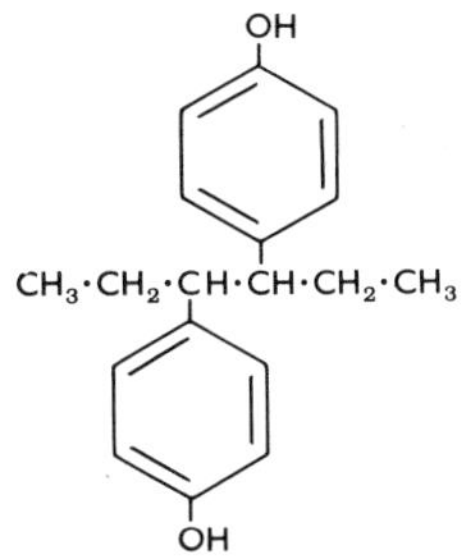

Colourless crystals or crystalline powder. M.p. 185° to 188°.

Solubility. Almost insoluble in water; soluble in ethanol and ether; slightly soluble in chloroform.

HEXOESTROL DIPROPIONATE

Proprietary Name: Retalon.

A white crystalline powder. M.p. 127° to 128°.

Solubility. Sparingly soluble in water; soluble in warm ethanol and ether.

Extraction. Hexoestrol is extracted from neutral solutions with freshly distilled ethyl acetate.

Chromatography. PAPER: system P15—Rf 0·85 (*diazotised* p-*nitroaniline spray*, brown; *Pauly's reagent*, red-brown).

Ultraviolet Absorption Spectrum. Hexoestrol in ethanol, maxima at 230 mμ (E1%, 1cm 775) and 280 mμ (E1%, 1cm 140); in 0·1N sodium hydroxide, maxima at 242 mμ (E1%, 1cm 965) and 295 mμ (E1%, 1cm 175).

Metabolism. Hexoestrol is a synthetic oestrogen which is not a steroid but has actions and uses similar to those of oestradiol. It is excreted chiefly as the glucuronide conjugate.

Dose. Up to 5 mg daily.

HEXYLCAINE

Local Anaesthetic

Synonym: D 109.

2-Cyclohexylamino-1-methylethyl benzoate
$C_{16}H_{23}NO_2$ = 261·4

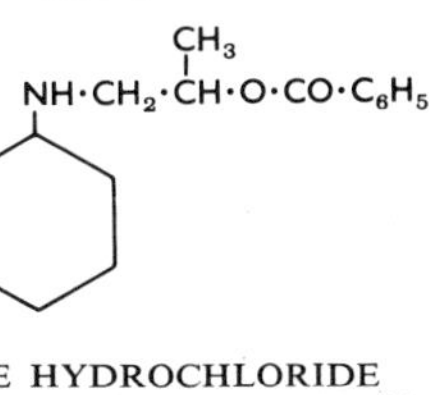

HEXYLCAINE HYDROCHLORIDE

Proprietary Name: Cyclaine Hydrochloride.

A white powder. M.p. 182° to 184°.
Solubility. Soluble 1 in about 17 of water; freely soluble in ethanol and chloroform; almost insoluble in ether.

Extraction. Hexylcaine is extracted by organic solvents from aqueous alkaline solutions.

Chromatography. PAPER: system P1—Rf 0·81 (location under ultraviolet light, absorption; location reagents: *iodoplatinate spray*, strong reaction; *bromocresol green spray*, weak reaction).

THIN-LAYER: system T1—Rf 0·01 (location reagent *acidified iodoplatinate spray*, positive reaction).

GAS: system G 2/225—retention time 1·4 relative to diphenhydramine.

Crystal Tests. MICRO: *gold bromide solution*—four-pointed stars (*sensitivity:* 1 in 1000); *potassium permanganate solution*—serrated plates and needles (*sensitivity:* 1 in 1000).

Ultraviolet Absorption Spectrum. Hexylcaine hydrochloride in 0·1N hydrochloric acid, maxima at about 232 mμ (E1%, 1cm about 422) and 275 mμ.

Use. Solutions of 1 to 5% are employed; single injections of up to 30 mg may be given for general surgical procedures.

Toxicity. The maximum safe amount for injection or topical application is stated to be 500 mg.

HEXYLRESORCINOL *Anthelmintic*

Synonym: Hexylresorcin.

4-Hexylbenzene-1,3-diol
$C_{12}H_{18}O_2$ = 194·3

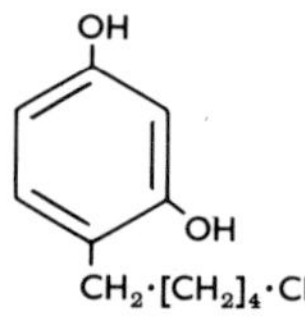

A white crystalline powder which turns brownish-pink on exposure to light and air. M.p. 66° to 68°.
Solubility. Soluble 1 in 2000 of water; readily soluble in ethanol, ether, and chloroform. Ethanolic solutions have vesicant properties.

Extraction. Hexylresorcinol is extracted by organic solvents from aqueous acid solutions.

Colour Tests. Add 0·2 ml of *ferric chloride solution* to an ethanolic solution—green. To 1 ml of a saturated solution, add 1 ml of 70% nitric acid—red.

Ultraviolet Absorption Spectrum. Hexylresorcinol in ethanol, maximum at 282 mμ (E1%, 1cm 134); in 0·1N sodium hydroxide, maximum at 297 mμ (E1%, 1cm 232).

Infra-red Absorption Spectrum. Potassium bromide disk. The principal peaks are: A 970, B 1185, C 1150 or 1453 or 1616 (p. 742).

Metabolism. When given by mouth in doses of 1 g, about 20 to 30% is excreted unchanged in the urine and 60 to 70% is eliminated in the faeces.

Dose. Up to 1 g as a single dose. Externally, a 0·1% solution of hexylresorcinol has been used as an antiseptic.

Toxicity. Hexylresorcinol is irritating to the respiratory tract and the skin. The lethal dose in man is about 5 g.

HISTAMINE *Gastric Secretion Indicator*

Synonym: Ergotidine.

4-(2-Aminoethyl)imidazole
$C_5H_9N_3$ = 111·1

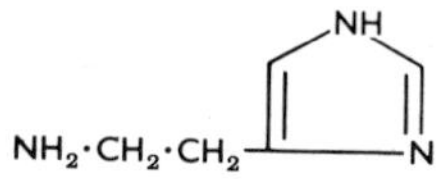

Deliquescent acicular crystals. M.p. 83° to 84°.
Solubility. Soluble in water and ethanol; sparingly soluble in ether; freely soluble in hot chloroform.

HISTAMINE ACID PHOSPHATE
Synonyms: Histamine Phosphate; Histamine Diphosphate.

Colourless crystals. M.p. 130° to 133°, after sintering at about 127°.
Solubility. Soluble 1 in 4 of water; slightly soluble in ethanol; almost insoluble in ether.

HISTAMINE DIHYDROCHLORIDE
Synonym: Histamine Hydrochloride.

Hygroscopic colourless crystals or a white crystalline powder.
Solubility. Very soluble in water; soluble in ethanol; slightly soluble in ether and chloroform.

Chromatography. PAPER: system P1—Rf 0·00 (location reagent *iodoplatinate spray*, white).

THIN-LAYER: system T1—Rf 0·13 (location reagent *acidified iodoplatinate spray*, positive reaction).

Crystal Tests. MICRO: *picric acid*—irregular blades (*sensitivity:* 1 in 1500); *platinic iodide solution*—plates, forming overnight (*sensitivity:* 1 in 3000).

Ultraviolet Absorption Spectrum. Histamine in 0·1N sulphuric acid, maximum at 269 mμ (E1%, 1cm 1).

Quantitative Estimation. Histamine in blood (Lowry *et al.*, 1954) and in tissue (Norn, 1965) may be determined spectrophotometrically following column chromatography and coupling with 2,4-dinitrofluorobenzene.

Metabolism. Exogenous histamine is metabolised by two routes. One involves *N*-methylation of the imidazole ring to form *N*,1-methylhistamine which may then be deaminated to *N*,1-methylimidazoleacetic acid; the other involves deamination directly to imidazoleacetic acid which is then conjugated to form imidazole-acetic acid riboside. *N*-acetylation of the side-chain to *N*-acetylhistamine may also occur. In man, the methylating pathway predominates. Histamine may be found in putrefied biological material as the decarboxylation product of histidine and it is present in a bound and inactive form in the tissues of all mammals, the highest concentration being in the lungs; leucocytes also contain appreciable amounts. Histamine is destroyed in the gastro-intestinal tract and has little effect when given by mouth. It is usually employed in the form of the acid phosphate as a subcutaneous injection.

Dose. The usual diagnostic dose is up to 1 mg subcutaneously; 5 mg after the administration of an antihistamine.

Toxicity. 0·5 mg administered parenterally may produce serious symptoms in the susceptible individual.

HISTAPYRRODINE *Antihistamine*

N - Phenyl - *N* - 2 - pyrrolidin - 1′ - ylethylbenzylamine

$C_{19}H_{24}N = 266{\cdot}4$

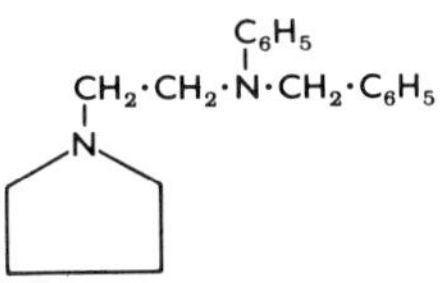

Histapyrrodine occurs as an oil.

HISTAPYRRODINE HYDROCHLORIDE

Proprietary Names: Domistan; Luvistin. It is an ingredient of Calcistin.

A white powder. M.p. 196°.

Extraction. Histapyrrodine is extracted by organic solvents from aqueous alkaline solutions.

Chromatography. PAPER: system P1—Rf 0·74 (location under ultraviolet light, dark blue fluorescence; location reagents: *iodoplatinate spray*, strong reaction; *bromocresol green spray*, strong reaction); system RP1a—Rf 0·43 (location under ultraviolet light, absorption; location reagent *iodoplatinate spray*, positive reaction); system RP1b—Rf 0·02 (location as for RP1a).
THIN-LAYER: system T1—Rf 0·60 (location reagent *acidified iodoplatinate spray*, positive reaction).

Colour Tests. MICRO: ammonium vanadate test—red-purple (*sensitivity:* 0·1 μg); Vitali's test — (yellow) -/yellow/yellow-brown (*sensitivity:* 0·25 μg).

Crystal Tests. MICRO: *gold bromide–hydrochloric acid solution*—needles (*sensitivity:* 1 in 400); *platinic iodide solution*—needles and plates (*sensitivity:* 1 in 200).

Ultraviolet Absorption Spectrum. Histapyrrodine in 0·1N sulphuric acid, maxima at 250 mμ (E1%, 1 cm 141) and 295 mμ (E1%, 1 cm 74).

Dose. Up to 150 mg daily.

HOMATROPINE *Parasympatholytic*

The tropine ester of (±)-mandelic acid

$C_{16}H_{21}NO_3 = 275{\cdot}4$

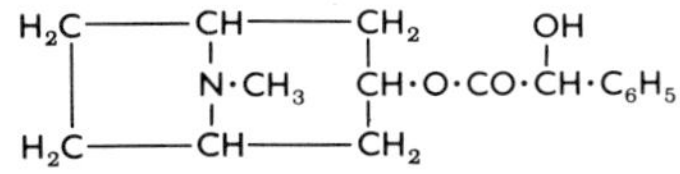

Small white prismatic crystals. M.p. 99° to 100°.

Solubility. Almost insoluble in water; soluble in ethanol, ether, and chloroform.

HOMATROPINE HYDROBROMIDE

A colourless crystalline powder. M.p. 214° to 217°, with partial decomposition.

Solubility. Soluble 1 in 6 of water, 1 in 60 of ethanol, and 1 in 420 of chloroform; insoluble in ether.

Extraction. Homatropine is extracted by organic solvents from aqueous alkaline solutions.

Chromatography. PAPER: system P1—Rf 0·30 (location under ultraviolet light, absorption; location reagent *iodoplatinate spray*, strong reaction); system RP1a—Rf 0·96 (location reagent *iodoplatinate spray*, positive reaction); system RP1b—Rf 0·00.
THIN-LAYER: system T1—Rf 0·15 (location reagent *acidified iodoplatinate spray*, positive reaction).
GAS: system G2/225—retention time 0·36 relative to codeine; system G4—retention time 0·39 relative to codeine; system G6—retention time 0·44 relative to codeine.

Crystal Tests. MICRO: *gold chloride solution*—plates and prisms (*sensitivity:* 1 in 1500); *potassium tri-iodide solution* (*3*)—plates, some serrated (*sensitivity:* 1 in 1500).

Ultraviolet Absorption Spectrum. Homatropine in 0·1N sulphuric acid, maxima at 252 mμ (E1%, 1 cm 4·8), 258 mμ (E1%, 1 cm 6·1), 264 mμ (E1%, 1 cm 5), and about 267 mμ (E1%, 1 cm 3).

Infra-red Absorption Spectrum. Homatropine (base). Potassium bromide disk. The principal peaks are: A 1172 or 1730 or 1032 (p. 742).

Use. Chiefly used as a mydriatic in solutions containing 1 or 2%.

Toxicity. The lethal dose in man is probably in the range 10 to 100 mg/kg.

HOMATROPINE METHOBROMIDE *Parasympatholytic*

Synonyms: Homatropine Methylbromide; Methylhomatropinium Bromatum.

Proprietary Names: Malcotran; Mesopin; Novatrin; Novatropine.

N-Methylhomatropine bromide
$C_{16}H_{21}NO_3,CH_3Br = 370{\cdot}3$

A white powder. M.p. 190° to 198°.
Solubility. Very soluble in water; freely soluble in ethanol; almost insoluble in ether.

Extraction. Homatropine methobromide is a quaternary ammonium compound (see p. 29).

Chromatography. PAPER: system P1—Rf 0·20 (location under ultraviolet light, absorption; location reagent *iodoplatinate spray*, strong reaction); system RP1a—Rf 0·94 (location reagent *iodoplatinate spray*, positive reaction); system RP1b—Rf 0·93 (location as for RP1a).
THIN-LAYER: system T1—Rf 0·02 (location reagent *acidified iodoplatinate spray*, positive reaction).

Crystal Tests. MICRO: *gold chloride solution*—small needles, often in crosses or snowflakes, best viewed under polarised light (*sensitivity:* 1 in 3000); *potassium permanganate solution*—long plates, sometimes in rosettes (*sensitivity:* 1 in 1000).

Ultraviolet Absorption Spectrum. Homatropine methobromide in ethanol, maxima at 252 mμ (E1%, 1cm 4), 258 mμ (E1%, 1cm 5), and 264 mμ (E1%, 1cm 4).

Dose. Up to 20 mg daily.

Toxicity. LD50 (oral): in mice 1·4 g/kg.

HOMIDIUM BROMIDE

Trypanocide (Veterinary)

Synonym: RD 1572.
Proprietary Name: Ethidium.

3,8 - Diamino - 5 - ethyl - 6 - phenylphenanthridinium bromide
$C_{21}H_{20}BrN_3 = 394{\cdot}3$

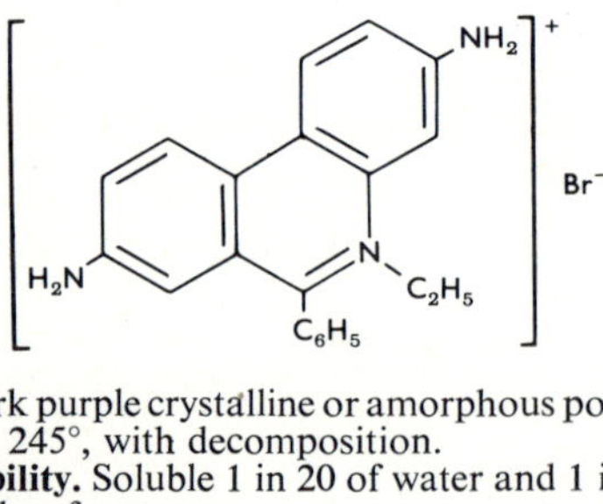

A dark purple crystalline or amorphous powder. M.p. 245°, with decomposition.
Solubility. Soluble 1 in 20 of water and 1 in 750 of chloroform.

Chromatography. PAPER: system P1—Rf 0·39 (location under ultraviolet light, bright orange fluorescence; location reagents: *iodoplatinate spray*, weak reaction; *potassium permanganate spray*, strong reaction); system RP1a—Rf 0·30 (location under ultraviolet light, orange fluorescence); system RP1b—Rf 0·31 (location as for RP1a).
THIN-LAYER: system T1—Rf 0·55 (location reagent *potassium permanaganate spray*, positive reaction).

Colour Tests. MICRO: the following tests are performed on homidium nitrate (see p. 134): sulphuric acid–formaldehyde test—(purple) colourless; ammonium vanadate test—(purple) yellow; Vitali's test—(purple) yellow/purple/brown.

Crystal Tests. MICRO: *gold cyanide solution*—small needles, best viewed under polarised light (*sensitivity:* 1 in 1000); *picric acid*—small rosettes, best viewed under polarised light (*sensitivity:* 1 in 400).

Ultraviolet Absorption Spectrum. Homidium bromide in 0·1N hydrochloric acid, maxima at 242 mμ (E1%, 1cm 720) and 283 mμ (E1%, 1cm 760).

Infra-red Absorption Spectrum. Potassium bromide disk. The principal peaks are: A 1629, B 1492, C 1259 (p. 787).

Dose. 1 mg/kg, intramuscularly or subcutaneously.

Toxicity. Doses of 10 mg/kg may cause transient liver damage in animals.

HOMOCHLORCYCLIZINE *Antihistamine*

Synonym: SA 97.

1 - (*p* - Chlorodiphenylmethyl) - 4 - methyl - 1,4-diazacycloheptane
$C_{19}H_{23}ClN_2 = 314{\cdot}9$

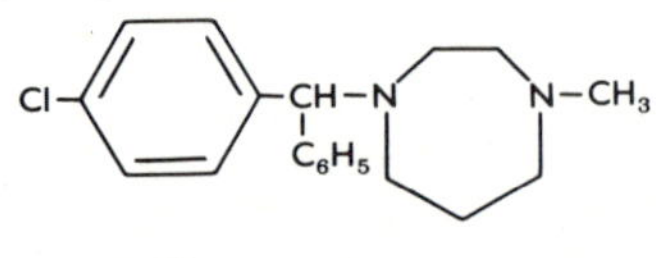

A white crystalline powder.
Solubility. Soluble in dilute acetic acid.

Extraction. Homochlorcyclizine is extracted by organic solvents from aqueous alkaline solutions.

Chromatography. PAPER: system P1—Rf 0·58 (location under ultraviolet light, absorption; location reagents: *iodoplatinate spray*, strong reaction; *bromocresol green spray*, weak reaction).
THIN-LAYER: system T1—Rf 0·28 (location reagent *acidified iodoplatinate spray*, positive reaction).

Colour Test. MICRO: ammonium molybdate test—faint blue (*sensitivity:* 1·0 μg).

Crystal Tests. MICRO: *picrolonic acid*—fans or rosettes of small needles (*sensitivity:* 1 in 1000); *styphnic acid*—rosettes (*sensitivity:* 1 in 1000).

Ultraviolet Absorption Spectrum. Homochlorcyclizine in 0·1N sulphuric acid, maxima at 233 mμ (E1%, 1cm 457), 258·5 mμ (E1%, 1cm 20·4), 263·5 mμ (E1%, 1cm 21·4), 270 mμ (E1%, 1cm 17·0), and about 276 mμ (E1%, 1cm 7·3).

HORDENINE *Sympathomimetic*
p-(2-Dimethylaminoethyl)phenol
$C_{10}H_{15}NO = 165{\cdot}2$

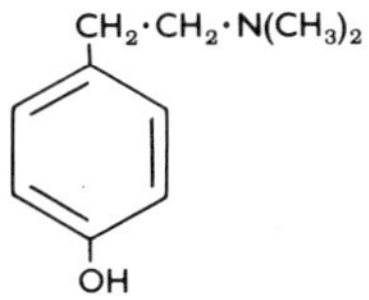

Hordenine occurs naturally in germinating barley and other Gramineae and may be prepared synthetically. It forms orthorhombic prisms from ethanol and needles from water. M.p. 117° to 118°.
Solubility. Slightly soluble in water; very soluble in ethanol, ether, and chloroform.

HORDENINE SULPHATE
Hordenine sulphate occurs as prisms or plates. M.p. 197° and 210° after drying at 100°.
Solubility. Soluble in water; slightly soluble in ethanol; insoluble in ether.

Extraction. Hordenine is extracted by organic solvents from aqueous ammoniacal solutions.

Chromatography. PAPER: system P1—Rf 0·23 (location under ultraviolet light, absorption; location reagents: *iodoplatinate spray*, weak reaction; *bromocresol green spray*, weak reaction); system RP1a—Rf 1·00 (location reagent *iodoplatinate spray*, positive reaction); system RP1b—Rf 0·58 (location as for RP1a).
THIN-LAYER: system T1—Rf 0·32 (location reagent *potassium permanganate spray*, positive reaction).

Colour Tests. MICRO: sulphuric acid–formaldehyde test—brown → green (*sensitivity:* 0·1 μg); ammonium molybdate test—blue → green → yellow (*sensitivity:* 0·025 μg); ammonium vanadate test—grey-green (*sensitivity:* 0·1 μg); Vitali's test—yellow/–/bright orange (*sensitivity:* 0·1 μg).

Crystal Tests. MICRO: *gold bromide solution*—long needles (*sensitivity:* 1 in 1000); *potassium bismuth iodide solution*—needles or rhomboids (*sensitivity:* 1 in 1500).

Ultraviolet Absorption Spectrum. Hordenine in 0·1N sulphuric acid, maximum at 274 mμ (E 1%, 1 cm 226) and inflexion at about 279 mμ.

Infra-red Absorption Spectrum. Hordenine (base). Potassium bromide disk. The principal peaks are: A 1252, B 820 or 1469 or 1512 (p. 787).

Metabolism. Its expected metabolites *in vivo* are *p*-hydroxyphenylacetic acid and breakdown products of dimethylamine.

HYDRALLAZINE *Antihypertensive*
Synonym: Hydralazine.
1-Hydrazinophthalazine
$C_8H_8N_4 = 160{\cdot}2$

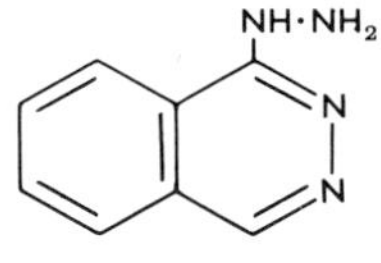

Hydrallazine melts at 172° to 173°.

HYDRALLAZINE HYDROCHLORIDE
Proprietary Names: Apresoline; Hydro-apresoline.
A white crystalline powder. M.p. about 275°, with decomposition.
Solubility. Soluble 1 in 25 of water and 1 in 500 of ethanol; very slightly soluble in ether.

Chromatography. PAPER: system P1—Rf 0·12 (location under ultraviolet light, absorption; location reagents: *iodoplatinate spray*, strong reaction; *bromocresol green spray*, weak reaction).
THIN-LAYER: system T1—Rf 0·48 (location reagent *acidified iodoplatinate spray*, positive reaction).

Colour Tests. MICRO: ammonium molybdate test—(brown) orange (*sensitivity:* 0·5 μg); Vitali's test— –/–/faint orange (*sensitivity:* 0·5 μg).

Crystal Tests. MICRO: *lead iodide solution*—dense rosettes (*sensitivity:* 1 in 1000); *potassium tri-iodide solution* (*3*)—clusters or masses of needles (*sensitivity:* 1 in 1000).

Ultraviolet Absorption Spectrum. Hydrallazine hydrochloride in water, maxima at 240 mμ (E 1%, 1 cm 711), 260 mμ (E 1%, 1 cm 662), 303 mμ (E 1%, 1 cm 331), and 315 mμ (E 1%, 1 cm 258).

Infra-red Absorption Spectrum. Hydrallazine (base). Potassium bromide disk. The principal peaks are: A 750 or 1529, B 1439, C 1142 or 1585 or 1625 (p. 788).

Metabolism. In man, only small proportions of oral or parenteral doses of hydrallazine are excreted in the urine unchanged and similar amounts are apparently bound to sulphydryl groups; there is evidence that the compound can be acetylated (Perry *et al.*, 1962). Studies in rats and rabbits have shown that hydroxylation and conjugation with glucuronic acid is the major metabolic pathway of hydrallazine. *N*-Acetylation accounted for 18% of a dose. Small but significant amounts of unchanged drug and its pyruvic hydrazone were also excreted. Excretion of the metabolites was rapid, a total of 75% of the dose appearing in the urine in 24 hours (McIsaac and Kanda, 1964).

Dose. Up to a maximum of 200 mg daily, according to the patient's needs.

Toxicity. The incidence of serious toxic reactions from continued administration is between 10 and 20%; fatalities have been rare.

LD50 (oral): in mice 213 mg/kg.

CASE EXAMPLE. The death of a 72-year-old woman is reported following treatment with 100 mg daily of hydrallazine for 2 years. No post-mortem levels are given (Bendersky and Ramirez, 1960).

HYDRASTINE *Alkaloid*

$C_{21}H_{21}NO_6 = 383{\cdot}4$

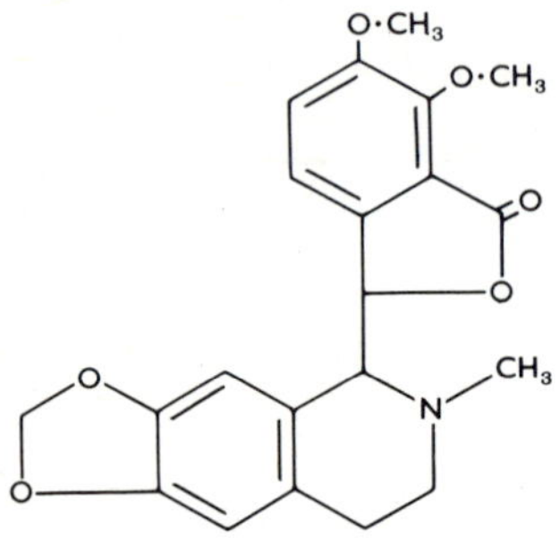

An alkaloid obtained from the rhizome and roots of golden seal, *Hydrastis canadensis* (Ranunculaceae).

It occurs as prisms which melt at 132°.

Solubility. Insoluble in water; soluble 1 in 210 of ethanol, 1 in 245 of ether, and 1 in 1 of chloroform.

HYDRASTINE HYDROCHLORIDE

A white hygroscopic powder. M.p. about 116°.

Solubility. Soluble in water and ethanol; very slightly soluble in ether; slightly soluble in chloroform.

Extraction. Hydrastine is extracted by organic solvents from aqueous alkaline solutions.

Chromatography. PAPER: system P1—Rf 0·38 (location under ultraviolet light, blue fluorescence; location reagent *iodoplatinate spray*, strong reaction); system RP1a—Rf 0·21 (location under ultraviolet light, blue fluorescence; location reagent *iodoplatinate spray*, positive reaction); system RP1b—Rf 0·07 (location as for RP1a).

THIN-LAYER: system T1—Rf 0·61 (location reagent *acidified iodoplatinate spray*, positive reaction).

GAS: system G6—retention time 1·18 relative to codeine.

Colour Tests. MICRO: ammonium molybdate test—grey-green → blue → pale green (*sensitivity:* 0·05 μg); ammonium vanadate test—reddish-brown → red (*sensitivity:* 0·1 μg).

Crystal Tests. MICRO: *potassium ferrocyanide–hydrochloric acid solution*—dense or feathery rosettes (*sensitivity:* 1 in 200); *sodium carbonate solution*—rosettes, best viewed under polarised light (*sensitivity:* 1 in 200).

Ultraviolet Absorption Spectrum. Hydrastine in ethanol:water (1:1), maximum at 295 mμ (E1%, 1cm 140).

Infra-red Absorption Spectrum. Hydrastine (base). Potassium bromide disk. The principal peaks are: A 1037 or 1501 or 1760, B 1260 (p. 788).

Dose. Up to 60 mg has been given.

HYDRASTININE *Alkaloid*

$C_{11}H_{13}NO_3 = 207{\cdot}2$

An alkaloid produced by oxidative hydrolysis of hydrastine.

A white crystalline substance which melts at 117°.

Solubility. Slightly soluble in hot water; soluble in ethanol, ether, and chloroform.

HYDRASTININE HYDROCHLORIDE

Pale yellow crystals or crystalline powder. M.p. 212°, with decomposition.

Solubility. Very soluble in water and ethanol; sparingly soluble in ether and chloroform.

Extraction. Hydrastinine is extracted by organic solvents from aqueous alkaline solutions.

Chromatography. PAPER: system P1—Rf 0·14 (location under ultraviolet light, bright blue fluorescence; location reagents: *iodoplatinate spray*, strong reaction; *bromocresol green spray*, weak reaction); system RP1a—Rf 0·87 (location under ultraviolet light, pale blue fluorescence; location reagent *iodoplatinate spray*, positive reaction); system RP1b—Rf 0·87 (location under ultraviolet light, blue fluorescence; location reagent *iodoplatinate spray*, positive reaction).

THIN-LAYER: system T1—Rf 0·00 (location reagent *acidified iodoplatinate spray*, positive reaction).

Colour Tests. MICRO: ammonium molybdate test—yellow → green (*sensitivity:* 0·25 μg); ammonium vanadate test—orange → pale green (*sensitivity:* 0·05 μg); Vitali's test—yellow/yellow/brown.

Crystal Tests. MICRO: *mercuric chloride solution*—branching needles or prisms (*sensitivity:* 1 in 1500); *potassium permanganate solution*—serrated blades (*sensitivity:* 1 in 1500).

Ultraviolet Absorption Spectrum. Hydrastinine in 0·1N sulphuric acid, maxima at 249 mμ (E1%, 1cm 3665), 306 mμ (E1%, 1cm 746), and 363 mμ (E1%, 1cm 976).

Infra-red Absorption Spectrum. Hydrastinine (base). Potassium bromide disk. The principal peaks are: A 1032 or 1235 or 1480, B 925 or 1499 (p. 788).

Dose. Up to 60 mg has been given.

HYDROCHLOROTHIAZIDE *Diuretic*

Synonyms: Chlorosulthiadil; Hydrochlorthiazide.

Proprietary Names: Aquarius; Dichlotride; Direma; Esidrex; Esidrix; Hydrid; Hydril; Hydro-Aquil; Hydrodiuril; Hydrosaluric; Hydrothide; Neo-Codema; Neo-Flumen; Oretic; Urazide; Vetidrex.

6-Chloro-3,4-dihydro-7-sulphamoyl-2*H*-benzo-1,2,4-thiadiazine 1,1-dioxide
$C_7H_8ClN_3O_4S_2$ = 297·7

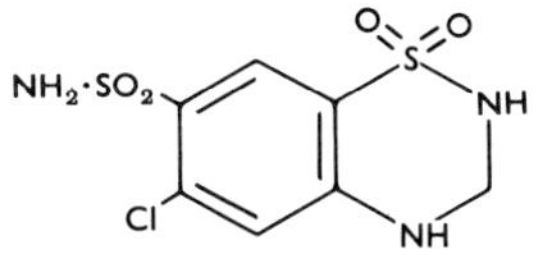

A white crystalline powder. M.p. about 267°, with decomposition.
Solubility. Almost insoluble in water, ether, and chloroform; soluble 1 in 200 of ethanol.

Extraction. Hydrochlorothiazide may be isolated in the A1 fraction (see p. 27); it is distinguished from the salicylates by chromatography (see below), by the fact that it does not react with *ferric chloride solution*, and by the presence of additional ultraviolet maxima in the region 270 to 330 mμ.

Chromatography. PAPER: system P16—Rf 0·08 (location under ultraviolet light, absorption; location reagent *sodium naphthaquinone spray*, strong reaction); system RP1b—Rf 0·62 (location as for P16).

Ultraviolet Absorption Spectrum. Hydrochlorothiazide in ethanol, maxima at 271 mμ (E1%, 1 cm about 660) and 317·5 mμ (E1%, 1 cm about 120).

Infra-red Absorption Spectrum. Potassium bromide disk. The principal peaks are: A 1175 or 1318 or 1336, B 1145 or 1160 or 1600 (p. 742).

Quantitative Estimation. Hydrochlorothiazide in urine may be determined by extracting with ethyl acetate followed by direct complexing with chromotropic acid or by alkaline hydrolysis, diazotisation, and coupling with *N*-(1-naphthyl)ethylenediamine (Sheppard *et al.*, 1960).

Dose. Up to 200 mg daily.

Toxicity. LD50 (oral): in rats, more than 2·75 g/kg.

HYDROCODONE

Narcotic Analgesic/Antitussive

Synonyms: Dihydrocodeinone; Hydrocone.

4,5 - Epoxy - 3 - methoxy - *N* - methyl - 6 - oxomorphinan
$C_{18}H_{21}NO_3$ = 299·4

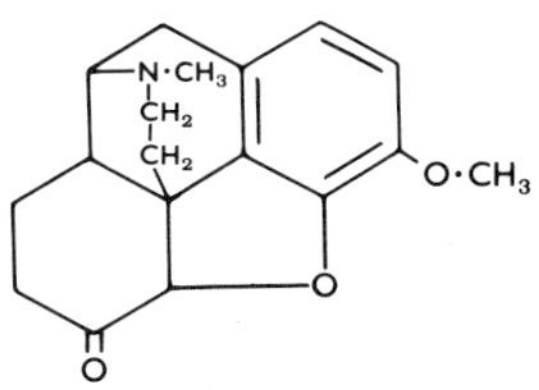

Hydrocodone melts at 198°.

Solubility. Insoluble in water; soluble in ethanol.

HYDROCODONE ACID TARTRATE
Synonyms: Hydrocodone Bitartrate; Dihydrocodeinone Hydrogen Tartrate.
Proprietary Names: Biocodone; Broncodid; Dicodid; Dicodinon; Hycodan Bitartrate; Mercodinone; Nyodid; Synkonin; Tucodil.

A fine white crystalline powder affected by light.
Solubility. Soluble 1 in 10 of water and 1 in 150 of ethanol; insoluble in ether and chloroform.

HYDROCODONE HYDROCHLORIDE
Proprietary Names: Codinovo Hydrochloride; Cofacodide Hydrochloride; Dicodid Hydrochloride.

A white crystalline powder.
Solubility. Soluble 1 in 2 of water; soluble in ethanol.

HYDROCODONE PHOSPHATE
A white crystalline powder.
Solubility. Soluble in water; almost insoluble in ethanol, ether, and chloroform.

Extraction. Hydrocodone is extracted by organic solvents from aqueous alkaline solutions; hydrolysis of biological material is required in order to improve the yield.

Chromatography. PAPER: system P1—Rf 0·22 (location under ultraviolet light, strong absorption; location reagents: *iodoplatinate spray*, strong reaction; *bromocresol green spray*, weak reaction); system RP1a—Rf 0·89 (location reagent *iodoplatinate spray*, positive reaction); system RP1b—Rf 0·13 (location as for RP1a).

THIN-LAYER: system T1—Rf 0·27 (location reagent *acidified iodoplatinate spray*, positive reaction).

GAS: system G2/225—retention time 1·16 relative to codeine; system G6—retention time 1·18 relative to codeine.

Colour Tests. MICRO: sulphuric acid–formaldehyde test—yellow → brown → purple (*sensitivity:* 0·25 μg); ammonium molybdate test—green → blue (*sensitivity:* 0·1 μg); Vitali's test—-/-/orange-red (*sensitivity:* 1·0 μg).

Crystal Tests. MICRO: *mercuric chloride solution*—dense rosettes (*sensitivity:* 1 in 1500); *potassium bismuth iodide solution*—rhomboidal plates (*sensitivity:* 1 in 400).

Ultraviolet Absorption Spectrum. Hydrocodone in ethanol, maximum at 280 mμ (E1%, 1 cm 44); in 0·1N sulphuric acid, maximum at 280 mμ (E1%, 1 cm 37): hydrocodone acid tartrate in water, maximum at 280 mμ (E1%, 1 cm 22·4); minimum at 262 mμ.

Dose. Usually up to 15 mg; max. in 24 hours 60 mg.

Toxicity. The estimated minimum lethal dose in adults is 100 mg. Hydrocodone has greater dependence-producing properties than codeine. Rosenwald and Russell (1961) have reported a form of drug addiction among 45 young men who took a cough syrup containing hydrocodone acid tartrate.

LD50 (subcutaneous): in mice 8·57 mg/kg.

HYDROCORTISONE *Corticosteroid*

Synonyms: Compound F; Cortisol; 17-Hydroxycorticosterone.

Proprietary Names: Cobadex; Cortef; Cortifoam; Cortril; Efcortelan; Genacort; Hydro-Adreson; Hydrocortistab; HydroCortisyl; Hydrocortone. Hydrocortisone is an ingredient of many proprietary preparations—see Extra Pharmacopoeia (Martindale), 25th Edn, p. 450.

NOTE. Many proprietary names used for preparations of hydrocortisone are also applied to preparations of hydrocortisone acetate.

11β, 17α, 21-Trihydroxypregn-4-ene-3,20-dione

$C_{21}H_{30}O_5 = 362·5$

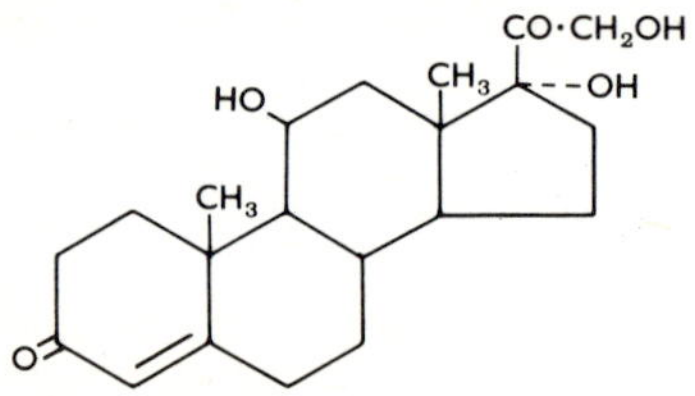

A white crystalline powder. M.p. about 214°, with decomposition. Specific rotation of a 1% solution in dioxan, +150° to +156°.

Solubility. Soluble 1 in 3500 of water, 1 in 40 of ethanol, and 1 in 80 of acetone; slightly soluble in chloroform; almost insoluble in ether.

HYDROCORTISONE ACETATE

21 - Acetoxy - 11β,17α - dihydroxypregn - 4 - ene - 3,20 - dione.

Synonym: Hydrocortisone 21-Acetate.

Proprietary Names: See under Hydrocortisone above.

A white crystalline powder. M.p. about 220°, with decomposition. Specific rotation of a 1% solution in dioxan, +157° to +167°.

Solubility. Insoluble in water; soluble 1 in 230 of ethanol and 1 in 150 of chloroform; almost insoluble in ether.

HYDROCORTISONE HYDROGEN SUCCINATE

21 - (β - Carboxypropionyloxy) - 11β,17α - dihydroxypregn-4-ene-3,20-dione.

Synonym: Hydrocortisone Hemisuccinate.

A white crystalline powder. M.p. about 168°; it may also occur in a form which melts at about 200°. Specific rotation of a 1% solution in ethanol, +147° to +153°.

Solubility. Almost insoluble in water; soluble 1 in 40 of ethanol and 1 in 7 of dehydrated ethanol. Soluble, with decomposition, in sodium hydroxide solution.

HYDROCORTISONE SODIUM SUCCINATE

Sodium 21 - (β - carboxypropionyloxy) - 11β,17α - dihydroxypregn-4-ene-3,20-dione.

Synonym: Hydrocortisone 21-Sodium Succinate.

Proprietary Names: Corlan Pellets; Efcortelan Soluble; Solu-Cortef.

A white hygroscopic crystalline powder or amorphous solid. M.p. 169° to 171°. Specific rotation of a 1% solution in ethanol, +134° to +146°.

Solubility. Soluble 1 in 3 of water, 1 in 34 of ethanol, and 1 in 200 of dehydrated ethanol; very slightly soluble in acetone; insoluble in chloroform and ether. It is unstable in aqueous solution.

Extraction. Hydrocortisone may be extracted from neutral solutions with freshly distilled ethyl acetate.

Chromatography. PAPER, for hydrocortisone: system P13—Rf 0·26 (location reagent *DPST solution*, violet on yellow); for hydrocortisone acetate: system P14—Rf 0·59 (location as for P13).

THIN-LAYER, for hydrocortisone acetate: system T18—Rf 0·66 (location reagent *DPST spray*); for hydrocortisone hydrogen succinate: system T19—Rf 0·18 (location as for T18).

Ultraviolet Absorption Spectrum. Hydrocortisone in ethanol, maximum at 240 mμ (E1%, 1 cm about 435); hydrocortisone acetate in ethanol, maximum at 240 mμ (E1%, 1 cm about 390).

Infra-red Absorption Spectrum. Hydrocortisone. Potassium bromide disk. The principal peaks are: A 1640, B 1702, C 1042 or 1232 (p. 743).

Metabolism. Hydrocortisone is the main glucocorticoid secreted by the human adrenal cortex. It is used for replacement therapy in adrenal insufficiency, as an anti-inflammatory agent, and occasionally as an anti-allergic agent.

Hydrocortisone is probably metabolised mainly in the liver to a number of physiologically inactive compounds. The metabolites may be excreted in the faeces and urine, largely as conjugates of glucuronic acid or sulphuric acid. Three main metabolic reactions seem to occur: reduction of the 4,5-double bond to dihydrocortisone, reduction of the 20-carbonyl group, and loss of the ketol side-chain at position 17.

Hydrocortisone is readily absorbed after oral administration, the effects being manifest in 3 to 10 hours. It has been found to be systemically absorbed when applied topically; Feldmann and Maibach (1965) found that between 0·2 and 1% of hydrocortisone appeared in the urine over a period of 10 days and that stripping the skin doubled the amount excreted and significantly enhanced the absorption; Feinblatt *et al.* (1966) recovered between 9·4 and 44·2% of hydrocortisone in the urine of 10 patients with normal skin who were treated with topical hydrocortisone.

Dose. The dose varies according to the patient's needs; the equivalent of between 2·5 and 100 mg of hydrocortisone may be administered as a single dose. Creams, ointments, or lotions usually contain between 0·25 and 2·5%.

HYDROFLUMETHIAZIDE *Diuretic*

Synonym: Trifluoromethylhydrothiazide.

Proprietary Names: Di-Ademil; Hydrenox; NaClex; Rontyl; Saluron.

3,4 - Dihydro - 7 - sulphamoyl - 6 - trifluoro -

methyl - 2*H* - benzo - 1,2,4 - thiadiazine 1,1 - dioxide

$C_8H_8F_3N_3O_4S_2$ = 331·3

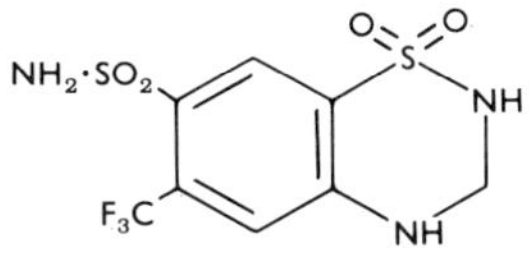

White glistening crystals or crystalline powder. M.p. about 271°.
Solubility. Soluble 1 in 3000 of water and 1 in 50 of ethanol; almost insoluble in ether and chloroform.

Extraction. Hydroflumethiazide may be isolated in the A1 fraction (see p. 27); it is distinguished from the salicylates by chromatography (see below), by the fact that it does not react with ferric chloride solution, and by the presence of additional ultraviolet maxima in the region 270 to 330 mμ.

Chromatography. PAPER: system P16—Rf 0·62 (location under ultraviolet light, fluorescence; location reagent *sodium naphthaquinone spray*, weak reaction); system RP1b—Rf 0·06 (location as for P16).

Ultraviolet Absorption Spectrum. Hydroflumethiazide in 0·01N sodium hydroxide, maxima at 274 mμ (E1%, 1cm about 460) and 333 mμ (E1%, 1cm about 95).

Infra-red Absorption Spectrum. Potassium bromide disk. The principal peaks are: A 1151 or 1180, B 1324 or 1341 (p. 743).

Dose. Up to 100 mg daily.

HYDROMORPHINOL *Narcotic Analgesic*

Proprietary Name: Numorphan Oral.

4,5 - Epoxy - 3,6,14 - trihydroxy - *N* - methylmorphinan

$C_{17}H_{21}NO_4$ = 303·4

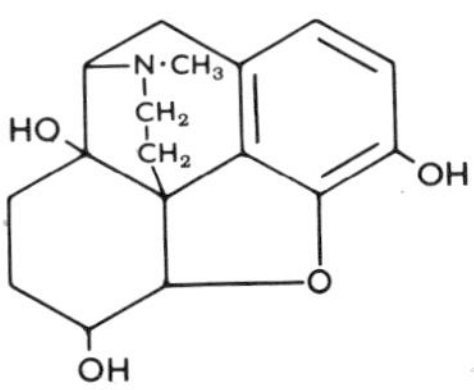

A creamy-white crystalline powder.
Solubility. Insoluble in water.

Extraction. Hydromorphinol is extracted by organic solvents from aqueous ammoniacal solutions; hydrolysis of biological material is required in order to improve the yield.

Chromatography. PAPER: system P1—Rf 0·08 (location under ultraviolet light, absorption; location reagents: *iodoplatinate spray*, weak reaction; *bromocresol green spray*, weak reaction).

THIN-LAYER: system T1—Rf 0·48 (location reagent *acidified iodoplatinate spray*, positive reaction).

Colour Tests. MICRO: sulphuric acid–formaldehyde test—purple (*sensitivity:* 0·1 μg); ammonium molybdate test—purple → blue → yellow (*sensitivity:* 0·1 μg); ammonium vanadate test—grey (*sensitivity:* 0·1 μg); Vitali's test—yellow/yellow/orange.

Crystal Test. MICRO: *gold bromide–hydrochloric acid solution*—very small plates (*sensitivity:* 1 in 200).

Ultraviolet Absorption Spectrum. Hydromorphinol in 0·1N sulphuric acid, maximum at 284 mμ (E1%, 1cm 54) and an inflexion at about 278 mμ.

Infra-red Absorption Spectrum. Potassium bromide disk. The principal peaks are: A 1086 or 1111 or 1318 or 1327 (p. 743).

Dose. Usually 15 mg.

HYDROMORPHONE *Narcotic Analgesic*

Synonyms: Dihydromorphinone; Dimorphone.

4,5 - Epoxy - 3 - hydroxy - *N* - methyl - 6 -oxomorphinan

$C_{17}H_{19}NO_3$ = 285·3

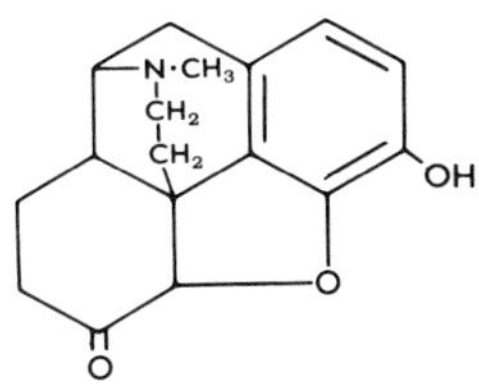

Hydromorphone occurs as crystals which melt at 265° to 267°, with decomposition.

HYDROMORPHONE HYDROCHLORIDE

Synonyms: Laudaconum; Morphodid.
Proprietary Names: Biomorphyl; Cofalaudide; Dilaudid; Dimorphinon; Hymorphan; Novolaudon.

A fine white crystalline powder which is affected by light. M.p. 305° to 315°, with decomposition.
Solubility. Soluble 1 in 3 of water and 1 in 100 of ethanol; almost insoluble in ether and chloroform.

Extraction. Hydromorphone is extracted by organic solvents from aqueous ammoniacal solutions; hydrolysis of biological material is required in order to improve the yield.

Chromatography. PAPER: system P1—Rf 0·15 (location under ultraviolet light, strong absorption; location reagent *iodoplatinate spray*, strong reaction); system RP1a—Rf 0·88 (location under ultraviolet light, absorption; location reagent *iodoplatinate spray*, positive reaction);

system RP1b—Rf 0·82 (location reagent *iodoplatinate spray*, positive reaction).
THIN-LAYER: system T1—Rf 0·24 (location reagent *acidified iodoplatinate spray*, positive reaction); system T7—Rf 0·17 (location reagent *iodoplatinate spray*, positive reaction); system T8—Rf 0·21 (location as for T7).
GAS: system G2/225—retention time 1·29 relative to codeine; system G6—retention time 1·47 relative to codeine.

Colour Tests. MICRO: sulphuric acid–formaldehyde test—yellow → red → purple (*sensitivity:* 0·05 μg); ammonium molybdate test—purple → blue → green (*sensitivity:* 0·05 μg); ammonium vanadate test—(green) dull purple → orange (*sensitivity:* 1·0 μg); Vitali's test—yellow/yellow /orange (*sensitivity:* 0·5 μg).

Crystal Test. MICRO: *sodium nitroprusside solution*—rods or prisms (*sensitivity:* 1 in 200).

Ultraviolet Absorption Spectrum. Hydromorphone in 0·1N sulphuric acid, maximum at 281 mμ (E1%, 1 cm 50).

Dose. Up to 5 mg.

Toxicity. The estimated minimum lethal dose of hydromorphone in adults is 100 mg. Addiction and tolerance are no less likely to occur than with morphine.
LD50 (intravenous): in mice 80 to 96 mg/kg.

HYDROQUINIDINE *Alkaloid*

Synonyms: Dihydroquinidine; Hydrocinchonine.
$C_{20}H_{26}N_2O_2 = 326{\cdot}4$

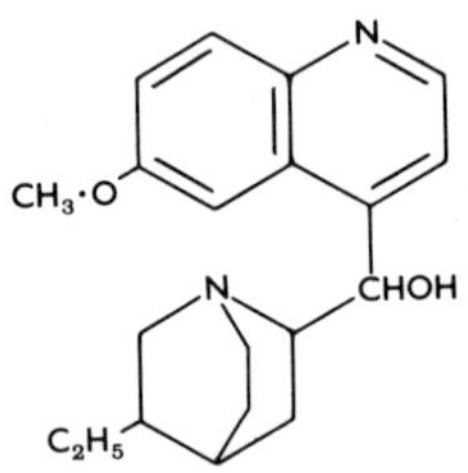

An alkaloid present in the bark of species of *Cinchona* (Rubiaceae). Quinidine (p. 531), as commercially available, contains 20 to 30% of hydroquinidine. Hydroquinidine is dextrorotatory and melts at 169·5°.
Solubility. Soluble in ethanol and ether.

Extraction. Hydroquinidine is extracted by organic solvents from aqueous alkaline solutions.

Chromatography. PAPER: system P1—Rf 0·53 (location under ultraviolet light, bright blue fluorescence; location reagents: *iodoplatinate spray*, strong reaction; *bromocresol green spray*, weak reaction); system RP1a—Rf 0·68 (location under ultraviolet light, blue fluorescence; location reagent *iodoplatinate spray*, positive reaction); system RP1b—Rf 0·13 (location as for RP1a).
THIN-LAYER: system T1—Rf 0·44 (location reagent *acidified iodoplatinate spray*, positive reaction).
GAS: system G2/225—retention time 3·26 relative to codeine.

Colour Test. Thalleioquin test—green (see p. 131).

Crystal Tests. MICRO: *gold bromide–hydrochloric acid solution*—branching needles (*sensitivity:* 1 in 3000); *gold chloride solution*—branching needles (*sensitivity:* 1 in 3000).

Ultraviolet Absorption Spectrum. Hydroquinidine in 0·1N sulphuric acid, maxima at 250 mμ (E1%, 1 cm 1242), 316 mμ (E1%, 1 cm 145), and 345 mμ (E1%, 1 cm 178).

Infra-red Absorption Spectrum. Potassium bromide disk. The principal peaks are: A 1509, B 1261, C 1620 (p. 788).

HYDROQUININE *Alkaloid*

Synonym: Dihydroquinine.
$C_{20}H_{26}N_2O_2 = 326{\cdot}4$

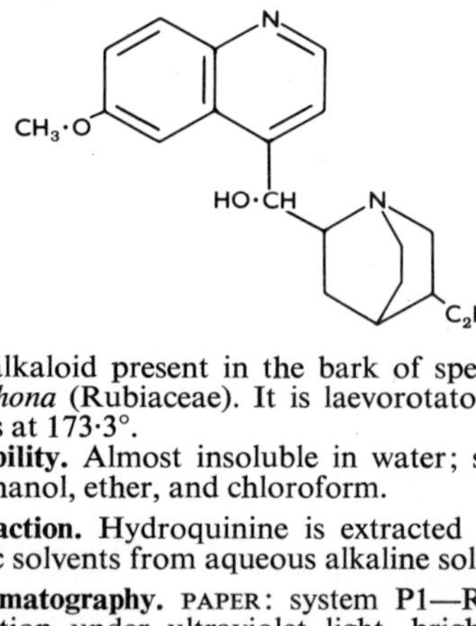

An alkaloid present in the bark of species of *Cinchona* (Rubiaceae). It is laevorotatory and melts at 173·3°.
Solubility. Almost insoluble in water; soluble in ethanol, ether, and chloroform.

Extraction. Hydroquinine is extracted by organic solvents from aqueous alkaline solutions.

Chromatography. PAPER: system P1—Rf 0·48 (location under ultraviolet light, bright blue fluorescence; location reagents: *iodoplatinate spray*, strong reaction; *bromocresol green spray*, weak reaction); system RP1a—Rf 0·67 (location under ultraviolet light, blue fluorescence; location reagent *iodoplatinate spray*, positive reaction); system RP1b—Rf 0·12 (location as for RP1a).
THIN-LAYER: system T1—Rf 0·42 (location reagent *acidified iodoplatinate spray*, positive reaction).

Colour Test. Thalleioquin test—green (see p. 131).

Crystal Tests. MICRO: *mercuric chloride solution*—large needles (*sensitivity:* 1 in 3000); *platinic bromide solution*—bunches of plates (*sensitivity:* 1 in 1500).

Ultraviolet Absorption Spectrum. Hydroquinine in 0·1N sulphuric acid, maxima at 250 mμ

(E1%, 1cm 915), 316 mμ (E1%, 1cm 133), and 345 mμ (E1%, 1cm 167).

Toxicity. It is more toxic than quinine (p. 532).

HYDROQUINONE *Antoxidant*

Synonyms: Hydroquinol; Quinol.
Proprietary Name: Tecquinol.

Benzene-1,4-diol
$C_6H_6O_2$ = 110·1

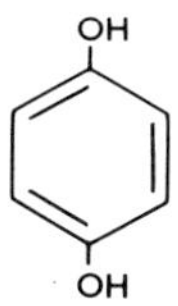

Colourless crystals or a white powder; solutions exposed to air become brown. M.p. 170° to 171°.

Solubility. Soluble 1 in 20 of water, 1 in 4 of ethanol, and 1 in 8 of ether.

Extraction. Hydroquinone is extracted by organic solvents from aqueous acid solutions.

Colour Test. With *ferric chloride solution*—transient green. Treat a chloroform solution with a little solid potassium hydroxide and warm—yellow-red to red-brown.

Ultraviolet Absorption Spectrum. Hydroquinone in ethanol, maxima at 225 mμ (E1%, 1cm 518) and 295 mμ (E1%, 1cm 282).

Metabolism. Hydroquinone is a reducing agent and there is evidence to suggest that on ingestion it produces its toxic effects after being oxidised to the more irritant quinone (Corby and Camps, 1960).
Hydroquinone has been found in the urine of rabbits as a metabolite of benzene.

Use. It is chiefly employed in photographic developers and as an antoxidant. It has been used as a 2 to 5% ointment for depigmentation of the skin.

Toxicity. The lethal dose in man is stated to be 2 g.
LD50 (oral): in rats 320 mg/kg.

NOTE. Hydroquinone is the toxic principle present in the seeds and young seedlings of cockleburs, *Xanthium* spp. (Compositae).

HYDROXOCOBALAMIN *Haemopoietic Vitamin*

Synonyms: Hydroxocobalamine; Vitamin B_{12a}; Vitamin B_{12b}.
Proprietary Names: Alpha Redisol; Hydrovit; Neo-Cytamen; Novobédouze.

Hydroxocobalamin occurs either as aquocobalamin chloride [α-(5,6-dimethylbenzimidazolyl)-aquocobamide chloride], $C_{62}H_{90}ClCoN_{13}O_{15}P$, or as aquocobalamin sulphate, $C_{124}H_{180}Co_2N_{26}O_{34}P_2S$.

NOTE. In acid solutions, hydroxocobalamin takes up a hydrogen ion which converts the hydroxyl to a co-ordinated water molecule. In this form, aquocobalamin, it is basic and forms salts with acids. Thus in solution it exists as an equilibrium mixture with hydroxocobalamin and, since it is more stable at acid pH values, commercial products are likely to be mainly in the aquocobalamin form (Smith *et al.*, 1962).

Both forms occur as dark red crystals or crystalline powder.

Solubility. Soluble in water.

Extraction. Biological material must be dehydrated and extracted with ethanol (see p. 29).

Ultraviolet Absorption Spectrum. Hydroxocobalamin in acetic acid, maxima at 274 mμ (E1%, 1cm 162), 351 mμ (E1%, 1cm 190), and 525 mμ (E1%, 1cm 57).

Quantitative Estimation. Martin and Shaw (1963) describe a method of determination of hydroxocobalamin in parenteral injection solutions by paper chromatography and spectrophotometry.

Metabolism. Hydroxocobalamin is more readily bound to serum protein than cyanocobalamin and so a higher initial level and more prolonged serum levels of vitamin B_{12} may be obtained. Following injections of 1 mg in normal subjects, 54 to 63% of hydroxocobalamin was excreted compared with 80 to 89% of cyanocobalamin.
Hydroxocobalamin has been used experimentally in animals as an antidote to cyanide poisoning, the detoxification presumably occurring by conversion of hydroxocobalamin to cyanocobalamin.

Dose. Up to 2 mg weekly, intramuscularly.

HYDROXYAMPHETAMINE *Sympathomimetic*

Synonym: Oxamphetamin.

4-(2-Aminopropyl)phenol
$C_9H_{13}NO$ = 151·2

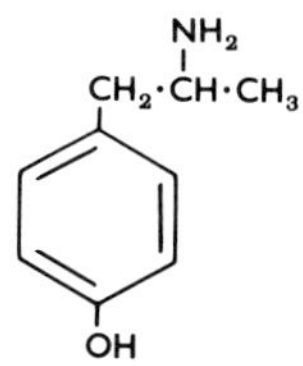

It occurs as crystals from benzene. M.p. 125° to 126°.

Solubility. Soluble in water, ethanol, and chloroform.

HYDROXYAMPHETAMINE HYDROBROMIDE
Proprietary Name: Paredrine Hydrobromide.

A white crystalline powder. M.p. 189° to 192°.
Solubility. Soluble 1 in 1 of water and 1 in 2·5 of ethanol; almost insoluble in ether; slightly soluble in chloroform.

Extraction. Hydroxyamphetamine is extracted

by organic solvents from aqueous ammoniacal solutions.

Chromatography. PAPER: system P1—Rf 0·36 (location under ultraviolet light, absorption; location reagent *potassium permanganate spray*, strong reaction).

THIN-LAYER: system T1—Rf 0·25 (location reagent *potassium permanganate spray*, positive reaction).

Colour Tests. MICRO: ammonium molybdate test—green (*sensitivity:* 0·5 μg); Vitali's test—yellow/yellow/orange (*sensitivity:* 0·5 μg).

Ultraviolet Absorption Spectrum. Hydroxyamphetamine in 0·1N sulphuric acid, maxima at 222 mμ (E1%, 1cm 623), and 274 mμ (E1%, 1cm 111), and an inflexion at about 279 mμ.

Infra-red Absorption Spectrum. Hydroxyamphetamine (base). Potassium bromide disk. The principal peaks are: A 1259, B 1517, C 1102 or 1599 (p. 788).

Metabolism. Studies in dogs following the intravenous administration of hydroxyamphetamine have shown that the plasma levels decline much more rapidly than those of dexamphetamine. About 30% of the drug was found in the urine in the free form and 30% as conjugated hydroxyamphetamine (Axelrod, 1954). Hydroxyamphetamine may be found as a metabolite of amphetamine and dexamphetamine.

Dose. Up to 180 mg daily; a 1 to 3% solution is used as a mydriatic; a 1% solution or spray is used as a nasal decongestant.

Toxicity. The estimated minimum lethal dose in children up to 2 years of age is 200 mg intranasally but the adult lethal dose may be at least 10 times as high.

HYDROXYCHLOROQUINE *Antimalarial*

Synonyms: SN 16168; Win 1258-2.

7 - Chloro - 4 - [4 - (*N* - ethyl - *N* - 2 - hydroxyethylamino)-1-methylbutylamino]quinoline

$C_{18}H_{26}ClN_3O = 335{\cdot}9$

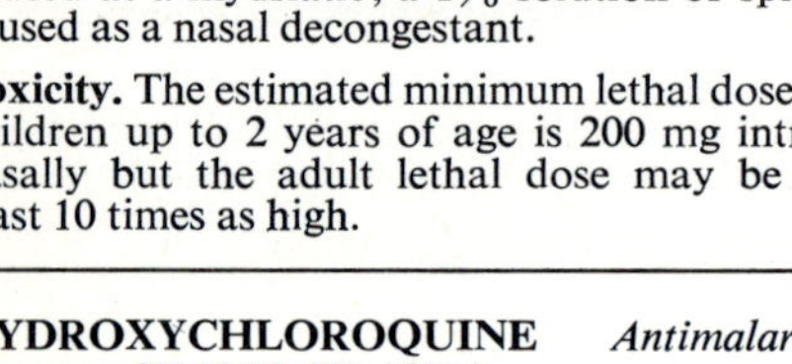

Hydroxychloroquine occurs as crystals. M.p. 89° to 91°.

HYDROXYCHLOROQUINE SULPHATE

Proprietary Name: Plaquenil.

A white crystalline powder. M.p. about 198° or about 240°

Solubility. Soluble 1 in 5 of water; almost insoluble in ethanol, ether, and chloroform.

Extraction. Hydroxychloroquine is extracted by organic solvents from aqueous alkaline solutions.

Chromatography. PAPER: system P1—Rf 0·12 (location under ultraviolet light, blue fluorescence; location reagents: *iodoplatinate spray*, strong reaction; *bromocresol green spray*, strong reaction); system RP1a—Rf 0·85 (location under ultraviolet light, blue fluorescence; location reagent *iodoplatinate spray*, positive reaction); system RP1b—Rf 0·30 (location as for RP1a).

THIN-LAYER: system T1—Rf 0·42 (location reagent *acidified iodoplatinate spray*, positive reaction).

Crystal Tests. MICRO: *picric acid*—small irregular plates, best viewed under polarised light (*sensitivity:* 1 in 1000); *styphnic acid*—snowflake rosettes or burrs (*sensitivity:* 1 in 400).

Ultraviolet Absorption Spectrum. Hydroxychloroquine in 0·1N sulphuric acid, maxima at 221 mμ (E1%, 1cm 746), 236 mμ (E1%, 1cm 427), about 250 mμ (E1%, 1cm 353), 256·5 mμ (E1%, 1 cm 385), 329 mμ (E1%, 1cm 399), and 343 mμ (E1%, 1cm 439).

Infra-red Absorption Spectrum. Hydroxychloroquine (base). Potassium bromide disk. The principal peaks are: A 1579, B 1447, C 1372 or 1608 (p. 788).

Quantitative Estimation. Hydroxychloroquine in blood and urine may be determined spectrophotometrically (Dalley and Hainsworth, 1965); similarly, in biological tissues (Bonnichsen and Maehly, 1965). McChesney *et al.* (1962) have described a spectrofluorimetric method of estimation in plasma.

Metabolism. Hydroxychloroquine is rapidly metabolised. McChesney and McAuliff (1961) found that 60 to 70% of ingested oral doses could not be accounted for. About 25% of daily doses has been found to be excreted unchanged in the urine. The drug is absorbed rapidly and completely from the gastro-intestinal tract.

After therapeutic doses, normal plasma levels are in the range 1 to 2·6 μg% with peak levels shortly after ingestion of about 20 μg%. The pattern of distribution in the tissues is similar to that seen after the administration of chloroquine, with the greatest concentrations occurring in the liver, spleen, kidney, lungs, skin, and leucocytes.

Dose. Up to 800 mg in malaria; up to 1·2 g daily in the treatment of discoid lupus erythematosus and rheumatoid arthritis.

Toxicity. Hydroxychloroquine is stated to be less toxic than chloroquine.

LD50 (oral): in mice about 3·1 g/kg.

CASE EXAMPLES. A man recovered following the ingestion of 7·2 g of hydroxychloroquine sulphate. At least an hour later he was found to have a plasma level of 0·61 mg%;

and 2 days later the plasma level was 0·27 mg% (Graham, 1960).
A 16-year-old boy died a few hours after ingestion of 12 g of hydroxychloroquine sulphate. Post-mortem levels: heart blood, 6·1 mg%; peripheral blood, 4·8 mg%; small intestine, 4·2 g; large intestine, 0·84 g; stomach contents, 0·07 g; liver, 7·1 mg%; urine, 97 mg% (Dalley and Hainsworth, 1965).
A 42-year-old diabetic woman ingested an unknown quantity of hydroxychloroquine. At post-mortem examination the liver contained 18 mg% of hydroxychloroquine (Bonnichsen and Maehly, 1965).

HYDROXYPETHIDINE *Narcotic*

Synonyms: 446; 10446; Hoechst 10446; Oxypetidin; Win 771.

Ethyl 4 - (3 - hydroxyphenyl) - 1 - methylpiperidine-4-carboxylate
$C_{15}H_{21}NO_3 = 263{\cdot}3$

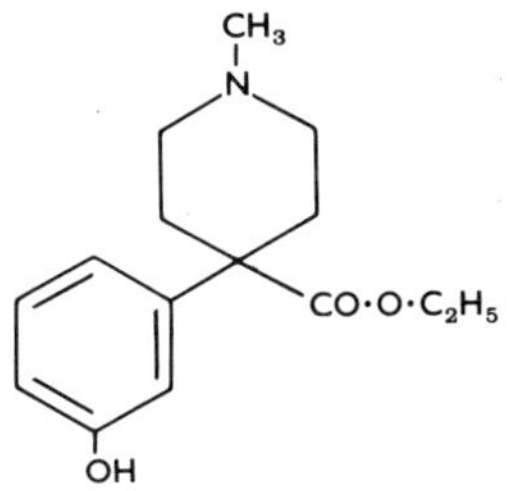

Extraction. Hydroxypethidine is extracted by organic solvents from aqueous ammoniacal solutions; hydrolysis of biological material is required in order to improve the yield.

Chromatography. PAPER: system P1—Rf 0·48 (location under ultraviolet light, absorption; location reagent *iodoplatinate spray*, weak reaction); system RP1a—Rf 0·53 (location under ultraviolet light, absorption); system RP1b—Rf 0·13 (location as for RP1a).

THIN-LAYER: system T1—Rf 0·47 (location reagent *potassium permanganate spray*, positive reaction).

GAS: system G2/225—retention time 1·75 relative to diphenhydramine; system G4—retention time 0·56 relative to codeine.

Colour Tests. MICRO: sulphuric acid–formaldehyde test—dull orange (*sensitivity:* 0·1 μg); ammonium molybdate test—bright blue, fading (*sensitivity:* 0·25 μg); ammonium vanadate test—dark green (*sensitivity:* 0·5 μg); Vitali's test— -/-/yellow (*sensitivity:* 0·25 μg).

Crystal Tests. MICRO: *gold bromide solution*—small plates and prisms (*sensitivity:* 1 in 1000); *styphnic acid*—blades, sometimes in rosettes, forming overnight (*sensitivity:* 1 in 200).

HYDROXYPHENAMATE *Tranquilliser*

Synonyms: Al 0361; Oxyfenamate; P 301.
Proprietary Name: Listica.

2-Hydroxy-2-phenylbutyl carbamate
$C_{11}H_{15}NO_3 = 209{\cdot}2$

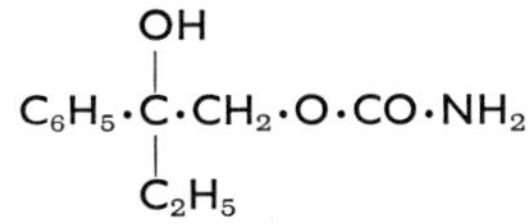

A white crystalline powder.
Solubility. Soluble 1 in 40 of water; soluble in ethanol and chloroform.

Extraction. Hydroxyphenamate is extracted by organic solvents from aqueous acid or alkaline solutions.

Chromatography. THIN-LAYER: system T1—Rf 0·74 (location reagent p-*dimethylaminobenzaldehyde spray*, positive reaction).
GAS: system G1/180—retention time 0·74 relative to diphenhydramine; system G2/225—retention time 0·63 relative to diphenhydramine; system G3—retention time 0·57 relative to diphenhydramine; system G4—retention time 0·50 relative to diphenhydramine; system G5—retention time 2·50 relative to barbitone.

Ultraviolet Absorption Spectrum. Hydroxyphenamate in 0·1N sulphuric acid, maxima at about 246·5 mμ (E1%, 1 cm 4·8), 250·5 mμ (E1%, 1 cm 6·8), 256·5 mμ (E1%, 1 cm 8·7), and 262·5 mμ (E1%, 1 cm 6·7).

Dose. Up to 800 mg daily.

Toxicity. The lethal dose in man is estimated to be between 100 and 500 mg/kg.

HYDROXYQUINOLINE *Antimicrobial*

Synonyms: Oxine; Oxyquinoline; 8-Quinolinol.
8-Hydroxyquinoline
$C_9H_7NO = 145{\cdot}2$

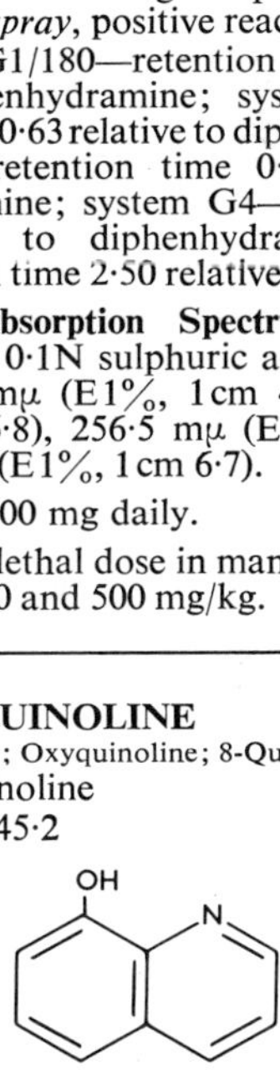

A white or faintly yellow crystalline powder. M.p. 76°. B.p. about 267°.
Solubility. Soluble 1 in 1500 of water; soluble in ethanol and chloroform; almost insoluble in ether.

HYDROXYQUINOLINE SULPHATE

Synonym: Chinosol.

A light yellow powder. M.p. 175° to 178°.
Solubility. Soluble 1 in 1 of water and 1 in 100 of ethanol; insoluble in ether.

POTASSIUM HYDROXYQUINOLINE SULPHATE

Synonym: Potassium Oxyquinoline Sulphate.

An equimolecular mixture of potassium sulphate and 8-hydroxyquinoline sulphate, containing the equivalent of 50% of 8-hydroxyquinoline.
It occurs as a pale yellow powder.
Solubility. Soluble 1 in 2 of water; partly soluble in ethanol; insoluble in ether.

Extraction. Hydroxyquinoline is extracted by organic solvents from aqueous ammoniacal solutions.

Chromatography. PAPER: system P1—Rf 0·64 (location under ultraviolet light, pale yellow fluorescence; location reagents: *iodoplatinate spray*, strong reaction; *potassium permanganate spray*, strong reaction).
THIN-LAYER: system T1—Rf 0·32, streaking (location reagent *acidified iodoplatinate spray*, positive reaction).
GAS: system G5—retention time 0·98 relative to barbitone.

Colour Tests. MICRO: ammonium molybdate test—(yellow) blue → green (*sensitivity:* 0·1 μg); ferric chloride test—deep emerald green.

Crystal Tests. MICRO: *gold bromide–hydrochloric acid solution*—feathery rosettes (*sensitivity:* 1 in 1000); *styphnic acid*—fine curved needles (*sensitivity:* 1 in 1000).

Ultraviolet Absorption Spectrum. Hydroxyquinoline in ethanol, maxima at 242 mμ (E1%, 1cm 2950) and 315 mμ (E1%, 1cm 175); in 0·1N hydrochloric acid, maxima at 252 mμ (E1%, 1cm 2750), 309 mμ (E1%, 1cm 73), 319 mμ (E1%, 1cm 74), and 365 mμ (E1%, 1cm 77).

Infra-red Absorption Spectrum. Hydroxyquinoline (base). Potassium bromide disk. The principal peaks are: A 1509, B 779, C 1409 (p. 788).

Metabolism. Hydroxyquinoline is excreted as glucuronide or ethereal sulphate conjugates.

HYDROXYZINE *Tranquilliser*

1-(*p*-Chlorodiphenylmethyl)-4-[2-(2-hydroxyethoxy)ethyl]piperazine
$C_{21}H_{27}ClN_2O_2$ = 374·9

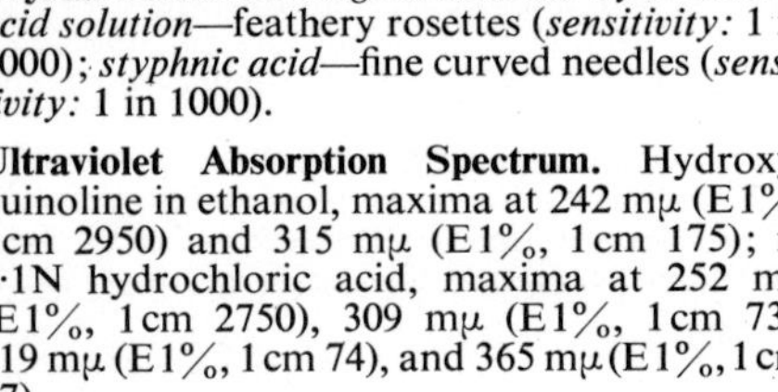

HYDROXYZINE EMBONATE
Synonym: Hydroxyzine Pamoate.
Proprietary Names: Paxistil; Vistaril (tablets).

A pale yellow crystalline powder.

HYDROXYZINE HYDROCHLORIDE
Proprietary Names: Atarax; Masmoran; Vistaril (injection).

A white powder. M.p. 196° to 204°, with decomposition.
Solubility. Very soluble in water; soluble in ethanol; almost insoluble in ether; soluble 1 in 11 of chloroform.

Extraction. Hydroxyzine is extracted by organic solvents from aqueous alkaline solutions.

Chromatography. PAPER: system P1—Rf 0·67 (location under ultraviolet light, absorption; location reagent *iodoplatinate spray*, strong reaction); system RP1a—Rf 0·28 (location under ultraviolet light, absorption; location reagent *iodoplatinate spray*, positive reaction); system RP1b—Rf 0·00 (location as for RP1a).
THIN-LAYER: system T1—Rf 0·66 (location reagent *acidified iodoplatinate spray*, positive reaction); system T2—Rf 0·84 (location reagent *iodoplatinate spray*, positive reaction); system T3—Rf 0·27 (location as for T2).
GAS: system G2/225—retention time 3·6 relative to codeine; system G4—retention time 1·6 relative to codeine.

Crystal Tests. MICRO: *gold bromide–hydrochloric acid solution*—dense rosettes, forming overnight (*sensitivity:* 1 in 200); *gold chloride solution*—dense rosettes, forming overnight (*sensitivity:* 1 in 200).

Ultraviolet Absorption Spectrum. Hydroxyzine in 0·1N sulphuric acid, maxima at 232 mμ (E1%, 1cm 420), 257 mμ (E1%, 1cm 19), 263 mμ (E1%, 1cm 20), and 269 mμ (E1%, 1cm 16).

Infra-red Absorption Spectrum. Hydroxyzine (base). Potassium bromide disk. The principal peaks are: A 1082 or 1130, B 1005 (p. 788).

Dose. Up to 400 mg daily.

Toxicity. The estimated lethal dose in man is between 25 and 250 mg/kg.
LD50 (oral): in mice 515 mg/kg.

HYOSCINE *Parasympatholytic*

Synonyms: (−)-Hyoscine; Scopolamine.

Scopine ester of (−)-tropic acid
$C_{17}H_{21}NO_4$ = 303·4

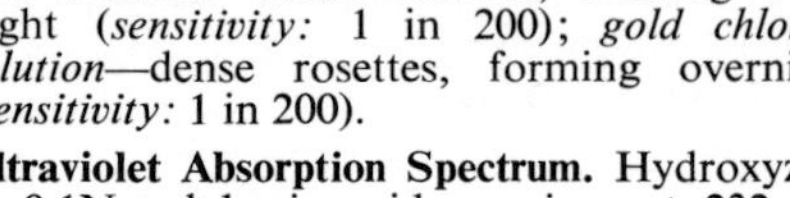

An alkaloid found in various solanaceous plants, particularly species of *Datura*, *Scopolia*, and *Duboisia*.
It is a viscous liquid which forms a crystalline monohydrate with a m.p. at 59°.
Solubility. Soluble 1 in 10 of water; freely soluble in ethanol, ether, and chloroform.

HYOSCINE HYDROBROMIDE
Synonym: Scopolamine Bromhydrate.
Proprietary Name: It is the active ingredient of Kwells.

A white crystalline powder which effloresces slightly in dry air. M.p. 195° to 198°.
Solubility. Soluble 1 in 3·5 of water and 1 in 30 of ethanol; almost insoluble in ether and chloroform.

HYOSCINE HYDROCHLORIDE
A white crystalline powder.
Solubility. Soluble in water and ethanol.

Extraction. Hyoscine is extracted by organic solvents from aqueous alkaline solutions.

Chromatography. PAPER: system P1—Rf 0·23

(location under ultraviolet light, absorption; location reagent *iodoplatinate spray*, strong reaction); system RP1a—Rf 0·93 (location reagent *iodoplatinate spray*, positive reaction); system RP1b—Rf 0·57 (location as for RP1a).

THIN-LAYER: system T1—Rf 0·54 (location reagent *acidified iodoplatinate spray*, positive reaction).

GAS: system G1/250—retention time 0·89 relative to codeine; system G2/225—retention time 0·84 relative to codeine; system G3—retention time 10·7 relative to diphenhydramine; system G4—retention time 1·39 relative to codeine; system G6—retention time 0·84 relative to codeine.

Colour Test. MICRO: Vitali's test— –/–/purple (*sensitivity:* 0·1 μg).

Crystal Tests. MICRO: *gold bromide–hydrochloric acid solution*—curving plates (*sensitivity:* 1 in 400); *potassium bismuth iodide solution*—rosettes of plates, forming overnight (*sensitivity:* 1 in 1500).

Ultraviolet Absorption Spectrum. Hyoscine in 0·1N sulphuric acid, maxima at 251 mμ (E1%, 1 cm 12), 257·5 mμ (E1%, 1 cm 14), and 263·5 mμ (E1%, 1 cm 11·2); hyoscine hydrochloride in water, maxima at 247 mμ (E1%, 1 cm 3), 252 mμ (E1%, 1 cm 4), 258 mμ (E1%, 1 cm 4), and 265 mμ (E1%, 1 cm 3).

Infra-red Absorption Spectrum. Hyoscine (base). Capillary film between potassium bromide windows. The principal peaks are: A 1725, B 1041 or 1165, C 1060 (p. 789).

Metabolism. Little is known about the fate of hyoscine; it is possible that small amounts are hydrolysed in the serum. It is readily absorbed from the gastro-intestinal tract and is tightly bound to plasma proteins. In rabbits, 2% of an oral dose and 30% of an intravenous dose are excreted in 3 days.

Dose. Usually up to 0·6 mg. Much larger doses (up to 24 mg daily) have been used in the treatment of Parkinson's syndrome.

Toxicity. Poisoning by hyoscine differs from that by atropine in that the cardiac rate is rarely increased and cerebral excitement is of short duration. Toxic symptoms may be manifest in about 10 minutes after the drug has been taken. In fatal cases death usually occurs within 3 or 4 hours; in non-fatal cases recovery takes a day or two. The lethal dose may be as low as 10 mg.

CASE EXAMPLES. A case of hyoscine intoxication is described in a 54-year-old woman who developed an addiction to 'Kwells' (tablets for motion-sickness, each containing 0·3 mg of hyoscine hydrobromide) over a period of 2 years, working up to a dosage of 12 tablets daily (Harper and Oakley, 1960).

Six cases of severe poisoning are reported in patients who took from 12 to 20, and in 1 case 'a handful', of tablets each containing 0·25 mg of hyoscine (Beach *et al.*, 1964).

Two cases of suicide attempts by taking tablets each containing 0·25 mg of hyoscine are described. The acute toxic effects of overdosage are described (Bernstein and Leff, 1967).

HYOSCINE BUTYLBROMIDE

Parasympatholytic

Synonyms: (–)-Hyoscine Butobromide; Scopolamine *N*-Butyl Bromide.

Proprietary Name: Buscopan.

(–)-*N*-Butylhyoscine bromide

$C_{21}H_{30}BrNO_4 = 440{\cdot}4$

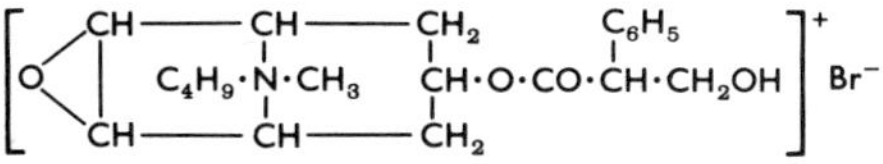

Hyoscine butylbromide melts at 143° to 144°.

Extraction. Hyoscine butylbromide is a quaternary ammonium compound (see p. 29).

Chromatography. PAPER: system P1—Rf 0·93 (location reagents: *iodoplatinate spray*, strong reaction; *bromocresol green spray*, strong reaction).

THIN-LAYER: system T1—Rf 0·79 (location reagent *acidified iodoplatinate spray*, positive reaction).

Crystal Tests. MICRO: *potassium tri-iodide solution (2)*—bundles of rods (*sensitivity:* 1 in 400); *sodium phosphate solution*—masses of rods (*sensitivity:* 1 in 400).

Ultraviolet Absorption Spectrum. Hyoscine butylbromide in 0·1N sulphuric acid, maximum at 276 mμ (E1%, 1 cm 292).

Metabolism. Following the subcutaneous injection of 190 mg of hyoscine butylbromide in 3 divided doses over 4 hours, the urine collected contained the equivalent of 26 mg of the drug (Herxheimer and Haefeli, 1966); thin-layer chromatography of urine samples, following injection, demonstrated the presence of hyoscine butylbromide and a possible metabolite.

Dose. Usually up to 100 mg daily; doses of 160 to 200 mg daily have been given.

Toxicity. LD50 (oral): in mice 3 g/kg.

HYOSCINE METHOBROMIDE

Parasympatholytic

Synonyms: Hyoscine Methylbromide; Methscopolamine Bromide; *N*-Methylscopolammonium Bromide; Scopolamine Methylbromide.

Proprietary Names: Lescopine Bromide; Pamine Bromide; Proscomide; Scopolate.

N-Methylhyoscine bromide

$C_{18}H_{24}BrNO_4 = 398{\cdot}3$

White crystals or a crystalline powder. M.p. 222° to 228°.

Solubility. Freely soluble in water; slightly soluble in ethanol; insoluble in chloroform.

For analytical data see Hyoscine Methonitrate, p. 378.

Dose. Up to 10 mg daily may be given.

Toxicity. The lethal dose in man is probably in the range 10 to 100 mg/kg.

HYOSCINE METHONITRATE

Parasympatholytic

Synonyms: Hyoscine Methylnitrate; Methscopolamine Nitrate; *N*-Methylscopolammonium Nitrate; Scopolamine Methylnitrate.
Proprietary Name: Skopyl.

N-Methylhyoscine nitrate
$C_{18}H_{24}N_2O_7$ = 380·4

A white microcrystalline powder.
Solubility. Soluble 1 in less than 2 of water and 1 in 50 of ethanol; almost insoluble in ether and chloroform.

Extraction. Hyoscine methonitrate is a quaternary ammonium compound (see p. 29).

Chromatography. PAPER: system P1—Rf 0·20 (location reagent *iodoplatinate spray*, strong reaction); system RP1a—Rf 0·96 (location under ultraviolet light, absorption; location reagent *iodoplatinate spray*, positive reaction); system RP1b—Rf 0·93 (location as for RP1a). THIN-LAYER: system T1—Rf 0·02 (location reagent *acidified iodoplatinate spray*, positive reaction).

Colour Test. MICRO: Vitali's test— -/-/purple (*sensitivity:* 0·025 μg).

Crystal Tests. MICRO: *gold bromide–hydrochloric acid solution*—plates, often in bunches (*sensitivity:* 1 in 1500); *mercuric chloride solution*—plates, sometimes in rosettes (*sensitivity:* 1 in 1500).

Ultraviolet Absorption Spectrum. Hyoscine methonitrate in 0·1N sulphuric acid, maxima at 251 mμ (E1%, 1 cm 4), 257·5 mμ (E1%, 1 cm 5), and 263·5 mμ (E1%, 1 cm 3).

Dose. Usually up to 4 mg; max. in 24 hours 12 mg.

Toxicity. The lethal dose in man is probably in the range 10 to 100 mg/kg.

HYOSCYAMINE

Parasympatholytic

Synonym: (−)-Hyoscyamine.

Tropine ester of (−)-tropic acid
$C_{17}H_{23}NO_3$ = 289·4

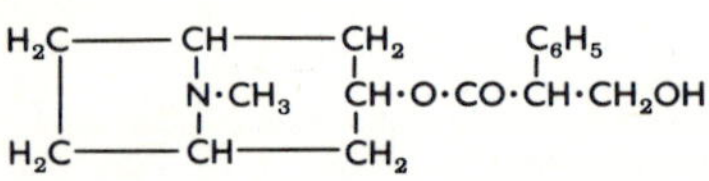

An alkaloid obtained from various solanaceous plants, *Hyoscyamus muticus* and *Duboisia myoporoides* being the best sources.
It is the laevo-isomer of atropine, (±)-hyoscyamine, and it may be differentiated from atropine by the shape of the crystals obtained with *potassium tri-iodide solution* (*3*)—see also Microcrystal Tests, p. 140.
A white crystalline powder. M.p. 108°.
Solubility. Soluble 1 in 280 of water and 1 in 48 of ether; very soluble in ethanol and chloroform.

HYOSCYAMINE HYDROBROMIDE

Synonym: Hyoscyamine Bromhydrate.

White deliquescent crystals or crystalline powder. M.p. not below 149°.
Solubility. Freely soluble in water; soluble 1 in about 2·5 of ethanol and 1 in about 1·7 of chloroform; very slightly soluble in ether.

HYOSCYAMINE SULPHATE

Proprietary Name: Levsin.

White crystals or a crystalline deliquescent powder which is affected by light. M.p. not below 200°.
Solubility. Soluble 1 in 0·5 of water and 1 in 5 of ethanol; very slightly soluble in ether and chloroform.

Extraction. Hyoscyamine is extracted by organic solvents from aqueous alkaline solutions.

Chromatography. PAPER: system P1—Rf 0·37 (location under ultraviolet light, absorption; location reagents: *iodoplatinate spray*, strong reaction; *bromocresol green spray*, weak reaction); system RP1a—Rf 0·94 (location reagent *iodoplatinate spray*, positive reaction). THIN-LAYER: system T1—Rf 0·18 (location reagent *acidified iodoplatinate spray*, positive reaction).
GAS: system G6—retention time 0·59 relative to codeine.

Colour Test. MICRO: Vitali's test— -/-/purple (*sensitivity:* 0·1 μg).

Crystal Tests. MICRO: *picric acid*—rosettes of needles, or plates (*sensitivity:* 1 in 400); *potassium tri-iodide solution* (*3*)—small plates and prisms, often in crosses and arrowheads (*sensitivity:* 1 in 1000).

Ultraviolet Absorption Spectrum. Hyoscyamine in ethanol, maxima at 247·5 mμ (E1%, 1 cm 4·5), 252 mμ (E1%, 1 cm 5), 255 mμ (E1%, 1 cm 5·4), and 264 mμ (E1%, 1 cm 5).

Infra-red Absorption Spectrum. Hyoscyamine (base). Potassium bromide disk. The principal peaks are: A 1712, B 1154, C 1032 (p. 743).

Dose. Usually up to 0·6 mg, but much higher doses have been given.

Toxicity. The toxic effects of hyoscyamine are similar to those of atropine.

IBOMAL

Barbiturate

Synonym: Isopropyl-bromallyl-barbituric Acid.
Proprietary Names: Noctal; Nostal; Propaldon.

5-(2-Bromoallyl)-5-isopropylbarbituric acid
$C_{10}H_{13}BrN_2O_3$ = 289·1

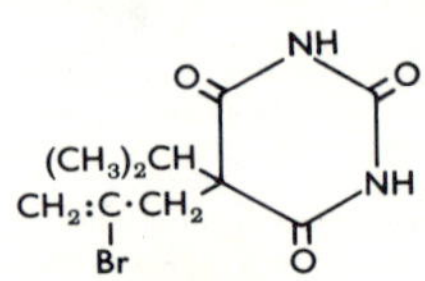

A white crystalline powder.
Solubility. Very slightly soluble in water; soluble in ethanol; slightly soluble in ether.

Extraction. Ibomal may be isolated in the A2 fraction (see p. 27).

Screening Tests. See under Barbiturates, p. 208.

Chromatography. PAPER: system P2—Rf 0·29 relative to amylobarbitone (location under ultraviolet light, dark spot).

GAS: system G5—retention time 5·10 relative to barbitone.

Colour Test. Zwikker's test—violet-blue.

Ultraviolet Absorption Spectrum. Ibomal is a 5,5-derivative—see Screening Test 3 under Barbiturates, p. 208.

Quantitative Estimation. See under Barbiturates, p. 208.

Metabolism. Ibomal is an intermediate-acting barbiturate—see under Barbiturates, p. 207. Following the oral administration of ibomal, 5-(2-acetonyl)-5-isopropylbarbituric acid, formed by side-chain oxidation, may be recovered from the urine in an amount corresponding to 6 to 16% of the dose administered, together with 1 to 3% of unchanged drug. The presence of this metabolite has been verified in human urine as long as 9 days after a single dose.

Dose. Up to 200 mg.

IDOXURIDINE *Antiviral Agent*

Synonyms: IDU; 5 IDUR; SKF 14287.
Proprietary Names: Dendrid; Herplex; Kerecid; Stoxil.

2′-Deoxy-5-iodouridine

$C_9H_{11}IN_2O_5 = 354{\cdot}1$

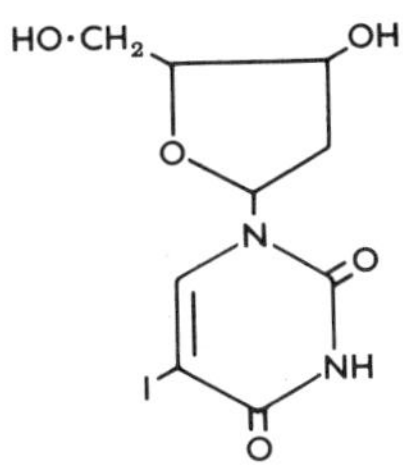

A white crystalline powder. A 1% solution in 1N sodium hydroxide solution is dextrorotatory. At 180° to 185°, iodoxuridine darkens and then decomposes with evolution of iodine vapour.

Solubility. Soluble 1 in 500 of water and 1 in 400 of ethanol; practically insoluble in ether and chloroform.

Ultraviolet Absorption Spectrum. Idoxuridine in 0·1N sodium hydroxide, maximum at about 280 mμ (E1%, 1cm 160); minimum at about 253 mμ.

Use. Idoxuridine is employed as a 0·1% ophthalmic solution.

IMIPRAMINE *Antidepressant*

5-(3-Dimethylaminopropyl)-10,11-dihydro-5*H*-dibenz[*b,f*]azepine

$C_{19}H_{24}N_2 = 280{\cdot}4$

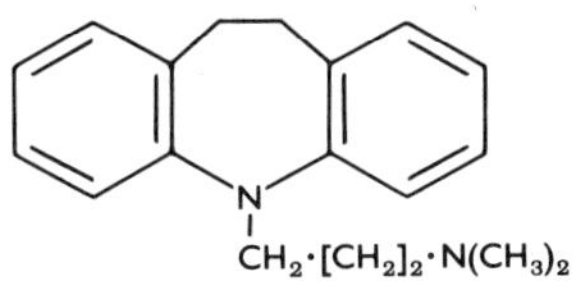

IMIPRAMINE HYDROCHLORIDE
Synonym: Imizine.
Proprietary Names: Berkomine; Tofranil.

A white crystalline powder. M.p. 170° to 174°.
Solubility. Soluble 1 in 2 of water and 1 in 1·5 of ethanol; almost insoluble in ether; readily soluble in chloroform.

Screening Test. See under Screening Tests, p. 13.

Extraction. Imipramine is extracted by organic solvents from aqueous alkaline solutions; hydrolysis of biological material is required in order to improve the yield.

Chromatography. PAPER: system P1—Rf 0·63 (location under ultraviolet light, dark blue fluorescence; location reagents: *iodoplatinate spray*, strong reaction; *bromocresol green spray*, weak reaction); system RP1a—Rf 0·44 (location reagent *iodoplatinate spray*, positive reaction); system RP1b—Rf 0·00 (location as for RP1a).

THIN-LAYER: system T1—Rf 0·43 (location reagent *acidified iodoplatinate spray*, positive reaction); system T3—Rf 0·86 (location reagent *iodoplatinate spray*, positive reaction); system T4—Rf 0·77 (location as for T3).

GAS: system G2/225—retention time 0·75 relative to codeine.

Colour Tests. MICRO: ammonium vanadate test—yellow → blue (*sensitivity:* 0·5 μg); Vitali's test—green/brown/brown (*sensitivity:* 0·5 μg).

Crystal Tests. MICRO: *styphnic acid*—feathery crystals (*sensitivity:* 1 in 100); *zinc chloride solution*—plates (*sensitivity:* 1 in 400).

Ultraviolet Absorption Spectrum. Imipramine in 0·1N sulphuric acid, maximum at 251 mμ (E1%, 1cm 238) and an inflexion at about 273 mμ (E1%, 1cm 189).

Infra-red Absorption Spectrum. Imipramine (base). Potassium bromide disk. The principal peaks are: A 1485, B 1452, C 745 or 1225 (p. 789).

Quantitative Estimation. Imipramine in biological tissues and fluids may be estimated, following extraction, by direct spectrophotometry (Denton, 1962) or by a spectrophotometric modification (Curry, 1963d) of the urinary screening test involving the potassium dichromate–perchloric acid reagent (Forrest *et al.*, 1960). However, neither of these methods will distinguish imipramine from its metabolite, desipramine.

Metabolism. Imipramine is rapidly metabolised in the body by *N*-demethylation to yield desipramine and by hydroxylation followed by glucuronide conjugation. After the administration of large doses, only small amounts of unchanged drug are excreted. It has been suggested that the antidepressant action of imipramine is due to desipramine.

Imipramine is rapidly absorbed from the gastro-intestinal tract and is largely bound to plasma proteins. It accumulates rapidly in the tissues where the levels are usually much greater than in the blood.

Dose. Up to 200 mg daily.

Toxicity. Fatalities have occurred after the ingestion of 750 mg of imipramine; in children, as little as 75 mg may cause severe toxic symptoms. In contrast, recoveries have occurred after the ingestion of 4·7 g (Rasmussen, 1965) and 5·4 g (Harthorne *et al.*, 1963). When imipramine is ingested in gramme quantities, blood-levels of about 0·1 mg% may be found, although the liver may contain much higher levels. The ingestion of imipramine together with monoamine oxidase inhibitors is dangerous.

CASE EXAMPLES. (1) A 36-year-old woman died about 6 hours after ingesting about 750 mg of imipramine. At post-mortem examination the stomach contents contained 150 mg and the liver 1·9 mg%. (2) A 15-month-old girl recovered following the ingestion of 200 mg of imipramine; 150 mg was recovered from the stomach contents. (3) A 29-year-old woman died very shortly after ingesting 1·75 g of imipramine. At post-mortem examination the stomach contents contained 19 mg and the liver 1·25 mg% (Denton, 1962).

Seven fatal cases involving imipramine are described; 4 were caused by acute overdosage and 3 involved high therapeutic doses in conjunction with other drugs. Post-mortem levels are given following analysis by 2 methods (Curry, 1964b).

IMOLAMINE *Coronary Vasodilator*

4 - (2 - Diethylaminoethyl) - 5 - imino - 3 - phenyl-2-1,2,4-oxadiazoline

$C_{14}H_{20}N_4O = 260{\cdot}3$

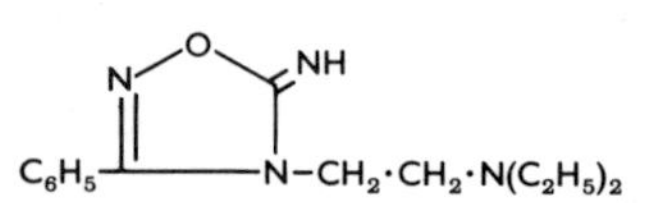

IMOLAMINE HYDROCHLORIDE

Synonym: LA 1211.

Proprietary Names: Angolon; Irrigor.

A white powder.

Solubility. Soluble 1 in 1 of water and 1 in 500 of ethanol; slightly soluble in chloroform.

Extraction. Imolamine is extracted by organic solvents from aqueous alkaline solutions.

Chromatography. PAPER: system P1—Rf 0·58 (location under ultraviolet light, absorption; location reagent *iodoplatinate spray*, strong reaction, white); system RP1a—Rf 0·69 (location under ultraviolet light, absorption; location reagent *iodoplatinate spray*, positive reaction); system RP1b—Rf 0·05 (location as for RP1a).

THIN-LAYER: system T1—Rf 0·56 (location reagent *acidified iodoplatinate spray*, positive reaction).

Colour Test. MICRO: ammonium molybdate test—very faint blue (*sensitivity:* 1·0 µg).

Crystal Tests. MICRO: *potassium mercuric iodide solution*—feathery crystals, best viewed under polarised light (*sensitivity:* 1 in 1000); *styphnic acid*—bunches of prisms, best viewed under polarised light (*sensitivity:* 1 in 1000).

Ultraviolet Absorption Spectrum. Imolamine in 0·1N sulphuric acid, maximum at 230 mµ (E1%, 1 cm 655).

Dose. Up to 60 mg daily.

Toxicity. LD50 (oral): in mice 475 and in rats 650 mg/kg.

INDOMETHACIN *Anti-inflammatory Agent*

Synonyms: Indométacine; MK 615.

Proprietary Names: Inacid; Indocid; Indocin.

(1 - *p* - Chlorobenzoyl - 5 - methoxy - 2 - methylindol-3-yl)acetic acid

$C_{19}H_{16}ClNO_4 = 357{\cdot}8$

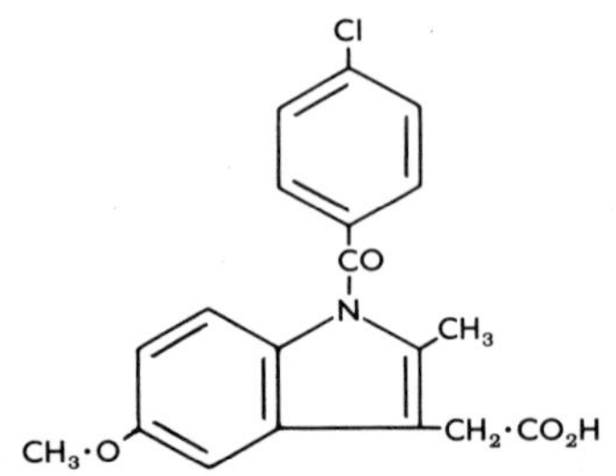

A yellowish-white powder. M.p. 153° to 154°.

Solubility. Insoluble in water; soluble in ethanol and ether.

Extraction. Indomethacin is extracted by organic solvents from aqueous acid solutions.

Ultraviolet Absorption Spectrum. Indomethacin in ethanol, maxima at 208 mµ, 235 mµ, and 325 mµ.

Quantitative Estimation. Holt and Hawkins (1965) describe a spectrofluorimetric method of determination of indomethacin in serum.

Metabolism. In man, no evidence of metabolic breakdown of indomethacin has been found. About 66% of the dose appears in the urine as indomethacin glucuronide and 33% appears unchanged in the faeces. Indomethacin is well-absorbed in man following oral administration, peak plasma levels occurring within 4 hours.

Dose. Usually up to 150 mg daily; up to 600 mg

daily has been given but with a higher incidence of side-effects.

Toxicity. Jacobs (1967b) has reported the sudden death of 4 arthritic children receiving indomethacin; 2 of the children received doses of 100 to 180 mg daily for more than a year, one took 50 mg daily for a month, and the fourth was given 100 mg daily for 2 months. LD50 (oral): in mice 50 and in rats 12 mg/kg.

IPRONIAZID

Antidepressant/Monoamine Oxidase Inhibitor

N'-Isopropylpyridine-4-carboxyhydrazine

$C_9H_{13}N_3O = 179{\cdot}2$

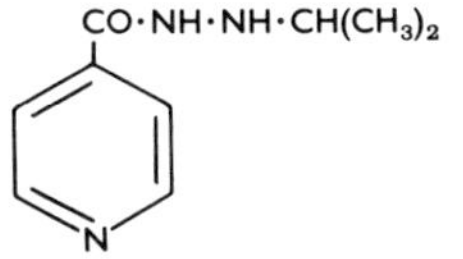

Iproniazid melts at 112·5° to 113·5°.
Solubility. Soluble in water and ethanol.

IPRONIAZID PHOSPHATE
Proprietary Name: Marsilid.

A white crystalline powder.
Solubility. Soluble 1 in 5 of water and 1 in 90 of ethanol; almost insoluble in ether; insoluble in chloroform.

Extraction. Iproniazid is extracted by organic solvents from aqueous alkaline solutions.

Chromatography. PAPER: system P1—Rf 0·75 (location under ultraviolet light, absorption; location reagent *iodoplatinate spray*, white); system RP1a—Rf 0·83 (location under ultraviolet light, absorption); system RP1b—Rf 0·79 (location under ultraviolet light, absorption; location reagent *iodoplatinate spray*, positive reaction).
THIN-LAYER: system T1—Rf 0·64 (location reagent *potassium permanganate spray*, positive reaction).

Colour Test. MICRO: ammonium molybdate test—(grey) pale yellow (*sensitivity:* 1·0 μg).

Crystal Tests. MICRO: *picrolonic acid*—fans of fine needles (*sensitivity:* 1 in 400); *potassium bismuth iodide solution*—bunches of plates (*sensitivity:* 1 in 400).

Ultraviolet Absorption Spectrum. Iproniazid in ethanol, maximum at 263·5 mμ (E1%, 1 cm 300); in 0·1N sulphuric acid, maximum at about 267 mμ (E1%, 1 cm 147·5).

Infra-red Absorption Spectrum. Iproniazid (base). Potassium bromide disk. The principal peaks are: A 961, B 1081, C 1414 or 1665 (p. 743).

Metabolism. Iproniazid is metabolised and excreted more slowly than isoniazid (p. 383); about 65% of a dose is excreted in 48 hours either unchanged or as metabolites, one of which appears to be isonicotinic acid which is excreted as its glycine conjugate. It is rapidly absorbed from the gastro-intestinal tract, peak plasma levels being reached in 1 to 2 hours.

Dose. Usually up to 150 mg daily.

Toxicity. See under Phenelzine, p. 482. Deaths have occurred with single doses of 25 to 100 mg/kg while 50 mg of iproniazid daily has caused fatal liver necrosis. Liver damage has occurred in about 0·1% of patients; 25% of these cases have ended fatally. Iproniazid has tuberculostatic properties but owing to the frequent occurrence of side-effects it is rarely used for this purpose.

ISOBUTYL AMINOBENZOATE

Local Anaesthetic

Synonym: Isobutylcaine.
Proprietary Names: Cyclocaine; Cycloform; Cyclogesin.

Isobutyl *p*-aminobenzoate

$C_{11}H_{15}NO_2 = 193{\cdot}2$

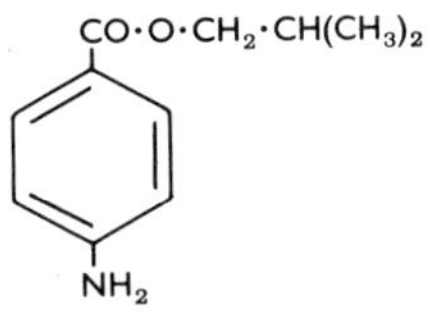

White scales or a white crystalline powder. M.p. 65°.
Solubility. Slightly soluble in water; soluble in ethanol and ether.

Extraction. Isobutyl aminobenzoate is extracted by organic solvents from aqueous alkaline solutions.

Chromatography. PAPER: system P1—Rf 0·96 (location under ultraviolet light, blue fluorescence; location, diazotisation followed by *alkaline betanaphthol spray*, red); system RP1a—Rf 0·04 (location under ultraviolet light, blue fluorescence); system RP1b—Rf 0·04 (location as for RP1a).
THIN-LAYER: system T1—Rf 0·77 (location reagents: diazotisation followed by *alkaline betanaphthol spray*, red; p-*dimethylaminobenzaldehyde spray*, positive reaction).

Colour Tests. MICRO: diazotisation test—red (*sensitivity:* 1·0 μg); *p*-dimethylaminobenzaldehyde test—bright yellow (*sensitivity:* 0·1 μg); Vitali's test— –/yellow-brown/bright yellow (*sensitivity:* 1·0 μg).

Crystal Tests. MICRO: *platinic chloride solution*—tufts of fine needles (*sensitivity:* 1 in 200); *potassium chromate solution*—plates (*sensitivity:* 1 in 200).

Ultraviolet Absorption Spectrum. Isobutyl aminobenzoate in ethanol, maxima at 223 mμ (E1%, 1 cm 371) and 294 mμ (E1%, 1 cm 1150).

Infra-red Absorption Spectrum. Potassium bromide disk. The principal peaks are: A 1278 or 1607, B 1172 or 1683, C 1109 or 1313 (p. 789).

ISOCARBOXAZID

Antidepressant/Monoamine Oxidase Inhibitor

Synonym: Ro 50831.
Proprietary Name: Marplan.

N - Benzyl - *N* '- (5 - methylisoxazol - 3 - yl - carbonyl)hydrazine

$C_{12}H_{13}N_3O_2$ = 231·3

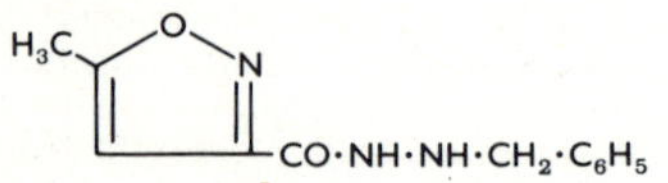

A white crystalline powder. M.p. 105° to 107°.
Solubility. Slightly soluble in water; soluble 1 in 150 of ethanol, 1 in 50 of ether, and 1 in 3 of chloroform.

Chromatography. PAPER: system P1—Rf 0·94 (location under ultraviolet light, strong absorption; location reagent *iodoplatinate spray*, white); system RP1a—Rf 0·17 (location under ultraviolet light, absorption; location reagent *iodoplatinate spray*, positive reaction); system RP1b—Rf 0·20 (location as for RP1a).

THIN-LAYER: system T1—Rf 0·72 (location reagent *potassium permanganate spray*, positive reaction).

Crystal Tests. MICRO: *potassium bismuth iodide solution*—rosettes or sheaves of needles (*sensitivity:* 1 in 200); *potassium chromate solution*—long branching needles (*sensitivity:* 1 in 200).

Ultraviolet Absorption Spectrum. Isocarboxazid in 0·1N sodium hydroxide, maximum at 272 mμ (E1%, 1cm 320).

Infra-red Absorption Spectrum. Potassium bromide disk. The principal peaks are: A 756 or 1670, B 710 (p. 743).

Metabolism. Isocarboxazid is hydrolysed and the benzyl fragment is oxidised to benzoic acid which is excreted as hippuric acid.

Dose. Up to 40 mg daily.

Toxicity. See under Phenelzine, p. 482; 300 mg has caused serious but non-fatal poisoning (Vlahakis, 1964).

ISOETHARINE

Bronchodilator

Synonyms: Etyprenaline; *N*-Isopropylethylnoradrenaline.
Proprietary Name: Dilabron.

1 - (3,4 - Dihydroxyphenyl) - 2 - isopropylaminobutan-1-ol

$C_{13}H_{21}NO_3$ = 239·3

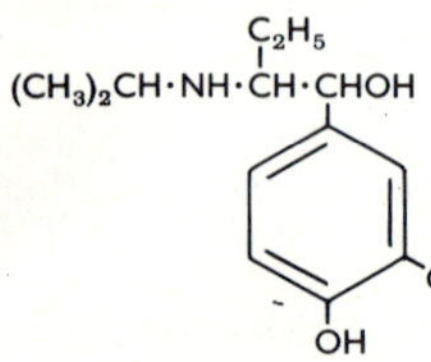

ISOETHARINE MESYLATE
Proprietary Name: It is an ingredient of Bronchilator.

Extraction. Isoetharine is extracted by organic solvents from aqueous ammoniacal solutions.

Chromatography. PAPER: system P1—Rf 0·39 (location under ultraviolet light, absorption; location reagent *bromocresol green spray*, weak reaction).

THIN-LAYER: system T1—Rf 0·24, streaking (location reagent *potassium permanganate spray*, positive reaction).

Colour Tests. Chen's test—grey-green → red-brown → yellow-brown.

MICRO: sulphuric acid–formaldehyde test—yellow → orange (*sensitivity:* 0·5 μg); ammonium molydbate test—(brown) green (*sensitivity:* 0·25 μg); ammonium vanadate test—(dark green) light brown (*sensitivity:* 0·1 μg); Vitali's test—yellow/orange/brown (*sensitivity:* 0·5 μg).

Crystal Tests. MICRO: *gold bromide solution*—small irregular plates (*sensitivity:* 1 in 200); *gold chloride solution*—purple, very small plates (*sensitivity:* 1 in 200).

Ultraviolet Absorption Spectrum. Isoetharine in 0·1N sulphuric acid, maxima at 222 mμ (E1%, 1cm 190) and 278 mμ (E1%, 1cm 100).

ISOMETHADONE

Narcotic

Synonyms: Isoadanone; Isoamidone; Win 1783.

6 - Dimethylamino - 5 - methyl - 4,4 - diphenylhexan-3-one

$C_{21}H_{27}NO$ = 309·5

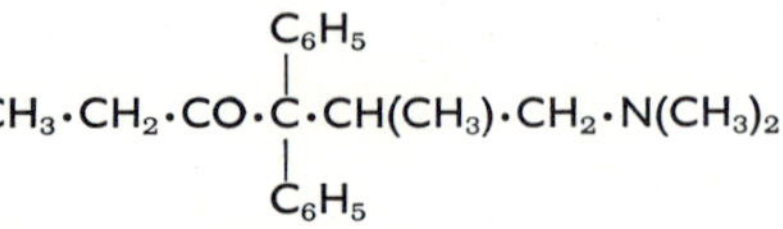

Isomethadone occurs as an oil.

Extraction. Isomethadone is extracted by organic solvents from aqueous alkaline solutions.

Chromatography. PAPER: system P1—Rf 0·73 (location reagent *iodoplatinate spray*, weak reaction).

THIN-LAYER: system T1—Rf 0·61 (location reagent *acidified iodoplatinate spray*, positive reaction).

Colour Test. MICRO: ammonium vanadate test—brown-purple → violet-blue (*sensitivity:* 0·1 μg).

Crystal Tests. MICRO: *picric acid*—dense rosettes of rods (*sensitivity:* 1 in 400); *platinic chloride solution*—dense rosettes of small plates (*sensitivity:* 1 in 1000).

Ultraviolet Absorption Spectrum. Isomethadone in ethanol, maxima at about 259 mμ, 265 mμ, and 298 mμ.

ISOMETHEPTENE *Sympathomimetic*

Synonym: N-Methyl Isoöctenylamine.
Proprietary Name: Octin.

N,1,5-Trimethylhex-4-enylamine
$C_9H_{19}N = 141{\cdot}3$

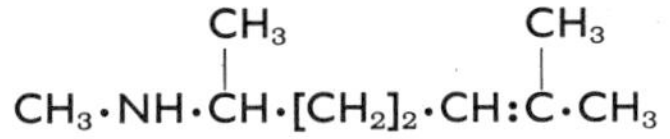

A colourless or slightly yellow oily liquid. B.p. 176° to 178°.
Solubility. Insoluble in water; soluble in ethanol, ether, and chloroform.

ISOMETHEPTENE HYDROCHLORIDE
A white hygroscopic powder. M.p. 68° to 69°.
Solubility. Readily soluble in water and ethanol.

ISOMETHEPTENE MUCATE
A white crystalline powder. M.p. 148°, with decomposition.
Solubility. Readily soluble in water; soluble 1 in 20 of ethanol; almost insoluble in ether and chloroform.

Extraction. Isometheptene is extracted by organic solvents from aqueous alkaline solutions.

Chromatography. PAPER: system P1—Rf 0·70 (location reagents: *iodoplatinate spray*, weak reaction; *bromocresol green spray*, weak reaction).

THIN-LAYER: system T1—Rf 0·24 (location reagent *potassium permanganate spray*, positive reaction).

GAS: system G2/120—retention time 0·21 relative to ephedrine.

Colour Test. MICRO: ammonium vanadate test —faint brown (*sensitivity:* 1·0 μg).

Crystal Tests. MICRO: *picrolonic acid*—small irregular grains (*sensitivity:* 1 in 200); *trinitrobenzoic acid solution*—long plates, sometimes in rosettes (*sensitivity:* 1 in 200).

Ultraviolet Absorption Spectrum. Isometheptene in 0·1N sulphuric acid, maximum at 276 mμ (E1%, 1cm 4·5).

Dose. Usually 100 to 130 mg every 30 minutes for 4 doses.

Toxicity. The estimated minimum lethal dose in children is 200 mg.

ISONIAZID *Tuberculostatic*

Synonyms: INH; Isonicotinic Acid Hydrazide; Isonicotinoylhydrazine; Isonicotinylhydrazide; Isonicotinylhydrazine; Tubazid.
Proprietary Names: Cotinazin; Mybasan; Neumandin; Nicetal; Nydrazid; Pycazide; Rimifon; Vazadrine.

Pyridine-4-carboxyhydrazide
$C_6H_7N_3O = 137{\cdot}1$

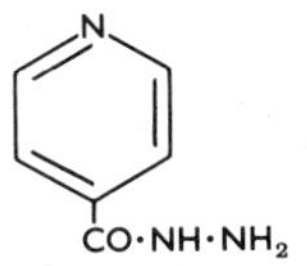

A white crystalline powder. M.p. 170° to 173°.
Solubility. Soluble 1 in 8 of water, 1 in 45 of ethanol, and 1 in 1000 of chloroform; almost insoluble in ether.

ISONIAZID AMINOSALICYLATE
Synonym: GEWO 339.
Proprietary Name: Dipasic.
Yellow crystals. M.p. 140° to 142°.
Solubility. Soluble in water and methanol.

Extraction. Isoniazid may be extracted from blood and urine with an iso-amyl alcohol–ether mixture in the presence of ammonium sulphate and sodium hydroxide, followed by re-extraction with dilute hydrochloric acid (Elmendorf *et al.*, 1952).

Chromatography. PAPER: system P1—Rf 0·32 (location under ultraviolet light, absorption; location reagents: *iodoplatinate spray*, strong reaction; *bromocresol green spray*, weak reaction).

THIN-LAYER: system T1—Rf 0·51 (location reagent *acidified iodoplatinate spray*, positive reaction).

Colour Test. MICRO: ammonium molybdate test —(grey) pale yellow (*sensitivity:* 1·0 μg).

Crystal Tests. MICRO: *mercuric chloride solution* —branching needles or blades (*sensitivity:* 1 in 400); *potassium bismuth iodide solution*—dense rosettes of plates (*sensitivity:* 1 in 400).

Ultraviolet Absorption Spectrum. Isoniazid in water, maximum at 266 mμ (E1%, 1cm 378); minimum at 234 mμ; in 0·01N hydrochloric acid, maximum at 265 mμ (E1%, 1cm about 420). Isoniazid may be differentiated from its major metabolite acetylisoniazid by the fact that the maximum at 265 mμ, which occurs with both in acid solution, will shift to 300 mμ at distinctly different pH values. Acetylisoniazid shows a complete shift to 300 mμ at pH10 whereas isoniazid itself does not shift until a pH of 12 is obtained (Belles and Littleman, 1960).

Infra-red Absorption Spectrum. Isoniazid (base). Potassium bromide disk. The principal peaks are: A 1659, B 1552, C 1335 or 1628 (p. 744).

Quantitative Estimation. Isoniazid may be estimated spectrophotometrically after treatment with *p*-dimethylaminobenzaldehyde (Elmendorf *et al.*, 1952). Wagner *et al.* (1955) describe a method of determination of isoniazid in serum based on its reaction with potassium mercuric iodide.
Venkataraman *et al.* (1968) describe a specific and sensitive spectrophotometric method for the direct estimation of acetylisoniazid, the principal metabolite of isoniazid, in urine; a modified procedure is described for use when isoniazid itself is present in high concentrations.

Metabolism. The major metabolic pathway of isoniazid in man is acetylation to yield acetylisoniazid; between 5 and 76% may be excreted in the urine as acetylisoniazid and between 4 and 32% may be excreted in the unchanged form. Hydrolysis to isonicotinic acid and subsequent formation of the glycine conjugate may also occur. The excretion of isoniazid reaches a peak between 2 and 4 hours after ingestion, nearly 50% of a dose being excreted within 6 hours and up to 86% within 24 hours. Isoniazid is almost completely absorbed from the gastro-intestinal tract and diffuses freely into the body tissues and fluids. Peak blood concentrations occur 1 to 3 hours after oral administration and detectable concentrations persist for up to 24 hours. The saliva has been found to contain concentrations comparable to those in the blood. Intramuscular injection produces blood concentrations approximately equal to those obtained with the same oral dose. Following injection, isoniazid is excreted more rapidly in the urine.

Dose. Usually up to 600 mg daily.

Toxicity. Serious toxic symptoms may occur with doses of 5 to 10 mg/kg or more daily. LD50 (oral): in mice 190 and in rats 650 mg/kg.

CASE EXAMPLES. A 20-year-old woman attempted suicide by taking 200 tablets (10 g) of isoniazid but recovered within 48 hours after treatment (Hadnagy *et al.*, 1964).

A 19-year-old woman ingested 7·5 g of isoniazid and recovered after 24 hours. A 21-year-old woman, who had been treated with isoniazid for a long time, ingested 3 g and went into a coma which persisted for 3 days. A 67-year-old woman took 6 g of isoniazid and on the third day the blood-level was 138 mg% and the urine concentration 59·6 mg% (Jeannerod *et al.*, 1965).

A 2-year-old child weighing 10·2 kg swallowed 4·6 g of isoniazid and recovered consciousness within 36 hours. The isoniazid level was 8 mg% in the serum after 10 hours and 56 mg% in the urine after 12 hours. Metabolites were detected in the blood (Holeček *et al.*, 1956).

A 15-year-old girl died 71 hours after ingestion of about 5 g of isoniazid. Peritoneal dialysis was started 43 hours after ingestion and continued for 16 hours with the collection of 22 litres of dialysate. The following isoniazid levels were found: peritoneal dialysis fluid, 5·1 mg% (representing more than 20% recovery of the ingested dose); post-mortem serum, 0·08 mg%; urine, 16·3 mg%. No barbiturates or alkaloids, both of which were used during treatment, could be detected (Kelso *et al.*, 1965).

ISOPRENALINE *Sympathomimetic*

Synonyms: Isopropylarterenol: Isopropylnoradrenaline; Isoproterenol.

1 - (3,4 - Dihydroxyphenyl) - 2 - isopropylaminoethanol

$C_{11}H_{17}NO_3 = 211{\cdot}3$

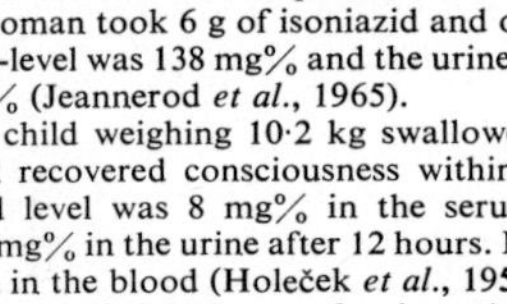

Isoprenaline melts at 155·5°.

ISOPRENALINE HYDROCHLORIDE

Proprietary Names: Aerotrol; Aludrine Hydrochloride; Asdrin; Isuprel Hydrochloride; Isupren; Isovon; Proternol; Saventrine; Suscardia.

A white crystalline powder which darkens on exposure to air; solutions become pink to brownish-pink on exposure to air. M.p. 167° to 172°.

Solubility. Soluble 1 in 3 of water and 1 in 50 of ethanol; insoluble in ether and chloroform.

ISOPRENALINE SULPHATE

Proprietary Names: Aleudrine; Bronchomister; Dyspnoesan; Isomist; Medihaler-Iso; Meterdos-iso; Neo-Epinine; Norisodrine; Prenomiser.

A white crystalline powder which darkens on exposure to air and light. M.p. about 128°, with decomposition.

Solubility. Soluble 1 in 4 of water; almost insoluble in ethanol, ether, and chloroform.

Extraction. Isoprenaline is extracted by organic solvents from aqueous ammoniacal solutions.

Chromatography. PAPER: system P1—Rf 0·22 (location under ultraviolet light, blue fluorescence; location reagent *bromocresol green spray*, weak reaction).

THIN-LAYER: system T1—Rf 0·33, streaking (location reagent *potassium permanganate spray*, positive reaction).

Colour Tests. Chen's test—green → brown.

MICRO: sulphuric acid–formaldehyde test—brown → dull purple (*sensitivity:* 0·5 μg); ammonium molybdate test—(brown) deep brown (*sensitivity:* 0·5 μg); ammonium vanadate test—(grey) brown (*sensitivity:* 0·5 μg); Vitali's test—yellow/orange/olive (*sensitivity:* 1·0 μg).

Crystal Tests. MICRO: *gold bromide solution*—small irregular plates (*sensitivity:* 1 in 400); *gold bromide–hydrochloric acid solution*—small plates or rosettes (*sensitivity:* 1 in 1500).

Ultraviolet Absorption Spectrum. Isoprenaline in 0·1N sulphuric acid, maxima at 222 mμ (E1%, 1 cm 228), 278·5 mμ (E1%, 1 cm 107), and 280 mμ (E1%, 1 cm about 132); minimum at 249·5 mμ.

Metabolism. Isoprenaline is probably metabolised similarly to adrenaline (p. 176) by deamination and *O*-methylation. It is readily absorbed after oral or parenteral administration.

Dose. Up to 20 mg sublingually or by inhalation of a solution by means of an atomiser.

Toxicity. For children the minimum lethal dose is 100 mg when applied to mucous membranes. LD50 (oral): in mice more than 2 g/kg.

ISOPROPAMIDE IODIDE *Parasympatholytic*

Synonyms: R79; SKF 4740.

Proprietary Names: Darbid; Priamide; Tyrimide.

(3 - Carbamoyl - 3,3 - diphenylpropyl)di - isopropylmethylammonium iodide

$C_{23}H_{33}IN_2O = 480{\cdot}4$

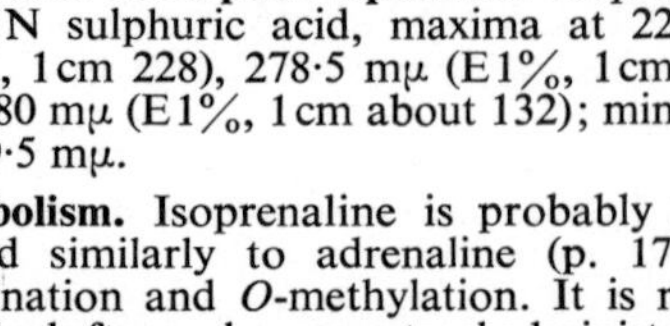

A white crystalline powder. M.p. 198° to 201°.

Solubility. Soluble in water.

Extraction. Isopropamide iodide is a quaternary ammonium compound (see p. 29).

Chromatography. PAPER: system P1—Rf 0·55 (location reagents: *iodoplatinate spray*, weak reaction; *bromocresol green spray*, weak reaction); system RP1a—Rf 0·87 (location reagent *iodoplatinate spray*, positive reaction); system RP1b—Rf 0·00.

THIN-LAYER: system T1—Rf 0·05 (location reagent *acidified iodoplatinate spray*, positive reaction).

Colour Test. MICRO: the following test is performed on isopropamide nitrate (see p. 134): Vitali's test—grey, fading/–/faint brown (*sensitivity:* 1·0 μg).

Crystal Tests. MICRO: *gold bromide–hydrochloric acid solution*—branching oily needles, forming overnight (*sensitivity:* 1 in 100); *potassium permanganate solution*—fans of needles (*sensitivity:* 1 in 100).

Ultraviolet Absorption Spectrum. Isopropamide iodide in 0·1N sulphuric acid, maxima at 259 mμ (E1%, 1 cm 19·8) and 265 mμ (E1%, 1 cm 15·5), and an inflexion at about 270 mμ.

Infra-red Absorption Spectrum. Potassium bromide disk. The principal peaks are: A 1650, B 1576, C 705 (p. 744).

Dose. 5 mg (base) every 12 hours.

Toxicity. The lethal dose is probably in the range 10 to 100 mg/kg.

ISOPROPANOL *Industrial Solvent*

Synonyms: Dimethyl Carbinol; Isopropyl Alcohol; Secondary Propyl Alcohol.
Proprietary Names: Avantine. It is an ingredient of CF15.

Propan-2-ol
$(CH_3)_2CHOH = 60{\cdot}10$

A clear colourless inflammable liquid. B.p. 81° to 83°. Refractive index, at 20°, 1·377 to 1·380.
Solubility. Miscible with water, ethanol, ether, and chloroform.

Extraction. Isopropanol is volatile and may be isolated by distillation (see p. 29).

Chromatography. GAS: system G8/100—retention time 0·62 relative to n-propanol; system G8/160—retention time 0·76 relative to n-propanol.

Colour Tests. *Acidified potassium dichromate solution*—green, on warming; iodoform test—positive reaction.

Quantitative Estimation. Ginther and Finch (1960) have described a method for determining isopropanol and acetone in distillates from biological materials.

Metabolism. Isopropanol is not used internally but it may be used topically. It is rapidly absorbed from the gastro-intestinal tract but only slowly absorbed through the skin. It is metabolised more slowly than ethanol, being largely oxidised to acetone (p. 171) which may be excreted in the urine and exhaled in the expired air, or further oxidised to acetate, formate, and carbon dioxide. Some isopropanol is excreted unchanged and some conjugated with glucuronic acid. Acetone may be detected in the urine within 1 hour and in the expired air within 15 minutes of ingestion of isopropanol. After the ingestion of large doses, there may be an increased excretion of the unchanged alcohol and its glucuronide.

Toxicity. Isopropanol is nearly twice as toxic and narcotic as ethanol due probably to its being metabolised much more slowly. The symptoms of intoxication appear to be similar to those produced by ethanol. A dose of 16 ml has been ingested daily for 3 days without discomfort but marked depression has been observed following a dose of 22·8 ml. The lethal dose in man is stated to be about 240 ml. The use of a cheap alcoholic beverage known as 'scrap iron' containing mainly isopropanol and naphthalene (moth balls) has caused serious toxic psychoses (Gadsden *et al.*, 1958).

LD50 (oral): in rats 5·8 g/kg.

CASE EXAMPLES. A 59-year-old man was admitted to hospital in coma following the ingestion of 1 litre of isopropanol. On admission, the blood-level of isopropanol was 346 mg% and of acetone 117 mg%; the urine contained 371 mg% of isopropanol and 127 mg% of acetone. Haemodialysis was instituted 7 hours later when the blood-level of isopropanol was 212 mg% and of acetone 188 mg%. Dialysis was discontinued about 3 hours later, blood-levels being 60 mg% of isopropanol and 150 mg% of acetone, and urine levels 90 mg% of isopropanol and 154 mg% of acetone. By the 2nd day after admission the blood-levels had dropped to 3 mg% of isopropanol and 61 mg% of acetone and the urine levels were 3 mg% and 66 mg% respectively (Freireich *et al.*, 1967).

ISOTHIPENDYL *Antihistamine*

Synonyms: D 201; Thypendyl.

9 - (2 - Dimethylaminopropyl) - 10 - thia - 1, 9 - diaza-anthracene
$C_{16}H_{19}N_3S = 285{\cdot}4$

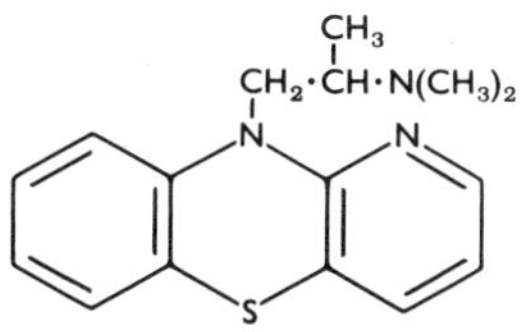

ISOTHIPENDYL HYDROCHLORIDE
Proprietary Names: Andantol; Nilergex; Theruhistin.

A fine white crystalline powder. M.p. about 212°, with decomposition.
Solubility. Soluble 1 in 5 of water, 1 in 60 of ethanol, and 1 in 10 of chloroform; insoluble in ether.

Extraction. Isothipendyl is extracted by organic solvents from aqueous alkaline solutions.

Chromatography. PAPER: system P1—Rf 0·58 (location under ultraviolet light, pale green fluorescence; location reagents: *iodoplatinate* *spray*, strong reaction; *bromocresol green spray*, weak reaction).

THIN-LAYER: system T1—Rf 0·48 (location reagent *acidified iodoplatinate spray*, positive reaction).

GAS: system G2/225—retention time 3·5 relative to diphenhydramine; 0·76 relative to codeine; system G4—retention time 0·53 relative to codeine.

Colour Tests. MICRO: sulphuric acid–formaldehyde test—dull orange (*sensitivity:* 0·5 μg); ammonium molybdate test—purple-brown → green (*sensitivity:* 0·5 μg); Vitali's test—grey/grey/pale brown (*sensitivity:* 0·5 μg).

Crystal Tests. MICRO: *lead iodide solution*—dendrites (*sensitivity:* 1 in 400); *mercuric chloride solution*—feathery rosettes (*sensitivity:* 1 in 400).

Ultraviolet Absorption Spectrum. Isothipendyl in 0·1N sodium hydroxide, maxima at 249 mμ (E1%, 1cm 981) and 315 mμ (E1%, 1cm 169); in 0·1N sulphuric acid, maxima at 244·5 mμ (E1%, 1cm 959) and 315 mμ (E1%, 1cm 180).

Dose. Up to 30 mg daily by mouth; up to 10 mg daily, by intramuscular or slow intravenous injection.

Toxicity. LD50 (oral): in mice 222 mg/kg.

ISOXSUPRINE *Vasodilator*

Synonyms: Caa 40; Compound 5029; Phenoxyisopropyl-nor-suprifen.

1 - (*p* - Hydroxyphenyl) - 2 - (1 - methyl - 2 - phenoxyethylamino)propan-1-ol

$C_{18}H_{23}NO_3 = 301{\cdot}4$

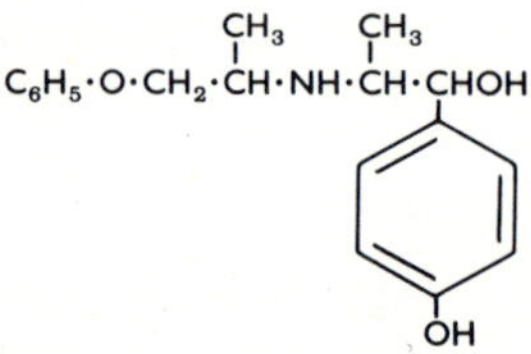

ISOXSUPRINE HYDROCHLORIDE

Proprietary Names: Dilavase; Duvadilan; Vasodilan.

A crystalline solid. M.p. 201° to 208°.

Solubility. Sparingly soluble in water; soluble in ethanol.

Extraction. Isoxsuprine is extracted by organic solvents from aqueous ammoniacal solutions.

Chromatography. PAPER: system P1—Rf 0·79 (location under ultraviolet light, absorption; location reagents: *iodoplatinate spray*, weak reaction; *bromocresol green spray*, weak reaction); system RP1a—Rf 0·67 (location under ultraviolet light, absorption); system RP1b—Rf 0·06 (location as for RP1a).

THIN-LAYER: system T1—Rf 0·74 (location reagent *potassium permanganate spray*, positive reaction).

Colour Tests. MICRO: sulphuric acid–formaldehyde test—red-purple (*sensitivity:* 0·5 μg); ammonium molybdate test—blue (*sensitivity:* 1·0 μg); ammonium vanadate test—dull green (*sensitivity:* 0·5 μg); Vitali's test—–/pale yellow/bright orange (*sensitivity:* 0·5 μg).

Crystal Tests. MICRO: *gold bromide–hydrochloric acid solution*—small plates and prisms (*sensitivity:* 1 in 100); *lead iodide solution*—small rosettes of rods or plates (*sensitivity:* 1 in 200).

Ultraviolet Absorption Spectrum. Isoxsuprine in 0·1N sulphuric acid, maxima at 219 mμ (E1%, 1cm 184), 269 mμ (E1%, 1cm 61), and 274 mμ (E1%, 1cm 59).

Metabolism. Isoxsuprine is found in the blood unchanged and as a conjugate, both being excreted in the urine; faecal excretion is insignificant. Isoxsuprine is slowly absorbed from the stomach and rapidly from the small intestine. After oral or subcutaneous administration, maximum blood-levels are attained within 1 hour and are maintained for 3 hours.

Dose. Up to 80 mg daily.

KANAMYCIN *Antibiotic*

An antibiotic produced by strains of *Streptomyces kanamyceticus*

$C_{18}H_{36}N_4O_{11} = 484{\cdot}5$

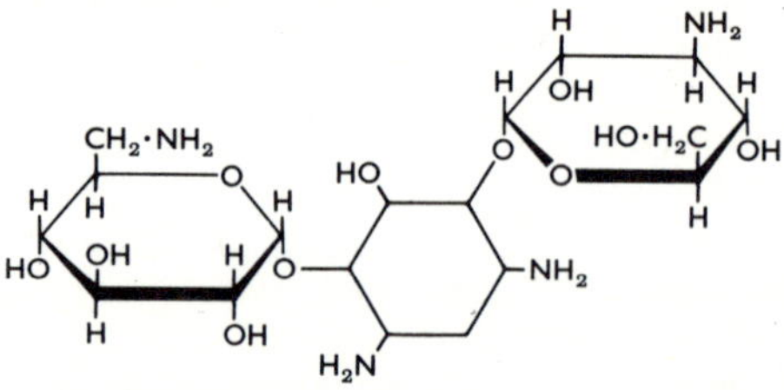

Kanamycin is a whitish powder.

KANAMYCIN SULPHATE

Proprietary Names: Kaminex; Kanabiol; Kanamitrex; Kanecidin; Kannasyn; Kantrex; Ophthalmokalixan; Resistomycin.

A white hygroscopic powder.

Solubility. Soluble 1 in 3 of water; insoluble in ethanol; very slightly soluble in ether and chloroform.

Extraction. Kanamycin is very soluble in water; special extraction methods are required (see p. 28).

Chromatography. PAPER: system P1—Rf 0·00 (location reagents: *bromine–starch–potassium iodide*, strong reaction; *ninhydrin spray*, dull purple).

THIN-LAYER: system T1—Rf 0·01 (location reagent *potassium permanganate spray*, positive reaction).

Metabolism. Kanamycin does not seem to be metabolised; during the 24 hours after administration 50 to 80% of the dose may be recovered from the urine unchanged.

Kanamycin sulphate is poorly absorbed from the gastro-intestinal tract but after intramuscular injection it is well absorbed and distributed in tissue fluids. The peak serum concentration occurs about 1 hour after administration; after an intramuscular dose of 1 g the peak serum level is usually in the range 2 to 3·5 mg% and the level then drops rapidly to negligible amounts at 24 hours.

Dose. The equivalent of up to 2 g of kanamycin base, intramuscularly, daily; for children, the equivalent of 15 mg/kg of the base, intramuscularly, daily.

Toxicity. The most serious toxic effect which may occur is irreversible loss of hearing. The possibility of this may be greatly reduced if the dose is adjusted so that the concentration in the serum does not exceed 3 mg% and the total dose administered in one course of treatment is not more than 50 g.

KETAMINE *Analgesic/Anaesthetic*

Synonym: CI 581.

2 - *o* - Chlorophenyl - 2 - methylaminocyclohexanone

$C_{13}H_{16}ClNO = 237·7$

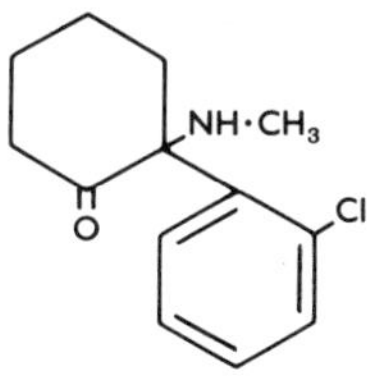

Extraction. Ketamine is extracted by organic solvents from aqueous alkaline solutions.

Chromatography. PAPER: system P1—Rf 0·55 (location under ultraviolet light, absorption; location reagents: *iodoplatinate spray*, strong reaction, white; *bromocresol green spray*, weak reaction).

THIN-LAYER: system T1—Rf 0·72 (location reagent *acidified iodoplatinate spray*, positive reaction).

GAS: system G2/225—retention time 1·0 relative to diphenhydramine; system G4—retention time 1·7 relative to diphenhydramine.

Crystal Tests. MICRO: *platinic iodide solution*—rhomboidal plates (*sensitivity:* 1 in 1000); *potassium bismuth iodide solution*—small plates (*sensitivity:* 1 in 1000).

Ultraviolet Absorption Spectrum. Ketamine in 0·1N sulphuric acid, maxima at about 264 mμ (E1%, 1 cm 16·6), 269 mμ (E1%, 1 cm 23·2), and 276 mμ (E1%, 1 cm 20·3).

KETOBEMIDONE *Narcotic Analgesic*

Synonym: Cétobémidone.

Proprietary Name: Cliradon.

4 - (3 - Hydroxyphenyl) - 1 - methyl - 4 - propionylpiperidine

$C_{15}H_{21}NO_2 = 247·3$

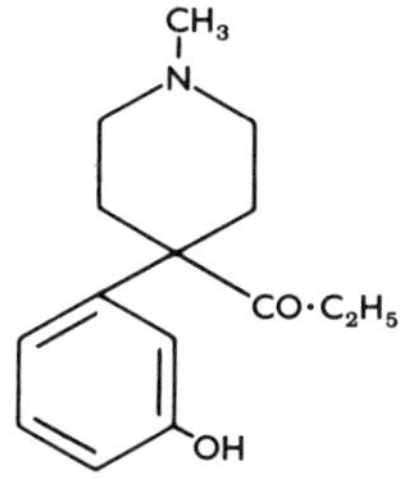

Extraction. Ketobemidone is extracted by organic solvents from aqueous ammoniacal solutions.

Chromatography. PAPER: system P1—Rf 0·50 (location under ultraviolet light, absorption; location reagents: *iodoplatinate spray*, weak reaction; *bromocresol green spray*, weak reaction); system RP1a—Rf 0·53 (location under ultraviolet light, absorption).

THIN-LAYER: system T1—Rf 0·42 (location reagent *acidified iodoplatinate spray*, positive reaction).

GAS: system G2/225—retention time 0·40 relative to codeine; system G4—retention time 1·28 relative to codeine.

Colour Tests. MICRO: sulphuric acid–formaldehyde test—dull orange (*sensitivity:* 1·0 μg); ammonium molybdate test—bright blue, fading (*sensitivity:* 0·25 μg); ammonium vanadate test—blue-green (*sensitivity:* 0·25 μg); Vitali's test— -/-/yellow (*sensitivity:* 0·25 μg).

Crystal Tests. MICRO, performed on a phosphoric acid solution: *gold bromide solution*—serrated plates (*sensitivity:* 1 in 3000); *gold bromide–hydrochloric acid solution*—serrated plates (*sensitivity:* 1 in 1500); *gold chloride solution*—serrated plates and needles (*sensitivity:* 1 in 100).

Ultraviolet Absorption Spectrum. Ketobemidone in 0·1N sulphuric acid, maximum at 279 mμ (E1%, 1 cm 75).

Metabolism. Ketobemidone has been reported to be *N*-demethylated to its corresponding nor-derivative (Vidic, 1957).

Toxicity. Ketobemidone has very marked dependence-producing properties.

LACHESINE CHLORIDE *Parasympatholytic*

Synonyms: E3; Lachesine.

(2 - Benziloyloxyethyl)ethyldimethylammonium chloride

$C_{20}H_{26}ClNO_3 = 363·9$

A white amorphous powder which darkens and shrinks at 2° to 3° below the melting-point. M.p. 212° to 216°.

Solubility. Soluble 1 in 3 of water and 1 in 10 of ethanol; almost insoluble in ether and chloroform.

Extraction. Lachesine chloride is a quaternary ammonium compound (see p. 29).

Chromatography. PAPER: system P1—Rf 0·44 (location under ultraviolet light, absorption; location reagents: *iodoplatinate spray*, strong reaction; *bromocresol green spray*, weak reaction); system RP1a—Rf 0·91 (location reagent *iodoplatinate spray*, positive reaction).
THIN-LAYER: system T1—Rf 0·02 (location reagent *acidified iodoplatinate spray*, positive reaction).
GAS: system G2/225—retention time 1·0 relative to diphenhydramine; system G4—retention time 1·5 relative to diphenhydramine. Both systems produce poor peaks, with tailing.

Colour Tests. MICRO: sulphuric acid–formaldehyde test—orange → green → blue (*sensitivity:* 0·025 μg); ammonium molybdate test—orange → green → blue (*sensitivity:* 0·05 μg); ammonium vanadate test—orange → olive (*sensitivity:* 0·05 μg).

Crystal Tests. MICRO: *gold chloride solution*—rods and needles (*sensitivity:* 1 in 3000); *lead iodide solution*—small needles in bundles (*sensitivity:* 1 in 3000).

Ultraviolet Absorption Spectrum. Lachesine chloride in 0·1N sulphuric acid, maxima at 252 mμ (E1%, 1cm 15·5), 258 mμ (E1%, 1cm 18·3), 262 mμ (E1%, 1cm 15·8), 264 mμ (E1%, 1cm 15·9), and about 268 mμ (E1%, 1cm 11·6).

Use. Lachesine is used as a mydriatic in eye-drops, usually containing 1%.

LANATOSIDE C *Cardiac Glycoside*

Proprietary Names: Cedilanid; Ceglunat; Celadigal; Cetosanol; Lanimerck.

NOTE. The name Cedilanid is applied also to a preparation of deslanoside.

3-Acetylglucosyltridigitoxoside of digoxigenin

$C_{49}H_{76}O_{20}$ = 985·1

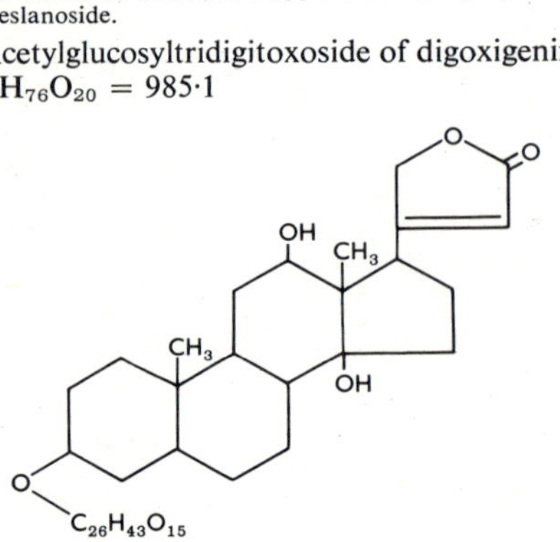

A glycoside obtained from the leaves of the woolly foxglove *Digitalis lanata* (Scrophulariaceae).

Colourless or white hygroscopic crystals or crystalline powder. It melts above 240°, indistinctly and with decomposition. Specific rotation of a 2% solution in methanol, +32° to +34·5°.

Solubility. Insoluble in water; sparingly soluble in ethanol; almost insoluble in ether; soluble 1 in 2000 of chloroform.

Extraction. Lanatoside C may be isolated by continuous extraction under reduced pressure with ethanol (see p. 29).

Chromatography. THIN-LAYER: system T14—Rf 0·36 (location reagents: *perchloric acid spray*, followed by examination under ultraviolet light, blue fluorescence; p-*anisaldehyde spray*, blue).

Colour Tests. Dissolve 2 to 3 mg in 5 ml of a solution containing 0·5 ml of 9% ferric chloride solution and 100 ml of glacial acetic acid; underlay with 5 ml of sulphuric acid—an intense blue colour forms in the glacial acetic acid layer and a brown ring free from red at the junction of the two liquids (see also Deslanoside, p. 286).

Ultraviolet Absorption Spectrum. Lanatoside C in *sulphuric acid*, maxima at 230 mμ (E1%, 1cm 235), 390 mμ (E1%, 1cm 295), and 480 mμ (E1%, 1cm 160); minima at 255 mμ and 430 mμ.

Metabolism. In the rat, following intravenous injection, lanatoside C is excreted predominantly in the bile, about 70% of a dose appearing unchanged. Only small amounts appear unchanged in the urine in the first 24 hours. Digoxin and an unidentified derivative of digoxigenin have been found as metabolites.

Lanatoside C is not as well absorbed from the gastro-intestinal tract as digitoxin, only 10% of a dose being absorbed; however, it is less cumulative. It is generally administered intravenously as deslanoside (p. 286).

Dose. Usually up to 1 mg.

Toxicity. The range between the therapeutic dose and the toxic dose of lanatoside C is wider than that of the other digitalis glycosides. The lethal dose is probably 20 to 50 times the maintenance dose.

LAUDEXIUM METHYLSULPHATE *Muscle Relaxant*

Synonym: Curarexium Methylsulphate.
Proprietary Name: Laudolissin.

Decamethylenebis[1 - (3,4 - dimethoxybenzyl) - 1,2,3,4 - tetrahydro - 6,7 - dimethoxy - 2 - methylisoquinolinium methyl sulphate]

$C_{52}H_{74}N_2O_8, C_2H_6O_8S_2 = 1077{\cdot}4$

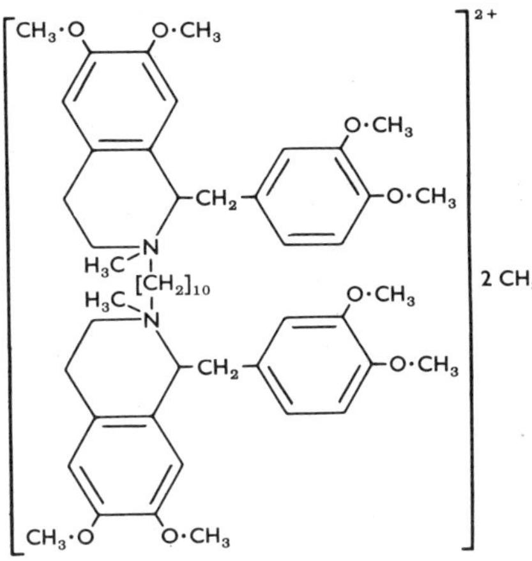

Extraction. Laudexium methylsulphate is a quaternary ammonium compound (see p. 29).

Chromatography. PAPER: system P1—Rf 0·18 (location under ultraviolet light, blue fluorescence; location reagent *iodoplatinate spray*, weak reaction); system RP1a—Rf 0·71 (location reagent *iodoplatinate spray*, positive reaction); system RP1b—Rf 0·58 (location as for RP1a). THIN-LAYER: system T1—Rf 0·01 (location reagent *acidified iodoplatinate spray*, positive reaction).

Colour Tests. MICRO: sulphuric acid–formaldehyde test—dull purple (*sensitivity:* 1·0 μg); ammonium molybdate test—blue→purple→brown (*sensitivity:* 0·1 μg); ammonium vanadate test—blue→purple→brown (*sensitivity:* 0·1 μg); Vitali's test—yellow/brown/brown (*sensitivity:* 1·0 μg).

Ultraviolet Absorption Spectrum. Laudexium methylsulphate in 0·1N sulphuric acid, maxima at 231 mμ (E1%, 1 cm 223) and 280 mμ (E1%, 1 cm 85).

LEPTAZOL *Analeptic*

Synonyms: Corazol; Pentamethazol; Pentetrazol.
Proprietary Names: Cardiazol(e); Centrazol(e); Diovascol; Gewazol; Metrazol; Pemetesan; Pentrazol.

1,5-Pentamethylenetetrazole
$C_6H_{10}N_4 = 138{\cdot}2$

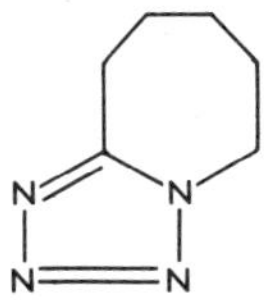

A white crystalline powder. M.p. 57° to 60°.

Solubility. Soluble 1 in less than 0·5 of water, of ethanol, and of chloroform; soluble 1 in less than 4 of ether.

Extraction. Leptazol is extracted by organic solvents from aqueous alkaline solutions.

Chromatography. PAPER: system P1—Rf 0·85 (location reagent *iodoplatinate spray*, white). THIN-LAYER: system T1—Rf 0·64 (location reagent *acidified iodoplatinate spray*, positive reaction).
GAS: system G2/120—retention time 1·9 relative to ephedrine.

Crystal Tests. MICRO: *mercuric chloride solution*—plates or tablets, often in bundles (*sensitivity:* 1 in 200); *potassium bismuth iodide solution*—small rods in bundles (*sensitivity:* 1 in 200).

Ultraviolet Absorption Spectrum. Leptazol in 0·1N sulphuric acid, maximum at 265 mμ (E1%, 1 cm 3·7).

Infra-red Absorption Spectrum. Potassium bromide disk. The principal peaks are: A 1435 or 1475, B 1115 or 1250 or 1535 (p. 744).

Metabolism. Studies in rats have shown that leptazol is metabolised in the liver to an inactive compound which is excreted in the urine and faeces but which apparently reverts to leptazol in the process of isolation (Esplin and Woodbury, 1956).
Leptazol is rapidly absorbed from the gastro-intestinal tract and from all injection sites; after a single intravenous injection it is rapidly and uniformly distributed throughout the tissues.

Dose. Usually 100 mg by mouth or by injection.

Toxicity. The estimated lethal dose is 1 to 2 g orally. Suicide by ingestion of 10 g has been reported.

LEUCINOCAINE *Local Anaesthetic*

2-Diethylamino-5-methylpentyl *p*-aminobenzoate
$C_{17}H_{28}N_2O_2 = 292{\cdot}4$

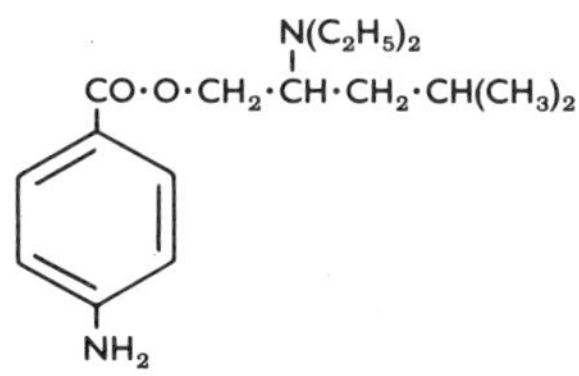

LEUCINOCAINE MESYLATE

Synonym: Leucinocaine Methanesulphonate.
Proprietary Names: Panthesin(e). It is an ingredient of Hypacom.

Leucinocaine mesylate is a powder with a melting-point of 157° to 159°.
Solubility. Soluble 1 in 3 of water; soluble in ethanol.

Extraction. Leucinocaine is extracted by organic solvents from aqueous alkaline solutions.

Chromatography. PAPER: system P1—Rf 0·62 (location under ultraviolet light, blue fluorescence; location reagents: *iodoplatinate spray*, strong reaction; *bromocresol green spray*, weak reaction); system RP1a—Rf 0·48 (location reagent *iodoplatinate spray*, positive reaction); system RP1b—Rf 0·09 (location as for RP1a). THIN-LAYER: system T1—Rf 0·62 (location reagent *acidified iodoplatinate spray*, positive reaction).

Colour Tests. MICRO: *p*-dimethylaminobenzaldehyde test—yellow; Vitali's test— –/yellow/bright yellow (*sensitivity:* 1·0 μg).

Crystal Tests. MICRO: *sodium carbonate solution*—branching needles (*sensitivity:* 1 in 400); *trinitrobenzoic acid solution*—burrs (*sensitivity:* 1 in 200).

Ultraviolet Absorption Spectrum. Leucinocaine in 0·1N sulphuric acid, maximum at 279 mμ (E1%, 1cm 114), and inflexions at about 273 mμ and about 290 mμ.

LEVALLORPHAN *Narcotic Antagonist*

(–)-*N*-Allyl-3-hydroxymorphinan

$C_{19}H_{25}NO$ = 283·4

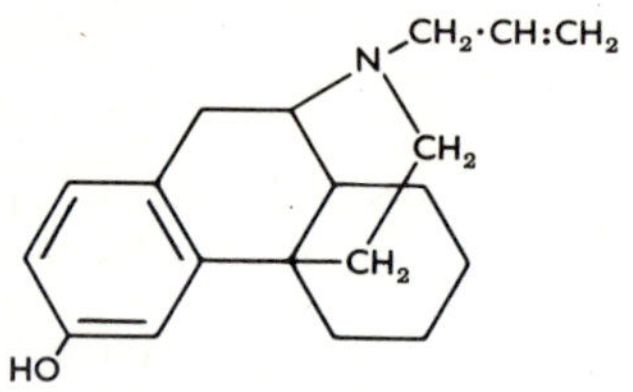

White crystals which melt at 180° to 182°. Specific rotation of a 3% solution in methanol, –88·9°.

LEVALLORPHAN TARTRATE

Proprietary Name: Lorfan.

A white crystalline powder. M.p. about 176°. Specific rotation of a 2% aqueous solution, –37·5° to –39·0°. **Solubility.** Soluble 1 in 20 of water and 1 in 100 of ethanol; very slightly soluble in ether; insoluble in chloroform.

Extraction. Levallorphan is extracted by organic solvents from aqueous ammoniacal solutions.

Chromatography. PAPER: system P1—Rf 0·73 (location reagents: *iodoplatinate spray*, strong reaction; *bromocresol green spray*, weak reaction); system RP1a—Rf 0·74 (location reagent *iodoplatinate spray*, positive reaction); system RP1b—Rf 0·06 (location as for RP1a). THIN-LAYER: system T1—Rf 0·63 (location reagent *acidified iodoplatinate spray*, positive reaction); system T7—Rf 0·98 (location reagent *iodoplatinate spray*, positive reaction); system T8—Rf 0·70 (location as for T7). GAS: system G2/225—retention time 0·95 relative to codeine.

Colour Test. MICRO: Vitali's test—yellow/yellow/orange (*sensitivity:* 0·25 μg).

Crystal Tests. MICRO: *potassium cyanide solution*—bunches of rods (*sensitivity:* 1 in 100); *potassium iodide solution*—needles and plates, forming overnight (*sensitivity:* 1 in 200).

Ultraviolet Absorption Spectrum. Levallorphan in ethanol, maxima at 229 mμ (E1%, 1cm 148) and 281·5 mμ (E1%, 1cm 54·5); in 0·1N hydrochloric acid, maxima at 226 mμ (E1%, 1cm 165) and 278 mμ (E1%, 1cm 74); in 0·1N sodium hydroxide, maxima at 240 mμ (E1%, 1cm 312) and 299 mμ (E1%, 1cm 107).

Metabolism. Levallorphan is metabolised by *N*-dealkylation and conjugation with glucuronic acid.

Dose. Up to 2 mg intravenously.

Toxicity. The estimated minimum lethal dose in man is 100 mg.

LEVAMPHETAMINE *Anorectic*

Synonyms: (–)-Amphetamine; Laevo-amphetamine.

(–)-α-Methylphenethylamine

$C_9H_{13}N$ = 135·2

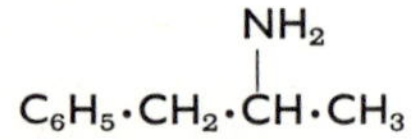

NOTE. For a microcrystalline method of differentiation of levamphetamine from amphetamine and dexamphetamine see Microcrystal Tests, p. 140.

LEVAMPHETAMINE SUCCINATE

Proprietary Names: Amodril; Cydril; Maigret.

LEVAMPHETAMINE SULPHATE

Proprietary Names: Ad-nil; Lavabo.

Extraction. Levamphetamine is extracted by organic solvents from aqueous alkaline solutions or by steam distillation.

For analytical data see under Dexamphetamine, p. 287.

LEVOMETHORPHAN *Narcotic*

(–)-3-Methoxy-*N*-methylmorphinan

$C_{18}H_{25}NO$ = 271·4

NOTE. Levomethorphan and the (±)-form, racemethorphan, are subject to international control but the (+)-isomer, dextromethorphan, is not. For a microcrystalline method of differentiation of levomethorphan from dextromethorphan see Microcrystal Tests, p. 140.

A white crystalline powder.

Solubility. Soluble 1 in 65 of water and 1 in 10 of ethanol; freely soluble in chloroform; insoluble in ether.

Extraction. Levomethorphan is extracted by organic solvents from aqueous alkaline solutions.

Chromatography. PAPER: system P1—Rf 0·60 (location reagents: *iodoplatinate spray*, strong reaction; *bromocresol green spray*, weak reaction); system RP1a—Rf 0·76 (location reagent *iodoplatinate spray*, positive reaction); system RP1b—Rf 0·09 (location as for RP1a).

THIN-LAYER: system T1—Rf 0·24 (location reagent *acidified iodoplatinate spray*, positive reaction).

GAS: system G2/225—retention time 0·70 relative to codeine.

Colour Test. MICRO: ammonium molybdate test—blue→green (*sensitivity:* 0·25 μg).

Crystal Tests. MICRO: *lead iodide solution*—bunches of serrated plates (*sensitivity:* 1 in 400); *platinic chloride solution*—feathery rosettes (*sensitivity:* 1 in 400).

Ultraviolet Absorption Spectrum. Levomethorphan in 0·1N sulphuric acid, maximum at 278 mμ (E1%, 1cm 78) and an inflexion at 283 mμ (E1%, 1cm 71·3).

LEVOMORAMIDE *Narcotic*

(−)-1-(3-Methyl-4-morpholino-2,2-diphenylbutyryl)pyrrolidine

$C_{25}H_{32}N_2O_2$ = 392·5

NOTE. For a microcrystalline method of differentiation of levomoramide from dextromoramide and racemoramide see Microcrystal Tests, p. 140.

Levomoramide melts at 190°.

Extraction. Levomoramide is extracted by organic solvents from aqueous alkaline solutions.

Chromatography. PAPER: system P1—Rf 0·61 (location reagent *iodoplatinate spray*, weak reaction); system RP1a—Rf 0·13 (location reagent *iodoplatinate spray*, positive reaction); system RP1b—Rf 0·00 (location reagent *iodoplatinate spray*, positive reaction).

THIN-LAYER: system T1—Rf 0·70 (location reagent *acidified iodoplatinate spray*, positive reaction).

Crystal Tests. MICRO: *gold chloride solution*—oily needles, some serrated, forming overnight (*sensitivity:* 1 in 1000); *picrolonic acid*—dense rosettes or rosettes of rods (*sensitivity:* 1 in 200).

Ultraviolet Absorption Spectrum. Levomoramide in 0·1N sulphuric acid, maxima at 254 mμ (E1%, 1cm 9·4), 259 mμ (E1%, 1cm 10·3), and 265 mμ (E1%, 1cm 8·6).

LEVOPHENACYLMORPHAN *Narcotic*

Synonym: NIH 7525.

(−)-3-Hydroxy-*N*-phenacylmorphinan

$C_{24}H_{27}NO_2$ = 361·5

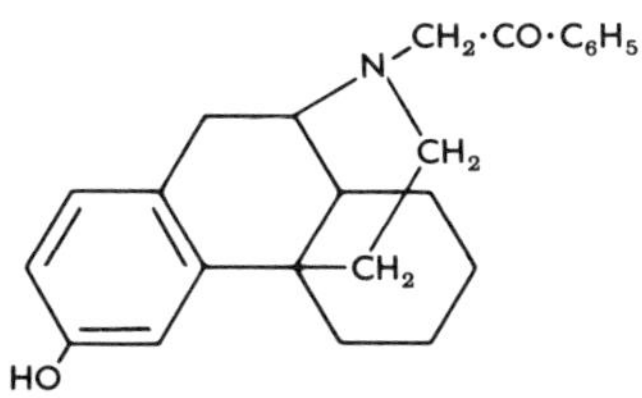

Extraction. Levophenacylmorphan is extracted by organic solvents from aqueous ammoniacal solutions.

Chromatography. PAPER: system P1—Rf 0·84 (location under ultraviolet light, absorption; location reagent *iodoplatinate spray*, weak reaction); system RP1a—Rf 0·10 (location under ultraviolet light, absorption); system RP1b—Rf 0·00 (location as for RP1a).

THIN-LAYER: system T1—Rf 0·15, streaking (location reagent *acidified iodoplatinate spray*, positive reaction).

Colour Tests. MICRO: sulphuric acid–formaldehyde test—faint purple→grey (*sensitivity:* 1·0 μg); ammonium molybdate test—blue, fading (*sensitivity:* 1·0 μg); ammonium vanadate test—faint grey (*sensitivity:* 1·0 μg); Vitali's test—yellow/faint yellow/orange (*sensitivity:* 1·0 μg).

Ultraviolet Absorption Spectrum. Levophenacylmorphan in 0·1N sulphuric acid, maximum at 251 mμ (E1%, 1cm 317) and inflexions at 275 mμ and 286 mμ.

LEVOPROPOXYPHENE *Antitussive*

(−)-α-4-Dimethylamino-3-methyl-1,2-diphenylbut-2-yl propionate

$C_{22}H_{29}NO_2$ = 339·5

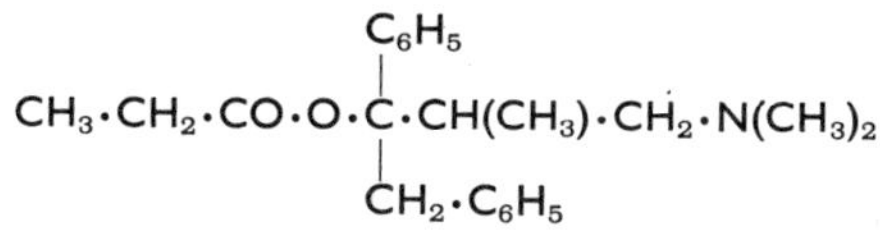

NOTE. For a microcrystalline method of differentiation of levopropoxyphene from dextropropoxyphene see Microcrystal Tests, p. 140.

LEVOPROPOXYPHENE NAPSYLATE

Synonym: Levopropoxyphene Naphthalene-2-sulphonate.

Proprietary Names: Letusin; Novrad.

Extraction. Levopropoxyphene is extracted by organic solvents from aqueous alkaline solutions.

For analytical data see under Dextropropoxyphene, p. 290.

Dose. Up to 600 mg daily has been given. Levopropoxyphene, unlike dextropropoxyphene, is said to have no analgesic activity.

LEVORPHANOL *Narcotic Analgesic*

Synonyms: Levorphan; Methorphinan.

(−)-3-Hydroxy-*N*-methylmorphinan

$C_{17}H_{23}NO$ = 257·4

NOTE. Levorphanol and the (±)-form, racemorphan (p. 534), are subject to international control but the (+)-isomer, dextrorphan (p. 291), is not. For a microcrystalline method of differentiation of levorphanol from dextrorphan see Microcrystal Tests, p. 140.

LEVORPHANOL TARTRATE

Proprietary Names: Dromoran; Levo-Dromoran.

A white crystalline powder. M.p. about 116°.

Solubility. Soluble 1 in 45 of water, 1 in 110 of ethanol, and 1 in 50 of ether.

Extraction. Levorphanol is extracted by organic solvents from aqueous ammoniacal solutions; hydrolysis of biological material is required in order to improve the yield.

Chromatography. PAPER: system P1—Rf 0·60 (location reagents: *iodoplatinate spray*, strong reaction; *bromocresol green spray*, weak reaction); system RP1a—Rf 0·86 (location reagent *iodoplatinate spray*, positive reaction); system RP1b—0·49 (location as for RP1a).
THIN-LAYER: system T1—Rf 0·24 (location reagent *acidified iodoplatinate spray*, positive reaction); system T7—Rf 0·80 (location reagent *iodoplatinate spray*, positive reaction); system T8—Rf 0·47 (location as for T7).
GAS: system G2/225—retention time 0·65 relative to codeine.

Colour Tests. MICRO: ammonium molybdate test—blue→green (*sensitivity:* 0·25 μg); Vitali's test—yellow/yellow/orange (*sensitivity:* 0·25 μg).

Crystal Tests. MICRO: *platinic bromide solution*—bunches of small irregular plates (*sensitivity:* 1 in 400); *platinic chloride solution*—masses of small irregular crystals (*sensitivity:* 1 in 400).

Ultraviolet Absorption Spectrum. Levorphanol in 0·1N sodium hydroxide, maxima at 240 mμ (E1%, 1 cm about 198) and 299 mμ (E1%, 1 cm about 70); in 0·1N sulphuric acid, maximum at 279 mμ (E1%, 1 cm 48) and an inflexion at about 285 mμ (E1%, 1 cm 44).

Metabolism. Levorphanol and dextrorphan (p. 291) appear to be metabolised *in vivo* in a similar manner. Studies in dogs have shown that both are excreted chiefly in the urine as conjugates of glucuronic acid; only insignificant amounts are excreted in the faeces in either the free or bound form. In certain species both compounds may be *N*-demethylated to some extent.

Dose. Up to 6 mg daily.

Toxicity. The estimated minimum lethal dose in adults is in the range 60 to 120 mg. It is dangerous to administer levorphanol with a barbiturate.

LIGNOCAINE *Local Anaesthetic*

Synonym: Lidocaine.

N-Diethylaminoacetyl-2,6-xylidine
$C_{14}H_{22}N_2O = 234{\cdot}3$

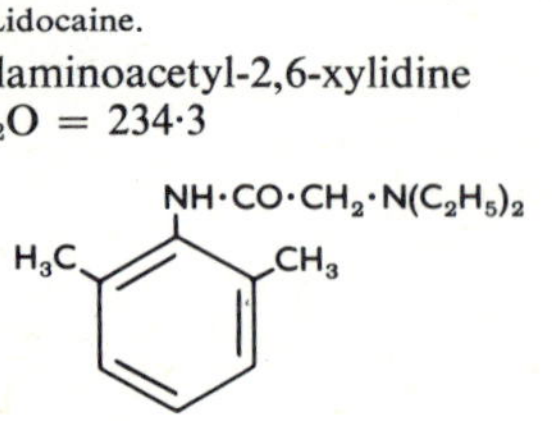

A white or slightly yellow crystalline powder. M.p. 66° to 69°
Solubility. Practically insoluble in water; very soluble in ethanol, ether, and chloroform.

LIGNOCAINE HYDROCHLORIDE

Proprietary Names: Duncaine; Lignostab; Xylocaine; Xylotox.

A white crystalline powder. M.p. 76° to 79°.
Solubility. Soluble 1 in 0·7 of water, 1 in 1·5 of ethanol, and 1 in 40 of chloroform; insoluble in ether.

Extraction. Lignocaine is extracted by organic solvents from aqueous alkaline solutions.

Chromatography. PAPER: system P1—Rf 0·62 (location under ultraviolet light, strong absorption; location reagents: *iodoplatinate spray*, strong reaction; *bromocresol green spray*, strong reaction); system RP1a—Rf 0·64 (location under ultraviolet light, absorption; location reagent *iodoplatinate spray*, positive reaction); system RP1b—Rf 0·04 (location as for RP1a).
THIN-LAYER: system T1—Rf 0·71 (location reagent *acidified iodoplatinate spray*, positive reaction).
GAS: system G1/180—retention time 1·03 relative to diphenhydramine; system G2/225—retention time 1·0 relative to diphenhydramine; system G3—retention time 3·90 relative to diphenhydramine; system G4—retention time 2·30 relative to diphenhydramine.

Colour Test. To a 2% solution in water, add 1 ml of dilute nitric acid and 3 ml of *mercuric nitrate solution* and heat to boiling—yellow or yellow-green.

Crystal Tests. MICRO: *potassium permanganate solution*—mass of needles (*sensitivity:* 1 in 1500); *potassium tri-iodide solution* (*1*)—yellow hexagonal crystals, forming overnight (*sensitivity:* 1 in 1500).

Ultraviolet Absorption Spectrum. Lignocaine in ethanol, maxima at 263 mμ (E1%, 1 cm 13·5) and 278 mμ (E1%, 1 cm 2·2), and an inflexion at about 270 mμ.

Infra-red Absorption Spectrum. Lignocaine (base). Potassium bromide disk. The principal peaks are: A 1490 or 1662, B 762 (p. 789).

Quantitative Estimation. Beckett *et al.* (1965a) describe a gas chromatographic determination of lignocaine in blood and urine.

Metabolism. Dealkylation is a major metabolic pathway in man; 3 to 5% of the dose is excreted as monoethylglycinexylidide (the monodealkylated derivative); only about 12% is excreted unchanged. Further dealkylation of monoethylglycinexylidide to glycinexylidide has not been demonstrated; however, it may occur slowly. The very low blood-levels of lignocaine 45 minutes after an intravenous injection indicate a high extravascular concentration of the drug (Beckett *et al.*, 1966).

Dose. The total dose should not exceed 500 mg in 24 hours if adrenaline has been added, or 200 mg if it has not.

Toxicity. Concentrations of lignocaine below 0·5% have about the same toxicity as similar concentrations of procaine hydrochloride, but stronger solutions of lignocaine hydrochloride are relatively more toxic.

LD50 (intravenous): in rabbits 15 mg/kg.

CASE EXAMPLE. A young woman died following infiltration of the right side of her face, head, and neck with about 100 ml of a 2% lignocaine solution. Post-mortem levels of lignocaine were as follows: blood, 1·2 mg%; brain, 6·6 mg%; kidney, 8·4 mg%; liver, 9·6 mg%; stomach contents, 44·0 mg%; urine, 1·8 mg%. The presence of a salicylate was indicated in the urine to the extent of 7·6 mg%, and phenacetin and dextropropoxyphene hydrochloride were found in the stomach contents (Sunshine and Fike, 1964).

LINCOMYCIN *Antibiotic*

Methyl 6,8-dideoxy-6-(1-methyl-4-propylpyrrolidine-2-carboxamido)-1-thio-D-*erythro*-α-D-*galacto*-octopyranoside

$C_{18}H_{34}N_2O_6S = 406·5$

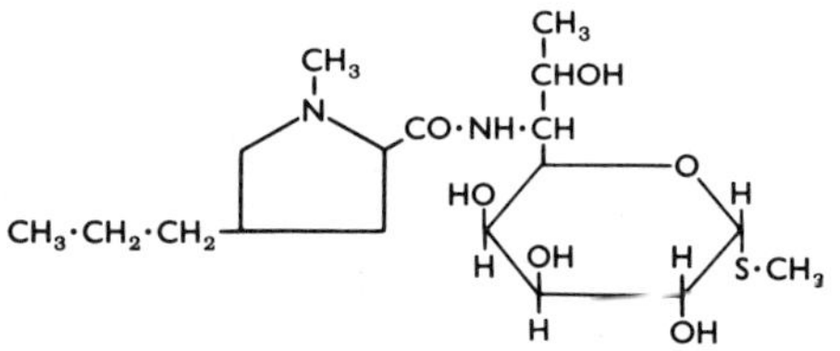

Solubility. Soluble in water and most organic solvents.

LINCOMYCIN HYDROCHLORIDE
Proprietary Names: Lincocin; Mycivin.

A white crystalline powder.
Solubility. Very soluble in water; soluble in ethanol.

Extraction. Lincomycin is extracted by organic solvents from aqueous alkaline solutions.

Chromatography. PAPER: system P1—Rf 0·18 (location reagents: *iodoplatinate spray*, white; *bromocresol green spray*, strong reaction; *iodine vapour*, weak reaction; *potassium permanganate spray*, strong reaction).
THIN-LAYER: system T1—Rf 0·67 (location reagent *potassium permanganate spray*, positive reaction).

Colour Test. MICRO: ammonium molybdate test—blue (*sensitivity:* 1·0 μg).

Infra-red Absorption Spectrum. Lincomycin (base). Potassium bromide disk. The principal peaks are: A 1645, B 1050 or 1075 or 1523 (p. 789).

Metabolism. Lincomycin is well-absorbed from the gastro-intestinal tract and is excreted in the urine and bile. It is widely distributed in the tissues. Following a 500-mg oral dose, lincomycin is absorbed rapidly, reaching peak plasma levels of 0·07 to 0·57 mg% after 2 to 4 hours, and within 24 hours between 4 and 13% is recovered unchanged in the urine. Following a single intramuscular injection of 600 mg of lincomycin, peak plasma concentrations of about 0·8 to 1·2 mg% appear after 1 to 2 hours, the level gradually decreasing over the following 22 hours. Approximately 30 to 60% of a parenteral dose is excreted unchanged in the urine within 24 hours.

Dose. Up to 2 g daily.

Toxicity. LD50 (oral): in rats more than 4 g/kg.

LOBELINE *Alkaloid*

Synonym: Alpha-lobeline.

2-(2-Hydroxy-2-phenylethyl)-*N*-methyl-6-phenacylpiperidine

$C_{22}H_{27}NO_2 = 337·5$

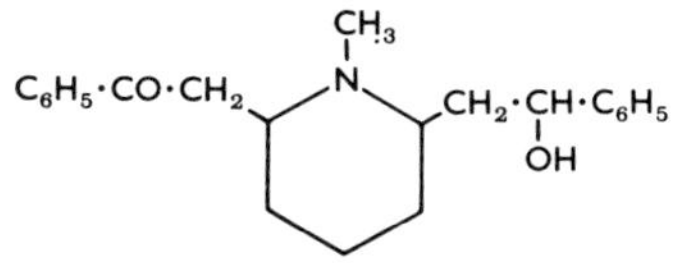

An alkaloid obtained from *Lobelia inflata* (Lobeliaceae). M.p. 130° to 131°.

Solubility. Sparingly soluble in water; soluble in hot ethanol, ether, and chloroform.

LOBELINE HYDROCHLORIDE
Proprietary Names: Lobeline-Sandoz. It is the main ingredient of Lobidan, a smoking deterrent.

A white crystalline powder. M.p. not lower than 180°.
Solubility. Soluble 1 in 40 of water and 1 in 12 of ethanol; very slightly soluble in ether; very soluble in chloroform.

Extraction. Lobeline is extracted by organic solvents from aqueous alkaline solutions.

Chromatography. PAPER: system P1—Rf 0·82 (location under ultraviolet light, strong absorption; location reagents: *iodoplatinate spray*, weak reaction; *bromocresol green spray*, weak reaction).
THIN-LAYER: system T1—Rf 0·55 (location reagent *acidified iodoplatinate spray*, positive reaction).

Colour Tests. MICRO: sulphuric acid–formaldehyde test—red-purple (*sensitivity:* 0·1 μg); ammonium molybdate test—grey → purple (*sensitivity:* 1·0 μg); ammonium vanadate test—grey (*sensitivity:* 0·5 μg).

Crystal Tests. MICRO: *potassium cyanide solution*—rosettes (*sensitivity:* 1 in 3000); *sodium carbonate solution*—rosettes (*sensitivity:* 1 in 3000).

Ultraviolet Absorption Spectrum. Lobeline in 0·1N hydrochloric acid, maximum at 249 mμ ($E^{1\%}_{1cm}$ 416); minimum at about 222 mμ; in 0·1N sulphuric acid, maximum at 249 mμ ($E^{1\%}_{1cm}$ 421).

Infra-red Absorption Spectrum. Lobeline (base). Potassium bromide disk. The principal peaks are: A 1687, B 700, C 1115 or 1211 (p. 789).

Dose. Up to 10 mg, intramuscularly, as a respiratory stimulant.

Toxicity. Lobeline has a peripheral action very closely resembling that of nicotine (p. 440).

LUCANTHONE *Filaricide*

Synonyms: BW 57-233; NSC 14574.

1 - (2 - Diethylaminoethylamino) - 4 - methylthiaxanthen-9-one

$C_{20}H_{24}N_2OS = 340{\cdot}5$

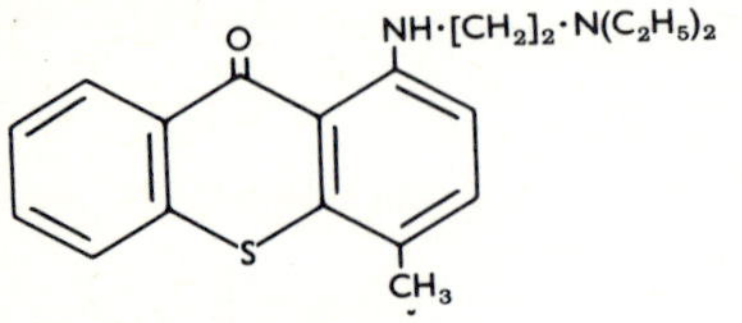

Lucanthone melts at 66°.

LUCANTHONE HYDROCHLORIDE

Proprietary Names: Miracil D; Nilodin.

A yellowish-orange crystalline powder. M.p. 195° to 198°. **Solubility.** Soluble 1 in 110 of water, 1 in 85 of ethanol, and 1 in 20 of chloroform; readily soluble in warm water and warm ethanol; insoluble in ether.

Extraction. Lucanthone is extracted by organic solvents from aqueous alkaline solutions.

Chromatography. PAPER: system P1—Rf 0·72 (location under ultraviolet light, orange fluorescence; location reagents: *iodoplatinate spray*, weak reaction; *potassium permanganate spray*, strong reaction).

THIN-LAYER: system T1—Rf 0·53 (location reagent *acidified iodoplatinate spray*, positive reaction).

Colour Tests. MICRO: sulphuric acid–formaldehyde test—(yellow) orange→purple→blue (*sensitivity:* 0·1 µg); Vitali's test—(yellow) yellow/yellow/red (*sensitivity:* 0·1 µg).

Crystal Tests. MICRO: *mercuric chloride solution*—bunches of oily needles (*sensitivity:* 1 in 1000); *potassium iodide solution*—branching needles (*sensitivity:* 1 in 1000).

Ultraviolet Absorption Spectrum. Lucanthone in 0·1N sulphuric acid, maxima at 223 mµ (E1%, 1 cm 566), 257 mµ (E1%, 1 cm 1325), and 331 mµ (E1%, 1 cm 236), and an inflexion at 280 mµ.

Infra-red Absorption Spectrum. Lucanthone (base). Potassium bromide disk. The principal peaks are: A 1616, B 1224 or 1512 or 1591 (p. 789).

Metabolism. Lucanthone hydrochloride is readily absorbed from the gastro-intestinal tract. Most of it is metabolised in the body, only 7% to 10% appearing unchanged in the urine.

Dose. Usually 1 g twice daily for 3 days.

Toxicity. Lucanthone is more toxic when given by injection than when given by mouth. The skin may turn yellow or orange and remain so for about 4 weeks. Hepatic or renal damage has resulted from chronic poisoning.

LD50 (oral): in mice 140 mg/kg.

LYMECYCLINE *Antibiotic*

Synonym: Tetracycline-L-methylenelysine.

Proprietary Names: Armyl; Mucomycin; Tetralysal.

N^2-{[(+)-5-Amino-5-carboxypentylamino]-methyl}tetracycline

$C_{29}H_{38}N_4O_{10} = 602{\cdot}6$

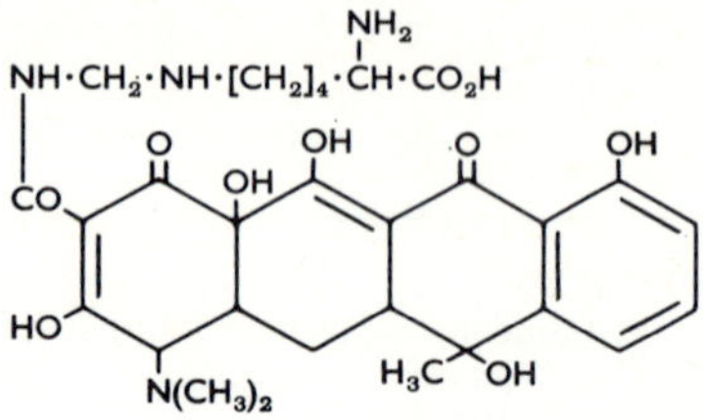

A yellow hygroscopic powder which darkens on exposure to light. M.p. above 200°, with slow decomposition. It is very unstable and, in solution, splits into tetracycline and methylenelysine; spots of these two substances appear on chromatograms.

Solubility. Soluble 1 in less than 1 of water; slightly soluble in ethanol; insoluble in ether and chloroform.

Chromatography. PAPER: system P1—Rf (for tetracycline) 0·25 (location under ultraviolet light, orange fluorescence; location reagents: *bromocresol green spray*, weak reaction; *potassium permanganate spray*, weak reaction); Rf (for methylenelysine) 0·00 (location reagent *ninhydrin spray*, purple).

THIN-LAYER: system T1—Rf 0·05, streaking (location under ultraviolet light, orange fluorescence; location reagent *potassium permanganate spray*, positive reaction).

Colour Tests. MICRO: sulphuric acid–formaldehyde test—(yellow) dull orange (*sensitivity:* 1·0 µg); ammonium molybdate test—(yellow) dull purple→yellow (*sensitivity:* 1·0 µg); ammonium vanadate test—(yellow) purple-brown→yellow (*sensitivity:* 1·0 µg); sulphuric acid test—purple→yellow; Vitali's test—(yellow) bright yellow/yellow/orange (*sensitivity:* 1·0 µg).

Crystal Tests. MICRO: *platinic iodide solution*—dense rosettes, forming overnight (*sensitivity:* 1 in 100); *potassium mercuric iodide solution*—gelatinous rosettes, forming overnight (*sensitivity:* 1 in 100); *potassium tri-iodide solution (2)*—shell-like rosettes, forming overnight (*sensitivity:* 1 in 100).

Ultraviolet Absorption Spectrum. Lymecycline in 0·1N sulphuric acid, maxima at 268·5 mµ (E1%, 1 cm 280) and 356 mµ (E1%, 1 cm 160).

Metabolism. Lymecycline is rapidly absorbed after oral administration and widely distributed in body tissues including the cerebrospinal fluid. Maximum blood-levels are soon reached and maintained for long periods. It is excreted in the urine and bile.

Dose. Usually 204 mg, the equivalent of 150 mg of tetracycline base, every 6 hours.

Toxicity. LD50 (oral): in mice 3 g/kg.

LYSERGAMIDE *Hallucinogen*

Synonyms: Lysergic Acid Amide; Ergine.

$C_{16}H_{17}N_3O = 267{\cdot}3$

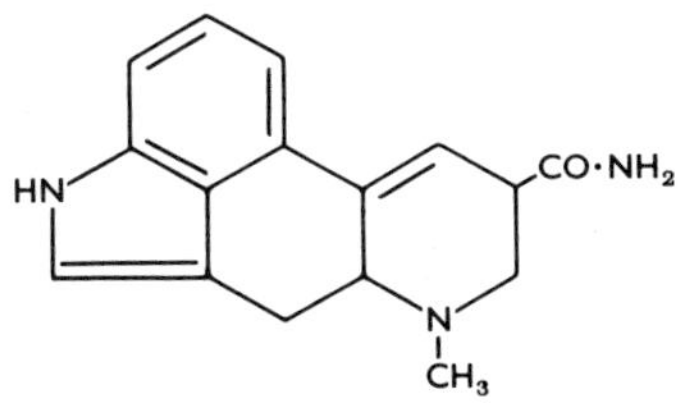

Lysergamide is found in *Rivea corymbosa*, *Ipomoea* spp. (Convolvulaceae), and ergot.

Chromatography. PAPER: system P1—Rf 0·11 (location under ultraviolet light, blue fluorescence; location reagents: *iodoplatinate spray*, weak reaction; *bromocresol green spray*, weak reaction; p-*dimethylaminobenzaldehyde spray*, purple).

THIN-LAYER: system T1—Rf 0·60 (location reagent p-*dimethylaminobenzaldehyde spray*, blue); system T9—Rf 0·18 (location as for T1).

Colour Tests. MICRO: sulphuric acid–formaldehyde test—brown (*sensitivity:* 1·0 μg); ammonium molybdate test—grey-blue→green (*sensitivity:* 1·0 μg); Vitali's test—brown/brown/purple-brown (*sensitivity:* 1·0 μg).

LYSERGIC ACID *Hallucinogen*

$C_{16}H_{16}N_2O_2 = 268{\cdot}3$

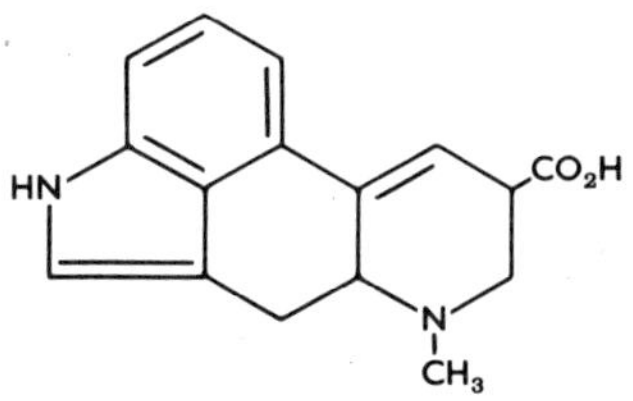

A white crystalline powder. M.p. 240°, with decomposition.

Solubility. Slightly soluble in water; soluble in dilute acids and alkalis.

Chromatography. PAPER: system P1—Rf 0·19 (location under ultraviolet light, blue fluorescence; location reagents: *iodoplatinate spray*, weak reaction; p-*dimethylaminobenzaldehyde spray*, purple); system RP1a—Rf 0·56 (location under ultraviolet light, purple fluorescence); system RP1b—Rf 0·61 (location as for RP1a).

THIN-LAYER: system T1—Rf 0·58 (location reagent p-*dimethylaminobenzaldehyde spray*, blue); system T9—Rf 0·05 (location under ultraviolet light, blue fluorescence; location reagent p-*dimethylaminobenzaldehyde spray*, blue).

Colour Tests. MICRO: sulphuric acid–formaldehyde test—brown (*sensitivity:* 1·0 μg); ammonium molybdate test—greenish-brown (*sensitivity:* 1·0 μg); ammonium vanadate test—greenish-brown (*sensitivity:* 1·0 μg); Vitali's test—brown/brown/brown (*sensitivity:* 1·0 μg).

Crystal Tests. MICRO: *potassium tri-iodide solution* (*2*)—dense rosettes (*sensitivity.* 1 in 400); *sodium carbonate solution*—rosettes (*sensiitivity:* 1 in 200).

Ultraviolet Absorption Spectrum. Lysergic acid in 0·1N sulphuric acid, maxima at 222 mμ (E1%, 1 cm 620), 281·5 mμ (E1%, 1 cm 140), and about 290 mμ (E1%, 1 cm 134).

Infra-red Absorption Spectrum. Potassium bromide disk. The principal peaks are: A 1592, B 1352 or 1372, C 1445 (p. 789).

LYSERGIDE *Hallucinogen*

Synonyms: LSD; LSD 25; Lysergic Acid Diethylamide.
Proprietary Name: Delysid.

(+)-*NN*-Diethyl-lysergamide

$C_{20}H_{25}N_3O = 323{\cdot}4$

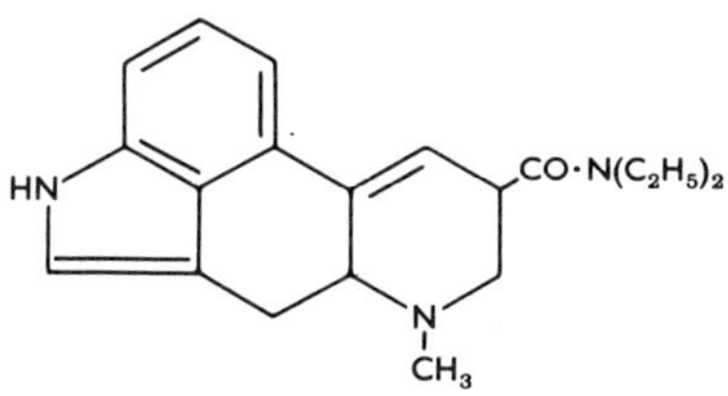

A crystalline substance. M.p. 80° to 85°.

Extraction. Lysergide is extracted by organic solvents from aqueous alkaline solutions.

Chromatography. PAPER: system P1—Rf 0·47 (location under ultraviolet light, blue fluorescence; location reagents: *iodoplatinate spray*, weak reaction; p-*dimethylaminobenzaldehyde spray*, deep purple).

THIN-LAYER: system T1—Rf 0·66 (location reagent p-*dimethylaminobenzaldehyde spray*, blue); system T9—Rf 0·60 (location under ultraviolet light, blue fluorescence; location reagent p-*dimethylaminobenzaldehyde spray*, blue).

Genest and Farmilo (1964) have described a thin-layer chromatographic system which separates lysergide from the barbiturates.

Colour Tests. MICRO: sulphuric acid–formaldehyde test—grey (*sensitivity:* 1·0 μg); ammonium molybdate test—grey-green→grey-blue (*sensitivity:* 1·0 μg); ammonium vanadate test—grey (*sensitivity:* 1·0 μg); Vitali's test—brown/brown/purple-brown.

Quantitative Estimation. Methods of detection and estimation of lysergide involving thin-layer chromatography, elution, and subsequent spectrofluorimetry have been described by Genest and Farmilo (1964) and Dal Cortivo and Broich (1966). Radecka and Nigam (1966) have described a gas chromatographic method of detection of lysergide and Cromp and Turney (1967) have described an infra-red spectrophotometric method.

Martin and Alexander (1967; 1968) describe methods of analysis of preparations containing lysergide, including extraction procedures, fluorescence tests, thin-layer chromatography, and infra-red identification.

Metabolism. Studies in animals have shown that lysergide is metabolised in the liver to 3 or 4 different compounds which are excreted in the bile to the extent that 60 to 80% of the radioactivity of injected lysergide is found in the gastro-intestinal tract. One route appears to be hydroxylation in the 12-position and conjugation with glucuronic acid.

Lysergide is rapidly absorbed after both oral and parenteral administration. Following the intravenous administration of 2 μg/kg bodyweight of lysergide in human subjects, the plasma levels fall steeply and then begin to level off after 30 minutes when a concentration of between 4 and 6 μg/ml may be obtained. After 8 hours, only a small amount remains in the plasma. Studies in rats have shown that lysergide is not present in the bound form in the blood and that it is widely distributed in most organs. Only 7 to 8% of the radioactivity is excreted in 12 hours.

Dose. A dose of 1 μg/kg is said to produce a hallucinatory psychosis of short duration; in psychotic patients, up to 4 μg/kg has been given.

Toxicity. Large doses have produced vomiting, dizziness, increased intestinal paralysis, ataxia, and paralysis of the arms and legs; death may occur from respiratory failure. A single dose of 1·5 mg has been tolerated.

Tolerance to lysergide can develop rapidly but is usually lost in 2 or 3 days. The usual dose taken by a non-tolerant person is 200 to 400 μg, but some physical effects are experienced when doses of as little as 30 μg are taken (Council on Mental Health and Committee on Alcoholism and Drug Dependence of the American Medical Association, 1967, *J. Am. med. Ass.*, **202**, 47).

MALATHION *Pesticide*

Synonyms: Carbofos; Malathon.

Proprietary Names: Cidial; Kypfos; Malastan; Malaphos; Malathexo. It is an ingredient of Malacon.

S-1,2-Di(ethoxycarbonyl)ethyl dimethyl phosphorothiolothionate

$C_{10}H_{19}O_6PS_2$ = 330·4

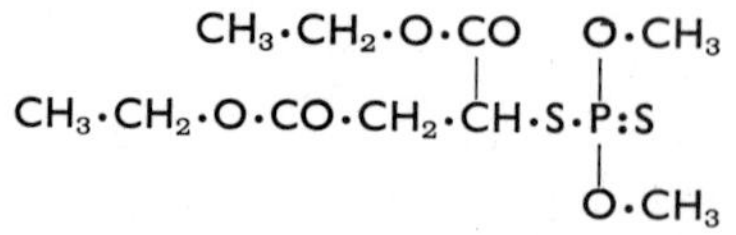

The pure product is a very pale straw-yellow oil which decomposes in strong acid or high humidity. Although stable in light, it decomposes at high temperatures. It corrodes iron, tinplate, lead, and copper. M.p. 2·85°. B.p. 156° to 157° at 0·7 mm Hg. Refractive index 1·4985.

Solubility. Soluble 1 in 6800 of water; miscible with ethanol, ether, and chloroform.

Screening Test. Fisk *et al.* (1965) have described a rapid qualitative screening test involving extraction into n-heptane and subsequent spectrophotometric determination.

Extraction. Malathion is extracted by organic solvents from aqueous acid or alkaline solutions.

Chromatography. PAPER: system P11—Rf 0·90 (location reagent *bromine vapour* followed by *congo red spray*, clear blue against a red background).

THIN-LAYER: system T15—Rf 0·29 (location reagent *palladium chloride spray*); system T16—Rf 0·45 (location reagent *bromophenol blue spray* followed by *5% aqueous acetic acid spray*, mauve).

GAS: see under Parathion, p. 469.

Quantitative Estimation. Malathion may be determined spectrophotometrically in cereals and oilseeds following extraction with carbon tetrachloride, hydrolysis with sodium hydroxide and conversion to the cupric salt (Report by the Malathion Panel, 1960).

Use. Malathion is employed as a dusting-powder in concentrations of 1, 4, and 5%, as a dispersible powder containing 25%, and as an emulsifiable concentrate containing 56%. It is also employed in sprays of varying concentrations. It is active both as a stomach and as a contact poison.

Toxicity. Malathion is one of the least toxic organophosphorus pesticides; it is said to be 100 times less toxic to man than parathion. The estimated mammalian lethal dose is said to be about 1 g/kg. Skin absorption is slow and slight. Ingestion of 4 g and 14 g has caused severe illness in a child and adult respectively, and 5 g has proved fatal in an old man (Gitelson *et al.*, 1966).

The quoted LD50 values vary very greatly, being dependent upon the purity of the product.

CASE EXAMPLES. A 42-year-old woman ingested at least 120 ml of a 50% malathion spray with suicidal intent, corresponding to 1 g/kg. She became unconscious and developed bronchial hypersecretion and cyanosis but recovered after treatment. Reference is made to 11 cases of accidental poisoning and 4 attempts at suicide reported in the literature. No analyses are given (Goldin *et al.*, 1964).

A 17-year-old boy accidentally drank at least 30 ml of a pesticide, consisting of a 1:1 mixture of malathion and xylene, and became unconscious. In hospital, a large amount of malathion in an aromatic solvent was recovered from the gastric contents. Following tracheostomy and administration of atropine and pralidoxime, the boy recovered within 20 days (Gitelson *et al.*, 1966).

MEBEZONIUM IODIDE *Muscle Relaxant*

Proprietary Name: It is an ingredient of T61, a preparation used for veterinary euthanasia.

4,4′ - Methylenedi(cyclohexyltrimethylammonium iodide)

$C_{19}H_{40}I_2N_2 = 550{\cdot}4$

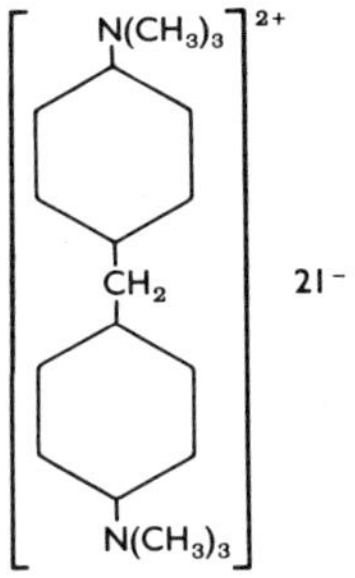

A white crystalline powder.
Solubility. Soluble in water.

Extraction. Mebezonium iodide is a quaternary ammonium compound (see p. 29).

Chromatography. PAPER: system P1—Rf 0·02 (location reagents: *iodoplatinate spray*, strong reaction; *bromocresol green spray*, strong reaction).

THIN-LAYER: system T1—Rf 0·00 (location reagent *acidified iodoplatinate spray*, positive reaction).

Crystal Tests. MICRO: *styphnic acid*—blades or plates, some serrated, best viewed under polarised light (*sensitivity:* 1 in 1000); *picric acid*—blades, some serrated, best viewed under polarised light (*sensitivity:* 1 in 1000).

MEBHYDROLIN *Antihistamine*

5 - Benzyl - 1,2,3,4 - tetrahydro - 2 - methyl - γ - carboline

$C_{38}H_{40}N_4 = 552{\cdot}8$

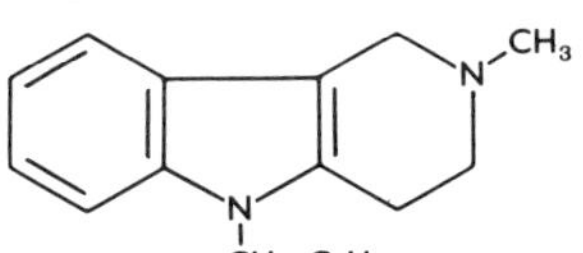

A white crystalline powder. M.p. 95°.
Solubility. Insoluble in water; soluble in ethanol, ether, and chloroform.

MEBHYDROLIN NAPADISYLATE

Synonym: Mebhydrolin Naphthalenedisulphonate.
Proprietary Names: Fabahistin; Incidal; Omeril.

A white powder.
Solubility. Very slightly soluble in water, ethanol, ether, and chloroform.

Extraction. Mebhydrolin is extracted by organic solvents from aqueous alkaline solutions.

Chromatography. PAPER: system P1—Rf 0·55 (location under ultraviolet light, blue fluorescence; location reagents: *iodoplatinate spray*, strong reaction; *bromocresol green spray*, strong reaction).

THIN-LAYER: system T1—Rf 0·58 (location reagent *acidified iodoplatinate spray*, positive reaction).
GAS: system G2/225—retention time 1·26 relative to codeine.

Colour Tests. MICRO: sulphuric acid–formaldehyde test—grey-blue (*sensitivity:* 1·0 μg); ammonium molybdate test—bright blue (*sensitivity:* 0·5 μg); ammonium vanadate test—bright blue (*sensitivity:* 0·5 μg); Vitali's test—green→yellow/yellow/yellow (*sensitivity:* 1·0 μg).

Crystal Tests. MICRO: *mercuric chloride solution*—rosettes of needles, sometimes dense (*sensitivity:* 1 in 400); *potassium cyanide solution*—rosettes (*sensitivity:* 1 in 200).

Dose. Up to 300 mg (base) daily.

MECAMYLAMINE *Antihypertensive*

Synonym: Dimécamine.

3-Methylaminoisocamphane

$C_{11}H_{21}N = 167{\cdot}3$

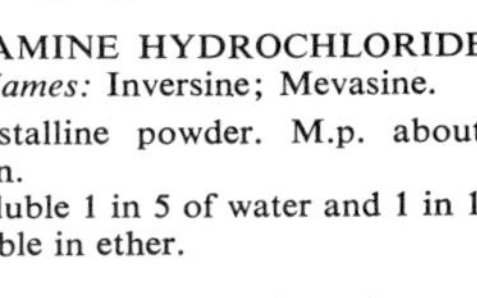

An oily liquid. B.p. 72°.
Solubility. Slightly soluble in water.

MECAMYLAMINE HYDROCHLORIDE

Proprietary Names: Inversine; Mevasine.

A white crystalline powder. M.p. about 246°, with decomposition.
Solubility. Soluble 1 in 5 of water and 1 in 12 of ethanol; almost insoluble in ether.

Extraction. Mecamylamine is extracted by organic solvents from aqueous alkaline solutions.

Chromatography. PAPER: system P1—Rf 0·64 (location under ultraviolet light, blue fluorescence; location reagents: *iodoplatinate spray*, weak reaction; *bromocresol green spray*, weak reaction).

THIN-LAYER: system T1—Rf 0·22, streaking (location reagent *iodine vapour*, positive reaction).

Crystal Tests. MICRO: *potassium permanganate solution*—small cubes (*sensitivity:* 1 in 1000); *potassium mercuric iodide solution*—long rhomboidal prisms (*sensitivity:* 1 in 1000).

Ultraviolet Absorption Spectrum. Mecamylamine

in 0·1N sulphuric acid, maximum at 228 mμ (E1%, 1 cm 24·4).

Metabolism. Mecamylamine appears to be metabolised, although metabolic products have not yet been identified; only 40 to 60% of the drug is excreted unchanged in the urine during 24 hours. The rate of excretion of mecamylamine is influenced by the pH of the urine, being greater in acid and less in alkaline urine. It is well absorbed from the gastro-intestinal tract, and, due to slow excretion, is very long-acting.

Dose. Up to 60 mg daily.

MECLOFENOXATE *Central Stimulant*

Synonyms: Centrophenoxine; Clophenoxate; Deanol 4-chlorophenoxyacetate; Meclofenoxane.

2-Dimethylaminoethyl *p*-chlorophenoxyacetate

$C_{12}H_{16}ClNO_3 = 257{\cdot}7$

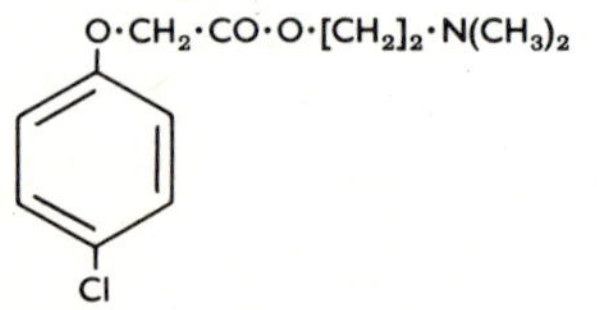

MECLOFENOXATE HYDROCHLORIDE

Proprietary Names: ANP 235; Lucidril.

A white powder which rapidly hydrolyses in aqueous solutions. M.p. 136°.

Solubility. Very soluble in water; insoluble in ether and chloroform.

Extraction. Meclofenoxate is extracted by organic solvents from aqueous alkaline solutions.

Chromatography. PAPER: system P1—Rf 0·38 (location under ultraviolet light, absorption; location reagent *iodoplatinate spray*, strong reaction).

THIN-LAYER: system T1—Rf 0·19 (location reagent *potassium permanganate spray*, positive reaction).

GAS: system G2/225—retention time 0·75 relative to diphenhydramine; system G4—retention time 1·30 relative to diphenhydramine.

Crystal Tests. MICRO: *gold bromide solution*—serrated plates (*sensitivity:* 1 in 1000); *styphnic acid*—clusters of long needles (*sensitivity:* 1 in 1000).

Ultraviolet Absorption Spectrum. Meclofenoxate in 0·1N sulphuric acid, maxima at 225 mμ (E1%, 1 cm 345) and 277 mμ (E1%, 1 cm 40), and an inflexion at about 283 mμ.

Dose. Usually up to 800 mg daily.

Toxicity. LD50 (intravenous): in mice 330 mg/kg.

MECLOZINE *Antihistamine*

Synonyms: Histamethizine; Meclizine.

1-(*p*-Chlorodiphenylmethyl)-4-(*m*-methylbenzyl)piperazine

$C_{25}H_{27}ClN_2 = 391{\cdot}0$

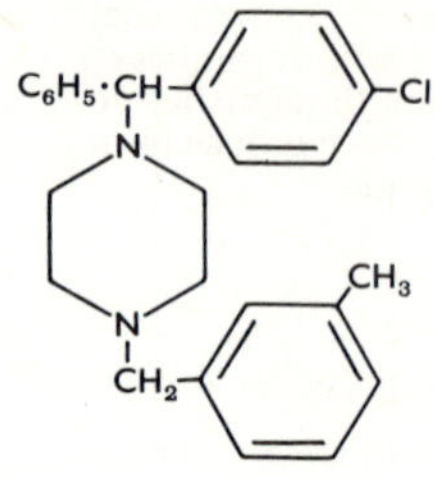

Meclozine has a boiling-point of 230° at 2 mm Hg.

MECLOZINE HYDROCHLORIDE

Proprietary Names: Ancolan; Antivert; Bonadettes; Bonamine Hydrochloride; Bonadoxin; Bonine; Postafene; Sea-Legs. It is an ingredient of Ancofen, Ancoloxin, and Ancovert.

A white crystalline powder. M.p. about 224°, with decomposition.

Solubility. Soluble 1 in 1000 of water, 1 in 25 of ethanol, and 1 in 5 of chloroform; soluble in glacial acetic acid.

Extraction. Meclozine is extracted by organic solvents from aqueous alkaline solutions.

Chromatography. PAPER: system P1—Rf 0·92 (location reagents: *iodoplatinate spray*, weak reaction; *bromocresol green spray*, strong reaction); system RP1a—Rf 0·00 (location under ultraviolet light, absorption; location reagent *iodoplatinate spray*, positive reaction); system RP1b—Rf 0·00 (location as for RP1a).

THIN-LAYER: system T1—Rf 0·80 (location reagent *acidified iodoplatinate spray*, positive reaction).

GAS: system G1/250—retention time 3·44 relative to codeine.

Colour Test. MICRO: ammonium molybdate test—yellow.

Ultraviolet Absorption Spectrum. Meclozine in 0·1N sulphuric acid, maxima at 230 mμ (E1%, 1 cm 330), about 261 mμ (E1%, 1 cm 32), 265·5 mμ (E1%, 1 cm 34), and 272·5 mμ (E1%, 1 cm 23); meclozine hydrochloride in ethanol, maximum at 230 mμ (E1%, 1 cm about 330).

Infra-red Absorption Spectrum. Meclozine (base). Potassium bromide disk. The principal peaks are: A 1489, B 1001, C 799 or 1081 or 1130 (p. 790).

Metabolism. Meclozine is an antihistamine which is used mainly for its anti-emetic action which is potent and prolonged. Studies in rats have shown meclozine to be metabolised, one of the metabolites being norchlorcyclizine which is found in the urine and in a large variety of tissues (Narrod *et al.*, 1965).

Dose. The usual dose of the hydrochloride is up to 50 mg daily.

Toxicity. There have been reports which suggest a possibility of human foetal abnormalities resulting from the administration of meclozine, but a causal relationship has not been confirmed. The estimated lethal dose in man is in the range 25 to 250 mg/kg.

MEFENAMIC ACID *Analgesic/Antipyretic*

Synonyms: CI 473; INF 3355; *N*-2,3-Xylylanthranilic Acid.
Proprietary Names: Coslan; Parkemed; Ponstan.

o-(2,3-Xylylamino)benzoic acid
$C_{15}H_{15}NO_2$ = 241·3

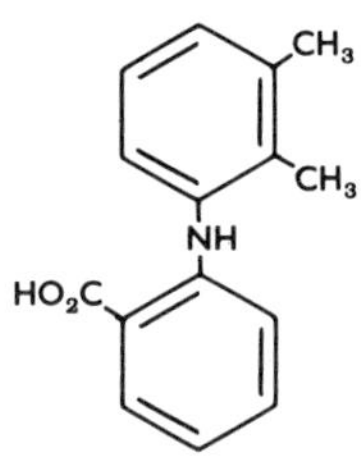

A white powder. M.p. 230° to 231°, with effervescence.
Solubility. Practically insoluble in water; slightly soluble in ethanol; sparingly soluble in ether and chloroform.

Extraction. Mefenamic acid is extracted by organic solvents from aqueous acid solutions.

Chromatography. PAPER: system P12—Rf 0·80 (location under ultraviolet light, pale green fluorescence).
GAS: system G2/225—retention time 0·64 relative to codeine (poor peak, with tailing).

Colour Test. To about 10 mg of mefenamic acid add 1 drop of a 4·5% sodium hydroxide solution, dilute to 10 ml with water and mix. To the resultant solution add 1 drop of 10% copper sulphate solution—a beige precipitate.

Ultraviolet Absorption Spectrum. Mefenamic acid in 0·1N sodium hydroxide, maximum at about 285 mμ (E1%, 1cm about 420); minimum at about 255 mμ.

Infra-red Absorption Spectrum. Potassium bromide disk. The principal peaks are: A 1253, B 1644, C 1575 (p. 744).

Dose. Usually up to 1·25 g daily.

Toxicity. Agranulocytosis, thrombocytopenic purpura, and megaloblastic anaemia have occurred in patients taking mefenamic acid, but no causal connexion has been established (*Med. Lett.*, 1967, **9**, 77).

MENAPHTHONE *Vitamin-K Analogue*

Synonyms: Menadione; Menaphthene; Vitamin K_3.
Proprietary Names: Kappaxin(e); Kayklot; Kayquinone; Thyloquinone.

2-Methyl-1,4-naphthaquinone
$C_{11}H_8O_2$ = 172·2

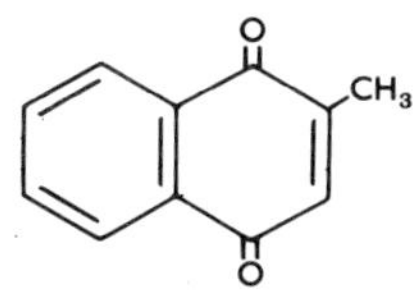

A bright yellow, crystalline powder, irritating to the mucous membranes and skin. M.p. 105° to 107°. On exposure to light, it decomposes, darkening to light brown.
Solubility. Insoluble in water; soluble 1 in 60 of ethanol, 1 in 50 of fixed oils, and 1 in 10 of benzene.

MENAPHTHONE SODIUM BISULPHITE

Synonyms: Kavitanum; Vikasol.
Proprietary Names: Hykinone; Vitavel K.

A white hygroscopic crystalline powder which should be protected from light.
Solubility. Soluble 1 in 2 of water; slightly soluble in ethanol; almost insoluble in ether and chloroform.

Extraction. Menaphthone is extracted by organic solvents from aqueous acid solutions.

Colour Test. Dissolve about 0·5 mg of menaphthone in 5 ml of ethanol and add 2 ml of strong ammonia solution and a few drops of ethyl cyanoacetate—violet; add 5 ml of a 20% sodium hydroxide solution—brownish-yellow. The violet colour is destroyed on the addition of acid or on exposure to sunlight.

Ultraviolet Absorption Spectrum. Menaphthone in ethanol, maxima at 245 mμ (E1%, 1cm 1080), 250 mμ (E1%, 1cm 1100), 263 mμ (E1%, 1cm 800), and 333 mμ (E1%, 1cm 160).

Quantitative Estimation. A colorimetric method of determination in serum, plasma, and urine is described by Kofler (1945).

Metabolism. Studies in rats show that menaphthone is partly reduced to 1,4-dihydroxy-2-methylnaphthalene and that, after oral or intravenous administration, both glucuronide and ethereal sulphate conjugates of the metabolite are excreted in the urine and some is excreted in the faeces. In man, some oxidation to phthalic acid has been shown to occur.

Dose. Menaphthone, up to 10 mg daily intramuscularly; or menaphthone sodium bisulphite, up to 2 mg daily intramuscularly or subcutaneously, in accordance with the patient's prothrombin activity.

MENTHOL

p-Menthan-3-ol

$C_{10}H_{20}O$ = 156·3

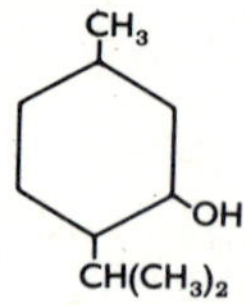

Menthol is natural (−)-menthol, obtained from the volatile oils of various species of *Mentha* (Labiatae), or synthetic(−)-menthol or (±)-menthol.

Colourless acicular or prismatic crystals. M.p. of the (−)- isomer, 42° to 44°, and of the (±)- isomer, 27° to 28° (30° to 32° on prolonged stirring). Specific rotation of the (−)-isomer in a 10% solution in ethanol, −49° to −50°.

Solubility. Almost insoluble in water; soluble 1 in 0·2 of ethanol, 1 in 0·4 of ether, and 1 in 0·25 of chloroform.

Extraction. Menthol is extracted by organic solvents from aqueous acid solutions.

Chromatography. GAS: system G5—retention time 0·32 relative to barbitone.

Colour Test. Dissolve 10 mg in 1 ml of *sulphuric acid* and add 1 ml of *vanillin in sulphuric acid solution*—orange-yellow; addition of 1 ml of water—violet (this test distinguishes menthol from thymol).

Metabolism. Menthol is excreted in the bile and urine as a glucuronide conjugate; the various isomers differ quantitatively in the extent to which they conjugate with glucuronic acid. In dogs and rabbits some degradation of the menthol molecule appears to take place. Menthol may occur in the conjugated form as a metabolite of pulegone which is a constituent of pulegium oil.

Toxicity. The estimated lethal dose in man is about 2 g.

The application of drops or ointments containing menthol to the nostrils of infants is dangerous and may cause instant collapse.

MEPACRINE *Antimalarial/Taenifuge*

Synonyms: Acrichinum; Acrinamine; Atebrinum; Chinacina; Erion; Quinacrine.

3-Chloro-9-(4-diethylamino-1-methylbutylamino)-7-methoxyacridine

$C_{23}H_{30}ClN_3O$ = 400·0

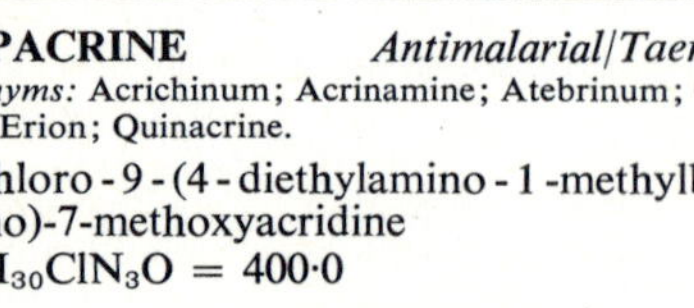

MEPACRINE HYDROCHLORIDE

Proprietary Names: Atabrine Hydrochloride; Atebrin; Metoquin(e); Quinacrine.

A bright yellow crystalline powder. M.p. 250°, with decomposition.

Solubility. Soluble 1 in 40 of water and 1 in 60 of ethanol; almost insoluble in ether; very slightly soluble in chloroform.

MEPACRINE MESYLATE

Synonym: Mepacrine Methanesulphonate.

Proprietary Name: Quinacrine Soluble.

Bright yellow crystals.

Solubility. Soluble 1 in 3 of water and 1 in 36 of ethanol.

Extraction. Mepacrine is extracted by organic solvents from aqueous alkaline solutions.

Chromatography. PAPER: system P1—Rf 0·27 (location under ultraviolet light, green fluorescence; location reagents: *iodoplatinate spray*, strong reaction; *bromocresol green spray*, strong reaction).

THIN-LAYER: system T1—Rf 0·36 (location reagent *acidified iodoplatinate spray*, positive reaction).

Colour Tests. MICRO: sulphuric acid–formaldehyde test—bright yellow (*sensitivity:* 1·0 μg); ammonium molybdate test—yellow-green (*sensitivity:* 0·25 μg); ammonium vanadate test—purple → bright yellow (*sensitivity:* 0·25 μg); Vitali's test—yellow/yellow/purple → grey (*sensitivity:* 0·5 μg).

Crystal Tests. MICRO: *gold cyanide solution*—clumps of hair-like needles (*sensitivity:* 1 in 1000); *potassium tri-iodide solution* (2)—dense rosettes of needles (*sensitivity:* 1 in 200).

Ultraviolet Absorption Spectrum. Mepacrine in water, maximum at 279 mμ (E1%, 1 cm 1020); in 0·1N sulphuric acid, maxima at 222 mμ (E1%, 1 cm 517) and 279·5 mμ (E1%, 1 cm 1282).

Infra-red Absorption Spectrum. Mepacrine (base). Potassium bromide disk. The principal peaks are: A 1225, B 1462 or 1557, C 1625 (p. 790).

Metabolism. Mepacrine is excreted slowly over the course of weeks in the bile and urine. Several metabolites are excreted, one of which appears to be demethylated in the acridine ring and others in which the side-chain may be degraded. These metabolites account for not more than 5% of the dose.

Mepacrine is rapidly absorbed after oral administration; it appears in the blood within 2 hours, and reaches a peak concentration in 8 hours. On discontinuing administration, the plasma level decreases rapidly during the first week but mepacrine does not disappear from the plasma for several weeks. Mepacrine is widely distributed throughout the body, high concentrations being found in the liver, lungs, and spleen; it also persists in the skin and finger-nails. The urine and skin may become yellow in colour.

Dose. For malaria, up to 500 mg daily; for tapeworm infestation, 1 g in divided doses.

Toxicity. Large doses may give rise to nausea

and vomiting and occasionally to transient mental disturbances. Attempts at suicide with massive doses have not been successful.

MEPENZOLATE BROMIDE

Parasympatholytic

Proprietary Name: Cantil.

3-Benziloyloxy-1,1-dimethylpiperidinium bromide

$C_{21}H_{26}BrNO_3 = 420{\cdot}4$

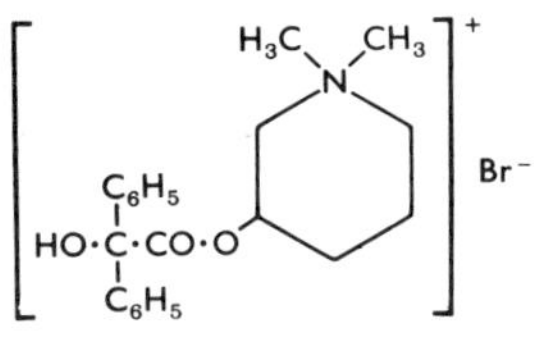

A white crystalline powder.

Solubility. Soluble in water.

Extraction. Mepenzolate is a quaternary ammonium compound (see p. 29).

Chromatography. PAPER: system P1—Rf 0·45 (location under ultraviolet light, absorption; location reagent *iodoplatinate spray*, strong reaction); system RP1a—Rf 0·87 (location reagent *iodoplatinate spray*, positive reaction); system RP1b—Rf 0·90 (location as for RP1a).
THIN-LAYER: system T1—Rf 0·01 (location reagent *acidified iodoplatinate spray*, positive reaction).

Colour Tests. MICRO: the following tests are performed on the nitrate (see p. 134): sulphuric acid–formaldehyde test—orange flash (*sensitivity:* 1·0 μg); ammonium molybdate test—orange → green → blue (*sensitivity:* 1·0 μg).

Crystal Tests. MICRO: *potassium permanganate solution*—bunches of blades (*sensitivity:* 1 in 1000); *styphnic acid*—irregular rosettes (*sensitivity:* 1 in 1000).

Dose. Usually up to 100 mg daily, increased if necessary.

MEPHENESIN

Muscle Relaxant

Synonyms: Cresoxydiol; Glykresin.
Proprietary Names: Dioloxol; Lissephen; Myanesin; Oranixon; Tolserol.

3-(2-Methylphenoxy)propane-1,2-diol

$C_{10}H_{14}O_3 = 182{\cdot}2$

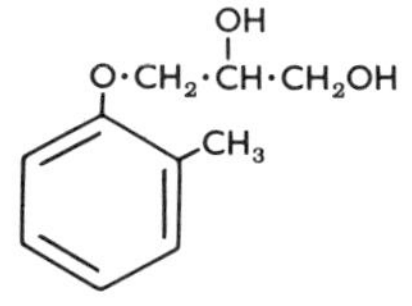

White crystals or crystalline aggregates. M.p. 70° to 73°.

Solubility. Soluble 1 in 100 of water, 1 in 8 of ethanol, and 1 in 12 of chloroform; soluble in ether.

MEPHENESIN CARBAMATE
Proprietary Name: Tolseram.

White crystals. M.p. 93°.
Solubility. Soluble 1 in 300 of water and 1 in 50 of chloroform; very soluble in ethanol.

Extraction. Mephenesin and mephenesin carbamate are extracted by organic solvents from aqueous acid or alkaline solutions.

Chromatography. PAPER, for the carbamate: system P1—Rf 0·89 (location reagent *Marquis reagent*, red); for the carbamate: system P6—Rf 0·83 (location under ultraviolet light, absorption; location reagent *furfural–hydrochloric acid spray*, positive reaction); for the carbamate: system P7—Rf 0·64 (location as for P6) and system RP1b—Rf 0·46 (location reagent *furfural–hydrochloric acid spray*).
THIN-LAYER: system T1—Rf 0·77 (location reagent *Marquis reagent*, positive reaction).
GAS: system G5—retention time 1·40 (3·80) relative to barbitone.

Colour Tests. MICRO, for the carbamate: sulphuric acid–formaldehyde test—red (*sensitivity:* 0·1 μg); ammonium molybdate test—blue-grey (*sensitivity:* 0·1 μg); ammonium vanadate test—grey-brown (*sensitivity:* 1·0 μg); Vitali's test—–/–/red (*sensitivity:* 0·1 μg).

Ultraviolet Absorption Spectrum. Mephenesin in ethanol, maxima at about 272 mμ (E1%, 1 cm 90) and 277 mμ (E1%, 1 cm 80).

Infra-red Absorption Spectrum. Mephenesin (base). Potassium bromide disk. The principal peaks are: A 1245, B 1041, C 745 (p. 744).

Metabolism. Mephenesin is very rapidly metabolised to β-(*o*-toloxy)lactic acid and β-(2-methyl-4-hydroxyphenoxy)lactic acid and these metabolites may be detected in the urine within 15 minutes of oral administration; very little unchanged mephenesin is excreted. Hence the duration of action is relatively short, about 3 hours; a more prolonged effect is obtained when it is given by injection.

Dose. Up to 6 g of mephenesin or 15 g of mephenesin carbamate daily, by mouth.

Toxicity. Intravenous administration of solutions containing more than 5% of mephenesin may cause intravascular haemolysis and haemoglobinuria; fatalities due to renal anoxia and anuria have been reported.
LD50 (oral) for mephenesin: in mice 890 mg/kg.
LD50 (intraperitoneal) for mephenesin carbamate: in mice 7·7 mg/kg.

CASE EXAMPLE. A 43-year-old woman, who ingested between 5·5 and 11 g of mephenesin, recovered within about 10 hours following treatment (Barron and Milliken, 1960).

MEPHENTERMINE

Sympathomimetic

Synonyms: Mephenterdrine; Mephetedrine.

$N\alpha\alpha$-Trimethylphenethylamine
$C_{11}H_{17}N = 163{\cdot}3$

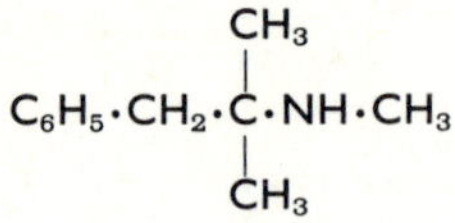

A colourless to pale yellow liquid.
Solubility. Insoluble in water; soluble in ethanol and ether.

MEPHENTERMINE SULPHATE
Proprietary Names: Mephine Sulphate; Wyamine Sulfate. It is an ingredient of Neo-Endrine.

Colourless crystals or a white crystalline powder.
Solubility. Soluble 1 in 20 of water and 1 in 150 of ethanol; insoluble in chloroform.

Extraction. Mephentermine is extracted by organic solvents from aqueous alkaline solutions.

Chromatography. PAPER: system P1—Rf 0·62 (location under ultraviolet light, absorption; location reagents: *iodoplatinate spray*, white; *bromocresol green spray*, weak reaction; *Marquis reagent*, orange).

THIN-LAYER: system T1—Rf 0·24 (location reagents: *acidified iodoplatinate spray*, positive reaction; *Marquis reagent*, positive reaction).

GAS: system G2/120—retention time 0·51 relative to ephedrine.

Colour Test. MICRO: sulphuric acid–formaldehyde test—orange → brown (*sensitivity:* 0·5 μg).

Crystal Tests. MICRO: *gold bromide solution*—rhomboidal plates (*sensitivity:* 1 in 1000); *picrolonic acid*—curved needles (*sensitivity:* 1 in 1000).

Ultraviolet Absorption Spectrum. Mephentermine in 0·1N sulphuric acid, maxima at 247·5 mμ (E1%, 1cm 4), 252 mμ (E1%, 1cm 5·5), 258 mμ (E1%, 1cm 6·9), and 264 mμ (E1%, 1cm 5·3).

Infra-red Absorption Spectrum. Mephentermine (base). Potassium bromide disk. The principal peaks are: A 1111, B 711, C 696 or 1394 (p. 790).

Metabolism. Mephentermine is a sympathomimetic amine which is rapidly metabolised in the body. Studies in animals have indicated that mephentermine is metabolised by demethylation, then subsequent hydroxylation may take place. Some unchanged drug may be excreted in the faeces.

Dose. Up to 80 mg (base) by mouth, daily; up to 80 mg (base) by intramuscular or slow intravenous injection.

Toxicity. The estimated minimum lethal dose in children up to 2 years of age is 200 mg.

LD50 (intraperitoneal) of base: in mice 89 mg/kg.

MEPIVACAINE *Local Anaesthetic*

(±)-1,2′,6′-Trimethylpipecolanilide
$C_{15}H_{22}N_2O = 246{\cdot}4$

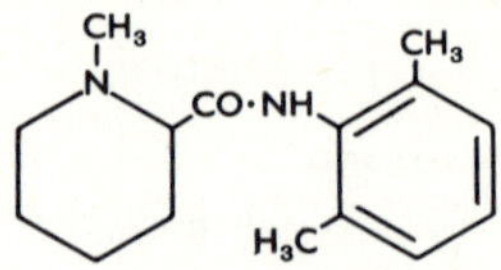

Yellow-white crystals. M.p. 149° to 153°.

MEPIVACAINE HYDROCHLORIDE
Proprietary Names: Carbocaine; Scandicain(e).

A white crystalline solid. M.p. 255° to 262°, with decomposition.
Solubility. Freely soluble in water; soluble 1 in 12 of ethanol; almost insoluble in ether; very slightly soluble in chloroform.

Extraction. Mepivacaine is extracted by organic solvents from aqueous alkaline solutions.

Chromatography. PAPER: system P1—Rf 0·62 (location under ultraviolet light, absorption; location reagents: *iodoplatinate spray*, strong reaction; *bromocresol green spray*, weak reaction); system RP1a—Rf 0·79 (location under ultraviolet light, absorption; location reagent *iodoplatinate spray*, positive reaction); system RP1b—Rf 0·12 (location as for RP1a).

THIN-LAYER: system T1—Rf 0·70 (location reagent *acidified iodoplatinate spray*, positive reaction).

GAS: system G2/225—retention time 1·9 relative to diphenhydramine.

Crystal Tests. MICRO: *lead iodide solution*—burrs or sheaves (*sensitivity:* 1 in 200); *platinic iodide solution*—needles and plates (*sensitivity:* 1 in 400).

Ultraviolet Absorption Spectrum. Mepivacaine in 0·1N hydrochloric acid, maxima at 263 mμ (E1%, 1cm 17) and 271 mμ (E1%, 1cm 13); minima at 254 mμ and 270 mμ.

Infra-red Absorption Spectrum. Mepivacaine (base). Potassium bromide disk. The principal peaks are: A 1650, B 1523, C 760 (p. 790).

Metabolism. Studies in rats with ^{14}C-labelled mepivacaine indicated that 2 routes of metabolism occurred, *N*-demethylation and *p*-hydroxylation; the *p*-hydroxy-derivative was identified in the urine. Following intravenous injection 55% of the radioactivity appeared in the urine in 24 hours but only a small amount of this consisted of unchanged drug. The glucuronide conjugate of the *p*-hydroxy-derivative was excreted into the bile to the extent of 50% of administered mepivacaine but only a small percentage was found in the faeces, hence resorption into the stomach must have occurred (Hansson *et al.*, 1965).

CASE EXAMPLE. Mepivacaine had been given as a local anaesthetic to a young woman who died while undergoing cosmetic surgery. Between 75 and 150 ml of a 2% mepivacaine solution was used. Post-mortem levels of mepivacaine were: bile, 5·0 mg%; blood, 5·0 mg%; brain, 5·1 mg%; kidney, 5·1 mg%; liver, 7·5 mg%; spleen, 7·2 mg%; stomach contents, a trace. Salicylate and glutethimide were also found in the blood and urine (Sunshine and Fike, 1964).

MEPROBAMATE *Tranquilliser*

Synonym: Procalmadiol.
Proprietary Names: Equanil; Mepavlon; Meprospan; Meprotabs; Miltown; Pensive; Setran; Vio-Bamate.

2,2-Di(carbamoyloxymethyl)pentane
$C_9H_{18}N_2O_4$ = 218·3

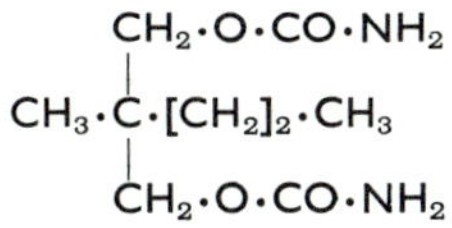

A white crystalline powder or white granular crystalline aggregates. M.p. 103° to 107°.
Solubility. Soluble 1 in 240 of water, 1 in 7 of ethanol, and 1 in 70 of ether.

Screening Test. See Screening Tests, p. 13.

Extraction. Meprobamate is extracted by organic solvents from aqueous acid or alkaline solutions.

Chromatography. PAPER: system P6—Rf 0·86 (location reagent *furfural–hydrochloric acid spray*, positive reaction); system P7—Rf 0·71 (location as for P6); system RP1b—Rf 0·64 (location reagent *furfural–hydrochloric acid spray*). Another method is described by Cann (1962).
THIN-LAYER: a method is described by Lindfors (1963).
GAS: system G1/180—retention time 1·01 relative to diphenhydramine; system G5—retention time 2·3 relative to barbitone.

Colour and **Crystal Tests.** Lucas and Korczak-Fabierkiewicz (1964) have described colour and crystal tests for meprobamate.

Infra-red Absorption Spectrum. Potassium bromide disk. The principal peaks are: A 1688, B 1069, C 1408 (p. 744).

Quantitative Estimation. Several methods have been reported: a thin-layer chromatographic method of estimation (Olesen, 1966); a spectrophotometric method of determination in urine (Renault *et al.*, 1966); gas chromatographic methods for the estimation of meprobamate in blood, liver, and urine (Goldbaum and Domanski, 1966; Skinner, 1967).

Metabolism. Meprobamate is excreted slowly in man, about 20% appearing in the urine as free drug or metabolites; a hydroxy-derivative has been detected in the urine. *N*-glucuronide formation also occurs. A single dose of 400 mg is detectable in the urine for 48 hours and maximum serum levels occur approximately 2 hours after ingestion. Blood-levels after the ingestion of 1·6 g are between 1 and 2 mg%.

Dose. Usually 1·2 g daily.

Toxicity. Fatalities have been reported following the ingestion of 17 and 24 g; recoveries have occurred after the ingestion of between 10 and 40 g. Meprobamate possesses marked dependence-producing properties.

CASE EXAMPLES. A 43-year-old woman died probably 7 hours after the ingestion of about 12 g of meprobamate. Post-mortem levels: liver, 30 mg%; stomach contents, 800 mg; urine, 34 mg%. A 25-year-old woman died about 7 hours after the ingestion of 20 g of meprobamate. Post-mortem levels: liver, 22 mg%; stomach contents, 393 mg%; urine, 83 mg% (Powell *et al.*, 1958).

MEPRYLCAINE *Local Anaesthetic*

2-Methyl-2-propylaminopropyl benzoate
$C_{14}H_{21}NO_2$ = 235·3

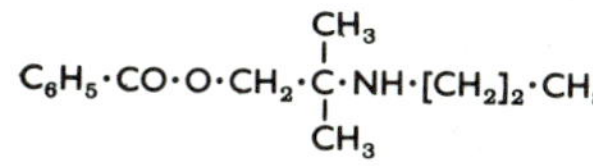

MEPRYLCAINE HYDROCHLORIDE
Proprietary Name: Oracaine Hydrochloride.

A white crystalline solid. M.p. 150° to 152°.
Solubility. Freely soluble in water, ethanol, and chloroform.

Extraction. Meprylcaine is extracted by organic solvents from aqueous alkaline solutions.

Chromatography. THIN-LAYER: Sunshine and Fike (1964) have described 3 systems which separate meprylcaine and other local anaesthetics.

Ultraviolet Absorption Spectrum. Meprylcaine in 0·1N sulphuric acid, maximum at 232 mμ (E1%, 1 cm 422).

MEPYRAMINE *Antihistamine*

Synonyms: Pyranisamine; Pyrilamine.

N-(*p*-Methoxybenzyl)-*N′N′*-dimethyl-*N*-(pyrid-2-yl)ethylenediamine
$C_{17}H_{23}N_3O$ = 285·4

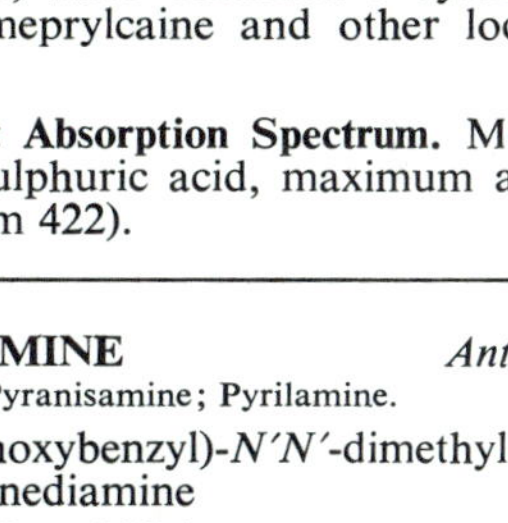

MEPYRAMINE MALEATE
Proprietary Names: Antallergan; Anthisan; Copsamine; Histacap; Histalon; Neo-Antergan Maleate; Paraminyl Maleate; Stangen Maleate; Statomin Maleate.

A white powder. M.p. 98° to 101°.
Solubility. Soluble 1 in 0·5 of water, 1 in 2·5 of ethanol, and 1 in 1·5 of chloroform; slightly soluble in ether.

Extraction. Mepyramine is extracted by organic solvents from aqueous alkaline solutions.

Chromatography. PAPER: system P1—Rf 0·32 (location under ultraviolet light, bright blue fluorescence; location reagents: *iodoplatinate spray*, strong reaction; *bromocresol green spray*, weak reaction); system RP1a—Rf 0·71 (location under ultraviolet light, purple fluorescence; location reagent *iodoplatinate spray*, positive reaction); system RP1b—Rf 0·05 (location as for RP1a).

THIN-LAYER: system T1—Rf 0·49 (location reagent *acidified iodoplatinate spray*, positive reaction); system T2—Rf 0·56 (location reagent *iodoplatinate spray*, positive reaction); system T3—Rf 0·82 (location as for T2).

GAS: system G2/225—retention time 0·65 relative to codeine.

Colour Tests. MICRO: sulphuric acid–formaldehyde test—purple (*sensitivity:* 1·0 μg); ammonium molybdate test—purple → brown (*sensitivity:* 0·1 μg); ammonium vanadate test—purple (*sensitivity:* 0·25 μg).

Crystal Tests. MICRO: *gold bromide–hydrochloric acid solution*—serrated needles and rods (*sensitivity:* 1 in 1000); *platinic chloride solution*—rosettes or fans of needles (*sensitivity:* 1 in 400).

Ultraviolet Absorption Spectrum. Mepyramine maleate in 0·01N hydrochloric acid, maxima at 239 mμ (E1%, 1cm about 633) and 316 mμ (E1%, 1cm about 288).

Infra-red Absorption Spectrum. Mepyramine (base). Potassium bromide disk. The principal peaks are: A 1490 or 1512 or 1598, B 1247 or 1441 (p. 790).

Dose. Up to 50 mg by injection; maximum daily dose by mouth 1 g.

Toxicity. LD50 (oral): in guinea-pigs 290 and in mice 325 mg/kg.

CASE EXAMPLES. A 21-month-old child lost consciousness 2 hours after swallowing 0·6 g of mepyramine maleate and died ¾ hour later. Post-mortem examination showed toxic changes throughout the body (Tobias, 1949).

At post-mortem examination, performed on a 16-month-old child who, unconscious and twitching, died 3 hours after ingesting about 0·6 g of mepyramine maleate, only the stomach contents produced evidence of the presence of the drug. The stomach contents and gastro-intestinal tract showed a greenish tinge (Miller and Pedley, 1950).

A 13-month-old child became unconscious 10 minutes after ingesting one or two 100-mg tablets of mepyramine and showed twitching of the face and limbs, frothing, and cyanosis. Despite treatment she died some 7 hours later. Mepyramine was identified in the gastro-intestinal contents and urine only (Prain, 1950).

(1) A 3½-year-old boy died following the ingestion of between 0·5 and 0·7 g of mepyramine maleate. At post-mortem examination the liver contained 690 mg%; the vomit contained traces of the drug. (2) A 2-year-old boy died following the ingestion of 1·1 g of mepyramine maleate. At post-mortem examination the gastro-intestinal tract contained 940 mg of mepyramine; the kidney, liver, spleen, and some blood were analysed as one sample, 210 mg% being recovered; the heart, thymus, lungs, and trachea were also analysed as one sample, 140 mg% being recovered (Oliver, 1951).

MESCALINE *Hallucinogen*

3,4,5-Trimethoxyphenethylamine

$C_{11}H_{17}NO_3 = 211{\cdot}3$

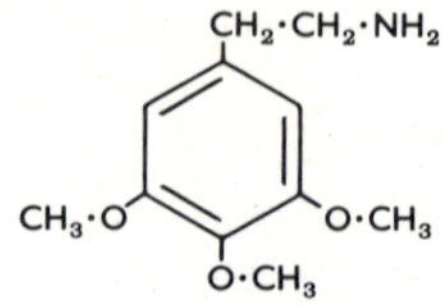

An alkaloid obtained from the cactus *Lophophora williamsii* (=*Anhalonium williamsii* = *A. lewinii*) (Cactaceae), known also as peyote or peyotl.

Crystals which take up carbon dioxide from the air. M.p. 35° to 36°. B.p. 180°.

Solubility. Soluble in water, ethanol, and chloroform; almost insoluble in ether.

Extraction. Mescaline is extracted by organic solvents from aqueous alkaline solutions.

Chromatography. PAPER: system P1—Rf 0·25 (location under ultraviolet light, absorption; location reagents: *iodoplatinate spray*, strong reaction; *bromocresol green spray*, weak reaction); system RP1a—Rf 0·90 (location under ultraviolet light, absorption); system RP1b—Rf 0·94 (location as for RP1a).

THIN-LAYER: system T1—Rf 0·22 (location reagent *acidified iodoplatinate spray*, positive reaction).

GAS: system G2/225—retention time 0·58 relative to diphenhydramine; system G6—retention time 0·21 relative to codeine.

Colour Tests. MICRO: sulphuric acid–formaldehyde test—orange (*sensitivity:* 0·1 μg); ammonium molybdate test—green → blue (*sensitivity:* 0·025 μg); Vitali's test—(dull red) purple/dull red/brown (*sensitivity:* 0·1 μg).

Crystal Tests. MICRO: *potassium bismuth iodide solution*—dense rosettes (*sensitivity:* 1 in 3000); *styphnic acid*—small needles (*sensitivity:* 1 in 3000).

Ultraviolet Absorption Spectrum. Mescaline in ethanol, maximum at 269 mμ (E1%, 1cm 75) and an inflexion at about 225 mμ; in 0·2N sulphuric acid, maximum at 268 mμ (E1%, 1cm 39).

Metabolism. Mescaline is metabolised partly by oxidative deamination to 3,4,5-trimethoxyphenylacetic acid; another metabolite, 3,4-dihydroxy-5-methoxyphenylacetic acid, is found to be excreted as a glutamine conjugate—see under The Metabolism of Drugs, pp. 145 and 149. Charalampous *et al.* (1964) found that human subjects given mescaline orally excreted an average of 81·9% of the administered dose in the urine during the first 12 hours; an average of 26·2% of the dose is excreted as free 3,4,5-trimethoxyphenylacetic acid which is inactive.

Mescaline is readily absorbed from the gastro-intestinal tract and it occurs in the highest concentrations in the kidneys, liver, and spleen. Some mescaline is bound to the plasma proteins and to the proteins of the liver (Jacobsen, 1963).

Dose. The average dose required to produce hallucinations in man is 400 to 700 mg by injection.

Toxicity. Mescaline induces psychotic changes similar to those produced by lysergide, but it is less potent. The effects of a single full dose of mescaline may persist for about 12 hours. The lethal intraperitoneal dose in mice is 500 mg/kg.

MESTRANOL *Oestrogen*

Synonyms: EE3ME; Ethinyloestradiol-3-methyl Ether.
Proprietary Names: It is an ingredient of many proprietary oral contraceptive preparations—see Extra Pharmacopoeia (Martindale), 25th Edn, p. 1291.

3 - Methoxy - 19 - nor - 17α - pregna - 1,3,5(10) - trien-20-yn-17-ol

$C_{21}H_{26}O_2 = 310{\cdot}4$

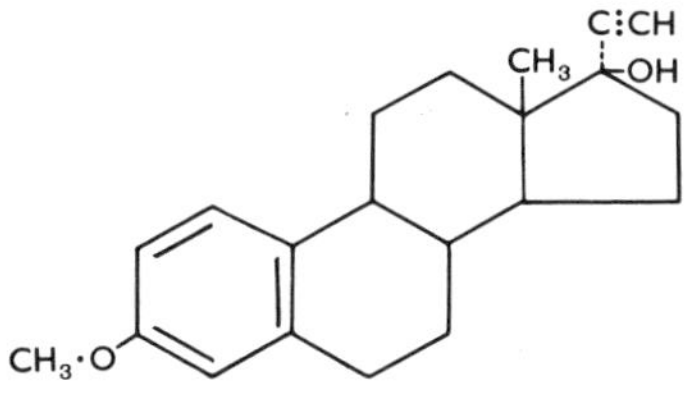

A white crystalline powder. M.p. about 150° to 154°.

Solubility. Almost insoluble in water; soluble 1 in 44 of ethanol, 1 in 23 of ether, and 1 in 4·5 of chloroform.

Extraction. Mestranol is extracted from neutral solutions with freshly distilled ethyl acetate.

Ultraviolet Absorption Spectrum. Mestranol in methanol, maxima at 279 mμ (E1%, 1cm 82) and 287·5 mμ (E1%, 1cm 14·4).

Quantitative Estimation. Bastow (1967) describes a method of spectrophotometric estimation of mestranol in tablets containing norethynodrel. Keay (1968) has devised an analytical scheme involving thin-layer chromatography and ultra-violet and infra-red spectrophotometry which enables mestranol to be identified and assayed, particularly when present in an oral contraceptive preparation.

Metabolism. Mestranol is a synthetic oestrogen which is more potent than oestradiol. It is readily absorbed from the gastro-intestinal tract.

Use. In conjunction with a progestational agent such as ethynodiol, lynoestrenol, norethisterone, or norethynodrel, it is taken by mouth as a contraceptive.

METABUTETHAMINE *Local Anaesthetic*

2-Isobutylaminoethyl *m*-aminobenzoate

$C_{13}H_{20}N_2O_2 = 236{\cdot}3$

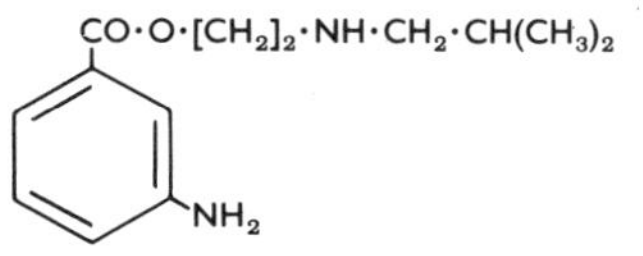

NOTE. Metabutethamine is an isomer of butethamine (p. 230).

METABUTETHAMINE HYDROCHLORIDE
Proprietary Name: Unacaine Hydrochloride.

A white crystalline solid or powder. M.p. 181° to 184°.
Solubility. Soluble in water; slightly soluble in ethanol and chloroform.

Extraction. Metabutethamine is extracted by organic solvents from aqueous alkaline solutions.

Chromatography. PAPER: system P1—Rf 0·35 (location under ultraviolet light, bright blue fluorescence; location reagents: *iodoplatinate spray*, strong reaction; *bromocresol green spray*, strong reaction).
THIN-LAYER: system T1—Rf 0·60 (location reagents: *acidified iodoplatinate spray*, positive reaction; p-*dimethylaminobenzaldehyde spray*, yellow).

Colour Tests. MICRO: diazotisation test—red (*sensitivity:* 0·1 μg); Vitali's test— –/yellow/ yellow (*sensitivity:* 1·0 μg).

Crystal Tests. MICRO: *gold bromide solution*—dense rosettes (*sensitivity:* 1 in 200); *platinic iodide solution*—rosettes of branching needles (*sensitivity:* 1 in 1000).

Ultraviolet Absorption Spectrum. Metabutethamine in 0·1N sulphuric acid, maxima at 228 mμ (E1%, 1cm 452) and 274 mμ (E1%, 1 cm 31), and an inflexion at about 280 mμ.

Toxicity. Metabutethamine is used by injection in dentistry, usually as a 3·8% solution with adrenaline. It provides a relatively short duration of anaesthesia and is considerably less toxic than procaine hydrochloride when injected subcutaneously or intraperitoneally but has about the same toxicity when injected intravenously.

METABUTOXYCAINE *Local Anaesthetic*

2′-Diethylaminoethyl 3-amino-2-butoxybenzoate

$C_{17}H_{28}N_2O_3 = 308{\cdot}4$

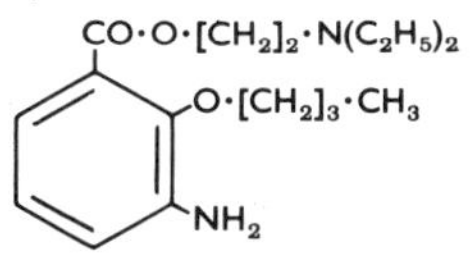

METABUTOXYCAINE HYDROCHLORIDE
Synonym: Primacaine Hydrochloride.

A white crystalline powder. M.p. 117° to 120°.
Solubility. Very soluble in water and ethanol; very slightly soluble in ether; sparingly soluble in chloroform.

Extraction. Metabutoxycaine is extracted by organic solvents from aqueous alkaline solutions.

Chromatography. THIN-LAYER: Sunshine and Fike (1964) have described 3 systems which separate metabutoxycaine and other local anaesthetics.

Ultraviolet Absorption Spectrum. Metabutoxycaine in 0·1N sulphuric acid, maximum at 313 mμ (E1%, 1cm 67).

Toxicity. Metabutoxycaine is used in dentistry as a 1·5% solution with adrenaline. Its potency is somewhat greater than that of procaine hydrochloride in the same concentration.

METALDEHYDE

Proprietary Names: It is an ingredient of many proprietary preparations used for the destruction of slugs. As a compressed fuel, it is known as Meta.

A polymer of acetaldehyde
A white crystalline solid which burns readily with a non-luminous carbon-free flame and which sublimes at 100°. In the presence of acids it decomposes slowly to acetaldehyde.
Solubility. Insoluble in water.

Extraction. Metaldehyde may be recovered as acetaldehyde (p. 169) by steam distillation of viscera acidified with sulphuric acid.

Colour Test. Add 1 drop of *sulphuric acid* to a small amount of solid, then add a trace of pyrocatechol—violet-red.

Toxicity. The toxic dose in dogs is very variable, around 0·4 g/kg. The lethal dose in chickens is 2 and in ducks 0·5 g/kg.
Children and young animals have died from eating Meta fuel. Post-mortem findings include hyperaemia of the liver and kidneys, liver-cell and brain ganglion-cell degeneration, and interstitial haemorrhages of the lungs.

METANEPHRINE

Synonym: Metadrenaline.

(−)-1-(4-Hydroxy-3-methoxyphenyl)-2-methylaminoethanol
$C_{10}H_{15}NO_3$ = 197·2

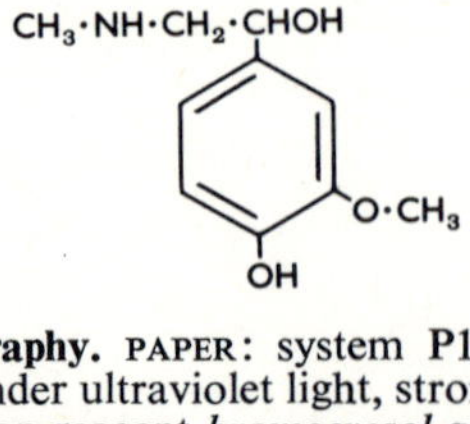

Chromatography. PAPER: system P1—Rf 0·15 (location under ultraviolet light, strong absorption; location reagent *bromocresol green spray*, weak reaction).
THIN-LAYER: system T1—Rf 0·21 (location reagent *potassium permanganate spray*, positive reaction).

Colour Tests. Chen's test—purple.
MICRO: sulphuric acid–formaldehyde test—dull orange→purple-brown (*sensitivity:* 0·5 μg); ammonium molybdate test—grey-blue→dull green (*sensitivity:* 0·25 μg); ammonium vanadate test—olive-green (*sensitivity:* 1·0 μg); Vitali's test — yellow/yellow-brown/yellow-brown (*sensitivity:* 0·5 μg).

Crystal Tests. MICRO: *gold bromide solution*—very small rosettes or plates, forming overnight (*sensitivity:* 1 in 100); *gold bromide–hydrochloric acid solution*—small plates, forming overnight (*sensitivity:* 1 in 1000).

Ultraviolet Absorption Spectrum. Metanephrine in 0·1N sulphuric acid, maxima at 226 mμ and 278 mμ.

Metabolism. After adrenaline has been metabolised by *O*-methylation and oxidative deamination, it is excreted as the inactivated compounds metanephrine and 3-methoxy-4-hydroxymandelic acid. Most of the metanephrine is excreted as sulphate or glucuronide conjugates but small portions are deaminated and excreted as 3-methoxy-4-hydroxymandelic acid.

METARAMINOL *Sympathomimetic*

*Synonym: l-m-*Hydroxynorephedrine.

(−)-2-Amino-1-(3-hydroxyphenyl)propan-1-ol
$C_9H_{13}NO_2$ = 167·2

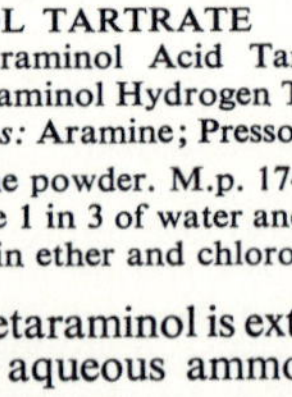

NOTE. Metaraminol is an isomer of phenylephrine.

METARAMINOL TARTRATE

Synonyms: Metaraminol Acid Tartrate; Metaraminol Bitartrate; Metaraminol Hydrogen Tartrate.
Proprietary Names: Aramine; Pressorol.

A white crystalline powder. M.p. 174° to 178°.
Solubility. Soluble 1 in 3 of water and 1 in 100 of ethanol; almost insoluble in ether and chloroform.

Extraction. Metaraminol is extracted by organic solvents from aqueous ammoniacal solutions.

Chromatography. PAPER: system P1—Rf 0·31 (location under ultraviolet light, strong absorption; location reagents: p-*dimethylaminobenzaldehyde spray*, yellow; *ninhydrin spray*, purple; *potassium permanganate spray*, weak reaction).
THIN-LAYER: system T1—Rf 0·47 (location reagent *potassium permanganate spray*, positive reaction).

Colour Tests. Chen's test—purple.
MICRO: ammonium molybdate test—light brown (*sensitivity:* 1·0 μg); ammonium vanadate test—

pale blue (*sensitivity:* 1·0 μg); Vitali's test—–/pale yellow/orange (*sensitivity:* 1·0 μg).

Crystal Tests. MICRO: *potassium bismuth iodide solution*—rods and tablets (*sensitivity:* 1 in 400); *potassium tri-iodide solution* (*3*)—tablets and prisms (*sensitivity:* 1 in 100).

Ultraviolet Absorption Spectrum. Metaraminol tartrate in water, maximum at 272 mμ (E1%, 1 cm about 58).

Infra-red Absorption Spectrum. Metaraminol (base). Potassium bromide disk. The principal peaks are: A 1263 or 1304, B 1216 or 1591 (p. 790).

Dose. Up to 5 mg (base) by intravenous injection; up to 100 mg (base) by slow intravenous infusion.

Toxicity. The estimated minimum lethal dose in children is 60 mg intranasally or intramuscularly.

METAZOCINE *Narcotic*

Synonym: NIH 7410.

1,2,3,4,5,6 - Hexahydro - 8 - hydroxy - 3,6,11 - trimethyl-2,6-methano-3-benzazocine

$C_{15}H_{21}NO = 231·3$

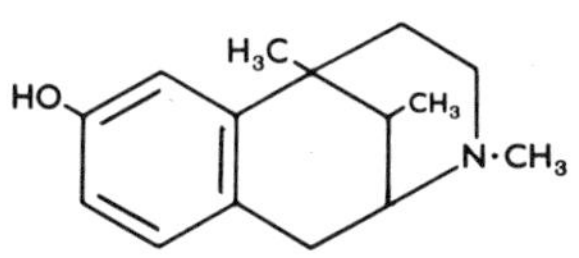

It occurs as crystals from methanol. M.p. 232° to 235°.

Extraction. Metazocine is extracted by organic solvents from aqueous alkaline solutions.

Chromatography. PAPER: system P1—Rf 0·48 (location under ultraviolet light, absorption; location reagent *iodoplatinate spray*, weak reaction).

THIN-LAYER: system T1—Rf 0·21 (location reagents: *acidified iodoplatinate spray*, positive reaction; *potassium permanganate spray*, positive reaction).

Colour Tests. MICRO: sulphuric acid–formaldehyde test—brown → greenish-grey → dull grey (*sensitivity:* 1·0 μg); ammonium molybdate test—bright blue → green (*sensitivity:* 1·0 μg); ammonium vanadate test—greenish-brown (*sensitivity:* 1·0 μg); Vitali's test—yellow/yellow/bright orange (*sensitivity:* 1·0 μg).

Crystal Tests. MICRO: *picrolonic acid*—curving needles (*sensitivity:* 1 in 400); *platinic chloride solution*—bunches of small plates (*sensitivity:* 1 in 400).

METFORMIN *Antidiabetic*

Synonym: LA 6023.

N^1N^1-Dimethyldiguanide

$C_4H_{11}N_5 = 129·2$

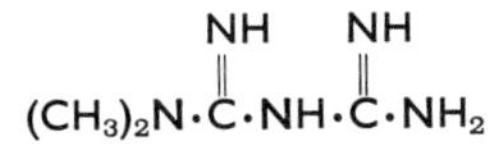

METFORMIN HYDROCHLORIDE

Proprietary Names: Diabefagos; Glucophage.

A white hygroscopic crystalline powder.

Solubility. Freely soluble in water and ethanol; insoluble in ether and chloroform.

Extraction. Metformin is extracted by organic solvents from aqueous alkaline solutions.

Chromatography. PAPER: system P1—Rf 0·07 (location under ultraviolet light, strong absorption; location reagent *iodoplatinate spray*, weak reaction); system RP1a—Rf 0·95 (location under ultraviolet light, absorption); system RP1b—Rf 0·95 (location as for RP1a).

THIN-LAYER: system T1—Rf 0·09 (location reagent *acidified iodoplatinate spray*, white).

Crystal Tests. MICRO: *picric acid*—branching rods (*sensitivity:* 1 in 400); *platinic iodide solution*—rhomboids (*sensitivity:* 1 in 400).

Ultraviolet Absorption Spectrum. Metformin in 0·1N sulphuric acid, maximum at 208 mμ (E1%, 1 cm 225).

Infra-red Absorption Spectrum. Metformin (base). Potassium bromide disk. The principal peaks are: A 1580, B 1620, C 1474 or 1487 (p. 790).

Dose. Up to 3 g daily.

METHACHOLINE BROMIDE *Parasympathomimetic*

Proprietary Names: Amechol Bromide; Mecholyl Bromide.

(2-Acetoxypropyl)trimethylammonium bromide

$C_8H_{18}BrNO_2 = 240·1$

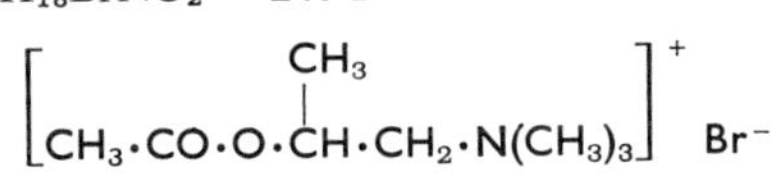

A white, very hygroscopic, crystalline powder. M.p. 147° to 150°.

Solubility. Freely soluble in water and ethanol; almost insoluble in ether; soluble 3 in 4 of chloroform.

METHACHOLINE CHLORIDE

Proprietary Name: Amechol Chloride.

A white deliquescent crystalline powder. M.p. 170° to 173°.

Solubility. Soluble 1 in less than 1 of water, and 1 in less than 2 of ethanol; freely soluble in chloroform.

Extraction. The methacholine salts are quaternary ammonium compounds (see p. 29).

Chromatography. PAPER: system P1—Rf 0·10 (location reagent *iodoplatinate spray*, weak reaction).

THIN-LAYER: system T1—Rf 0·02 (location reagent *acidified iodoplatinate spray*, positive reaction).

Crystal Tests. MICRO: *gold bromide solution*—serrated plates (*sensitivity:* 1 in 400); *lead iodide solution*—branching needles (*sensitivity:* 1 in 400).

Dose. Up to 2 g daily by mouth; up to 25 mg (chloride) subcutaneously.

Toxicity. Methacholine is 10 to 20 times more potent than acetylcholine by subcutaneous injection.
LD50 (oral): in rats 750 mg/kg.

METHACYCLINE *Antibiotic*

Synonyms: GS 2876; 6-Methyleneoxytetracycline.

4 - Dimethylamino - 1,4,4a,5,5a,6,11,12a - octahydro - 3,5,10,12,12a - pentahydroxy - 6 - methylene - 1,11 - dioxonaphthacene - 2 - carboxyamide
$C_{22}H_{22}N_2O_8$ = 442·4

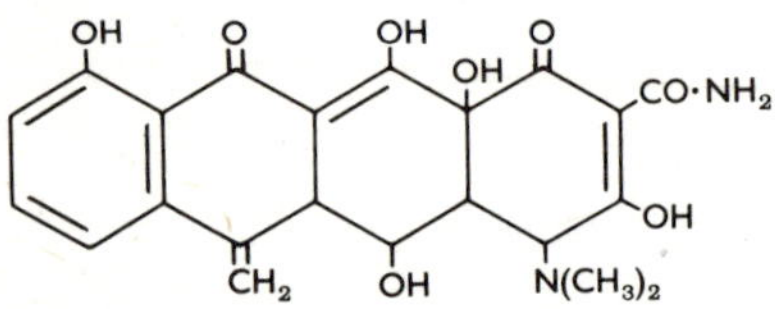

METHACYCLINE HYDROCHLORIDE
Proprietary Name: Rondomycin.

A dark yellow crystalline powder. M.p. about 205°, with decomposition.
Solubility. Soluble in water; sparingly soluble in ethanol; almost insoluble in ether and chloroform.

Chromatography. PAPER: system P1—Rf 0·35 (location under ultraviolet light, orange fluorescence; location reagents: *ninhydrin spray*, orange; *potassium permanganate spray*, strong reaction).
THIN-LAYER: system T1—Rf 0·05, streaking (location under ultraviolet light, orange fluorescence; location reagent *potassium permanganate spray*, positive reaction).

Colour Tests. MICRO: sulphuric acid–formaldehyde test—(yellow) dull orange (*sensitivity:* 1·0 μg); ammonium molybdate test—(yellow) yellow→brown (*sensitivity:* 1·0 μg); ammonium vanadate test—(yellow)yellow→orange→purple (*sensitivity:* 1·0 μg); sulphuric acid test—yellow→orange→red; Vitali's test—(yellow) yellow/yellow/brown (*sensitivity:* 1·0 μg).

Ultraviolet Absorption Spectrum. Methacycline in 0·1N sulphuric acid, maxima at 243 mμ (E1%, 1 cm about 552) and 340 mμ (E1%, 1 cm 361).

Quantitative Estimation. A spectrophotometric method of estimation is described in *Drugs of Today*, 1965, **1**, 14.

Metabolism. After oral administration, methacycline is more rapidly absorbed than demethylchlortetracycline but the blood-level is less persistently maintained. About 75 to 80% of an absorbed dose is bound to protein. It is excreted more slowly than tetracycline, partly in the urine and partly unchanged in the faeces.

Dose. Up to 1·2 g daily.

METHADONE *Narcotic Analgesic*

Synonyms: Amidon(e); Hoechst 10820; Phenadon(e).

(±) - 6 - Dimethylamino - 4,4 - diphenylheptan - 3-one
$C_{21}H_{27}NO$ = 309·5

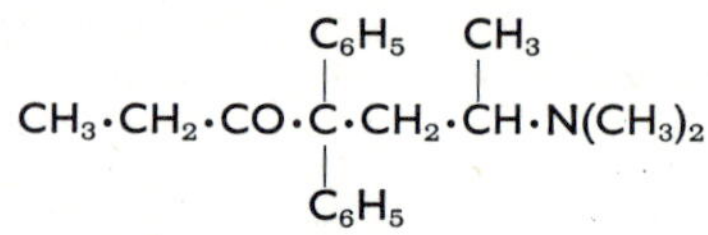

METHADONE HYDROCHLORIDE.
Proprietary Names: Adanon(e) Hydrochloride; Butalgin; Diadone; Diaminone Hydrochloride; Dolophine; Eptadone; Mecodin; Mephenon; Miadone; Polamidon; Physeptone; Symoron; Zefalgin.

A white crystalline powder. M.p. 233° to 236°.
Solubility. Soluble 1 in 12 of water, 1 in 7 of ethanol, and 1 in 3 of chloroform; insoluble in ether.

Extraction. Methadone is extracted by organic solvents from aqueous alkaline solutions.

Chromatography. PAPER: system P1—Rf 0·74 (location under ultraviolet light, absorption; location reagent *iodoplatinate spray*, weak reaction); system RP1a—Rf 0·59 (location reagent *iodoplatinate spray*, positive reaction); system RP1b—Rf 0·00 (location under ultraviolet light, absorption; location reagent *iodoplatinate spray*, positive reaction).
THIN-LAYER: system T1—Rf 0·37 (location reagent *acidified iodoplatinate spray*, positive reaction).
GAS: system G1/180—retention time 2·78 relative to diphenhydramine; system G2/225—retention time 0·55 relative to codeine; system G6—retention time 0·49 relative to codeine.

Colour Test. MICRO: ammonium vanadate test—faint green→blue (*sensitivity:* 0·5 μg).

Crystal Tests. MICRO: *mercuric chloride solution*—rosettes of branching rods (*sensitivity:* 1 in 3000); *platinic bromide solution*—bunches of prisms (*sensitivity:* 1 in 400).

Ultraviolet Absorption Spectrum. Methadone in ethanol:water (1:1), maxima at 259 mμ (E1%, 1 cm 22) and 295 mμ (E1%, 1 cm 22); in 0·1N sulphuric acid, maxima at 253 mμ (E1%, 1 cm 16·5), 259 mμ (E1%, 1 cm 17·7), 265 mμ (E1%, 1 cm 16·7), and 292 mμ (E1%, 1 cm 16·8).

Metabolism. Methadone is rapidly and extensively metabolised; *N*-demethylation has been established to be a metabolic pathway.
Some 10 minutes after subcutaneous injection, methadone is to be found in blood

plasma and soon in the liver, lungs, kidneys, and spleen. Peak levels in the brain are reached in 1 to 2 hours. Methadone is bound to tissue protein. It is excreted in the urine and faeces in the form of metabolites, less than 10% being excreted unchanged.

Dose. As an analgesic, usually up to 60 mg daily.

Toxicity. The minimum lethal dose in man is stated to be in the range 60 to 120 mg. Methadone has marked addiction-producing properties; addicts have been known to take as much as 1·2 g daily, intravenously.

CASE EXAMPLES. Details are given of 7 fatal cases involving methadone in which the drug was found in the stomach contents, small intestine, and urine. Four other cases are described in which methadone was thought to be a contributory cause of death (Alha and Ohela, 1955).

METHANOL *Industrial Solvent*

Synonym: Methyl Alcohol.

$CH_3OH = 32{\cdot}04$

A colourless highly inflammable liquid. B.p. 64·5° to 65·5°. Refractive index 1·328 to 1·329.

Solubility. Miscible with water, ethanol, ether, and chloroform.

NOTE. The commercial substance known as wood naphtha (pyroxylic acid; wood spirit) is 60 to 90% pure and contains acetone and other empyreumatic impurities. The variety used for denaturing alcohol (see under Ethanol, p. 332) contains 72% v/v of methanol.

Screening Tests. See under Screening Tests, p. 6.

Extraction. Methanol is volatile and may be isolated by distillation (see p. 18).

Chromatography. GAS: system G8/100—retention time 0·1 relative to n-propanol; system G8/160—retention time 0·22 relative to n-propanol.

Colour Test. *Acidified potassium dichromate solution*—green, on warming.

Quantitative Estimation. Feldstein and Klendshoj (1954) have described a spectrophotometric method of determination of methanol in biological fluids involving diffusion, oxidation with permanganate, and treatment with chromotropic acid. Williams *et al.* (1961) describe a very similar spectrophotometric method but diffusion is not involved.

Metabolism. Methanol is metabolised and excreted much more slowly than ethanol. The main metabolic route of methanol is oxidation to formaldehyde (p. 349) and then to formic acid (p. 349). Formic acid may be eventually oxidised to carbon dioxide which is exhaled. After large doses of methanol, formic acid is found in the blood and urine and severe acidosis may result. Both unchanged methanol and methylglucuronide may also be excreted via the lungs and kidneys.
The high oral and inhalation toxicity of methanol is thought to be due to the localised action of formaldehyde and formic acid, either of which may inhibit cellular metabolism.
Methanol is distributed in the body according to the water content of the tissues. The aqueous and vitreous humour and the optic nerve have a high water content and for this reason the optic nerve and the retina specifically may be damaged.

Toxicity. Methanol is the least acutely toxic of the lower aliphatic alcohols in animals but due to its slow rate of metabolism it exerts characteristic and severe chronic toxic effects. The onset of symptoms may be delayed up to 36 hours and the symptoms may include severe upper abdominal pain, visual disturbance, often proceeding to incurable blindness, severe acidosis, and prolonged coma, which may terminate in death from respiratory failure.
The fatal dose varies greatly but is usually from 100 to 200 ml; permanent blindness has been caused by as little as 10 ml. Blood-levels of 80 mg% and above must be considered extremely dangerous. It has been suggested that concurrent administration of ethanol with methanol may reduce the toxicity of the latter.

CASE EXAMPLES. Poisoning of 23 persons who had been drinking Korean saké containing 16% methanol; 5 died of respiratory arrest after several hours of coma and another was brought into hospital in profound shock and died within 4 hours. Autopsy revealed cerebral and pulmonary oedema, gastritis and fatty livers. Of the other 17, all were treated with 6 to 8 g of sodium bicarbonate 2-hourly, fluids were forced, and they were encouraged to eat heartily. One of these patients died but the rest recovered with no visual impairment (Keeney and Mellinkoff, 1951).

In October, 1951, a large consignment of contraband whisky was distributed in the city of Atlanta, Georgia. During a 5-day period thereafter 323 patients with acute methanol poisoning were admitted to hospital and 41 of them died. The whisky contained 35 to 40% of methanol and only 4% of ethanol. A latent period, usually of about 24 hours, followed ingestion of the whisky and thereafter patients complained of headache, dizziness, anorexia, nausea, weakness, and visual disturbance. The outstanding feature in all severe cases was acidosis. Of the 323 cases, 115 were found to have plasma-bicarbonate levels below 20 mEq per litre. Of 30 patients in whom this figure was below 10 mEq per litre, 15 died; 4 patients, all moribund, had bicarbonate levels of zero (Bennett, 1953).

METHANTHELINIUM BROMIDE *Parasympatholytic*

Synonyms: Dixamone Bromide; Methantheline Bromide; Methanthine Bromide.

Proprietary Names: Avagal; Banthine.

2 - Diethylaminoethyl xanthen - 9 - carboxylate methobromide

$C_{21}H_{26}BrNO_3 = 420{\cdot}4$

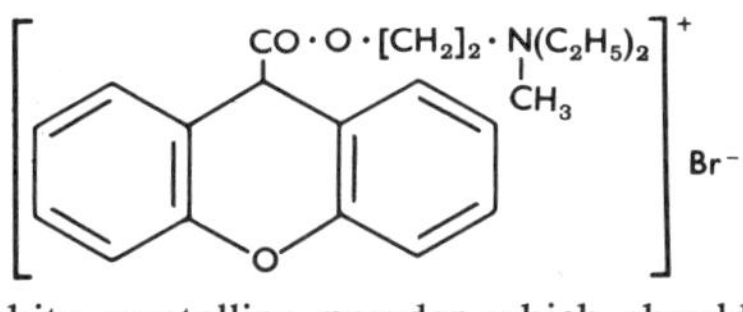

A white crystalline powder which should be

protected from moisture. Aqueous solutions decompose on standing. M.p. 171° to 177°.
Solubility. Very soluble in water; freely soluble in ethanol and chloroform; almost insoluble in ether.

Extraction. Methanthelinium bromide is a quaternary ammonium compound (see p. 29).

Chromatography. PAPER: system P1—Rf 0·53 (location under ultraviolet light, pale blue fluorescence; location reagent *iodoplatinate spray*, strong reaction); system RP1a—Rf 0·77 (location under ultraviolet light, blue fluorescence; location reagent *iodoplatinate spray*, positive reaction); system RP1b—Rf 0·75 (location under ultraviolet light, blue fluorescence).

THIN-LAYER: system T1—Rf 0·02 (location reagent *acidified iodoplatinate spray*, positive reaction).

Colour Tests. MICRO: the following tests are performed on the nitrate (see p. 134): sulphuric acid–formaldehyde test—orange (*sensitivity:* 0·25 μg); ammonium molybdate test—blue-grey (*sensitivity:* 0·25 μg); ammonium vanadate test—orange (*sensitivity:* 0·1 μg); Vitali's test—yellow/–/green (*sensitivity:* 0·5 μg).

Crystal Tests. MICRO: *lead iodide solution*—bunches of plates, forming overnight (*sensitivity:* 1 in 200); *zinc chloride solution*—coarse needles (*sensitivity:* 1 in 100).

Ultraviolet Absorption Spectrum. Methanthelinium bromide in ethanol, maxima at 246 mμ (E1%, 1 cm 135) and 282 mμ (E1%, 1 cm 69).

Metabolism. Methanthelinium bromide is poorly absorbed from the gastro-intestinal tract and is rapidly degraded in the blood. Urinary excretion is very rapid; faecal excretion may also occur.

Dose. Usually up to 400 mg daily, adjusted as necessary.

Toxicity. Methanthelinium bromide is much more toxic than propantheline bromide (p. 519) which has largely replaced it.
LD50 (oral): in mice about 460 and in rats about 1660 mg/kg.

METHAPHENILENE *Antihistamine*

Synonym: Methaphenylene.

NN - Dimethyl - *N′* - phenyl - *N′* - then - 2 - ylethylenediamine
$C_{15}H_{20}N_2S = 260{\cdot}4$

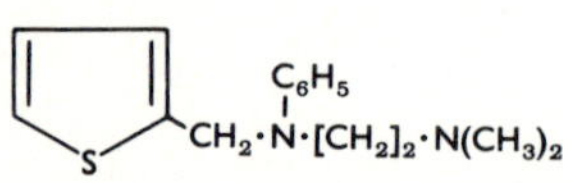

A dark yellow oil. B.p. 183° to 185° at 7 mm Hg.

METHAPHENILENE HYDROCHLORIDE
Proprietary Names: Diatrin(e); Nilistine.
A white crystalline powder. M.p. 184° to 189°.
Solubility. Soluble in water; sparingly soluble in ethanol and chloroform; almost insoluble in ether.

Extraction. Methaphenilene is extracted by organic solvents from aqueous alkaline solutions.

Chromatography. PAPER: system P1—Rf 0·67 (location under ultraviolet light, strong absorption; location reagent *iodoplatinate spray*, strong reaction).

THIN-LAYER: system T1—Rf 0·53 (location reagent *acidified iodoplatinate spray*, positive reaction).

GAS: system G2/225—retention time 1·30 relative to diphenhydramine.

Colour Tests. MICRO: sulphuric acid–formaldehyde test—dull purple (*sensitivity:* 1·0 μg); ammonium molybdate test—grey-blue (*sensitivity:* 1·0 μg); ammonium vanadate test—orange→purple (*sensitivity:* 0·1 μg); Vitali's test—red-brown/greenish-brown/brown (*sensitivity:* 0·5 μg).

Crystal Tests. MICRO: *platinic bromide solution*—small plates (*sensitivity:* 1 in 1000); *platinic chloride solution*—serrated plates (*sensitivity:* 1 in 400).

Ultraviolet Absorption Spectrum. Methaphenilene in ethanol, maximum at 243 mμ (E1%, 1 cm 582).

Dose. Usually up to 200 mg daily.

Toxicity. The estimated lethal dose in man is 25 to 250 mg/kg.
LD50 (intraperitoneal): in mice 117 mg/kg.

METHAPYRILENE *Antihistamine*

Synonym: Thenylpyramine.

NN - Dimethyl - *N′* - pyrid - 2 - yl - *N′* - then - 2-ylethylenediamine
$C_{14}H_{19}N_3S = 261{\cdot}4$

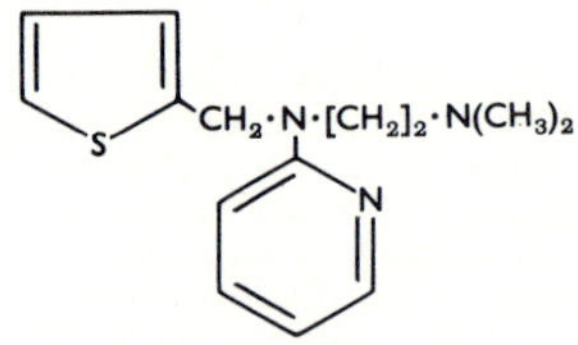

NOTE. Methapyrilene is an isomer of thenyldiamine (p. 566).

A liquid which boils at 173° to 175°.

METHAPYRILENE FUMARATE
A white crystalline powder. M.p. 133° to 136°.
Solubility. Soluble in water; slightly soluble in ethanol; insoluble in ether.

METHAPYRILENE HYDROCHLORIDE
Proprietary Names: Allergin; Driliton; Dormin; Dozar; Dylhista; Histadyl; Lullamin; Pyrathyn; Pyrteen; Semikon Hydrochloride; Sleepwell; Somnicaps; Thenylene; Thionylan.

A white crystalline powder which should be protected from light. M.p. 159° to 163°.

Solubility. Soluble 1 in 0·5 of water, 1 in 5 of ethanol, and 1 in 3 of chloroform; almost insoluble in ether.

Extraction. Methapyrilene is extracted by organic solvents from aqueous alkaline solutions.

Chromatography. PAPER: system P1—Rf 0·32 (location under ultraviolet light, bright blue fluorescence; location reagents: *iodoplatinate spray*, strong reaction; *bromocresol green spray*, strong reaction); system RP1a—Rf 0·71 (location under ultraviolet light, blue fluorescence; location reagent *iodoplatinate spray*, positive reaction); system RP1b—Rf 0·05 (location as for RP1a).

THIN-LAYER: system T1—Rf 0·48 (location reagent *acidified iodoplatinate spray*, positive reaction); system T2—Rf 0·56 (location reagent *iodoplatinate spray*, positive reaction); system T3—Rf 0·83 (location as for T2).

GAS: system G1/180—retention time 1·56 relative to diphenhydramine.

Colour Tests. MICRO: sulphuric acid–formaldehyde test—black-purple (*sensitivity:* 0·1 μg); ammonium molybdate test—purple-brown→greenish-brown (*sensitivity:* 0·1 μg); ammonium vanadate test—black-purple (*sensitivity:* 0·1 μg); Vitali's test—purple/brown-purple/yellow-green (*sensitivity:* 0·1 μg).

Crystal Tests. MICRO: *platinic chloride solution*—branching needles (*sensitivity:* 1 in 1000); *styphnic acid*—stout blades in bunches (*sensitivity:* 1 in 1000).

Ultraviolet Absorption Spectrum. Methapyrilene in 0·1N sodium hydroxide, maxima at 237 mμ (E1%, 1 cm 600) and 308 mμ (E1%, 1 cm 100); in 0·1N sulphuric acid, maxima at about 237 mμ (E1%, 1 cm 764) and 313 mμ (E1%, 1 cm 342).

Metabolism. Following oral administration in man, only about 10% is excreted in the urine, the maximum excretion occurring between 1½ and 4½ hours after ingestion.

Dose. Usually up to 400 mg daily.

Toxicity. The lethal dose in man is in the range 10 to 100 mg/kg.

LD50 (oral): in mice 190 and in rats 450 mg/kg.

CASE EXAMPLES. Death of a 16-month-old girl after swallowing 100 mg of methapyrilene hydrochloride: symptoms were vomiting, drowsiness, rapidly followed by excitation, convulsions, and tremors (Rives *et al.*, 1949).

A suicide took '2 bottles' of 25-mg capsules of methapyrilene hydrochloride and died 1½ hours later. Post-mortem examination showed the stomach to contain 720 mg of the drug and the blood 1·2 mg% (O'Dea and Liss, 1953).

In a case of fatal poisoning in a young woman the stomach contents contained 3·0 mg%, the blood 38 mg%, and the spleen 83 mg% (Jackson, 1967).

METHAQUALONE *Hypnotic*

Synonyms: QZ2; TR 495; Tuazolon.

Proprietary Names: Dormutil; Omnyl; Quaalude. It is the main ingredient of Mandrax.

3,4 - Dihydro - 2 - methyl - 4 - oxo - 3 - *o* - tolylquinazoline

$C_{16}H_{14}N_2O = 250{\cdot}3$

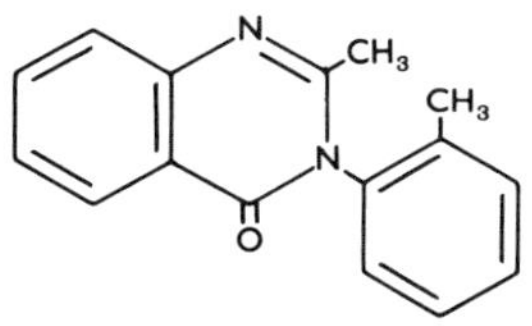

A white crystalline powder. M.p. about 115°.

Solubility. Insoluble in water; soluble in ethanol, ether, and chloroform.

METHAQUALONE HYDROCHLORIDE

Proprietary Names: Melsedin; Revonal; Sedaquin; Somnium; Toquilon; Toraflon; Tuazol(e).

A white crystalline powder. M.p. 255° to 265°.

Solubility. Insoluble in water; soluble in ethanol and ether.

Screening Test. See Screening Tests, p. 13.

Extraction. Methaqualone is extracted by organic solvents from aqueous alkaline solutions.

Methaqualone may be extracted from blood and tissues as follows. The material is made alkaline with 0·1N sodium hydroxide and extracted with 10 times its volume of chloroform; the chloroform layer is filtered and washed with 0·1 of its volume of 0·1N hydrochloric acid. Finally, the chloroform layer is filtered, dried, and evaporated (Bogan, 1967).

Chromatography. PAPER: system P1—Rf 0·94 (location under ultraviolet light, strong absorption; location reagent *iodine vapour*, weak reaction); system RP1a—Rf 0·06 (location under ultraviolet light, absorption); system RP1b—Rf 0·04 (location as for RP1a).

THIN-LAYER: system T1—Rf 0·70 (location reagent *acidified iodoplatinate spray*, positive reaction).

GAS: system G2/225—retention time 0·51 relative to codeine; system G4—retention time 0·53 relative to codeine.

Crystal Tests. MICRO: *potassium permanganate solution*—serrated plates (*sensitivity:* 1 in 200); *sodium carbonate solution*—bunches of prisms (*sensitivity:* 1 in 200).

Ultraviolet Absorption Spectrum. Methaqualone in ethanol, maxima at 225 mμ, 263 mμ, 304 mμ, and 316 mμ; in 0·01N hydrochloric acid, maxima at about 234 mμ (E1%, 1cm 1280 to 1340) and about 269 mμ (E1%, 1 cm 290 to 320).

Infra-red Absorption Spectrum. Methaqualone (base). Potassium bromide disk. The principal peaks are: A 1682, B 1599, C 1335 or 1465 or 1565 (p. 790).

Quantitative Estimation. Akagi *et al.* (1963) have described 2 spectrophotometric methods of estimation of methaqualone in biological fluids and tissues. Maehly and Bonnichsen (1966) also describe a method.

Metabolism. Methaqualone is readily absorbed

from the gastro-intestinal tract. It is concentrated primarily in the liver and body fat. Daily ingestion of 500 mg of methaqualone leads to blood-levels of about 0·5 mg%.

Dose. Up to 300 mg as a hypnotic.

Toxicity. Plasma levels greater than 3 mg%, corresponding to the ingestion of 5 g of methaqualone, are indicative of dangerous poisoning, at least in those not habituated to the drug (Lawson and Brown, 1966), although recoveries have occurred following the ingestion of about 16 g (Young, 1967).

LD50 (oral): in mice 400 and in rats 250 mg/kg.

CASE EXAMPLES. At post-mortem examination, liver and kidney specimens from an elderly woman, who died after ingesting at least 7 g of methaqualone and 700 mg of diphenhydramine, were found to contain methaqualone metabolites, estimated at 25 mg% and 37 mg% respectively (Sanderson *et al.*, 1966).

In 19 mildly poisoned patients, the plasma levels of methaqualone on admission to hospital ranged from 0·2 to 2 mg%. The mean plasma level in 9 more severe cases was 2·7 mg%, reached within 12 hours of admission. Methaqualone was readily detected in the urine of these patients (Lawson and Brown, 1966).

In 5 suicide cases due to methaqualone, at post-mortem examination the blood-levels ranged from 0·5 to 3·2 mg% and concentrations in the liver were 3·8 to 5·8 mg% and in the kidneys 2·2 to 9·2 mg% (Maehly and Bonnichsen, 1966).

A 58-year-old woman was admitted to hospital in a coma some hours after taking between 5 and 7·5 g of methaqualone and 500 to 750 mg of diphenhydramine. On admission, the serum-methaqualone level was 10·5 mg%. After 12 hours of forced diuresis, haemodialysis was instituted, and at the end of 6 hours the level was 5·8 mg%. After 24 hours the woman was fully conscious (Caridis *et al.*, 1967).

A 49-year-old man ingested 6 g of methaqualone and 600 mg of diphenhydramine. The following levels of methaqualone were measured: blood, 1·8 mg%; liver, 3·8 mg%; urine, 0·5 mg% (Bogan, 1967).

METHARBITONE *Barbiturate*

Synonyms: Endiemal; Metharbital.
Proprietary Name: Gemonil.

5,5-Diethyl-1-methylbarbituric acid
$C_9H_{14}N_2O_3 = 198{\cdot}2$

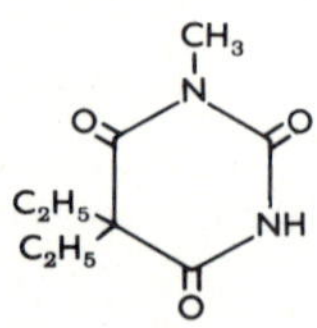

A white crystalline powder. M.p. 151° to 155°.

Solubility. Soluble 1 in 830 of water, 1 in 23 of ethanol, and 1 in 40 of ether.

Screening Tests. See under Barbiturates, p. 208.

Extraction. Metharbitone may be isolated in the A2 fraction (see p. 27).

Chromatography. PAPER: system P2—Rf 1·35 relative to amylobarbitone (location under ultraviolet light, dark spot).

THIN-LAYER: system T10—Rf 0·55 (location reagents: *mercurous nitrate spray*, black; *Zwikker's reagent spray*, faint pink); system T11—Rf 0·53 (location reagent *mercurous nitrate spray*, white on grey); system T12—Rf 0·66 (location as for T11); system T13—Rf 0·85 (location as for T11).

GAS: system G7—retention time 0·76 relative to barbitone.

Colour Test. Zwikker's test—violet-blue.

Ultraviolet Absorption Spectrum. Metharbitone is a 1,5,5-derivative—see Screening Test 3 under Barbiturates, p. 208.

Infra-red Absorption Spectrum. Potassium bromide disk. The principal peaks are: A 1655 or 1699, B 1326 (p. 745).

Quantitative Estimation. See under Barbiturates, p. 208.

Metabolism. Metharbitone is a long-acting barbiturate—see under Barbiturates, p. 207. After a therapeutic dose, only 0·6% was excreted unchanged in the urine and 1·72% as the demethylated metabolite, barbitone. After 48 hours 1·18% of the dose had been excreted unchanged and 9·37% as barbitone. Metharbitone is much less rapidly demethylated than methylphenobarbitone (Svendsen and Brochmann-Hanssen, 1962).

Dose. Up to 300 mg daily, increasing gradually if necessary.

Toxicity. The estimated minimum lethal dose in man is 2 g.

METHDILAZINE *Antihistamine*

10-(1-Methylpyrrolidin-3-ylmethyl)phenothiazine
$C_{18}H_{20}N_2S = 296{\cdot}4$

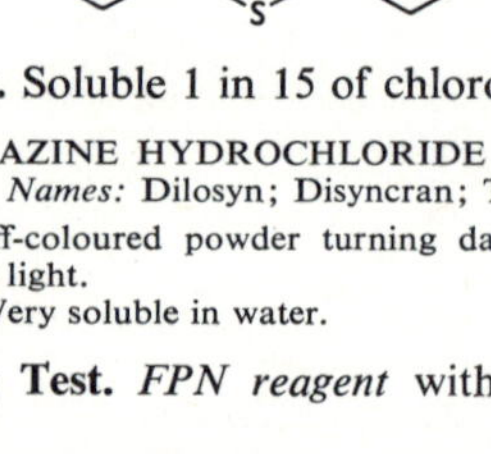

Solubility. Soluble 1 in 15 of chloroform.

METHDILAZINE HYDROCHLORIDE
Proprietary Names: Dilosyn; Disyncran; Tacaryl.

A pale buff-coloured powder turning dark brown on exposure to light.

Solubility. Very soluble in water.

Screening Test. *FPN reagent* with urine (see p. 10).

Extraction. Methdilazine is extracted by organic solvents from aqueous alkaline solutions; hydrolysis of biological material is required in order to improve the yield.

Chromatography. PAPER: system P1—Rf 0·64 (location under ultraviolet light, blue fluorescence; location reagents: *iodoplatinate spray*, strong reaction; *bromocresol green spray*, weak reaction).
THIN-LAYER: system T1—Rf 0·27 (location reagent *acidified iodoplatinate spray*, positive reaction); system T3—Rf 0·40 (location reagent *iodoplatinate spray*, positive reaction); system T4—Rf 0·61 (location as for T3); system T6—Rf 0·64 (the spot may be converted on the plate to the sulphoxide, Rf 0·43; location of both spots under ultraviolet light).
GAS: system G2/225—retention time 1·22 relative to codeine.

Colour Tests. MICRO: sulphuric acid–formaldehyde test—red-purple (*sensitivity:* 0·1 µg); ammonium molybdate test—green → dull purple (*sensitivity:* 0·25 µg); ammonium vanadate test—green → purple (*sensitivity:* 0·5 µg); Vitali's test—purple → yellow/yellow/yellow (*sensitivity:* 0·5 µg).

Crystal Test. MICRO: *gold bromide–hydrochloric acid solution*—oily needles, forming overnight (*sensitivity:* 1 in 100).

Ultraviolet Absorption Spectrum. Methdilazine in ethanol, maxima at 254 mµ (E 1%, 1 cm 1054) and 304 mµ (E 1%, 1 cm 136).

Metabolism. Studies in animals have shown that methdilazine is absorbed slowly from the stomach and very rapidly from the small intestine. About a quarter of the dose is excreted in the urine as methdilazine sulphoxide; it is more readily oxidised than some of the other phenothiazines. Methdilazine is distributed throughout the body tissues, but no accumulation is observed after repeated daily doses.

Dose. Usually up to 16 mg daily.

Toxicity. The acute lethal dose in man of the phenothiazine derivatives appears to be in the range 15 to 150 mg/kg, although severe toxic symptoms have occurred with doses of less than 1 mg/kg. Recovery has followed the ingestion of 280 mg of methdilazine.
LD50 (oral): in mice 225 and in rats 448 mg/kg.

METHICILLIN *Antibiotic*

Synonyms: BRL 1241; P 35; X 1497.

6-(2,6-Dimethoxybenzamido)penicillanic acid
$C_{17}H_{20}N_2O_6S$ = 380·4

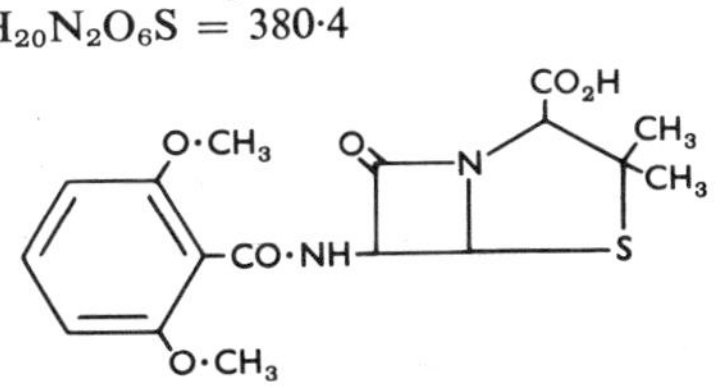

METHICILLIN SODIUM
Synonyms: Dimethoxyphenecillin Sodium; Dimethoxyphenyl Penicillin Sodium.
Proprietary Names: Celbenin; Dimocillin; Penistaph; Staphcillin; Synticillin.

A white microcrystalline powder. Methicillin sodium is unstable in acid solutions. Specific rotation of a 5% aqueous solution, +225° to +233°.
Solubility. Soluble 1 in 0·6 of water and 1 in 35 of ethanol; insoluble in ether; slightly soluble in chloroform.

Ultraviolet Absorption Spectrum. Methicillin sodium in water, maximum at 280 mµ (E 1%, 1 cm about 55).

Metabolism. Since methicillin is inactivated in acid media it must be given by injection. It is rapidly absorbed following intramuscular injection; 30 minutes after the intramuscular injection of 1 g the blood-level ranges from 1·8 to 2·1 mg% and by the fourth hour the level has gradually declined to 0·2 mg%. Excretion is rapid; 20% or more may be excreted in the bile and 50% or more may appear in the urine within 6 hours of a single dose of 1 g.

Dose. Up to 6 g daily.

METHIMAZOLE *Antithyroid Agent*

Synonyms: Mercazole; Thiamazole.
Proprietary Name: Tapazole.

2-Mercapto-1-methylimidazole
$C_4H_6N_2S$ = 114·2

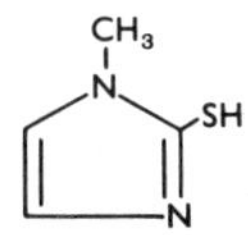

A white to pale buff crystalline powder. M.p. 144° to 147°. B.p. 280°, with decomposition.
Solubility. Soluble 1 in 5 of water, 1 in 5 of ethanol, 1 in 125 of ether, and 1 in 4·5 of chloroform.

Extraction. Methimazole is extracted from neutral solutions by chloroform.

Chromatography. PAPER: system P1—Rf 0·72 (location under ultraviolet light, absorption; location reagents: *iodoplatinate spray*, white; *potassium permanganate spray*, strong reaction); system RP1a—Rf 0·27 (location under ultraviolet light, absorption; location reagent *iodoplatinate spray*, positive reaction); system RP1b—Rf 0·00 (location as for RP1a).
THIN-LAYER: system T1—Rf 0·67 (location reagent *acidified iodoplatinate spray*, positive reaction).
GAS: system G2/225—retention time 0·43 relative to diphenhydramine.

Colour Test. MICRO: ammonium molybdate test—(grey) blue (*sensitivity:* 0·1 µg).

Crystal Tests. MICRO: *gold bromide–hydrochloric acid solution*—plates, often in crosses (*sensitivity:* 1 in 1000); *potassium tri-iodide solution (1)*—bunches of rods or needles (*sensitivity:* 1 in 1000).

Ultraviolet Absorption Spectrum. Methimazole in 0·1N sulphuric acid, maxima at 211 mµ

(E1%, 1 cm 593) and 251·5 mμ (E1%, 1 cm 1528).

Infra-red Absorption Spectrum. Potassium bromide disk. The principal peaks are: A 1466, B 1570, C 1271 (p. 745).

Metabolism. Methimazole depresses the formation of thyroid hormone and so lowers the basal metabolic rate. It is the active agent released by carbimazole (p. 238).

Dose. Usually up to 30 mg daily.

Toxicity. Fatal agranulocytosis has been reported but no deaths from acute toxicity.

METHIXENE *Parasympatholytic*

Synonym: SJ 1977.

9-(1-Methylpiperid-3-ylmethyl)thiaxanthen

$C_{20}H_{23}NS = 309{\cdot}5$

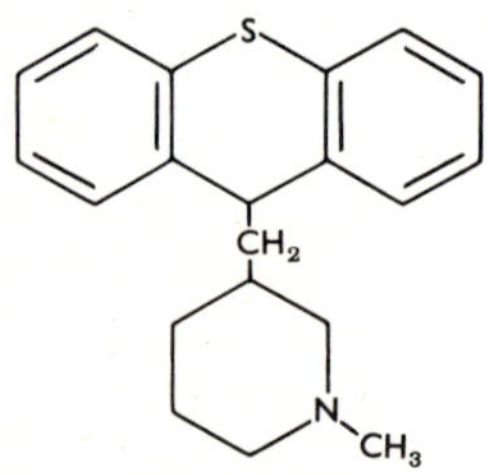

METHIXENE HYDROCHLORIDE

Proprietary Names: Tremaril; Tremonil; Trest.

A white crystalline powder.

Solubility. Soluble in water, ethanol, and chloroform.

Extraction. Methixene is extracted by organic solvents from aqueous alkaline solutions.

Chromatography. PAPER: system P1—Rf 0·66 (location under ultraviolet light, absorption; location reagents: *iodoplatinate spray*, strong reaction; *bromocresol green spray*, strong reaction); system RP1a—Rf 0·27 (location reagent *iodoplatinate spray*, positive reaction); system RP1b—Rf 0·00 (location as for RP1a). THIN-LAYER: system T1—Rf 0·48 (location reagent *acidified iodoplatinate spray*, positive reaction).

GAS: system G2/225—retention time 1·4 relative to codeine.

Colour Tests. MICRO: ammonium molybdate test—black → purple → orange (*sensitivity:* 0·5 μg); ammonium vanadate test—bright orange (*sensitivity:* 0·25 μg).

Crystal Tests. MICRO: *potassium iodide solution*—clusters of plates or prisms (*sensitivity:* 1 in 1000); *zinc chloride solution*—small needles in bunches (*sensitivity:* 1 in 1000).

Infra-red Absorption Spectrum. Methixene (base). Potassium bromide disk. The principal peaks are: A 750, B 1462, C 1439 (p. 791).

Metabolism. Methixene is excreted in the urine partly unchanged, partly as its two isomeric sulphoxides, and partly as the stereoisomeric sulphoxides of *N*-demethylated methixene (Lehner *et al.*, 1964).
Studies in mice have shown that 5 minutes after intravenous administration, unchanged methixene and its two isomeric sulphoxides are present in the liver, gastro-intestinal tract, and brain; the unchanged methixene remains longer than the 2 sulphoxides in these organs (Aebi *et al.*, 1964).

Dose. Up to 60 mg daily.

Toxicity. The lethal dose in man is probably in the range 10 to 100 mg/kg.

METHOCARBAMOL *Muscle Relaxant*

Synonym: AHR 85.

Proprietary Names: Neuraxin; Robaxin; Tresortil.

2-Hydroxy-3-*o*-methoxyphenoxypropyl carbamate

$C_{11}H_{15}NO_5 = 241{\cdot}2$

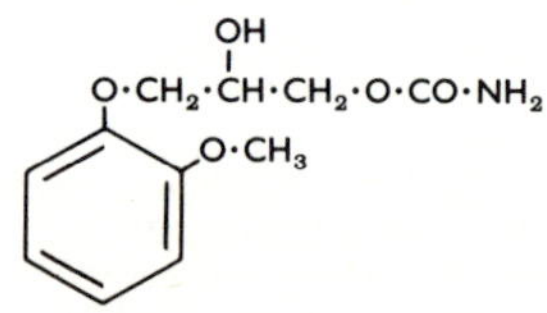

A white crystalline powder. M.p. 92° to 94°.

Solubility. Soluble 1 in 40 of water; soluble in ethanol.

Extraction. Methocarbamol is extracted by organic solvents from aqueous acid or alkaline solutions.

Chromatography. PAPER: systems P6 and P7 separate carbamate drugs and they should therefore be applicable to methocarbamol.
THIN-LAYER: system T1—Rf 0·70 (location reagent *strongly acid iodoplatinate spray*, positive reaction).

Colour Tests. MICRO: sulphuric acid–formaldehyde test—blue-purple (*sensitivity:* 0·1 μg); ammonium molybdate test—greenish-blue (*sensitivity:* 0·5 μg); ammonium vanadate test—green (*sensitivity:* 0·1 μg); Vitali's test—yellow/yellow/yellow (*sensitivity:* 1·0 μg).

Ultraviolet Absorption Spectrum. Methocarbamol in methanol, maximum at 274 mμ (E1%, 1 cm 98).

Infra-red Absorption Spectrum. Potassium bromide disk. The principal peaks are: A 1248 or 1667, B 1119 or 1215 (p. 745).

Metabolism. Following ingestion of methocarbamol for 3 consecutive days, less than 1% of the drug was detected in the urine before hydrolysis and about 10% after hydrolysis. Urinary excretion of the drug ceased almost completely within 2 days after methocarbamol was discontinued (Campbell *et al.*, 1961).

Dose. Up to 8 g daily initially; subsequently reduced.

METHOHEXITONE *Barbiturate*

Synonym: Methohexital.

α-(±)-5-Allyl-1-methyl-5-(1-methylpent-2-ynyl)barbituric acid

$C_{14}H_{18}N_2O_3 = 262{\cdot}3$

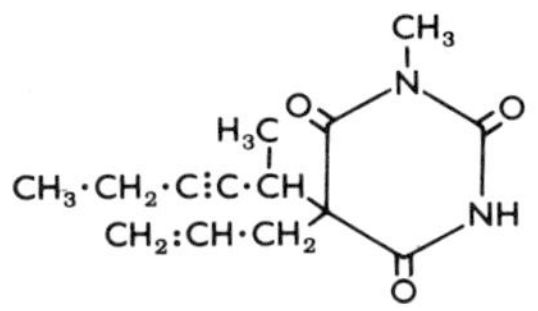

METHOHEXITONE SODIUM

Synonym: Enallynymalnatrium.

Proprietary Names: Brevital Sodium; Brietal Sodium.

A white crystalline substance.

Solubility. Soluble in water.

Screening Tests. See under Barbiturates, p. 208.

Extraction. Methohexitone may be isolated in the A2 fraction (see p. 27).

Chromatography. PAPER: system P2—Rf 1·68 relative to amylobarbitone (location under ultraviolet light, dark spot); system RP1b—Rf 0·03 (location under ultraviolet light after exposure to ammonia; location reagent *potassium permanganate spray*, yellow on pink).

THIN-LAYER: system T10—Rf 0·67 (location reagents: *mercurous nitrate spray*, black; *potassium permanganate spray*, yellow-brown on purple; *Zwikker's reagent spray*, faint pink); system T11—Rf 0·75 (location reagents: *mercurous nitrate spray*, white on grey; *potassium permanganate spray*, yellow on purple); system T12—Rf 0·78 (location as T11); system T13—Rf 0·92 (location as T11).

GAS: system G5—retention time 2·3 relative to barbitone.

Colour Test. Zwikker's test—violet-blue.

Ultraviolet Absorption Spectrum. See Screening Test 3 under Barbiturates, p. 208.

Quantitative Estimation. See under Barbiturates, p. 208.

Metabolism. Methohexitone is a very short-acting barbiturate—see Barbiturates, p. 207.

In the dog and the rat the major route of metabolism is by hydroxylation of the side-chain to yield 5-allyl-1-methyl-5-(4-hydroxy-1-methylpent-2-ynyl)barbituric acid. *N*-Demethylation seems to be of minor importance. The excretion of the metabolites is very rapid; the combined urinary and biliary excretion is 21·5% of the dose after 5 hours and 52·7% after 8 hours (Welles *et al.*, 1963).

Dose. For the induction of anaesthesia, up to 120 mg by slow intravenous injection.

Toxicity. The estimated minimum lethal dose in man is 1 g.

CASE EXAMPLE. A 41-year-old woman was found dead with an 'intravenous drip' bottle attached to a hypodermic needle introduced into her right arm. The bottle contained an aqueous solution of methohexitone. Post-mortem levels: blood, 10·3 mg%; kidney, 4·5 mg%; liver, 4·1 mg%; spleen, 4·1 mg%. The blood also contained alcohol (Finkle, 1967a).

METHOIN *Anticonvulsant*

Synonyms: Mephenetoin; Mephenytoin; Methantoin; Phenantoin.

Proprietary Names: Mesantoin; Mesontoin; Sedantoinal. It is an ingredient of Hydantal-Sandoz.

5-Ethyl-3-methyl-5-phenylhydantoin

$C_{12}H_{14}N_2O_2 = 218{\cdot}3$

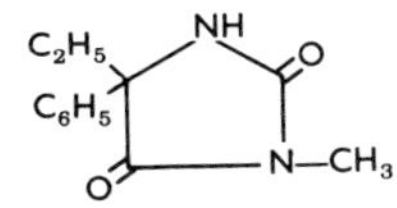

Colourless lustrous plates. M.p. 137° to 138°.

Solubility. Soluble 1 in 1500 of water, 1 in 13 of ethanol, 1 in 2·5 of chloroform, and 1 in 85 of ether.

Extraction. Methoin is extracted by organic solvents from aqueous acid or alkaline solutions.

Colour Tests. Spot a drop of an aqueous solution of methoin on filter paper impregnated with a 10% aqueous solution of trisodium orthophosphate and locate with *mercurous nitrate spray*—black. *Liebermann's reagent*—orange.

Metabolism. Methoin is demethylated and excreted in the urine largely as phenylethylhydantoin but this may be further metabolised by hydroxylation and ring fission.

Dose. Usually up to 100 mg daily initially, increasing as necessary up to 600 mg daily. It may be administered in conjunction with phenobarbitone.

Toxicity. Methoin gives rise to toxic symptoms more frequently than phenytoin sodium. Cases of pancytopenia, agranulocytosis, and aplastic anaemia have been reported. The minimum estimated lethal dose is 5 g.

CASE EXAMPLES. A 10-year-old girl died as a result of fulminating dermatitis after being treated with methoin 300 mg daily for 12 days (Ruskin, 1948).

A fatal case of acute aplastic anaemia during the treatment of epilepsy (England and McEachern, 1949).

A patient died after taking methoin 100 mg with phenobarbitone daily for 6 months (Weller and Metcalfe, 1949).

METHOSERPIDINE *Antihypertensive*

Synonym: 10-Methoxydeserpidine.

Proprietary Name: Decaserpyl.

Methyl 11-demethoxy-10-methoxy-18-(3,4,5-trimethoxybenzoyl)reserpate

$C_{33}H_{40}N_2O_9 = 608{\cdot}7$

A white microcrystalline powder. M.p. about 171°, with decomposition. Specific rotation of a 1% solution in dioxan, −144° to −154°.

Solubility. Very slightly soluble in water; soluble 1 in 60 of ethanol and 1 in 5 of chloroform.

Extraction. Methoserpidine is extracted by organic solvents from aqueous alkaline solutions.

Chromatography. PAPER: system P1—Rf 0·73 (location under ultraviolet light, white fluorescence; location reagents: *iodoplatinate spray*, weak reaction; *bromocresol green spray*, weak reaction; *potassium permanganate spray*, weak reaction).

THIN-LAYER: system T1—Rf 0·77 (location reagent *acidified iodoplatinate spray*, positive reaction).

Colour Tests. MICRO: sulphuric acid–formaldehyde test—grey (*sensitivity:* 0·25 µg); ammonium molybdate test—blue-green (*sensitivity:* 0·25 µg); ammonium vanadate test—grey-purple (*sensitivity:* 1·0 µg); Vitali's test—brown/yellow/purple-brown (*sensitivity:* 0·25 µg).

Crystal Tests. MICRO: *platinic chloride solution*—small irregular needles (*sensitivity:* 1 in 400); *potassium iodide solution*—small branching needles (*sensitivity*: 1 in 200).

Ultraviolet Absorption Spectrum. Methoserpidine in ethanol, maxima at 273 mµ (E1%, 1 cm 640) and 295 mµ (E1%, 1 cm 400).

Dose. Usually 30 mg daily, initially, adjusted as necessary; max. in 24 hours 60 mg.

Toxicity. LD50 (intraperitoneal): in mice 2 g/kg.

METHOTRIMEPRAZINE *Tranquilliser*

Synonyms: Levomepromazine; RP 7044; SKF 5116.
Proprietary Name: Levoprome.

(−) - 10 - (3 - Dimethylamino - 2 - methylpropyl)-2-methoxyphenothiazine
$C_{19}H_{24}N_2OS$ = 328·5

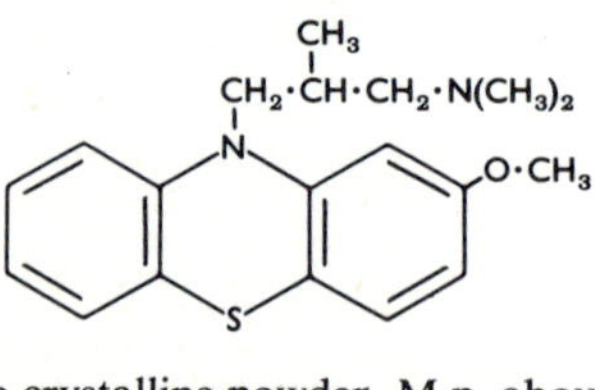

A white crystalline powder. M.p. about 125·5°. Specific rotation of a 5% solution in chloroform, −17°.

Solubility. Very slightly soluble in water; freely soluble in ethanol, ether, and chloroform.

METHOTRIMEPRAZINE HYDROCHLORIDE
Proprietary Name: Veractil (injection).
Solubility. Very soluble in water and ethanol.

METHOTRIMEPRAZINE MALEATE
Synonym: Methotrimeprazine Acid Maleate.
Proprietary Names: Neuractil; Neurocil; Nozinan; Veractil (tablets).

A fine white powder. M.p. 190°.
Solubility. Slightly soluble in water and ethanol.

Screening Test. *FPN reagent* with urine—blue-violet (see p. 10).

Extraction. Methotrimeprazine is extracted by organic solvents from aqueous alkaline solutions; hydrolysis of biological material is required in order to improve the yield.

Chromatography. PAPER: system P1—Rf 0·65 (location under ultraviolet light, blue fluorescence; location reagents: *iodoplatinate spray*, weak reaction; *FPN spray*, blue); system RP1a—Rf 0·13 (location under ultraviolet light, blue fluorescence; location reagent *iodoplatinate spray*, positive reaction); system RP1b—Rf 0·04 (location as for RP1a).

THIN-LAYER: system T1—Rf 0·28 (location reagent *acidified iodoplatinate spray*, positive reaction).

GAS: system G2/225—retention time 1·56 relative to codeine; system G4—retention time 1·10 relative to codeine.

Colour Tests. MICRO: sulphuric acid–formaldehyde test—blue-purple (*sensitivity:* 0·1 µg); ammonium molybdate test—blue-purple (*sensitivity:* 0·1 µg); ammonium vanadate test—blue-purple (*sensitivity:* 0·1 µg); Vitali's test—purple → yellow/brown/yellow (*sensitivity:* 0·5 µg).

Ultraviolet Absorption Spectrum. Methotrimeprazine in ethanol, maxima at 255 mµ (E1%, 1 cm 822) and 310 mµ (E1%, 1 cm 162); in 0·1N hydrochloric acid, maxima at 251·5 mµ (E1%, 1 cm 987) and 302 mµ (E1%, 1 cm 176).

Infra-red Absorption Spectrum. Methotrimeprazine (base). Potassium bromide disk. The principal peaks are: A 1460, B 1446 or 1587, C 1269 (p. 791).

Quantitative Estimation. Allgén *et al.* (1963) have described methods for the determination of methotrimeprazine in serum and urine; Afifi and Way (1967) have described a method of estimating methotrimeprazine in the brain.

Metabolism. Following the administration of methotrimeprazine in doses of 100 to 450 mg daily, about 1% of the daily dose appeared in the urine as unchanged drug and about 10% as the sulphoxide metabolite. Glucuronide conjugates also appeared in the urine. About 14% of the daily dose appeared unchanged in the faeces (Allgén *et al.*, 1963). See also *J. Am. med. Ass.*, 1968, **204**, 159.

Dose. For ambulatory patients, up to 50 mg daily, initially; for patients in bed, up to 200 mg daily, initially.

Toxicity. The acute lethal dose in man of the phenothiazine derivatives appears to be in the range 15 to 150 mg/kg, although severe toxic symptoms have occurred with doses of less than 1 mg/kg.

CASE EXAMPLE. A 54-year-old woman died by falling from a sixth-floor window whilst under the influence of drugs. At post-mortem examination the following levels of methotrimeprazine were found: liver, 0·1 mg%; contents of small intestine, 1·5 mg%; stomach contents, 0·9 mg% (Heyndrickx *et al.*, 1965).

METHOXAMINE *Sympathomimetic*

2-Amino-1-(2,5-dimethoxyphenyl)propan-1-ol

$C_{11}H_{17}NO_3 = 211{\cdot}3$

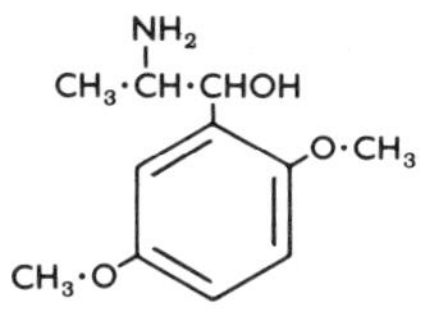

METHOXAMINE HYDROCHLORIDE

Proprietary Names: Pressomin; Vasoxine; Vasoxyl; Vasylox.

A white crystalline powder. M.p. 212° to 216°.

Solubility. Soluble 1 in 2·5 of water and 1 in 12 of ethanol; very slightly soluble in ether and chloroform.

Extraction. Methoxamine is extracted by organic solvents from aqueous alkaline solutions.

Chromatography. PAPER: system P1—Rf 0·43 (location under ultraviolet light, absorption; location reagents: *diazotised* p-*nitroaniline–sodium hydroxide spray*, purple; *ninhydrin spray*, purple).

THIN-LAYER: system T1—Rf 0·55 (location reagent *potassium permanganate spray*, positive reaction).

GAS: system G2/225—retention time 0·7 relative to diphenhydramine.

Colour Tests. MICRO: sulphuric acid–formaldehyde test—purple-brown → green (*sensitivity:* 0·5 μg); ammonium molybdate test—green (*sensitivity:* 0·1 μg); ammonium vanadate test—greenish-yellow (*sensitivity:* 0·5 μg); Vitali's test—yellow/yellow/olive (*sensitivity:* 0·5 μg).

Crystal Test. MICRO: *picrolonic acid*—dendrites (*sensitivity:* 1 in 400).

Ultraviolet Absorption Spectrum. Methoxamine hydrochloride in water, maximum at 290 mμ (E1%, 1 cm 156); minimum at 251 mμ.

Infra-red Absorption Spectrum. Methoxamine (base). Potassium bromide disk. The principal peaks are: A 1496, B 1215, C 1044 (p. 791).

Dose. Usually up to 20 mg intramuscularly. A solution containing 0·25% is used as nasal drops or as a nasal spray.

Toxicity. LD50 (oral): in mice 234 mg/kg.

METHOXYAMPHETAMINE *Hallucinogen*

Synonyms: *p*-Methoxyamphetamine; PMA.

α-Methyl-*p*-methoxyphenethylamine

$C_{10}H_{15}NO = 165{\cdot}2$

Colourless oil.

Solubility. Insoluble in water; soluble in chloroform and dilute acids.

METHOXYAMPHETAMINE HYDROCHLORIDE

White crystals.

Solubility. Soluble in water.

Extraction. Methoxyamphetamine is extracted by organic solvents from aqueous ammoniacal solutions.

Chromatography. PAPER: system P1—Rf 0·50 (location under ultraviolet light, absorption; location reagents: *bromocresol green spray*, strong reaction; *ninhydrin spray*, dull purple).

THIN-LAYER: system T1—Rf 0·40 (location reagent *acidified iodoplatinate spray*, positive reaction).

Colour Tests. MICRO: ammonium molybdate test—blue; ammonium vanadate test—green.

Crystal Tests. MICRO: *platinic chloride solution*—irregular rosettes; *platinic iodide solution*—bunches of irregular plates.

NOTE. Behavioural studies in rats involving the trimethoxy-, dimethoxy-, and monomethoxyamphetamines, lysergide, and mescaline showed *p*-methoxyamphetamine to be the most potent hallucinogen tested, with the exception of lysergide. The severe and prolonged disruption of behaviour produced by *p*-methoxyamphetamine suggests that it might cause an irreversible inhibition of an enzyme, possibly catechol *o*-methyl transferase (Smythies *et al.*, 1967).

METHOXYCHLOR *Pesticide*

Synonyms: DMDT; Dimethoxy-DT; Methoxy-DDT.

Proprietary Name: Marlate.

1,1,1-Trichloro-2,2-di-(4-methoxyphenyl)-ethane

$C_{16}H_{15}Cl_3O_2 = 345{\cdot}7$

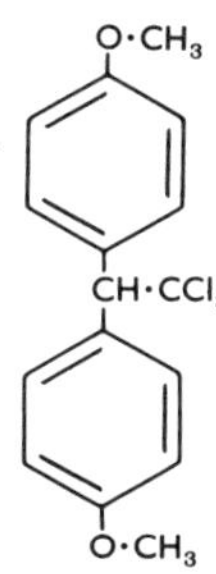

Colourless crystals. M.p. about 89°.

Solubility. Insoluble in water; soluble in ethanol and aromatic solvents; very soluble in ether.

Extraction. Methoxychlor is extracted by organic solvents from aqueous acid or alkaline solutions.

Ultraviolet Absorption Spectrum. Methoxychlor in ethanol, maximum at 228 mμ (E1%, 1 cm 480).

Metabolism. Methoxychlor is eliminated very rapidly in the faeces; only small amounts appear in the urine. At least 3 metabolites have been detected. Methoxychlor is stored in the fat to a very limited extent and disappears in 2 to 4 weeks after cessation of exposure.

Toxicity. Methoxychlor is the least toxic of the chlorinated hydrocarbon insecticides. The

maximum permissible atmospheric concentration is 14 p.p.m.
LD50 (oral): in rats 5 to 7 g/kg.

METHOXYPHENAMINE *Sympathomimetic*

Synonyms: Methoxiphenadrin; Mexyphamine.

o-Methoxy-*N*α-dimethylphenethylamine

$C_{11}H_{17}NO = 179{\cdot}3$

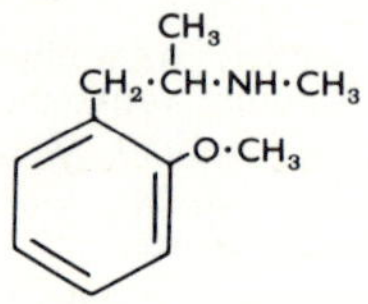

METHOXYPHENAMINE HYDROCHLORIDE
Proprietary Names: Orthoxine. It is an ingredient of Orthoxicol.

A white crystalline powder. M.p. 124° to 128°.
Solubility. Soluble in water, ethanol, and chloroform; slightly soluble in ether.

Extraction. Methoxyphenamine is extracted by organic solvents from aqueous alkaline solutions.

Chromatography. PAPER: system P1—Rf 0·58 (location under ultraviolet light, absorption; location reagents: *iodoplatinate spray*, weak reaction; *bromocresol green spray*, weak reaction).

THIN-LAYER: system T1—Rf 0·24 (location reagent *acidified iodoplatinate spray*, positive reaction).

GAS: system G2/120—retention time 0·91 relative to ephedrine.

Colour Tests. MICRO: sulphuric acid–formaldehyde test—red (*sensitivity:* 0·25 μg); ammonium molybdate test—green (*sensitivity:* 0·25 μg); ammonium vanadate test—blue-green (*sensitivity:* 0·25 μg).

Crystal Tests. MICRO: *platinic chloride solution*—rhomboids (*sensitivity:* 1 in 400); *platinic iodide solution*—rods or long plates (*sensitivity:* 1 in 1000).

Dose. Up to 600 mg daily; single doses of up to 200 mg have been given.

METHOXYPROMAZINE *Tranquilliser*

Synonyms: Methopromazine; RP 4632.

10 - (3 - Dimethylaminopropyl) - 2 - methoxyphenothiazine

$C_{18}H_{22}N_2OS = 314{\cdot}5$

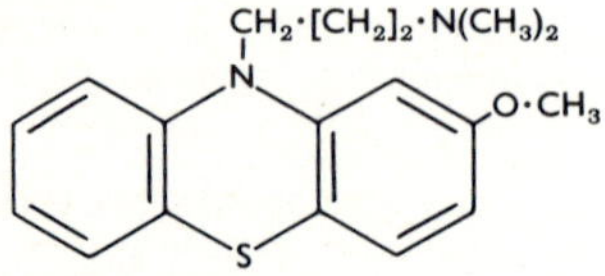

METHOXYPROMAZINE MALEATE
Proprietary Name: Tentone.

A crystalline powder.
Solubility. Soluble 1 in 330 of water; very slightly soluble in ethanol; insoluble in ether; soluble in chloroform.

Extraction. Methoxypromazine is extracted by organic solvents from aqueous alkaline solutions; hydrolysis of biological material is required in order to improve the yield.

Chromatography. PAPER: system P1—Rf 0·62 (location under ultraviolet light, blue fluorescence; location reagents: *iodoplatinate spray*, strong reaction; *bromocresol green spray*, weak reaction).

THIN-LAYER: system T1—Rf 0·39 (location reagent *acidified iodoplatinate spray*, positive reaction); system T3—Rf 0·74 (location reagent *iodoplatinate spray*, positive reaction); system T4—Rf 0·58 (location as for T3); system T6—Rf 0·67 (the spot may be converted on the plate to the sulphoxide, Rf 0·35; location of both spots under ultraviolet light).

Colour Tests. MICRO: sulphuric acid–formaldehyde test—purple (*sensitivity:* 0·1 μg); ammonium molybdate test—purple (*sensitivity:* 0·1 μg); ammonium vanadate test—purple (*sensitivity:* 0·5 μg); Vitali's test—purple flash → brown/brown/yellow (*sensitivity:* 0·1 μg).

Crystal Test. MICRO: *platinic chloride solution*—dense rosettes (*sensitivity:* 1 in 1000).

Ultraviolet Absorption Spectrum. Methoxypromazine in 0·1N sulphuric acid, maxima at 250 mμ (E1%, 1 cm 571), 278 mμ (E1%, 1 cm 64), and 303 mμ (E1%, 1 cm 95).

Infra-red Absorption Spectrum. Methoxypromazine maleate. Potassium bromide disk. The principal peaks are: A 1470, B 1356, C 748 or 1152 or 1582 (p. 745).

Dose. Up to 500 mg daily.

Toxicity. The acute lethal dose in man of the phenothiazine derivatives appears to be in the range 15 to 150 mg/kg, although severe toxic symptoms have occurred with doses of less than 1 mg/kg.

METHSUXIMIDE *Anticonvulsant*

Synonyms: Mesuximide; PM 396.
Proprietary Name: Celontin.

*N*α-Dimethyl-α-phenylsuccinimide

$C_{12}H_{13}NO_2 = 203{\cdot}2$

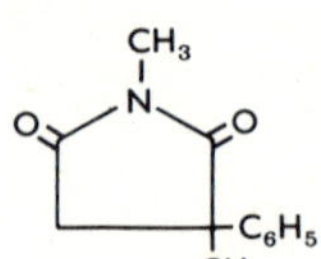

A white to greyish-white crystalline powder. M.p. 50° to 56°.
Solubility. Slightly soluble in hot water; freely soluble in ethanol and ether; very soluble in chloroform.

Extraction. Methsuximide is extracted by organic solvents from aqueous acid or alkaline solutions.

Chromatography. PAPER: system P1—Rf 0·94 (location under ultraviolet light, absorption; location reagent *iodine vapour*, positive reaction).

THIN-LAYER: system T1—Rf 0·76 (location reagent *iodine–carbon tetrachloride spray*, positive reaction).

Ultraviolet Absorption Spectrum. Methsuximide in 0·1N sulphuric acid, maximum at 256 mμ (E1%, 1 cm 18), and an inflexion at about 263 mμ (E1%, 1 cm 10).

Infra-red Absorption Spectrum. Potassium bromide disk. The principal peaks are: A 1705, B 1435, C 1282 (p. 791).

Dose. Up to 1·2 g daily.

Toxicity. The estimated lethal dose in man is 5 g.

METHYCLOTHIAZIDE *Diuretic*

Synonym: Methyclothizide.
Proprietary Names: Duretic; Enduron.

6 - Chloro - 3 - chloromethyl - 3,4 - dihydro - 2 - methyl - 7 - sulphamoyl - 2*H* - benzo - 1,2,4 - thiadiazine 1,1-dioxide

$C_9H_{11}Cl_2N_3O_4S_2$ = 360·2

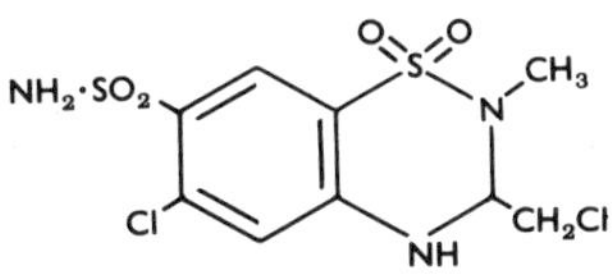

A colourless crystalline solid. M.p. 216°.

Solubility. Soluble in water and in solutions of alkali hydroxides and carbonates.

Extraction. Methyclothiazide may be isolated in the A2 fraction (see p. 27). It may be distinguished from the barbiturates by chromatography (see below), and by the presence of additional ultraviolet maxima in the region 270 to 330 mμ.

Chromatography. PAPER: system P16—Rf 0·73 (location under ultraviolet light, absorption; location reagent *sodium naphthaquinone spray*, strong reaction); system RP1b—Rf 0·20 (location as for P16).

Ultraviolet Absorption Spectrum. Methyclothiazide in distilled water made alkaline to pH 10 with 2N ammonium hydroxide, maxima at 264 mμ (E1%, 1 cm 420) and 318 mμ (E1%, 1 cm 60); in distilled water made acid to pH 2 with *sulphuric acid*, maxima at 270 mμ (E1%, 1 cm 525) and 315 mμ (E1%, 1 cm 120). These spectra may be confused with those of polythiazide.

Infra-red Absorption Spectrum. Potassium bromide disk. The principal peaks are: A 1158, B 1595, C 1320 (p. 745).

Metabolism. Methyclothiazide is completely absorbed after oral administration. The diuretic action is maintained for more than 5 hours but for less than 24 hours.

Dose. Up to 10 mg daily.

Toxicity. LD50 (intraperitoneal): in mice 870 mg/kg.

METHYL NICOTINATE *Vasodilator*

Methyl pyridine-3-carboxylate

$C_7H_7NO_2$ = 137·1

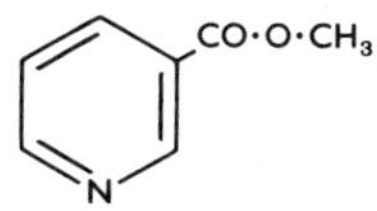

White to straw-coloured crystals which darken to a reddish colour on keeping. M.p. 39°.

Solubility. Soluble in water and ethanol.

Extraction. Methyl nicotinate is extracted by organic solvents from aqueous alkaline solutions.

Infra-red Absorption Spectrum. Potassium bromide disk. The principal peaks are: A 1284 or 1720, B 737 or 1110 (p. 745).

Use. Methyl nicotinate in concentrations of up to 5% is used in ointments and creams for topical application as a rubefacient.

METHYL PHENIDATE *Central Stimulant*

Synonym: Methylphenidylacetate.

Methyl α-phenyl-α-piperid-2-ylacetate

$C_{14}H_{19}NO_2$ = 233·3

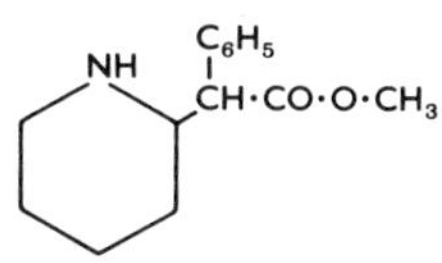

It occurs as crystals which melt at 74° to 75°.

Solubility. Insoluble in water; soluble in ethanol and ether.

METHYL PHENIDATE HYDROCHLORIDE

Proprietary Name: Ritalin.

A fine white crystalline powder.

Solubility. Freely soluble in water; soluble in ethanol; slightly soluble in chloroform.

Extraction. Methyl phenidate is extracted by organic solvents from aqueous alkaline solutions.

Chromatography. PAPER: system P1—Rf 0·63 (location reagents: *iodoplatinate spray*, strong reaction; *bromocresol green spray*, strong reaction; *ninhydrin spray*, purple).

THIN-LAYER: system T1—Rf 0·60 (location reagents: *acidified iodoplatinate spray*, positive reaction; *potassium permanganate spray*, positive reaction).

GAS: system G2/120—retention time 5·5 relative to ephedrine; system G2/225—retention time 2·2 (1·9) relative to diphenhydramine.

Crystal Tests. MICRO: *lead iodide solution*—dense rosettes or rosettes of needles (*sensitivity:* 1 in 400); *picric acid*—bunches of plates or needles (*sensitivity:* 1 in 400).

Ultraviolet Absorption Spectrum. Methyl phenidate in 0·1N sulphuric acid, maxima at 246·5 mμ (E1%, 1 cm 5), 251 mμ (E1%, 1 cm 6), 257 mμ (E1%, 1 cm 8), and 263 mμ (E1%, 1 cm 6).

Infra-red Absorption Spectrum. Methyl phenidate (base). Potassium bromide disk. The principal peaks are: A 1728, B 1165 or 1431, C 1140 or 1200 (p. 746).

Toxicity. Methyl phenidate has actions similar to those of amphetamine but its toxic effects are less pronounced and occur less frequently.

Dose. Usually 30 mg daily.

CASE EXAMPLE. A 42-year-old woman took 1·2 g of methyl phenidate hydrochloride daily for 6 months with no untoward effects, signs of addiction, or alteration in blood count and blood chemistry (Pollack, 1964).

METHYL SALICYLATE *Analgesic*

Synonyms: Betula Oil; Gaultheria Oil; Sweet Birch Oil; Teaberry Oil; Wintergreen Oil.

Methyl *o*-hydroxybenzoate

$C_8H_8O_3$ = 152·2

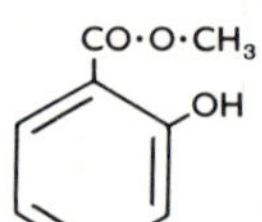

A colourless or pale yellow oily liquid. M.p. −8·6°. B.p. 219° to 224°, with some decomposition. Refractive index at 20°, 1·536 to 1·538.

Solubility. Slightly soluble in water; miscible with ethanol; soluble in ether and chloroform.

Screening Test. *Ferric chloride solution* with urine—blue-violet, after hydrolysis (see p. 8).

Extraction. Methyl salicylate is extracted by organic solvents from aqueous acid or alkaline solutions.

Ultraviolet Absorption Spectrum. Methyl salicylate in ethanol, maxima at 238 mμ (E1%, 1 cm about 570) and 306 mμ (E1%, 1 cm about 280).

Quantitative Estimation. Methyl salicylate may be estimated as salicylic acid by the spectrophotometric methods of Trinder (1954) or Stevenson (1960)—see under Salicylic Acid, p. 593.

Metabolism. Methyl salicylate is found to be completely hydrolysed shortly after oral administration to rats and dogs but in man hydrolysis is not complete. The major site of hydrolysis in animals is the liver, although the intestines, spleen, kidneys, and pancreas may play a minor role in such breakdown. In man, the small proportion of unhydrolysed ester may have a more toxic action than that of salicylic acid (Davison *et al.*, 1961).

Use. Methyl salicylate has the actions of the salicylates but is seldom given by mouth. It is readily absorbed through the skin and is applied in liniments and ointments as an analgesic.

Toxicity. 30 ml is usually fatal but deaths have occurred in children after as little as 4 ml.

LD50 (oral): in rats 1·25 g/kg.

CASE EXAMPLE. A 20-month-old child swallowed about 5 ml of wintergreen oil. On admission to hospital 22 hours later the blood salicylate level was 72·7 mg%. Recovery followed an exchange blood transfusion which reduced the salicylate level by 59% (Adams *et al.*, 1957).

METHYLAMINOHEPTANE *Sympathomimetic*

N,1-Dimethylhexylamine

$C_8H_{19}N$ = 129·2

$$CH_3{\cdot}[CH_2]_4{\cdot}\underset{}{\overset{\displaystyle CH_3 \atop |}{C}}H{\cdot}NH{\cdot}CH_3$$

An oily liquid. B.p. 155°.

Solubility. Slightly soluble in water.

METHYLAMINOHEPTANE HYDROCHLORIDE

Proprietary Name: Oenethyl.

A crystalline solid.

Solubility. Readily soluble in water.

Extraction. Methylaminoheptane is extracted by organic solvents from aqueous alkaline solutions.

Chromatography. PAPER: system P1—Rf 0·58 (location reagent *bromocresol green spray*, weak reaction).

Crystal Tests. MICRO: *gold bromide solution*—leaflike plates (*sensitivity:* 1 in 100); *platinic iodide solution*—plates, some hexagonal (*sensitivity:* 1 in 200).

Dose. Usually up to 100 mg intramuscularly.

Toxicity. LD50 (oral): in rats 538 mg/kg.

METHYLAMPHETAMINE *Central Stimulant*

Synonyms: *d*-Deoxyephedrine; Desoxyephedrine; Methamphetamine; Phenylmethylaminopropane.

(+)-*N*α-Dimethylphenethylamine

$C_{10}H_{15}N$ = 149·2

$$C_6H_5{\cdot}CH_2{\cdot}\overset{\displaystyle CH_3 \atop |}{C}H{\cdot}NH{\cdot}CH_3$$

NOTE. Methylamphetamine is an isomer of phentermine (p. 491).

A colourless mobile liquid. B.p. about 214°.
Solubility. Slightly soluble in water; miscible with ethanol, ether, and chloroform.

METHYLAMPHETAMINE HYDROCHLORIDE
Proprietary Names: Amphedroxyn; Desoxyn; Dexoval; Doxyfed; Isophen; Metamsustac; Methedrine; Pervitin.

A white crystalline powder. M.p. 172° to 174°. Specific rotation of a 5% aqueous solution, +16° to +18°.
Solubility. Soluble 1 in 2 of water, 1 in 4 of ethanol, and 1 in 5 of chloroform; almost insoluble in ether.

Extraction. Methylamphetamine is extracted by organic solvents from aqueous alkaline solutions; it is volatile and may be isolated by distillation (see p. 18).

Chromatography. PAPER: system P1—Rf 0·56 (location under ultraviolet light, absorption; location reagents: *iodoplatinate spray*, strong reaction; *bromocresol green spray*, strong reaction; *Marquis reagent*, orange; *ninhydrin spray*, purple).
THIN-LAYER: system T1—Rf 0·28 (location reagents: *acidified iodoplatinate spray*, positive reaction; *Marquis reagent*, positive reaction; *potassium permanganate spray*, positive reaction).
GAS: system G2/120—retention time 0·4 relative to ephedrine.

Colour Test. MICRO: sulphuric acid–formaldehyde test—orange (*sensitivity:* 0·5 μg).

Crystal Tests. MICRO: *platinic iodide solution*—blades, some serrated (*sensitivity:* 1 in 400); *potassium bismuth iodide solution*—elongated plates, forming overnight (*sensitivity:* 1 in 200).

Ultraviolet Absorption Spectrum. Methylamphetamine in 0·1N sulphuric acid, maxima at 251·5 mμ (E1%, 1cm 8), 257 mμ (E1%, 1cm 10), and 263 mμ (E1%, 1cm 8), and an inflexion at 266 mμ; methylamphetamine hydrochloride in water, maxima at 251 mμ (E1%, 1cm 8), 257 mμ (E1%, 1cm 10), 263 mμ (E1%, 1cm 8); minima at 226·5 mμ, 254 mμ, and 261 mμ.

Infra-red Absorption Spectrum. Methylamphetamine hydrochloride. Potassium bromide disk. The principal peaks are: A 747, B 698, C 1475 (p. 746).

Metabolism. The excretion of methylamphetamine is found to be significantly influenced by changes in the urinary pH. Under normal conditions most of the methylamphetamine is excreted unchanged, only a small amount of *N*-demethylation occurring. Subjective effects are more prolonged under alkaline urine conditions, indicating resorption and longer retention of the drug in the body. Under acid urine conditions there is a 40-fold increase in the 16-hour excretion of unchanged methylamphetamine over that found under alkaline urine conditions. In these circumstances excretion of unchanged drug is the major route of elimination of methylamphetamine from the body (Beckett and Rowland, 1965).

Dose. Usually up to 15 mg daily by mouth; up to 30 mg intravenously.

Toxicity. The estimated minimum lethal dose in children is 100 mg; in adults at least 1 g.

CASE EXAMPLES. A 1-year-old girl swallowed an unknown quantity of methylamphetamine and phenobarbitone. Prompt peritoneal dialysis removed 66·6 mg of methylamphetamine and 140 mg of phenobarbitone from her circulation and she recovered without complications (Wallace *et al.*, 1964a).
A 22-year-old man died following ingestion of 140 mg of methylamphetamine. Toxic effects included acute renal failure, hyperpyrexia, jaundice, and vascular collapse. Peritoneal dialysis was effective in removing the drug from the body (Zalis and Parmley, 1963).

METHYLCHLOROPHENOXYACETIC ACID *Herbicide*

Synonyms: MCPA; Mephanac.
Proprietary Names: Agritox; Agroxone; Ardox M; Empal; Farmon A; Phenoxylene Plus; Shell M25; Vigon-P. It is an ingredient of Verdone.

4-Chloro-2-methylphenoxyacetic acid
$C_9H_9ClO_3 = 200{\cdot}6$

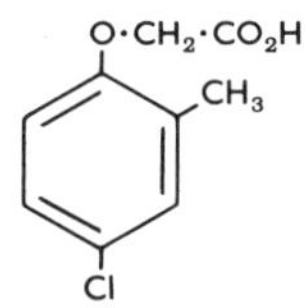

Methylchlorophenoxyacetic acid, as commercially available, melts at 99° to 107°; the pure compound melts at 118° to 119°.
Solubility. Slightly soluble in water; soluble 1 in 160 of ethanol and 1 in 80 of ether.

Extraction. Methylchlorophenoxyacetic acid is extracted by organic solvents from aqueous acid solutions.

Ultraviolet Absorption Spectrum. Methylchlorophenoxyacetic acid in ethanol, maxima at 279 mμ (E1%, 1cm 90) and 286 mμ (E1%, 1 cm 76).

Quantitative Estimation. Johnson and Koumides (1965) have described a method of estimation of methylchlorophenoxyacetic acid from biological fluids and tissues involving column chromatographic purification of the extract and subsequent spectrophotometric determination.

Toxicity. The chronic toxicity of methylchlorophenoxyacetic acid is low for farm animals but it is best to keep them away from sprayed areas for 2 weeks.
LD50 (oral): in rats about 700 mg/kg.

CASE EXAMPLES. An Indian, aged 32, with a long history of pulmonary tuberculosis, was found comatose and in epileptiform fits an hour after swallowing about 85 ml of Verdone (a 25% aqueous solution of methylchlorophenoxyacetic acid as the potassium salt) which is stated to be equivalent to a dose of about 440 mg/kg. He died some 20 hours later. Analysis showed methylchlorophenoxyacetic acid in the following amounts: brain,

0·038 g; gastric washings, 0·3 g; heart, 0·037 g; liver, 0·158 g; stomach, 0·041 g. The blood contained 23 mg% (Popham and Davies, 1964).

A 65-year-old man died 20½ hours after being found unconscious. He had taken, in a fit of depression, probably 57 ml of Verdone (a 25% aqueous solution of methylchlorophenoxyacetic acid as the potassium salt) which is stated to be equivalent to a dose of about 250 mg/kg, and also about 20 compound codeine tablets (equivalent to 5 g of aspirin, 5 g of phenacetin, and 0·16 g of codeine phosphate). The following post-mortem methylchlorophenoxyacetic-acid levels were found: blood, 18 mg%; stomach contents, 17 mg%; stomach washings, 250 mg%; urine, 80 mg%. Salicylate analysis showed: blood, 13 mg%; stomach contents, 17 mg%; stomach washings, 8 mg%; urine, 38 mg%. Tests for barbiturates and codeine proved negative. Despite the patient's severe respiratory disease, there was no doubt that death was due to methylchlorophenoxyacetic-acid poisoning. A dose of 250 mg/kg which proved fatal casts doubt on the previously accepted belief that methylchlorophenoxyacetic acid is of low toxicity (Johnson and Koumides, 1965).

METHYLDESORPHINE *Narcotic*

Synonym: MK 57.

6,7 - Dehydro - 4,5 - epoxy - 3 - hydroxy - *N*,6 - dimethylmorphinan

$C_{18}H_{20}NO_2$ = 282·4

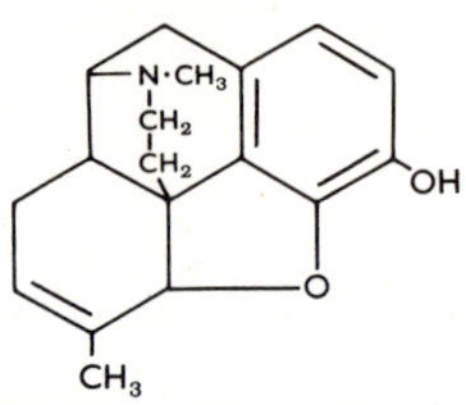

Extraction. Methyldesorphine is extracted by organic solvents from aqueous ammoniacal solutions; hydrolysis of biological material is required in order to improve the yield.

Chromatography. PAPER: system P1—Rf 0·44 (location reagent *iodoplatinate spray*, strong reaction).

THIN-LAYER: system T1—Rf 0·35 (location reagent *acidified iodoplatinate spray*, positive reaction).

GAS: system G2/225—retention time 0·81 relative to codeine.

Colour Tests. MICRO: sulphuric acid–formaldehyde test—dull purple (*sensitivity:* 0·1 μg); ammonium molybdate test—black-purple → greenish-brown (*sensitivity:* 0·1 μg); ammonium vanadate test—brown (*sensitivity:* 0·25 μg); Vitali's test—yellow/yellow/orange (*sensitivity:* 0·25 μg).

Crystal Tests. MICRO: *potassium bismuth iodide solution*—small blades (*sensitivity:* 1 in 1000); *sodium phosphate solution*—long needles (*sensitivity:* 1 in 1000).

Ultraviolet Absorption Spectrum. Methyldesorphine in 0·1N sulphuric acid, inflexion at about 278 mμ (E1%, 1cm 40) and maximum at 283 mμ (E1%, 1cm 42).

METHYLDIHYDROMORPHINE *Narcotic*

Synonym: Methydromorphine.

4,5 - Epoxy - 3,6 - dihydroxy - *N*,6 - dimethylmorphinan

$C_{18}H_{23}NO_3$ = 301·4

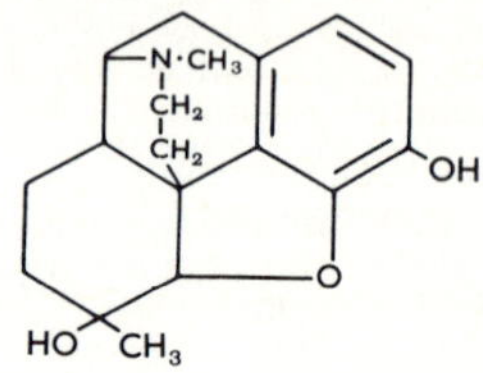

Extraction. Methyldihydromorphine is extracted by organic solvents from aqueous ammoniacal solutions; hydrolysis of biological material is required in order to improve the yield.

Chromatography. PAPER: system P1—Rf 0·25 (location under ultraviolet light, absorption; location reagents: *iodoplatinate spray*, weak reaction; *bromocresol green spray*, weak reaction).

THIN-LAYER: system T1—Rf 0·28 (location reagent *acidified iodoplatinate spray*, positive reaction).

GAS: system G2/225—retention time 1·0 relative to codeine.

Colour Tests. MICRO: sulphuric acid–formaldehyde test—purple (*sensitivity:* 0·1 μg); ammonium molybdate test—violet-blue → green (*sensitivity:* 0·1 μg); ammonium vanadate test—grey-purple → brown (*sensitivity:* 0·5 μg); Vitali's test—yellow/yellow/orange (*sensitivity:* 1·0 μg).

Crystal Tests. MICRO: *potassium cadmium iodide solution*—plates, some serrated (*sensitivity:* 1 in 400); *potassium mercuric iodide solution*—feathery rosettes (*sensitivity:* 1 in 1000).

METHYLDOPA *Antihypertensive*

Synonyms: Alpha-methyldopa; MK 351.

Proprietary Names: Aldomet (tablets); Hyperpax; Presinol; Sembrina; it is an ingredient of Hydromet.

(−) - α - Amino - β - (3,4 - dihydroxyphenyl) - α - methylpropionic acid sesquihydrate

$C_{10}H_{13}NO_4,1\frac{1}{2}H_2O$ = 238·2

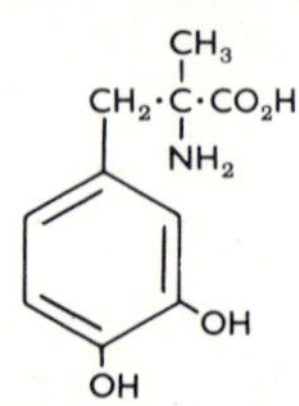

A fine white powder. M.p. 290°. Specific rotation of a 4·4% solution in *aluminium chloride solution*, −25° to −28°.

Solubility. Soluble 1 in 100 of water and 1 in 400 of ethanol; almost insoluble in ether; soluble 1 in 0·5 of dilute hydrochloric acid.

Chromatography. PAPER: system P1—Rf 0·07 (location under ultraviolet light, absorption; location reagent *ninhydrin spray*, purple).
THIN-LAYER: system T1—Rf 0·26, streaking (location reagent *potassium permanganate spray*, positive reaction).

Colour Tests. MICRO: sulphuric acid–formaldehyde test—yellow → dull purple (*sensitivity:* 0·25 μg); ammonium molybdate test—(dull orange) dull purple → grey-blue → yellow-green (*sensitivity:* 0·25 μg); ammonium vanadate test—(dull green) orange (*sensitivity:* 0·25 μg); Vitali's test—yellow/olive/olive (*sensitivity:* 0·25 μg).

Crystal Tests. MICRO: *gold chloride solution*—very small plates (*sensitivity:* 1 in 400); *mercuric chloride solution*—small crosses or rosettes, forming overnight (*sensitivity:* 1 in 200).

Ultraviolet Absorption Spectrum. Methyldopa in 0·1N sulphuric acid, maxima at about 220 mμ (E1%, 1 cm 300) and 279 mμ (E1%, 1 cm 138).

Infra-red Absorption Spectrum. Potassium bromide disk. The principal peaks are: A 1600, B 1288, C 1374 or 1402 (p. 791).

Metabolism. After oral administration, about 50% of an oral dose was absorbed and peak plasma levels occurred in 3 to 6 hours. About 30% was present in the plasma as methyldopa mono-*O*-sulphate. From 80 to 90% of the dose was excreted in the urine in 48 hours, 24% as unchanged methyldopa, 64% as the mono-*O*-sulphate, 4% as 3-*O*-methyl-methyldopa, and 2 further fractions, one of which contained α-methyldopamine.
It is considered that methyldopa inhibits the conversion of dopa to dopamine by competing for the enzyme dopa decarboxylase and in consequence there is a reduction in the amount of noradrenaline formed from dopamine and released at sympathetic nerve endings. Methyldopa also inhibits the formation of serotonin.

Dose. Usually up to 3 g daily.

Toxicity. Abnormal results in liver function tests have been noted in some cases during early treatment but there is a return to normal on discontinuance of the drug. Methyldopa may occasionally cause urine to darken due to the presence of metabolites.
LD50 (oral): in mice 5·3 to 15 g/kg.

CASE EXAMPLES. Examination was made of the methyldopa levels in 2 cases of suspected overdosage; the serum contained 0·72 and 0·94 mg% respectively and the urine 12·6 and 12·9 mg%. A procedure for the estimation is described (Tompsett, 1967b).

METHYLDOPATE *Antihypertensive*

The ethyl ester of methyldopa

Ethyl (−)-α-amino-β-(3,4-dihydroxyphenyl)-α-methylpropionate
$C_{12}H_{17}NO_4 = 239{\cdot}3$

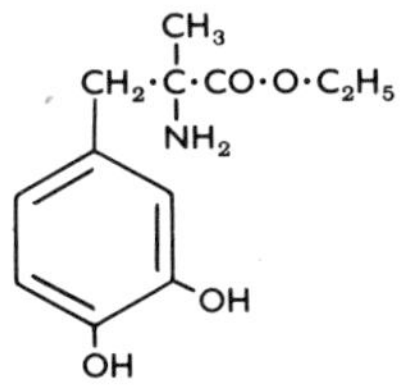

METHYLDOPATE HYDROCHLORIDE
Proprietary Name: Aldomet (injection).

Chromatography. PAPER: system P1—Rf 0·40 (location under ultraviolet light, absorption; location reagent *ninhydrin spray*, yellow).
THIN-LAYER: system T1—Rf 0·65 (location reagent *potassium permanganate spray*, positive reaction).

Colour Tests. MICRO: sulphuric acid–formaldehyde test—dull yellow → dull purple (*sensitivity:* 0·25 μg); ammonium molybdate test—(dull orange) dull purple → grey-blue → yellow-green (*sensitivity:* 0·25 μg); ammonium vanadate test—(dull green) orange (*sensitivity:* 0·25 μg); Vitali's test—yellow/olive/olive (*sensitivity:* 0·25 μg).

Crystal Tests. MICRO: *gold chloride solution*—very small plates, forming overnight (*sensitivity:* 1 in 400); *mercuric chloride solution*—small crosses or rosettes, forming overnight (*sensitivity:* 1 in 200).

Ultraviolet Absorption Spectrum. Methyldopate in 0·1N sulphuric acid, maxima at about 220 mμ (E1%, 1 cm 213) and 280 mμ (E1%, 1 cm 100).

Infra-red Absorption Spectrum. Methyldopate. Potassium bromide disk. The principal peaks are: A 1527, B 1726, C 1290 or 1516 (p. 791).

Dose. Usually up to 500 mg, intravenously, every 6 hours; maximum intravenous dose 1 g every 6 hours. Single doses of 3 g have been given.

METHYLEPHEDRINE *Sympathomimetic*

Synonym: *l*-*N*-Methylephedrine.

(−)-2-Dimethylamino-1-phenylpropan-1-ol
$C_{11}H_{17}NO = 179{\cdot}3$

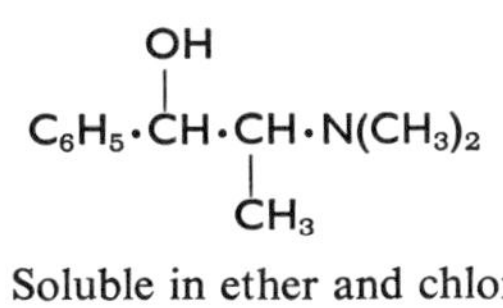

Solubility. Soluble in ether and chloroform.

METHYLEPHEDRINE HYDROCHLORIDE
Proprietary Name: Metheph.

A white crystalline powder.
Solubility. Soluble in water and ethanol; almost insoluble in ether.

Extraction. Methylephedrine is extracted by organic solvents from aqueous alkaline solutions.

Chromatography. PAPER: system P1—Rf 0·46 (location under ultraviolet light, absorption; location reagents: *iodoplatinate spray*, weak reaction; *bromocresol green spray*, strong reaction).

THIN-LAYER: system T1—Rf 0·32 (location reagent *acidified iodoplatinate spray*, positive reaction).

GAS: system G2/120—retention time 1·13 relative to ephedrine.

Colour Test. Chen's test—purple.

Crystal Tests. MICRO: *gold bromide–hydrochloric acid solution*—small plates, often serrated, best viewed under polarised light (*sensitivity:* 1 in 400); *gold chloride solution*—plates or coarse needles (*sensitivity:* 1 in 400).

Ultraviolet Absorption Spectrum. Methylephedrine in 0·1N sulphuric acid, maxima at 251 mμ (E1%, 1 cm 9), 257 mμ (E1%, 1 cm 11·3), and 263 mμ (E1%, 1 cm 9), and inflexions at about 247 mμ and about 266·5 mμ.

Infra-red Absorption Spectrum. Methylephedrine (base). Potassium bromide disk. The principal peaks are: A 702 or 742 or 1039, B 1447 (p. 791).

Quantitative Estimation. Beckett and Wilkinson (1965) describe a method of ether extraction from urine followed by gas chromatographic analysis.

Metabolism. Following the administration of a 10-mg dose of methylephedrine hydrochloride in man, 32% was excreted unchanged in the urine and 8% was excreted as the demethylated metabolite, ephedrine. The rate of excretion fluctuated with changes in the urinary pH. This is consistent with the concept of resorption of the non-ionised drug in the kidney tubules (Beckett and Wilkinson, 1965).

Dose. Up to 200 mg daily.

METHYLERGOMETRINE *Ergot Alkaloid*

Synonym: Methylergonovine.

(+)-*N*-[1-(Hydroxymethyl)propyl]lysergamide

$C_{20}H_{25}N_3O_2$ = 339·4

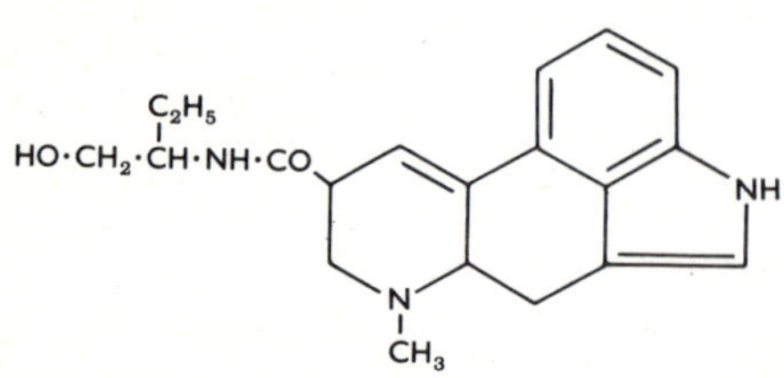

Methylergometrine occurs as crystals. M.p. 172°, with decomposition.

Solubility. Slightly soluble in water; very soluble in ethanol.

METHYLERGOMETRINE MALEATE

Proprietary Name: Methergin.

A white crystalline powder. M.p. 185° to 195°, with decomposition. Specific rotation of a 0·5% solution, +44° to +50°.

Solubility. Soluble 1 in 200 of water and 1 in 140 of ethanol; very slightly soluble in ether and chloroform.

Extraction. Methylergometrine is extracted by organic solvents from aqueous alkaline solutions.

Chromatography. PAPER: system P1—Rf 0·40 (location under ultraviolet light, bright blue fluorescence; location reagent p-*dimethylaminobenzaldehyde spray*, blue).

THIN-LAYER: system T1—Rf 0·70 (location reagent p-*dimethylaminobenzaldehyde spray*, blue); system T9—Rf 0·23 (location under ultraviolet light, absorption; location reagent p-*dimethylaminobenzaldehyde spray*, blue).

Colour Tests. MICRO: sulphuric acid–formaldehyde test—grey-brown (*sensitivity:* 0·25 μg); ammonium molybdate test—green → brown (*sensitivity:* 0·25 μg); ammonium vanadate test—purple-brown (*sensitivity:* 0·5 μg); Vitali's test—yellow-brown/dull orange/purple-brown (*sensitivity:* 0·1 μg).

Crystal Tests. MICRO: *picric acid*—rosettes or fans of needles (*sensitivity:* 1 in 200); *trinitrobenzoic acid solution*—feathery rosettes (*sensitivity:* 1 in 200).

Ultraviolet Absorption Spectrum. Methylergometrine in 0·1N sulphuric acid, maxima at 226 mμ (E1%, 1 cm 699) and 313 mμ (E1%, 1 cm 255).

Infra-red Absorption Spectrum. Methylergometrine maleate. Potassium bromide disk. The principal peaks are: A 1573, B 1643, C 1383 (p. 746).

Dose. Usually up to 0·5 mg by mouth; up to 0·2 mg by injection.

METHYLHEXANEAMINE *Sympathomimetic*

Synonym: Methylhexamine.

Proprietary Name: Forthane.

1,3-Dimethylpentylamine

$C_7H_{17}N$ = 115·2

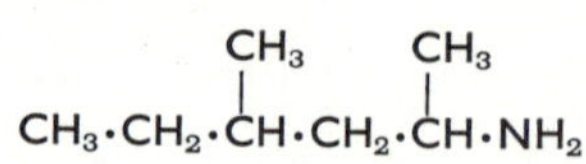

A colourless to pale yellow liquid. B.p. 130° to 135°.

Solubility. Slightly soluble in water; very soluble in ethanol, ether, and chloroform.

Extraction. Methylhexaneamine is volatile and may be isolated by distillation (see p. 18).

Chromatography. PAPER: system P1—Rf 0·60

(location reagents: *bromocresol green spray*, strong reaction; *ninhydrin spray*, orange).

Crystal Tests. MICRO: *gold bromide solution*—long hexagonal plates, unstable (*sensitivity:* 1 in 200); *platinic iodide solution*—irregular plates, unstable (*sensitivity:* 1 in 400).

Use. As the carbonate, it is used in inhalers for the temporary relief of nasal congestion.

Toxicity. Excessive use of methylhexaneamine inhalers may produce headache, nervousness, mental overactivity, and tremors.
The estimated minimum lethal dose in children up to 2 years of age is 200 mg.

METHYLPENTYNOL *Hypnotic*

Synonyms: Meparfynol; Methylparafynol.
Proprietary Names: Atempol; Dormison; Insomnol; Oblivon; Riposon; Util.

3-Methylpent-1-yn-3-ol
$C_6H_{10}O = 98{\cdot}15$

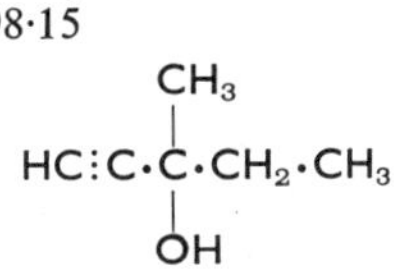

A colourless or pale yellow liquid. B.p. about 120°. Refractive index at 20°, 1·430 to 1·432.
Solubility. Soluble 1 in 10 of water; miscible with ethanol, ether, and chloroform.

METHYLPENTYNOL CARBAMATE
3-Carbamoyloxy-3-methylpent-1-yne.
Proprietary Names: *N*-Oblivon; Oblivon C.

A white powder. M.p. 53° to 56°.
Solubility. Soluble 1 in less than 200 of water, 1 in 1 of ethanol, and 1 in 2 of chloroform.

Extraction. Methylpentynol is extracted by organic solvents from aqueous acid or alkaline solutions.

Chromatography. PAPER, for the carbamate: system P6—Rf 0·88 (location reagent *furfural-hydrochloric acid spray*, positive reaction); system P7—Rf 0·72 (location as for P6).

Ultraviolet Absorption Spectrum. Methylpentynol in 0·1N sulphuric acid, maximum at 296 mμ (E1%, 1 cm 3·3).

Infra-red Absorption Spectrum. Methylpentynol (base). Capillary film between potassium bromide windows. The principal peaks are: A 917, B 1126 or 1156, C 995 (p. 746).

Metabolism. Methylpentynol appears to be almost completely metabolised, no unaltered drug being found in the urine after an oral dose of 100 mg and 15% or less after doses of 0·5 to 3 g (Perlman *et al.*, 1953b). It is largely conjugated with glucuronic acid although oxidation also takes place. It is present in blood and milk within 90 minutes after ingestion of 2 g, can be found in amniotic fluid after the mother has taken 1 g by mouth, and can be recovered from foetal liver and heart. If more than 2 g is ingested daily, accumulation occurs. It has been detected in the cerebrospinal fluid, after the intravenous infusion of 1·1 g.

Dose. Up to 1 g, as a hypnotic.

Toxicity. Death has been recorded from a dose of 5 g although recoveries have been reported after the ingestion of 6·25, 8·75, and 10 g. Repeated medication may cause toxic reactions in the liver and skin.
LD50 (oral): in mice 698, guinea-pigs 534, and rats 300 to 900 mg/kg.

CASE EXAMPLE. In a fatal case of poisoning, 3·2 g was recovered from the stomach contents. The liver contained 110 mg% and the urine 41 mg% (Jackson, 1967).

METHYLPHENOBARBITONE *Barbiturate*

Synonyms: Enphenemalum; Mephobarbital; Phemitone.
Proprietary Names: Isonal; Mebaral; Prominal.

5-Ethyl-1-methyl-5-phenylbarbituric acid
$C_{13}H_{14}N_2O_3 = 246{\cdot}3$

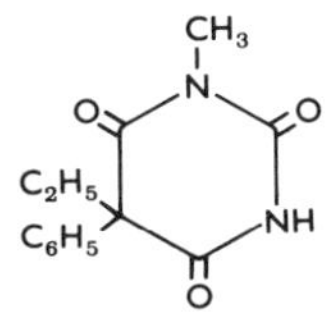

A white crystalline powder. M.p. 178° to 181°.
Solubility. Very slightly soluble in water; soluble 1 in 240 of ethanol, 1 in 200 of ether, and 1 in 40 of chloroform.

Screening Tests. See under Barbiturates, p. 208.

Extraction. Methylphenobarbitone may be isolated in the A2 fraction (see p. 27).

Chromatography. PAPER: system P2—Rf 2·00 relative to amylobarbitone (location under ultraviolet light, dark spot); system P3—Rf 0·63 (location reagent *silver nitrate spray*, white); system P4—Rf 0·90 (location as for P3).
THIN-LAYER: system T10—Rf 0·59 (location reagents: *mercurous nitrate spray*, black; *Zwikker's reagent spray*, faint pink); system T11—Rf 0·85 (location reagent *mercurous nitrate spray*, white on grey); system T12—Rf 0·60 (location as for T11); system T13—Rf 0·98 (location as to T11).
GAS: system G1/180—retention time 1·20 relative to diphenhydramine; system G5—retention time 4·60 relative to barbitone; system G7—retention time 3·30 relative to barbitone.

Colour Test. Zwikker's test—violet-blue.

Ultraviolet Absorption Spectrum. Methylphenobarbitone is a 1,5,5-substituted derivative—see Screening Test 3 under Barbiturates, p. 208.

Infra-red Absorption Spectrum. Potassium bromide disk. The principal peaks are: A 1684 or 1707, B 1365 (p. 746).

Quantitative Estimation. See under Barbiturates, p. 208.

Metabolism. Methylphenobarbitone is a long-acting barbiturate—see under Barbiturates, p. 207.

Nine hours after administration of a 150-mg dose of methylphenobarbitone, 0·8% of the dose was excreted unchanged and 4·3% as the *N*-demethylated metabolite, phenobarbitone; after 24 and 32 hours, only traces of methylphenobarbitone were excreted and 8·5% and 13% respectively of phenobarbitone. At each urine examination significant amounts of *p*-hydroxyphenobarbitone were also present (Svendsen and Brochmann-Hanssen, 1962).

Dose. In the treatment of epilepsy, up to 800 mg daily.

Toxicity. The estimated lethal dose in man is 2 g. In 2 non-fatal cases of poisoning, blood-levels of 90 and 26 mg% were found; in the latter case phenobarbitone was also present.

METHYLTESTOSTERONE *Androgen*

Proprietary Names: Glosso-Sterandryl; Metandren; Micryston Testosterone; Neo-Hombreol-M; Oreton-M; Pantestin Oral; Perandren Linguets; Testosid; Virormone-Oral.

17β-Hydroxy-17-methylandrost-4-en-3-one
$C_{20}H_{30}O_2 = 302{\cdot}5$

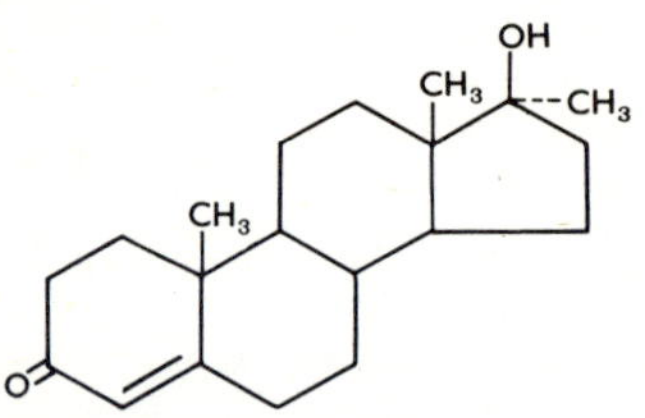

A white, slightly hygroscopic, crystalline powder. M.p. 162° to 167°. Specific rotation of a 1% solution in ethanol, +79° to +85°.
Solubility. Almost insoluble in water; soluble 1 in 5 of ethanol; soluble in ether and chloroform.

Extraction. Methyltestosterone is extracted from neutral solutions with freshly distilled ethyl acetate.

Chromatography. THIN-LAYER: thin-layer chromatography on starch-bound silica gel layers involving several solvent systems is described for the separation of methyltestosterone and other steroids by Smith and Foell (1962).

GAS: system G2/225—retention time 2·04 relative to codeine; system G4—retention time 3·3 relative to codeine.

Ultraviolet Absorption Spectrum. Methyltestosterone in ethanol, maximum at about 240 mμ (E1%, 1 cm 535).

Infra-red Absorption Spectrum. Potassium bromide disk. The principal peaks are: A 1657, B 1149, C 1375 (p. 746).

Metabolism. Methyltestosterone differs from testosterone in that it does not increase the excretion of 17-ketosteroids in the urine. It is absorbed from the gastro-intestinal tract and through intact skin.

Dose. Up to 50 mg for men and up to 20 mg for women, daily; in mammary carcinoma, up to 100 mg daily.

METHYPRYLONE *Hypnotic*

Synonyms: Methyprylon; Ro 1-6463.
Proprietary Name: Noludar.

3,3-Diethyl-5-methyl-2,4-dioxopiperidine
$C_{10}H_{17}NO_2 = 183{\cdot}3$

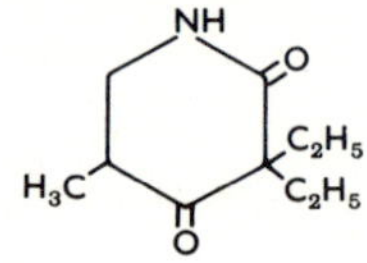

A white crystalline powder. M.p. 74° to 77°.
Solubility. Soluble 1 in 14 of water, 1 in 0·7 of ethanol, 1 in 3·5 of ether, and 1 in 0·6 of chloroform.

Extraction. Methyprylone is extracted by organic solvents from aqueous acid or alkaline solutions.

Chromatography. PAPER: system P1—Rf 0·94 (location reagent *bromine–starch–potassium iodide*, weak reaction); system RP1b—Rf 0·55 (location reagent *bromine–starch–potassium iodide*).

THIN-LAYER: system T1—Rf 0·58 (location reagent *potassium permanganate spray*, positive reaction); system T11—Rf 0·81 (location reagents: *mercurous nitrate spray*, white on grey; *potassium permanganate spray*, yellow on purple); system T12—Rf 0·45 (location as for T11); system T13—Rf 0·50 (location as for T11).

GAS: system G1/180—retention time 0·40 relative to diphenhydramine; system G3—retention time 1·40 relative to diphenhydramine; system G5—retention time 1·30 relative to barbitone.

Colour Test. MICRO: ammonium molybdate test—faint blue (*sensitivity:* 0·1 μg).

Ultraviolet Absorption Spectrum. Methyprylone in ethanol, maximum at 290 mμ (E1%, 1 cm about 2).

Infra-red Absorption Spectrum. Potassium bromide disk. The principal peaks are: A 1655, B 1688, C 1463 (p. 747).

Quantitative Estimation. Methyprylone in serum and urine may be determined colorimetrically (Xanthaky *et al.*, 1966). Goldbaum and Domanski (1966) have described a procedure for extraction and quantitative determination, involving gas chromatography, applicable to methyprylone in biological fluids and tissues.

Metabolism. In man, 60% of an ingested dose

of methyprylone is excreted as metabolites in the urine; only 3% is excreted unchanged (Xanthaky *et al.*, 1966). One urinary metabolite of methyprylone has been identified as 3,3-diethyl-5-methyl-2,4,6-trioxopiperidine (Bösche and Schmidt, 1966).
In the dog, about 3% has been found to be excreted as a dehydrogenated derivative (Randall *et al.*, 1956).

Dose. Up to 400 mg, as a hypnotic.

Toxicity. The estimated minimum lethal dose in man is 5 g. Recoveries have occurred following the ingestion of up to 9 g. Addiction to methyprylone has been reported.

CASE EXAMPLES. A 36-year-old woman recovered after taking about 30 g of methyprylone. About 80% of the drug was removed by gastric lavage (Burnstein and Stauss, 1965).
Four hours after swallowing 30 g of methyprylone a 39-year-old woman was admitted to hospital; on admission, the blood-level of methylprylone was 8·6 mg%. Dialysis was performed for 15 hours and 1 g of the drug recovered, 263 mg of it from the urine. The patient recovered (Xanthaky *et al.*, 1966).
In a fatal case of poisoning in an elderly woman, the blood-level of methyprylone was 114 mg%. Pentobarbitone was also present (Jackson, 1967).

METHYRIDINE *Anthelmintic (Veterinary)*

Proprietary Names: Mintic; Promintic.

2-(2-Methoxyethyl)pyridine
$C_8H_{11}NO = 137{\cdot}2$

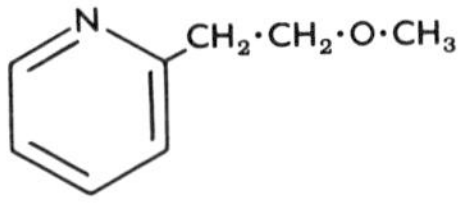

A colourless or pale yellow to pale brown liquid which should be stored in airtight containers protected from light.
Solubility. Miscible with water and ethanol.

Extraction. Methyridine is extracted by organic solvents from aqueous alkaline solutions.

Chromatography. PAPER: system P1—Rf 0·52 (location under ultraviolet light, absorption; location reagent *iodoplatinate spray*, white).
THIN-LAYER: system T1—Rf 0·65 (location reagent *acidified iodoplatinate spray*, positive reaction).
GAS: system G5—retention time 1·09 (2·18) relative to barbitone.

Crystal Tests. MICRO: *gold bromide solution*—irregular rhomboids (*sensitivity:* 1 in 1000); *platinic iodide solution*—small rectangular plates (*sensitivity:* 1 in 1000).

Ultraviolet Absorption Spectrum. Methyridine in cyclohexane, maxima at 256 mμ (E1%, 1 cm 780) and 262 mμ (E1%, 1 cm 770).

Metabolism. Methyridine is rapidly absorbed into the blood-stream and distributed throughout the tissues. It may be absorbed through the skin.

Dose. Usually 200 mg/kg. Maximum doses: cattle, 54 g; sheep and goats, 9 g.

Toxicity. Twice the therapeutic dose may cause death from respiratory depression except in birds in whom the margin of safety is much greater. Because methyridine is absorbed from the skin, any spillage should be washed off at once with cold water.

METHYSERGIDE *Migraine Prophylactic*

Synonyms: 1-Methyl-D-lysergic Acid Butanolamide; UML 491.

N-[1-(Hydroxymethyl)propyl]-4-methyl-(+)-lysergamide
$C_{21}H_{27}N_3O_2 = 353{\cdot}5$

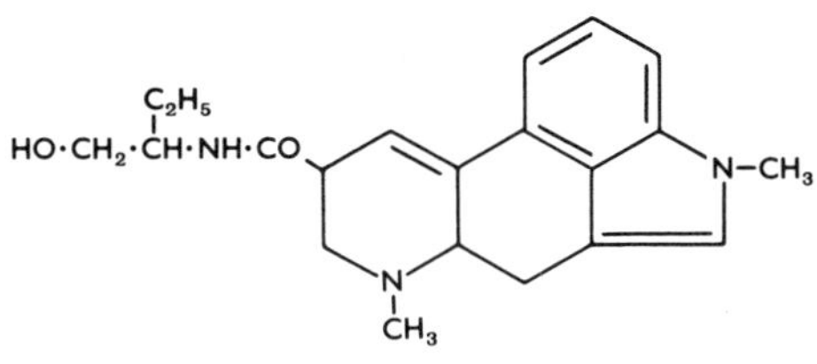

METHYSERGIDE MALEATE
Proprietary Names: Deseril; Desernil; Sansert.
A white to reddish-yellow crystalline powder.
Solubility. Soluble 1 in 250 of water and 1 in 125 of methanol.

Extraction. Methysergide is extracted by organic solvents from aqueous alkaline solutions.

Chromatography. PAPER: system P1—Rf 0·45 (location under ultraviolet light, blue fluorescence; location reagents: *iodoplatinate spray*, weak reaction; *bromocresol green spray*, weak reaction; p-*dimethylaminobenzaldehyde spray*, blue); system RP1a—Rf 0·46 (location under ultraviolet light, blue fluorescence; location reagent *iodoplatinate spray*, positive reaction); system RP1b—Rf 0·16 (location as for RP1a).
THIN-LAYER: system T1—Rf 0·66 (location reagent p-*dimethylaminobenzaldehyde spray*, blue); system T9—Rf 0·35 (location under ultraviolet light, absorption; location reagent p-*dimethylaminobenzaldehyde spray*, blue).

Colour Tests. MICRO: sulphuric acid–formaldehyde test—faint grey (*sensitivity:* 1·0 μg); ammonium molybdate test—(blue) green-blue (*sensitivity:* 0·25 μg); ammonium vanadate test—faint brown (*sensitivity:* 1·0 μg); Vitali's test—yellow/yellow/dull purple (*sensitivity:* 0·25 μg).

Crystal Test. MICRO: *picric acid*—irregular plates or prisms (*sensitivity:* 1 in 1000).

Infra-red Absorption Spectrum. Methysergide maleate. Potassium bromide disk. The principal peaks are: A 1566, B 1466, C 1343 or 1650 (p. 747).

Dose. The usual therapeutic dose is the equivalent of 2 to 6 mg of methysergide daily; 1 mg of methysergide is approximately equivalent to 1·33 mg of methysergide maleate.

Toxicity. Toxic effects are frequent and may necessitate withdrawal of methysergide in up to 30% of patients.

LD50 (oral): in mice 0·581 and in rats 2·1 g/kg.

METOCLOPRAMIDE *Anti-emetic*

4-Amino-5-chloro-*N*-(2-diethylaminoethyl)-2-methoxybenzamide

$C_{14}H_{22}ClN_3O_2$ = 299·8

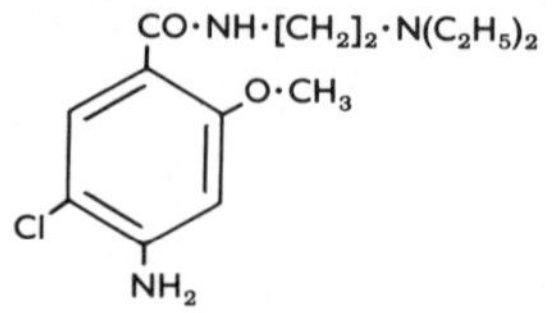

A white crystalline powder. M.p. about 148°.

Solubility. Almost insoluble in water; soluble 1 in 45 of ethanol and 1 in 15 of chloroform.

METOCLOPRAMIDE HYDROCHLORIDE

Proprietary Names: Imperan; Maxolon; Paspertin; Primperan.

A white crystalline powder.

Solubility. Soluble 1 in 10 of water and 1 in 5 of ethanol; almost insoluble in ether and chloroform.

Extraction. Metoclopramide is extracted by organic solvents from aqueous alkaline solutions.

Chromatography. PAPER: system P1—Rf 0·45 (location under ultraviolet light, blue fluorescence; location reagents: *iodoplatinate spray*, strong reaction; *bromocresol green spray*, weak reaction; *potassium permanganate spray*, weak reaction); system RP1a—Rf 0·77 (location under ultraviolet light, absorption; location reagent *iodoplatinate spray*, positive reaction); system RP1b—Rf 0·36 (location as for RP1a). THIN-LAYER: system T1—Rf 0·40 (location reagent *acidified iodoplatinate spray*, positive reaction).

Colour Tests. MICRO: ammonium vanadate test—light brown (*sensitivity:* 1·0 μg); Vitali's test—pale yellow/light brown/light brown (*sensitivity:* 1·0 μg).

Crystal Tests. MICRO: *gold cyanide solution*—needles, sometimes in rosettes (*sensitivity:* 1 in 1000); *lead iodide solution*—feathery rosettes (*sensitivity:* 1 in 1000).

Ultraviolet Absorption Spectrum. Metoclopramide hydrochloride in water, maximum at about 275 mμ.

Metabolism. In man, within 12 hours of a single dose, 50% is excreted unchanged in the urine, the remainder being metabolised in a manner which has not yet been elucidated.

Dose. Up to 30 mg daily.

METOFOLINE *Analgesic*

Synonyms: Methopholine; Ro 4-1778.

1-*p*-Chlorophenethyl-1,2,3,4-tetrahydro-6,7-dimethoxy-2-methylisoquinoline

$C_{20}H_{24}ClNO_2$ = 345·9

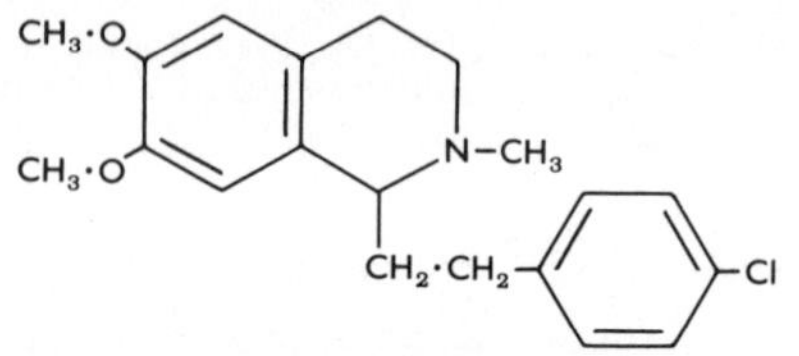

METOFOLINE HYDROCHLORIDE

Proprietary Name: Versidyne.

Extraction. Metofoline is extracted by organic solvents from aqueous alkaline solutions.

Chromatography. PAPER: system P1—Rf 0·68 (location reagents: *iodoplatinate spray*, strong reaction; *bromocresol green spray*, weak reaction).

THIN-LAYER: system T1—Rf 0·57 (location reagent *acidified iodoplatinate spray*, positive reaction).

Colour Tests. MICRO: sulphuric acid–formaldehyde test—pale yellow (*sensitivity:* 1·0 μg); ammonium molybdate test—dull green (*sensitivity:* 1·0 μg); ammonium vanadate test—pale green (*sensitivity:* 1·0 μg); Vitali's test—yellow/yellow/yellow (*sensitivity:* 1·0 μg).

Crystal Tests. MICRO: *lead iodide solution*—feathery rosettes (*sensitivity:* 1 in 1000); *trinitrobenzoic acid solution*—dense rosettes (*sensitivity:* 1 in 400).

Dose. Up to 240 mg daily.

Toxicity. It has been reported to have a depressive effect on respiration.

Tests in former opiate addicts have shown that metofoline has substantially less addiction-producing properties than morphine and codeine and even less than dextropropoxyphene (Fraser *et al.*, 1961).

METOPON *Narcotic Analgesic*

Synonyms: Dihydromethylmorphinone; Methyldihydromorphinone.

4,5-Epoxy-3-hydroxy-*N*,5-dimethyl-6-oxomorphinan

$C_{18}H_{21}NO_3$ = 299·4

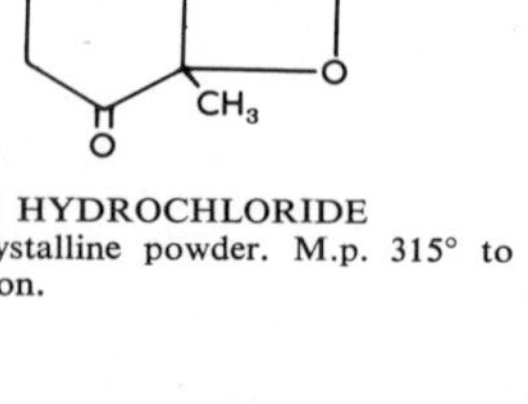

METOPON HYDROCHLORIDE

A white crystalline powder. M.p. 315° to 318°, with decomposition.

Solubility. Soluble 1 in 2 of water; sparingly soluble in ethanol; insoluble in ether; slightly soluble in chloroform.

Extraction. Metopon is extracted by organic solvents from aqueous ammoniacal solutions; hydrolysis of biological material is required in order to improve the yield.

Chromatography. PAPER: system P1—Rf 0·24 (location under ultraviolet light, strong absorption; location reagents: *iodoplatinate spray*, strong reaction; *bromocresol green spray*, weak reaction).
THIN-LAYER: system T1—Rf 0·25 (location reagent *acidified iodoplatinate spray*, positive reaction).
GAS: system G2/225—retention time 1·0 relative to codeine.

Colour Tests. MICRO: sulphuric acid–formaldehyde test—purple (*sensitivity:* 0·5 μg); ammonium molybdate test—blue-violet → blue → green (*sensitivity:* 0·1 μg); ammonium vanadate test—dull purple (*sensitivity:* 0·25 μg); Vitali's test—yellow/yellow/orange (*sensitivity:* 0·25 μg).

Crystal Tests. MICRO: *picrolonic acid*—serrated needles (*sensitivity:* 1 in 200); *potassium bismuth iodide solution*—very small rods (*sensitivity:* 1 in 1000).

Ultraviolet Absorption Spectrum. Metopon in ethanol, maximum at 284·5 mμ, minimum at 267 mμ; in 0·1N sulphuric acid, maximum at 280 mμ (E1%, 1 cm 0·5) and an inflexion at about 225 mμ.

Dose. Usually up to 6 mg.

Toxicity. Metopon is about twice as potent an analgesic as morphine and has a similar duration of action. The estimated minimum lethal dose is 100 mg. Metopon may cause addiction. LD50 (subcutaneous): in mice 25 mg/kg.

METRONIDAZOLE *Trichomonacide*

Synonyms: Bayer 5360; RP 8823.
Proprietary Names: Clont; Flagyl; Trichazol.

1-(2-Hydroxyethyl)-2-methyl-5-nitroimidazole
$C_6H_9N_3O_3$ = 171·2

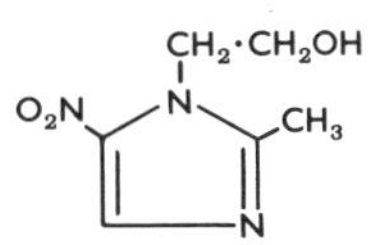

A white crystalline powder. M.p. 159° to 162°.
Solubility. Soluble 1 in 100 of water, 1 in 200 of ethanol, and 1 in 250 of chloroform; slightly soluble in ether.

Chromatography. PAPER: system P1—Rf 0·80 (location under ultraviolet light, strong absorption; location reagents: *iodoplatinate spray*, white; *potassium permanganate spray*, weak reaction); system RP1a—Rf 0·84 (location under ultraviolet light, absorption); system RP1b—Rf 0·81 (location as for RP1a).
THIN-LAYER: system T1—Rf 0·64 (location reagent *potassium permanganate spray*, positive reaction).
GAS: system G2/225—retention time 0·44 relative to diphenhydramine; system G4—retention time 0·35 relative to codeine.

Crystal Tests. MICRO: *gold bromide–hydrochloric acid solution*—rhomboids (*sensitivity:* 1 in 200); *potassium bismuth iodide solution*—irregular dense rhomboids (*sensitivity:* 1 in 1000).

Ultraviolet Absorption Spectrum. Metronidazole in 0·1N hydrochloric acid, maximum at 277 mμ (E1%, 1 cm 380).

Infra-red Absorption Spectrum. Potassium bromide disk. The principal peaks are: A 1187 or 1535, B 1365 or 1485, C 1070 or 1467 (p. 791).

Quantitative Estimation. A method of estimation by spectrophotometry is described by Ings *et al.* (1966). Durel *et al.* (1967) describe a method for the rapid detection and determination of metronidazole in urine which involves diazotisation and coupling with *p*-dimethylaminobenzaldehyde.

Metabolism. In man and dogs, 60 to 70% of a dose of metronidazole is found to be excreted unchanged in the urine. The major metabolic pathway involves oxidation of the hydroxyl group, producing 2-methyl-5-nitroimidazol-1-ylacetic acid; a second metabolite appears to be the glucuronide of metronidazole (Ings *et al.*, 1966).
The concentration of the drug in serum and urine reaches a trichomonacidal level within an hour, attains its maximum in 2 to 3 hours, and persists in the serum for at least 12 hours.

Dose. Usually 600 mg daily.

Toxicity. A pregnant woman ingested 4·2 g of metronidazole but no ill effects resulted in either mother or foetus (Fluker, 1961).

METYRAPONE

Diagnostic Aid (pituitary function)

Synonyms: Methopyrapone; SU 4885.
Proprietary Name: Metopirone.

2-Methyl-1,2-di(pyrid-3-yl)propan-1-one
$C_{14}H_{14}N_2O$ = 226·3

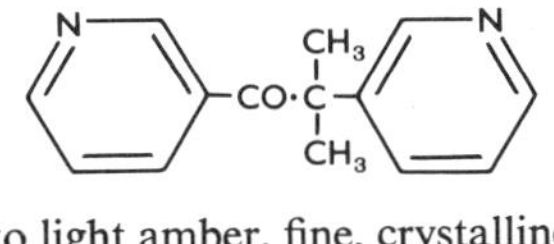

A white to light amber, fine, crystalline powder which darkens on exposure to light. M.p. 50° to 52°.
Solubility. Soluble in chloroform and methanol.

Extraction. Metyrapone is extracted by organic solvents from aqueous alkaline solutions.

Chromatography. PAPER: system P1—Rf 0·75 (location under ultraviolet light, strong absorption; location reagent *iodoplatinate spray*, strong reaction); system RP1a—Rf 0·38 (location under ultraviolet light, absorption; location reagent *iodoplatinate spray*, positive reaction); system RP1b—Rf 0·28 (location as for RP1a).

THIN-LAYER: system T1—Rf 0·65 (location reagent *acidified iodoplatinate spray*, positive reaction).

Crystal Tests. MICRO: *lead iodide solution*—dense rosettes or rods (*sensitivity:* 1 in 400); *picric acid*—clusters of irregular crystals (*sensitivity:* 1 in 1000).

Ultraviolet Absorption Spectrum. Metyrapone in 0·1N sulphuric acid, maximum at 260 mμ (E1%, 1cm 597) and an inflexion at about 265 mμ (E1%, 1cm 553).

Infra-red Absorption Spectrum. Potassium bromide disk. The principal peaks are: A 1672, B 1578, C 1255 or 1417 (p. 747).

Metabolism. Metyrapone selectively inhibits the enzyme 11β-hydroxylase which affects the 11β-hydroxylation of steroids in the adrenal cortex; it thus prevents the synthesis of cortisone and hydrocortisone. The inhibition results in an increased urinary excretion of 17-hydroxycorticosteroids and 17-ketogenic steroids and their measurement may be used as a test of glandular function.

Dose. The usual diagnostic dose is 750 mg every 4 hours for 6 doses.

Toxicity. Metyrapone may precipitate acute adrenal failure in patients with gross hypopituitarism.

6-MONOACETYLMORPHINE

Synonym: Alpha-acetylmorphine.

6-Acetoxy-7,8-dehydro-4,5-epoxy-3-hydroxy-*N*-methylmorphinan

$C_{18}H_{20}NO_4$ = 314·4

6-MONOACETYLMORPHINE HYDROCHLORIDE

6-Monoacetylmorphine hydrochloride occurs as crystals. **Solubility.** Soluble in water.

Extraction. 6-Monoacetylmorphine is extracted by organic solvents from aqueous ammoniacal solutions.

Chromatography. PAPER: system P1—Rf 0·29 (location under ultraviolet light, absorption; location reagents: *iodoplatinate spray*, strong reaction; *bromocresol green spray*, weak reaction).

THIN-LAYER: system T1—Rf 0·44 (location reagent *acidified iodoplatinate spray*, positive reaction); system T7—Rf 0·64 (location reagent *iodoplatinate spray*, positive reaction); system T8—Rf 0·40 (location as for T7).

GAS: system G2/225—retention time 1·45 relative to codeine.

Colour Tests. MICRO: sulphuric acid–formaldehyde test—purple (*sensitivity:* 0·1 μg); Vitali's test—yellow/yellow/orange (*sensitivity:* 1·0 μg).

Ultraviolet Absorption Spectrum. 6-Monoacetylmorphine in ethanol, maximum at 287 mμ; minimum at 262 mμ: in 0·5N hydrochloric acid, maximum at 284 mμ; minimum at 259 mμ: in 0·5N sodium hydroxide, maximum at 298 mμ; minimum at 276·5 mμ.

Metabolism. 6-Monoacetylmorphine is the first hydrolysis product of diamorphine (p. 292); it is then slowly hydrolysed to morphine.

NOTE. In forensic investigations where diamorphine ingestion is suspected the blood should be tested for the presence of 6-monoacetylmorphine. However, the blood must be collected within 30 minutes of the suspected ingestion of diamorphine (Nakamura and Ukita, 1967).

MONOSULFIRAM *Parasiticide*

Proprietary Name: Tetmosol.

Tetraethylthiuram monosulphide

$C_{10}H_{20}N_2S_3$ = 264·5

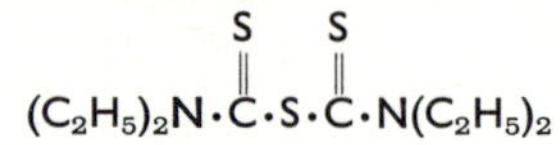

A yellowish or yellowish-brown, soft, crystalline powder. M.p. 28·5° to 32°.

Solubility. Insoluble in water; very soluble in ethanol.

Extraction. Monosulfiram is extracted by organic solvents from aqueous acid or alkaline solutions.

Chromatography. PAPER: system P1—Rf 0·95 (location under ultraviolet light, absorption; location reagents: *iodoplatinate spray*, weak reaction (yellow); *potassium permanganate spray*, strong reaction).

THIN-LAYER: system T1—Rf 0·75 (location reagent *acidified iodoplatinate spray*, positive reaction).

Colour Test. MICRO: ammonium molybdate test—grey (*sensitivity:* 1·0 μg).

Ultraviolet Absorption Spectrum. Monosulfiram in ethanol, maximum at 280 mμ (E1%, 1cm 673).

Use. Monosulfiram is generally used as a 25% alcoholic solution or as a soap containing 5%.

MORPHERIDINE *Narcotic*

Synonyms: Morpholinoethylnorpethidine; Ta 1.

Ethyl 1-(2-morpholinoethyl)-4-phenylpiperidine-4-carboxylate

$C_{20}H_{30}N_2O_3$ = 346·5

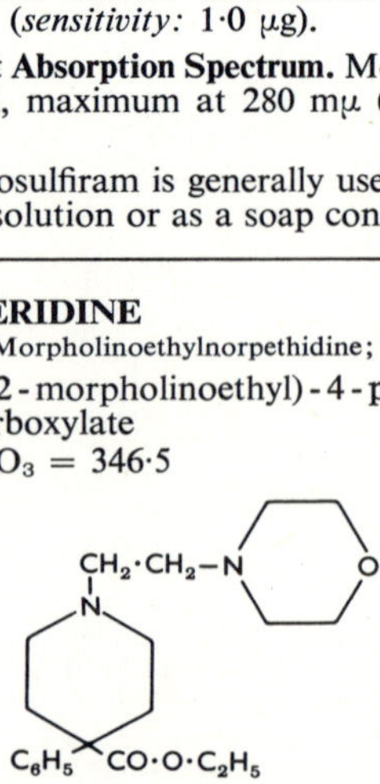

Extraction. Morpheridine is extracted by

organic solvents from aqueous alkaline solutions; hydrolysis of biological material is required in order to improve the yield.

Chromatography. PAPER: system P1—Rf 0·22 (location reagents: *iodoplatinate spray*, strong reaction; *bromocresol green spray*, weak reaction); system RP1a—Rf 0·76 (location reagent *iodoplatinate spray*, positive reaction); system RP1b—Rf 0·13 (location as for RP1a).

THIN-LAYER: system T1—Rf 0·56 (location reagent *acidified iodoplatinate spray*, positive reaction).

GAS: system G2/225—retention time 1·54 relative to codeine.

Colour Test. MICRO: sulphuric acid–formaldehyde test—dull orange (*sensitivity:* 1·0 μg).

Crystal Tests. MICRO: *potassium bismuth iodide solution*—small rosettes and fans of needles, forming overnight (*sensitivity:* 1 in 1000); *potassium cadmium iodide solution*—plates, often in bunches (*sensitivity:* 1 in 1000).

MORPHINE *Narcotic Analgesic*

Synonyms: Morphia; Morphina.

7,8 - Dehydro - 4,5 - epoxy - 3,6 - dihydroxy - *N* - methylmorphinan

$C_{17}H_{19}NO_3 = 285·3$

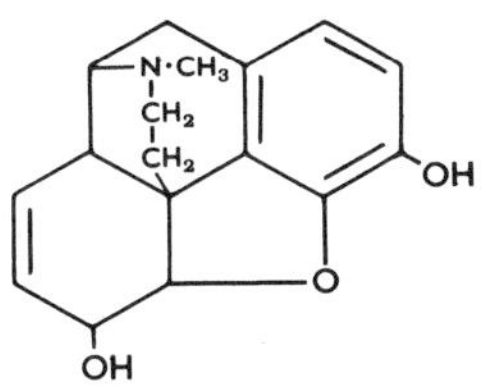

Morphine is the principal alkaloid of opium. Morphine (anhydrous base) consists of short rhombic prisms; the monohydrate is a white crystalline powder. M.p. of the anhydrous base 254°, with decomposition; m.p. of the monohydrate 254° to 256°, with decomposition.

Solubility. Soluble 1 in 5000 of water, 1 in 400 of boiling water, 1 in 250 of ethanol, 1 in 1500 of chloroform; almost insoluble in ether.

NOTE. The solubility can vary according to the method of preparation and the crystalline state.

MORPHINE ACETATE

A white amorphous or crystalline powder.

Solubility. Soluble 1 in 2·5 of water and 1 in 100 of ethanol; insoluble in ether.

MORPHINE HYDROCHLORIDE

Synonyms: Morphinum Chloratum; Morphinum Muriaticum.

Colourless glistening needles or a white crystalline powder.

Solubility. Soluble 1 in 23 of water and 1 in 100 of ethanol; insoluble in ether and chloroform.

MORPHINE SULPHATE

White acicular crystals, cubical masses, or crystalline powder. M.p. 250°, with decomposition.

Solubility. Soluble 1 in 21 of water and 1 in 1000 of ethanol; insoluble in ether and chloroform. When exposed to air it gradually loses water of crystallisation.

MORPHINE TARTRATE

Minute, colourless, acicular, efflorescent crystals.

Solubility. Soluble 1 in 10 of water and 1 in 1000 of ethanol; almost insoluble in ether and chloroform.

Extraction. Morphine may be isolated in the D3 fraction; hydrolysis of biological material is required in order to improve the yield.

Chromatography. PAPER: system P1—Rf 0·14 (location under ultraviolet light, strong absorption; location reagents: *iodoplatinate spray*, strong reaction; *bromocresol green spray*, weak reaction; *Marquis reagent*, purple); system RP1a—Rf 0·88 (location reagent *iodoplatinate spray*, positive reaction); system RP1b—Rf 0·81 (location as for RP1a).

THIN-LAYER: system T1—Rf 0·34 (location reagent *acidified iodoplatinate spray*, positive reaction); system T7—Rf 0·11 (location reagent *iodoplatinate spray*, positive reaction); system T8—Rf 0·27 (location as for T7).

GAS: system G1/250—retention time 1·28 relative to codeine; system G2/225—retention time 1·15 relative to codeine; system G6—retention time 1·21 relative to codeine.

Colour Tests. MICRO: sulphuric acid–formaldehyde test—purple (*sensitivity:* 0·05 μg); ammonium molybdate test—purple → blue → light green (*sensitivity:* 0·05 μg); ammonium vanadate test—blue-grey (*sensitivity:* 1·0 μg); Vitali's test—yellow/yellow/orange (*sensitivity:* 0·5 μg).

Crystal Tests. MICRO: *potassium cadmium iodide solution*—sheaves of fine needles (*sensitivity:* 1 in 3000); *potassium tri-iodide solution* (*I*)—plates (*sensitivity:* 1 in 1000).

Ultraviolet Absorption Spectrum. Morphine in ethanol, maximum at 287 mμ (E1%, 1 cm 55); minimum at 263 mμ (E1%, 1 cm 22): in 0·1N sodium hydroxide, maxima at 250·5 mμ (E1%, 1 cm 255) and 296 mμ (E1%, 1 cm 116): in 0·1N sulphuric acid, maximum at 284 mμ (E1%, 1 cm 43·4) and an inflexion at 279 mμ. Morphine hydrochloride and morphine sulphate in water, maximum at 285 mμ (E1%, 1 cm about 41); minimum at 261 mμ.

Infra-red Absorption Spectrum. Morphine (base). Potassium bromide disk. The principal peaks are: A 805, B 1243 or 1448, C 945 or 1118 or 1475 (p. 747).

Quantitative Estimation. Siminoff and Saunders (1958) and Way *et al.* (1960) have described methods of extraction and of spectrophotometric estimation of free and conjugated morphine in biological tissues.

Metabolism. The main metabolic pathway of morphine is conjugation in the liver with glucuronic acid to form morphine-3-glucuronide. *N*-Demethylation and *O*-methylation may also occur; in 5 subjects given 10 to 15 mg of *N*-methyl-^{14}C-labelled morphine sulphate intramuscularly, the pulmonary excretion of labelled carbon dioxide ranged from 3·5 to 6% of the injected dose in 24 hours.

Morphine is excreted in the urine largely as the glucuronide conjugate, over 50% appearing within 8 hours; by 24 hours, roughly 90% has been excreted but traces are still detectable after 48 hours. Nearly all the excreted free morphine can be found in the urine within 8 hours after intravenous or subcutaneous administration; the average amount excreted within a 24-hour period is about 7%.

Morphine is promptly absorbed after parenteral administration, peak levels being attained after 1 hour; gastro-intestinal absorption is poor. It leaves the blood-stream rapidly and concentrates in the lungs, spleen, and kidneys. However, accumulation does not occur in these tissues. Both free and conjugated morphine may be found in the plasma.

NOTE. Morphine is slowly converted to pseudomorphine in cadavers and it is found as such on exhumation.

Dose. The usual analgesic dose is up to 20 mg.

Toxicity. The estimated minimum lethal dose in man is 200 mg but it may be up to 10 times higher in addicts and much lower in infants.

Morphine leaves the blood-stream very rapidly and if it is detected in a blood-sample considerably more than a single therapeutic dose has been taken; 0·1 mg% found in a blood-sample represents a very large dose. Concentrations of total morphine in urine greater than 5 mg% suggest excessive overdosage.

Villandy (1967) in a statistical study of 133 deaths due to acute morphine intoxication suggests that blood is the tissue of choice for morphine determination, especially when the history indicates that death followed shortly after injection; the mere presence of morphine in the bile or urine, if not correlated by good history and good pathology, is poor prima facie evidence of acute morphine poisoning. It must be borne in mind that the average urinary morphine level of diamorphine addicts is generally higher than the urinary morphine level found in acute morphine poisoning.

LD50 (subcutaneous): in mice 700 mg/kg.

CASE EXAMPLES. In a fatal case of poisoning by morphine sulphate, the levels of base found were: blood, 4 mg%; brain, 2 mg%; heart, 3 mg%; kidneys, 1 mg%; liver, 8 mg%; lungs, 4 mg%; pancreas, 1 mg%; and spleen 4 mg%. Morphine tartrate, 2 mg%, was recovered from the liver of a body which had been decomposing for about a month (Jackson, 1967).

Death followed the subcutaneous administration of morphine. The drug was found only in the urine, 5 mg% before hydrolysis and 12·7 mg% after hydrolysis. None was found in the blood, liver, stomach contents or intestines. None could be found in the liver even after strong hydrolysis (Zwikker and Steenhauer, 1942).

Seventeen fatal cases are described very completely in which death is ascribed to injection of therapeutic doses of morphine or morphine and hyoscine where the persons were seriously affected by alcohol or bromides, or under the influence of moderate but toxic quantities of barbiturates (Møller, 1953).

MORPHINE *N*-OXIDE *Narcotic*

Synonyms: Genomorphine; Morphine Aminoxide; *N*-Oxymorphine.

$C_{17}H_{19}NO_4 = 301{\cdot}3$

Morphine *N*-oxide melts at 275°. It is stated to be bimolecular.

Solubility. Slightly soluble in water; insoluble in chloroform.

Chromatography. PAPER: system P1—Rf 0·14 (location under ultraviolet light, strong absorption; location reagents: *iodoplatinate spray*, weak reaction; *bromocresol green spray*, weak reaction).

THIN-LAYER: system T1—Rf 0·23 (location reagent *acidified iodoplatinate spray*, positive reaction).

Colour Tests. MICRO: sulphuric acid–formaldehyde test—purple (*sensitivity:* 0·1 μg); ammonium molybdate test—deep purple → blue → green (*sensitivity:* 0·1 μg); ammonium vanadate test—dull purple → brown (*sensitivity:* 0·25 μg).

Crystal Tests. MICRO: *platinic chloride solution*—small oily rosettes, forming overnight (*sensitivity:* 1 in 200); *potassium tri-iodide solution* (*3*)—dense rosettes (*sensitivity:* 1 in 200).

Ultraviolet Absorption Spectrum. Morphine *N*-oxide in 0·1N sulphuric acid, maximum at 284·5 mμ (E1%, 1 cm 46·4) and an inflexion at about 279 mμ.

MUSTINE *Antineoplastic*

Synonyms: Chlorethazine; Chlormethine; HN 2; Mechlorethamine; Methchlorethamine; Nitrogen Mustard.

2,2′-Dichloro-*N*-methyldiethylamine

$C_5H_{11}Cl_2N = 156{\cdot}1$

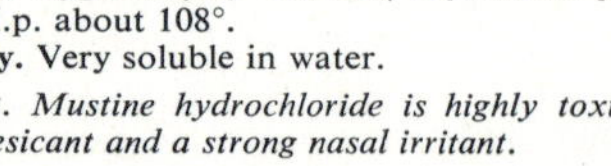

An oily substance.

Solubility. Relatively insoluble in water.

MUSTINE HYDROCHLORIDE

Proprietary Name: Mustargen Hydrochloride.

A white, hygroscopic, vesicant, crystalline powder or mass. M.p. about 108°.

Solubility. Very soluble in water.

CAUTION. *Mustine hydrochloride is highly toxic; it is a strong vesicant and a strong nasal irritant.*

Chromatography. A paper chromatographic method for detecting nitrogen mustard derivatives is based on their reaction with compounds having a mercapto-group (Sakurai and Ito, 1960).

Metabolism. In neutral or alkaline solutions mustine rapidly undergoes intramolecular transformation with release of a chloride ion to form a cyclic ethyleneimmonium derivative which is highly reactive chemically.

Some of the physiological effects of mustine

may be due to deactivation of crucial enzymes but it is more likely that mustine acts mainly on proliferating cells by alkylating the nucleic acids of the chromosomes.
Mustine is only active when given parenterally and it is rapidly removed from the blood-stream. Metabolism is so rapid that less than 0·01% of the drug may be recovered in the urine.

Dose. The usual dose is 0·4 mg/kg intravenously.

Toxicity. Severe haemopoietic depression may follow the administration of even therapeutic doses. Bone-marrow changes may lead to severe anaemia and thrombocytopenic purpura. Skin reactions may also occur.
LD50 (oral): in rats 10 mg/kg.

MYRISTICIN

1-Allyl-3-methoxy-4,5-methylenedioxybenzene
$C_{11}H_{12}O_3 = 192·2$

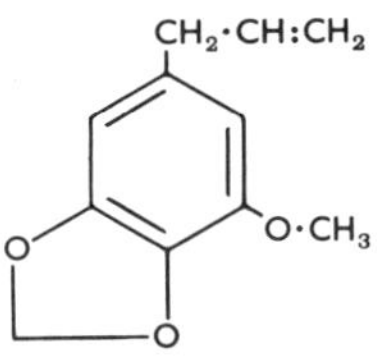

The most toxic principle of nutmeg (see below) and nutmeg oil. M.p. below −20°. B.p. 276° to 277°. Refractive index 1·5403.
Solubility. Slightly soluble in ethanol; soluble in ether.

NUTMEG
Synonyms: Muscade; Myristica; Nux Moschata.
The dried, light brown kernels of the seeds of *Myristica fragrans* (Myristicaceae) containing not less than 5% of volatile oil.

NUTMEG OIL
Synonyms: Essence de Muscade; Myristica Oil.
A colourless or pale yellow, volatile oil obtained by distillation from nutmeg and containing up to 4% of myristicin. Refractive index, at 20°, 1·472 to 1·488.
Solubility. Fairly soluble in ethanol; soluble in glacial acetic acid.

Toxicity. Severe symptoms of poisoning have been caused by the ingestion of 1 to 1½ nutmegs, and doses of 5 g or more of nutmeg or nutmeg powder will produce a marked depressive action on the central nervous system.
CASE EXAMPLES. A 28-year-old woman took 18·3 g of powdered nutmeg. Following a period of disorientation, delirium, and excitement, the patient became semi-stuporous for 12 hours. For some days she complained of numbness, dizziness and nausea, and there were further periods of excitement. No specific therapy was given and she was discharged after 7 days (Green, 1959).
Two young women consumed 15 and 25 g respectively of ground nutmeg in order to experience its hallucinogenic action. Both became intoxicated but recovered within 2 weeks and 10 days respectively. Analyses of the blood and urine were normal in both cases (Åkesson and Wålinder, 1965).

MYROPHINE *Narcotic*

Synonyms: C 5; Myricodine; Myristylbenzylmorphine; NIH 5986.

3-Benzyloxy-7,8-dehydro-4,5-epoxy-*N*-methyl-6-myristoyloxymorphinan
$C_{38}H_{51}NO_4 = 585·8$

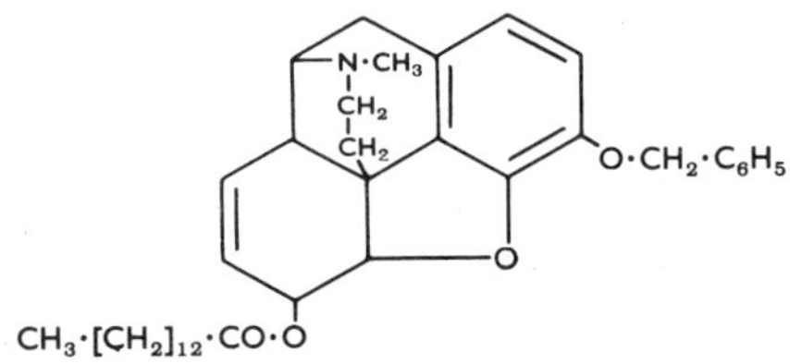

Myrophine melts at 33° to 34°.

Extraction. Myrophine is extracted by organic solvents from aqueous alkaline solutions.

Chromatography. PAPER: system P1—Rf 0·83 (location under ultraviolet light, absorption; location reagent *iodoplatinate spray*, strong reaction); system RP1a—Rf 0·00 (location under ultraviolet light, absorption; location reagent *iodoplatinate spray*, positive reaction); system RP1b—Rf 0·00 (location as for RP1a).
THIN-LAYER: system T1—Rf 0·52 (location reagent *acidified iodoplatinate spray*, positive reaction).

Colour Tests. MICRO: sulphuric acid–formaldehyde test—brown-purple (*sensitivity:* 0·25 µg); ammonium molybdate test—blue-violet (*sensitivity:* 0·25 µg); Vitali's test—yellow/yellow/orange (*sensitivity:* 1·0 µg).

Crystal Tests. MICRO: *picrolonic acid*—bunches of needles (*sensitivity:* 1 in 400); *potassium tri-iodide solution* (2)—oily needles (*sensitivity:* 1 in 400).

Ultraviolet Absorption Spectrum. Myrophine in 0·1N hydrochloric acid, maximum at 283 mµ (E 1%, 1 cm 29); minimum at 261 mµ.

NAEPAINE *Local Anaesthetic*

2-Pentylaminoethyl *p*-aminobenzoate
$C_{14}H_{22}N_2O_2 = 250·3$

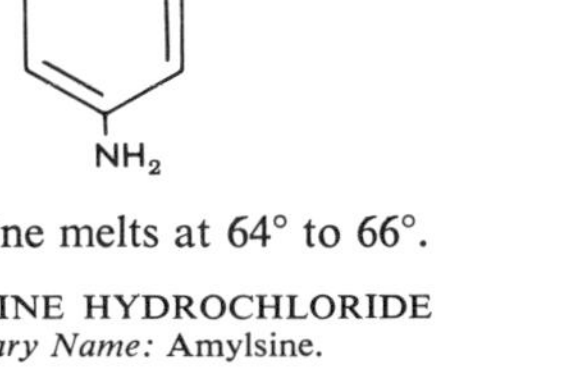

Naepaine melts at 64° to 66°.

NAEPAINE HYDROCHLORIDE
Proprietary Name: Amylsine.
Fine white crystals, or a fine powder. M.p. of one form 153° and of the other form 175° to 177°.
Solubility. Soluble in water; sparingly soluble in ethanol; insoluble in ether and chloroform.

Extraction. Naepaine is extracted by organic solvents from aqueous alkaline solutions.

Chromatography. PAPER: system P1—Rf 0·66 (location under ultraviolet light, blue fluorescence; location reagents: *iodoplatinate spray*, strong reaction; *bromocresol green spray*, strong reaction).

THIN-LAYER: system T1—Rf 0·63 (location reagent *acidified iodoplatinate spray*, positive reaction).

Colour Test. MICRO: Vitali's test— -/yellow/orange (*sensitivity:* 1·0 μg).

Crystal Tests. MICRO: *gold bromide–hydrochloric acid solution*—fans or rosettes of needles (*sensitivity:* 1 in 1000); *potassium tri-iodide solution* (*3*)—irregular needles, best viewed under polarised light (*sensitivity:* 1 in 1000).

Ultraviolet Absorption Spectrum. Naepaine in 0·1N sulphuric acid, maxima at 273 mμ (E1%, 1cm 83), 278·5 mμ (E1%, 1cm 84), and about 290 mμ (E1%, 1cm 61).

Infra-red Absorption Spectrum. Naepaine (base). Potassium bromide disk. The principal peaks are: A 1605, B 1277, C 1170 or 1685 (p. 792).

Toxicity. Naepaine hydrochloride is about 1½ times as toxic as procaine hydrochloride systemically. The maximum amount which is safe for surface use is 100 mg of the hydrochloride. The minimum intravenous lethal dose in guinea-pigs is 10 to 40, in rabbits 28·5, and in rats 25 to 30 mg/kg.

NALIDIXIC ACID *Antibacterial*

Synonym: Win 18320.
Proprietary Names: Negram; Nogram.

1 - Ethyl - 7 - methyl - 4 - oxo - 1,8 - naphthyridine-3-carboxylic acid

$C_{12}H_{12}N_2O_3 = 232{\cdot}2$

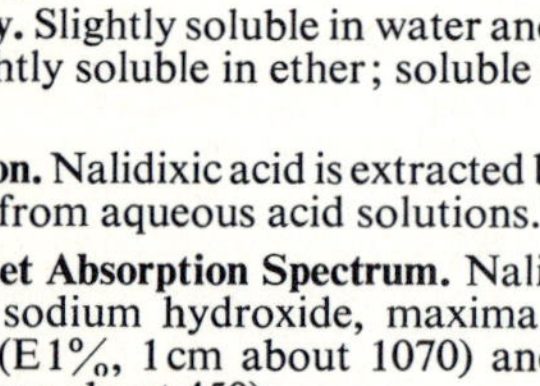

A pale buff-yellow crystalline powder. M.p. 225° to 231°.
Solubility. Slightly soluble in water and ethanol; very slightly soluble in ether; soluble in chloroform.

Extraction. Nalidixic acid is extracted by organic solvents from aqueous acid solutions.

Ultraviolet Absorption Spectrum. Nalidixic acid in 0·1N sodium hydroxide, maxima at about 259 mμ (E1%, 1cm about 1070) and 338 mμ (E1%, 1cm about 450).

Quantitative Estimation. Nalidixic acid may be estimated spectrophotometrically (Murgu, 1964) and spectrofluorimetrically (McChesney *et al.*, 1964).

Metabolism. Nalidixic acid is readily absorbed from the gastro-intestinal tract and about 80% of a dose is rapidly excreted in the urine. Of the 4 metabolites which have been isolated, hydroxynalidixic acid is the only one which has shown biological activity. The other 3 metabolites are nalidixic acid glucuronide, hydroxynalidixic acid glucuronide, and the 3,7-dicarboxylic acid (Portmann *et al.*, 1966).

Dose. Usually 4 g daily.

NALORPHINE *Narcotic Antagonist*

Synonym: N-Allylnormorphine.

N - Allyl - 7,8 - dehydro - 4,5 - epoxy - 3,6- dihydroxymorphinan

$C_{19}H_{21}NO_3 = 311{\cdot}4$

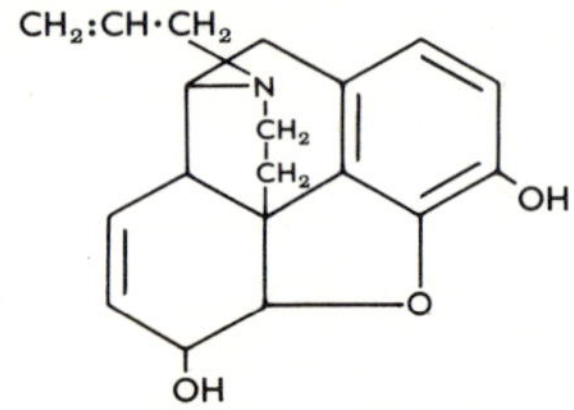

Nalorphine melts at 208°.
Solubility. Slightly soluble in water and ether; soluble in ethanol and chloroform.

NALORPHINE HYDROBROMIDE
Proprietary Name: Lethidrone.

A white crystalline powder. M.p. about 260°, with decomposition.
Solubility. Soluble 1 in 24 of water and 1 in 35 of ethanol. Aqueous solutions may deposit crystals of the dihydrate, which is readily soluble in dehydrated ethanol but the solution rapidly yields a deposit of the anhydrous salt.

NALORPHINE HYDROCHLORIDE
Proprietary Names: Anarcon; Nalline Hydrochloride.

A white crystalline powder which slowly darkens on exposure to air and light. M.p. 260° to 263°.
Solubility. Soluble 1 in 8 of water and 1 in 35 of ethanol; insoluble in ether and chloroform.

Extraction. Nalorphine is extracted by organic solvents from aqueous alkaline solutions.

Chromatography. PAPER: system P1—Rf 0·30 (location under ultraviolet light, absorption; location reagent *iodoplatinate spray*, weak reaction); system RP1a—Rf 0·87 (location under ultraviolet light, absorption; location reagent *iodoplatinate spray*, positive reaction); system RP1b—Rf 0·36 (location as for RP1a).

THIN-LAYER: system T1—Rf 0·62 (location reagent *acidified iodoplatinate spray*, positive reaction); system T7—Rf 0·35 (location as for T1); system T8—Rf 0·55 (location as for T1).

GAS: system G2/225—retention time 1·76 relative to codeine; system G6—retention time 1·85 relative to codeine.

Colour Tests. MICRO: sulphuric acid–formaldehyde test—purple (*sensitivity:* 0·25 μg); ammonium molybdate test—violet-blue → green (*sensitivity:* 0·25 µg); Vitali's test—yellow/yellow/orange (*sensitivity:* 0·5 µg).

Crystal Tests. MICRO: *potassium chromate solution*—four-pointed stars (*sensitivity:* 1 in 200); *potassium mercuric iodide solution*—smudge rosettes or fibres (*sensitivity:* 1 in 400).

Ultraviolet Absorption Spectrum. Nalorphine in 0·1N hydrochloric acid, inflexion at about 241 mµ and maximum at 283·5 mµ (E1%, 1cm 51); in 0·1N sulphuric acid, maximum at 285 mµ (E1%, 1cm 38) and an inflexion at 278 mµ. Nalorphine hydrobromide in water, maximum at 285 mµ (E1%, 1cm about 39); minimum at 260 mµ.

Infra-red Absorption Spectrum. Nalorphine hydrobromide. Potassium bromide disk. The principal peaks are: A 1505, B 1466, C 1121 or 1155 or 1304 (p. 747).

Metabolism. After intravenous injection of nalorphine, normorphine has been demonstrated in the brain of rats and evidence has been obtained that this *N*-dealkylation occurs in the brain itself although not so readily as in the case of morphine (Milthers, 1962).
Studies in dogs have shown that after subcutaneous injection nalorphine is more rapidly absorbed than morphine, maximum plasma levels being obtained after 30 to 60 minutes. The free drug disappears very rapidly from the blood but conjugated nalorphine is present in the plasma for more than 6 to 7 hours after injection (Woods, 1956).
Between 2 and 6% of unchanged nalorphine is recovered in the urine and 79 to 84% is recovered as a glucuronide conjugate (Hug and Woods, 1963).

Dose. Up to a total of 40 mg intravenously.

Toxicity. The estimated minimum lethal dose in man is 200 mg. The administration of nalorphine to morphine addicts may be followed by a typical withdrawal syndrome.
LD50 (subcutaneous): in mice 600 mg/kg.

NANDROLONE *Anabolic Steroid*

Synonyms: 19-Norandrostenolone; Norandrosterone; 19-Nortestosterone.

17β-Hydroxyoestr-4-en-3-one
$C_{18}H_{26}O_2$ = 274·4

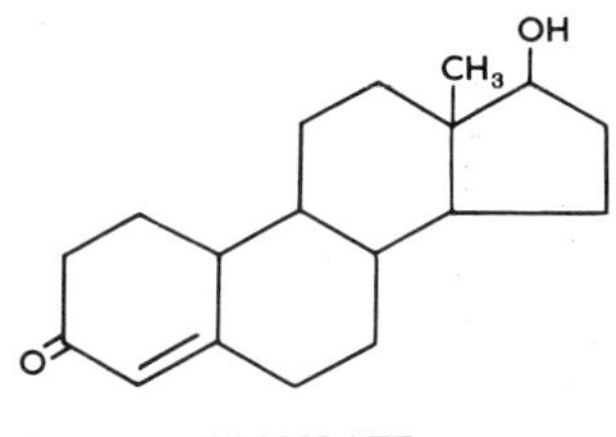

NANDROLONE DECANOATE
17β-Decanoyloxyoestr-4-en-3-one.
Proprietary Name: Deca-Durabolin.

A white crystalline powder. M.p. about 35°. Specific rotation of a 2% solution in dioxan, +32° to +36°.
Solubility. Almost insoluble in water; soluble 1 in 1 of ethanol; readily soluble in ether and chloroform.

NANDROLONE PHENYLPROPIONATE
17β-(β-Phenylpropionyloxy)oestr-4-en-3-one.
Synonym: Nandrolone Phenpropionate.
Proprietary Name: Durabolin.

A white crystalline powder. M.p. 95° to 99°. Specific rotation of a 1% solution in dioxan, +48° to +51°.
Solubility. Almost insoluble in water; soluble 1 in 20 of ethanol.

Extraction. Nandrolone is extracted from neutral solutions with freshly distilled ethyl acetate.

Ultraviolet Absorption Spectrum. Nandrolone decanoate in ethanol, maximum at about 239 mµ (E1%, 1cm about 400); nandrolone phenylpropionate in ethanol, maximum at about 240 mµ (E1%, 1cm 430).

Dose. Intramuscular: up to 100 mg of the decanoate every 3 weeks; up to 50 mg of the phenylpropionate weekly.

NAPHAZOLINE *Sympathomimetic*

2-(1-Naphthylmethyl)-2-imidazoline
$C_{14}H_{14}N_2$ = 210·3

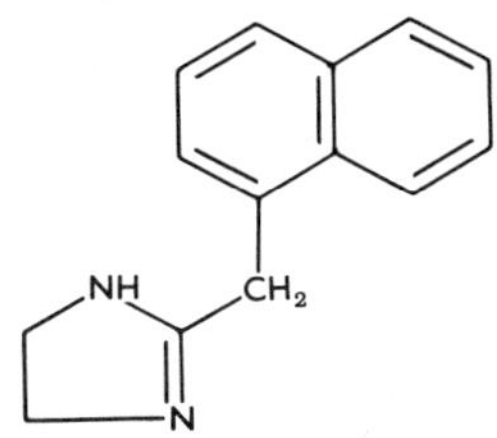

Naphazoline has a melting-point of about 120°.

NAPHAZOLINE HYDROCHLORIDE
Proprietary Names: Antan; Privine Hydrochloride.

A white crystalline powder. M.p. about 257°, with decomposition.
Solubility. Soluble 1 in 6 of water and 1 in 15 of ethanol; very slightly soluble in ether and chloroform.

NAPHAZOLINE NITRATE
Proprietary Name: Privine.

A white crystalline powder. M.p. about 168°.
Solubility. Soluble 1 in 36 of water and 1 in 16 of ethanol; almost insoluble in ether; very slightly soluble in chloroform.

Extraction. Naphazoline is extracted by organic solvents from aqueous alkaline solutions.

Chromatography. PAPER: system P1—Rf 0·51 (location under ultraviolet light, pale blue fluorescence; location reagents: *iodoplatinate spray*, strong reaction; *bromocresol green spray*, weak reaction); system RP1a—Rf 0·81 (location reagent *iodoplatinate spray*, positive reaction); system RP1b—Rf 0·76 (location reagent *iodoplatinate spray*, positive reaction).
THIN-LAYER: system T1—Rf 0·13 (location reagent *acidified iodoplatinate spray*, positive reaction).

GAS: system G2/225—retention time 0·36 relative to codeine.

Colour Tests. MICRO: sulphuric acid–formaldehyde test—grey-green (*sensitivity:* 1·0 μg); ammonium molybdate test—grey-purple → green (*sensitivity:* 0·5 μg); ammonium vanadate test—brown-purple (*sensitivity:* 0·5 μg); Vitali's rest— –/pale yellow/orange (*sensitivity:* 0·25 μg).

Crystal Tests. MICRO: *picric acid*—feathery rosettes (*sensitivity:* 1 in 400); *potassium permanganate solution*—masses of blades (*sensitivity:* 1 in 400).

Ultraviolet Absorption Spectrum. Naphazoline in 0·01N hydrochloric acid, maxima at 271 mμ (E1%, 1 cm 270), 281 mμ (E1%, 1 cm 311), 288 mμ (E1%, 1 cm 217), and 291 mμ (E1%, 1 cm about 217).

Infra-red Absorption Spectrum. Naphazoline (base). Potassium bromide disk. The principal peaks are: A 780 or 1615, B 791 or 1499, C 1211 (p. 792).

Metabolism. Naphazoline is very poorly absorbed through mucous membranes and therefore it exerts little or no systemic effect on local application.

Dose. The usual maximum dose is 3 drops of a 0·1% solution, intranasally.

Toxicity. LD50 (intravenous): in mice 170 and in rabbits 0·8 mg/kg.

NAPHTHALENE

$C_{10}H_8$ = 128·2

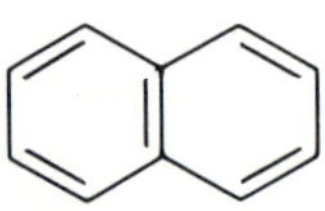

Colourless transparent scales. M.p. 80°. B.p. 218°.

Solubility. Insoluble in water; soluble in ethanol; soluble 1 in 1·5 of chloroform; very soluble in ether.

Extraction. Naphthalene is extracted by organic solvents from aqueous acid or alkaline solutions.

Chromatography. GAS: system G5—retention time 0·45 relative to barbitone.

Ultraviolet Absorption Spectrum. Naphthalene in ethanol, maxima at 220 mμ (E1%, 1 cm 7670), 266 mμ (E1%, 1 cm 411), 275 mμ (E1%, 1 cm 454), and 286 mμ (E1%, 1 cm 307).

Metabolism. Studies on the urine of various species have revealed the formation of a great many metabolites from naphthalene including 1-naphthol, 1-naphthylsulphuric acid, 1-naphthylglucuronide, 2-naphthol, 1,2-dihydroxynaphthalene, 1,2-dihydronaphthalene-1,2-diol, 1,2-dihydro-2-hydroxy-1-naphthylglucuronide, and 1-naphthylmercapturic acid.

Uses. A 10% oily solution has been used as a parasiticide in scabies and pediculosis. In the form of mothballs or flakes, it is employed to keep moths away from articles of clothing.

Toxicity. The lethal dose by ingestion is approximately 2 g. The maximum permissible atmospheric concentration is 10 p.p.m.

CASE EXAMPLES. Naphthalene vapour inhaled by 21 infants from their clothes and blankets, which had been stored with mothballs, caused serious poisoning. There were 2 fatalities (Valaes *et al.*, 1963). See also Picchioni (1960).

NARCEINE *Alkaloid*

$C_{23}H_{27}NO_8,3H_2O$ = 499·5

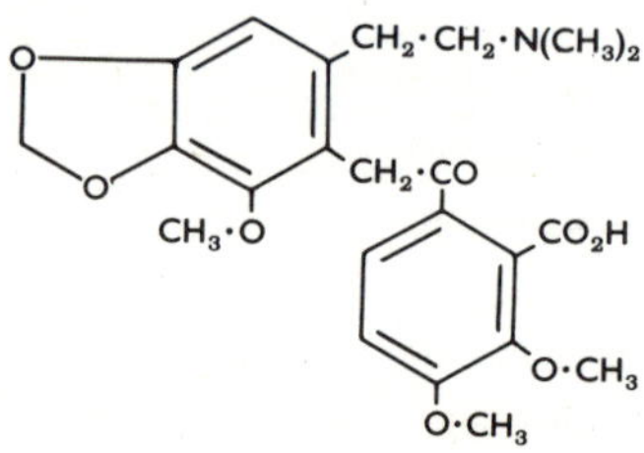

Narceine is an alkaloid of opium.

White silky crystals. M.p. 170° to 171°. The anhydrous substance melts at about 138° and is very hygroscopic.

Solubility. Slightly soluble in cold water; soluble in boiling water and ethanol; insoluble in ether; almost insoluble in chloroform.

NARCEINE HYDROCHLORIDE

Prismatic crystals. The anhydrous salt melts at 192° to 193°.

Solubility. Slightly soluble in hot water and ether; soluble in hot ethanol.

Extraction. Narceine is extracted by organic solvents from aqueous acid or alkaline solutions.

Chromatography. PAPER: system P1—Rf 0·46 (location under ultraviolet light, strong absorption; location reagent *iodoplatinate spray*, weak reaction).

THIN-LAYER: system T1—Rf 0·33 (location reagent *acidified iodoplatinate spray*, positive reaction).

Colour Tests. MICRO: sulphuric acid–formaldehyde test—brown → deep brown → green (*sensitivity:* 0·05 μg); ammonium molybdate test—brown → green (*sensitivity:* 0·05 μg); ammonium vanadate test—greenish-brown (*sensitivity:* 0·1 μg); Vitali's test—yellow/orange/orange (*sensitivity:* 0·5 μg).

Crystal Tests. MICRO: *lead iodide solution*—threadlike needles (*sensitivity:* 1 in 1500); *potassium tri-iodide solution (2)*—needles (*sensitivity:* 1 in 3000).

Ultraviolet Absorption Spectrum. Narceine in 0·1N hydrochloric acid, maximum at 277 mμ (E1%, 1 cm 291).

NARCOBARBITAL *Barbiturate*

Synonym: Enibomal.

Proprietary Names: Eunarcon; Narcodorm; Narkotal; Venopan.

5 - (2 - Bromoallyl) - 5 - isopropyl - 1 - methyl - barbituric acid

$C_{11}H_{15}BrN_2O_3 = 303{\cdot}2$

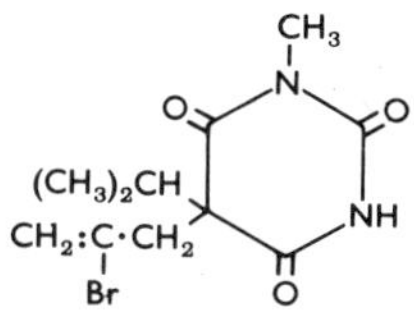

A white powder.

Solubility. Slightly soluble in water; soluble 1 in 20 of ethanol; soluble in ether and chloroform.

Screening Tests. See under Barbiturates, p. 208.

Extraction. Narcobarbital may be isolated in the A2 fraction (see p. 27).

Ultraviolet Absorption Spectrum. A 1,5,5-derivative—see Screening Test 3, p. 208.

Quantitative Estimation. See under Barbiturates, p. 208.

Metabolism. Narcobarbital is a very short-acting barbiturate—see Barbiturates, p. 207.

Dose. Up to 1 g intravenously.

NEALBARBITONE *Barbiturate*

Synonyms: Alneobarbital; Nealbarbital; Neallymalum.

Proprietary Names: Censedal; Nevental.

5-Allyl-5-neopentylbarbituric acid

$C_{12}H_{18}N_2O_3 = 238{\cdot}3$

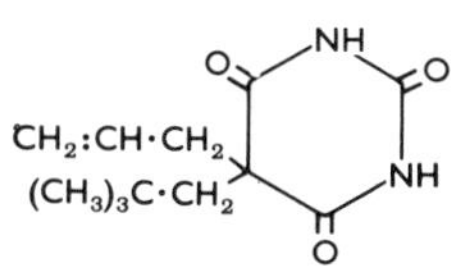

A white crystalline powder. M.p. 155° to 157°.

Solubility. Slightly soluble in water; soluble 1 in 4 of ethanol, 1 in 5 of ether, and 1 in 80 of chloroform.

Screening Tests. See under Barbiturates, p. 208.

Extraction. Nealbarbitone may be isolated in the A2 fraction (see p. 27).

Chromatography. PAPER: system P2—Rf 0·72 relative to amylobarbitone (location under ultraviolet light, dark spot).

THIN-LAYER: system T10—Rf 0·38 (location reagents: *mercurous nitrate spray*, black; *potassium permanganate spray*, yellow-brown; *Zwikker's reagent spray*, pink).

GAS: system G5—retention time 2·35 relative to barbitone.

Ultraviolet Absorption Spectrum. A 5,5-derivative—see Screening Test 3, p. 208.

Infra-red Absorption Spectrum. Potassium bromide disk. The principal peaks are: A 1695 or 1719, B 1364 or 1430, C 1320 or 1752 (p. 747).

Quantitative Estimation. See under Barbiturates, p. 208.

Dose. Usually up to 600 mg daily; up to 2·4 g daily has been given. It is an intermediate-acting barbiturate—see Barbiturates, p. 207.

NEOMYCIN *Antibiotic*

Neomycin, obtained from a selected strain of *Streptomyces fradiae*, consists of 2 isomers, neomycin B and neomycin C, the latter comprising about 10 to 15%. Neomycin A has been shown to be neamine, an inactive component and degradation product of neomycins B and C.

NEOMYCIN SULPHATE

A mixture of the sulphates of neomycin.

Synonyms: Fradiomycin; Neomycin.

Proprietary Names: Mycifradin; Neobiotic; Neolate; Neomin; Nivemycin.

A white hygroscopic powder which discolours at temperatures exceeding 30°.

Solubility. Readily soluble 1 in 3 of water and slowly soluble 1 in 1; very slightly soluble in ethanol; insoluble in ether and chloroform. A solution is dextrorotatory.

Chromatography. PAPER: system P1—Rf 0·00 (location reagents: *bromine–starch–potassium iodide*, strong reaction; *ninhydrin spray*, dull purple).

THIN-LAYER: system T1—Rf 0·00 (location reagent *potassium permanganate spray*, positive reaction).

Quantitative Estimation. Majumdar and Majumdar (1967) describe a method of quantitative estimation of the constituents of neomycin involving conversion to their *N*-acetyl derivatives, separation by paper chromatography, subsequent conversion to *N*-chloro-derivatives, and final spectrophotometric determination; assays of neomycin sulphate involving thin-layer chromatography are described by Foppiano and Brown (1965) and Vickers (1966).

Metabolism. Neomycin is poorly absorbed from the gastro-intestinal tract; demonstrable levels occur in the serum after 1 to 8 hours following oral administration of 4 g, the average peak level at 1 hour being 0·4 mg%. Only about 0·6% of the dose may be recovered unchanged from the urine in 24 hours (Kunin *et al.*, 1960). About 97% of an oral dose may be excreted unchanged in the faeces. However, neomycin is rapidly absorbed after intramuscular injection, 1 g producing peak blood-levels of about 2 mg% which are maintained for some 4 to 8 hours. Neomycin does not accumulate in the tissues but some passes into the cerebrospinal fluid; it is rapidly excreted unchanged in the urine.

Dose. As an intestinal antiseptic, up to 12 g daily, by mouth; for systemic infections, up to 1 g daily, intramuscularly.

Toxicity. Serious kidney damage and irreversible deafness may occur following parenteral administration for several days. Blood-levels of 20 mg% may be regarded as toxic and they can be attained very rapidly. Neomycin is relatively non-toxic when given orally or applied locally.

NEOPINE *Alkaloid*

Synonym: β-Codeine. It has been incorrectly called hydroxycodeine.

$C_{18}H_{21}NO_3 = 299{\cdot}4$

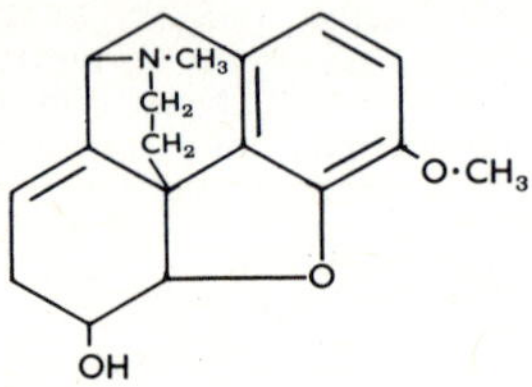

Neopine is an alkaloid of opium; it differs from codeine only in the position of the double bond which is between $C_{(8)}$ and $C_{(14)}$ instead of $C_{(7)}$ and $C_{(8)}$.

Long needle-shaped crystals. M.p. about 127°.

Solubility. Slightly soluble in water; soluble in chloroform.

NEOPINE HYDROBROMIDE.

The crystals darken at about 240° and decompose at about 283°.

Solubility. Almost insoluble in water hence ease of separation from other opium alkaloids.

Extraction. Neopine is extracted by organic solvents from aqueous alkaline solutions.

Chromatography. PAPER: system P1—Rf 0·18 (location under ultraviolet light, strong absorption; location reagents: *iodoplatinate spray*, strong reaction; *bromocresol green spray*, weak reaction).

THIN-LAYER: system T1—Rf 0·32 (location reagent *acidified iodoplatinate spray*, positive reaction).

Colour Tests. MICRO: sulphuric acid–formaldehyde test—blue-purple (*sensitivity:* 0·1 μg); ammonium molybdate test—blue → green (*sensitivity:* 0·05 μg); Vitali's test—yellow/yellow/orange (*sensitivity:* 1·0 μg).

Crystal Tests. MICRO: *mercuric chloride solution*—bunches of rods (*sensitivity:* 1 in 100); *potassium tri-iodide solution* (*3*)—large orange crystals (*sensitivity:* 1 in 100).

Ultraviolet Absorption Spectrum. Neopine in 0·1N sulphuric acid, maximum at 284 mμ (E 1%, 1 cm 39) and an inflexion at 277 mμ.

NEOSTIGMINE BROMIDE *Anticholinesterase*

Synonym: Synstigmine Bromide.

Proprietary Names: Leostigmin; Prostigmin (tablets).

(3 - Dimethylcarbamoyloxyphenyl)trimethyl - ammonium bromide

$C_{12}H_{19}BrN_2O_2 = 303{\cdot}2$

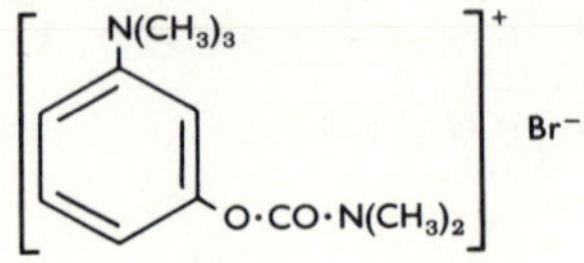

Colourless crystals or a white crystalline powder. M.p. 167°, with decomposition.

Solubility. Soluble 1 in 0·5 of water, 1 in 8 of ethanol, and 1 in 5 of chloroform; insoluble in ether.

NEOSTIGMINE METHYLSULPHATE

Synonym: Proserine.

Proprietary Name: Prostigmin (injection).

Colourless crystals or a white crystalline powder. M.p. 142° to 145°.

Solubility. Soluble 1 in 0·5 of water and 1 in 6 of ethanol.

Extraction. The neostigmine salts are quaternary ammonium compounds (see p. 29).

Chromatography. PAPER: system P1—Rf 0·20 (location under ultraviolet light, absorption; location reagents: *iodoplatinate spray*, weak reaction; *bromocresol green spray*, weak reaction); system RP1a—Rf 1·00 (location under ultraviolet light, absorption); system RP1b—Rf 0·66 (location as for RP1a).

THIN-LAYER: system T1—Rf 0·02 (location reagent *acidified iodoplatinate spray*, positive reaction).

Crystal Tests. MICRO: *lead iodide solution*—branching needles (*sensitivity:* 1 in 400); *platinic iodide solution*—bunches of curved needles (*sensitivity:* 1 in 400).

Ultraviolet Absorption Spectrum. Neostigmine methylsulphate in 1N sulphuric acid, maxima at 260 mμ (E 1%, 1 cm 20) and 266 mμ (E 1%, 1 cm 18).

Infra-red Absorption Spectrum. Neostigmine bromide. Potassium bromide disk. The principal peaks are: A 1711, B 1215, C 1154 (p. 748).

Metabolism. After oral administration of neostigmine, no unchanged drug was found in the urine on examination by paper chromatography but 2 metabolites were detected, one being identified as 3-hydroxyphenyltrimethylammonium bromide. After intramuscular injection, however, only unchanged neostigmine was found, no metabolites being detected (Scott *et al.*, 1962).

Studies in rats (Roberts *et al.*, 1967) have shown that 24 hours after intramuscular injection nearly 50% of the dose is excreted in the urine unchanged, the remainder being excreted as 3-hydroxyphenyltrimethylammonium bromide and its glucuronide conjugate in equal proportions.

Dose. Up to 30 mg by mouth; up to 2 mg by injection.

Toxicity. LD50 (oral): in mice 7·5 (bromide) and 14·4 (methylsulphate) mg/kg.

NIALAMIDE

Antidepressant/Monoamine Oxidase Inhibitor

Synonym: BEIH.

Proprietary Names: Espril; Niamid.

N - Benzyl - *β* - pyridine - 4 - carboxyhydrazidopropionamide

$C_{16}H_{18}N_4O_2 = 298{\cdot}3$

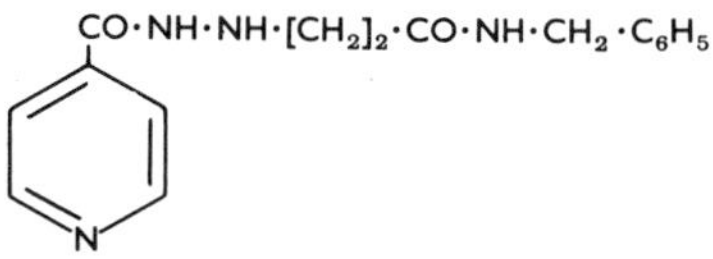

A white crystalline powder. M.p. 151° to 153°.

Solubility. Soluble 1 in 400 of water, 1 in 40 of ethanol, and 1 in 150 of chloroform.

Extraction. Nialamide is extracted by organic solvents from aqueous alkaline solutions.

Chromatography. PAPER: system P1—Rf 0·78 (location under ultraviolet light, absorption; location reagents: *iodoplatinate spray*, white; *potassium permanganate spray*, weak reaction); system RP1a—Rf 0·78 (location under ultraviolet light, absorption; location reagent *iodoplatinate spray*, positive reaction); system RP1b—Rf 0·77 (location as for RP1a).

THIN-LAYER: system T1—Rf 0·48 (location reagent *acidified iodoplatinate spray*, positive reaction).

Colour Tests. MICRO: ammonium molybdate test—(brown) light brown (*sensitivity:* 0·1 μg); ammonium vanadate test—red (*sensitivity:* 0·25 μg); Vitali's test— –/–/yellow (*sensitivity:* 0·5 μg).

Crystal Tests. MICRO: *gold bromide–hydrochloric acid solution*—feathery rosettes (unstable) (*sensitivity:* 1 in 400); *platinic chloride solution*—bunches of plates form at the edge of the drop (*sensitivity:* 1 in 100).

Ultraviolet Absorption Spectrum. Nialamide in 0·1N sodium hydroxide, maxima at 238 mμ (E1%, 1 cm 185) and 305 mμ (E1%, 1 cm 230); in 0·1N sulphuric acid, maximum at 264·5 mμ (E1%, 1 cm 250).

Dose. Up to 300 mg daily.

Toxicity. See under Phenelzine, p. 482.

NICOCODINE

Narcotic/Antitussive

Synonym: 6-Nicotinoylcodeine.

Proprietary Name: Lyopect.

7,8 - Dehydro - 4,5 - epoxy - 3 - methoxy - *N* - methyl-6-nicotinoyloxymorphinan

$C_{24}H_{24}N_2O_4 = 404{\cdot}5$

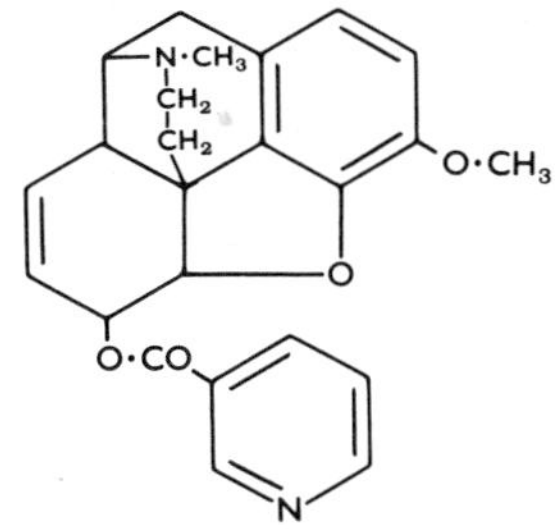

Extraction. Nicocodine is extracted by organic solvents from aqueous alkaline solutions.

Chromatography. PAPER: system P1—Rf 0·31 (location under ultraviolet light, absorption; location reagents: *iodoplatinate spray*, strong reaction; *bromocresol green spray*, weak reaction); system RP1a—Rf 0·66 (location reagent *iodoplatinate spray*, positive reaction); system RP1b—Rf 0·06 (location under ultraviolet light, absorption; location reagent *iodoplatinate spray*, positive reaction).

THIN-LAYER: system T1—Rf 0·36 (location reagent *acidified iodoplatinate spray*, positive reaction).

Colour Tests. MICRO: sulphuric acid–formaldehyde test—purple → blue-purple (*sensitivity:* 1 in 1000); ammonium molybdate test—green → blue → green (*sensitivity:* 1 in 1000); Vitali's test—yellow/yellow/orange (*sensitivity:* 1 in 1000).

Crystal Tests. MICRO: *potassium cadmium iodide solution*—blades, often serrated (*sensitivity:* 1 in 3000); *potassium iodide solution*—fine needles (*sensitivity:* 1 in 400).

Ultraviolet Absorption Spectrum. Nicocodine in 0·1N sulphuric acid, maxima at 261 mμ (E1%, 1 cm 251) and 267 mμ (E1%, 1 cm 230), and an inflexion at about 256 mμ.

NICOMORPHINE

Narcotic Analgesic

Synonyms: 3,6-Dinicotinylmorphine; Nicophin.

7,8 - Dehydro - 4,5 - epoxy - *N* - methyl - 3,6 - di(nicotinoyloxy)morphinan

$C_{29}H_{25}N_3O_5 = 495{\cdot}5$

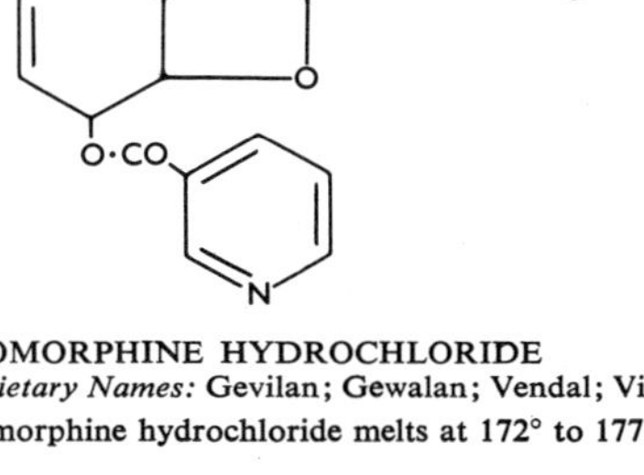

NICOMORPHINE HYDROCHLORIDE

Proprietary Names: Gevilan; Gewalan; Vendal; Vilan.

Nicomorphine hydrochloride melts at 172° to 177°.

Extraction. Nicomorphine is extracted by organic solvents from aqueous alkaline solutions.

Chromatography. PAPER: system P1—Rf 0·25 (location under ultraviolet light, absorption; location reagents: *iodoplatinate spray*, strong reaction; *bromocresol green spray*, weak reaction); system RP1a—Rf 0·56 (location under ultraviolet light, absorption; location reagent *iodoplatinate spray*, positive reaction); system RP1b—Rf 0·00 (location as for RP1a).

THIN-LAYER: system T1—Rf 0·36 (location reagent *acidified iodoplatinate spray*, positive reaction).

Colour Tests. MICRO: ammonium vanadate test—purple flash → olive (*sensitivity:* 0·25 μg); Vitali's test— -/-/orange (*sensitivity:* 1·0 μg).

Crystal Tests. MICRO: *picrolonic acid*—gelatinous rosettes, forming overnight (*sensitivity:* 1 in 400); *potassium iodide solution*—burrs, forming overnight (*sensitivity:* 1 in 400).

Ultraviolet Absorption Spectrum. Nicomorphine in 0·1N sulphuric acid, inflexion at about 256 mμ and maxima at 261·5 mμ (E1%, 1 cm 163) and about 268 mμ (E1%, 1 cm 138). Nicomorphine hydrochloride in 50% ethanol, maximum at 263 mμ; minimum at 247 mμ: in 0·1N sodium hydroxide, maxima at 256 mμ (E1%, 1 cm 222) and 298 mμ (E1%, 1 cm 56); minima at 243 mμ and 283 mμ.

NICOTINAMIDE *Vitamin*

Synonyms: Niacinamide; Nicotinic Acid Amide; Nicotylamide; Vitamin B_3; Vitamin PP.

Proprietary Names: Benicot; Nicamina; Nicobion; Nicosedine; Nicovel; Nicovit; Vi-nicotyl.

Pyridine-3-carboxyamide

$C_6H_6N_2O = 122{\cdot}1$

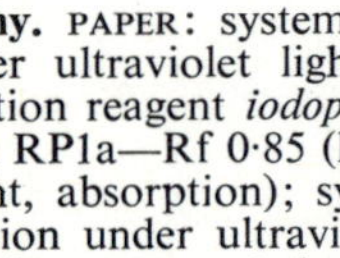

A white crystalline powder. M.p. 128° to 131°.

Solubility. Soluble 1 in 1 of water and 1 in 1·5 of ethanol; slightly soluble in ether and chloroform.

Chromatography. PAPER: system P1—Rf 0·47 (location under ultraviolet light, strong absorption; location reagent *iodoplatinate spray*, white); system RP1a—Rf 0·85 (location under ultraviolet light, absorption); system RP1b—Rf 0·79 (location under ultraviolet light, absorption; location reagent *iodoplatinate spray*, positive reaction).

THIN-LAYER: system T1—Rf 0·54, streaking (location reagent *iodine vapour*, positive reaction).

Colour Test. To 2 ml of a 0·1% solution add 6 ml of *cyanogen bromide solution* and 1 ml of a 2·5% v/v solution of aniline—golden-yellow.

Crystal Tests. MICRO: *gold chloride solution*—dense rosettes (*sensitivity:* 1 in 400); *platinic iodide solution*—masses of hairlike needles (*sensitivity:* 1 in 400).

Ultraviolet Absorption Spectrum. Nicotinamide in ethanol, maximum at 262 mμ (E1%, 1 cm 238), and inflexions at 257 mμ and 269 mμ; in 0·1N hydrochloric acid, maximum at 261 mμ (E1%, 1 cm 454).

Infra-red Absorption Spectrum. Potassium bromide disk. The principal peaks are: A 1300 or 1324, B 744 (p. 748).

Metabolism. Nicotinamide is the form in which nicotinic acid is generally found in nature. It is a component of the pyridine nucleotides which are essential co-enzymes for biochemical oxidations. The free amide and the free acid are interchangeable in the nutrition of higher animals; the normal daily human requirement is probably in the range 15 to 20 mg, depending on the protein intake. Nicotinamide lacks the vasodilating activity of nicotinic acid. Nicotinamide may be found unchanged in the urine together with nicotinic acid, *N*-methylnicotinamide, and nicotinuric acid.

Dose. The usual therapeutic dose is up to 250 mg daily.

Toxicity. LD50 (subcutaneous): in rats 1·68 g/kg.

NICOTINE *Pesticide*

1-Methyl-2-(3-pyridyl)pyrrolidine

$C_{10}H_{14}N_2 = 162{\cdot}2$

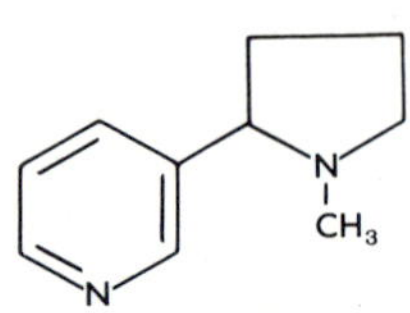

An alkaloid obtained from the leaves of the tobacco plant, *Nicotiana tabacum* (Solanaceae). A colourless to pale yellow, volatile, very hygroscopic, oily liquid which gradually becomes brown on exposure to air or light.

B.p. 247°, with decomposition. Refractive index 1·5280.

Solubility. Soluble in water, ethanol, ether, and chloroform.

Extraction. Nicotine is extracted by organic solvents from aqueous alkaline solutions; it is volatile and may be isolated by distillation from alkaline solutions (see p. 18).

NOTE. Great care must be exercised in the evaporation of solutions of nicotine in ether or chloroform; the final stages are best done at room temperature.

Chromatography. PAPER: system P1—Rf 0·07 (location under ultraviolet light, strong absorption; location reagents: *iodoplatinate spray*, strong reaction; *bromocresol green spray*, weak reaction); system RP1a—Rf 0·99 (location under ultraviolet light, absorption; location reagent *iodoplatinate spray*, positive reaction); system RP1b—Rf 0·39 (location reagent *iodoplatinate spray*, positive reaction).

THIN-LAYER: system T1—Rf 0·57 (location reagent *acidified iodoplatinate spray*, positive reaction).

GAS: system G2/120—retention time 0·84 relative to ephedrine; system G5—retention time 0·71 relative to barbitone; system G6—retention time 0·08 relative to codeine.

Crystal Tests. MICRO: *mercuric chloride solution*—rosettes of blades (*sensitivity:* 1 in 1500); *picric acid*—branching needles (*sensitivity:* 1 in 3000).

Ultraviolet Absorption Spectrum. Nicotine in 0·1N sulphuric acid, maximum at 260 mμ (E 1%, 1 cm 490).

Infra-red Absorption Spectrum. Capillary film between potassium bromide windows. The principal peaks are: A 712, B 1429, C 810 or 1022 (p. 748).

Quantitative Estimation. Beckett and Triggs (1966) describe a method of extraction of nicotine and its primary metabolite, cotinine, from urine, followed by gas chromatographic determination.

Metabolism. Nicotine is metabolised in man and various animal species by oxidation at position 5 of the pyrrolidine ring to yield cotinine, which may be further metabolised by hydroxylation or demethylation or cleavage of the pyrrolidine ring to yield γ-(3-pyridyl)-β-oxo-*N*-methylbutyramide (Bowman and McKennis, 1962; Hansson and Schmiterlöw, 1962).

Nicotine is readily absorbed from the gastro-intestinal tract, the respiratory tract, and the intact skin. When cigarette smoke is inhaled, 90 to 98% of the nicotine in the smoke is retained in the respiratory tract. The nicotine blood-level of smokers is usually less than 0·03 mg%. Nicotine is readily distributed throughout the tissues and it is also in the milk of lactating women who smoke.

Urinary excretion of unchanged nicotine accounts for only a small percentage of the administered dose but it is greater when the urine is acid. Under normal conditions, subjects who simultaneously smoked 2 cigarettes after abstaining from smoking for a period of 24 hours excreted in the following 24 hours, 0·1 to 0·5 mg of nicotine and 0·25 to 0·6 mg of cotinine; when the urine was acidified by oral ingestion of ammonium chloride the values were 0·5 to 0·8 mg of nicotine in 8 hours and 0·3 to 0·9 mg of cotinine in 22 hours (Beckett and Triggs, 1966).

Use. Nicotine is mainly used as a horticultural pesticide either as a vapour or as a spray.

Toxicity. Nicotine is one of the most toxic substances known. The lethal dose in man is from 40 to 60 mg. It is rapidly absorbed through the skin and most cases of posioning are due to its careless handling when employed as a horticultural insecticide.

Lethal concentrations of nicotine were found in organs which had been preserved for 1 year at about 0° or −20° and also in others which had been preserved for 1 year in formaldehyde at 10° to 15° (Tiess, 1966a).

LD50 (oral): in rats 55 mg/kg.

CASE EXAMPLES. The nicotine levels in 3 fatal cases were: blood, 0·5 to 5·2 mg%; liver, 10 to 20 mg%; stomach contents, 60 to 2000 mg (Turner, 1964a).

Post-mortem examination of a 55-year-old chronic alcoholic revealed the following nicotine levels: blood (heart), 10 mg%; blood (venous), 0·4 mg%; brain, 1·1 mg%; duodenal contents, 305 mg; faeces, 32 mg%; intestine (small), 225 mg; kidney, 4·5 mg%; stomach contents, 396 mg; urine, a trace. The possibility of post-mortem contamination of heart and spleen samples with those of the gastro-intestinal tract cannot be excluded (Tiess, 1966a).

In a series of cases of poisoning the following levels of nicotine were found: bile, 9·5 to 250 mg%; blood, 53 to 60 mg%; kidney, 2·5 to 25 mg%; liver, 45 to 500 mg%; stomach contents, 23 to 5850 mg; urine, 1·7 to 5·8 mg% (Jackson, 1967).

NICOTINIC ACID *Vitamin/Vasodilator*

Synonyms: Niacin; Vitamin PP.

Proprietary Names: Efacin; Nicamin; Niconazid; Niconacid; Nico-Span; Nicovel; Nicyl; Pelonin.

Pyridine-3-carboxylic acid

$C_6H_5NO_2 = 123{\cdot}1$

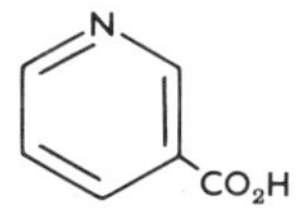

White crystals or a crystalline powder. M.p. 234° to 237°.

Solubility. Soluble 1 in 55 of water and 1 in 100 of ethanol; freely soluble in boiling water and boiling ethanol; almost insoluble in ether and chloroform.

Extraction. Nicotinic acid is extracted by organic solvents from aqueous acid solutions.

Chromatography. PAPER: system P1—Rf 0·55 (location under ultraviolet light, absorption; location reagent *iodoplatinate spray*, white); system RP1a—Rf 0·89 (location under ultraviolet light, absorption; location reagent *iodoplatinate spray*, positive reaction); system RP1b—Rf 0·87 (location as for RP1a).

THIN-LAYER: system T1—Rf 0·58 (location reagent *iodine vapour*, positive reaction).

Colour Test. To 2 ml of a 0·1% solution, add 6 ml of *cyanogen bromide solution* and 1 ml of a 2·5% v/v solution of aniline—golden-yellow → red-orange.

Crystal Tests. MICRO: *picrolonic acid*—bunches of needles (*sensitivity:* 1 in 400); *potassium bismuth iodide solution*—plates or rods (*sensitivity:* 1 in 400).

Ultraviolet Absorption Spectrum. Nicotinic acid in ethanol, maxima at about 257 mμ (E1%, 1cm 221) and 262 mμ (E1%, 1cm 237); in 0·1N sulphuric acid, inflexion at about 255 mμ (E1%, 1cm 470), and maxima at 260·5 mμ (E1%, 1cm 559) and about 266·5 mμ (E1%, 1cm 441).

Infra-red Absorption Spectrum. Potassium bromide disk. The principal peaks are: A 1300 or 1324, B 744 (p. 748).

Metabolism. Nicotinic acid is an essential growth factor in animals. In the form of nicotinamide it is a component of the pyridine nucleotides which are essential co-enzymes for biochemical oxidations. The free acid and the free amide are interchangeable in the nutrition of higher animals; the normal daily human requirement is probably in the range 15 to 20 mg, depending on the protein intake. Nicotinic acid may be found unchanged in the urine together with nicotinamide, *N*-methylnicotinamide, and nicotinuric acid.

Dose. The usual therapeutic dose is up to 250 mg daily.

Toxicity. LD50 (oral): in rats 7 g/kg.

NICOTINYL ALCOHOL *Vasodilator*

Synonyms: 3-Hydroxymethylpyridine; Nicotinic Alcohol; NU 2121; 3-Pyridinemethanol; β-Pyridylcarbinol.
Proprietary Names: Roniacol; Ronicol (injection).

Pyrid-3-ylmethanol

$C_6H_7NO = 109{\cdot}1$

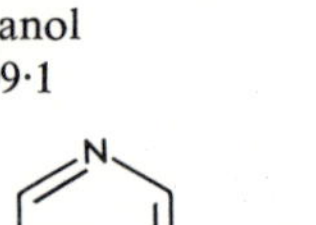

A very hygroscopic liquid. B.p. 144° to 145° at 16 mm Hg. Refractive index 1·5425.
Solubility. Very soluble in water and ether.

NICOTINYL TARTRATE
Proprietary Names: Niacol; Roniacol; Ronicol (tablets).
A crystalline solid.
Solubility. Freely soluble in water and ethanol; soluble in ether.

Extraction. Nicotinyl alcohol is extracted by organic solvents from aqueous alkaline solutions.

Chromatography. PAPER: system P1—Rf 0·16 (location under ultraviolet light, strong absorption; location reagent *iodoplatinate spray*, weak reaction); system RP1a—Rf 0·89 (location under ultraviolet light, absorption; location reagent *iodoplatinate spray*, positive reaction); system RP1b—Rf 0·81 (location as for RP1a).

THIN-LAYER: system T1—Rf 0·65 (location reagent *iodine–carbon tetrachloride spray*, positive reaction).

GAS: system G5—retention time 0·31 relative to barbitone.

Crystal Tests. MICRO: *picrolonic acid*—bunches of fine hairlike needles (*sensitivity:* 1 in 400); *potassium bismuth iodide solution*—rhomboidal plates and prisms (*sensitivity:* 1 in 1000).

Ultraviolet Absorption Spectrum. Nicotinyl alcohol in 0·1N sulphuric acid, maximum at 260 mμ (E1%, 1cm 254).

Infra-red Absorption Spectrum. Nicotinyl alcohol. Potassium bromide disk. The principal peaks are: A 675 or 1215 or 1262 or 1305, B 1556, C 788 (p. 792).

Dose. Usually up to 200 mg daily.

NICOUMALONE *Anticoagulant*

Synonyms: Acenocoumarin; Acenocoumarol; G 23350.
Proprietary Names: Sinthrome; Sintrom.

3-(α-Acetonyl-4-nitrobenzyl)-4-hydroxycoumarin

$C_{19}H_{15}NO_6 = 353{\cdot}3$

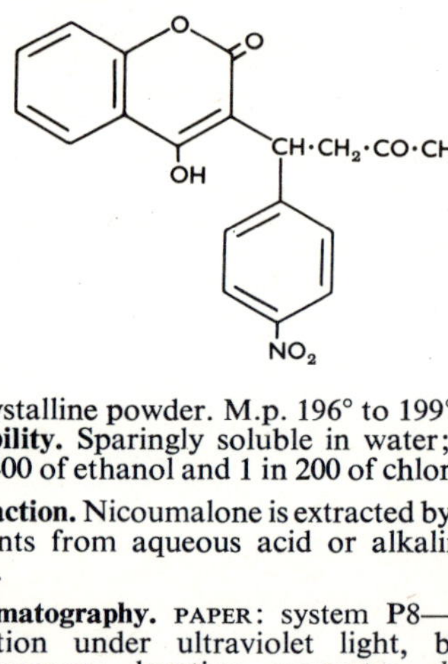

A crystalline powder. M.p. 196° to 199°.
Solubility. Sparingly soluble in water; soluble 1 in 400 of ethanol and 1 in 200 of chloroform.

Extraction. Nicoumalone is extracted by organic solvents from aqueous acid or alkaline solutions.

Chromatography. PAPER: system P8—Rf 0·88 (location under ultraviolet light, brownish fluorescence; location reagents: *diazotised o-dianisidine spray*, white; *diazotised sulphanilic acid spray*, white); system P9—Rf 0·28 (location as for P8); system P10—Rf 0·80 (location as for P8).

Ultraviolet Absorption Spectrum. Nicoumalone in 0·1N sulphuric acid, maxima at 283 mμ E1%, 1cm 660) and 304 mμ (E1%, 1cm 620).

Metabolism. Nicoumalone is excreted largely unchanged in the urine.

Dose. 2 to 16 mg daily, according to the prothrombin activity of the blood.

NIFENAZONE *Analgesic/Anti-inflammatory*

Synonym: Nicotinylamidoantipyrine.
Proprietary Names: Dolongan; Nicopyron; Thylin.

1,5 - Dimethyl - 4 - nicotinamido - 3 - oxo - 2 - phenylpyrazoline
$C_{17}H_{16}N_4O_2 = 308{\cdot}3$

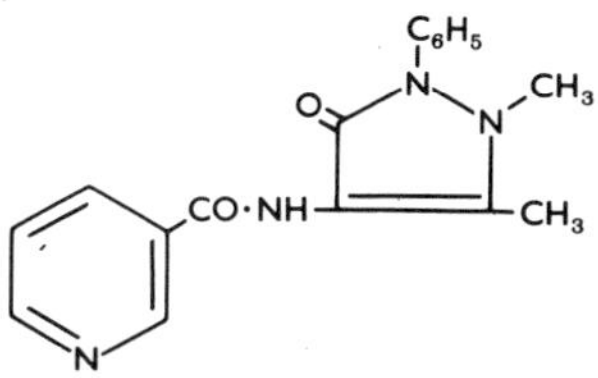

Extraction. Nifenazone is extracted by organic solvents from aqueous acid or alkaline solutions.

Chromatography. PAPER: system P1—Rf 0·73 (location under ultraviolet light, strong absorption; location reagent *iodoplatinate spray*, weak reaction).

THIN-LAYER: system T1—Rf 0·57 (location reagent *potassium permanganate spray*, positive reaction).

GAS: system G2/225—retention time 0·50 relative to diphenhydramine.

Colour Test. MICRO: ammonium molybdate test—faint grey-blue (*sensitivity:* 1·0 μg).

Crystal Tests. MICRO: *potassium cyanide solution*—irregular tablets (*sensitivity:* 1 in 100); *sodium carbonate solution*—irregular tablets (*sensitivity:* 1 in 100).

Ultraviolet Absorption Spectrum. Nifenazone in 0·1N sulphuric acid, maximum at 261 mμ (E 1%, 1 cm 496).

Metabolism. Nifenazone is rapidly absorbed from the gastro-intestinal tract. It is excreted practically unchanged in the urine, only small amounts being excreted as 4-aminophenazone and nicotinic acid. Excretion continues for several days so that 40 to 90% of a dose may be detected in the urine within a period of 4 days (Hoffmann and Roller, 1964).

Dose. Usually up to 1·5 g daily; doses of up to 3 g daily have been given.

Toxicity. LD50 (subcutaneous): in mice 3·75 g/kg.

NIKETHAMIDE *Central Stimulant*

Synonyms: Aminocordine; Cardiamide; Diethylamide Nicotinic Acid; Nicethamidum; Nicorine; Nikethylamide.
Proprietary Names: Anacardone; Cardiamina; Coramine; Cordiamin; Cormed; Corvotone; Nicamide; Niketharol; Nikorin.

Pyridine-3-carboxydiethylamide
$C_{10}H_{14}N_2O = 178{\cdot}2$

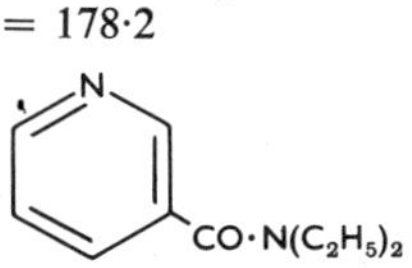

A colourless or yellowish oily liquid or crystalline solid. B.p. 280°. F.p. 23° to 25°. Refractive index, at 20°, 1·524 to 1·526.

Solubility. Miscible with water, ethanol, ether, and chloroform.

Extraction. Nikethamide is extracted by organic solvents from aqueous acid or alkaline solutions.

Chromatography. PAPER: system P1—Rf 0·86 (location under ultraviolet light, strong absorption; location reagent *iodoplatinate spray*, strong reaction); system RP1a—Rf 0·65 (location under ultraviolet light, absorption); system RP1b—Rf 0·68 (location under ultraviolet light, absorption; location reagent *iodoplatinate spray*, positive reaction).

THIN-LAYER: system T1—Rf 0·67 (location reagent *iodine vapour*, positive reaction).

GAS: system G2/120—retention time 1·9 relative to ephedrine.

Crystal Test. MICRO: *gold bromide–hydrochloric acid solution*—serrated rods or prisms (*sensitivity:* 1 in 200).

Ultraviolet Absorption Spectrum. Nikethamide in 0·1N sodium hydroxide, maxima at 255 mμ (E 1%, 1 cm 840) and 260 mμ (E 1%, 1 cm 860); in 0·1N sulphuric acid, maximum at 263·5 mμ (E 1%, 1 cm 273).

Infra-red Absorption Spectrum. Capillary film between potassium bromide windows. The principal peaks are: A 1627, B 1437, C 1285 or 1412 or 1460 (p. 748).

Metabolism. Nikethamide is rapidly absorbed and converted in the body to nicotinamide; it is also rapidly excreted.

Dose. Up to 2 g intravenously.

NITRAZEPAM *Hypnotic*

Synonym: Ro 4-5360.
Proprietary Names: Megadon; Mogadon.

1,2 - Dihydro - 7 - nitro - 2 - oxo - 5 - phenyl - 3*H*-1,4-benzodiazepine
$C_{15}H_{11}N_3O_3 = 281{\cdot}3$

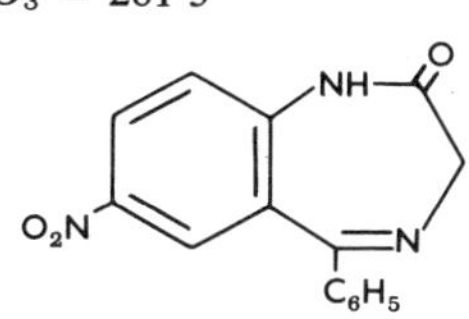

A yellow crystalline powder. M.p. 224° to 226°.

Solubility. Insoluble in water and ether; soluble in ethanol and chloroform.

Screening Tests. See under Screening Tests, p. 13.

Extraction. Nitrazepam is extracted by organic solvents from aqueous alkaline solutions.

Chromatography. PAPER: system P1—Rf about 0·92 (location under ultraviolet light, strong absorption).

THIN-LAYER: system T1—Rf 0·74 (location reagent *Dragendorff spray*, positive reaction).
GAS: system G2/225—retention time 2·94 relative to codeine.

Ultraviolet Absorption Spectrum. Nitrazepam in ethanol, maxima at 218 mμ and 260 mμ; minimum at about 242 mμ; in 0·1N sulphuric acid, maximum at 277·5 mμ (E1%, 1cm 1500) and an inflexion at about 340 mμ.

Infra-red Absorption Spectrum. Potassium bromide disk. The principal peaks are: A 1352 or 1692, B 702 or 1615 (p. 748).

Metabolism. Nitrazepam is a rapidly acting non-barbiturate hypnotic whose action is similar to that of the intermediate-acting barbiturates. It may accumulate since only 23% of a dose is excreted in the urine within 48 hours of administration—4·8% as unchanged drug, 8·2% as a 7-amino-metabolite, and 9·8% as a 7-acetylamino-metabolite. Some nitrazepam may be excreted in the faeces, as it is incompletely absorbed.

Dose. Usually 5 mg; doses of up to 20 mg have been given.

Toxicity. Doses of up to 300 mg have been taken without harmful effect.
LD50 (oral): in mice 1·8 and in rats 2 g/kg.

NITROBENZENE

Synonyms: Nitrobenzol; Oil of Mirbane.

$C_6H_5{\cdot}NO_2$ = 123·1

A pale yellow oily liquid. B.p. between 210° and 211°.
Solubility. Almost insoluble in water; miscible with ethanol, ether, and benzene.

Extraction. Nitrobenzene is volatile and may be isolated by distillation; it may also be isolated in the A2 fraction (see p. 27).

Chromatography. PAPER and THIN-LAYER: Bonnichsen *et al.* (1966) describe a paper system and a thin-layer system, both of which will detect nitrobenzene.

Ultraviolet Absorption Spectrum. Nitrobenzene in ethanol, maximum at 258·5 mμ (E1%, 1cm 697).

Quantitative Estimation. A spectrophotometric method of determination is described by Bonnichsen *et al.* (1966).

Metabolism. Nitrobenzene is metabolised fairly slowly in man and animals to a variety of products, some of which are very toxic. The 2 main routes of metabolism are oxidation to the *o*-, *m*-, and *p*-nitrophenols and reduction to aniline and *p*-aminophenol. *p*-Aminophenol is the chief urinary metabolite, being excreted largely as the glucuronide conjugate. The nitrophenols may be oxidised further to 4-nitrocatechol and nitroquinol. The conversion of nitrobenzene into the conjugated forms of these various phenols results in its detoxication.

The main toxic effect of nitrobenzene, the formation of methaemoglobin, is probably due to *p*-nitrophenol and *p*-aminophenol, both very toxic, and to the intermediates involved in the conversion of nitrobenzene to aniline (Brodie and Axelrod, 1949; Kiese, 1965).
Some unchanged nitrobenzene may be excreted in the expired air, and a small quantity of metabolites may be found in the faeces.

Toxicity. In man, 1 g may be fatal. The maximum permissible atmospheric concentration is 1 p.p.m.

CASE EXAMPLES. Reports of 2 deaths probably due to accidental ingestion of nitrobenzene with alcohol—(1) a man, aged 55, at post-mortem examination, had nitrobenzene levels: in blood, 0·05 mg%; in brain, 0·14 mg%; in kidney, 1·05 mg%; (2) a 42-year-old man had levels: in brain, 0·47 mg%; in kidney, 1·25 mg% (Bonnichsen *et al.*, 1966).

NITROFURANTOIN *Antibacterial (Urinary)*

Proprietary Names: Berkfurin; Furadantin; Furadoine; Furan; Furina; N-Fur; Nitoin.

1-(5-Nitrofurfurylideneamino)hydantoin
$C_8H_6N_4O_5$ = 238·2

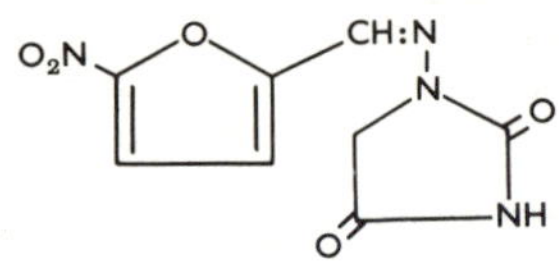

Yellow crystals.
Solubility. Soluble 1 in 5000 of water and 1 in 2000 of ethanol.

Extraction. Nitrofurantoin is extracted by organic solvents from acid or alkaline solutions.

Colour Test. Dissolve 5 mg in 5 ml of 0·1N sodium hydroxide—deep yellow→deep orange-red.

Ultraviolet Absorption Spectrum. Nitrofurantoin in *dimethylformamide–sodium acetate trihydrate solution*, maxima at 266 mμ and 367 mμ (E1%, 1cm 765).

Infra-red Absorption Spectrum. Potassium bromide disk. The principal peaks are: A 1345 or 1716, B 1239, C 1200 or 1435 (p. 749).

Quantitative Estimation. Conklin and Hollifield (1965) describe a spectrophotometric estimation of nitrofurantoin in urine. Jones *et al.* (1965) give methods for the polarographic and microbiological determination of nitrofurantoin in urine.

Metabolism. After oral ingestion, nitrofurantoin is readily absorbed and about 50% excreted unchanged in the urine. No antibacterial activity is detected in the blood, perhaps because the drug is bound to plasma protein. In 12 patients receiving 100 mg of nitrofurantoin thrice daily, the mean plasma level was found to be 0·18 mg% (Loughridge, 1962).

Dose. Up to 600 mg daily.

Toxicity. According to the Report of the U.S. Registry on Blood Dyscrasias for 1962, haemolytic anaemia occurred in 3 patients given nitrofurantoin alone and 6 other reports of toxicity were made where nitrofurantoin was given with other drugs (Best, 1963).
Polyneuropathy developed in 5 patients treated for long periods, up to 7 months, with nitrofurantoin (Rubenstein, 1964).

NITROFURAZONE *Antibacterial*

Synonyms: Furacilin; Nitrofural.
Proprietary Names: Furacin; Furalone; Nefco; Nifuzon.

5-Nitrofurfuraldehyde semicarbazone
$C_6H_6N_4O_4 = 198{\cdot}1$

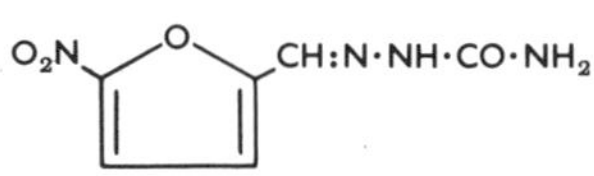

A lemon-yellow crystalline powder which turns brownish-black on heating at high temperatures and decomposes between 236° and 240°.
Solubility. Very slightly soluble in water; soluble 1 in 600 of ethanol; almost insoluble in ether and chloroform.

Extraction. Nitrofurazone is extracted by organic solvents from aqueous acid or alkaline solutions.

Colour Test. Dissolve 10 mg in 10 ml of a 5% sodium hydroxide solution—dark orange-red.

Ultraviolet Absorption Spectrum. Nitrofurazone in ethanol diluted to 0·005% with water, maxima at 260 mμ and 375 mμ (E1%, 1 cm 810); minimum at 306 mμ.

Quantitative Estimation. Nitrofurazone may be estimated spectrophotometrically following its conversion to the phenylhydrazone derivative (Herrett and Buzard, 1960).
Cross *et al.* (1960) have developed a spectrophotometric method for determining nitrofurazone in feed mixes.

Metabolism. Nitrofurazone is extensively metabolised in the body.

Dose. Although mainly used for topical application, usually as a 0·2% ointment or solution, nitrofurazone has been given by mouth in doses of up to 500 mg daily.

Toxicity. Toxic effects, including polyneuritis, which may be irreversible, jaundice, and leucopenia may follow oral ingestion. Sensitisation may be produced by continuous local application.
LD50 (oral): in mice 580 mg/kg.

NORACYMETHADOL *Narcotic Analgesic*

Synonym: ARC I-C-25.

α - (±) - 1 - Ethyl - 4 - methylamino - 2,2 - diphenylpentyl acetate
$C_{22}H_{29}NO_2 = 339{\cdot}5$

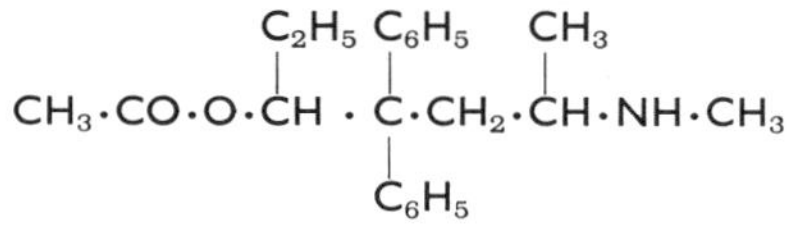

Solubility. Soluble in dilute acetic acid.

NORACYMETHADOL HYDROCHLORIDE

Synonym: NIH 7667.

Extraction. Noracymethadol is extracted by organic solvents from aqueous alkaline solutions.

Chromatography. PAPER: system P1—Rf 0·79 (location reagents: *iodoplatinate spray*, weak reaction; *bromocresol green spray*, strong reaction).
THIN-LAYER: system T1—Rf 0·51 (location reagent *acidified iodoplatinate spray*, positive reaction).

Colour Tests. MICRO: sulphuric acid–formaldehyde test—brown-purple (*sensitivity:* 0·25 μg); ammonium molybdate test—dull purple (*sensitivity:* 0·25 μg); ammonium vanadate test—dull purple→grey-green (*sensitivity:* 0·25 μg); Vitali's test— –/–/brown (*sensitivity:* 0·25 μg).

Crystal Tests. MICRO: *potassium chromate solution*—dense rosettes (*sensitivity:* 1 in 1500); *potassium iodide solution*—rosettes of plates (*sensitivity:* 1 in 400).

Ultraviolet Absorption Spectrum. Noracymethadol in 0·1N sulphuric acid, maxima at 253 mμ (E1%, 1 cm 12·7), 258 mμ (E1%, 1 cm 14·3), 264 mμ (E1%, 1 cm 12·3), and about 269 mμ (E1%, 1 cm 8).

NORADRENALINE *Sympathomimetic*

Synonyms: *l*-Arterenol; Levarterenol; *l*-Norepinephrine; Norepirenamine.

(–)-2-Amino-1-(3,4-dihydroxyphenyl)ethanol
$C_8H_{11}NO_3 = 169{\cdot}2$

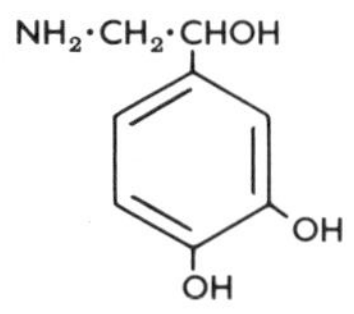

Noradrenaline occurs as microcrystals which melt at 217°, with decomposition.
Solubility. Slightly soluble in water, ethanol, and ether.

NORADRENALINE ACID TARTRATE

Synonyms: Noradrenaline Bitartrate; Noradrenaline Hydrogen Tartrate.
Proprietary Names: Adrenor; Aktamin; Levophed; Noradrec.

A white crystalline powder. M.p. about 102°.
Solubility. Soluble 1 in 2·5 of water and 1 in 300 of ethanol; almost insoluble in ether and chloroform.

NORADRENALINE HYDROCHLORIDE
Noradrenaline hydrochloride occurs as crystals which melt at about 145° to 146°.
Solubility. Freely soluble in water.

Chromatography. PAPER: system P1—Rf 0·04 (location under ultraviolet light, absorption; location reagents: *Marquis reagent*, red-brown; *potassium permanganate spray*, strong reaction).
THIN-LAYER: system T1—Rf 0·23 (location reagent *potassium permanganate spray*, positive reaction).

Colour Tests. Chen's test—green→greenish-brown.
MICRO: sulphuric acid–formaldehyde test—faint brown (*sensitivity:* 1·0 μg); ammonium molybdate test—(brown) grey (*sensitivity:* 0·5 μg); ammonium vanadate test—(grey) orange (*sensitivity:* 0·5 μg); Vitali's test—yellow/orange/olive (*sensitivity:* 0·5 μg).

Ultraviolet Absorption Spectrum. Noradrenaline in 0·01N hydrochloric acid, maximum at 279 mμ (E1%, 1 cm about 84).

Infra-red Absorption Spectrum. Noradrenaline acid tartrate. Potassium bromide disk. The principal peaks are: A 1300, B 1210, C 1412 or 1602 (p. 749).

Quantitative Estimation. Noradrenaline and adrenaline may be estimated spectrofluorimetrically in urine following column chromatographic separation (Pekkarinen and Pitkänen, 1955).
Choulis (1967) describes a method of separation of adrenaline from dopamine and noradrenaline involving thin-layer chromatography and subsequent determination by spectrophotometry.

Metabolism. Noradrenaline is present in the adrenal glands from which it is liberated together with adrenaline but, unlike adrenaline, it has little or no bronchodilator or vasodilator action. It is not absorbed from the gastro-intestinal tract but when injected it disappears rapidly from the circulation into the tissues.
When infused intravenously only 3 to 6% is excreted in the urine unchanged, the remainder being deactivated by oxidative deamination or *O*-methylation in the intestine and the liver. The resulting compounds, 3,4-dihydroxymandelic acid and the 3-*O*-methylated amine, normetanephrine (p. 449), are excreted free, as sulphate or glucuronide conjugates, or as a further metabolite, 3-methoxy-4-hydroxymandelic acid.

Dose. Up to 20 micrograms (μg) per minute, by intravenous infusion, according to the patient's blood-pressure.

Toxicity. The estimated minimum lethal dose in children is 10 mg by intramuscular or subcutaneous injection.

Extravasation of the solution may cause serious local ischaemia and skin necrosis.

NORBORMIDE *Rodenticide*

Synonym: McN 1025.
Proprietary Names: Shoxin. It is the main ingredient of the rat-bait, RATicate.

5 - (α - Hydroxy - α - pyrid - 2′ - ylbenzyl) - 7 - (α - pyrid - 2′ - ylbenzylidene)bicyclo[2,2,1]hept-5-ene-2,3-dicarboximide
$C_{33}H_{25}N_3O_3$ = 511·6

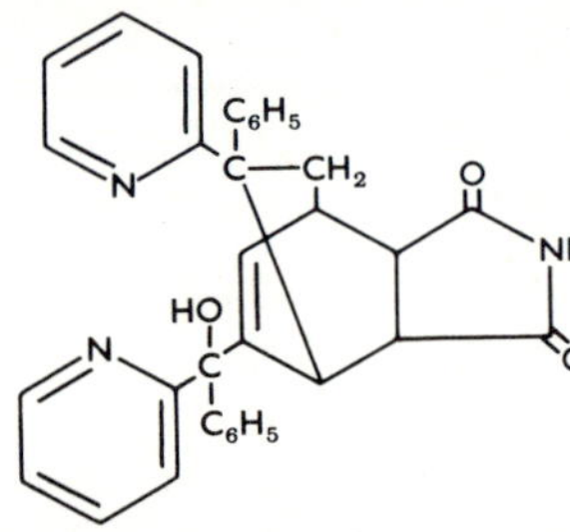

Norbormide is a mixture of stereoisomers. It is a white crystalline solid. M.p. 190° to 198°.
Solubility. Almost insoluble in water; slightly soluble in ethanol; very slightly soluble in ether; soluble in chloroform.

Extraction. Norbormide is extracted by organic solvents from aqueous alkaline solutions.

Chromatography. PAPER: system P1—Rf 0·87 (location under ultraviolet light, bright blue fluorescence; location reagents: *iodoplatinate spray*, strong reaction; *potassium permanganate spray*, weak reaction).
THIN-LAYER: system T1—Rf 0·72 (location reagent *acidified iodoplatinate spray*, positive reaction).
GAS: system G2/225—retention time 0·49 (0·44) relative to codeine.

Colour Test. MICRO: ammonium molybdate test—blue, forming slowly (*sensitivity:* 0·5 μg).

Crystal Test. MICRO: *platinic chloride solution*—dense yellow rosettes, forming slowly (*sensitivity:* 1 in 400).

Ultraviolet Absorption Spectrum. Norbormide in 4% methanol in 0·1N hydrochloric acid, maxima at 238 mμ and 300 mμ (E1%, 1 cm 136); minimum at 287 mμ.

Infra-red Absorption Spectrum. Potassium bromide disk. The principal peaks are: A 1708, B 701, C 751 (p. 792).

Quantitative Estimation. The stereoisomers may be separated by thin-layer chromatography and estimated spectrophotometrically (Janicki *et al.*, 1966).

Toxicity. Norbormide is a rodenticide which is specific for the *Rattus* genus. The lethal dose in man is probably about 10 g.

LD50 (oral): in mice 2·25 g/kg; in rats (albino) 5·3, (wild Norway) 12, (roof) 30 to 40 mg/kg.

NORBUTRINE *Bronchodilator*

Synonyms: *N*-Cyclobutylnoradrenaline; Norbudrine.

2-Cyclobutylamino-1-(3,4-dihydroxyphenyl)-ethanol

$C_{12}H_{17}NO_3 = 223{\cdot}3$

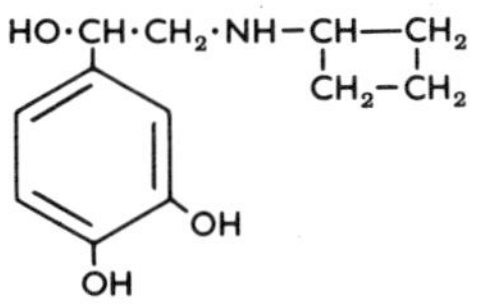

NORBUTRINE HYDROCHLORIDE

Synonym: RD 9338.

Norbutrine hydrochloride melts at 170°, with decomposition.

Solubility. Very soluble in water; soluble 1 in 10 of ethanol.

Chromatography. PAPER: system P1—Rf 0·30 (location under ultraviolet light, absorption; location reagents: *bromocresol green spray*, weak reaction; *potassium permanganate spray*, strong reaction).

THIN-LAYER: system T1—Rf 0·57 (location reagent *potassium permanganate spray*, positive reaction).

Colour Tests. MICRO: sulphuric acid–formaldehyde test—orange (*sensitivity:* 0·5 μg); ammonium molybdate test—(yellow) grey-blue (*sensitivity:* 0·1 μg); ammonium vanadate test —(blue-green) light brown (*sensitivity:* 0·1 μg); Vitali's test—orange/orange/brown (*sensitivity:* 0·5 μg).

Ultraviolet Absorption Spectrum. Norbutrine in 0·1N sulphuric acid, maxima at 253·5 mμ (E1%, 1 cm 128) and 285 mμ (E1%, 1 cm 6).

Infra-red Absorption Spectrum. Norbutrine (base). Potassium bromide disk. The principal peaks are: A 1247 or 1437, B 1614, C 1192 (p. 792).

NORCODEINE

Synonyms: *N*-Demethylcodeine; Normorphine 3-Methyl Ether.

7,8 - Dehydro - 4,5 - epoxy - 6 - hydroxy - 3 - methoxymorphinan

$C_{17}H_{19}NO_3 = 285{\cdot}3$

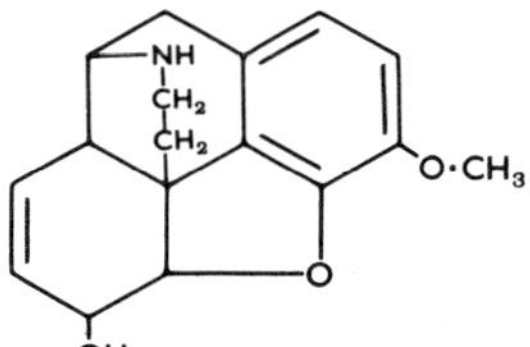

Norcodeine occurs as plates or needles. M.p. 185°.

Solubility. Slightly soluble in water and ether; soluble in ethanol.

NORCODEINE HYDROCHLORIDE

It forms needles from water; the anhydrous form decomposes at 309°.

Solubility. Sparingly soluble in cold water but more soluble in hot water; freely soluble in ethanol.

Extraction. Norcodeine is extracted by organic solvents from aqueous alkaline solutions.

Chromatography. PAPER: system P1—Rf 0·18 (location under ultraviolet light, absorption; location reagent *iodoplatinate spray*, weak reaction).

THIN-LAYER: system T7—Rf 0·21 (location reagent *iodoplatinate spray*, positive reaction); system T8—Rf 0·50 (location as for T7).

Colour Tests. MICRO: sulphuric acid–formaldehyde test—yellow → purple (*sensitivity:* 0·1 μg); ammonium molybdate test—blue-green → blue → green (*sensitivity:* 0·1 μg); Vitali's test—yellow/yellow/orange (*sensitivity:* 0·5 μg).

Crystal Tests. MICRO: *potassium chromate solution*—needles (*sensitivity:* 1 in 400); *zinc chloride solution*—needles (*sensitivity:* 1 in 1000).

Metabolism. Norcodeine may be found in the urine, both free and conjugated, as a metabolite of codeine.

NORETHISTERONE *Progestational Steroid*

Synonyms: Anhydrohydroxy-19-norprogesterone; Ethinylnortestosterone; Norethindrone.

Proprietary Names: Norluten; Norlutin; Primolut N. It is an ingredient of Norinyl and Ortho-Novum.

17-Hydroxy-19-nor-17α-pregn-4-en-20-yn-3-one

$C_{20}H_{26}O_2 = 298{\cdot}4$

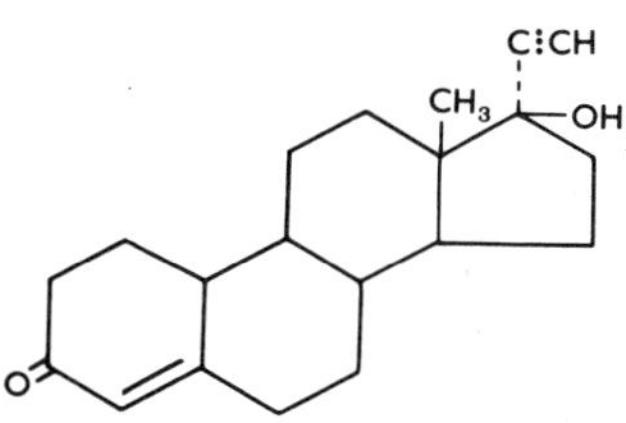

A white crystalline powder. M.p. 201° to 206°. Specific rotation of a 1% solution in chloroform, −23° to −27°.

Solubility. Insoluble in water; soluble 1 in 150 of ethanol and 1 in 30 of chloroform.

NORETHISTERONE ACETATE

Proprietary Names: Norlutate; Norlutin-A; SH 420. It is an ingredient of Anovlar 21, Gestest, Gynovlar 21, Norlestrin, and Primodos.

A white crystalline powder. M.p. about 163°. Specific rotation of a 2% solution in dioxan, −32° to −38°.

Solubility. Almost insoluble in water; soluble 1 in 12·5 of ethanol; sparingly soluble in ether; soluble in chloroform.

Extraction. Norethisterone may be extracted from neutral solutions with freshly distilled ethyl acetate.

Chromatography. Golab and Layne (1962) describe 2 thin-layer systems using a solvent consisting of cyclohexane and ethyl acetate in differing proportions which separates norethisterone from norethynodrel.

Ultraviolet Absorption Spectrum. Norethisterone in ethanol, maximum at about 240 mμ (E1%, 1cm 571); norethisterone acetate in ethanol, maximum at 240 mμ (E1%, 1cm 490 to 520).

Quantitative Estimation. Keay (1968) has devised an analytical scheme involving thin-layer chromatography and ultraviolet and infra-red absorption spectrophotometry which enables norethisterone to be identified and assayed.

Dose. Up to 20 mg (acetate) or 30 mg (base) daily.
Norethisterone is frequently administered in conjunction with ethinyloestradiol (p. 335) or mestranol (p. 405).

NORETHYNODREL *Progestational Steroid*

Proprietary Names: Norethynodrel is an ingredient of Conovid, Enavid, Enovid, Norone, and Previson.

17-Hydroxy-19-nor-17α-pregn-5(10)-en-20-yn-3-one

$C_{20}H_{26}O_2 = 298{\cdot}4$

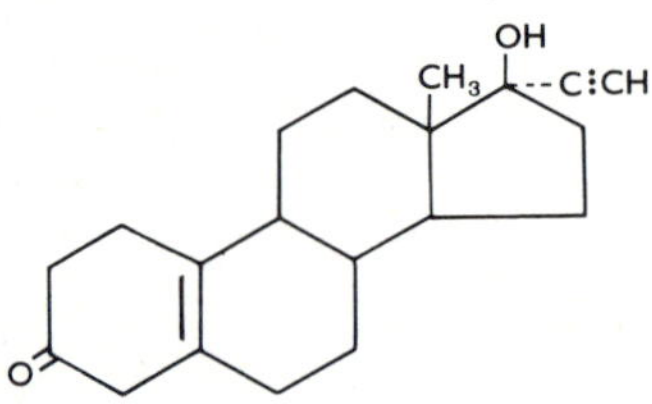

NOTE. As normally manufactured, it contains up to 1·5% of mestranol (p. 405).

A white crystalline powder. M.p. about 175°. Specific rotation of a 1% solution in dioxan, +120° to +125°.

Solubility. Insoluble in water; soluble 1 in 30 of ethanol, 1 in 60 of ether, and 1 in 7 of chloroform.

Extraction. Norethynodrel is extracted from neutral solutions with freshly distilled ethyl acetate.

Chromatography. Golab and Layne (1962) describe 2 thin-layer systems using a solvent consisting of cyclohexane and ethyl acetate in differing proportions which separate norethynodrel from norethisterone.

Colour Test. Dissolve 2 mg in 0·3 ml of a 0·5% solution of dinitrobenzene in ethanol and add 2 drops of *benzalkonium chloride solution*. Mix, and add 2 ml of *dilute ammonia solution*—intense magenta immediately, changing to reddish-brown in about 5 minutes.

Ultraviolet Absorption Spectrum. Norethynodrel in ethanol, maximum at 240 mμ (E1%, 1cm about 560).

Quantitative Estimation. Chissell (1964) and Bastow (1967) describe methods of spectrophotometric estimation of norethynodrel in tablets containing mestranol. Keay (1968) has devised an analytical scheme involving thin-layer chromatography and ultraviolet and infra-red absorption spectrophotometry which enables norethynodrel to be identified and assayed.

Dose. Up to 30 mg daily. It is usually administered in conjunction with mestranol (p. 405).

NORHARMAN *Putrefactive Base*

Synonym: β-Carboline.

9-Pyrid[3,4-*b*]indole

$C_{11}H_8N_2 = 168{\cdot}2$

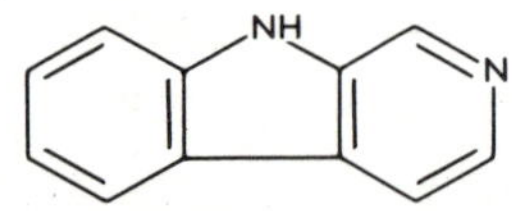

Colourless crystals. M.p. 198·5°.

Solubility. Soluble in hot water, ethanol, and ether.

Extraction. Norharman is extracted by organic solvents from aqueous alkaline solutions.

Chromatography. PAPER: system P1—Rf 0·33 (location under ultraviolet light, bright blue fluorescence; location reagents: *iodoplatinate spray*, strong reaction; *bromocresol green spray*, strong reaction); system RP1a—Rf 0·31 (location under ultraviolet light, blue fluorescence; location reagent *iodoplatinate spray*, positive reaction); system RP1b—Rf 0·08 (location as for RP1a).

THIN-LAYER: system T1—Rf 0·68 (location reagent *acidified iodoplatinate spray*, positive reaction).

Colour Tests. MICRO: sulphuric acid–formaldehyde test—green (*sensitivity:* 0·1 μg); ammonium vanadate test—green→yellow (*sensitivity:* 0·1 μg); Vitali's test—yellow/yellow/red (*sensitivity:* 0·1 μg).

Crystal Tests. MICRO: *potassium permanganate solution*—fine needles (*sensitivity:* 1 in 1000); *trinitrobenzoic acid solution*—masses of curved needles (*sensitivity:* 1 in 1000).

Ultraviolet Absorption Spectrum. Norharman in 0·1N sulphuric acid, maxima at 247 mμ (E1%, 1cm 1726) and 300 mμ (E1%, 1cm 910).

Infra-red Absorption Spectrum. Potassium bromide disk. The principal peaks are: A 1247, B 1450, C 731 or 747 (p. 792).

NOTE. Norharman may be found as a putrefactive base, particularly in cases where embalming has taken place. It is a condensation product of tryptophan and formaldehyde. It has also been found in tobacco smoke and in home-made wine; 1-hydroxymethylnorharman has also been found in autopsy material (Kaempe, 1967).

NORLEVORPHANOL *Narcotic Analgesic*

Synonym: Ro 1-7686.

(−)-3-Hydroxymorphinan

$C_{16}H_{21}NO = 243{\cdot}4$

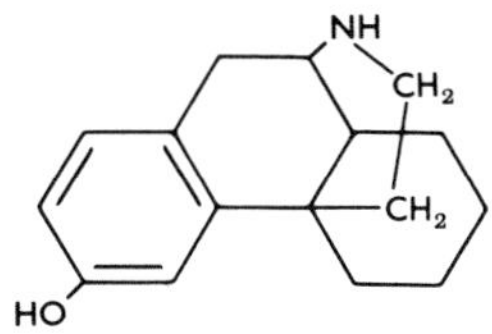

NORLEVORPHANOL HYDROBROMIDE

Synonym: NIH 7539.

Extraction. Norlevorphanol is extracted by organic solvents from aqueous ammoniacal solutions.

Chromatography. PAPER: system P1—Rf 0·60 (location under ultraviolet light, absorption; location reagents: *iodoplatinate spray*, strong reaction; *bromocresol green spray*, weak reaction).

THIN-LAYER: system T1—Rf 0·12, streaking (location reagent *acidified iodoplatinate spray*, positive reaction).

Colour Tests. MICRO: sulphuric acid–formaldehyde test—olive-green (*sensitivity:* 1·0 μg); ammonium molybdate test—blue→yellow-green (*sensitivity:* 0·25 μg); Vitali's test—faint yellow/faint yellow/orange (*sensitivity:* 1·0 μg).

Crystal Tests. MICRO: *gold bromide–hydrochloric acid solution*—rosettes of rods (*sensitivity:* 1 in 1000); *platinic chloride solution*—irregular blades (*sensitivity:* 1 in 1000).

NORMETANEPHRINE

Synonym: Normetadrenaline.

(−)-2-Amino-1-(4-hydroxy-3-methoxyphenyl)ethanol

$C_9H_{13}NO_3 = 183{\cdot}2$

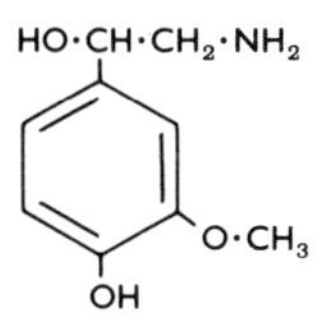

Chromatography. PAPER: system P1—Rf 0·11 (location under ultraviolet light, absorption; location reagent *bromocresol green spray*, weak reaction).

THIN-LAYER: system T1—Rf 0·33 (location reagent *potassium permanganate spray*, positive reaction).

Colour Tests. Chen's test—purple.

MICRO: sulphuric acid–formaldehyde test—dull orange→purple-brown (*sensitivity:* 0·5 μg); ammonium molybdate test—grey-blue→dull green (*sensitivity:* 0·25 μg); ammonium vanadate test—green (*sensitivity:* 1·0 μg); Vitali's test—yellow/yellow-brown/yellow-brown (*sensitivity:* 0·5 μg).

Crystal Test. MICRO: *gold chloride solution*—very small plates (*sensitivity:* 1 in 100).

Ultraviolet Absorption Spectrum. Normetanephrine in 0·1N sulphuric acid, maxima at 227 mμ (E1%, 1 cm 218) and 277·5 mμ (E1%, 1 cm 85), and an inflexion at 284 mμ.

Infra-red Absorption Spectrum. Normetanephrine hydrochloride. Potassium bromide disk. The principal peaks are: A 1162 or 1529, B 1037 or 1250 (p. 749).

Quantitative Estimation. Taniguchi *et al.* (1964) describe a method of extraction and spectrofluorimetric determination of normetanephrine.

Metabolism. After noradrenaline has been metabolised by *O*-methylation and oxidative deamination, it is excreted as the inactivated compounds normetanephrine and 3-methoxy-4-hydroxymandelic acid. Most of the normetanephrine is excreted as sulphate or glucuronide conjugates but small portions are deaminated to the major excretory product, 3-methoxy-4-hydroxymandelic acid.

NORMETHADONE

Narcotic Analgesic/Antitussive

Synonyms: Hö 10582; Phenyldimazone; U 9558.

Proprietary Names: Mepidon; Normedon.

6-Dimethylamino-4,4-diphenylhexan-3-one

$C_{20}H_{25}NO = 295{\cdot}4$

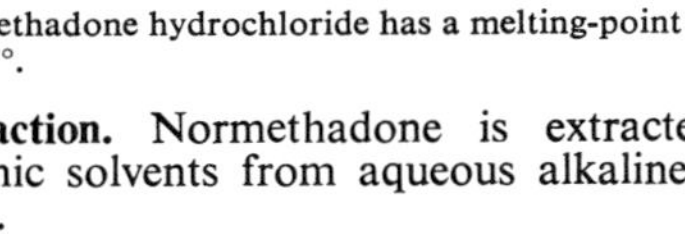

NORMETHADONE HYDROCHLORIDE

Synonym: NIH 2820.

Proprietary Names: Ticarda; Tikapect. It is an ingredient of Cophylac.

Normethadone hydrochloride has a melting-point of 175° to 177°.

Extraction. Normethadone is extracted by organic solvents from aqueous alkaline solutions.

Chromatography. PAPER: system P1—Rf 0·67 (location reagent *iodoplatinate spray*, strong reaction); system RP1b—Rf 0·00 (location under ultraviolet light, absorption; location reagent *iodoplatinate spray*, positive reaction).

THIN-LAYER: system T1—Rf 0·46 (location reagent *acidified iodoplatinate spray*, positive reaction).

Colour Test. MICRO: ammonium vanadate test—pale yellow-green (*sensitivity:* 1·0 μg).

Crystal Tests. MICRO: *gold bromide–hydrochloric acid solution*—small plates, often crosses (*sensitivity:* 1 in 1000); *lead iodide solution*—masses of blades (*sensitivity:* 1 in 1000).

Ultraviolet Absorption Spectrum. Normethadone hydrochloride in 0·1N hydrochloric acid, maxima at 253 mμ (E1%, 1 cm 17), 259 mμ (E1%, 1 cm 19), 265 mμ (E1%, 1 cm 16), and 292 mμ (E1%, 1 cm 19); minima at 251 mμ, 255 mμ, 263 mμ, and 274 mμ.

NORMORPHINE *Narcotic*

Synonyms: *N*-Demethylmorphine; Desmethylmorphine.

7,8 - Dehydro - 4,5 - epoxy - 3,6 - dihydroxymorphinan

$C_{16}H_{17}NO_3$ = 271·3

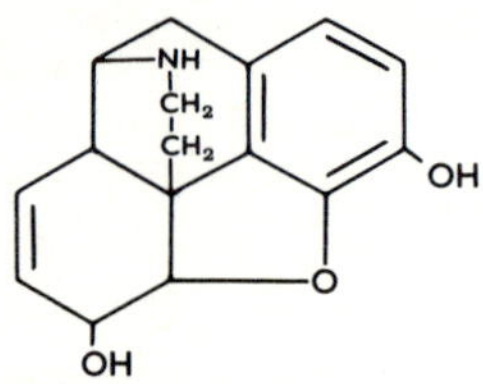

Crystals which melt between 273° and 277°.

Solubility. Slightly soluble in water and ethanol; insoluble in ether and chloroform.

Extraction. Milthers (1961) has described a method of extraction from blood and tissues involving deproteinisation using uranyl chloride and extraction into a mixture of chloroform and isopropanol.

Chromatography. PAPER: system P1—Rf 0·12 (location under ultraviolet light, strong absorption; location reagents: *iodoplatinate spray*, weak reaction; *bromocresol green spray*, weak reaction); system RP1b—Rf 0·82 (location reagent *iodoplatinate spray*, positive reaction).

THIN-LAYER: system T1—Rf 0·17 (location reagent *acidified iodoplatinate spray*, positive reaction); system T7—Rf 0·40 (location reagent *iodoplatinate spray*, positive reaction); system T8—Rf 0·48 (location as for T7).

Colour Tests. MICRO: sulphuric acid–formaldehyde test—purple (*sensitivity:* 0·1 μg); ammonium molybdate test—purple→blue (*sensitivity:* 0·1 μg); ammonium vanadate test—grey-green (*sensitivity:* 0·5 μg); Vitali's test—yellow/yellow/orange (*sensitivity:* 0·25 μg).

Crystal Tests. MICRO: *potassium bismuth iodide solution*—rosettes of plates or rods (*sensitivity:* 1 in 1000); *potassium cadmium iodide solution*—bunches of plates (*sensitivity:* 1 in 1000).

Ultraviolet Absorption Spectrum. Normorphine in 0·1N sulphuric acid, maximum at 285 mμ (E1%, 1 cm 56·5) and an inflexion at 279 mμ.

Metabolism. *N*-Demethylation of morphine to normorphine has been postulated as a fairly important metabolic pathway of morphine but so far normorphine, either free or conjugated, has not been detected in the urine of man. Misra *et al.* (1961a), however, have reported the recovery of normorphine from the urine of the rat after the administration of morphine. Studies in dogs and monkeys (Misra *et al.*, 1961b) have shown that after subcutaneous injection of normorphine, 34 to 40% may be recovered in the urine in the free form and 34 to 37% in the conjugated form in dogs; in monkeys 18 to 22% was recovered in the urine in the free form and 56 to 60% in the conjugated form.

NORPSEUDOEPHEDRINE *Sympathomimetic*

Synonyms: Cathine; Katine; Pseudonorephedrine.

(+)-2-Amino-1-phenylpropan-1-ol

$C_9H_{13}NO$ = 151·2

$$C_6H_5{\cdot}\underset{}{\overset{OH}{\overset{|}{C}}}H{\cdot}\underset{\underset{NH_2}{|}}{C}H{\cdot}CH_3$$

An alkaloid found in the leaves of *Catha edulis* (Celastraceae). The fresh or dried leaves (known as Catha; Kat; Kath; Khat; Miraa; Abyssinian, African, or Arabian Tea) are chewed or used as an infusion in northern and eastern Africa as a stimulant.

It crystallises as plates from methanol. M.p. 77·5° to 78°.

Solubility. Soluble in ethanol, chloroform, and ether.

Extraction. Norpseudoephedrine is extracted by organic solvents from aqueous alkaline solutions.

Chromatography. PAPER: system P1—Rf 0·37 (location under ultraviolet light, weak absorption; location reagent *bromocresol green spray*, strong reaction).

THIN-LAYER: system T1—Rf 0·48 (location reagent *potassium permanganate spray*, positive reaction).

GAS: system G2/120—retention time 0·82 relative to ephedrine.

Colour Test. Chen's test—purple.

Ultraviolet Absorption Spectrum. Norpseudoephedrine in 0·1N sulphuric acid, maxima at about 246·5 mμ (E1%, 1 cm 5), 250·5 mμ (E1%, 1 cm 8), 256·5 mμ (E1%, 1 cm 10), 262·5 mμ (E1%, 1 cm 8), and about 266 mμ (E1%, 1 cm 4).

Toxicity. Addiction to catha has been reported; addicts experience a dreamy euphoria with loquacity, followed by apathy, depression, and anorexia.

NORTRIPTYLINE *Antidepressant*

Synonym: L 38489.

10,11-Dihydro-5-(3-methylaminopropylidene)-5*H*-dibenzo[*a*,*d*]cycloheptene
$C_{19}H_{21}N = 263{\cdot}4$

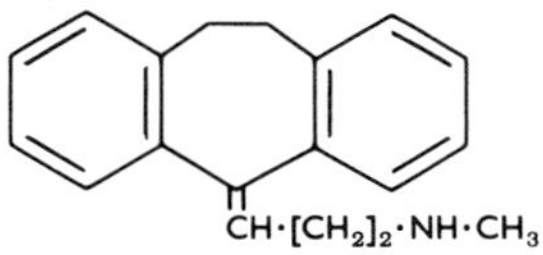

NORTRIPTYLINE HYDROCHLORIDE
Proprietary Names: Acetaxa; Allegron; Aventyl; Nortrilen.

A white powder. M.p. about 218°.
Solubility. Soluble 1 in 50 of water, 1 in 10 of ethanol, and 1 in 5 of chloroform; almost insoluble in ether.

Screening Tests. See under Screening Tests, p. 7.

Extraction. Nortriptyline is extracted by organic solvents from aqueous alkaline solutions.

Chromatography. PAPER: system P1—Rf 0·74 (location under ultraviolet light, absorption; location reagent *iodoplatinate spray*, weak reaction); system RP1a—Rf 0·55 (location under ultraviolet light, absorption); system RP1b—Rf 0·04 (location as for RP1a).

THIN-LAYER: system T1—Rf 0·28 (location reagent *acidified iodoplatinate spray*, positive reaction).

GAS: system G2/225—retention time 0·63 relative to codeine.

Colour Tests. MICRO: sulphuric acid–formaldehyde test—orange-brown (*sensitivity:* 0·1 μg); ammonium molybdate test—orange-brown (*sensitivity:* 0·1 μg); ammonium vanadate test —brown→green (*sensitivity:* 0·25 μg); Vitali's test—faint red flash/–/faint brown (*sensitivity:* 1·0 μg).

Crystal Tests. MICRO: *picric acid*—large irregular crystals, forming overnight (*sensitivity:* 1 in 400); *platinic iodide solution*—plates and needles, forming overnight (*sensitivity:* 1 in 1000).

Ultraviolet Absorption Spectrum. Nortriptyline hydrochloride in water, maximum at about 240 mμ (E1%, 1 cm about 470); minimum at about 230 mμ: in methanol, maximum at 239 mμ (E1%, 1 cm about 480).

Infra-red Absorption Spectrum. Nortriptyline hydrochloride. Potassium bromide disk. The principal peaks are: A 756, B 742, C 768 or 1488 (p. 792).

Quantitative Estimation. Amundson and Manthey (1966) describe the extraction, thin-layer chromatographic separation, and spectrophotometric determination of nortriptyline and its hydroxy-metabolite from urine.
Wallace and Dahl (1967) describe a rapid and specific spectrophotometric method of determination of nortriptyline and its principal metabolite in biological materials; the procedure involves extraction into n-hexane and oxidation of the compounds with alkaline potassium permanganate to yield carbonyl derivatives which have a characteristic ultraviolet spectrum.

Metabolism. The major metabolite of nortriptyline in man has been tentatively identified as 10-hydroxynortriptyline (Amundson and Manthey, 1966).
In 8 patients on a chronic dosage regimen an average of about 58% of the administered dose was excreted in the urine in a 24-hour period; only small amounts of unchanged nortriptyline were excreted and more of the hydroxy-derivative was excreted in the free than in the conjugated form. Following single doses the maximum excretion rate was found to occur within 4 to 8 hours but excretion was slow and substantial levels of the drug were found 2 to 3 days after dosing.

Dose. The usual therapeutic dose is up to 100 mg of base, daily.

Toxicity. LD50 (oral): in mice 327 and in rats 502 mg/kg.
CASE EXAMPLE. A woman recovered after taking 600 mg of nortriptyline; toxic symptoms were present for 24 hours after ingestion (Stinnett *et al.*, 1968).

NOSCAPINE *Antitussive*

Synonyms: α-Gnoscopine; Narcotine; *l*-Narcotine.
Proprietary Names: Coscopin; Coscotabs; Longatin; Nectadon; Nicolane.

(−)-α-(1,2,3,4-Tetrahydro-8-methoxy-2-methyl-6,7-methylenedioxyisoquinol-1-yl)-5,6-dimethoxyphthalide
$C_{22}H_{23}NO_7 = 413{\cdot}4$

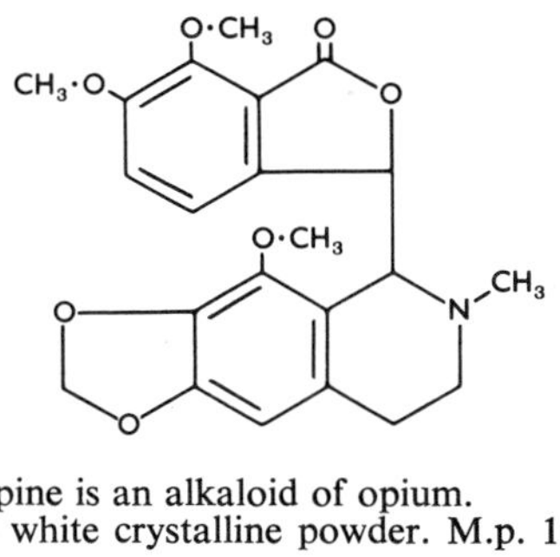

Noscapine is an alkaloid of opium.
A fine white crystalline powder. M.p. 174° to 176°.
Solubility. Insoluble in water; slightly soluble in ethanol and ether; freely soluble in chloroform.

NOSCAPINE HYDROCHLORIDE
A fine white crystalline powder.
Solubility. Soluble 1 in 4 of water and 1 in 8 of ethanol; almost insoluble in ether; freely soluble in chloroform.

Extraction. Noscapine is extracted by organic solvents from aqueous acid or alkaline solutions.

Chromatography. PAPER: system P1—Rf 0·40 (location under ultraviolet light, bright blue fluorescence; location reagent *iodoplatinate spray*, strong reaction).

THIN-LAYER: system T1—Rf 0·62 (location reagent *acidified iodoplatinate spray*, positive reaction).

Colour Tests. MICRO: sulphuric acid–formaldehyde test—bluish-purple, quickly fading (*sensitivity:* 0·1 μg); ammonium molybdate test—brown→green→blue→pale green (*sensitivity:* 0·05 μg); Vitali's test—red → yellow/yellow/yellow (*sensitivity:* 0·5 μg).

Crystal Tests. MICRO: *potassium chromate solution*—feathery rosettes or bunches of blades (*sensitivity:* 1 in 1500); *sodium carbonate solution*—rosettes and bunches of needles (*sensitivity:* 1 in 1500).

Ultraviolet Absorption Spectrum. Noscapine in ethanol, maxima at 291 mμ (E1%, 1 cm about 100) and 310 mμ (E1%, 1 cm about 120): noscapine hydrochloride in water, maximum at about 313 mμ; minimum at about 268 mμ.

Infra-red Absorption Spectrum. Noscapine (base). Potassium bromide disk. The principal peaks are: A 1745, B 1276, C 1038 (p. 749).

Quantitative Estimation. Vedsø (1961) describes a spectrofluorimetric method of determination of noscapine in plasma and urine.
Fairbairn and El-Masry (1967) describe a spectrophotometric method following thin-layer chromatographic separation from the other opium alkaloids.

Metabolism. Following the ingestion of single oral doses of between 250 and 500 mg of noscapine hydrochloride, peak plasma concentrations are obtained after about 1 hour. Noscapine disappears rapidly from the blood-stream and is deposited in the tissues, only about 1% of the dose being excreted during the first 6 hours. Initially, free noscapine is excreted almost exclusively but, after 6 hours, it is excreted almost entirely in the conjugated form. It is not known whether or not conjugated noscapine is present in the plasma (Vedsø, 1961).

Dose. Up to 120 mg daily; single doses of 60 mg may be given.

Toxicity. Noscapine has no analgesic or narcotic action and it is unlikely to lead to addiction. The lethal dose in man is probably between 100 and 500 mg/kg.

LD50 (oral): in rats 800 mg/kg.

OCTATROPINE METHYLBROMIDE

Parasympatholytic

Synonym: Anisotropine Methobromide.
Proprietary Name: Valpin.

N-Methyl-*O*-(2-propylpentanoyl)tropinium bromide

$C_{17}H_{32}BrNO_2 = 362{\cdot}4$

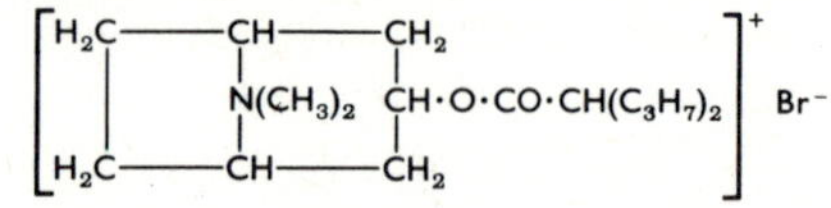

A white glistening hygroscopic powder.

Solubility. Soluble in water; freely soluble in ethanol and chloroform; almost insoluble in ether.

Extraction. Octatropine methylbromide is a quaternary ammonium compound (see p. 29).

Chromatography. PAPER: system P1—Rf 0·56 (location reagent *iodoplatinate spray*, strong reaction).

THIN-LAYER: system T1—Rf 0·02 (location reagent *acidified iodoplatinate spray*, positive reaction).

Crystal Tests. MICRO: *picric acid*—plates and needles, best viewed under polarised light (*sensitivity:* 1 in 1000); *potassium iodide solution*—plates and needles (*sensitivity:* 1 in 1000).

Quantitative Estimation. Pfeffer *et al.* (1968) describe a spectrophotometric method of estimation of octatropine in urine.

Metabolism. Octatropine methylbromide is incompletely absorbed from the gastro-intestinal tract, but a substantial amount remains in the body for an appreciable length of time. Pfeffer *et al.* (1968) administered 20 mg of octatropine methylbromide to each of 6 subjects; only between 3·5 and 11·4% of the dose was recovered in the urine within 4 days.

Dose. Up to 15 mg.

Toxicity. The lethal dose is probably in the range 10 to 100 mg/kg.

OCTAVERINE

Antispasmodic

1 - (3,4,5 - Triethoxyphenyl) - 6,7 - dimethoxyisoquinoline

$C_{23}H_{27}NO_5 = 397{\cdot}5$

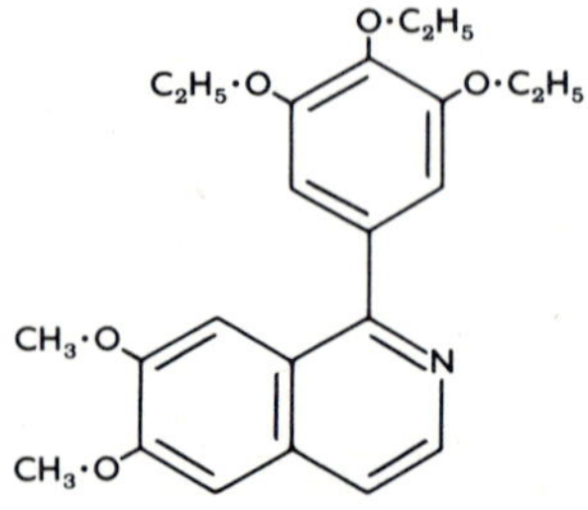

Solubility. Insoluble in water.

OCTAVERINE HYDROCHLORIDE
Octaverine hydrochloride occurs as crystals which melt at 199° to 200°.
Solubility. Sparingly soluble in water.

Extraction. Octaverine is extracted by organic solvents from aqueous alkaline solutions.

Chromatography. PAPER: system P1—Rf 0·77 (location under ultraviolet light, green fluorescence; location reagent *iodoplatinate spray*, weak reaction); system RP1a—Rf 0·06 (locarion reagent *iodoplatinate spray*, positive reaction); system RP1b—Rf 0·00 (location as for RP1a).
THIN-LAYER: system T1—Rf 0·75 (location reagent *potassium permanganate spray*, positive reaction).

Colour Tests. MICRO: sulphuric acid–formaldehyde test—green→brown (*sensitivity:* 0·1 μg); ammonium molybdate test—green (*sensitivity:* 0·1 μg); ammonium vanadate test—red (*sensitivity:* 0·1 μg); Vitali's test—red-brown/brown/red-orange (*sensitivity:* 0·1 μg).

Crystal Tests. MICRO: *platinic bromide solution*—bunches of small needles (*sensitivity:* 1 in 1000); *sodium carbonate solution*—small rosettes with some fine needles (*sensitivity:* 1 in 1000).

Ultraviolet Absorption Spectrum. Octaverine in ethanol, maxima at 247 mμ (E1%, 1 cm 976), 321 mμ (E1%, 1 cm 239), and 358 mμ (E1%, 1 cm 213).

OESTRADIOL *Oestrogen*

Synonyms: Beta-oestradiol; Dihydrofolliculine; Dihydrotheelin; Dihydroxyoestrin; Estradiol.
Proprietary Names: Diogyn; Femestral; Oestroform; Progynon.

Oestra-1,3,5(10)-triene-3,17β-diol
$C_{18}H_{24}O_2$ = 272·4

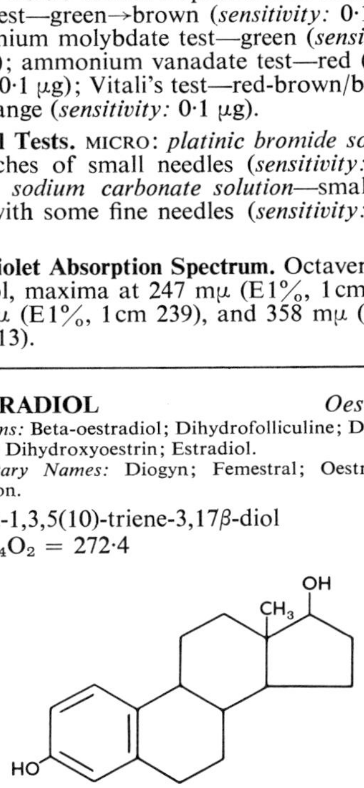

A white crystalline powder. M.p. 175° to 178°. Specific rotation of a 1% solution in dioxan, +75° to +82°.
Solubility. Very slightly soluble in water; soluble 1 in 30 of ethanol; soluble in chloroform.

OESTRADIOL BENZOATE
3-Benzoyloxyoestra-1,3,5(10)-trien-17β-ol.
Synonym: Oestradiol Monobenzoate.
Proprietary Names: Benztrone; Dimenformon; Follicormon; Glandubolin-Monobenz; Oestrin; Oestroform; Ovocyclin-M; Progynon-B; Solestro.

A white crystalline powder. M.p. 191° to 195°. Specific rotation of a 1% solution in dioxan, +57° to +63°.
Solubility. Insoluble in water; soluble 1 in 150 of ethanol; sparingly soluble in ether; soluble in chloroform.

OESTRADIOL BUTYRYLACETATE
17β-(3-Oxohexanoyl)oestra-1,3,5(10)-trien-3-ol.
Proprietary Name: Follicosid.

OESTRADIOL CYPIONATE
17β-(3-Cyclopentyl)propionyloxyoestra-1,3,5(10)-trien-3-ol.
Synonyms: Oestradiol Cyclopentylpropionate.
Proprietary Name: Depo-Estradiol.

A white crystalline powder. M.p. 149° to 153°. Specific rotation of a 2% solution in dioxan, +39° to +44°.
Solubility. Insoluble in water; soluble in ethanol, ether, and chloroform.

OESTRADIOL DIPROPIONATE
3,17β-Dipropionyloxyoestra-1,3,5(10)-triene.
Proprietary Names: Ovocyclin Dipropionate; Ovocyclin-P; Progynon-DP.

Small white crystals or crystalline powder. M.p. 104° to 109°. Specific rotation of a 1% solution in dioxan, +37° to +41°.
Solubility. Almost insoluble in water; soluble in ethanol and ether.

OESTRADIOL VALERATE
17β-Valeryloxyoestra-1,3,5(10)-trien-3-ol.
Proprietary Names: Delestrogen; Primogyn-Depot.

A white crystalline powder. M.p. 143° to 150°. Specific rotation of a 2·5% solution in dioxan, +41° to +47°.
Solubility. Almost insoluble in water; soluble in methanol, benzyl benzoate, and dioxan.

Extraction. Oestradiol is extracted from neutral solutions with freshly distilled ethyl acetate.

Chromatography. PAPER: Axelrod (1953b) describes a paper chromatographic method for the separation and identification of oestradiol and other oestrogens.
THIN-LAYER: system T20—Rf 0·37 (location under ultraviolet light, greenish-yellow fluorescence; location reagent *50% sulphuric acid spray*, pink). Smith and Foell (1962) describe several solvent systems which may be used to separate oestradiol and other steroids by thin-layer chromatography on starch-bound silica gel layers.

Colour Tests. Heat 0·05 mg with 1 ml of a 2·5% w/w solution of betanaphthol in *sulphuric acid* for 2 minutes at 100°. Cool, and add 1 ml of water—orange-yellow which changes to red when the solution is heated for 90 seconds at 100°.
2 mg of oestradiol in 2 ml of *sulphuric acid*—greenish-yellow.

Ultraviolet Absorption Spectrum. Oestradiol in isopropanol, maximum at 281 mμ (E1%, 1 cm 78); oestradiol cypionate in ethanol, maximum at about 280 mμ.

Quantitative Estimation. Brown and Matthew (1962) have developed a method for the accurate determination of oestradiol in urine.

Metabolism. Oestradiol is the most active of the naturally occurring oestrogenic hormones. Following oral administration it is rapidly absorbed from the gastro-intestinal tract and converted in the liver to oestrone and oestriol. Injected oestradiol is almost entirely destroyed in the liver; only a very small amount, 3% to 12%, can be recovered unchanged in the urine. Oestradiol and its metabolites appear in the urine conjugated with glucuronic or sulphuric acid.

The esters of oestradiol become less and less polar as the size of the substituents increases; correspondingly, the rate of absorption is progressively slowed and the duration of action prolonged.

Therapeutic doses of oestradiol benzoate are effective for several days; oestradiol dipropionate is absorbed over several weeks.

In the normal menstrual cycle the mean daily excretion at the midcycle ovulatory maximum has been found to be 8 μg of oestradiol, 21 μg of oestrone, and 29 μg of oestriol; the second rise during the luteal phase is broader and more prolonged, but the maximal rates of excretion are somewhat smaller.

OESTRIOL *Oestrogen*

Synonyms: Estriol; Theelol.
Proprietary Name: Ovestin.

Oestra-1,3,5(10)-triene-3,16α,17β-triol
$C_{18}H_{24}O_3$ = 288·4

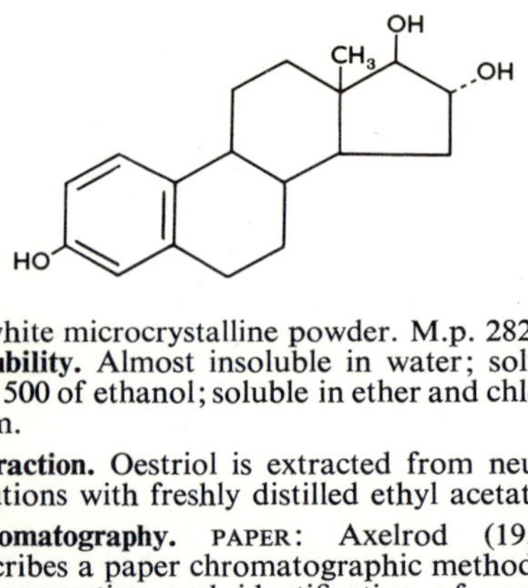

A white microcrystalline powder. M.p. 282°.
Solubility. Almost insoluble in water; soluble 1 in 500 of ethanol; soluble in ether and chloroform.

Extraction. Oestriol is extracted from neutral solutions with freshly distilled ethyl acetate.

Chromatography. PAPER: Axelrod (1953b) describes a paper chromatographic method for the separation and identification of oestriol and other oestrogens.

THIN-LAYER: system T20—Rf 0·07 (location under ultraviolet light, greenish-yellow fluorescence, with a purple tinge; location reagent *50% sulphuric acid spray*, purple). Smith and Foell (1962) have described several solvent systems which may be used to separate oestriol and other steroids by thin-layer chromatography on starch-bound silica gel layers.

Ultraviolet Absorption Spectrum. Oestriol in ethanol, maxima at 280 mμ (E 1%, 1 cm 74) and 281 mμ (E 1%, 1 cm 66).

Quantitative Estimation. Brown and Matthew (1962) have developed a method for the accurate determination of oestriol in urine.

Metabolism. Oestriol is a naturally occurring oestrogen which is less potent than oestradiol. Following the intravenous administration of ^{14}C-labelled oestriol, 20% was excreted in the bile, the remainder being found in the urine within 72 hours. This excretion rate is much faster than that of oestrone or oestradiol. ^{14}C-Labelled oestriol glucuronide was rapidly excreted in the urine and there was no evidence to show that the conjugate was split to any extent in the body. No biliary excretion of the glucuronide occurred (Sandberg and Slaunwhite, 1965).

Dose. Up to 1 mg daily.

OESTRONE *Oestrogen*

Synonyms: Estrone; Folliculin; Ketohydroxyoestrin; Oestroform; Theelin.
Proprietary Names: Estromone; Estrugenone; Estrusol; Glandubolin; Kolpon; Menagen; Menformon; Micryston Oestrone; Perlatan; Thelestrin; Wynestron.

3-Hydroxyoestra-1,3,5(10)-trien-17-one
$C_{18}H_{22}O_2$ = 270·4

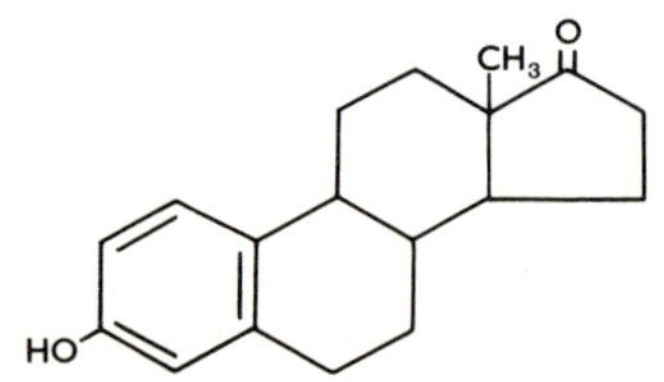

Colourless plate-like crystals, or a white crystalline powder. M.p. 256° to 262°. Specific rotation of a 1% solution in dioxan, +158° to +165°.
Solubility. Almost insoluble in water; soluble 1 in 400 of ethanol; slightly soluble in ether; soluble in chloroform.

OESTRONE BENZOATE
White plate-like crystals.
Solubility. Almost insoluble in water; soluble in ethanol.

Extraction. Oestrone is extracted from neutral solutions with freshly distilled ethyl acetate.

Chromatography. PAPER: Axelrod (1953b) describes a paper chromatographic method for the separation and identification of oestrone and other oestrogens.

THIN-LAYER: system T20—Rf 0·58 (location under ultraviolet light, greenish-yellow fluorescence; location reagent *50% sulphuric acid spray*, pink). Smith and Foell (1962) have described several solvent systems which may be used to separate oestrone and other steroids by thin-layer chromatography on starch-bound silica gel layers.

Crystal Test. MICRO: *potassium tri-iodide solution (3)*—serrated plates.

Ultraviolet Absorption Spectrum. Oestrone in ethanol, maximum at 287 mμ (E 1%, 1 cm 80).

Quantitative Estimation. Brown and Matthew (1962) have developed a method for the accurate determination of oestrone in urine.

Metabolism. Oestrone is a naturally occurring oestrogen. It may be found in the urine as an oxidation product of oestradiol.

Dose. Up to 10 mg by mouth daily, or up to 1 mg intramuscularly once or twice weekly.

OLEANDOMYCIN *Antibiotic*

Synonym: PA 105.
Proprietary Names: Matromycin; Romicil.

An antibiotic obtained from *Streptomyces antibioticus.*
$C_{35}H_{61}NO_{12} = 687{\cdot}9$

OLEANDOMYCIN PHOSPHATE
Proprietary Name: It is an ingredient of Sigmamycin.

A white crystalline powder.
Solubility. Soluble 1 in 2·5 of water and 1 in 3 of ethanol; slightly soluble in ether.

Chromatography. PAPER: system P1—Rf 0·60 (location reagent *iodoplatinate spray*, white). THIN-LAYER: system T1—Rf 0·45 (location reagent *potassium permanganate spray*, positive reaction).

Colour Tests. MICRO: sulphuric acid–formaldehyde test—olive-green (*sensitivity:* 1·0 μg); ammonium molybdate test—olive (*sensitivity:* 1·0 μg); ammonium vanadate test—olive (*sensitivity:* 1·0 μg); Vitali's test— –/faint brown/brown (*sensitivity:* 1·0 μg).

Ultraviolet Absorption Spectrum. Oleandomycin in 0·1N sulphuric acid, maximum at 242 mμ (E1%, 1cm 6·9).

Metabolism. Oleandomycin is incompletely absorbed from the gastro-intestinal tract. High concentrations are attained in the bile; it is excreted in the urine. Serum concentrations have been reported to range from 0·4 to 1·6 μg/ml 1 to 4 hours after a dose of 250 or 500 mg.

Dose. Up to 3 g daily.

Toxicity. LD50 (intravenous): in mice 550 mg/kg.

OPIPRAMOL *Antidepressant*

Synonym: G 33040.

5-{3-[4-(2-Hydroxyethyl)piperazin-1-yl]-propyl}-5*H*-dibenz[*b*,*f*]azepine
$C_{23}H_{29}N_3O = 363{\cdot}5$

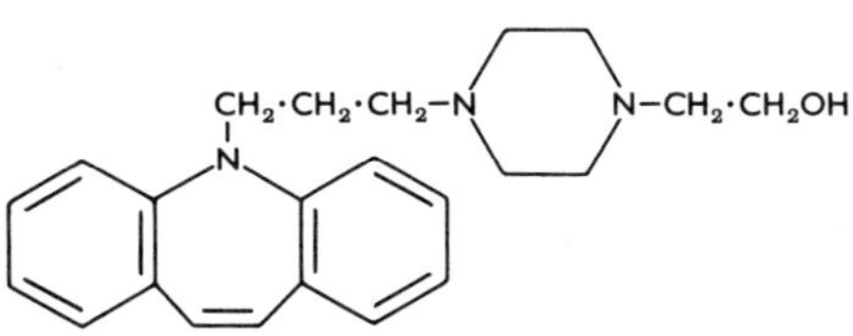

OPIPRAMOL HYDROCHLORIDE
Proprietary Names: Dinsidon; Ensidon; Insidon; Nisidana.

A light yellow, crystalline powder which develops a reddish tinge on prolonged exposure to light. M.p. 210° to 211°, with decomposition.
Solubility. Very soluble in water; soluble in ethanol; almost insoluble in acetone.

Extraction. Opipramol is extracted by organic solvents from aqueous alkaline solutions.

Chromatography. PAPER: system P1—Rf 0·20 (location under ultraviolet light, yellow fluorescence; location reagents: *iodoplatinate spray*, strong reaction; *bromocresol green spray*, weak reaction); system RP1a—Rf 0·47 (location under ultraviolet light, yellow fluorescence; location reagent *iodoplatinate spray*, positive reaction); system RP1b—Rf 0·04 (location as for RP1a).

THIN-LAYER: system T1—Rf 0·53 (location reagent *acidified iodoplatinate spray*, positive reaction).

Colour Tests. MICRO: ammonium molybdate test—blue → blue-green (*sensitivity:* 0·1 μg); ammonium vanadate test—yellow-green (*sensitivity:* 1·0 μg); Vitali's test—yellow-green/yellow/dull orange (*sensitivity:* 0·1 μg).

Crystal Tests. MICRO: *potassium cadmium iodide solution*—masses of very small plates and needles (*sensitivity:* 1 in 1000); *potassium tri-iodide solution* (*3*)—serrated plates (*sensitivity:* 1 in 1000).

Ultraviolet Absorption Spectrum. Opipramol in 0·1N sulphuric acid, maxima at 255 mμ (E1%, 1cm 734) and about 280 mμ (E1%, 1cm 142).

Quantitative Estimation. Herrmann (1964) describes colorimetric, spectrophotometric, and spectrofluorimetric methods of determination of opipramol in biological fluids and tissues.

Metabolism. Studies in rabbits and rats (Herrmann, 1964) have indicated that opipramol is well absorbed after oral and parenteral administration. It is rapidly metabolised and only low concentrations appear in the blood. About 1% of the dose is excreted unchanged in the urine.

Dose. Up to 150 mg daily, but it should not be administered in conjunction with monoamine oxidase inhibitors.

Toxicity. LD50 (oral): in mice 0·7 and in rats 1·9 g/kg.

CASE EXAMPLE. An epileptic, aged 6 years, died after ingesting about 49 tablets of Insidon, equivalent to 2·45 g of opipramol. Toxicological examination of the viscera disclosed the presence of 66 mg/kg of opipramol (Breton *et al.*, 1964).

ORCIPRENALINE *Sympathomimetic*

Synonyms: Metaproterenol; Résorcinéthanolamine; TH 152.

1-(3,5-Dihydroxyphenyl)-2-isopropylaminoethanol

$C_{11}H_{17}NO_3 = 211{\cdot}3$

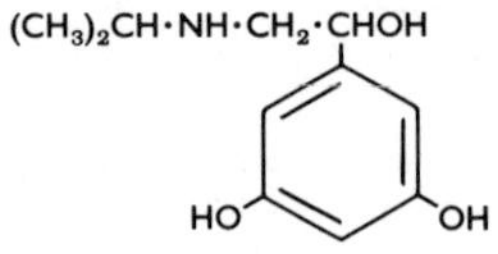

ORCIPRENALINE SULPHATE
Proprietary Name: Alupent.

A white crystalline powder. M.p. about 205°.
Solubility. Soluble 1 in 2 of water and 1 in 1 of ethanol; sparingly soluble in most organic solvents.

Extraction. It is soluble in water; special extraction methods are required (see p. 28).

Chromatography. PAPER: system P1—Rf 0·26 (location under ultraviolet light, absorption; location reagents: *iodoplatinate spray*, weak reaction; *bromocresol green spray*, weak reaction); system RP1a—Rf 0·87 (location reagent *iodoplatinate spray*, positive reaction); system RP1b—Rf 0·88 (location as for RP1a).
THIN-LAYER: system T1—Rf 0·56 (location reagent *potassium permanganate spray*, positive reaction).

Colour Tests. Chen's test—purple → green.
MICRO: sulphuric acid–formaldehyde test—yellow (*sensitivity:* 0·5 μg); ammonium molybdate test—pale blue (*sensitivity:* 1·0 μg); Vitali's test—faint yellow/faint yellow/yellow (*sensitivity:* 1·0 μg).

Crystal Test. MICRO: *gold bromide solution*—small dense rosettes (*sensitivity:* 1 in 100).

Ultraviolet Absorption Spectrum. Orciprenaline in 0·1N sulphuric acid, maxima at 276 mμ (E1%, 1 cm 87) and 280 mμ (E1%, 1 cm 80); orciprenaline sulphate in 0·01N hydrochloric acid, maximum at 328 mμ (E1%, 1 cm 0·3).

Dose. Up to 80 mg daily by mouth; the usual intramuscular or subcutaneous dose is 0·5 mg.

Toxicity. LD50 (oral): in mice 4·8 g/kg.

ORPHENADRINE *Parasympatholytic*

Synonyms: BS 5930; Mephenamine.

NN - Dimethyl - 2 - (α - *o* - tolylbenzyloxy)-ethylamine

$C_{18}H_{23}NO = 269{\cdot}4$

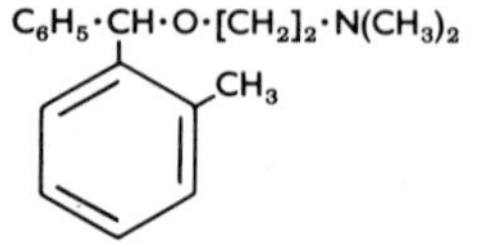

ORPHENADRINE CITRATE
Proprietary Names: Norflex. It is an ingredient of Norgesic.

A white crystalline powder. M.p. 135° to 138°.
Solubility. Soluble 1 in 70 of water; slightly soluble in ethanol; insoluble in ether and chloroform.

ORPHENADRINE HYDROCHLORIDE
Proprietary Name: Disipal.

A white crystalline powder. M.p. 159° to 162°.
Solubility. Soluble 1 in 1 of water, 1 in 1 of ethanol, and 1 in 2 of chloroform; almost insoluble in ether.

Extraction. Orphenadrine is extracted by organic solvents from aqueous alkaline solutions.

Chromatography. PAPER: system P1—Rf 0·67 (location reagents: *iodoplatinate spray*, strong reaction; *bromocresol green spray*, weak reaction); system RP1a—Rf 0·71 (location under ultraviolet light, absorption; location reagent *iodoplatinate spray*, positive reaction); system RP1b—Rf 0·00 (location as for RP1a).
THIN-LAYER: system T1—Rf 0·51 (location reagent *acidified iodoplatinate spray*, positive reaction).
GAS: system G2/225—retention time 1·28 relative to diphenhydramine.

Colour Tests. MICRO: sulphuric acid–formaldehyde test—yellow-orange (*sensitivity:* 0·25 μg); ammonium molybdate test—yellow-orange (*sensitivity:* 0·25 μg); ammonium vanadate test—orange (*sensitivity:* 0·25 μg); Vitali's test —-/-/grey-brown (*sensitivity:* 1·0 μg).

Crystal Tests. MICRO: *gold bromide–hydrochloric acid solution*—small blades or plates (*sensitivity:* 1 in 1000); *lead iodide solution*—sheaves or masses of oily needles (*sensitivity:* 1 in 1000).

Ultraviolet Absorption Spectrum. Orphenadrine in 0·01N hydrochloric acid, maximum at about 264 mμ (E1%, 1 cm 24).

Infra-red Absorption Spectrum. Orphenadrine citrate. Potassium bromide disk. The principal peaks are: A 1718, B 1216, C 1108 (p. 749).

Metabolism. Orphenadrine is an analogue of diphenhydramine but it has a very weak antihistaminic action. Studies in rats have indicated that it may be metabolised by *O*-dealkylation and *N*-demethylation (Hespe *et al.*, 1965). It is rapidly absorbed from the gastro-intestinal tract and 30 to 50% is excreted unchanged in the urine.

Dose. Up to 400 mg daily.

Toxicity. The maximum safe dose of orphenadrine is stated to be 450 mg, administered cautiously.

CASE EXAMPLES. A 22-year-old woman died about 4 hours after ingesting thirty-two 50-mg tablets of orphenadrine hydrochloride. Post-mortem levels: blood, 0·5 mg%; liver, 2·5 mg%; and stomach contents, 163 mg (Kimber, 1965).

A fatal case of orphenadrine poisoning is recorded in which the total amount of drug recovered from the stomach contents was 715 mg; the blood contained 0·4 mg% and the liver 4 mg% (Jackson, 1967).

ORTHOCAINE *Local Anaesthetic*

Synonyms: Aminobenz; Methyl Aminoxybenzoate.
Proprietary Name: Orthoform.

Methyl 3-amino-4-hydroxybenzoate
$C_8H_9NO_3$ = 167·2

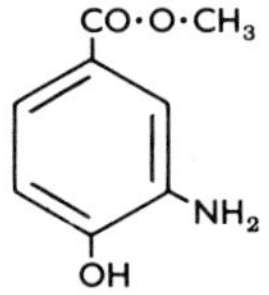

A white crystalline powder. M.p. 143°.
Solubility. Almost insoluble in water; soluble 1 in 7 of ethanol and 1 in 50 of ether.

Extraction. Orthocaine is extracted by organic solvents from aqueous alkaline solutions.

Chromatography. PAPER: system P1—Rf 0·79 (location under ultraviolet light, blue fluorescence; location reagents: *iodoplatinate spray*, weak reaction; *bromocresol green spray*, weak reaction; p-*dimethylaminobenzaldehyde spray*, yellow); system RP1a—Rf 0·52 (location under ultraviolet light, blue fluorescence; location reagent *iodoplatinate spray*, positive reaction); system RP1b—Rf 0·54 (location under ultraviolet light, blue fluorescence).
THIN-LAYER: system T1—Rf 0·71 (location reagents: p-*dimethylaminobenzaldehyde spray*, yellow; *potassium permanganate spray*, positive reaction).

Colour Tests. MICRO: ammonium molybdate test—(dull green) brown, fading (*sensitivity:* 1·0 μg); ammonium vanadate test—(grey-brown) brown (*sensitivity:* 1·0 μg); *p*-dimethylaminobenzaldehyde test—yellow (*sensitivity:* 1·0 μg); Vitali's test—yellow → blue-grey/brown/dark brown (*sensitivity:* 1·0 μg).

Crystal Tests. MICRO: *gold bromide–hydrochloric acid solution*—small plates (*sensitivity:* 1 in 1000); *mercuric chloride solution*—rosettes of rods (*sensitivity:* 1 in 1500).

Ultraviolet Absorption Spectrum. Orthocaine in 0·1N sulphuric acid, maximum at 253 mμ (E1%, 1cm 836).

Metabolism. Owing to its insolubility, orthocaine penetrates the tissues very slowly. It is excreted largely in the conjugated form; a certain amount may be acetylated at the amino-group.

Dose. Doses of up to 3 g daily have been given but considerable risk attends its internal administration. Externally, it is employed as a dusting-powder or as a 5 or 10% ointment.

Toxicity. The maximum amount stated to be safe for surface anaesthesia is 5 g.

OUABAIN *Cardiac Glycoside*

Synonyms: G-Strophanthin; Strophanthin-G; Strophanthoside-G; Uabaina; Ubaina.
Proprietary Names: Cardibaine; Purostrophan; Strophalen; Strophoperm.

A glycoside obtained from the seeds of *Strophanthus gratus* or from the wood of *Acokanthera schimperi* (Apocynaceae).
$C_{29}H_{44}O_{12},8H_2O$ = 728·8

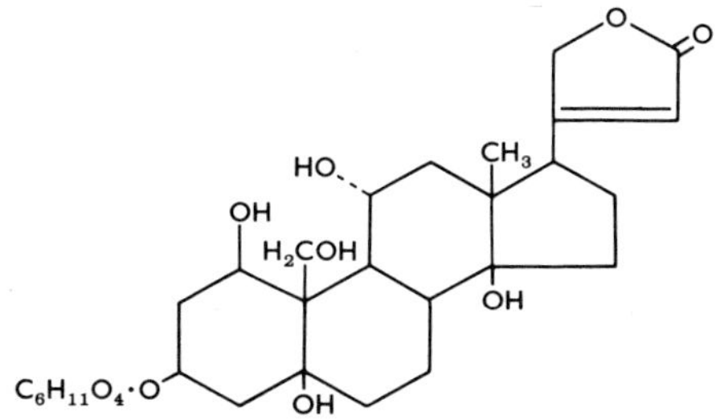

Small colourless crystals or a white crystalline powder. M.p. about 190°, indistinctly and with decomposition. Specific rotation of a 1·0% aqueous solution, −31° to −32·5°.
Solubility. Slowly soluble 1 in 75 of water; soluble 1 in 100 of ethanol; almost insoluble in ether and chloroform.

Extraction. Ouabain may be isolated by continuous extraction under reduced pressure with ethanol (p. 29).

Chromatography. THIN-LAYER: system T14—Rf 0·09 (location reagents: *perchloric acid spray*, followed by ultraviolet light, yellow-green fluorescence; p-*anisaldehyde spray*, yellow).

Colour Test. Dissolve 2 mg in 2 ml of *sulphuric acid*—dark red.

Ultraviolet Absorption Spectrum. Ouabain in sulphuric acid, maxima at 240 mμ (E1%, 1cm 450), 325 mμ (E1%, 1cm 215), and 515 mμ (E1%, 1cm 80); minima at 215 mμ, 295 mμ, and 365 mμ.

Metabolism. The absorption of ouabain from the gastro-intestinal tract is extremely poor. Following intravenous administration of tritium-labelled ouabain in man, excretion occurred primarily in the urine, only a small amount being excreted in the bile. No metabolites were detected (Marks *et al.*, 1964). Studies in rats (Dutta *et al.*, 1963) showed that following the intraperitoneal administration of 50 μg of tritium-labelled ouabain, approximately 12% of the drug was excreted in the urine in 72 hours, most of the remaining ouabain being recovered from the faeces. Other studies in rats (Farah, 1946; Cox *et al.*, 1959) have shown that the bile is an important route of elimination of ouabain.

Dose. Usually up to 0·25 mg intravenously.

Toxicity. Ouabain takes effect extremely rapidly when given by intravenous injection.
LD50 (intramuscular): in guinea-pigs 0·26 mg/kg.

OXALIC ACID

$HO_2C\cdot CO_2H,2H_2O$ = 126·1

Colourless, transparent, efflorescent crystals.

Solubility. Soluble 1 in 12 of water, 1 in 2 of boiling water, 1 in 3 of ethanol, and 1 in 100 of ether; insoluble in chloroform.

Extraction. Oxalic acid is extracted by organic solvents from aqueous acid solutions.

Colour Test. Add a few drops of a strong solution of ferrous sulphate to the acid or to a slightly acid solution of an oxalate—lemon-yellow.

Quantitative Estimation. Hodgkinson and Zarembski (1961) have described a method of determination of oxalic acid in urine. Rieders and Frere (1963) have described the detection and estimation of oxalic acid in biological material. Raekallio *et al.* (1967) have described a microscopic technique for the demonstration of calcium oxalate crystals in kidney sections.

Metabolism. Oxalic acid is rapidly converted *in vivo* to insoluble calcium oxalate. The calcium oxalate crystals are deposited in the renal tubules often causing oliguria or anuria and necrosis; the crystals may also be found in the brain and spinal cord at post-mortem examination.

Toxicity. In dilute solution oxalic acid and its salts are toxic owing to withdrawal of ionisable calcium from the blood and tissues. Strong solutions of the acid are toxic by corrosive action. The smallest recorded fatal dose of oxalic acid is 5 g. The normal oxalic acid content of biological fluids due to dietary effects is said seldom to exceed 1·0 mg%.
Farm stock, especially sheep, are sometimes poisoned by eating large quantities of plants containing oxalates.

CASE EXAMPLES. Following a case of suicide due to oxalic acid ingestion, the post-mortem levels were: blood, 6·5 mg%; stomach contents, 10·2 g%; urine, 44·4 mg% (Koumides, 1967).

In a case of fatal poisoning due to oxalic acid, the following levels were found: blood, 7·0 mg%; brain, 0·26 mg%; liver, 5·06 mg%. In 2 other cases blood-levels of 2·0 mg% and 6·6 mg% were recorded (Curry, 1967).

OXAZEPAM — *Tranquilliser*

Synonym: Wy 3498.
Proprietary Names: Adumbran; Praxiten; Serax; Serenid-D.

7 - Chloro - 1,2 - dihydro - 3 - hydroxy - 2 - oxo - 5-phenyl-3*H*-1,4-benzodiazepine
$C_{15}H_{11}ClN_2O_2$ = 286·7

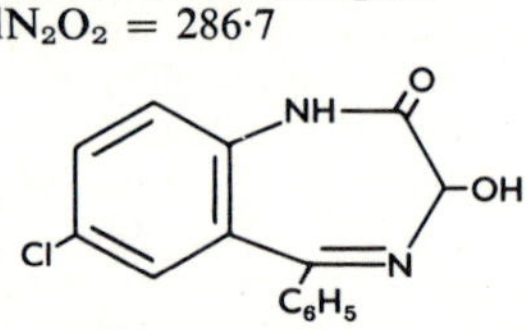

A white crystalline powder. M.p. 205° to 206°.
Solubility. Almost insoluble in water; soluble in ethanol and chloroform.

Extraction. Oxazepam is extracted by organic solvents from aqueous alkaline solutions.

Chromatography. GAS: system G2/225—retention time 0·9 relative to codeine; system G4—retention time 1·08 relative to codeine.

Ultraviolet Absorption Spectrum. Oxazepam in ethanol, maxima at 230 mμ (E1%, 1 cm about 1200) and 315 mμ (E1%, 1 cm about 85).

Infra-red Absorption Spectrum. Potassium bromide disk. The principal peaks are: A 1687, B 1706, C 693 or 830 (p. 749).

Quantitative Estimation. A method of quantitative determination in biological materials involving diazotisation is described in *Drugs of Today*, 1965, **1**, 102.

Metabolism. Following the administration of oxazepam in man, only the glucuronide conjugate of the unchanged drug is found in the urine; oxazepam does not seem to undergo further metabolism (Randall *et al.*, 1965).
After single oral doses of 60 mg in man, peak plasma levels are obtained after 4 hours and the drug persists in the plasma for at least 48 hours; a glucuronide conjugate has been detected in the plasma. The urine has been found to contain only oxazepam glucuronide and the faeces only unchanged drug (Walkenstein *et al.*, 1964). Oxazepam glucuronide is found as the main urinary metabolite of diazepam in man.

Dose. Usually up to 45 mg daily; max. in 24 hours 120 mg.

Toxicity. The lethal dose in man is probably in the range 100 to 500 mg/kg.

CASE EXAMPLE. A 2-year-old girl ingested 90 mg of oxazepam. Eighteen hours later, the serum oxazepam level was 0·05 mg% and the urine contained 0·13 mg% of unchanged drug and 1·95 mg% of oxazepam glucuronide. After 3 days none of the unchanged drug was detectable in the serum or urine but 0·12 mg% of the glucuronide was found in the urine. A test for phenothiazines was negative. The child recovered in 2 weeks (Shimkin and Shaivitz, 1966).

OXEDRINE — *Sympathomimetic*

Synonyms: Oxyphenylmethylaminoethanol; Sympaethaminum; Synephrine.

(±) - 1 - (*p* - Hydroxyphenyl) - 2 - methyl - aminoethanol
$C_9H_{13}NO_2$ = 167·2

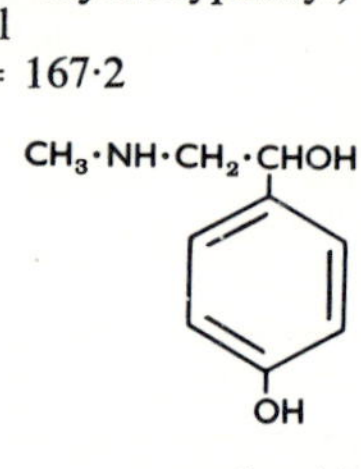

Oxedrine occurs as crystals which melt at 184° to 185°.

OXEDRINE TARTRATE
Synonym: Aetaphenum.
Proprietary Names: Analeptin; Corvasympton; Symcorthal; Sympatol; Synthenate; Vasocordrin.

A white crystalline powder.
Solubility. Soluble 1 in 2 of water and 1 in 400 of ethanol; almost insoluble in ether and chloroform.

Extraction. Oxedrine is extracted by organic solvents from aqueous ammoniacal solutions.

Chromatography. PAPER: system P1—Rf 0·15 (location under ultraviolet light, strong absorption; location reagents: *bromocresol green spray*, weak reaction; *potassium permanganate spray*, weak reaction).
THIN-LAYER: system T1—Rf 0·22 (location reagent *potassium permanganate spray*, positive reaction).

Colour Tests. Chen's test—purple.
MICRO: ammonium molybdate test—grey (*sensitivity:* 0·5 μg); Vitali's test—yellow/yellow/orange (*sensitivity:* 0·25 μg).

Crystal Test. MICRO: *gold bromide solution*—serrated plates (*sensitivity:* 1 in 200).

Ultraviolet Absorption Spectrum. Oxedrine in water, maximum at 272 mμ (E1%, 1cm 53); in 0·1N sulphuric acid, maximum at 273 mμ (E1%, 1cm 96) and an inflexion at 278 mμ.

Dose. Usually up to 300 mg daily by mouth; up to 150 mg subcutaneously or intramuscularly as a single dose.

OXELADIN *Antitussive*

2 - (2 - Diethylaminoethoxy)ethyl α - ethyl - α - phenylbutyrate
$C_{20}H_{33}NO_3$ = 335·5

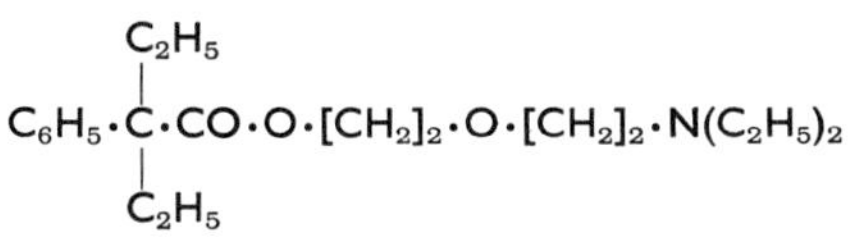

OXELADIN CITRATE
Proprietary Names: Pectamol; Tussimol.

A white crystalline powder.
Solubility. Soluble in water.

Extraction. Oxeladin is extracted by organic solvents from aqueous alkaline solutions.

Chromatography. PAPER: system P1—Rf 0·82 (location reagents: *iodoplatinate spray*, strong reaction; *bromocresol green spray*, weak reaction); system RP1a—Rf 0·42 (location reagent *iodoplatinate spray*, positive reaction); system RP1b—Rf 0·00 (location as for RP1a).
THIN-LAYER: system T1—Rf 0·45 (location reagent *acidified iodoplatinate spray*, positive reaction).

Colour Tests. MICRO: sulphuric acid–formaldehyde test—orange (*sensitivity:* 0·5 μg); ammonium molybdate test—faint blue (*sensitivity:* 1·0 μg).

Crystal Test. MICRO: *lead iodide solution*—sheaves of fine needles (*sensitivity:* 1 in 1000).

Ultraviolet Absorption Spectrum. Oxeladin in 0·1N sulphuric acid, maxima at 252·5 mμ (E1%, 1cm 6), 258·5 mμ (E1%, 1cm 7), and 264·5 mμ (E1%, 1cm 5).

Dose. Up to 80 mg daily.

OXETHAZAINE *Local Anaesthetic*

Synonyms: Oxetacaine; Wy 806.
Proprietary Names: It is an ingredient of Mucaine and Oxaine.

αα′ - (2 - Hydroxyethyl)iminobis[*N* - (αα - dimethylphenethyl)-*N*-methylacetamide]
$C_{28}H_{41}N_3O_3$ = 467·7

Oxethazaine melts at 104° to 104·5°.
Solubility. Insoluble in water.

OXETHAZAINE HYDROCHLORIDE
Oxethazaine hydrochloride melts at 146° to 147°.
Solubility. Soluble in water.

Extraction. Oxethazaine is extracted by organic solvents from aqueous alkaline solutions.

Chromatography. PAPER: system P1—Rf 0·87 (location reagents: *iodoplatinate spray*, weak reaction; *bromocresol green spray*, weak reaction); system RP1a—Rf 0·04 (location reagent *iodoplatinate spray*, positive reaction); system RP1b—Rf 0·00 (location as for RP1a).
THIN-LAYER: system T1—Rf 0·12, streaking (location reagent *acidified iodoplatinate spray*, positive reaction).

Colour Tests. MICRO: sulphuric acid–formaldehyde test—red-brown (*sensitivity:* 0·1 μg); ammonium molybdate test—purple-brown (*sensitivity:* 0·1 μg); ammonium vanadate test—purple-brown (*sensitivity:* 0·1 μg); Vitali's test—yellow, fading/faintly yellow/faintly yellow (*sensitivity:* 1·0 μg).

Crystal Tests. MICRO: *platinic bromide solution*—oily branching plates (*sensitivity:* 1 in 3000); *platinic chloride solution*—branching serrated needles, from dilute solutions only (*sensitivity:* 1 in 3000).

Ultraviolet Absorption Spectrum. Oxethazaine in 0·1N sulphuric acid, maxima at 248 mμ (E1%, 1cm 9), 252 mμ (E1%, 1cm 11), 258 mμ (E1%, 1cm 12·5), 264 mμ (E1%, 1cm 10), and about 267 mμ (E1%, 1cm 8).

Metabolism. Oxethazaine is a surface anaesthetic which is said to have a prolonged action after a somewhat slow onset. It is poorly absorbed from mucous membranes.

Use. It has been given by mouth, in conjunction with antacids, for the relief of pain and discomfort in dyspeptic patients.

Dose. Up to 100 mg daily, by mouth.

Toxicity. LD50 (oral): in mice 0·4 and in rats 0·63 g/kg.

OXYBUPROCAINE *Local Anaesthetic*

Synonym: Benoxinate.

2-Diethylaminoethyl 4-amino-3-butoxybenzoate

$C_{17}H_{28}N_2O_3 = 308{\cdot}4$

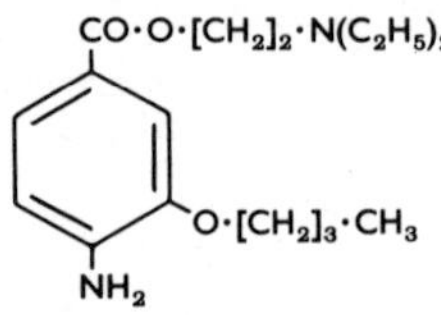

OXYBUPROCAINE HYDROCHLORIDE

Proprietary Names: Dorsacaine; Novesine.

White crystals or a crystalline powder. M.p. 155°.

Solubility. Very soluble in water, ethanol, and chloroform; very slightly soluble in ether.

Extraction. Oxybuprocaine is extracted by organic solvents from aqueous alkaline solutions.

Chromatography. PAPER: system P1—Rf 0·70 (location under ultraviolet light, blue fluorescence; location reagents: *iodoplatinate spray*, strong reaction; *bromocresol green spray*, weak reaction).

THIN-LAYER: system T1—Rf 0·63 (location reagent *acidified iodoplatinate spray*, positive reaction).

Colour Test. MICRO: diazotisation test—red.

Crystal Tests. MICRO: *gold bromide–hydrochloric acid solution*—small plates or needles, best viewed under polarised light (*sensitivity:* 1 in 1000); *potassium tri-iodide solution* (*3*)—irregular needles (*sensitivity:* 1 in 400).

Infra-red Absorption Spectrum. Oxybuprocaine hydrochloride. Potassium bromide disk. The principal peaks are: A 1215 or 1262 or 1698 (p. 750).

Use. A 0·4% solution is employed in ophthalmological procedures.

Toxicity. The maximum amount stated to be safe for surface anaesthesia is 100 mg.

OXYCODONE *Narcotic Analgesic*

Synonyms: Dihydrohydroxycodeinone; 7,8-Dihydro-14-hydroxycodeinone; Dihydrone; Oxycone; Thecodin.

4,5 - Epoxy - 14 - hydroxy - 3 - methoxy - *N* - methyl-6-oxomorphinan

$C_{18}H_{21}NO_4 = 315{\cdot}4$

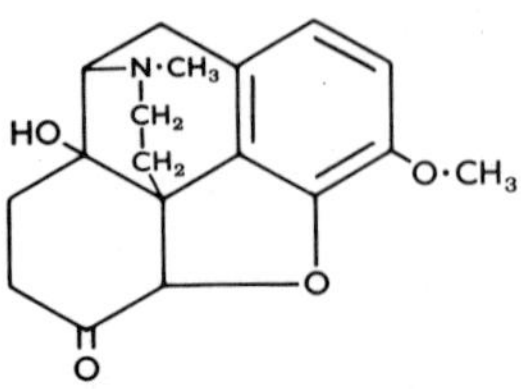

Oxycodone melts at 218° to 220°.

Solubility. Insoluble in water and ether; soluble in ethanol and chloroform.

OXYCODONE HYDROCHLORIDE

Proprietary Name: Eucodal.

A white crystalline powder.

Solubility. Soluble 1 in 6 of water, 1 in 60 of ethanol, and 1 in 600 of chloroform; almost insoluble in ether.

OXYCODONE PECTINATE

Proprietary Name: Proladone.

Extraction. Oxycodone may be isolated in the D2 fraction; hydrolysis of biological material is required in order to improve the yield.

Chromatography. PAPER: system P1—Rf 0·16 (location under ultraviolet light, strong absorption; location reagents: *iodoplatinate spray*, strong reaction; *bromocresol green spray*, weak reaction); system RP1a—Rf 0·90 (location reagent *iodoplatinate spray*, positive reaction); system RP1b—Rf 0·06 (location under ultraviolet light, absorption).

THIN-LAYER: system T1—Rf 0·53 (location reagent *acidified iodoplatinate spray*, positive reaction).

GAS: system G2/225—retention time 1·17 relative to codeine; system G4—retention time 2·05 relative to codeine.

Colour Tests. MICRO: sulphuric acid–formaldehyde test—yellow → brown → purple; ammonium molybdate test—yellow → brown → purple (*sensitivity:* 0·1 μg); Vitali's test—faint yellow/–/yellow (*sensitivity:* 1·0 μg).

Crystal Tests. MICRO: *potassium tri-iodide solution* (*1*)—small dark plates (*sensitivity:* 1 in 400); *sodium carbonate solution*—long thin needles (*sensitivity:* 1 in 3000).

Ultraviolet Absorption Spectrum. Oxycodone in 0·1N sulphuric acid, maximum at 280 mμ (E1%, 1 cm 31).

Infra-red Absorption Spectrum. Oxycodone (base). Potassium bromide disk. The principal peaks are: A 1719, B 1501, C 1033 or 1255 or 1448 (p. 750).

Dose. Up to 30 mg.

Toxicity. The estimated minimum lethal dose in man is 500 mg. Oxycodone possesses addiction-producing properties.

OXYMETAZOLINE *Vasoconstrictor*

Synonym: H 990.

2 - (3 - Hydroxy - 2,6 - dimethyl - 4 - t - butylbenzyl)-2-imidazoline

$C_{16}H_{24}N_2O = 260{\cdot}4$

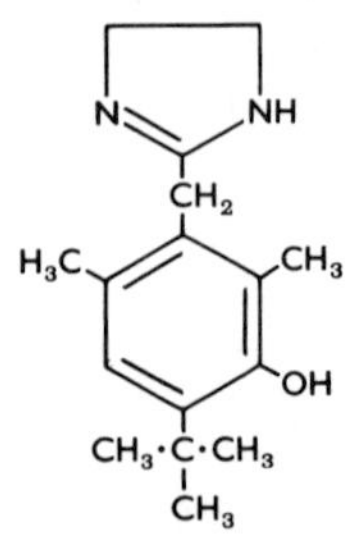

OXYMETAZOLINE HYDROCHLORIDE

Proprietary Names: Afrin; Atomol; Hazol; Nasivin.

A white crystalline powder.
Solubility. Readily soluble in water and ethanol; almost insoluble in ether and chloroform.

Extraction. Oxymetazoline is extracted by organic solvents from aqueous alkaline solutions.

Chromatography. PAPER: system P1—Rf 0·76 (location under ultraviolet light, absorption; location reagents: *iodoplatinate spray*, strong reaction; *bromocresol green spray*, weak reaction); system RP1a—Rf 0·89 (location reagent *iodoplatinate spray*, positive reaction); system RP1b—Rf 0·88 (location as for RP1a).
THIN-LAYER: system T1—Rf 0·14, streaking (location reagent *acidified iodoplatinate spray*, positive reaction).
GAS: system G2/225—retention time 0·60 relative to codeine.

Colour Tests. MICRO: ammonium molybdate test—blue → green (*sensitivity:* 0·25 μg); ammonium vanadate test—olive (*sensitivity:* 0·5 μg); Vitali's test—pale yellow/pale yellow/bright orange (*sensitivity:* 0·25 μg).

Crystal Tests. MICRO: *gold chloride solution*—oily needles (*sensitivity:* 1 in 200); *picric acid*—bunches of blades (*sensitivity:* 1 in 400).

Ultraviolet Absorption Spectrum. Oxymetazoline in water, maximum at 279 mμ (E1%, 1 cm 60).

Infra-red Absorption Spectrum. Oxymetazoline hydrochloride. Potassium bromide disk. The principal peaks are: A 1595, B 1199, C 1285 (p. 750).

Use. As a 0·05% solution in nasal sprays and drops.

OXYMORPHONE *Narcotic Analgesic*

Synonyms: Dihydrohydroxymorphinone; 7,8-Dihydro-14-hydroxymorphinone; Dimorphone; Oximorphone; Oxydimorphone.

4,5 - Epoxy - 3,14 - dihydroxy - *N* - methyl - 6 - oxomorphinan
$C_{17}H_{19}NO_4$ = 301·3

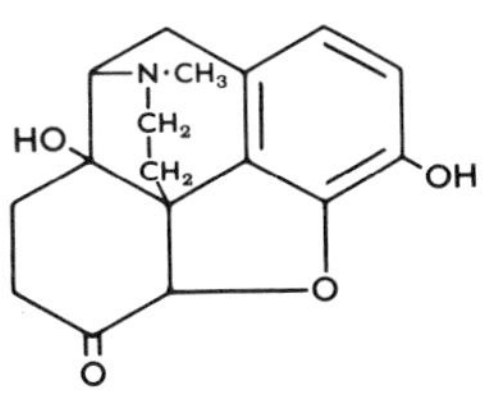

Oxymorphone occurs as crystals which melt at 248° to 249°.
Solubility. Soluble in boiling ethanol and in chloroform.

OXYMORPHONE HYDROCHLORIDE
Proprietary Name: Numorphan.

A white crystalline powder.
Solubility. Soluble in water; slightly soluble in ethanol.

Extraction. Oxymorphone may be isolated in the D3 fraction; hydrolysis of biological material is required in order to improve the yield (see p. 27).

Chromatography. PAPER: system P1—Rf 0·09 (location under ultraviolet light, dark blue fluorescence; location reagent *iodoplatinate spray*, weak reaction); system RP1a—Rf 0·94 (location under ultraviolet light, absorption); system RP1b—Rf 0·33 (location as for RP1a).
THIN-LAYER: system T1—Rf 0·50 (location reagent *acidified iodoplatinate spray*, positive reaction).
GAS: system G2/225—retention time 1·6 relative to codeine.

Colour Tests. MICRO: sulphuric acid–formaldehyde test—faint grey-purple (*sensitivity:* 0·5 μg); ammonium molybdate test—bright blue → green (*sensitivity:* 0·25 μg); Vitali's test—yellow/yellow/bright orange (*sensitivity:* 0·5 μg).

Crystal Tests. MICRO: *gold bromide solution*—dense rosettes (*sensitivity:* 1 in 1000); *mercuric chloride solution*—fans of needles, forming overnight (*sensitivity:* 1 in 1000).

Ultraviolet Absorption Spectrum. Oxymorphone in 0·1N sulphuric acid, maximum at 281 mμ (E1%, 1 cm 33·6).

Dose. Usually up to 5 mg by injection; up to 10 mg by mouth.

Toxicity. The estimated minimum lethal dose in man is 50 mg. Oxymorphone possesses marked addiction-producing properties.

OXYPERTINE *Tranquilliser*

Synonym: Win 18501.

5,6 - Dimethoxy - 2 - methyl - 3 - [2 - (4 - phenylpiperazin-1-yl)ethyl]indole
$C_{23}H_{29}N_3O_2$ = 379·5

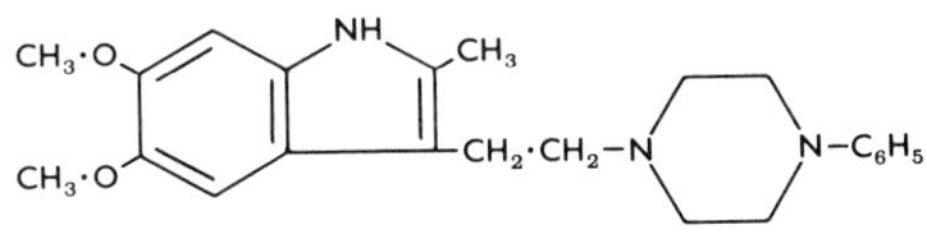

OXYPERTINE HYDROCHLORIDE
Proprietary Names: Forit; Integrin.

A white crystalline powder. M.p. 249° to 255°.

Extraction. Oxypertine is extracted by organic solvents from aqueous alkaline solutions.

Chromatography. PAPER: system P1—Rf 0·57 (location under ultraviolet light, blue fluorescence; location reagent *iodoplatinate spray*, weak reaction).
THIN-LAYER: system T1—Rf 0·73 (location reagent *acidified iodoplatinate spray*, positive reaction).
GAS: system G2/225—retention time 0·53 relative to codeine; system G4—retention time 2·25 relative to diphenhydramine.

Colour Tests. MICRO: sulphuric acid–formaldehyde test—grey-green (*sensitivity:* 0·1 μg); ammonium molybdate test—blue → green (*sensitivity:* 0·1 μg); ammonium vanadate test—grey (*sensitivity:* 0·25 μg); Vitali's test—orange/yellow-brown/orange (*sensitivity:* 0·1 μg).

Crystal Tests. MICRO: *ammonium thiocyanate solution*—irregular blades (*sensitivity:* 1 in 1000); *potassium iodide solution*—irregular blades (*sensitivity:* 1 in 1000).

Ultraviolet Absorption Spectrum. Oxypertine in 0·1N sulphuric acid, maxima at 225 mμ (E1%, 1 cm 851), 277 mμ (E1%, 1 cm 141), and 302 mμ (E1%, 1 cm 212).

Dose. Usually up to 120 mg; max. in 24 hours 300 mg.

OXYPHENBUTAZONE

Analgesic and Antipyretic

Synonyms: G 27202; Hydroxyphenylbutazone.
Proprietary Names: Tandearil; Tanderil.

4 - Butyl - 1 - *p* - hydroxyphenyl - 3,5 - dioxo - 2-phenylpyrazolidine monohydrate
$C_{19}H_{20}N_2O_3,H_2O$ = 342·4

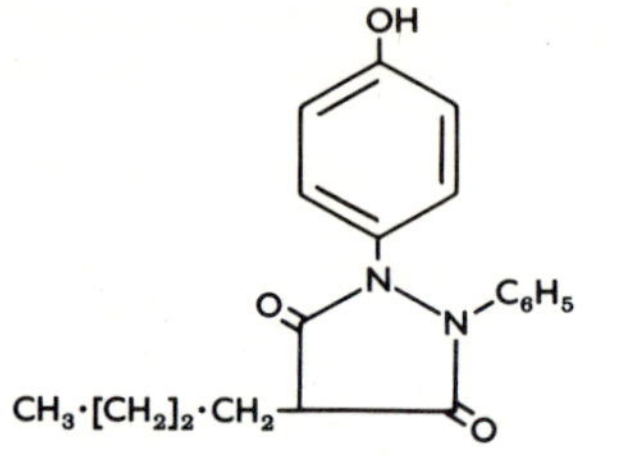

A white crystalline powder. M.p. about 96°.

Solubility. Almost insoluble in water; soluble 1 in 3 of ethanol, 1 in 20 of ether, and 1 in 20 of chloroform.

Extraction. Oxyphenbutazone is extracted by organic solvents from aqueous acid or alkaline solutions.

Chromatography. PAPER: system P1—Rf 0·96 (location under ultraviolet light, strong absorption; location reagents: p-*dimethylaminobenzaldehyde spray*, pale yellow; *potassium permanganate spray*, weak reaction); system RP1a—Rf 0·04 (location under ultraviolet light, absorption); system RP1b—Rf 0·58 (location as for RP1a).

THIN-LAYER: system T1—Rf 0·77 (location reagent *potassium permanganate spray*, positive reaction).

Colour Tests. MICRO: sulphuric acid–formaldehyde test—pale yellow (*sensitivity:* 1·0 μg); ammonium molybdate test—pale orange (*sensitivity:* 1·0 μg); Vitali's test—pale yellow/pale yellow/red (*sensitivity:* 0·25 μg).

Crystal Tests. MICRO: *platinic iodide solution*—rosettes of prisms, forming overnight (*sensitivity:* 1 in 100); *potassium iodide solution*—shell-like crystals, forming overnight (*sensitivity:* 1 in 100).

Ultraviolet Absorption Spectrum. Oxyphenbutazone in ethanol, maximum at 242 mμ (E1%, 1 cm 564) and an inflexion at 275 mμ; in 0·01N sodium hydroxide, maximum at 254 mμ (E1%, 1 cm 1500).

Infra-red Absorption Spectrum. Potassium bromide disk. The principal peaks are: A 1683, B 1725, C 1275 or 1518 (p. 750).

Quantitative Estimation. Oxyphenbutazone may be estimated quantitatively by the methods described under Phenylbutazone—see p. 493.

Metabolism. Oxyphenbutazone is slowly metabolised to unknown compounds. It is one of the 2 main metabolites of phenylbutazone and is considered to be more toxic than the latter. It may accumulate in the body since it is excreted very slowly.

Dose. Up to 600 mg daily.

Toxicity. Oxyphenbutazone may give rise to a wide variety of toxic side-effects even when the dosage does not exceed 400 mg daily. Untoward reactions occur in some 25 to 40% of patients and they are often sufficiently severe to necessitate withdrawal of the drug. Fatal cases of leukaemia and of agranulocytosis have occurred. The acute lethal dose is stated to be between 5 and 30 g.

OXYPHENCYCLIMINE *Parasympatholytic*

(1,4,5,6 - Tetrahydro - 1 - methylpyrimidin - 2 - yl)methyl α-cyclohexyl-α-phenylglycollate
$C_{20}H_{28}N_2O_3$ = 344·5

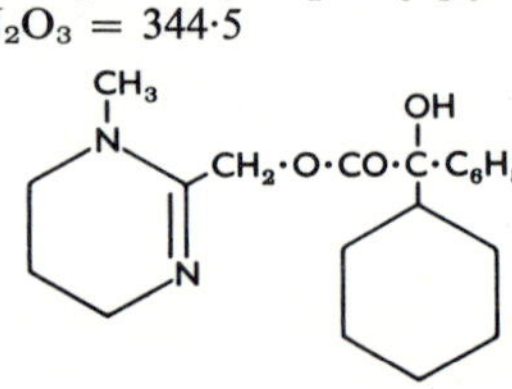

OXYPHENCYCLIMINE HYDROCHLORIDE
Proprietary Names: Daricon; Vio-thene.

A white crystalline powder. M.p. about 230°, with decomposition.

Solubility. Soluble 1 in 100 of water, 1 in 60 of ethanol, 1 in 3000 of ether, and 1 in 200 of chloroform.

Extraction. Oxyphencyclimine is extracted by organic solvents from aqueous alkaline solutions.

Chromatography. PAPER: system P1—Rf 0·72 (location reagent *iodoplatinate spray*, strong reaction).

THIN-LAYER: system T1—Rf 0·03 (location reagent *acidified iodoplatinate spray*, positive reaction).

Colour Tests. MICRO: ammonium molybdate test—faint blue (*sensitivity:* 0·5 μg); ammonium vanadate test—grey-green (*sensitivity:* 0·5 μg).

Crystal Tests. MICRO: *platinic bromide solution*—irregular dense rosettes, forming overnight (*sensitivity:* 1 in 100); *platinic chloride solution*—bunches of plates (*sensitivity:* 1 in 1000).

Dose. Usually up to 20 mg daily; max. in 24 hours 50 mg.

Toxicity. The lethal dose in man is probably in the range 10 to 100 mg/kg.

OXYPHENONIUM BROMIDE

Parasympatholytic

Proprietary Name: Antrenyl.

[2 - (2 - Cyclohexyl - 2 - hydroxy - 2 - phenyl - acetoxy)ethyl]diethylmethylammonium bromide

$C_{21}H_{34}BrNO_3$ = 428·4

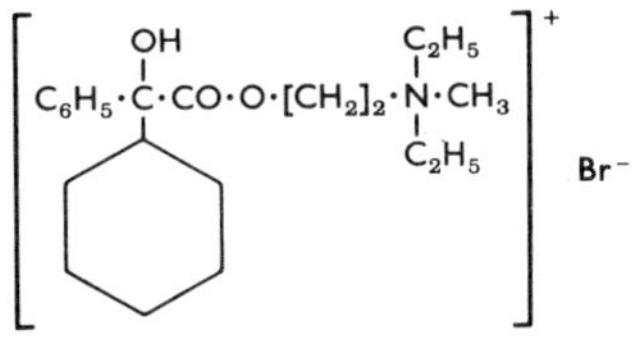

A white crystalline powder.

Solubility. Readily soluble in water.

Extraction. Oxyphenonium bromide is a quaternary ammonium compound (see p. 29).

Chromatography. PAPER: system P1—Rf 0·62 (location reagents: *iodoplatinate spray*, strong reaction; *bromocresol green spray*, weak reaction); system RP1a—Rf 0·86 (location reagent *iodoplatinate spray*, positive reaction); system RP1b—Rf 0·76 (location as for RP1a).

THIN-LAYER: system T1—Rf 0·03 (location reagent *acidified iodoplatinate spray*, positive reaction).

Crystal Tests. MICRO: *gold bromide–hydrochloric acid solution*—bunches of plates, often serrated (*sensitivity:* 1 in 3000); *gold chloride solution*—masses of needles and serrated plates (*sensitivity:* 1 in 3000).

Ultraviolet Absorption Spectrum. Oxyphenonium bromide in ethanol, maximum at 257·5 mμ (E1%, 1cm 5·4); in 0·1N sulphuric acid, maxima at 252 mμ (E1%, 1cm 417), 258 mμ (E1%, 1cm 513), 264 mμ (E1%, 1cm 4·2), and about 268 mμ (E1%, 1cm 2·3).

Infra-red Absorption Spectrum. Potassium bromide disk. The principal peaks are: A 1225, B 1719, C 729 (p. 750).

Dose. Up to 40 mg daily.

Toxicity. The lethal dose in man is probably in the range 10 to 100 mg/kg.

OXYTETRACYCLINE DIHYDRATE

Antibiotic

Synonyms: Oxytetracycline; Terrafungine.
Proprietary Names: Imperacin; Oxymycin; Terramycin.

4 - Dimethylamino - 1,4,4a,5,5a,6,11,12a - octahydro - 3,5,6,10,12,12a - hexahydroxy - 6 - methyl - 1,11 - dioxonaphthacene - 2 - carboxyamide dihydrate

$C_{22}H_{24}N_2O_9,2H_2O$ = 496·5

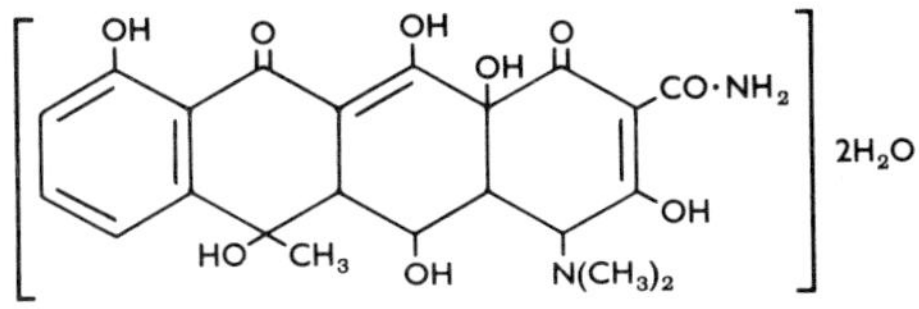

A tawny crystalline powder. Specific rotation of a 1·0% solution in 0·1N hydrochloric acid, −188° to −200°.

Solubility. Soluble 1 in 2000 of water and 1 in 100 of ethanol. It deteriorates in solutions having a pH of less than 2 and is rapidly destroyed by alkalis.

OXYTETRACYCLINE HYDROCHLORIDE

A yellow hygroscopic crystalline powder.

Solubility. Soluble 1 in 2 of water and 1 in 45 of ethanol; insoluble in ether and chloroform.

Extraction. Oxytetracycline is extracted by organic solvents from aqueous alkaline solutions.

Chromatography. PAPER: system P1—Rf 0·24 (location under ultraviolet light, orange fluorescence; location reagents: *bromine-starch–potassium iodide*, strong reaction; *potassium permanganate spray*, weak reaction).

Addison and Clark (1963) describe a paper chromatographic method of separation of tetracycline derivatives in blood and urine.

THIN-LAYER: system T1—Rf 0·05, streaking (location under ultraviolet light, orange fluorescence; location reagent *potassium permanganate spray*, positive reaction).

Colour Tests. MICRO: sulphuric acid–formaldehyde test—dull orange (*sensitivity:* 0·5 μg); ammonium molybdate test—black-purple (*sensitivity:* 0·5 μg); ammonium vanadate test—purple → red → orange (*sensitivity:* 0·5 μg); sulphuric acid test—purple → yellow; Vitali's test—yellow/yellow/brown (*sensitivity:* 0·5 μg).

Crystal Tests. MICRO: *gold bromide–hydrochloric acid solution*—dense rosettes (*sensitivity:* 1 in 440); *sodium phosphate solution*—rods, best viewed under polarised light (*sensitivity:* 1 in 100).

Ultraviolet Absorption Spectrum. Oxytetracycline dihydrate in *solution of standard pH 2·0*, maximum at 353 mμ (E1%, 1cm 270 to 280); in 0·1N sulphuric acid, maxima at 269 mμ (E1%, 1cm 400), about 320 mμ (E1%, 1cm 203), and 352 mμ (E1%, 1cm 272).

Metabolism. Both oxytetracycline and its hydrochloride are rapidly absorbed from the gastro-intestinal tract. After a single 2-g oral

dose, maximum levels are obtained in the serum within 2 to 4 hours and appreciable concentrations maintained for up to 24 hours. Intravenous administration of only 250 mg produces serum levels of 0·5 to 1·0 mg% within 1 hour.
Oxytetracycline readily diffuses through the body fluids and is widely distributed. High concentrations in a biologically active form are excreted in the bile, faeces, and urine.

Dose. Up to 3 g daily.

Toxicity. LD50 (oral): in mice 6·7 to 7·2 g/kg.

PAMAQUIN *Antimalarial*

Synonyms: Aminoquin; Gametocidum; Pamachin; Pamaquine Naphthoate; Plasmoquinum; RP 4516; SN 971.
Proprietary Names: Praequine; Plasmochin Naphthoate.

8 - (4 - Diethylamino - 1 - methylbutylamino) - 6 - methoxyquinoline 2,2′ - dihydroxy - 1,1′ - dinaphthylmethane-3,3′-dicarboxylate

$C_{19}H_{29}N_3O, C_{23}H_{16}O_6 = 703·8$

The following is the formula of the free base, 8 - (4 - diethylamino - 1 - methylbutylamino) - 6-methoxyquinoline:

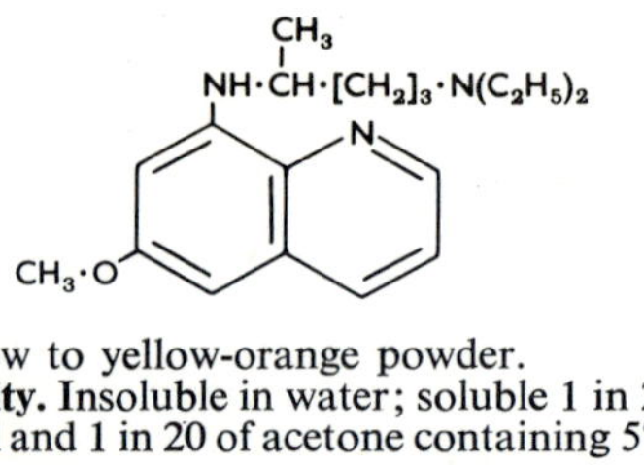

A yellow to yellow-orange powder.
Solubility. Insoluble in water; soluble 1 in 20 of ethanol and 1 in 20 of acetone containing 5% of water.

Extraction. Pamaquin is extracted by organic solvents from aqueous alkaline solutions.

Chromatography. PAPER: system P1—Rf 0·67 (location under ultraviolet light, orange fluorescence; location reagents: *iodoplatinate spray*, strong reaction; *bromocresol green spray*, weak reaction).
THIN-LAYER: system T1—Rf 0·22 (location reagent *diazotised* p-*nitroaniline–sodium hydroxide spray*, positive reaction).

Colour Tests. MICRO: the following tests are performed on the free base: sulphuric acid–formaldehyde test—orange (*sensitivity:* 0·25 μg); ammonium molybdate test—pale blue (*sensitivity:* 1·0 μg); ammonium vanadate test—purple-brown (*sensitivity:* 0·5 μg); Vitali's test—brown/yellow/orange (*sensitivity:* 1·0 μg).

Ultraviolet Absorption Spectrum. Pamaquin in 0·1N sodium hydroxide, maxima at 237·5 mμ (E1%, 1 cm 4775), 287·5 mμ (E1%, 1 cm 566), about 297·5 mμ (E1%, 1 cm 400), and 362 mμ (E1%, 1 cm 400).

Infra-red Absorption Spectrum. Potassium bromide disk. The principal peaks are: A 1458, B 1393, C 1355 (p. 750).

Metabolism. In man, pamaquin has been found to be metabolised fairly rapidly into 2 compounds which are excreted in the urine. One metabolite is unstable and can lead to methaemoglobinaemia, a toxic effect of pamaquin; it is suggested that this compound is 5-hydroxypamaquin which may undergo reversible conversion to the iminoquinone. About 3% of a daily dose is excreted as this metabolite. The second metabolite is a stable, highly fluorescent compound.
A 5,6-quinone metabolite of pamaquin has been found to be excreted by chickens; it is 16 times as active as pamaquin *in vitro*. The formation of this metabolite involves both demethylation and oxidation—see under The Metabolism of Drugs, p. 161.

Dose. Usually up to 20 mg daily.

Toxicity. The margin between therapeutic and toxic doses is small, 30 mg daily having caused serious toxic effects. Toxic reactions may include methaemoglobinaemia, jaundice, and intravascular haemolysis with passage of blood pigments in the urine.

PAPAVERINE

Muscle Relaxant/Antispasmodic

Proprietary Name: it is an ingredient of Monotrean.

6,7 - Dimethoxy - 1 - (3,4 - dimethoxybenzyl) - isoquinoline

$C_{20}H_{21}NO_4 = 339·4$

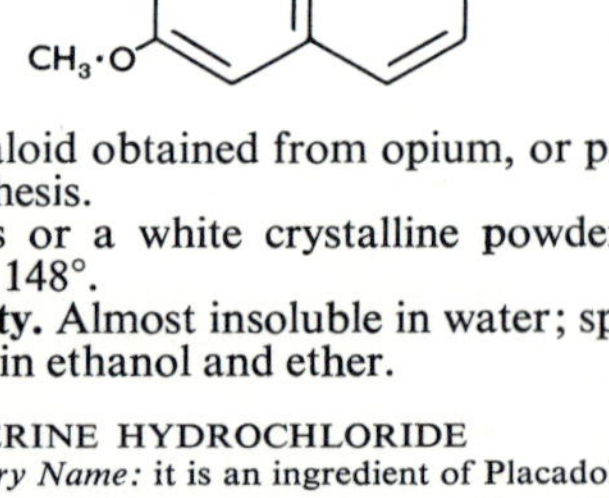

An alkaloid obtained from opium, or prepared by synthesis.
Crystals or a white crystalline powder. M.p. 146° to 148°.
Solubility. Almost insoluble in water; sparingly soluble in ethanol and ether.

PAPAVERINE HYDROCHLORIDE

Proprietary Name: it is an ingredient of Placadol.

A white crystalline powder. M.p. 215° to 225°, after drying at 105° for 30 minutes.
Solubility. Soluble 1 in 40 of water, 1 in 120 of ethanol, and 1 in 10 of chloroform; insoluble in ether.

PAPAVERINE SULPHATE

A white crystalline powder.
Solubility. Soluble 1 in 2 of water, 1 in 20 of ethanol, 1 in 5000 of ether, and 1 in 20 of chloroform.

Extraction. Papaverine is extracted by organic solvents from aqueous alkaline solutions.

Chromatography. PAPER: system P1—Rf 0·49 (location under ultraviolet light, pale yellow-green fluorescence; location reagent *iodoplatinate spray*, weak reaction); system RP1a—Rf 0·08 (location under ultraviolet light, pale yellow fluorescence; location reagent *iodoplatinate spray*, positive reaction); system RP1b—Rf 0·00 (location as for RP1a).

THIN-LAYER: system T1—Rf 0·66 (location reagent *acidified iodoplatinate spray*, positive reaction).

GAS: system G2/225—retention time 3·5 relative to codeine; system G6—retention time 3·17 relative to codeine.

Colour Tests. MICRO: ammonium molybdate test—(faint green) blue (*sensitivity:* 0·5 μg); ammonium vanadate test—grey-green (*sensitivity:* 1·0 μg); Vitali's test—faint yellow/orange/brown.

Crystal Tests. MICRO: *potassium cadmium iodide solution*—rosettes of blades (*sensitivity:* 1 in 1500); *zinc chloride solution*—bunches of plates (*sensitivity:* 1 in 3000).

Ultraviolet Absorption Spectrum. Papaverine in 1N hydrochloric acid, maxima at 250 mμ (E1%, 1 cm 1830), 284 mμ (E1%, 1 cm 193), and 310 mμ (E1%, 1 cm 253); papaverine sulphate in 1N hydrochloric acid, maxima at about 250 mμ (E1%, 1 cm 1440), about 254 mμ (E1%, 1 cm about 150), and about 310 mμ (E1%, 1 cm about 200).

Infra-red Absorption Spectrum. Papaverine (base). Potassium bromide disk. The principal peaks are: A 1507, B 1068, C 1273 (p. 751).

Quantitative Estimation. Fairbairn and El-Masry (1967) describe a spectrophotometric determination of papaverine following thin-layer chromatographic separation from the other opium alkaloids.

Metabolism. In man, papaverine has been shown to be metabolised by a selective demethylation at position 4. About 40% of administered papaverine is excreted as the 4-demethylated compound, 4-hydroxypapaverine, mostly in the form of a glucuronide conjugate.

Dose. Up to 300 mg by mouth; up to 100 mg by injection.

Toxicity. Occasional fatalities have resulted from intravenous administration which can cause cardiac arrhythmias. The lethal dose in man is said to be in the range 100 to 500 mg/kg.

LD50 (oral): in mice 2·5 and in rats 0·75 g/kg.

PARACETAMOL *Analgesic and Antipyretic*

Synonyms: Acetaminophen; *p*-Hydroxyacetanilide.
Proprietary Names: Calpol; Cetal; Eneril; Febrilix; PCM; Pamol; Panadol; Panaleve; Panasorb; Panets; Panok; Tabalgin; Tetmal; Tylenol. It is an ingredient of many proprietary preparations—see Extra Pharmacopoeia (Martindale), 25th Edn, p. 41.

p-Acetamidophenol
$C_8H_9NO_2 = 151{\cdot}2$

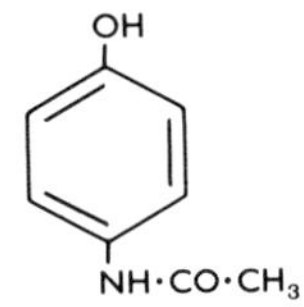

A white crystalline powder. M.p. 169° to 172°.

Solubility. Soluble 1 in 70 of water, 1 in 20 of boiling water, 1 in 7 of ethanol, and 1 in 50 of chloroform; insoluble in ether.

Screening Test. See under Screening Tests, p. 14.

Extraction. Paracetamol is extracted by organic solvents from aqueous acid solutions; hydrolysis of biological material is required in order to improve the yield.

Chromatography. PAPER: system RP1b—Rf 0·80 (location reagent *bromine–starch–potassium iodide*).

GAS: system G5—retention time 2·4 relative to barbitone.

Colour Tests. Ferric chloride test—blue. *Liebermann's reagent*—violet. Boil 0·1 g of paracetamol with 1 ml of concentrated hydrochloric acid for 3 minutes, add 10 ml of water and cool before adding 0·05 ml of 0·1N potassium dichromate solution—violet, developing slowly (which in contrast to phenacetin does not become red).

Ultraviolet Absorption Spectrum. Paracetamol in methanol, maximum at 249 mμ (E1%, 1 cm 900).

Infra-red Absorption Spectrum. Potassium bromide disk. The principal peaks are: A 1650, B 1563, C 1443 (p. 751).

Quantitative Estimation. Gwilt (1963) has described a method of determination of non-conjugated paracetamol in blood. Welch and Connery (1965) have described a spectrophotometric estimation of paracetamol in urine following acid hydrolysis.

Metabolism. Paracetamol is excreted fairly rapidly in the urine, about 67% in the form of an ethereal sulphate conjugate and about 33% as a glucuronide conjugate; up to 3% may be detected in the free form. Deacetylation occurs to yield *p*-aminophenol.

Absorption from the gastro-intestinal tract is rapid; after doses of 1 g, plasma levels may range from 0·45 to 2·6 mg% within 45 minutes of ingestion; after doses of 2 g, plasma levels of up to 5 mg% may be expected.

Paracetamol is found as one of the main metabolites of phenacetin (p. 477) and of acetanilide (p. 170).

Dose. Up to 1 g every 3 or 4 hours.

Toxicity. The lethal dose in man is stated to be between 5 and 20 g, although recoveries have occurred following the ingestion of 40 g (see below) and 35 g.

LD50 (oral): in rats 3·7 g/kg.

CASE EXAMPLES. (1) A 30-year-old female mental patient was admitted to hospital 2 hours after taking at least 50 paracetamol tablets. Death occurred after 4 days and acute liver necrosis was found at post-mortem examination. The patient had currently been taking 75 mg of nortriptyline daily and barbiturates for many years. On admission, the plasma *p*-aminophenol level was 22·4 mg% and the plasma barbiturate level 6·1 mg%, the latter decreasing to 4·1 mg% by the 4th day. (2) A 28-year-old male mental patient was admitted to hospital 7 hours after taking about 150 paracetamol tablets together with a gill of vodka. Death occurred within 4 days of admission and acute liver necrosis was found at post-mortem examination. For 18 months he had been treated with chlorpromazine and had also been taking 600 mg of amylobarbitone sodium daily. On admission, the plasma *p*-aminophenol level was 26·7 mg% and on the second day it had fallen to 14·4 mg% (Davidson and Eastham, 1966). A 47-year-old man was admitted to hospital 12 hours after taking 40 g of paracetamol. On admission, the blood *p*-aminophenol level was 32·7 mg% and the urine level 232 mg%. Treatment by forced alkaline diuresis was instituted and 18 hours later the blood-level was 3·6 mg% falling to less than 1 mg% within the next 24 hours, the corresponding urine levels being 36·5 mg% and 7·2 mg% (Jacobs, 1967a).

PARACHLOROPHENOL *Antibacterial*

Synonym: *p*-Chlorophenol.

4-Chlorophenol

$C_6H_5ClO = 128{\cdot}6$

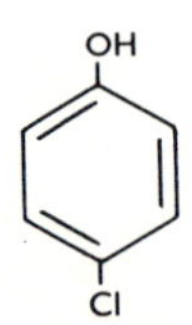

White or pink crystals. M.p. about 42°; it congeals between 42° and 44°.

Solubility. Soluble 1 in 60 of water; very soluble in ethanol, ether, and chloroform.

Extraction. Parachlorophenol may be isolated in the A2 fraction (see p. 27).

Colour Test. Ferric chloride test—violet.

Ultraviolet Absorption Spectrum. Parachlorophenol in ethanol, maximum at 284 mμ (E1%, 1 cm 149) and an inflexion at 291 mμ; in 0·1N sodium hydroxide, maximum at 298·5 mμ (E1%, 1 cm 194).

Metabolism. In the rabbit, 22% of a dose of parachlorophenol has been found to be excreted as an ethereal sulphate conjugate.

Toxicity. The estimated lethal dose in man is 5 g. The lethal oral dose in rats is 670 mg/kg.

PARADICHLOROBENZENE *Pesticide*

Synonyms: Dichlorbenzol; PDB.

$C_6H_4Cl_2 = 147{\cdot}0$

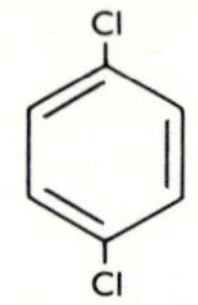

Colourless shining crystals. M.p. 53° to 54°.

Solubility. Insoluble in water; soluble in most organic solvents.

Extraction. Paradichlorobenzene is volatile and may be isolated by distillation (see p. 18); it is also extracted by organic solvents from aqueous acid or alkaline solutions.

Chromatography. GAS: system G5—retention time 0·21 relative to barbitone.

Ultraviolet Absorption Spectrum. Paradichlorobenzene in ethanol, maxima at 272·5 mμ (E1%, 1 cm 27), 275 mμ (E1%, 1 cm 20), and 282 mμ (E1%, 1 cm 17).

Metabolism. Studies in rabbits following oral ingestion of paradichlorobenzene show that it is metabolised slowly, mainly to 2,5-dichlorophenol, the latter being excreted to the extent of about 35% of the dose. The peak excretion of the phenol occurs on the second day after dosage. About 6% of a dose occurs as 2,5-dichloroquinol and some 63% of these 2 metabolites is excreted in the form of conjugates. In contrast to its *o*- and *m*-isomers, paradichlorobenzene is not metabolised to a mercapturic acid.

Toxicity. The maximum permissible concentration in the atmosphere is 75 p.p.m. and the estimated lethal dose is 25 g. Paradichlorobenzene vapour is very irritant to the eyes, mucous membranes, and skin, and it may cause narcosis.

PARALDEHYDE *Hypnotic*

Synonym: Paracetaldehyde.

$C_6H_{12}O_3 = 132{\cdot}2$

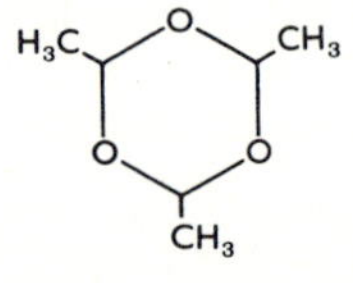

A colourless liquid, which decomposes on storage. M.p. not below 11°. B.p. 123° to 126°. At low temperatures it solidifies to form a crystalline mass.

Solubility. Soluble 1 in 9 of water and 1 in 17 of boiling water; miscible with ethanol, ether, and chloroform.

Extraction. Paraldehyde is volatile and may be isolated by distillation; distillation in the presence of dilute acid will cause depolymerisation of paraldehyde to acetaldehyde (p. 169).

Chromatography. GAS: as for Acetaldehyde, p. 170.

Colour Test. Paraldehyde reduces *silver ammonio-nitrate solution.*

Infra-red Absorption Spectrum. Capillary film between potassium bromide windows. The principal peaks are: A 1095 or 1170, B 946 (p. 751).

Quantitative Estimation. As for Acetaldehyde, p. 170.

Metabolism. When administered internally, paraldehyde imparts a strong characteristic odour to the breath which often persists for a whole day, even after a single dose. However, a large proportion of paraldehyde is destroyed in the body by depolymerisation to acetaldehyde followed by oxidation to acetic acid and final decomposition into carbon dioxide and water.
Studies in dogs have shown that up to 88% of a dose of paraldehyde is destroyed; up to 28% may be exhaled from the lungs and only about 2·5% is excreted in the urine.

Dose. Up to 10 ml by mouth or by intramuscular injection; up to 30 ml by rectal injection as a basal anaesthetic.

Toxicity. Fatalities are rare, although 25 ml by mouth and 12 ml by rectum have caused death. Blood-levels of 50 mg% of total acetaldehyde, or less when ethanol has also been ingested, are indicative of serious poisoning by paraldehyde. Tolerance to paraldehyde may be acquired and addiction is not infrequent.
On storage, paraldehyde may decompose to acetaldehyde and acetic acid; severe acidosis and even death may follow the use of partly decomposed material (Curry, 1962).
LD50 (oral): in mice 1·79 ml/kg.

CASE EXAMPLES. Nine cases of sudden death following paraldehyde therapy for acute alcohol intoxication are reported by Kaye and Haag (1964).

PARAMETHADIONE *Anticonvulsant*

Proprietary Name: Paradione.

5-Ethyl-3,5-dimethyloxazolidine-2,4-dione
$C_7H_{11}NO_3 = 157{\cdot}2$

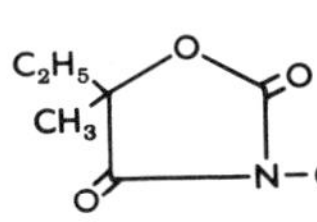

A clear colourless liquid. Refractive index, at 25°, 1·4485 to 1·4505.

Solubility. Sparingly soluble in water; freely soluble in ethanol, ether, and chloroform.

Extraction. Paramethadione is extracted by organic solvents from aqueous acid solutions.

Chromatography. GAS: system G5—retention time 0·17 relative to barbitone.

Ultraviolet Absorption Spectrum. Paramethadione in ethanol:water (1:1), maxima at 228 mμ and 280 mμ; minimum at 220 mμ.

Metabolism. Paramethadione is completely metabolised by *N*-demethylation to 5-ethyl-5-methyloxazolidine-2,4-dione. This metabolite may be found in the plasma and the urine. Continuous administration of the drug leads to accumulation of the metabolite in the plasma.

Dose. Up to 1·8 g daily.

Toxicity. The estimated minimum lethal dose in man is 5 g. Toxic effects may include neutropenia, renal damage, and thrombocytopenic purpura.

PARAPHENYLENEDIAMINE *Hair-dye*

Synonym: 'Para'.

1,4-Diaminobenzene
$C_6H_8N_2 = 108{\cdot}1$

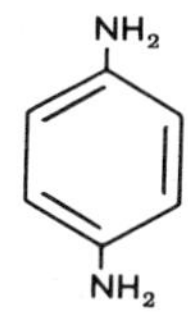

White to slightly red crystals. M.p. 145° to 147°. B.p. 267°.

Solubility. Soluble 1 in 100 of water; soluble in ethanol, ether, and chloroform.

Extraction. Paraphenylenediamine is extracted by organic solvents from aqueous alkaline solutions.

Chromatography. PAPER: system P1—Rf 0·08 (location under ultraviolet light, absorption; location reagents: *iodoplatinate spray*, strong reaction; *bromocresol green spray*, strong reaction).

THIN-LAYER: system T1—Rf 0·61 (location reagent *acidified iodoplatinate spray*, positive reaction).

Colour Tests. MICRO: ammonium vanadate test—(green) pale yellow (*sensitivity:* 0·1 μg); Vitali's test—-/grey/brown (*sensitivity:* 1·0 μg).

Crystal Tests. MICRO: *mercuric chloride solution*—dense rosettes (*sensitivity:* 1 in 1000); *platinic iodide solution*—serrated plates, often in crosses (*sensitivity:* 1 in 1000).

Ultraviolet Absorption Spectrum. Paraphenylenediamine in ethanol, maxima at 230 mμ (E1%, 1 cm 719) and 289 mμ (E1%, 1 cm 250); in 0·1N sulphuric acid, maxima at 240 mμ (E1%, 1 cm 22·5), 244 mμ (E1%, 1 cm 22·1), 248 mμ (E1%, 1 cm 21·4), 255 mμ (E1%, 1 cm 20·6), and 260 mμ (E1%, 1 cm 16·7).

Metabolism. Paraphenylenediamine is thought to be oxidised *in vivo* to a quinone di-imine and then acetylated to form a diacetyl derivative. The hair-dyeing action is stated to be due to the polymerisation of the quinone di-imine.

Toxicity. The lethal dose of paraphenylenediamine is stated to be about 10 g. It is estimated that about 4% of apparently normal subjects are sensitive to paraphenylenediamine and 1% acutely sensitive. The minimum lethal oral dose in rabbits is 250 mg/kg.

CASE EXAMPLE. A 22-month-old child died 3 hours after eating some paraphenylenediamine. The stomach contents gave qualitative tests for paraphenylenediamine. The remaining crystals were identified by their melting-point of about 140° (Bowen, 1963).

PARAQUAT *Herbicide*

1,1′-Dimethyl-4,4′-bipyridylium dichloride

$C_{12}H_{14}Cl_2N_2 = 257{\cdot}2$

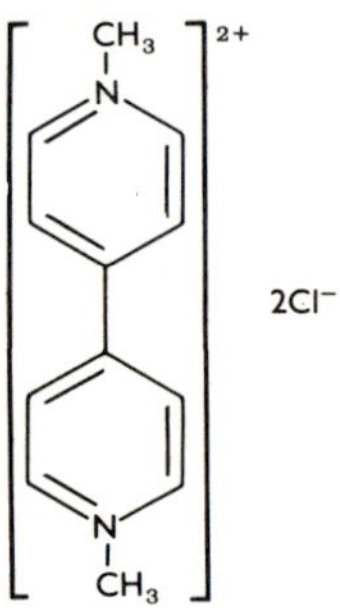

Solubility. Very soluble in water.

Extraction. Paraquat is a quaternary ammonium compound (see p. 29).

Chromatography. PAPER: system P1—Rf 0·00 (location under ultraviolet light, strong absorption; location reagents: *iodoplatinate spray*, strong reaction; *bromocresol green spray*, weak reaction); system RP1a—Rf 0·96 (location reagent *iodoplatinate spray*, positive reaction); system RP1b—Rf 0·93 (location as for RP1a). THIN-LAYER: system T1—Rf 0·00 (location reagent *acidified iodoplatinate spray*, positive reaction).

Colour Tests. *Alkaline sodium dithionite solution*—purple.

MICRO: Vitali's test—-/-/purple-brown → yellow-brown (*sensitivity:* 0·5 μg).

A rapid test for the detection of paraquat in gastric aspirate/lavage and urine has been devised by S. L. Tompsett and may be carried out as as follows. To 5 ml of fluid add 100 mg of sodium bicarbonate and 100 mg of sodium dithionite and mix. Paraquat gives a blue colour; 2 to 5 mg% can be detected without difficulty. Urine may require dilution, and gastric aspirate/lavage may require filtration and dilution before application of the test. Diquat gives a yellowish-green colour with this test (Kerr *et al.*, 1968).

Crystal Tests. MICRO: *potassium cadmium iodide solution*—irregular blades or plates, often serrated (*sensitivity:* 1 in 1000); *styphnic acid*—long curved needles (*sensitivity:* 1 in 3000).

Ultraviolet Absorption Spectrum. Paraquat in 0·1N sulphuric acid, maximum at 257·5 mμ (E1%, 1 cm 693).

Infra-red Absorption Spectrum. Potassium bromide disk. The principal peaks are: A 1174, B 1638, C 1064 or 1229 or 1284 (p. 792).

Metabolism. Studies in laboratory animals (Daniel and Gage, 1966) have shown that 96% of ^{14}C-labelled paraquat is excreted unchanged in the urine within 3 days of its subcutaneous administration.

Toxicity. Paraquat is extremely toxic to man; the estimated lethal dose is stated to be 5 g but death may occur after much lower doses.

CASE EXAMPLES. (1) A 28-year-old man who ingested about 110 ml of a 20% aqueous solution of paraquat died after 7 days, despite intensive treatment from the third day. (2) A 23-year-old man died 15 days after swallowing about a mouthful of a 20% aqueous solution of paraquat, although he vomited and rejected most of the paraquat and was admitted to hospital for intensive treatment after 6 days. Case (1) exhibited toxic changes in the heart, liver, and kidneys but these were not evident in case (2). In both cases, however, the lungs were congested, haemorrhagic, oedematous, and almost wholly solid (Bullivant, 1966).

A 30-year-old man injected himself subcutaneously with approximately 1 ml of a 20% aqueous solution of paraquat. He died 18 days later following progressive pulmonary failure. The main post-mortem findings were in the lungs (similar to the 2 cases reported above); the upper lung segments were swollen and emphysematous and there was evidence of intrapulmonary and subpleural petechial haemorrhages. No paraquat was found in the urine or sputum (Almog and Tal, 1967).

A 6-year-old boy was admitted to hospital in a serious condition 5 days after ingesting a quantity of undiluted paraquat. He died 2 days after admission. Soon after admission the urine level of paraquat was 0·36 mg% and at post-mortem examination the following levels of paraquat were found: kidneys, 0·18 mg%; liver, 0·21 mg% (Campbell, 1968).

PARATHION *Pesticide*

Other Names: Alkron; Aphamite; Corothion; E 605; Fosferno; Fosfex; Fosfive; Fosova; Genithion; Kilphos; Kypthion; Murfos; Niran; Nitrostigmine; Orthophos; Paraphos; Pestox Plus; Pethion; SNP; Thiophos 3422; Vapophos.

Diethyl *p*-nitrophenylphosphorothionate

$C_{10}H_{14}NO_5PS = 291{\cdot}3$

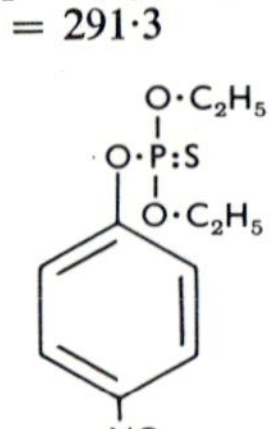

A pale yellow liquid which is decomposed by heat and darkens on exposure to light. M.p. 6°. B.p. 157° to 162° at 0·6 mm Hg and 360° to 375° at 760 mm Hg. Refractive index, at 25°, 1·5367.

Solubility. Soluble 1 in 50,000 of water; miscible

with organic solvents. Parathion is rapidly hydrolysed in alkaline solution.

Extraction. Parathion is extracted by organic solvents from aqueous acid solutions; it is volatile and may be isolated by distillation (see p. 18).

Chromatography. PAPER: system P11—Rf 0·71 (location reagent *congo red spray*, clear blue against a red background).

GAS: Dawson *et al.* (1964) and Lodi (1964) have described methods of determination of parathion involving gas chromatography.

The gas chromatographic examination of 23 organophosphorus pesticides and their oxidation products is described by Ruzicka *et al.* (1967).

Ultraviolet Absorption Spectrum. Parathion in ethanol, maximum at 274 mμ (E 1%, 1 cm 343).

Quantitative Estimation. Karlog (1957) has described a method of extraction of parathion and its metabolites from biological fluids and tissues and a method of determination involving paper chromatography and spectrophotometry. Vercruysse and Deslypere (1964) have described a method of extraction of parathion from biological fluids and tissues and qualitative and quantitative methods of identification. Heyndrickx *et al.* (1967) review 41 cases of organophosphorus pesticide poisoning and present a thin-layer chromatographic separation procedure and qualitative and quantitative methods of identification.

Metabolism. Parathion is a cholinesterase inhibitor and the symptoms of parathion poisoning resemble overstimulation of the parasympathetic nervous system. It is a much stronger cholinesterase inhibitor *in vivo* than *in vitro* because it is largely activated in the body to paraoxon which has a much greater inhibiting power than parathion. Paraoxon has been isolated from the livers of rats treated with parathion.

Parathion is finally excreted in the urine as *p*-nitrophenol; urinary *p*-nitrophenol levels may indicate the extent of exposure to parathion. Mild and moderate cases of exposure have been found to excrete amounts of *p*-nitrophenol ranging from 0·057 to 3·22 mg% and severe and fatal cases from 0·16 to 1·16 mg% (Arterberry *et al.*, 1961).

p-Nitrophenol is rapidly excreted in the urine but can no longer be detected 48 hours after the cessation of exposure, in contrast to the blood cholinesterase activity which remains depressed for about 30 days in the plasma and 80 to 100 days in the erythrocytes. A urinary *p*-nitrophenol level of 0·01 mg% or more is indicative of absorption of a dangerous quantity of parathion. A diurnal variation in *p*-nitrophenol excretion has been observed, the highest levels being detected during the middle of the day. Parathion seems to be much more toxic when absorbed through the lungs than when absorbed through the skin or when taken by mouth. Unchanged parathion has been found to be detectable in the gastro-intestinal contents of birds for up to 8 days after death.

Use. Parathion is employed in emulsifiable concentrates containing up to 20% and in water-dispersible powders containing less than 15%.

Toxicity. The estimated lethal dose in man is 20 to 100 mg; 0·5 ml in the eye may be fatal.

LD50 (oral): in mice 25 and in rats 3·5 to 12·5 mg/kg.

CASE EXAMPLES. Fifty-three cases of parathion poisoning, 9 of them fatal, occurred when parathion was accidentally spilled into sacks of barley which was later eaten (Kanagaratnam *et al.*, 1960).

A 29-year-old man was admitted to hospital about 4 hours after being found in a collapsed state. He had been loading 2% parathion dust for 4 hours. On the day after admission, 0·11 mg of *p*-nitrophenol was excreted in the urine per hour. He recovered (Funckes, 1960).

A one-year-old child suffered from chronic parathion poisoning after drinking the milk of cows that had been drinking water contaminated with parathion (Heyndrickx *et al.*, 1964).

PARGYLINE

Antihypertensive/Monoamine Oxidase Inhibitor

Synonyms: A 19120; MO 911.

N-Methyl-*N*-prop-2-ynylbenzylamine

$C_{11}H_{13}N = 159{\cdot}2$

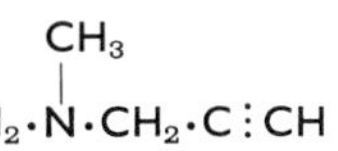

PARGYLINE HYDROCHLORIDE

Proprietary Names: Eudatime; Eutonyl.

A fine white crystalline powder. M.p. 158° to 162°, with sublimation.

Solubility. Very soluble but unstable in water; freely soluble in ethanol.

Extraction. Pargyline is extracted by organic solvents from aqueous alkaline solutions.

Chromatography. PAPER: system P1—Rf 0·55 (location under ultraviolet light, absorption; location reagents: *iodoplatinate spray*, strong reaction; *bromocresol green spray*, strong reaction).

THIN-LAYER: system T1—Rf 0·70 (location reagent *acidified iodoplatinate spray*, positive reaction).

GAS: system G2/120—retention time 0·43 relative to ephedrine.

Crystal Test. MICRO: *picrolonic acid*—burrs or rosettes, forming overnight (*sensitivity:* 1 in 200).

Ultraviolet Absorption Spectrum. Pargyline in 0·1N hydrochloric acid, maxima at 251 mμ (E 1%, 1 cm 11), 256 mμ (E 1%, 1 cm 15), 261 mμ (E 1%, 1 cm 16), and 268 mμ (E 1%, 1 cm 13); minima at about 229 mμ, about 253 mμ, about 259 mμ, and about 266 mμ.

Infra-red Absorption Spectrum. Pargyline (base). Potassium bromide disk. The principal peaks are: A 697, B 746, C 1458 (p. 793).

Metabolism. Studies in rats (Taylor and Krause, 1962) have shown that pargyline is slowly and steadily absorbed from the gastro-intestinal tract. The tissues attain maximum concentrations after 1 to 2 hours. Urinary excretion begins soon after ingestion, 30% of the dose being excreted after 4 hours and 90% after 24 hours. Most of the drug is excreted unchanged, although after 8 hours one metabolite has been detected, accounting for only 3% of the total dose.

Dose. Up to 50 mg daily, increasing as necessary.

Toxicity. LD50 (oral): in mice 680 and in rats about 250 mg/kg.

CASE EXAMPLE. A 2½-year-old girl who was admitted to hospital about 15 hours after ingesting 150 to 175 mg of pargyline hydrochloride eventually recovered and was discharged (Lipkin and Kushnick, 1967).

PECAZINE *Tranquilliser*

Synonyms: Mepazine; P 391.

10-(1-Methylpiperid-3-ylmethyl)phenothiazine

$C_{19}H_{22}N_2S = 310{\cdot}5$

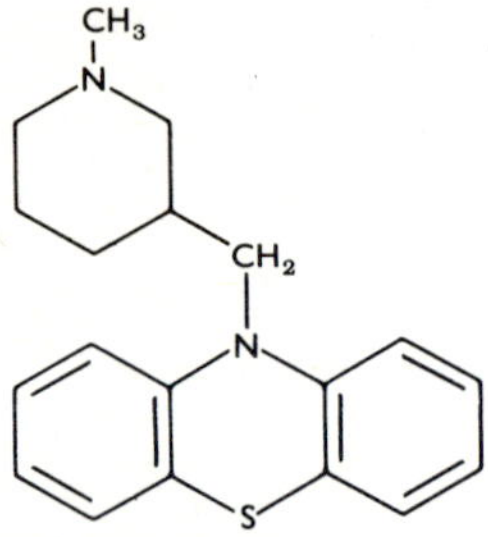

PECAZINE HYDROCHLORIDE

Proprietary Names: Lacumin; Pacatal.

A white crystalline powder. M.p. 171° to 174°, with decomposition.

Solubility. Very slightly soluble in water; freely soluble in dehydrated ethanol; almost insoluble in ether; soluble in chloroform.

Screening Test. *FPN reagent* with urine—orange-red (see p. 10).

Extraction. Pecazine is extracted by organic solvents from aqueous alkaline solutions.

Chromatography. PAPER: system P1—Rf 0·72 (location under ultraviolet light, pale blue fluorescence; location reagents: *iodoplatinate spray*, strong reaction; *bromocresol green spray*, weak reaction); system RP1a—Rf 0·31 (location under ultraviolet light, blue fluorescence; location reagent *iodoplatinate spray*, positive reaction); system RP1b—Rf 0·00 (location as for RP1a).

THIN-LAYER: system T1—Rf 0·52 (location reagent *acidified iodoplatinate spray*, positive reaction); system T4—Rf 0·57 (location reagents: *iodoplatinate spray*, positive reaction; *sulphuric acid–ethanol spray*, orange); system T5—Rf 0·29 (location as for T4).

GAS: system G2/225—retention time 1·58 relative to codeine; system G4—retention time 1·1 relative to codeine.

Colour Tests. MICRO: sulphuric acid–formaldehyde test—purple (*sensitivity:* 0·1 µg); ammonium molybdate test—purple (*sensitivity:* 0·1 µg); ammonium vanadate test—green → purple (*sensitivity:* 0·25 µg); Vitali's test—purple → yellow/yellow/yellow (*sensitivity:* 0·5 µg).

Crystal Tests. MICRO: *potassium iodide solution*—small irregular crystals (*sensitivity:* 1 in 1000); *ammonium thiocyanate solution*—small blades in bundles (*sensitivity:* 1 in 1000).

Ultraviolet Absorption Spectrum. Pecazine in 0·1N sulphuric acid, maxima at 253 mµ (E1%, 1 cm 950) and 300 mµ (E1%, 1 cm 115).

Infra-red Absorption Spectrum. Pecazine hydrochloride. Potassium bromide disk. The principal peaks are: A 1458, B 750, C 768 (p. 751).

Metabolism. Pecazine undergoes sulphoxide formation to a small extent in the body; only 4% is excreted unchanged or as sulphoxide and 11% is reported to be degraded in the liver following injection. When administered orally, only 7·7% is excreted, the major portion of the substance being destroyed in the body.
Pecazine is rapidly absorbed after oral and parenteral administration; considerable amounts are found in the brain, kidneys, liver, and spleen.

Dose. Up to 400 mg daily.

Toxicity. The lethal dose in man is probably in the range 15 to 150 mg/kg. Fatal blood dyscrasias and liver damage have occurred following the administration of pecazine.
LD50 (oral): in mice 700 mg/kg.

PEMOLINE *Central Stimulant*

Synonyms: LA 956; PIO; Phenilone; 5-Phenylisohydantoin.

Proprietary Names: Deltamine; Hyton; Kethamed; Pioxol; Ronyl; Stimul; Tradon; Volital.

2-Imino-4-oxo-5-phenyloxazolidine

$C_9H_8N_2O_2 = 176{\cdot}2$

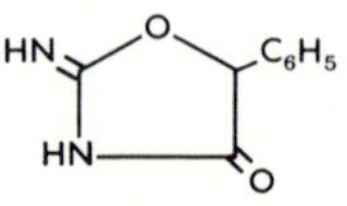

A white crystalline powder. M.p. 259°.

Solubility. Almost insoluble in water; insoluble in ether.

Extraction. Pemoline is extracted by organic solvents from aqueous alkaline solutions.

Chromatography. PAPER: system P1—Rf 0·04 (location under ultraviolet light, absorption; location reagents: *bromine–starch–potassium iodide*, weak reaction; *iodine vapour*, weak reaction; *ninhydrin spray*, purple; *potassium permanganate spray*, weak reaction).

THIN-LAYER: system T1—Rf 0·64 (location reagent *potassium permanganate spray*, positive reaction).

Crystal Tests. MICRO: *picric acid*—blades and serrated plates (*sensitivity:* 1 in 1000); *trinitrobenzoic acid solution*—long plates, best viewed under polarised light (*sensitivity:* 1 in 1000).

Ultraviolet Absorption Spectrum. Pemoline in 0·1N sulphuric acid, maxima at about 250 mμ (E1%, 1 cm 18), 256 mμ (E1%, 1 cm 18), 261·5 mμ (E1%, 1 cm 17), and 268 mμ (E1%, 1 cm 11·5).

Infra-red Absorption Spectrum. Potassium bromide disk. The principal peaks are: A 1218, B 1653, C 695 or 1450 (p. 751).

Dose. Up to 60 mg daily.

Toxicity. LD50 (oral): in mice 2·2 and in rats 0·56 g/kg.

PEMPIDINE *Antihypertensive*

1,2,2,6,6-Pentamethylpiperidine

$C_{10}H_{21}N = 155·3$

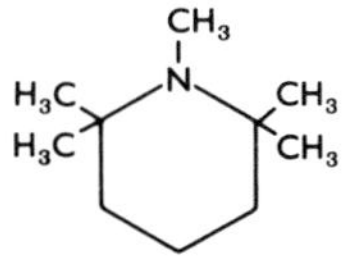

Pempidine occurs as a liquid.

PEMPIDINE TARTRATE

Synonym: Pempidine Hydrogen Tartrate.

Proprietary Names: Perolysen; Tenormal.

A white crystalline powder. M.p. about 160°.

Solubility. Soluble 1 in 2 of water and 1 in 14 of ethanol; insoluble in ether and chloroform.

Extraction. Pempidine is extracted by organic solvents from aqueous alkaline solutions.

Chromatography. PAPER: system P1—Rf 0·44 (location reagents: *iodoplatinate spray*, weak reaction; *bromocresol green spray*, weak reaction).

THIN-LAYER: system T1—Rf 0·17 (location reagent *acidified iodoplatinate spray*, positive reaction).

Crystal Tests. MICRO: *lead iodide solution*—masses of small stout needles (*sensitivity:* 1 in 1000); *styphnic acid*—masses of rods (*sensitivity:* 1 in 1000).

Ultraviolet Absorption Spectrum. Pempidine in 0·1N sulphuric acid, maximum at 265 mμ (E1%, 1 cm about 27).

Infra-red Absorption Spectrum. Pempidine tartrate. Potassium bromide disk. The principal peaks are: A 1261 or 1308 or 1400 (p. 751).

Metabolism. Pempidine is rapidly and completely absorbed from the gastro-intestinal tract. About 70% of a single dose is excreted in the urine within 24 hours, the excretion being more rapid when the urine is acid. Following a single oral dose the plasma concentration of the drug increased rapidly, reaching a maximum in 2 hours, and fell to very low levels within 6 hours (Dollery *et al.*, 1960).

Dose. Usually 2·5 mg every 6 hours, initially, increasing gradually to a maximum of 80 mg according to the patient's needs.

PENTACHLOROPHENOL *Preservative*

Synonyms: PCP; Penta.

Proprietary Names: Penchloral; Santophen 20. The sodium salt is marketed as Dowicide G and Santobrite.

2,3,4,5,6-Chlorophenol

$C_6HCl_5O = 266·3$

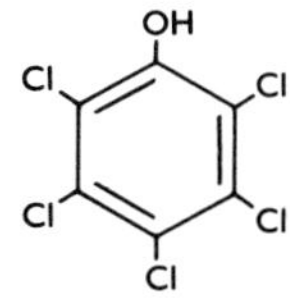

It occurs as white crystals. M.p. 190° to 191°. B.p. 309° to 310°.

Solubility. Very slightly soluble in water; freely soluble in ethanol and ether.

Extraction. Pentachlorophenol may be isolated in the A2 fraction (see p. 27); it may also be isolated by distillation from acid solutions.

Chromatography. PAPER: Erne (1958) describes a paper chromatographic system.

THIN-LAYER: Mason *et al.* (1965) describe a thin-layer chromatographic system.

GAS: a method of differentiation from other chlorinated benzenes and phenols is described by Barry *et al.* (1962).

Ultraviolet Absorption Spectrum. Pentachlorophenol in ethanol, maxima at about 295·5 mμ (E1%, 1 cm 89) and 303 mμ (E1%, 1 cm 114·6); in 0·1N sodium hydroxide, maximum at 319·5 mμ (E1%, 1 cm 194).

Quantitative Estimation. Erne (1958) describes a method of extraction of pentachlorophenol from biological fluids and tissues followed by paper chromatographic purification and spectrophotometric determination. Mason *et al.* (1965) describe a method of extraction from biological fluids and tissues followed by thin-layer chromatographic purification and spectrophotometric determination.

Metabolism. Pentachlorophenol may be absorbed by inhalation, ingestion, or absorption through intact skin. It is rapidly excreted, mainly in the urine in the unchanged form, and does not appear to be conjugated to any significant extent. It causes a rapid uncoupling of oxidation with a resulting increase in metabolic rate.

Toxicity. The lethal dose in man is stated to be about 2 g. Toxic symptoms occur at blood-levels of 4 to 8 mg%. The use of pentachlorophenol as a wood preservative in piggeries has led to fatalities on numerous occasions.

LD50 (oral): in rats 78 to 200 mg/kg.

CASE EXAMPLES. Two men died less than 24 hours after inhaling considerable amounts of pentachlorophenol dust particles. The corrected post-mortem levels were, in one case: blood, 11·3 mg%; brain, 1·4 mg%; liver, 9·4 mg%; in the second case: blood, 15·6 mg%; brain, 3·5 mg%; kidney, 12·3 mg%; liver, 13·4 mg%; urine, 52·0 mg%. These levels, giving a total body quantity of 2 to 4 g and 3 to 5 g respectively, indicate that both men had a massive exposure to the dust particles (Mason *et al.*, 1965).

A 3¾-year-old girl was admitted to hospital after washing for 13 days in water contaminated with pentachlorophenol. The urine contained acetone and acetoacetic acid; Fujiwara's test for halogenated hydrocarbons was weakly positive and the ferric nitrate reaction for phenolic compounds was positive. Forty hours after admission the urine still contained ketone bodies. The urine contained 6 mg% of pentachlorophenol but no dieldrin. The child recovered in a week (Chapman and Robson, 1965).

Levels recorded in a case of fatal pentachlorophenol poisoning were: blood, 10·3 mg%; brain, 2·0 mg%; kidney, 5·2 mg%; liver, 8·7 mg%; urine, 19·6 mg% (Jackson, 1967).

PENTAMIDINE *Trypanocide*

1,5-Di(4-amidinophenoxy)pentane

$C_{19}H_{24}N_4O_2$ = 340·4

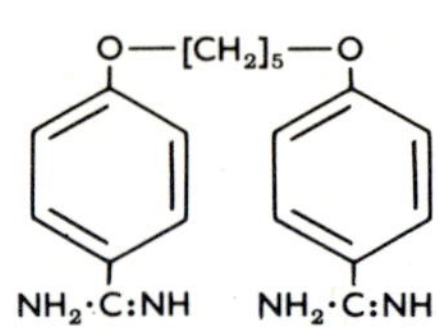

PENTAMIDINE ISETHIONATE

Synonyms: M & B 800; Pentamidine 2-Hydroxyethanesulphonate.

A white hygroscopic crystalline powder. M.p. about 190°.

Solubility. Soluble 1 in 10 of water; slightly soluble in ethanol; insoluble in ether and chloroform.

PENTAMIDINE MESYLATE

Synonyms: Pentamidine Dimethylsulphonate; Pentamidine Methanesulphonate; RP 2512.

Proprietary Name: Lomidine.

A white granular powder.

Solubility. Slightly soluble in water; almost insoluble in ethanol, ether, and chloroform.

Extraction. Pentamidine is extracted by organic solvents from aqueous alkaline solutions.

Chromatography. PAPER: system P1—Rf 0·17 (location under ultraviolet light, dark blue fluorescence; location reagent *iodoplatinate spray*, strong reaction); system RP1a—Rf tailing (location under ultraviolet light, purple fluorescence; location reagent *iodoplatinate spray*, positive reaction); system RP1b—Rf 0·72 (location as for RP1a).

THIN-LAYER: system T1—Rf 0·67 (location reagent *acidified iodoplatinate spray*, positive reaction).

Crystal Tests. MICRO: *potassium iodide solution*—hairlike needles (*sensitivity:* 1 in 1000); *potassium permanganate solution*—masses of small needles (*sensitivity:* 1 in 1000).

Ultraviolet Absorption Spectrum. Pentamidine in ethanol, maximum at 267 mμ (E1%, 1 cm 946).

Metabolism. Pentamidine is fairly well absorbed following parenteral administration. After a single dose the drug is detectable in the blood for only a very brief period. Studies in animals have shown that it may be stored in the liver and the kidneys for periods of months. The brain fixes only a small amount of the drug but stores it for several months.

In the treatment of advanced cases of trypanosomiasis involving the central nervous system, pentamidine is of little value since it does not attain sufficient concentration in the cerebrospinal fluid.

Dose. Up to 300 mg daily, intramuscularly.

Toxicity. Pentamidine sometimes causes hypoglycaemia and, if administered intravenously, it may produce sudden hypotension.

PENTAQUIN *Antimalarial*

Synonym: SN 13276.

8-(5-Isopropylaminopentylamino)-6-methoxyquinoline

$C_{18}H_{27}N_3O$ = 301·4

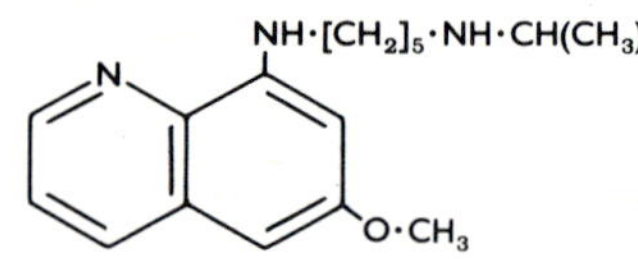

PENTAQUIN PHOSPHATE

A yellow crystalline powder.

Solubility. Soluble 1 in 25 of water; almost insoluble in ethanol; insoluble in ether and chloroform.

Extraction. Pentaquin is extracted by organic solvents from aqueous alkaline solutions.

Chromatography. PAPER: system P1—Rf 0·68 (location under ultraviolet light, orange fluorescence; location reagents: *iodoplatinate spray*, strong reaction; *bromocresol green spray*, weak reaction); system RP1a—Rf 0·61 (location reagent *iodoplatinate spray*, positive reaction); system RP1b—Rf 0·08 (location as for RP1a).

THIN-LAYER: system T1—Rf 0·20 (location reagent *diazotised* p-*nitroaniline–sodium hydroxide spray*, positive reaction).

GAS: system G2/225—retention time 1·7 relative to codeine.

Colour Tests. MICRO: sulphuric acid–formaldehyde test—orange (*sensitivity:* 0·25 μg); ammonium molybdate test—pale blue (*sensitivity:* 1·0 μg); ammonium vanadate test—purple (*sensitivity:* 0·5 μg); Vitali's test—grey-brown/yellow/yellow (*sensitivity:* 0·1 μg).

Crystal Tests. MICRO: *picrolonic acid*—dense

rosettes (*sensitivity:* 1 in 1000); *potassium cadmium iodide solution*—dendrites (*sensitivity:* 1 in 1000).

Ultraviolet Absorption Spectrum. Pentaquin in 0·1N sulphuric acid, maxima at 222 mμ (E1%, 1cm 835), 265 mμ (E1%, 1cm 624), about 277 mμ (E1%, 1cm 603), 331 mμ (E1%, 1cm 95), and 400 mμ (E1%, 1cm 58).

Metabolism. Studies in monkeys with radioactively labelled pentaquin have suggested that it is initially metabolised by demethylation to the 6-hydroxy-derivative. This is then hydroxylated to the 5,6-dihydroxy-compound which readily forms the 5,6-quinone. The latter is probably an active antimalarial. The side-chain seems to be completely degraded.

Dose. Up to 60 mg (base) daily.

Toxicity. The toxic effects of pentaquin are similar to those of pamaquin (p. 464) but are less likely to occur with therapeutic dosage.

PENTAZOCINE *Analgesic*

Synonyms: NIH 7958; Win 20228.
Proprietary Names: Fortral; Talwin.

1,2,3,4,5,6 - Hexahydro - 8 - hydroxy - 6,11 - dimethyl - 3 - (3 - methylbut - 2 - enyl) - 2,6 - methano-3-benzazocine
$C_{19}H_{27}NO = 285{\cdot}4$

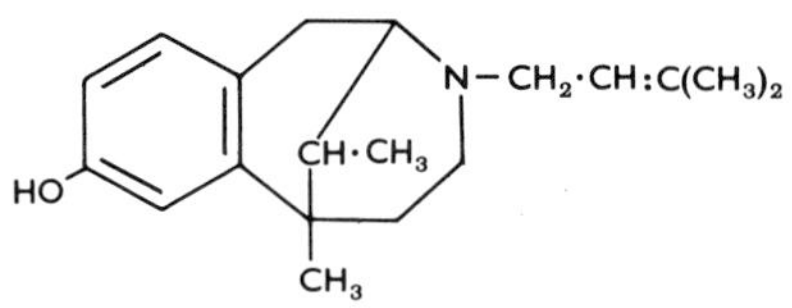

A white powder.
Solubility. Soluble in dilute acids.

Extraction. Pentazocine is extracted by organic solvents from aqueous alkaline solutions; hydrolysis of biological material is required in order to improve the yield.

Chromatography. PAPER: system P1—Rf 0·80 (location reagents: *iodoplatinate spray*, weak reaction; *bromocresol green spray*, strong reaction); system RP1a—Rf 0·84 (location under ultraviolet light, absorption; location reagent *iodoplatinate spray*, positive reaction); system RP1b—Rf 0·15 (location as for RP1a).
THIN-LAYER: system T1—Rf 0·60 (location reagent *acidified iodoplatinate spray*, positive reaction).
GAS: system G2/225—retention time 0·75 relative to codeine.

Colour Tests. MICRO: sulphuric acid–formaldehyde test—dull red → olive-green (*sensitivity:* 0·25 μg); ammonium molybdate test—bright blue (*sensitivity:* 0·1 μg); ammonium vanadate test—olive (*sensitivity:* 1·0 μg); Vitali's test—pale yellow/pale yellow/orange (*sensitivity:* 0·25 μg).

Ultraviolet Absorption Spectrum. Pentazocine in 0·1N hydrochloric acid, maximum at 298 mμ (E1%, 1cm 112); in 0·1N sodium hydroxide, maximum at 278 mμ (E1%, 1cm 67).

Dose. Up to 60 mg subcutaneously or intramuscularly.

Toxicity. Pentazocine is claimed to be free of addiction-producing properties.

PENTHIENATE METHOBROMIDE *Parasympatholytic*

Synonym: Penthienate Bromide.
Proprietary Name: Monodral.

Diethylmethyl [2 - (2 - cyclopentyl - 2 - thien - 2 - ylglycolloyloxy)ethyl]ammonium bromide
$C_{18}H_{30}BrNO_3S = 420{\cdot}4$

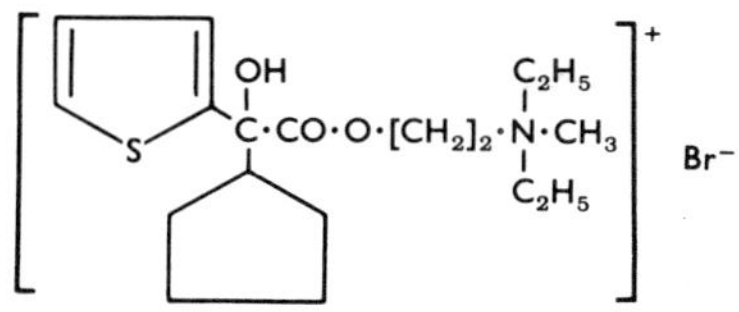

A white crystalline powder. M.p. 122° to 128°.
Solubility. Soluble in water and ethanol; almost insoluble in ether; freely soluble in chloroform.

Extraction. Penthienate methobromide is a quaternary ammonium compound (see p. 29).

Chromatography. PAPER: system P1—Rf 0·58 (location under ultraviolet light, strong absorption; location reagent *iodoplatinate spray*, strong reaction); system RP1a—Rf 0·90 (location under ultraviolet light, absorption; location reagent *iodoplatinate spray*, positive reaction); system RP1b—Rf 0·93 (location as for RP1a).
THIN-LAYER: system T1—Rf 0·02 (location reagent *acidified iodoplatinate spray*, positive reaction).

Colour Tests. MICRO, the following tests are performed on the nitrate (see p. 134): sulphuric acid–formaldehyde test—purple (*sensitivity:* 0·25 μg); ammonium molybdate test—purple (*sensitivity:* 0·1 μg); ammonium vanadate test—purple (*sensitivity:* 0·1 μg); Vitali's test—brown/brown/red-brown (*sensitivity:* 1·0 μg).

Crystal Test. MICRO: *lead iodide solution*—oily plates, best viewed under polarised light (*sensitivity:* 1 in 1500).

Ultraviolet Absorption Spectrum. Penthienate methobromide in 0·1N sulphuric acid, maximum at 238 mμ (E1%, 1cm 191).

Dose. Up to 40 mg daily.

Toxicity. The lethal dose in man is probably in the range 10 to 100 mg/kg.

PENTOBARBITONE *Barbiturate*

Synonyms: Ethaminal; Pentobarbital.

5-Ethyl-5-(1-methylbutyl)barbituric acid
$C_{11}H_{18}N_2O_3 = 226{\cdot}3$

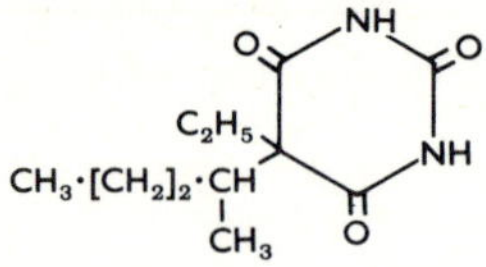

PENTOBARBITONE CALCIUM
A fine white crystalline powder.
Solubility. Slightly soluble in water and ethanol; almost insoluble in ether.

PENTOBARBITONE SODIUM
Synonyms: Mebumalnatrium; Soluble Pentobarbitone.
Proprietary Names: Nembutal; Pental; Sagatal. It is an ingredient of several proprietary preparations—see Extra Pharmacopoeia (Martindale), 25th Edn, p. 193.

A white crystalline powder or granules. A solution in water slowly decomposes.
Solubility. Very soluble in water and ethanol; almost insoluble in ether.

Screening Tests. See under Barbiturates, p. 208.

Extraction. Pentobarbitone may be isolated in the A2 fraction (see p. 27).

Chromatography. PAPER: system P2—Rf 1·16 relative to amylobarbitone (location under ultraviolet light, dark spot); system P3—Rf 0·41 (location reagent *silver nitrate spray*, white); system P4—Rf 0·64 (location as for P3); system P5—Rf 0·70 relative to quinalbarbitone (location under ultraviolet light after exposure to ammonia, absorption); system RP1b—Rf 0·16 (location under ultraviolet light after exposure to ammonia; location reagent *potassium permanganate spray*, yellow on pink).
THIN-LAYER: system T10—Rf 0·33 (location reagents: *mercurous nitrate spray*, black; *Zwikker's reagent spray*, pink); system T11—Rf 0·40 (location reagent *mercurous nitrate spray*, white on grey); system T12—Rf 0·49 (location as for T11); system T13—Rf 0·57 (location as for T11).
GAS: system G1/180—retention time 0·73 relative to diphenhydramine; system G3—retention time 2·07 relative to diphenhydramine; system G5—retention time 2·55 relative to barbitone; system G7—retention time 2·09 relative to barbitone.

Colour Test. Zwikker's test—violet-blue.

Ultraviolet Absorption Spectrum. Pentobarbitone is a 5,5-derivative—see Screening Test 3 under Barbiturates, p. 208.

Infra-red Absorption Spectrum. Pentobarbitone. Potassium bromide disk. The principal peaks are: A 1685, B 1719, C 1744 (p. 752).

Quantitative Estimation. See under Barbiturates, p. 208. Oroszlan and Maengwyn-Davies (1960) have described a spectrophotometric method of determination of pentobarbitone in blood.

Metabolism. Pentobarbitone is a short-acting barbiturate (see p. 207) which is metabolised in the liver by hydroxylation to 5-ethyl-5-(3-hydroxy-1-methylbutyl)barbituric acid and by oxidation to 5-ethyl-5-(3-carboxy-1-methylpropyl)barbituric acid. Both metabolites and unchanged pentobarbitone have been found in the urine.
Maynert (1965) states that after a 500-mg dose between 47 and 50% is excreted in the urine as the hydroxy-derivative but Brodie *et al.* (1953) isolated only 15% of the dose in this form. About 45% of the pentobarbitone present in post-mortem blood appears to be protein-bound (Turner, 1964b).

Dose. Up to 200 mg.

Toxicity. The estimated minimum lethal dose is stated to be 1 g.

LD50 (oral): in mice 280 mg/kg.

CASE EXAMPLE. The post-mortem examination of a man who was thought by his family to have committed suicide revealed the following levels of pentobarbitone: blood, 2·4 mg%; stomach contents, a total of 2·2 g; urine, 72 mg%. Two metabolites were present in the urine (Algeri and McBay, 1953).

PENTOLINIUM TARTRATE

Antihypertensive

Synonyms: M&B 2050A; Pentapyrrolidinium Bitartrate; Pentolonium Tartrate.
Proprietary Name: Ansolysen.

Pentamethylenebis(1-methylpyrrolidinium hydrogen tartrate)
$C_{23}H_{42}N_2O_{12} = 538{\cdot}6$

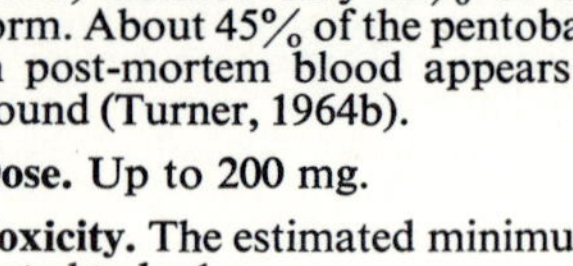

A white powder. M.p. about 206°, with decomposition.
Solubility. Soluble 1 in 0·4 of water and 1 in 800 of ethanol; insoluble in ether and chloroform.

Extraction. Pentolinium tartrate is a quaternary ammonium compound (see p. 29).

Chromatography. PAPER: system P1—Rf 0·00 (location reagent *iodoplatinate spray*, strong reaction); system RP1a—Rf 0·95 (location reagent *iodoplatinate spray*, positive reaction); system RP1b—Rf 1·00 (location as for RP1a).
THIN-LAYER: system T1—Rf 0·00 (location reagent *acidified iodoplatinate spray*, positive reaction).

Crystal Tests. MICRO: *potassium bismuth iodide solution*—rectangular or boat-shaped plates (*sensitivity:* 1 in 200); *styphnic acid*—small irregular prisms (*sensitivity:* 1 in 1000).

Dose. Usually up to 40 mg daily initially, increasing gradually to 100 to 900 mg daily according to the patient's needs. Initial subcutaneous dose usually up to 2·5 mg.

PERICYAZINE *Tranquilliser*

Synonyms: Propericiazine; RP 8909; SKF 20716.
Proprietary Names: Aolept; Neulactil; Neuleptil.

2 - Cyano - 10[3 - (4 - hydroxypiperidino)propyl] phenothiazine

$C_{21}H_{23}N_3OS = 365{\cdot}5$

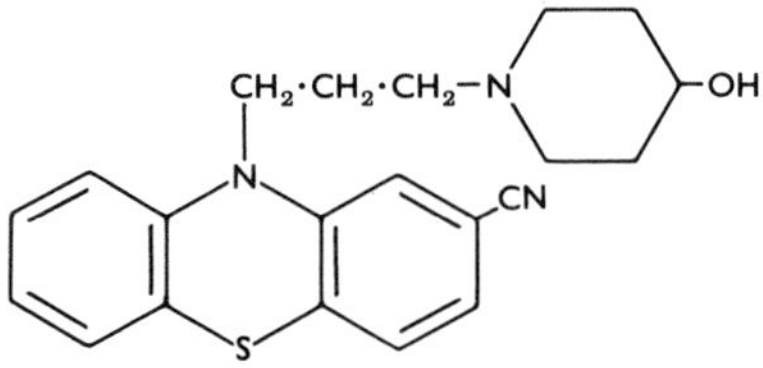

A yellow crystalline powder. M.p. 115°.

Solubility. Insoluble in water; soluble in ethanol; slightly soluble in ether; freely soluble in chloroform.

Screening Test. *FPN reagent* with urine—red (see p. 10).

Extraction. Pericyazine is extracted by organic solvents from aqueous alkaline solutions; hydrolysis of biological material is required in order to improve the yield.

Chromatography. PAPER: system P1—Rf 0·59 (location under ultraviolet light, pale green fluorescence; location reagents: *iodoplatinate spray*, strong reaction; *Dragendorff spray*, weak reaction).

THIN-LAYER: system T1—Rf 0·61 (location reagent *acidified iodoplatinate spray*, positive reaction).

Colour Tests. MICRO: sulphuric acid–formaldehyde test—red (*sensitivity:* 0·1 μg); ammonium molybdate test—deep purple (*sensitivity:* 0·1 μg); ammonium vanadate test—red (green may be seen first) (*sensitivity:* 0·25 μg); Vitali's test—red flash → yellow/light brown/light brown (*sensitivity:* 0·1 μg).

Crystal Tests. MICRO: *gold bromide solution*—masses of small needles (*sensitivity:* 1 in 1000); *gold bromide–hydrochloric acid solution*—masses of small needles (*sensitivity:* 1 in 1000).

Ultraviolet Absorption Spectrum. Pericyazine in 0·1N sulphuric acid, maxima at 233 mμ (E1%, 1 cm 684) and 268 mμ (E1%, 1 cm 800).

Infra-red Absorption Spectrum. Potassium bromide disk. The principal peaks are: A 1464, B 736, C 811 or 1066 (p. 752).

Dose. From 5 to 90 mg daily, according to the patient's condition.

Toxicity. The acute lethal dose of the phenothiazine tranquillisers is stated to be in the range 15 to 150 mg/kg.

LD50 (oral): in mice 530 and in rats about 395 mg/kg.

PERPHENAZINE *Tranquilliser*

Synonym: Chlorpiprazine.
Proprietary Names: Decentan; Fentazin; Trilafon.

2 - Chloro - 10{3 - [4 - (2 - hydroxyethyl)piperazin-1-yl]propyl}phenothiazine

$C_{21}H_{26}ClN_3OS = 404{\cdot}0$

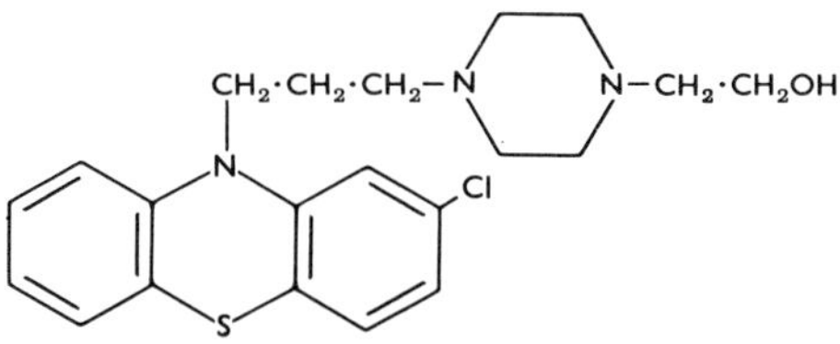

A white powder. M.p. 96° to 100°.

Solubility. Almost insoluble in water; soluble 1 in 20 of ethanol, 1 in 80 of ether, and 1 in 1 of chloroform.

Screening Test. *FPN reagent* with urine—red-purple (see p. 10).

Extraction. Perphenazine is extracted by organic solvents from aqueous alkaline solutions; hydrolysis of biological material is required in order to improve the yield.

Chromatography. PAPER: system P1—Rf 0·23 (location under ultraviolet light, blue fluorescence; location reagents: *iodoplatinate spray*, strong reaction; *bromocresol green spray*, weak reaction); system RP1a—Rf 0·19 (location under ultraviolet light, blue fluorescence; location reagent *iodoplatinate spray*, positive reaction); system RP1b—Rf 0·00 (location as for RP1a).

THIN-LAYER: system T1—Rf 0·58 (location reagent *acidified iodoplatinate spray*, positive reaction); system T3—Rf 0·36 (location reagents: *iodoplatinate spray*, strong reaction; *sulphuric acid–ethanol spray*, reddish-pink); system T4—Rf 0·44 (location as for T3); system T5—Rf 0·48 (location as for T3); system T6—Rf 0·65 (the spot may be converted on the plate to the sulphoxide, Rf 0·45; location of both spots under ultraviolet light).

Colour Tests. MICRO: sulphuric acid–formaldehyde test—purple (*sensitivity:* 0·5 μg); ammonium molybdate test—purple (*sensitivity:* 0·5 μg); ammonium vanadate test—purple (*sensitivity:* 0·5 μg); Vitali's test—purple → yellow/yellow/yellow (*sensitivity:* 0·5 μg).

Crystal Test. MICRO: *trinitrobenzoic acid solution*—blades, forming overnight (*sensitivity:* 1 in 100).

Ultraviolet Absorption Spectrum. Perphenazine in ethanol, maxima at 257 mμ (E1%, 1 cm 933) and 310 mμ (E1%, 1 cm 115); minima at 225 mμ and 280 mμ: in 0·1N sulphuric acid, maxima at 254·5 mμ (E1%, 1 cm 833) and 306 mμ (E1%, 1 cm 92).

Dose. Up to 8 mg as an anti-emetic; up to 64 mg daily in schizophrenia.

Toxicity. The acute lethal dose of the phenothiazine tranquillisers is stated to be in the range 15 to 150 mg/kg.

High dosage of perphenazine may cause

dystonia of the neck and shoulder muscles, drowsiness, blurred vision, and paraesthesias.

PETHIDINE *Narcotic Analgesic*

Synonyms: Isonipecaine; Meperidine.

Ethyl 1-methyl-4-phenylpiperidine-4-carboxylate

$C_{15}H_{21}NO_2 = 247{\cdot}3$

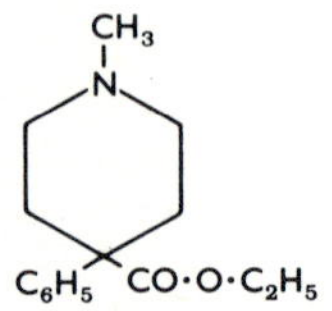

An oily liquid which slowly crystallises.

PETHIDINE HYDROCHLORIDE

Proprietary Names: Algil; Demerol; Dolantin; Dolantol; Dolosal; Mefedina; Pantalgine; Phytadon; Sauteralgyl; Suppolosal.

A white crystalline powder. M.p. 187° to 189°.

Solubility. Very soluble in water; soluble 1 in 20 of ethanol; sparingly soluble in ether; soluble in chloroform.

Extraction. Pethidine is extracted by organic solvents from aqueous alkaline solutions; hydrolysis of biological material is required in order to improve the yield.

Chromatography. PAPER: system P1—Rf 0·00 (location reagent *Dragendorff spray*, weak reaction); system RP1a—Rf 0·83 (location reagent *iodoplatinate spray*, positive reaction); system RP1b—Rf 0·03 (location as for RP1a).

THIN-LAYER: system T1—Rf 0·48 (location reagent *acidified iodoplatinate spray*, positive reaction); system T7—Rf 0·97 (location reagent *iodoplatinate spray*); system T8—Rf 0·41 (location as for T7).

GAS: system G1/180—retention time 0·69 relative to diphenhydramine ; system G2/225—retention time 0·78 relative to diphenhydramine; system G6—retention time 0·18 relative to codeine.

Colour Test. MICRO: sulphuric acid–formaldehyde test—dull orange (*sensitivity:* 1·0 μg).

Crystal Tests. MICRO: *picric acid*—feathery rosettes (*sensitivity:* 1 in 1000); *picrolonic acid*—feathery rosettes (*sensitivity:* 1 in 1000).

Ultraviolet Absorption Spectrum. Pethidine in ethanol, maxima at 252 mμ (E1%, 1cm 7·1), 258 mμ (E1%, 1cm 8·5), and 264 mμ (E1%, 1cm 6·3); minima at 250 mμ, 255 mμ, and 262 mμ. Pethidine hydrochloride in water, maxima at 251 to 252 mμ (E1%, 1cm 6·2), 257 mμ (E1%, 1cm 7·6), and 263 mμ (E1%, 1cm 6·1); minima at 248 mμ, 254 mμ, and 261 mμ.

NOTE. The ultraviolet spectra of amphetamine (p. 192) and phenethylamine (p. 482) bear many points of resemblance to that of pethidine. The 3 compounds, however, may be separated by paper or thin-layer chromatography.

Infra-red Absorption Spectrum. Pethidine hydrochloride. Potassium bromide disk. The principal peaks are: A 1708, B 1218, C 1148 or 1166 (p. 752).

Quantitative Estimation. A spectrophotometric method for the determination of pethidine in biological fluids and tissues following its conversion to the methyl orange complex is described by Burns *et al.* (1955).

Metabolism. Pethidine is metabolised in man by *N*-demethylation and hydrolysis; the latter appears to be the main route; only about 15% of the dose seems to be metabolised by *N*-demethylation. The metabolism of pethidine in normal subjects and in addicts does not differ significantly.

Following a dose of 175 mg administered to normal subjects over a period of 4 hours, 5% of the dose appeared in the urine in 24 hours in the unchanged form, 7% as norpethidine, 21% as free pethidinic acid, 16% as bound pethidinic acid, 7·5% as free norpethidinic acid, and 10% as bound norpethidinic acid. A total of 65% of the dose was recovered in 24 hours. None of the metabolites has any significant analgesic activity.

The excretion of pethidine has been shown to be influenced by the pH of the urine (Asatoor *et al.*, 1963); in highly acidic urine the excretion of unchanged pethidine and of the nor-derivative is significantly increased.

Dose. Up to 100 mg orally, intramuscularly, or subcutaneously; up to 50 mg intravenously.

Toxicity. The estimated minimum lethal dose in man is 1 g; a fatality has been reported following the ingestion of 1·2 g but recovery has occurred after the ingestion of 2 g.

Pethidine possesses marked addiction-producing properties; doses as large as 3 or 4 g daily may be taken by addicts.

In 2 fatal cases of pethidine poisoning, 0·1 mg% was found in the blood in one and 30 mg% in the liver in the second.

Serious toxic reactions have occurred in patients given pethidine while under treatment with monoamine oxidase inhibitors—see under Phenelzine, p. 482.

PHANQUONE *Anti-amoebic*

Synonyms: C 11925; Phenanthrolinquone; Pheninquone.

Proprietary Name: Entobex.

4,7-Phenanthroline-5,6-quinone

$C_{12}H_6N_2O_2 = 210{\cdot}2$

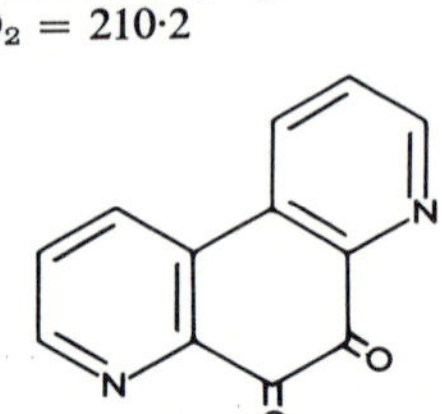

An orange crystalline powder. M.p. 295°, with decomposition.

Solubility. Slightly soluble in water; almost insoluble in ethanol and chloroform.

Chromatography. PAPER: system P1—Rf 0·37 (location under ultraviolet light, yellow fluorescence; location reagents: *iodoplatinate spray*, weak reaction; *Dragendorff spray*, strong reaction).

THIN-LAYER: system T1—Rf 0·22, streaking (location reagent *acidified iodoplatinate spray*, positive reaction).

Colour Tests. MICRO: sulphuric acid–formaldehyde test—faint yellow (*sensitivity:* 1·0 μg); Vitali's test— -/faint yellow/green (*sensitivity:* 0·5 μg).

Crystal Tests. MICRO: *gold bromide–hydrochloric acid solution*—fine needles (*sensitivity:* 1 in 400); *potassium mercuric iodide solution*—rods (*sensitivity:* 1 in 400).

Ultraviolet Absorption Spectrum. Phanquone in 1N sulphuric acid, maxima at 265 mμ (E1%, 1 cm about 500), 272 mμ (E1%, 1 cm about 500), and 292 mμ (E1%, 1 cm about 480).

Metabolism. Phanquone is absorbed from the intestines and excreted in active form in the bile and urine; hence it is active in cases of both intestinal and extra-intestinal amoebiasis. Phanquone metabolites excreted in the urine render it dark-coloured; one of the metabolites is claimed to possess amoebicidal activity.

Dose. Up to 300 mg daily.

Toxicity. LD50 (oral): in rats 3 g/kg.

PHENACEMIDE *Anticonvulsant*

Synonym: Carbamide Phenylacetate.
Proprietary Name: Phenurone.

Phenylacetylurea

$C_9H_{10}N_2O_2 = 178{\cdot}2$

$$C_6H_5{\cdot}CH_2{\cdot}CO{\cdot}NH{\cdot}CO{\cdot}NH_2$$

A white crystalline solid. M.p. 212° to 216°.

Solubility. Almost insoluble in water; slightly soluble in ethanol, ether, and chloroform.

Colour Test. *Liebermann's reagent*—orange.

Ultraviolet Absorption Spectrum. Phenacemide in methanol, maximum at 257 mμ (E1%, 1 cm 16).

Infra-red Absorption Spectrum. Potassium bromide disk. The principal peaks are: A 1660, B 1090, C 716 or 1410 or 1618 (p. 752).

Metabolism. Phenacemide is well-absorbed from the gastro-intestinal tract and has a long duration of action. It is metabolised to inactive compounds in the liver, the main route of metabolism being *p*-hydroxylation of the phenyl ring. Further degradation is uncertain. No unchanged phenacemide has been detected in the urine.

Dose. Up to 3 g daily.

Toxicity. Phenacemide may give rise to serious toxic effects including liver damage, bone-marrow depression which may cause aplastic anaemia or other blood disorders, and distressing personality changes. The estimated minimum lethal dose in man is 5 g.

CASE EXAMPLES. Eight cases of death associated with liver degeneration following phenacemide therapy, in terms of total dosage and intervals between start of treatment and death: (1) 152 g, 3½ months; (2) 51 g, 7 weeks; (3) 50 g, 7 weeks; (4) 72 g, 2 months; (5) 60 g, 7 months; (6) 42 g, 6 weeks; (7) 80 g, 3½ months; (8) 61 g, 10 weeks (Pfaff and Forbeck, 1961).

PHENACETIN *Analgesic and Antipyretic*

Synonyms: p-Acetophenetidide; Acetophenetidin; Acetylphenetidin; Paracetophenetidin.

N-p-Ethoxyphenylacetamide

$C_{10}H_{13}NO_2 = 179{\cdot}2$

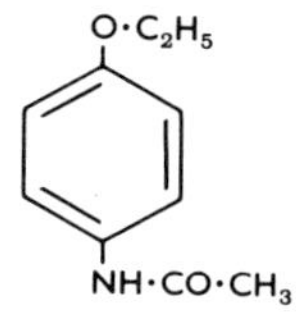

A white crystalline powder. M.p. 134° to 136·5°.

Solubility. Soluble 1 in 1700 of water, 1 in 20 of ethanol, and 1 in 15 of chloroform; slightly soluble in ether.

Screening Test. See under Screening Tests, p. 14.

Extraction. Phenacetin is extracted by organic solvents from aqueous acid or alkaline solutions.

Chromatography. PAPER: system RP1b—Rf 0·35 (location reagent *bromine–starch–potassium iodide*).

GAS: system G1/180—retention time 0·60 relative to diphenhydramine; system G3—retention time 1·57 relative to diphenhydramine; system G5—retention time 2·30 relative to barbitone.

Colour Tests. Boil 0·1 g of phenacetin with 1 ml of *hydrochloric acid* for 3 minutes, dilute with 10 ml of water, cool, filter, and add 1 drop of 0·1N potassium dichromate solution to the filtrate—violet→ruby-red. *Liebermann's reagent*—violet.

Ultraviolet Absorption Spectrum. Phenacetin in ethanol, maximum at 250 mμ (E1%, 1 cm 908).

Infra-red Absorption Spectrum. Potassium bromide disk. The principal peaks are: A 1243 or 1655, B 1513, C 1555 (p. 752).

Quantitative Estimation. Spectrophotometric methods of estimating phenacetin as free *p*-aminophenol following acid hydrolysis of the main metabolite, paracetamol, are described by Tompsett (1958) and Welch and Connery (1965). Methods of determination of 4-chloroacetanilide, a contaminant of phenacetin, are described by Jones and Page (1964) and Crummett *et al.* (1964).

Metabolism. Phenacetin is metabolised in the liver, the major route of degradation being de-ethylation to acetaldehyde (p. 169) and paracetamol (p. 465) which is the active agent; paracetamol is excreted in the urine in the form of the inactive glucuronide or ethereal sulphate conjugates, 80 to 90% of 1 to 2 g doses being excreted in these forms in 24 hours.
A minor pathway of degradation involves de-acetylation to *p*-ethoxyaniline; further metabolism of this compound may be responsible for the methaemoglobinaemia sometimes observed following phenacetin therapy. Two other metabolites have been detected, 2-hydroxyphenacetin and *S*-(1-acetamido-4-hydroxyphenyl)cysteine.
Phenacetin is well absorbed from the gastro-intestinal tract; it attains maximal effect 30 to 60 minutes after oral ingestion and the effect of a single dose usually lasts 2 to 3 hours.

Dose. Usually up to 600 mg.

Toxicity. The lethal dose in man is stated to be between 5 and 20 g.
When phenacetin has been taken in doses of 1 g or more daily, methaemoglobinaemia and haemolytic anaemia have occasionally ensued. In addition, there are many recent reports of the toxic action of phenacetin on the kidneys when the drug has been taken in large amounts over long periods; it has been suggested (*Br. med. J.*, 1960, **1**, 714) that 4-chloroacetanilide, a contaminant of phenacetin, may be responsible for the renal damage.
LD50 (oral): in rats 1·65 g/kg.
CASE EXAMPLES. In 4 cases of suspected or known overdosage with phenacetin, serum levels of 4·5, 7·5, 8·5, and 25·0 mg% of total *p*-aminophenol were detected (Tompsett, 1966).

PHENADOXONE *Narcotic Analgesic*

Synonyms: CB 11; Heptazone; Morphodone.

6-Morpholino-4,4-diphenylheptan-3-one
$C_{23}H_{29}NO_2 = 351·5$

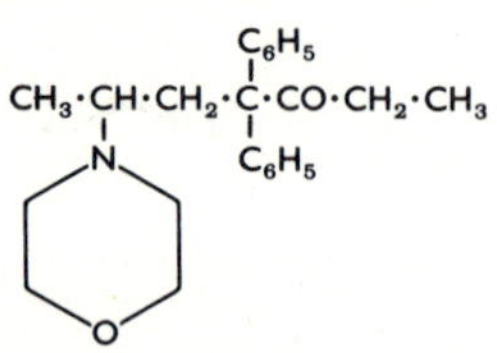

Phenadoxone melts at 75°.

PHENADOXONE HYDROCHLORIDE
Proprietary Name: Heptalgin.

A colourless crystalline powder. M.p. 224° to 225°, with decomposition.
Solubility. Soluble 1 in 25 of water and 1 in 10 of ethanol; very soluble in chloroform.

Extraction. Phenadoxone is extracted by organic solvents from aqueous alkaline solutions; hydrolysis of biological material is required in order to improve the yield.

Chromatography. PAPER: system P1—Rf 0·77 (location reagent *iodoplatinate spray*, strong reaction); system RP1a—Rf 0·00 (location under ultraviolet light, absorption); system RP1b—Rf 0·00 (location as for RP1a).
THIN-LAYER: system T1—Rf 0·77 (location reagent *acidified iodoplatinate spray*, positive reaction).
GAS: system G2/225—retention time 1·6 relative to codeine; system G4—retention time 0·96 relative to codeine.

Colour Test. MICRO: ammonium vanadate test —deep green→blue (*sensitivity:* 0·5 μg).

Crystal Tests. MICRO: *picrolonic acid*—dense oily rosettes, forming overnight (*sensitivity:* 1 in 1000); *potassium tri-iodide solution (1)*—rods and plates, forming overnight (*sensitivity:* 1 in 1000).

Ultraviolet Absorption Spectrum. Phenadoxone in ethanol, maxima at about 259 mμ (E1%, 1cm 12·0) and 296 mμ (E1%, 1cm 11·8); minima at 258 mμ and 279 mμ: in 0·1N sulphuric acid, maxima at 253 mμ (E1%, 1cm 14·9), 259 mμ (E1%, 1cm 16), 266 mμ (E1%, 1cm 15·3), and 292 mμ (E1%, 1cm 16·2).

Infra-red Absorption Spectrum. Phenadoxone hydrochloride. Potassium bromide disk. The principal peaks are: A 1699, B 698 or 704 or 1090 (p. 752).

Dose. Up to 50 mg by mouth; up to 15 mg subcutaneously or intramuscularly.

PHENAMIDINE *Antiprotozoal*

Di(*p*-amidinophenyl) ether
$C_{14}H_{14}N_4O = 254·3$

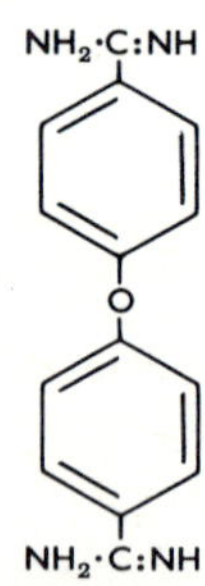

PHENAMIDINE ISETHIONATE
White crystals or powder. M.p. 225°, with decomposition.
Solubility. Soluble 1 in 1·4 of water and 1 in 300 of ethanol; insoluble in ether and chloroform.

Extraction. Phenamidine is extracted by organic solvents from aqueous alkaline solutions.

Chromatography. PAPER: system P1—Rf 0·04 (location under ultraviolet light, blue fluorescence; location reagents: *iodoplatinate spray*, weak reaction, white; *bromocresol green spray*, strong reaction); system RP1a—Rf 0·83 (location under ultraviolet light, blue fluorescence; location reagent *iodoplatinate spray*, positive reaction); system RP1b—Rf 0·79 (location as for RP1a).

THIN-LAYER: system T1—Rf 0·04, streaking (location reagent *acidified iodoplatinate spray*, positive reaction).

Crystal Tests. MICRO: *gold bromide–hydrochloric acid solution*—irregular plates (*sensitivity:* 1 in 1000); *potassium bismuth iodide solution*—plates and serrated blades (*sensitivity:* 1 in 1000).

Ultraviolet Absorption Spectrum. Phenamidine in 0·1N sulphuric acid, maximum at 265 mμ (E1%, 1 cm 914).

Dose. By subcutaneous injection, per kg body-weight: horses and cattle, 0·03 ml of a 40% solution; dogs, 0·3 ml of a 5% solution.

Toxicity. Phenamidine is usually well tolerated when used in single doses in the treatment of babesiasis in animals. The repeated use of large doses in the treatment of demodectic mange in dogs has caused toxic symptoms, probably associated with hepatic damage due to a cumulative effect.

PHENAMPROMIDE *Narcotic Analgesic*

N-(1-Methyl-2-piperidinoethyl)propionanilide

$C_{17}H_{26}N_2O$ = 274·4

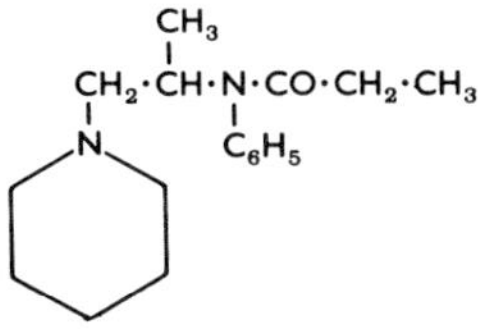

Phenampromide has a b.p. of 124° to 128° at 0·2 mm Hg. Refractive index 1·518.

Extraction. Phenampromide is extracted by organic solvents from aqueous alkaline solutions.

Chromatography. PAPER: system P1—Rf 0·68 (location reagents: *iodoplatinate spray*, strong reaction; *bromocresol green spray*, weak reaction); system RP1b—Rf 0·06 (location reagent *iodoplatinate spray*, positive reaction).

THIN-LAYER: system T1—Rf 0·73 (location reagent *acidified iodoplatinate spray*, positive reaction).

Crystal Tests. MICRO: *gold bromide solution*—serrated blades (*sensitivity:* 1 in 400); *gold bromide–hydrochloric acid solution*—plates or prisms, forming overnight (*sensitivity:* 1 in 400).

Ultraviolet Absorption Spectrum. Phenampromide in 0·1N sulphuric acid, maxima at about 250 mμ (E1%, 1 cm 8) and 256·5 mμ (E1%, 1 cm 8), and inflexions at about 260 mμ (E1%, 1 cm 7), about 262 mμ (E1%, 1 cm 6·7), and about 266 mμ (E1%, 1 cm 5).

PHENAZOCINE *Narcotic Analgesic*

Synonym: NIH 7519.

1,2,3,4,5,6 - Hexahydro - 8 - hydroxy - 2,6 - methano - 6,11 - dimethyl - 3 - phenethyl - 3 - benzazocine

$C_{22}H_{27}NO$ = 321·5

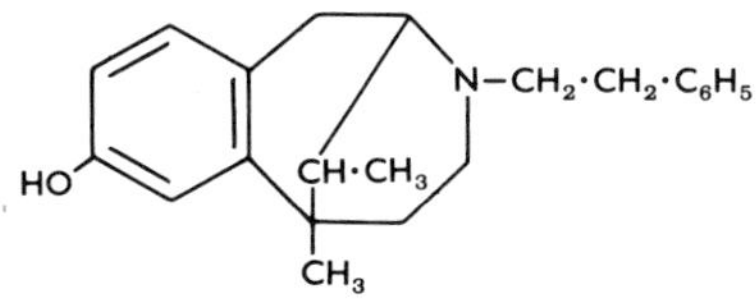

Phenazocine melts at 180° to 181°.

Solubility. Insoluble in water; sparingly soluble in chloroform.

PHENAZOCINE HYDROBROMIDE

Synonym: Phenethylazocine Bromide.

Proprietary Names: Narphen; Prinadol; Xenagol.

A white microcrystalline powder which can exist in 3 polymorphic forms. M.p. 164·5°.

Solubility. Soluble 1 in 350 of water, 1 in 45 of ethanol, and 1 in 140 of chloroform; insoluble in ether.

Extraction. Phenazocine is extracted by organic solvents from aqueous alkaline solutions; hydrolysis of biological material is required in order to improve the yield.

Chromatography. PAPER: system P1—Rf 0·86 (location reagents: *iodoplatinate spray*, strong reaction; *bromocresol green spray*, weak reaction); system RP1a—Rf 0·55 (location reagent *iodoplatinate spray*, positive reaction); system RP1b—Rf 0·00 (location under ultraviolet light, absorption).

THIN-LAYER: system T1—Rf 0·66 (location reagent *acidified iodoplatinate spray*, positive reaction); system T7—Rf 0·97 (location reagent *iodoplatinate spray*, positive reaction); system T8—Rf 0·87 (location as for T7).

GAS: system G2/225—retention time 2·15 relative to codeine.

Colour Tests. MICRO: sulphuric acid–formaldehyde test—brown (*sensitivity:* 0·25 μg); ammonium molybdate test—bright blue → green (*sensitivity:* 0·5 μg); Vitali's test—yellow/yellow/orange (*sensitivity:* 0·1 μg).

Crystal Tests. MICRO: *potassium iodide solution*—dense oily rosettes (*sensitivity:* 1 in 1500); *sodium carbonate solution*—bunches of irregular prisms (*sensitivity:* 1 in 1000).

Ultraviolet Absorption Spectrum. Phenazocine in 0·1N hydrochloric acid, maximum at 278 mμ (E1%, 1 cm 64); in 0·1N sulphuric acid, maximum at 277·5 mμ (E1%, 1 cm 48·5) and an inflexion at about 278 mμ (E1%, 1 cm 44·5). Phenazocine hydrobromide in 0·1N sodium hydroxide, maxima at 243 mμ and 299 mμ; minima at 226 mμ and 272 mμ.

Metabolism. Phenazocine is metabolised in the

liver. It is readily absorbed from the gastro-intestinal tract and from injection sites. It has an onset of action within 5 to 30 minutes of injection, peak activity occurring after 30 minutes. The duration of action is up to 6 hours.

Dose. 5 mg by mouth or up to 3 mg intramuscularly; max. in 24 hours 12 mg.

Toxicity. The estimated minimum lethal dose in man is 100 mg. Phenazocine is addictive although tolerance develops more slowly and less completely than with morphine.
LD50 (oral): in mice 630 mg/kg.

PHENAZONE *Analgesic and Antipyretic*

Synonyms: Antipyrin(e); Azophenum; Analgesine; Fenazona.
Proprietary Names: It is an ingredient of Auralgicin, Auraltone, Dismenol, Felsol, Otalgan, Rybronsol, Sedonan, and Tympalgin.

1,5-Dimethyl-3-oxo-2-phenylpyrazoline
$C_{11}H_{12}N_2O = 188{\cdot}2$

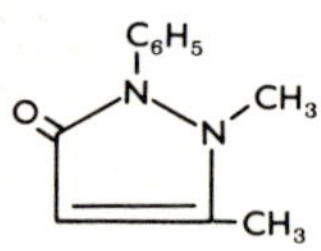

A white crystalline powder. M.p. 111° to 113°.
Solubility. Soluble 1 in 1 of water, 1 in 1 of ethanol, 1 in 50 of ether, and 1 in 1 of chloroform.

Extraction. Phenazone is extracted by organic solvents from aqueous acid solutions.

Chromatography. PAPER: system P1—Rf 0·87 (location under ultraviolet light, strong absorption; location reagent *iodoplatinate spray*, weak reaction); system RP1a—Rf 0·86 (location under ultraviolet light, absorption); system RP1b—Rf 0·79 (location as for RP1a).
THIN-LAYER: system T1—Rf 0·65 (location reagent *acidified iodoplatinate spray*, positive reaction).
GAS: system G3—retention time 6·10 relative to diphenhydramine; system G5—retention time 5·15 relative to barbitone.

Colour Tests. Dissolve 0·1 g of phenazone in 10 ml of water containing 0·1 g of 95% sodium nitrite solution; add 1 ml of dilute sulphuric acid—green.
MICRO: ammonium vanadate test—faint green (*sensitivity:* 1·0 μg); ferric chloride test—red-orange; Vitali's test—faint yellow/brown/bright yellow (*sensitivity:* 0·25 μg).

Crystal Tests. MICRO: *picric acid*—long plates (*sensitivity:* 1 in 200); *platinic chloride solution*—fine branching needles (*sensitivity:* 1 in 200).

Ultraviolet Absorption Spectrum. Phenazone in 0·1N sulphuric acid, maximum at 230 mμ (E1%, 1 cm 588) and inflexions at about 259 mμ and about 265 mμ.

Infra-red Absorption Spectrum. Potassium bromide disk. The principal peaks are: A 1660, B 770, C 1486 (p. 753).

Metabolism. Phenazone is slowly metabolised in man. Some 30 to 40% of a dose is excreted as the glucuronide conjugate of the 4-hydroxylated metabolite, about 5% is eliminated unchanged, and more than 50% is metabolised by an unknown route possibly involving cleavage of the ring. Phenazone is rapidly and completely absorbed from the gastro-intestinal tract, peak plasma levels occurring in 1 to 2 hours.

Dose. Up to 600 mg; max. in 24 hours 3 g.

Toxicity. The lethal dose in man is stated to be between 5 and 30 g. Large doses may cause nausea, fainting, and collapse; the prolonged administration of therapeutic doses of phenazone may give rise to agranulocytosis.
LD50 (oral): in rats 1·8 g/kg.

PHENAZOPYRIDINE *Urogenital Analgesic*

Proprietary Name: Gastrotest.

2,6-Diamino-3-phenylazopyridine
$C_{11}H_{11}N_5 = 213{\cdot}2$

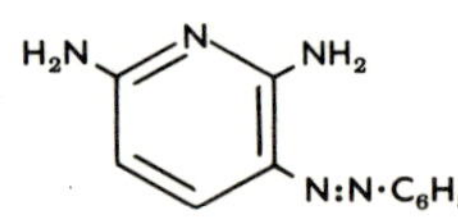

PHENAZOPYRIDINE HYDROCHLORIDE
Proprietary Names: Mallophene; Phenazodine; Pirid; Pyrazofen; Pyridium; Uridinal; Urodine.

A red microcrystalline powder.
Solubility. Soluble 1 in 300 of water and 1 in 20 of boiling water; slightly soluble in ethanol; insoluble in ether and chloroform. Phenazopyridine hydrochloride readily forms supersaturated aqueous solutions which deposit slowly on storage.

Extraction. Phenazopyridine is extracted by organic solvents from aqueous alkaline solutions.

Chromatography. PAPER: system P1—Rf 0·60 (location under ultraviolet light, red-brown fluorescence; location as a visible red spot).
THIN-LAYER: system T1—Rf 0·70 (location reagent *potassium permanganate spray*, positive reaction).

Colour Tests. MICRO: sulphuric acid-formaldehyde test—red (*sensitivity:* 0·1 μg); ammonium vanadate test—green (*sensitivity:* 0·1 μg); Vitali's test—(brown)red/orange/blue-purple→brown (*sensitivity:* 0·1 μg).

Crystal Tests. MICRO: *potassium chromate solution*—blades, often in sheaves (*sensitivity:* 1 in 400); *sodium carbonate solution*—blades, often in sheaves (*sensitivity:* 1 in 400).

Ultraviolet Absorption Spectrum. Phenazopyridine in ethanol, maxima at 238 mμ (E1%, 1 cm 423), about 267 mμ (E1%, 1 cm 243),

277 mμ (E1%, 1 cm 235), and 405 mμ (E1%, 1 cm 893).

Metabolism. Phenazopyridine is quickly eliminated by the kidneys and gives an orange-red colour to the urine.

Dose. Up to 600 mg daily.

Toxicity. Phenazopyridine in high dosage may give rise to methaemoglobinaemia. It should not be administered in the presence of kidney or liver disease.

CASE EXAMPLES. A 25-year-old woman, given 200 mg of phenazopyridine 3 times daily for urinary tract infection, had a transitory febrile attack which subsided after drug withdrawal. Three months later she was again given phenazopyridine and pain developed in her right upper abdominal quadrant, with diarrhoea and jaundice. Withdrawal of the drug produced recovery within 24 hours. On 3 later occasions jaundice appeared within 24 hours of taking phenazopyridine (Hood and Toth, 1966). Methaemoglobinaemia developed in a 15-month-old child who swallowed tablets containing 8 g of phenazopyridine—the condition was reversed with methylene blue given intravenously (*Am. J. Dis. Child.*, 1965, **110**, 105).

PHENCYCLIDINE *Analgesic/Anaesthetic*

Synonym: CI 395.

1-(1-Phenylcyclohexyl)piperidine

$C_{17}H_{25}N = 243{\cdot}4$

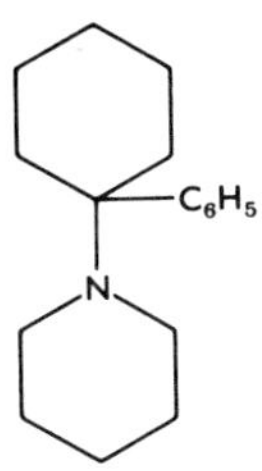

PHENCYCLIDINE HYDROCHLORIDE

Proprietary Names: Sernyl; Sernylan.

Phencyclidine hydrochloride is a white solid.

Solubility. Very soluble in water and ethanol.

Extraction. Phencyclidine is extracted by organic solvents from aqueous alkaline solutions.

Chromatography. PAPER: system P1—Rf 0·80 (location reagents: *iodoplatinate spray*, strong reaction; *bromocresol green spray*, weak reaction); system RP1a—Rf 0·53 (location under ultraviolet light, absorption); system RP1b—Rf 0·00 (location as for RP1a).

THIN-LAYER: system T1—Rf 0·59 (location reagent *acidified iodoplatinate spray*, positive reaction).

GAS: system G2/225—retention time 1·3 relative to diphenhydramine; system G4—retention time 0·84 relative to diphenhydramine.

Crystal Tests. MICRO: *gold bromide solution*—small oily crystals, best viewed under polarised light (*sensitivity:* 1 in 1000); *potassium permanganate solution*—small irregular plates (*sensitivity:* 1 in 1000).

Ultraviolet Absorption Spectrum. Phencyclidine in solution at pH2, maxima at 253 mμ, 258 mμ, 263 mμ (E1%, 1 cm 15), and 269 mμ; in 0·1N sulphuric acid, maxima at 252·5 mμ (E1%, 1 cm 8), 257·5 mμ (E1%, 1 cm 10·9), 262·5 mμ (E1%, 1 cm 12·3), and 269 mμ (E1%, 1 cm 9·2).

Infra-red Absorption Spectrum. Phencyclidine hydrochloride. Potassium bromide disk. The principal peaks are: A 1446, B 700, C 760 (p. 753).

Dose. As a single dose to assist psychotherapy, 10 mg by mouth; the usual anaesthetic dose is 0·2 mg/kg intravenously.

Toxicity. The range between the effective and toxic doses is narrow, the toxic effects including hallucinations, catatonic rigidity, incoordination, numbness, and rash.

PHENDIMETRAZINE *Anorectic*

(+)-3,4-Dimethyl-2-phenylmorpholine

$C_{12}H_{17}NO = 191{\cdot}3$

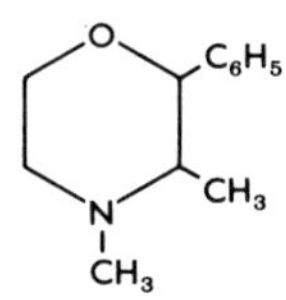

PHENDIMETRAZINE TARTRATE

Synonyms: Phendimetrazine Acid Tartrate; Phendimetrazine Bitartrate.

Proprietary Names: Dietrol; Plegine.

A white crystalline powder.

Solubility. Soluble in water and ethanol.

Extraction. Phendimetrazine is extracted by organic solvents from aqueous alkaline solutions.

Chromatography. PAPER: system P1—Rf 0·48 (location reagents: *iodoplatinate spray*, strong reaction; *bromocresol green spray*, strong reaction).

THIN-LAYER: system T1—Rf 0·50 (location reagents: *acidified iodoplatinate spray*, positive reaction; *potassium permanganate spray*, positive reaction).

GAS: system G2/120—retention time 1·4 relative to ephedrine; system G2/225—retention time 0·32 relative to diphenhydramine; system G5—retention time 1·0 relative to barbitone.

Crystal Tests. MICRO: *gold bromide solution*—curved needles (*sensitivity:* 1 in 1000); *picrolonic acid*—masses of small needles (*sensitivity:* 1 in 1000); *styphnic acid*—dendrites (*sensitivity:* 1 in 1000).

Ultraviolet Absorption Spectrum. Phendimetrazine in 0·1N sulphuric acid, maxima at 250·5 mμ (E1%, 1 cm 10), 256·5 mμ (E1%, 1 cm

13·4), 260·5 mμ (E1%, 1cm 12·5), and 267 mμ (E1%, 1cm 8·6).

Dose. Up to 200 mg daily.

PHENELZINE

Antidepressant/Monoamine Oxidase Inhibitor

2-Phenethylhydrazine

$C_8H_{12}N_2 = 136{\cdot}2$

$$C_6H_5{\cdot}[CH_2]_2{\cdot}NH{\cdot}NH_2$$

Solubility. Insoluble in water; soluble in ether and chloroform.

PHENELZINE SULPHATE

Synonym: Phenethylhydrazine Dihydrogen Sulphate.
Proprietary Names: Nardelzine; Nardil.

A white powder. M.p. 164° to 168°.

Solubility. Soluble 1 in 7 of water; almost insoluble in ethanol; insoluble in ether and chloroform.

Extraction. See under Chromatography (below).

Chromatography. PAPER, for the sulphate: system P1—Rf 0·38 (location under ultraviolet light, weak absorption; location reagent *iodoplatinate spray*, white).

NOTE. If an aqueous solution of the sulphate is made alkaline with *dilute ammonia solution* and extracted with ether, the extract gives 2 spots on system P1—Rf 0·60 (location reagent *iodoplatinate spray*, deep blue) and Rf 0·90 (location under ultraviolet light, strong absorption; location reagent *iodoplatinate spray*, yellow).

THIN-LAYER, for the sulphate: system T1—Rf 0·48 (location reagent *acidified iodoplatinate spray*, white).

GAS: system G5—retention time 0·25 relative to barbitone.

Colour Tests. MICRO: ammonium molybdate test—(grey) blue (*sensitivity:* 0·5 μg); ammonium vanadate test—(grey) brown (*sensitivity:* 0·5 μg); Vitali's test—very faint yellow/faint brown/dark brown (*sensitivity:* 1·0 μg).

Crystal Test. MICRO: *platinic iodide solution*—rhomboids or hexagons, which rapidly vanish (*sensitivity:* 1 in 100).

Ultraviolet Absorption Spectrum. Phenelzine in 0·1N sulphuric acid, maxima at 247·5 mμ (E1%, 1cm 7·4), 252 mμ (E1%, 1cm 10·1), 257·5 mμ (E1%, 1cm 12·6), and 262·5 mμ (E1%, 1cm 9·8), and an inflexion at about 267 mμ. Phenelzine sulphate in ethanol : water (1:1), maximum at 258 mμ (E1%, 1cm 80); minimum at 228 mμ.

Infra-red Absorption Spectrum. Phenelzine (base). Potassium bromide disk. The principal peaks are: A 1016, B 1108, C 1050 (p. 753).

Quantitative Estimation. A method of estimation of phenelzine in biological fluids and tissues is reported by Bian *et al.* (1964).

Metabolism. Phenelzine is an inhibitor of monoamine oxidase. Studies in mice (Bian *et al.*, 1964) have indicated that the peak plasma level after oral or intraperitoneal administration occurs in ½ to 1 hour; the drug is widely distributed, highest concentrations occurring in the liver and brain and lowest in the lungs. The drug disappears from tissues more slowly than from plasma.

Dose. Up to 60 mg of the base daily.

Toxicity. Jaundice, blurred vision, anxiety, and psychotic episodes may occur. More severe reactions, characterised by a rapid and prolonged rise in blood-pressure followed by intracranial haemorrhage, sometimes fatal, occur if a monoamine oxidase inhibitor is given at the same time as other antidepressants such as imipramine, desipramine, and amitriptyline, or with adrenaline, ephedrine, amphetamines, phenylpropanolamine and other smypathomimetic amines, pethidine, morphine, reserpine, guanethidine, antiparkinsonian drugs, antihistamines, atropine, cocaine, ethamivan, procaine, or chloroquine. Similarly, such reactions are likely to be induced if the patient concurrently takes alcohol or eats foods rich in tyramine (p. 592) or other pressor amines, e.g. cheese, yeast extract, and broad-bean pods.

CASE EXAMPLES. Many reports of toxic reactions of the types indicated under Toxicity, above, are given in Extra Pharmacopoeia (Martindale), 25th Edn, pp. 1039 to 1041.

PHENETHYLAMINE *Putrefactive Base*

Synonym: β-Aminoethylbenzene.

1-Amino-2-phenylethane

$C_8H_{11}N = 121{\cdot}2$

$$C_6H_5{\cdot}[CH_2]_2{\cdot}NH_2$$

A strongly basic liquid which absorbs carbon dioxide from the air. B.p. 194·5° to 195°.

Solubility. Soluble in water; freely soluble in ethanol and ether.

Extraction. Phenethylamine is extracted by organic solvents from aqueous alkaline solutions; it is volatile and may also be isolated by distillation from alkaline solutions.

Chromatography. PAPER: system P1—Rf 0·34 (location under ultraviolet light, absorption; location reagents: *iodoplatinate spray*, strong reaction; *bromocresol green spray*, strong reaction).

THIN-LAYER: system T1—Rf 0·33, streaking (location reagent *acidified iodoplatinate spray*, positive reaction).

Colour Test. MICRO: sulphuric acid–formaldehyde test—orange (*sensitivity:* 0·5 μg).

Crystal Test. MICRO: *trinitrobenzoic acid solution*—needles (*sensitivity:* 1 in 100).

Ultraviolet Absorption Spectrum. Phenethylamine in 0·1N sodium hydroxide, maxima at 257 mμ and 266 mμ; minimum at 233 mμ: in 0·1N sulphuric acid, maxima at 242 mμ (E1%, 1cm 15), 247 mμ (E1%, 1cm 17·2), 251·5 mμ (E1%, 1cm 19·8), 257·5 mμ (E1%, 1cm 21·3), and 263 mμ (E1%, 1cm 16), and an inflexion at about 266 mμ (E1%, 1cm 11·1).

NOTE. The ultraviolet spectrum of phenethylamine bears

many points of resemblance to those of amphetamine (p. 192) and pethidine (p. 476); the 3 compounds may be separated by paper or thin-layer chromatography.

Metabolism. Phenethylamine is the putrefactive base obtained from phenylalanine by decarboxylation. It is not generally detected in post-mortem liver tissue until after 5 days' storage (Kaempe, 1965).

Toxicity. The lethal dose in mice is about 300 mg/kg subcutaneously.

PHENETURIDE *Anticonvulsant*

Synonyms: Ethylphenacemide; S 46.
Proprietary Names: Benuride. It is an ingredient of Trinuride.

(α-Phenylbutyryl)urea
$C_{11}H_{14}N_2O_2 = 206{\cdot}2$

$$CH_3{\cdot}CH_2{\cdot}\underset{}{\overset{C_6H_5}{\overset{|}{C}}}H{\cdot}CO{\cdot}NH{\cdot}CO{\cdot}NH_2$$

A white crystalline powder.
Solubility. Almost insoluble in water and ether; slightly soluble in ethanol.

Chromatography. PAPER: system P1—Rf 0·94 (location under ultraviolet light, absorption; location reagent *iodine vapour*, positive reaction); system RP1a—Rf 0·18 (location under ultraviolet light, absorption); system RP1b—Rf 0·15 (location as for RP1a).
THIN-LAYER: system T1—Rf 0·76 (location reagent *iodine–carbon tetrachloride spray*, positive reaction).
GAS: system G2/225—retention time 0·33 relative to diphenhydramine; system G4—retention time 1·0 relative to diphenhydramine.

Ultraviolet Absorption Spectrum. Pheneturide in chloroform, maxima at 259 mμ (E1%, 1 cm 18) and 265 mμ (E1%, 1 cm 11).

Infra-red Absorption Spectrum. Potassium bromide disk. The principal peaks are: A 1672, B 1395, C 1093 (p. 753).

Dose. Usually up to 1 g daily.

Toxicity. Aplastic anaemia has been reported in a woman who took 1·2 g daily for 10 months. Pheneturide is less likely to cause toxic effects than phenacemide (p. 477) to which it is chemically related.

PHENFORMIN *Antidiabetic*

Synonym: Phenethylbiguanide.

N^1-Phenethyldiguanide
$C_{10}H_{15}N_5 = 205{\cdot}3$

$$C_6H_5{\cdot}[CH_2]_2{\cdot}NH{\cdot}\overset{NH}{\overset{\|}{C}}{\cdot}NH{\cdot}\overset{NH}{\overset{\|}{C}}{\cdot}NH_2$$

PHENFORMIN HYDROCHLORIDE
Synonym: PEDG.
Proprietary Names: DBI; Dibotin.

A white crystalline powder.
Solubility. Soluble in water.

Extraction. Phenformin is extracted by organic solvents from aqueous alkaline solutions.

Chromatography. PAPER: system P1—Rf 0·25 (location under ultraviolet light, strong absorption; location reagent *bromocresol green spray*, strong reaction); system RP1a—Rf 0·92 (location under ultraviolet light, absorption); system RP1b—Rf 0·94 (location as for RP1a).
THIN-LAYER: system T1—Rf 0·55 (location reagent *Marquis reagent*, positive reaction).

Colour Tests. MICRO: sulphuric acid–formaldehyde test—orange→brown (*sensitivity:* 0·5 μg); ammonium molybdate test—green (*sensitivity:* 0·5 μg); ammonium vanadate test—pale green (*sensitivity:* 1·0 μg).

Crystal Tests. MICRO: *picric acid*—bunches of prisms (*sensitivity:* 1 in 400); *platinic iodide solution*—irregular dense or feathery rosettes (*sensitivity:* 1 in 400).

Ultraviolet Absorption Spectrum. Phenformin in 0·1N sulphuric acid, maxima at 251 mμ (E1%, 1 cm 11), 257·5 mμ (E1%, 1 cm 11), 263·5 mμ (E1%, 1 cm 8), and about 267 mμ (E1%, 1 cm 5·8).

Infra-red Absorption Spectrum. Phenformin hydrochloride. Potassium bromide disk. The principal peaks are: A 1568, B 1537, C 1590 or 1625 (p. 753).

Quantitative Estimation. Phenformin in biological fluids and tissues may be determined spectrophotometrically (Freedman *et al.*, 1961).

Metabolism. Phenformin is a hypoglycaemic agent whose effects last for 4 to 5 hours. It is found to accumulate in the gastric juice and in the liver. Studies in animals with ^{14}C–labelled phenformin have shown that 95% of a dose is excreted in the urine within 24 hours (Wick *et al.*, 1960).

Dose. Usually up to 150 mg daily.

PHENGLUTARIMIDE *Parasympatholytic*

α - 2 - Diethylaminoethyl - α - phenylglutarimide
$C_{17}H_{24}N_2O_2 = 288{\cdot}4$

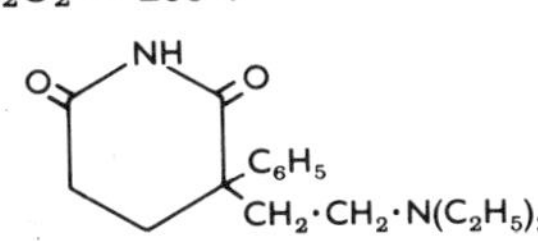

PHENGLUTARIMIDE HYDROCHLORIDE
Proprietary Name: Aturbane.

A white crystalline powder. M.p. about 177°, with decomposition.
Solubility. Soluble 1 in less than 1 of water and 1 in 1·5 of ethanol; very slightly soluble in ether.

Extraction. Phenglutarimide is extracted by organic solvents from aqueous acid solutions.

Chromatography. PAPER: system P1—Rf 0·35 (location under ultraviolet light, absorption; location reagent *iodoplatinate spray*, strong reaction).

THIN-LAYER: system T1—Rf 0·38 (location reagent *acidified iodoplatinate spray*, positive reaction).

Crystal Test. MICRO: *platinic iodide solution*—dense rosettes or hairlike crystals (*sensitivity:* 1 in 100).

Ultraviolet Absorption Spectrum. Phenglutarimide hydrochloride in 0·01N hydrochloric acid, maxima at 251 mμ (E1%, 1cm about 11·6), 257 mμ (E1%, 1cm about 11·8), and 263 mμ (E1%, 1cm about 9).

Infra-red Absorption Spectrum. Phenglutarimide hydrochloride. Potassium bromide disk. The principal peaks are: A 1698, B 1194, C 1181 (p. 753).

Dose. Usually up to 20 mg daily; up to 50 mg daily has been given.

Toxicity. The lethal dose is probably between 100 and 500 mg/kg.

PHENINDAMINE *Antihistamine*

1,2,3,4 - Tetrahydro - 2 - methyl - 9 - phenyl - 2 - azafluorene

$C_{19}H_{19}N = 261{\cdot}4$

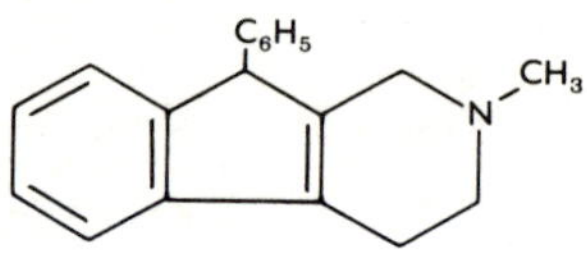

PHENINDAMINE TARTRATE

Synonym: Phenindamine Acid Tartrate.

Proprietary Name: Thephorin.

A white voluminous powder. M.p. 160° to 162°; it resolidifies at 163° and melts again at 168°, with decomposition.

Solubility. Soluble 1 in 70 of water and 1 in 300 of ethanol; almost insoluble in ether and chloroform.

Extraction. Phenindamine is extracted by organic solvents from aqueous alkaline solutions.

Chromatography. PAPER: system P1—Rf 0·63 (location under ultraviolet light, pale green fluorescence; location reagents: *iodoplatinate spray*, strong reaction; *bromocresol green spray*, weak reaction); system RP1a—Rf 0·37 (location reagent *iodoplatinate spray*, positive reaction); system RP1b—Rf 0·00 (location as for RP1a).

THIN-LAYER: system T1—Rf 0·57 (location reagent *acidified iodoplatinate spray*, positive reaction); system T2—Rf 0·65 (location reagent *iodoplatinate spray*, positive reaction); system T3—Rf 0·90 (location as for T2); system T4—Rf 0·67 (location as for T2); system T5—Rf 0·48 (location as for T2).

GAS: system G2/225—retention time 0·54 relative to codeine; system G4—retention time 0·3 relative to codeine.

Colour Tests. MICRO: sulphuric acid–formaldehyde test—grey-green (*sensitivity:* 0·1 μg); ammonium molybdate test—green (*sensitivity:* 0·1 μg); ammonium vanadate test—green (*sensitivity:* 0·1 μg); Vitali's test— –/–/green (*sensitivity:* 0·25 μg).

Crystal Tests. MICRO: *mercuric chloride solution*—rosettes, often dense (*sensitivity:* 1 in 100); *potassium tri-iodide solution* (*1*)—branching needles (*sensitivity:* 1 in 1000).

Ultraviolet Absorption Spectrum. Phenindamine in 0·1N sulphuric acid, maximum at 259·5 mμ (E1%, 1cm 316·5); phenindamine tartrate in water, maximum at 259 mμ (E1%, 1cm about 346).

Infra-red Absorption Spectrum. Phenindamine (base). Potassium bromide disk. The principal peaks are: A 1304, B 1412, C 1261 (p. 754).

Metabolism. Following a dose of 25 mg in man, only a very small amount of unchanged phenindamine was recovered from the urine extract; the major metabolite was thought to be a phenol. A second metabolite which was thought to be demethylated phenindamine was also recovered (Cochin and Daly, 1963b).

Dose. Up to 200 mg daily.

Toxicity. The estimated acute lethal dose in man is 25 to 250 mg/kg.
LD50 (oral): in rats 280 and in mice 255 mg/kg.

PHENINDIONE *Anticoagulant*

Synonym: Phenylindanedione.

Proprietary Names: Danilone; Dindevan; Eridione; Hedulin; Indema; Theradione.

2-Phenylindane-1,3-dione

$C_{15}H_{10}O_2 = 222{\cdot}2$

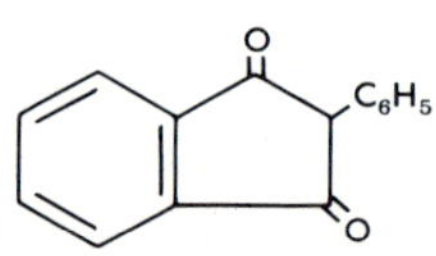

Soft white crystals. M.p. 148° to 151°.

Solubility. Very slightly soluble in water; soluble 1 in 125 of ethanol, 1 in 110 of ether, and 1 in 6·5 of chloroform.

Extraction. Phenindione is extracted by organic solvents from aqueous acid solutions.

Chromatography. PAPER: system P8—Rf 0·77 (location under ultraviolet light, absorption; location reagents: *diazotised* o-*dianisidine spray*, yellow-orange; *diazotised sulphanilic acid spray*, yellow); system P9—Rf 0·04 (location as for P8); system P10—Rf 0·96 (location as for P8).

Ultraviolet Absorption Spectrum. Phenindione in ethanol, maxima at 269 mμ (E1%, 1cm 1006) and 320 mμ (E1%, 1cm 154).

Infra-red Absorption Spectrum. Potassium

bromide disk. The principal peaks are: A 1700, B 700, C 766 or 1219 (p. 754).

Quantitative Estimation. Phenindione may be determined by extraction of deproteinised material with toluene from acid solution, purification and subsequent spectrophotometric estimation (Bose and Vijayvargiya, 1962).

Metabolism. Although the exact metabolic pathway of phenindione is unknown, a metabolic product excreted by the kidneys colours the urine red-orange.

Dose. Up to 300 mg daily.

Toxicity. Fatalities have occurred following doses of 200 mg.

PHENIRAMINE *Antihistamine*

Synonym: Prophenpyridamine.

NN-Dimethyl-3-phenyl-3-pyrid-2′-ylpropylamine

$C_{16}H_{20}N_2 = 240{\cdot}4$

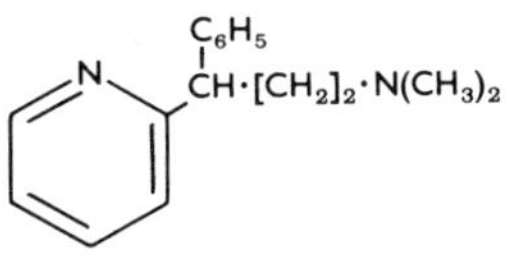

A slightly yellow oily liquid.

Solubility. Insoluble in water; soluble in ethanol, ether, and chloroform.

PHENIRAMINE AMINOSALICYLATE

Proprietary Names: Avil; Daneral.

It occurs as needles. M.p. 142°, with decomposition.

Solubility. Soluble 1 in 10 of water; freely soluble in ethanol; sparingly soluble in ether.

PHENIRAMINE MALEATE

Proprietary Names: Inhiston; Metron; Trimeton; Tripoton.

A white crystalline powder. M.p. 104° to 108°.

Solubility. Soluble 1 in 5 of water; very soluble in ethanol; slightly soluble in ether.

Extraction. Pheniramine is extracted by organic solvents from aqueous alkaline solutions.

Chromatography. PAPER: system P1—Rf 0·27 (location under ultraviolet light, dark blue fluorescence; location reagents: *iodoplatinate spray*, strong reaction; *bromocresol green spray*, weak reaction); system RP1a—Rf 0·92 (location under ultraviolet light, blue fluorescence; location reagent *iodoplatinate spray*, positive reaction); system RP1b—Rf 0·20 (location as for RP1a).

THIN-LAYER: system T1—Rf 0·32 (location reagent *acidified iodoplatinate spray*, positive reaction); system T2—Rf 0·63 (location reagent *iodoplatinate spray*, positive reaction); system T3—Rf 0·68 (location as for T2); system T4—Rf 0·38, tailing (location as for T2); system T5—Rf 0·19 (location as for T2).

GAS: system G1/180—retention time 0·83 relative to diphenhydramine; system G2/225—retention time 0·87 relative to diphenhydramine; system G3—retention time 0·92 relative to diphenhydramine; system G4—retention time 0·90 relative to diphenhydramine.

Crystal Tests. MICRO: *gold bromide–hydrochloric acid solution*—small stout needles (*sensitivity:* 1 in 1000); *gold chloride solution*—serrated blades, forming overnight (*sensitivity:* 1 in 1000).

Ultraviolet Absorption Spectrum. Pheniramine in water, maxima at 256 mμ and 262 mμ; in 0·1N sodium hydroxide, maxima at 261 mμ (E1%, 1cm 208), and 268 mμ (E1%, 1cm 163); in 0·1N sulphuric acid, maxima at 262 mμ (E1%, 1cm 318) and 266 mμ (E1%, 1cm 318), and an inflexion at about 271 mμ.

Infra-red Absorption Spectrum. Pheniramine maleate. Potassium bromide disk. The principal peaks are: A 1584, B 1481, C 1366 (p. 754).

Dose. Up to 200 mg daily.

Toxicity. The estimated acute lethal dose in man is 25 to 250 mg/kg.

LD50 (oral): in guinea-pigs 277 and in mice 185·1 mg/kg.

PHENISONONE *Bronchodilator*

3,4-Dihydroxy-α-(isopropylamino)propiophenone

$C_{12}H_{17}NO_3 = 223{\cdot}3$

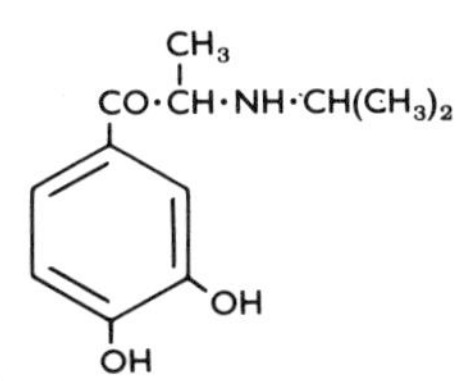

Solubility. Insoluble in water and organic solvents.

PHENISONONE HYDROBROMIDE

Proprietary Name: Dapanone.

Phenisonone hydrobromide occurs as crystals. M.p. 141° to 143°.

Solubility. Soluble 1 in 3·3 of water and 1 in 4 of ethanol; insoluble in ether and chloroform. Aqueous solutions are unstable.

Extraction. Phenisonone is extracted by organic solvents from aqueous alkaline solutions.

Chromatography. PAPER: system P1—Rf 0·51 (location under ultraviolet light, pale blue fluorescence; location reagent *bromocresol green spray*, weak reaction); system RP1a—Rf 0·91 (location under ultraviolet light, blue fluorescence); system RP1b—Rf 0·93 (location as for RP1a).

THIN-LAYER: system T1—Rf 0·30, streaking (location reagent *potassium permanganate spray*, positive reaction).

Colour Tests. MICRO: sulphuric acid–formaldehyde test—yellow (*sensitivity:* 0·5 μg); ammonium molybdate test—(yellow) blue-green (*sensitivity:* 0·5 μg); ammonium vanadate test—(green) yellow (*sensitivity:* 1·0 μg); Vitali's test—yellow/brown/brown (*sensitivity:* 1·0 μg).

Crystal Tests. MICRO: *gold bromide solution*—very small plates, forming overnight (*sensitivity:* 1 in 100); *gold chloride solution*—very small plates (*sensitivity:* 1 in 100).

Ultraviolet Absorption Spectrum. Phenisonone in 0·1N sulphuric acid, maxima at 233 mμ (E1%, 1cm 473), 284 mμ (E1%, 1cm 409), and 313 mμ (E1%, 1cm 350); phenisonone hydrobromide in water, maxima at 233 mμ (E1%, 1cm 38·2) and 284 mμ (E1%, 1cm 32·5).

PHENMETRAZINE *Anorectic*

3-Methyl-2-phenylmorpholine

$C_{11}H_{15}NO = 177{\cdot}2$

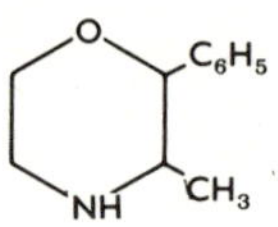

Phenmetrazine has a boiling-point of 138° at 12 mm Hg.

PHENMETRAZINE HYDROCHLORIDE

Proprietary Name: Preludin.

A white crystalline powder. M.p. about 174°.

Solubility. Soluble 1 in less than 1 of water, 1 in 2 of ethanol, and 1 in 2 of chloroform; slightly soluble in ether.

PHENMETRAZINE THEOCLATE

Synonyms: Phenmetrazine 8-Chlorotheophyllinate; R382.

Proprietary Name: It is an ingredient of Filon.

A white powder.

Solubility. Soluble in water and ethanol; slightly soluble in ether.

Extraction. Phenmetrazine is extracted by organic solvents from aqueous alkaline solutions.

Chromatography. PAPER: system P1—Rf 0·49 (location reagents: *iodoplatinate spray*, strong reaction; *bromocresol green spray*, weak reaction; *ninhydrin spray*, faint purple).

THIN-LAYER: system T1—Rf 0·50 (location reagent *potassium permanganate spray*, positive reaction).

GAS: system G2/120—retention time 1·25 relative to ephedrine.

Crystal Tests. MICRO: *gold bromide–hydrochloric acid solution*—jagged plates (*sensitivity:* 1 in 100); *picrolonic acid*—dense rosettes (*sensitivity:* 1 in 200).

Ultraviolet Absorption Spectrum. Phenmetrazine hydrochloride in 0·01N hydrochloric acid, maxima at 250 mμ (E1%, 1cm about 7·8), 256 mμ (E1%, 1cm about 10·6), 261 mμ (E1%, 1cm about 9·4), and 267 mμ (E1%, 1cm about 5·8).

Infra-red Absorption Spectrum. Phenmetrazine hydrochloride. Potassium bromide disk. The principal peaks are: A 1083, B 695 or 757 (p. 754).

Dose. Up to 75 mg daily.

Toxicity. Estimated minimum lethal dose in children up to 2 years of age, 200 mg. Recovery has occurred following the ingestion of 1400 25-mg tablets in 12 weeks.

Large doses and prolonged treatment may lead to severe mental depression and to addiction characterised by psychotic reactions.

CASE EXAMPLE. A report of 150 cases of addiction in Sweden where Preludin tablets were dissolved in water and injected intravenously. Each injection contained 200 to 500 mg, and in 24 hours the quantities injected were up to 1 to 2 g of phenmetrazine hydrochloride (Rylander, 1966).

PHENOBARBITONE *Barbiturate*

Synonyms: Fenobarbital; Phenemalum; Phenobarbital; Phenylethylmalonylurea.

Proprietary Names: Agrypnal; Barbenyl; Eskabarb; Fenemal; Gardenal; Luminal; Phenomet; T(h)eoloxin.

5-Ethyl-5-phenylbarbituric acid

$C_{12}H_{12}N_2O_3 = 232{\cdot}2$

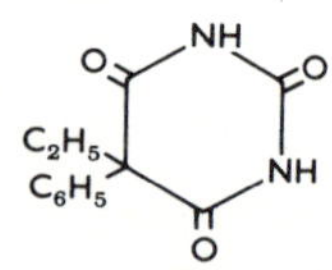

A white crystalline powder. M.p. 174° to 177°.

Solubility. Soluble 1 in 1000 of water, 1 in 15 of ethanol, 1 in 40 of ether, and 1 in 50 of chloroform.

PHENOBARBITONE SODIUM

Synonyms: Phenemalnatrium; Phenobarbital Sodium; Soluble Phenobarbitone; Sodium Phenylethylbarbiturate.

Proprietary Names: Gardenal Sodium; Luminal Sodium.

A white hygroscopic powder.

Solubility. Soluble 1 in 3 of water and 1 in 25 of ethanol; insoluble in ether and chloroform.

Screening Tests. See under Barbiturates, p. 208.

Extraction. Phenobarbitone may be isolated in the A2 fraction (see p. 27).

Chromatography. PAPER: system P2—Rf 0·09 relative to amylobarbitone (location under ultraviolet light, dark spot); system RP1b—Rf 0·48 (location under ultraviolet light after exposure to ammonia; location reagent *potassium permanganate spray*, yellow on pink).

THIN-LAYER: system T10—Rf 0·24 (location reagents: *mercurous nitrate spray*, black;

potassium permanganate spray, yellow-brown on purple; *Zwikker's reagent spray*, pink); system T11—Rf 0·36 (location reagent *mercurous nitrate spray*, white on grey); system T12—Rf 0·26 (location as for T11); system T13—Rf 0·50 (location as for T11).
GAS: system G1/180—retention time 1·80 relative to diphenhydramine; system G3—retention time 4·70 relative to diphenhydramine; system G5—retention time 6·90 relative to barbitone; system G7—retention time 4·80 relative to barbitone.

Colour Test. Zwikker's test—violet-blue.

Ultraviolet Absorption Spectrum. Phenobarbitone is a 5,5-derivative—see Screening Test 3 under Barbiturates, p. 208.
p-Hydroxyphenobarbitone in solution at pH 10, maximum at 244 mμ; in solution at pH 13, maximum at 249 mμ.

Infra-red Absorption Spectrum. Phenobarbitone. Potassium bromide disk. The principal peaks are: A 1703 or 1756, B 1406 (p. 754).

Quantitative Estimation. See under Barbiturates, p. 208.

Metabolism. Phenobarbitone is a long-acting barbiturate—see under Barbiturates, p. 207. The main metabolite in man is the *p*-hydroxy-derivative, 5-ethyl-5-*p*-hydroxyphenylbarbituric acid. About 50% is conjugated, less than 10%, however, as the glucuronide. The rest is thought to be conjugated as the ethereal sulphate.
The hydroxylation reaction of phenobarbitone to form this *p*-hydroxy-derivative appears to be a mechanism of major importance in the inactivation of phenobarbitone.
Curry (1955) has described a method of paper chromatographic separation of phenobarbitone and its *p*-hydroxy-derivative.
The ultraviolet spectrum of the metabolite shows a significant difference from that of phenobarbitone—see under Ultraviolet Absorption Spectrum (above).
Following the administration of phenobarbitone as a single dose of 300 mg in man, unchanged drug was detected in the urine by paper chromatography for 17 to 28 days and *p*-hydroxyphenobarbitone for 12 to 24 days.

Dose. Up to 120 mg; max. in 24 hours, 600 mg.

Toxicity. The estimated minimum lethal dose in man is 1·5 g. Blood-levels of 5 mg% have been found in fatal poisoning cases.
CASE EXAMPLES. In a survey based on 84 cases of fatal barbiturate poisoning including 12 cases involving phenobarbitone, the following mean post-mortem levels of phenobarbitone were found: brain, 14·4 mg%; liver, 17·8 mg%; solid organs (average), 19·6 mg%; urine, 41 mg%. The highest concentration of a long-acting barbiturate like phenobarbitone which can be reached in the tissues before death ensues appears to be about 40 to 50 mg% and there is probably a tendency for phenobarbitone to show a higher concentration than the body average in the liver and a lower concentration in the brain. Any possible correlation between the amount ingested and the period of survival seems to be obscured by variations in individual susceptibility (Walls, 1958).
A 46-year-old woman recovered 24 hours after taking 1230 mg of phenobarbitone. Twenty-four hours after ingestion of the drug the blood-level of phenobarbitone was 2·3 mg%; 130 mg of the drug was recovered from the stomach washings (Wright and Johns, 1953).
A 57-year-old man took 4 g of phenobarbitone and 500 mg of methotrimeprazine. Eight hours later, on admission to hospital, the phenobarbitone plasma level was 12 mg% and the urine level 6·8 mg%. After 3 haemoperfusions through charcoal during the subsequent 15 hours the plasma level of phenobarbitone was reduced to 3·7 mg%, and after 24 hours it had dropped to 3·4 mg%. During the 24 hours the patient voided 4 litres of urine containing only 230 mg of phenobarbitone (Yatzidis *et al.*, 1965).
A 25-year-old man was admitted to hospital in a deep coma. He had obviously ingested a large amount of phenobarbitone. Two hours and a half after admission the blood was found to contain 21·6 mg% and the urine 78·3 mg% of phenobarbitone, and 5½ hours later the urine was found to contain 51·3 mg%. A day after admission the blood contained 11·38 mg%. The patient recovered after 5 days (Jain and Forney, 1967).

PHENOL *Antiseptic*

Synonyms: Benzophenol; Carbolic Acid; Fenol; Phenyl Hydrate.

Hydroxybenzene
$C_6H_5 \cdot OH = 94{\cdot}11$

Colourless or faintly pink, deliquescent, needle-shaped crystals or crystalline masses. F.p. not below 40°. B.p. about 181°.
Solubility. Soluble 1 in 12 of water, 6 in 1 of ethanol, 5 in 1 of ether, and 2 in 1 of chloroform.

Extraction. Phenol is extracted by organic solvents from aqueous acid solutions.

Chromatography. GAS: system G5—retention time 0·12 relative to barbitone.

Colour Tests. *Liebermann's reagent*—blue-red. MICRO: ferric chloride test—violet.

Ultraviolet Absorption Spectrum. Phenol in ethanol, maximum at 272 mμ (E 1%, 1 cm 194·6) and an inflexion at about 279 mμ; in 0·1N sodium hydroxide, maximum at 286 mμ (E 1%, 1 cm 274).

Metabolism. Phenol is metabolised by conjugation to yield phenylglucuronide and phenyl sulphate; small amounts are oxidised to catechol and quinol which are also conjugated. Oxidation of these metabolites to quinones may tint the urine green.
Phenol is rapidly absorbed from the gastro-intestinal tract and readily penetrates the skin, mucous membranes, and other tissues. It denatures and precipitates cellular proteins and thus may rapidly cause poisoning, and so its use as an antiseptic has greatly declined.

Toxicity. The fatal dose by mouth varies between 8 and 15 g. Severe and even fatal poisoning may also arise from absorption of phenol from open wounds or even through the intact skin.

LD50 (oral): in rats 1·3 g/kg.

CASE EXAMPLES. Between 4 and 5 g of phenol was found in the stomach of a man who had committed suicide by drinking a phenol mouth-wash.—per *Pharm J.*, ii/1955, 48.

A workman fell into a vat of phenol and became submerged up to his thighs. He was immediately hauled out and hosed down, without removal of his clothing. Shortly afterwards he became drowsy and was nearly unconscious by the time his clothing was removed. He died within half an hour of the accident. At post-mortem examination the blood contained about 9 mg% of phenol (Consden, 1967).

PHENOLPHTHALEIN *Purgative*

Synonym: Dihydroxyphthalophenone.

αα-Di(*p*-hydroxyphenyl)phthalide
$C_{20}H_{14}O_4$ = 318·3

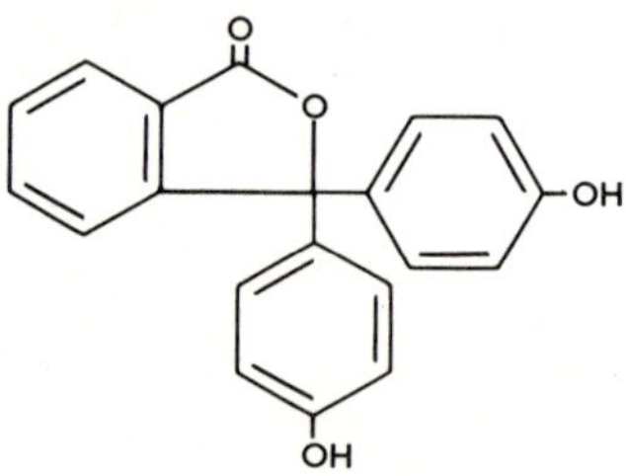

A white crystalline or amorphous powder. M.p. 258° to 263°.

Solubility. Almost insoluble in water; soluble 1 in 15 of ethanol and 1 in 100 of ether.

Extraction. Phenolphthalein is extracted by organic solvents from aqueous acid solutions.

Colour Test. To 1 ml of a solution add 1 ml of the *Folin–Ciocalteu reagent* followed by 2 ml of a 20% sodium carbonate solution—blue.

Ultraviolet Absorption Spectrum. Phenolphthalein in methanol, maximum at 276 mμ (E1%, 1 cm 145); in solution at pH 11·2, maximum at 555 mμ (E1%, 1 cm 1055).

Metabolism. Some phenolphthalein may be absorbed from the gastro-intestinal tract and excreted partly in the bile, so that purgative effects may continue for several days. It is excreted chiefly in the faeces but some may be excreted in the urine; if the urine is alkaline the excreted compound will colour it red. Small, 30- to 60-mg, doses of phenolphthalein are excreted entirely in the conjugated form, but doses of up to 300 mg result in the excretion of both free and conjugated phenolphthalein.

Dose. Up to 300 mg.

Toxicity. Phenolphthalein is usually non-toxic even in relatively large doses.

CASE EXAMPLE. Death from encephalitis of a girl aged 2½ years following ingestion of chocolate laxative tablets containing about 10 to 20 grains (0·6 to 1·2 g) of phenolphthalein (Kendall, 1954).

PHENOMORPHAN *Narcotic*

3-Hydroxy-*N*-phenethylmorphinan
$C_{24}H_{29}NO$ = 347·5

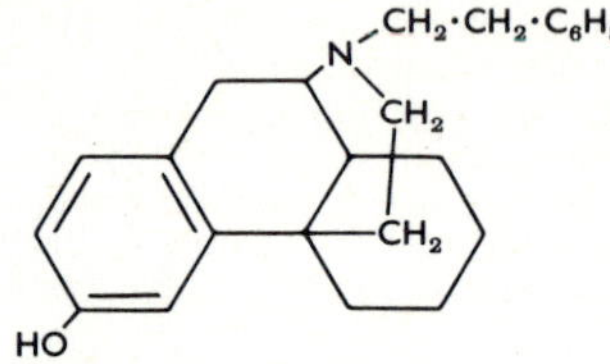

PHENOMORPHAN HYDROBROMIDE

Phenomorphan hydrobromide melts at 289° to 292°.

Extraction. Phenomorphan is extracted by organic solvents from aqueous ammoniacal solutions; hydrolysis of biological material is required in order to improve the yield.

Chromatography. PAPER: system P1—Rf 0·68 (location reagent *iodoplatinate spray*, weak reaction).

THIN-LAYER: system T1—Rf 0·72 (location reagent *acidified iodoplatinate spray*, positive reaction).

Colour Tests. MICRO: ammonium molybdate test—blue (*sensitivity:* 0·25 μg); Vitali's test—yellow/yellow/orange (*sensitivity:* 0·25 μg).

Crystal Tests. MICRO: *disodium methyl arsonate solution*—needles, some serrated (*sensitivity:* 1 in 1000); *sodium carbonate solution*—small irregular plates (*sensitivity:* 1 in 1000).

Ultraviolet Absorption Spectrum. Phenomorphan in ethanol, maximum at 280 mμ and inflexions at about 230 mμ and about 288 mμ; in 0·1N sodium hydroxide, maxima at 242 mμ and 300 mμ; in 0·1N sulphuric acid, maximum at 279 mμ (E1%, 1 cm 43·7) and an inflexion at about 284 mμ (E1%, 1 cm 41).

PHENOPERIDINE *Narcotic Analgesic*

Synonyms: Phenopridine; R 951; SC 9369.

Ethyl 1-(3-hydroxy-3-phenylpropyl)-4-phenylpiperidine-4-carboxylate
$C_{23}H_{29}NO_3$ = 367·5

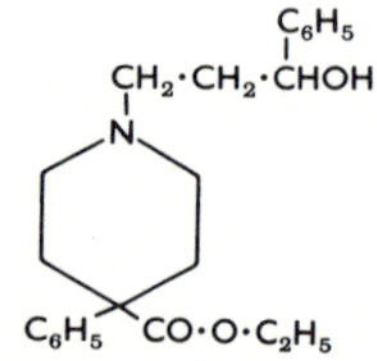

PHENOPERIDINE HYDROCHLORIDE

Synonym: R 1406.

Proprietary Names: Lealgin; Operidine.

A white crystalline powder.

Solubility. Soluble 1 in 50 of water, 1 in 10 of ethanol, and 1 in 3 of chloroform; insoluble in ether.

Extraction. Phenoperidine is extracted by organic solvents from aqueous alkaline solutions; hydrolysis of biological material is required in order to improve the yield.

Chromatography. PAPER: system P1—Rf 0·90 (location reagents: *iodoplatinate spray*, weak reaction; *bromocresol green spray*, weak reaction); system RP1a—Rf 0·20 (location reagent *iodoplatinate spray*, positive reaction); system RP1b—Rf 0·00 (location as for RP1a).

THIN-LAYER: system T1—Rf 0·75 (location reagent *acidified iodoplatinate spray*, positive reaction).

Colour Tests. MICRO: sulphuric acid–formaldehyde test—faint red (*sensitivity:* 1·0 μg); ammonium molybdate test—faint grey-purple (*sensitivity:* 1·0 μg).

Crystal Tests. MICRO: *potassium iodide solution*—rosettes of rods (*sensitivity:* 1 in 200); *potassium permanganate solution*—plates or blades (*sensitivity:* 1 in 1000).

Ultraviolet Absorption Spectrum. Phenoperidine in 0·1N sulphuric acid, maxima at 246 mμ (E1%, 1 cm 40·8) and 250 mμ (E1%, 1 cm 30·4), and an inflexion at about 256 mμ (E1%, 1 cm 26).

Dose. As an analgesic, up to 2 mg intramuscularly; in anaesthesia, up to 5 mg intravenously.

PHENOTHIAZINE *Anthelmintic (Veterinary)*

Synonym: Thiodiphenylamine.
Proprietary Names: Agrazine; Phenosan; Phenovis.

$C_{12}H_9NS = 199{\cdot}3$

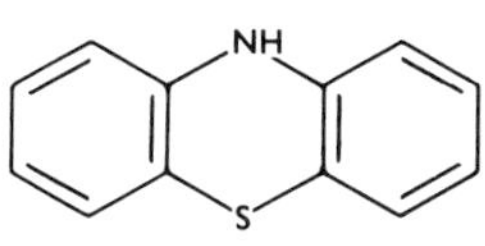

A greyish-brown powder which is slowly oxidised in air and darkens on exposure to light. M.p. 185·5° to 189°. B.p. 371°.

Solubility. Insoluble in water; soluble 1 in 60 of ethanol and 1 in 20 of chloroform.

Extraction. Phenothiazine is extracted by organic solvents from aqueous acid solutions.

Chromatography. THIN-LAYER: system T6—Rf 0·69 (the spot may be converted on the plate to the sulphoxide, Rf 0·37; location of both spots under ultraviolet light).

GAS: system G2/225—retention time 0·38 relative to codeine.

Colour Test. To 5 ml of a 0·05% solution in ethanol add 0·05 ml of a 5% ferric chloride solution—green.

Ultraviolet Absorption Spectrum. Phenothiazine in ethanol, maxima at 254 mμ (E1%, 1 cm 2160) and 317 mμ (E1%, 1 cm 266).

Infra-red Absorption Spectrum. Potassium bromide disk. The principal peaks are: A 735, B 1476, C 750 or 1445 (p. 754).

Metabolism. Phenothiazine is almost insoluble in water and about 30 to 50% of an oral dose passes through the gastro-intestinal tract unchanged. Some phenothiazine is converted within the gastro-intestinal tract to phenothiazine sulphoxide which is absorbed into the portal venous system. The sulphoxide is converted by the liver into leucophenothiazone and leucothionol. These derivatives are excreted in the urine and are responsible for its red colour when exposed to the air.
Urinary and faecal excretion of phenothiazine or its derivatives accounts for 80% of an oral dose in sheep; the fate of the remaining 20% is unknown.

Dose. In horses, up to 30 g; in cattle, up to 60 g; in sheep, up to 40 g; in poultry, up to 1 g.

Toxicity. Phenothiazine is too toxic to be used safely in human medicine; doses of 8 to 10 g, administered over a period of 5 to 6 days, have caused severe haemolytic anaemia in children. The toxicity of phenothiazine in animals varies widely. Animals have died after receiving the customary therapeutic dose, whereas others of the same species have survived many times this amount. Susceptibility to the toxic effects of phenothiazine is generally considered to be greatest in the horse. The toxicity is to some extent dependent on particle size, finely divided preparations being considerably more toxic than coarsely divided ones.
LD50 (oral): in rats 5 g/kg.

PHENOXYBENZAMINE *Anti-adrenergic*

Synonym: SKF 688A.

Benzyl(2-chloroethyl)(1-methyl-2-phenoxyethyl)amine

$C_{18}H_{22}ClNO = 303{\cdot}8$

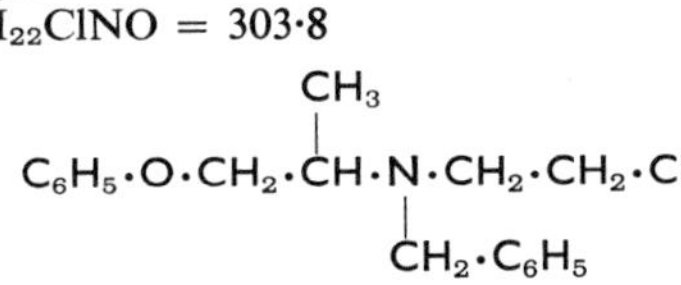

It occurs as crystals. M.p. 38° to 40°.

Solubility. Soluble in benzene.

PHENOXYBENZAMINE HYDROCHLORIDE

Proprietary Names: Dibenyline; Dibenzyline.

A white crystalline powder. M.p. 137·5° to 140°.

Solubility. Sparingly soluble in water; soluble 1 in 9 of ethanol and 1 in 9 of chloroform.

Extraction. Phenoxybenzamine is extracted by organic solvents from aqueous alkaline solutions.

Chromatography. PAPER: system P1—Rf 0·92 (location reagents: *iodoplatinate spray*, strong reaction).

THIN-LAYER: system T1—Rf 0·76 (location reagent *acidified iodoplatinate spray*, positive reaction).

GAS: system G2/225—retention time 0·68 relative to codeine.

Colour Tests. MICRO: sulphuric acid–formaldehyde test—purple (*sensitivity:* 0·25 μg); ammonium molybdate test—dull green → blue (*sensitivity:* 0·25 μg); ammonium vanadate test—dull green → purple (*sensitivity:* 0·25 μg); Vitali's test—-/-/faint red, fading (*sensitivity:* 1·0 μg).

Crystal Tests. MICRO: *gold chloride solution*—bunches of oily rods (*sensitivity:* 1 in 400); *potassium iodide solution*—bunches of plates or prisms, forming overnight (*sensitivity:* 1 in 200).

Ultraviolet Absorption Spectrum. Phenoxybenzamine in 0·1N sulphuric acid, maxima at 262 mμ (E1%, 1 cm 42), 268 mμ (E1%, 1 cm 50), and 274 mμ (E1%, 1 cm 36).

Infra-red Absorption Spectrum. Phenoxybenzamine (base). Potassium bromide disk. The principal peaks are: A 1242, B 1114 or 1497, C 1384 or 1600 (p. 793).

Metabolism. Studies of tissue distribution in mice with ^{14}C-labelled phenoxybenzamine demonstrated that the drug penetrated readily into most tissues. Although the liver, kidney, and fat initially contained the greatest amounts, the heart and central nervous system retained greater amounts after 4 days (Masuoka *et al.*, 1967).

Dose. Up to 20 mg daily initially, gradually increasing up to a total of 240 mg daily, according to the patient's response.

Toxicity. In therapeutic doses, phenoxybenzamine may cause orthostatic hypotension. Large doses sometimes produce tachycardia.

PHENOXYMETHYLPENICILLIN *Antibiotic*

Synonyms: Penicillin V; Phenoxymethyl Penicillin; Phénomycilline.
Proprietary Names: Calcipen; Distaquaine V; Oracilline; Oratren; Pen-Vee; V-Cillin; Viacillin.

6-Phenoxyacetamidopenicillanic acid
$C_{16}H_{18}N_2O_5S = 350·4$

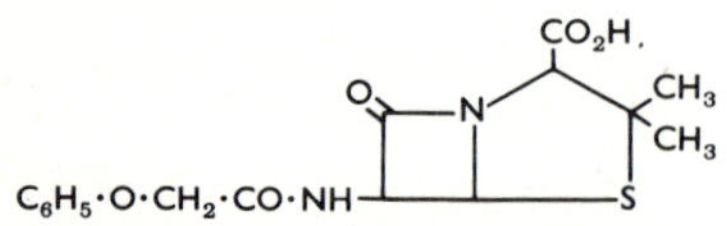

A white finely crystalline powder.
Solubility. Soluble 1 in 1700 of water and 1 in 7 of ethanol.

PHENOXYMETHYLPENICILLIN CALCIUM
Synonym: Penicillin V Calcium.
Proprietary Names: Calcipen-V; Crystapen V (suspension); Penicals.

A white finely crystalline powder.
Solubility. Slowly soluble 1 in 120 of water.

PHENOXYMETHYLPENICILLIN POTASSIUM
Synonym: Penicillin V Potassium.
Proprietary Names: Acocillin; Apsin VK; Compocillin-VK; Crystapen V (tablets and syrup); Distaquaine V-K; Econocil-VK; Econopen V; Fenoxypen; Icipen; Markacillin V-K; Penavlon V; Stabillin V-K; Tonsillin; V-Cil-K.

A white finely crystalline powder.
Solubility. Soluble 1 in 1·5 of water and 1 in 150 of ethanol; insoluble in ether.

Colour Test. Heat a small quantity of phenoxymethylpenicillin with a few crystals of chromotropic acid sodium salt and 2 ml of sulphuric acid in a bath of glycerin at 150° for 2 minutes—deep bluish-purple (distinction from benzylpenicillin).

Ultraviolet Absorption Spectrum. Phenoxymethylpenicillin in water, maxima at 268 mμ and 274 mμ; in methanol, maxima at 263 mμ (E1%, 1 cm 30·5), 268 mμ (E1%, 1 cm 39), and 275 mμ (E1%, 1 cm 32·5).

Metabolism. Phenoxymethylpenicillin is more resistant to inactivation by the acid gastric secretion and is more completely absorbed than benzylpenicillin from the gastro-intestinal tract following oral administration.
The blood-concentration of phenoxymethylpenicillin achieved after oral administration is higher than that after a corresponding oral dose of benzylpenicillin but is not so high as that obtained after parenteral administration of benzylpenicillin.
Serum concentrations of phenoxymethylpenicillin have been reported to range from 0·027 to 0·060 mg% two hours after a dose of 125 mg.
After oral administration, up to 25% may be excreted in 24 hours in the urine and after parenteral administration up to 60%.

Dose. Up to 1·5 g daily.

Toxicity. Phenoxymethylpenicillin is usually well tolerated but allergic reactions may occur.

PHENOXYPROPAZINE

Antidepressant/Monoamine Oxidase Inhibitor
(1-Methyl-2-phenoxyethyl)hydrazine
$C_9H_{14}N_2O = 166·2$

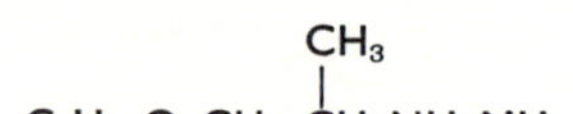

PHENOXYPROPAZINE MALEATE
Synonyms: HP 1275; Phenoxypropazine Hydrogen Maleate.
Proprietary Name: Drazine.

A white crystalline powder. M.p. 107° to 110°.
Solubility. Very soluble in water; soluble in ethanol.

Extraction. Phenoxypropazine is extracted by organic solvents from aqueous alkaline solutions.

Chromatography. PAPER: system P1—Rf 0·69 (location under ultraviolet light, absorption; location reagent *iodoplatinate spray*, white).
THIN-LAYER: system T1—Rf 0·52 (location reagent *acidified iodoplatinate spray*, white).

GAS: system G2/120—retention time 1·5 relative to ephedrine.

Colour Tests. MICRO: sulphuric acid–formaldehyde test—pale red (*sensitivity:* 0·5 μg); ammonium molybdate test—(grey) blue (*sensitivity:* 0·5 μg); ammonium vanadate test—(brown) brown (*sensitivity:* 0·5 μg); Vitali's test—brown → yellow/yellow/yellow (*sensitivity:* 1·0 μg).

Crystal Tests. MICRO: *gold bromide solution*—very small plates (*sensitivity:* 1 in 200); *mercuric chloride solution*—rods or very small needles (*sensitivity:* 1 in 100).

Ultraviolet Absorption Spectrum. Phenoxypropazine in 0·1N sulphuric acid, maxima at 263 mμ (E1%, 1 cm 44), 268 mμ (E1%, 1 cm 53), and 274·5 mμ (E1%, 1 cm 43).

Infra-red Absorption Spectrum. Phenoxypropazine maleate. Potassium bromide disk. The principal peaks are: A 1465 or 1500 or 1582, B 760 or 1353 (p. 755).

Dose. Up to 20 mg daily.

Toxicity. See under Phenelzine, p. 482.
LD50 (oral): in mice 460 mg/kg.

PHENPROBAMATE

Muscle Relaxant/Tranquilliser

Synonyms: MH 532; Proformiphen.
Proprietary Names: Gamaquil. It is an ingredient of Alutan.

3-Phenylpropyl carbamate
$C_{10}H_{13}NO_2 = 179{\cdot}2$

$$C_6H_5{\cdot}[CH_2]_3{\cdot}O{\cdot}CO{\cdot}NH_2$$

A fine white crystalline powder.
Solubility. Insoluble in water; soluble in ethanol and chloroform; slightly soluble in ether.

Extraction. Phenprobamate is extracted by organic solvents from aqueous acid or alkaline solutions.

Chromatography. PAPER: system RP1a—Rf 0·16 (location under ultraviolet light, absorption); system RP1b—Rf 0·11 (location as for RP1a).
THIN-LAYER: system T1—Rf 0·75 (location reagents: *strongly acid iodoplatinate spray*, positive reaction; *iodine–carbon tetrachloride spray*, positive reaction).
GAS: system G2/225—retention time 0·4 relative to diphenhydramine; system G5—retention time 1·3 relative to barbitone.

Colour Test. MICRO: sulphuric acid–formaldehyde test—red-brown (*sensitivity:* 1·0 μg).

Ultraviolet Absorption Spectrum. Phenprobamate in ethanol, maxima at about 248·5 mμ (E1%, 1 cm 6·6), 253·5 mμ (E1%, 1 cm 9·5), 259 mμ (E1%, 1 cm 11·6), 261·5 mμ (E1%, 1 cm 11·6), 265 mμ (E1%, 1 cm 9·5), and 268·5 mμ (E1%, 1 cm 9·6).

Quantitative Estimation. Schatz and Jahn (1966) have described a method of quantitative estimation of phenprobamate in blood and urine.

Metabolism. Phenprobamate is metabolised by oxidative degradation of the side chain (Schatz and Jahn, 1966). Partial *p*-hydroxylation of the phenyl ring may also occur.
Following oral doses of 2·4 and 3·2 g, 7% of a dose is excreted unchanged in the urine in 48 hours and 76% in the form of metabolites, 67% being hippuric acid. Phenprobamate is rapidly absorbed when taken by mouth.

Dose. Up to 2·4 g daily.

PHENSUXIMIDE

Anticonvulsant

Proprietary Names: Lifène; Milontin.
N-Methyl-α-phenylsuccinimide
$C_{11}H_{11}NO_2 = 189{\cdot}2$

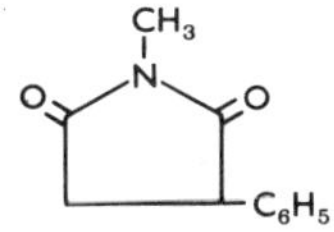

A white crystalline powder. M.p. 69° to 72°.
Solubility. Soluble 1 in 250 of water, 1 in 20 of ethanol, and 1 in 35 of ether; very soluble in chloroform.

Extraction. Phensuximide is extracted by organic solvents from aqueous acid or alkaline solutions.

Chromatography. THIN-LAYER: system T1—Rf 0·75 (location reagents: *iodine–carbon tetrachloride spray*, positive reaction; *potassium permanganate spray*, positive reaction).

Colour Test. MICRO: Vitali's test— –/–/purple (*sensitivity:* 1·0 μg).

Ultraviolet Absorption Spectrum. Phensuximide in ethanol:water (1:1), maxima at 251 mμ, 257 mμ (E1%, 1 cm 15), and 263 mμ.

Infra-red Absorption Spectrum. Potassium bromide disk. The principal peaks are: A 1686, B 1275, C 1439 or 1637 (p. 755).

Dose. Up to 3 g daily.

Toxicity. Phensuximide appears to be relatively non-toxic; periodic blood counts and urine analyses are advised for patients on long-term therapy. The estimated minimum lethal dose in man is stated to be 5 g.

PHENTERMINE

Anorectic

Proprietary Names: Duromine; Ionamin; Linyl.

αα-Dimethylphenethylamine
$C_{10}H_{15}N = 149{\cdot}2$

$$C_6H_5{\cdot}CH_2{\cdot}\underset{\displaystyle CH_3}{\overset{\displaystyle CH_3}{C}}{\cdot}NH_2$$

NOTE. Phentermine is an isomer of methylamphetamine (p. 420).

PHENTERMINE HYDROCHLORIDE
Proprietary Name: Wilpo.

Extraction. Phentermine is extracted by organic solvents from aqueous alkaline solutions.

Chromatography. PAPER: system P1—Rf 0·60 (location under ultraviolet light, absorption; location reagents: *bromocresol green spray*, strong reaction; *diazotised* p-*nitroaniline–sodium hydroxide spray*, purple; *Marquis reagent*, orange).

THIN-LAYER: system T1—Rf 0·56 (location reagent *acidified iodoplatinate spray*, positive reaction).

GAS: system G2/120—retention time 0·33 relative to ephedrine; system G5—retention time 1·36 relative to barbitone.

Colour Tests. MICRO: sulphuric acid–formaldehyde test—orange (*sensitivity:* 0·25 μg); ammonium molybdate test—faint grey-blue (*sensitivity:* 1·0 μg).

Crystal Tests. MICRO: *picrolonic acid*—long curved needles (*sensitivity:* 1 in 200); *platinic chloride solution*—plates and prisms (*sensitivity:* 1 in 200).

Ultraviolet Absorption Spectrum. Phentermine in 0·1N sulphuric acid, maxima at 252 mμ (E1%, 1cm 13·3), 257·5 mμ (E1%, 1cm 18·5), 264 mμ (E1%, 1cm 20·4), and 281 mμ (E1%, 1cm 23·8).

Dose. Up to 30 mg daily.

Toxicity. LD50 (oral): in mice 124 and rats 151 mg/kg.

PHENTOLAMINE *Anti-adrenergic*

2-[*N*-(*m*-Hydroxyphenyl)-*p*-toluidinomethyl]-2-imidazoline

$C_{17}H_{19}N_3O = 281{\cdot}4$

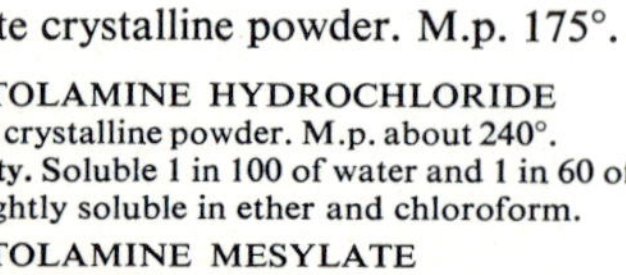

A white crystalline powder. M.p. 175°.

PHENTOLAMINE HYDROCHLORIDE
A white crystalline powder. M.p. about 240°.
Solubility. Soluble 1 in 100 of water and 1 in 60 of ethanol; very slightly soluble in ether and chloroform.

PHENTOLAMINE MESYLATE
Synonym: Phentolamine Methanesulphonate.
Proprietary Names: Regitine; Rogitine.

A white, slightly hygroscopic, crystalline powder. M.p. 177° to 181°.
Solubility. Soluble 1 in 1 of water, 1 in 5 of ethanol, and 1 in 700 of chloroform.

Extraction. Phentolamine is extracted by organic solvents from aqueous ammoniacal solutions.

Chromatography. PAPER: system P1—Rf 0·74 (location under ultraviolet light, strong absorption; location reagent *iodoplatinate spray*, weak reaction); system RP1a—Rf 0·80 (location under ultraviolet light, absorption); system RP1b—Rf 0·56 (location as for RP1a).

THIN-LAYER: system T1—Rf 0·29 (location reagent *acidified iodoplatinate spray*, positive reaction).

Colour Tests. MICRO: sulphuric acid–formaldehyde test—yellow (*sensitivity:* 0·1 μg); ammonium molybdate test—green-blue (*sensitivity:* 0·25 μg); ammonium vanadate test—blue-green (*sensitivity:* 0·1 μg); Vitali's test—green-brown/green-brown/olive (*sensitivity:* 0·25 μg).

Crystal Tests. MICRO: *potassium iodide solution*—branching rods, forming overnight (*sensitivity:* 1 in 100); *potassium mercuric iodide solution*—segmented rods with some rosettes, forming overnight, from dilute solutions only (*sensitivity:* 1 in 1000).

Ultraviolet Absorption Spectrum. Phentolamine in water, maximum at 278 mμ (E1%, 1cm 215); in 0·1N sulphuric acid, inflexion at about 228 mμ (E1%, 1cm 456) and maximum at 276 mμ (E1%, 1cm 326).

Metabolism. The metabolic fate of phentolamine is largely unknown. Studies in dogs have shown that it is excreted in the free form and in unknown conjugated forms; after oral administration 52 to 65% was excreted conjugated and after intravenous administration only 31 to 47%.
Phentolamine is very rapidly absorbed from the gastro-intestinal tract, peak plasma levels being obtained 15 to 30 minutes after oral administration. It disappears equally rapidly and cannot be detected after an hour.

Dose. Phentolamine hydrochloride: up to 600 mg by mouth daily; mesylate: up to 10 mg intravenously.

Toxicity. Phentolamine hydrochloride taken by mouth may give rise to nausea, vomiting, diarrhoea, gastro-intestinal disturbances, and anorexia. Phentolamine mesylate when given intravenously may cause tachycardia with anginal pain.

CASE EXAMPLES. A woman with a phaeochromocytoma was given a routine phentolamine test (5 mg intravenously), developed hypotension, was revived with noradrenaline, but died 30½ hours after the test (Emanuel *et al.*, 1956).

A pregnant woman, given a test for phaeochromocytoma, developed profound vasomotor shock and died immediately after administration of the phentolamine mesylate (Roland, 1959).

PHENYLBUTAZONE *Analgesic*

Synonyms: Butadion; Fenilbutazona; Pyrazolone.
Proprietary Names: Artrizin; Butazolidin; Butazone; Phebuzin. It is an ingredient of Irgapyrin and Parazolidin.

4-Butyl-3,5-dioxo-1,2-diphenylpyrazolidine
$C_{19}H_{20}N_2O_2$ = 308·4

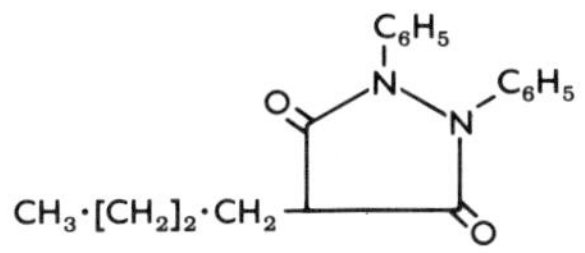

A fine white crystalline powder. M.p. 104° to 107°.
Solubility. Almost insoluble in water; soluble 1 in 28 of ethanol, 1 in 15 of ether, and 1 in 1·3 of chloroform.

Extraction. Phenylbutazone is extracted by organic solvents from aqueous acid solutions.

Chromatography. PAPER: system P1—Rf 0·96 (location under ultraviolet light, absorption; location reagent *potasium permanganate spray*, weak reaction); system RP1a—Rf 0·06 (location under ultraviolet light, absorption); system RP1b—Rf 0·43 (location as for RP1a).
THIN-LAYER: system T1—Rf 0·79 (location reagent *potassium permanganate spray*, positive reaction).
GAS: system G2/225—retention time 1·0 (1·25) relative to codeine.

Colour Tests. MICRO: ammonium vanadate test —dull purple (*sensitivity:* 1·0 μg); Vitali's test — -/-/red (*sensitivity:* 1·0 μg).

Ultraviolet Absorption Spectrum. Phenylbutazone in ethanol, maximum at 240 mμ (E1%, 1 cm 534); in 0·01N sodium hydroxide, maximum at 264 mμ (E1%, 1 cm about 660).

Infra-red Absorption Spectrum. Potassium bromide disk. The principal peaks are: A 1708, B 1300 or 1743, C 755 (p. 755).

Quantitative Estimation. Phenylbutazone may be estimated spectrophotometrically or colorimetrically after hydrolysis, diazotisation, and coupling with *N*-sulphatoethyl-*m*-toluidine (Moss, 1954). A modification of this method, involving coupling with *N*-(1-naphthyl)ethylenediamine, has been used by Tompsett (1967a).

Metabolism. Phenylbutazone is metabolised in 2 ways, by hydroxylation in the *p*-position of one of the benzene rings to yield oxyphenbutazone (p. 462) and by (ω-1)-hydroxylation of the butyl side-chain. Both metabolites have been isolated from human urine, oxyphenbutazone to the extent of 3% of a dose. It is unusually stable in the body and is apparently not conjugated. The second metabolite may account for 5% of a dose.
Phenylbutazone is metabolised unusually slowly in man, about 10 to 15% per day, but in mice, rabbits, dogs, guinea-pigs, and horses it disappears from the body in a few hours (Brodie, 1956).
Phenylbutazone is rapidly absorbed from the gastro-intestinal tract, peak plasma levels being reached in about 2 hours. Patients undergoing routine therapy with phenylbutazone may be expected to have blood-levels in the range 5 to 10 mg%.

Dose. Up to 400 mg daily.

Toxicity. Phenylbutazone may give rise to a wide variety of toxic side-effects even when the dosage does not exceed 400 mg daily. Untoward reactions, often sufficiently severe to cause withdrawal of the drug, occur in some 25 to 40% of patients.
A causative relationship between phenylbutazone administration and reported cases of leukaemia has not been fully established.
The acute lethal dose in man is reported to be between 5 and 30 g.
LD50 (intravenous): in mice 123 mg/kg.
CASE EXAMPLES. After taking 300 mg of phenylbutazone daily for 9 months, an 83-year-old woman developed pernicious anaemia and aplasia of the bone marrow from which she died (Lander and Bonnin, 1962).
After swallowing about 25 phenylbutazone tablets, a 19-month-old infant died.—per *Pharm. J.*, i/1965, 604.
Since early in 1964, 50 reports of serious complications with 18 deaths in patients given phenylbutazone have been made. Toxic effects included liver damage, peptic ulceration, and blood dyscrasias (Committee on Safety of Drugs, 1965).
A 16-month-old child ingested up to forty-five 100-mg tablets of phenylbutazone. One to 3 hours later gastric avage was performed, but the child died within 12 hours of consuming the tablets. Post-mortem phenylbutazone levels: blood, 6·2 mg%; liver, 16·6 mg%; muscles, 7 mg%; gastric contents, 2·1 mg. Considerable amounts of the metabolite, oxyphenbutazone, were also found: blood, 9·3 mg%; liver, 5·9 mg%; muscles, 1·5 mg%; gastric contents, 1·3 mg (Steentoft, 1967).

PHENYLEPHRINE *Sympathomimetic*

Synonyms: Metaoxedrine; Neosynephrine.
(−)-1-(*m*-Hydroxyphenyl)-2-methylaminoethanol
$C_9H_{13}NO_2$ = 167·2

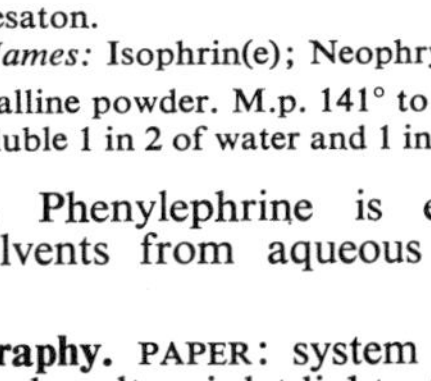

Phenylephrine melts at about 174°.

PHENYLEPHRINE HYDROCHLORIDE

Synonym: Mesaton.
Proprietary Names: Isophrin(e); Neophryn.
A white crystalline powder. M.p. 141° to 144°.
Solubility. Soluble 1 in 2 of water and 1 in 4 of ethanol.

Extraction. Phenylephrine is extracted by organic solvents from aqueous ammoniacal solutions.

Chromatography. PAPER: system P1—Rf 0·24 (location under ultraviolet light, strong absorption; location reagents: *bromocresol green spray*, weak reaction; *potassium permanganate spray*, weak reaction).

THIN-LAYER: system T1—Rf 0·28 (location reagent *potassium permanganate spray*, positive reaction).

Colour Tests. Chen's test—purple.

MICRO: sulphuric acid–formaldehyde test—dull red (*sensitivity:* 0·5 μg); ammonium molybdate test—blue, fading (*sensitivity:* 0·25 μg); ammonium vanadate test—faint brown (*sensitivity:* 0·5 μg); Vitali's test—yellow/brown/bright yellow (*sensitivity:* 0·5 μg).

Crystal Test. MICRO: *gold chloride solution*—dense rosettes, forming overnight (*sensitivity:* 1 in 100).

Ultraviolet Absorption Spectrum. Phenylephrine in 0·1N sodium hydroxide, maxima at 238 mμ (E1%, 1 cm 575) and 291 mμ (E1%, 1 cm 192); in 1N sulphuric acid, maximum at 273 mμ (E1%, 1 cm 96); in 0·1N sulphuric acid, maximum at 270 mμ (E1%, 1 cm 107).

Infra-red Absorption Spectrum. Phenylephrine hydrochloride. Potassium bromide disk. The principal peaks are: A 1592, B 1464, C 1268 (p. 755).

Quantitative Estimation. Phenylephrine may be determined colorimetrically (Kelly and Auerbach, 1961; Koshy and Mitchner, 1963).

Dose. Up to 10 mg by injection.

Toxicity. LD50 (oral): in mice, less than 500 mg/kg.

PHENYLMETHYLBARBITURIC ACID

Barbiturate

Synonym: Heptobarbital.
Proprietary Name: Rutonal.

5-Methyl-5-phenylbarbituric acid

$C_{11}H_{10}N_2O_3 = 218·2$

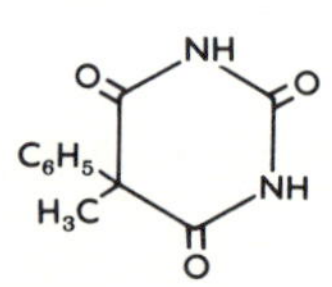

A white crystalline powder.
Solubility. Almost insoluble in water; soluble 1 in 60 of ethanol; soluble in ether.

Screening Tests. See under Barbiturates, p. 208.

Extraction. Phenylmethylbarbituric acid may be isolated in the A2 fraction (see p. 27).

Chromatography. PAPER: system P2—Rf 0·06, relative to amylobarbitone (location under ultraviolet light, dark spot).

THIN-LAYER: system T10—Rf 0·12 (location reagents: *mercurous nitrate spray*, black; *Zwikker's reagent spray*, pink).

GAS: system G5—retention time 5·60 relative to barbitone.

Ultraviolet Absorption Spectrum. A 5,5-derivative—see Screening Test 3, p. 208.

Quantitative Estimation. See under Barbiturates, p. 208.

Dose. Up to 1 g daily.

Toxicity. Phenylmethylbarbituric acid is a long-acting barbiturate—see under Barbiturates, p. 207.

PHENYLPROPANOLAMINE

Sympathomimetic

Synonym: dl-Norephedrine.

(±)-2-Amino-1-phenylpropan-1-ol

$C_9H_{13}NO = 151·2$

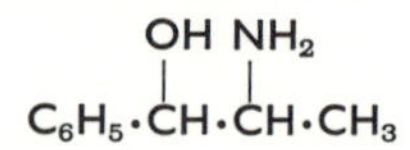

Phenylpropanolamine melts at 101°.

PHENYLPROPANOLAMINE HYDROCHLORIDE
Synonym: Mydriatin.
Proprietary Names: Panamine; Propadine. It is an ingredient of Eskornade, Triominic, and Triotussic.

A white crystalline powder. M.p. 193° to 196°.
Solubility. Soluble 1 in 2·5 of water and 1 in 9 of ethanol; insoluble in ether and chloroform.

Extraction. Phenylpropanolamine is extracted by organic solvents from aqueous alkaline solutions.

Chromatography. PAPER: system P1—Rf 0·44 (location under ultraviolet light, absorption; location reagent *bromocresol green spray*, weak reaction).

THIN-LAYER: system T1—Rf 0·52 (location reagent *potassium permanganate spray*, positive reaction).

Colour Test. Chen's test—purple.

Ultraviolet Absorption Spectrum. Phenylpropanolamine in 0·1N sulphuric acid, maxima at 251 mμ (E1%, 1 cm 7·6), 257 mμ (E1%, 1 cm 9·7), and 263 mμ (E1%, 1 cm 7·4), and inflexions at about 242 mμ, about 247 mμ, and about 267 mμ.

Infra-red Absorption Spectrum. Phenylpropanolamine hydrochloride. Potassium bromide disk. The principal peaks are: A 700, B 746 or 1030, C 1500 (p. 755).

Quantitative Estimation. Axelrod (1953a) describes a spectrophotometric method of determination of phenylpropanolamine in biological fluids and tissues involving the formation of a methyl-orange complex.

Metabolism. An average of at least 90% of single oral doses of phenylpropanolamine has been found to be excreted in the urine. Dogs and rats also excrete the drug mainly in the unchanged form; in the dog, a minor route of metabolism has been found to involve the hydroxylation of phenylpropanolamine to the corresponding *p*-hydroxy-derivative. Phenylpropanolamine has been found as a metabolite of ephedrine.

Dose. Up to 150 mg daily.

Toxicity. The intravenous lethal dose in rabbits is 75 mg/kg.

PHENYLPROPYLMETHYLAMINE

Sympathomimetic

Synonym: Phenpromethamine.

$N\beta$-Dimethylphenethylamine

$C_{10}H_{15}N = 149{\cdot}2$

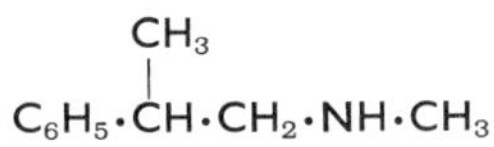

A volatile liquid. B.p. 205° to 210°. Refractive index 1·5102.

Solubility. Soluble 1 in 80 of water; very soluble in ethanol and ether.

PHENYLPROPYLMETHYLAMINE HYDROCHLORIDE

Proprietary Name: Vonedrine Hydrochloride.

It has a melting-point of 144° to 148°.

Extraction. Phenylpropylmethylamine is extracted by organic solvents from aqueous alkaline solutions.

Chromatography. PAPER: system P1—Rf 0·51 (location under ultraviolet light, absorption; location reagents: *iodoplatinate spray*, strong reaction; *bromocresol green spray*, weak reaction; *Marquis reagent*, orange; *ninhydrin spray*, purple).

THIN-LAYER: system T1—Rf 0·30 (location reagents: *Marquis reagent*, positive reaction; *ninhydrin spray*, positive reaction; *potassium permanganate spray*, positive reaction).

Colour Test. MICRO: sulphuric acid–formaldehyde test—orange → brown (*sensitivity:* 0·25 µg).

Crystal Tests. MICRO: *gold bromide–hydrochloric acid solution*—rods or elongated plates (*sensitivity:* 1 in 400); *mercuric chloride solution*—thin plates, best viewed under polarised light (*sensitivity:* 1 in 200).

Ultraviolet Absorption Spectrum. Phenylpropylmethylamine in 0·1N sulphuric acid, maxima at 251·5 mµ (E1%, 1 cm 11·6), 257 mµ (E1%, 1 cm 15·2), and 263 mµ (E1%, 1 cm 10·8).

PHENYLTOLOXAMINE

Antihistamine

Synonyms: C 5581; Phenyltolyloxamine; PRN.

2-(*o*-Benzylphenoxy)-*NN*-dimethylethylamine

$C_{17}H_{21}NO = 255{\cdot}4$

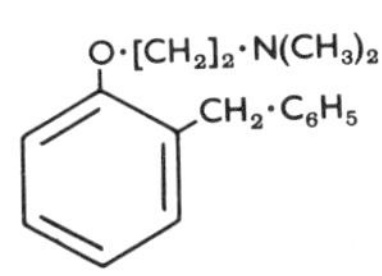

NOTE. Phenyltoloxamine is an isomer of diphenhydramine (p. 315).

An oily liquid. B.p. 141° to 144° at 0·1 mm Hg.

PHENYLTOLOXAMINE CITRATE

Proprietary Names: Bristamine; Britamin; Floxamine. It is an ingredient of Pholtex and Rinurel.

Phenyltoloxamine citrate occurs as crystals.

Solubility. Soluble in water.

Extraction. Phenyltoloxamine is extracted by organic solvents from aqueous alkaline solutions.

Chromatography. PAPER: system P1—Rf 0·62 (location reagent *iodoplatinate spray*, strong reaction).

THIN-LAYER: system T1—Rf 0·50 (location reagent *acidified iodoplatinate spray*, positive reaction).

GAS: system G2/225—retention time 1·30 relative to diphenhydramine.

Colour Tests. MICRO: sulphuric acid–formaldehyde test—purple (*sensitivity:* 0·05 µg); ammonium molybdate test—green → blue → yellow (*sensitivity:* 0·5 µg); ammonium vanadate test—green (*sensitivity:* 1·0 µg).

Crystal Tests. MICRO: *potassium tri-iodide solution (1)*—plates and needles (*sensitivity:* 1 in 400); *styphnic acid*—rods, often curved (*sensitivity:* 1 in 1000).

Ultraviolet Absorption Spectrum. Phenyltoloxamine in 0·1N sulphuric acid, maxima at 270 mµ (E1%, 1 cm 73·3) and 276 mµ (E1%, 1 cm 62·8).

Infra-red Absorption Spectrum. Phenyltoloxamine citrate. Potassium bromide disk. The principal peaks are: A 1722, B 1588, C 1235 (p. 755).

Dose. Up to 200 mg daily.

PHENYRAMIDOL

Analgesic

Synonym: IN 511.

1-Phenyl-2-(pyrid-2-ylamino)ethanol

$C_{13}H_{14}N_2O = 214{\cdot}3$

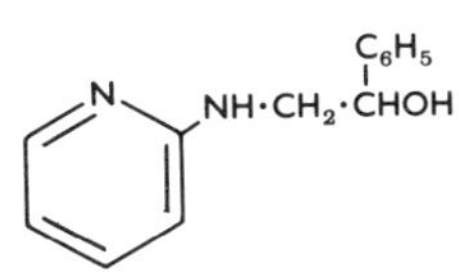

PHENYRAMIDOL HYDROCHLORIDE

Proprietary Names: Analexin; Evasprine.

A white crystalline powder.

Solubility. Freely soluble in water; soluble in ethanol.

Extraction. Phenyramidol is extracted by organic solvents from aqueous alkaline solutions.

Chromatography. PAPER: system P1—Rf 0·52 (location under ultraviolet light, blue fluorescence; location reagents: *iodoplatinate spray*, strong reaction; *bromocresol green spray*, strong reaction); system RP1a—Rf 0·86 (location under ultraviolet light, blue fluorescence; location reagent *iodoplatinate spray*, positive reaction); system RP1b—Rf 0·29 (location as for RP1a).

THIN-LAYER: system T1—Rf 0·72 (location reagent *potassium permanganate spray*, positive reaction).

GAS: system G2/225—retention time 1·35 relative to codeine.

Colour Tests. MICRO: sulphuric acid–formaldehyde test—yellow (*sensitivity:* 0·5 μg); ammonium molybdate test—blue → green (*sensitivity:* 0·5 μg); ammonium vanadate test—blue (*sensitivity:* 0·25 μg); Vitali's test — –/–/yellow (*sensitivity:* 1·0 μg).

Crystal Tests. MICRO: *potassium bismuth iodide solution*—hexagonal or rectangular plates (*sensitivity:* 1 in 3000); *potassium tri-iodide solution* (*1*)—needles or hexagons (*sensitivity:* 1 in 1000).

Ultraviolet Absorption Spectrum. Phenyramidol in 0·1N sodium hydroxide, maxima at 240 mμ (E1%, 1 cm 620) and 297 mμ (E1%, 1 cm 170); in 0·1N sulphuric acid, maxima at 236·5 mμ (E1%, 1 cm 580) and 308 mμ (E1%, 1 cm 300).

Dose. Up to 1·6 g daily.

PHENYTOIN *Anticonvulsant*

Synonyms: Diphenylhydantoin; Phenantoinum.
Proprietary Names: Di-Hydan; Glior.

5,5-Diphenylhydantoin
$C_{15}H_{12}N_2O_2 = 252·3$

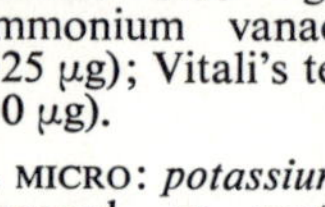

A white crystalline powder. M.p. 295° to 298°.
Solubility. Almost insoluble in water; soluble 1 in 70 of ethanol, 1 in 600 of ether, and 1 in 500 of chloroform.

PHENYTOIN SODIUM
Synonyms: Diphenin; Soluble Phenytoin.
Proprietary Names: Dilantin Sodium; Epanutin; Eptoin; Solantyl. It is an ingredient of Garoin.

A white hygroscopic powder.
Solubility. Soluble in water and ethanol; insoluble in ether and chloroform.

Screening Tests. For 2 tests which may be used to detect phenytoin—see Screening Tests 1 and 2 under Barbiturates, p. 208. See also under Screening Tests, p. 14.

Extraction. Phenytoin may be isolated in the A2 fraction (see p. 27).

Chromatography. THIN-LAYER: system T10—Rf 0·20 (location reagent *mercurous nitrate spray*, black).

GAS: system G1/250—retention time 1·05 relative to codeine.

Colour Test. Spot a drop of an ethanolic solution of phenytoin on filter paper impregnated with a 10% aqueous solution of trisodium orthophosphate and locate with *mercurous nitrate spray*—black.

Ultraviolet Absorption Spectrum. Phenytoin in methanol, maximum at 258 mμ (E1%, 1 cm 29·2).

Infra-red Absorption Spectrum. Phenytoin. Potassium bromide disk. The principal peaks are: A 1713 or 1747, B 1768, C 748 (p. 756).

Quantitative Estimation. Phenytoin may be estimated by hydrolysis followed by oxidation to benzophenone and subsequent determination by spectrophotometry (Wallace, 1966) or by thin-layer chromatography (Olesen, 1967).

Metabolism. Phenytoin is metabolised by two main routes. It undergoes aromatic hydroxylation to 5-*p*-hydroxyphenyl-5-phenylhydantoin and hydrolysis of the hydantoin ring to α-aminodiphenylacetic acid—see The Metabolism of Drugs, p. 159. Ring fission to hydantoic acid may also occur.
Over a 3-day period approximately 1 to 4% of a dose is excreted unchanged in the urine and about 10·5% in the faeces; approximately 44 to 62% of the dose appears in the urine as the conjugated hydroxy-metabolite and from 10 to 27% as α-aminodiphenylacetic acid.
Phenytoin is slowly absorbed from the gastro-intestinal tract; after absorption it is apparently concentrated in the bile, excreted into the gastro-intestinal tract, resorbed to a great extent, and then excreted via the kidneys. After oral administration in therapeutic doses, each mg/kg of phenytoin has been found to correspond to about 0·3 mg% in the serum.

Dose. Up to 600 mg daily by mouth.

Toxicity. Toxic effects frequently occur and are occasionally severe; they may occur at blood-levels of 2 to 4 mg% and above. Adults have recovered after ingesting 21 g and a child recovered after ingesting 900 mg. The estimated minimum lethal dose in man is 5 g.
LD50 (oral): in mice 490 mg/kg.

CASE EXAMPLES. A 16-year-old girl died some 50 hours after swallowing an unknown amount of phenytoin sodium. Chemical analysis of the stomach, stomach contents, liver, and kidneys was negative but the brain contained 6 mg% of phenytoin sodium (Tichner and Enselberg, 1951).

A 4½-year-old girl died 3 days after ingesting 2 g of phenytoin. A blood sample, drawn 24 hours after the onset of symptoms, revealed a hydantoin level of 9·4 mg%. Post-mortem levels: blood, 4·5 mg%; brain, 7·8 mg%; kidney, 11·2 mg%; liver, 27·2 mg% (Laubscher, 1966).

PHOLCODINE *Antitussive*

Synonyms: MEM; Morpholinylethylmorphine.
Proprietary Names: It is an ingredient of many proprietary cough preparations—see Extra Pharmacopoeia (Martindale), 25th Edn, pp. 1087–8.

7,8 - Dehydro - 4,5 - epoxy - 6 - hydroxy - *N* -

methyl - 3 - (2 - morpholinoethoxy)morphinan monohydrate

$C_{23}H_{30}N_2O_4, H_2O = 416{\cdot}5$

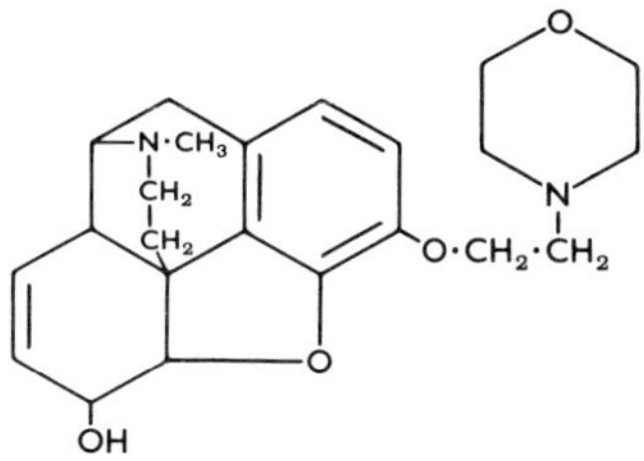

A white crystalline powder. M.p. about 99°. Specific rotation of a 2% solution in ethanol, −91° to −94°.

Solubility. Soluble 1 in 50 of water, 1 in 8·5 of boiling water, and 1 in 3 of dehydrated ethanol; slightly soluble in ether; very soluble in chloroform.

PHOLCODINE TARTRATE.
Synonym: Pholcodine Di(hydrogen tartrate) Trihydrate.

A white crystalline powder.
Solubility. Soluble 1 in 8 of water; very slightly soluble in ethanol; slightly soluble in ether and chloroform.

Extraction. Pholcodine is extracted by organic solvents from aqueous alkaline solutions; hydrolysis of biological material is required in order to improve the yield.

Chromatography. PAPER: system P1—Rf 0·02 (location under ultraviolet light, strong absorption; location reagent *iodoplatinate spray*, strong reaction); system RP1a—Rf 0·89 (location reagent *iodoplatinate spray*, positive reaction); system RP1b—Rf 0·29 (location as for RP1a).

THIN-LAYER: system T1—Rf 0·27 (location reagent *acidified iodoplatinate spray*, positive reaction).

Colour Tests. MICRO: sulphuric acid–formaldehyde test—purple (*sensitivity:* 0·25 μg); ammonium molybdate test—green → blue (*sensitivity:* 0·25 μg); Vitali's test—faint yellow/–/orange rim (*sensitivity:* 1·0 μg).

Crystal Tests. MICRO: *platinic chloride solution*—feathery rosettes (*sensitivity:* 1 in 400); *styphnic acid*—rosettes of plates, forming overnight, from dilute solutions only (*sensitivity:* 1 in 400).

Ultraviolet Absorption Spectrum. Pholcodine in ethanol, maximum at 284 mμ (E1%, 1cm 41); in 0·1N sulphuric acid, maximum at 283 mμ (E1%, 1cm 39) and an inflexion at about 277 mμ.

Infra-red Absorption Spectrum. Pholcodine (base). Potassium bromide disk. The principal peaks are: A 1118, B 969, C 1043 or 1250 or 1448 (p. 756).

Dose. Up to 60 mg daily.

Toxicity. The addiction-producing properties of pholcodine are no greater than those of codeine. The estimated minimum lethal dose is 500 mg.

PHOLEDRINE *Sympathomimetic*

Synonyms: Isodrine; Sympropaminum.

4-(2-Methylaminopropyl)phenol

$C_{10}H_{15}NO = 165{\cdot}2$

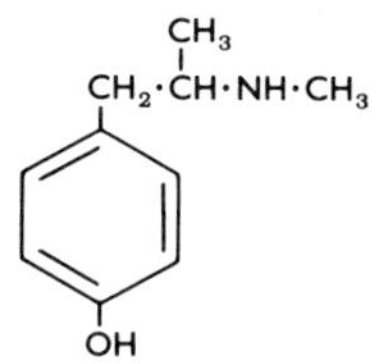

It occurs as crystals. M.p. 162°.

Solubility. Slightly soluble in water; soluble in ethanol and ether.

PHOLEDRINE SULPHATE
Proprietary Names: Veritain; Veritol.

A white powder. M.p. 320° to 323°, with decomposition.
Solubility. Soluble 1 in 20 of water; almost insoluble in ethanol, ether, and chloroform.

Extraction. Pholedrine is extracted by organic solvents from aqueous ammoniacal solutions.

Chromatography. PAPER: system P1—Rf 0·38 (location under ultraviolet light, absorption; location reagents: *iodoplatinate spray*, weak reaction; *bromocresol green spray*, weak reaction).

THIN-LAYER: system T1—Rf 0·24 (location reagent *potassium permanganate spray*, positive reaction).

Colour Tests. MICRO: sulphuric acid–formaldehyde test—grey → green (*sensitivity:* 0·5 μg); ammonium molybdate test—blue (*sensitivity:* 0·1 μg); Vitali's test—yellow/yellow/orange (*sensitivity:* 1·0 μg).

Ultraviolet Absorption Spectrum. Pholedrine in 0·1N sulphuric acid, maxima at 224 mμ (E1%, 1cm 332) and 275 mμ (E1%, 1cm 88), and an inflexion at about 280 mμ (E1%, 1cm 76).

Infra-red Absorption Spectrum. Pholedrine sulphate. Potassium bromide disk. The principal peaks are: A 1110, B 1519, C 1185 (p. 756).

Dose. Up to 30 mg intramuscularly or 15 mg intravenously.

PHTHALYLSULPHACETAMIDE *Sulphonamide*

Proprietary Names: Enterocid; Enterosulfon; Sterathal; Strycital; Thalamyd.

N - [*p* - (*o* - Carboxybenzamido)benzenesulphonyl]acetamide
$C_{16}H_{14}N_2O_6S = 362{\cdot}4$

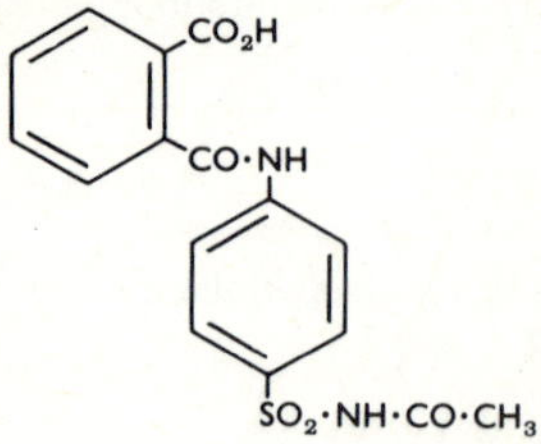

White crystals or crystalline powder. It decomposes with liquefaction between 186° and 202°.

Solubility. Very slightly soluble in water; slightly soluble in ethanol.

Extraction. Phthalylsulphacetamide may be extracted by ether from aqueous acid solutions; addition of an equal volume of acetone to the aqueous phase prior to extraction greatly increases the yield.

Chromatography. THIN-LAYER: system T23—Rf 0·51 (location under ultraviolet light, bright blue fluorescence; location reagent *bromocresol purple spray*, blue or purple, fading rapidly).

Colour Test. Copper sulphate test—blue.

Crystal Test. MICRO: *gold cyanide solution*—small dense rosettes, forming overnight (*sensitivity:* 1 in 100).

Metabolism. After oral administration, the systemic absorption of phthalylsulphacetamide is negligible but it attains a high concentration in the tissues of the intestinal wall and the lumen of the gut.

Dose. Up to 12 g daily.

PHTHALYLSULPHATHIAZOLE *Sulphonamide*

Synonyms: Ftalilsulfatiazol; Phthalazol.
Proprietary Names: Cremothalidine; Sulfathalidine; Taleudron; Talidine; Thalazole.

2 - [*p* - (*o* - Carboxybenzamido)benzenesulphonamido]thiazole
$C_{17}H_{13}N_3O_5S_2 = 403{\cdot}4$

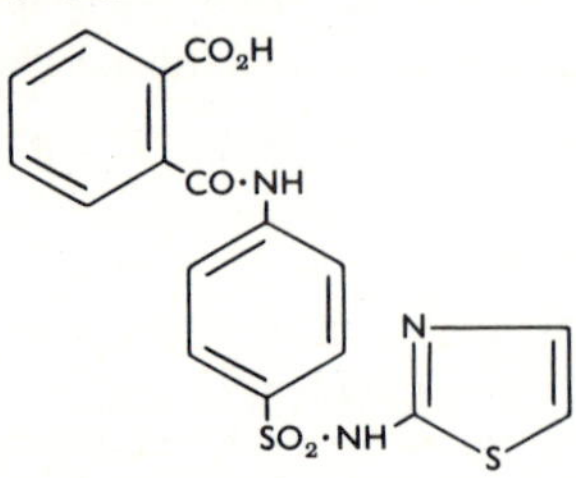

White or yellowish-white crystals or powder.

Solubility. Almost insoluble in water and chloroform; soluble 1 in 600 of ethanol; very slightly soluble in ether.

Extraction. Phthalylsulphathiazole is extracted by ether from aqueous acid solutions; addition of an equal volume of acetone to the aqueous phase prior to extraction greatly increases the yield.

Chromatography. THIN-LAYER: system T23—Rf 0·61 (location under ultraviolet light, faintly blue fluorescence; location reagent *bromocresol purple spray*, blue or purple on yellow).

Colour Test. Copper sulphate test—green.

Crystal Test. MICRO: *picrolonic acid*—bunches of plates (*sensitivity:* 1 in 100).

Ultraviolet Absorption Spectrum. Phthalylsulphathiazole in ethanol, maxima at 260 mμ (E1%, 1 cm 497) and 291 mμ (E1%, 1 cm 651).

Metabolism. Phthalylsulphathiazole is used for its bacteriostatic effect in the gastro-intestinal tract. Only about 5% is absorbed from the gastro-intestinal tract and this is rapidly excreted in the urine, hence blood-levels are very low, being not more than 1·5 mg% with normal doses. It occurs in the blood in both the free and acetylated forms.
Phthalylsulphathiazole is hydrolysed in the large intestine to sulphathiazole, which is believed to be the bacteriostatically active substance.

Dose. Up to 10 g daily.

Toxicity. Toxic effects following phthalylsulphathiazole administration are rare since very little is present in the blood and tissues.

PHYSOSTIGMINE *Anticholinesterase*

Synonym: Eserine.

An alkaloid obtained from the calabar bean, the seed of *Physostigma venenosum* (Leguminosae).
$C_{15}H_{21}N_3O_2 = 275{\cdot}4$

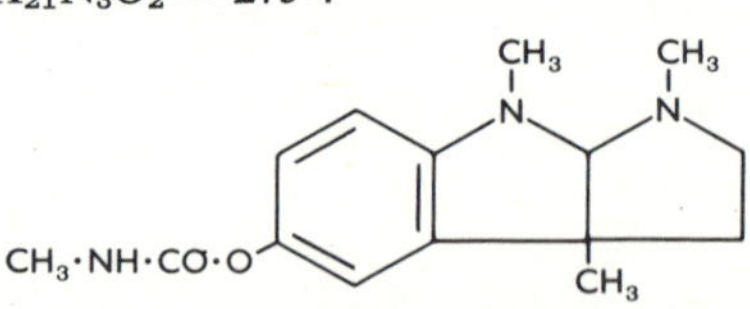

Colourless crystals. M.p. about 106°.
Physostigmine, its salts and their aqueous solutions become red on exposure to light and air owing to the formation of rubreserine; the change is less rapid in acid solution.

Solubility. Soluble 1 in 75 of water, 1 in 10 of ethanol, 1 in 30 of ether, and 1 in 1 of chloroform.

PHYSOSTIGMINE SALICYLATE
Colourless or faintly yellow crystals. M.p. 184° to 187°, after drying at 105°.
Solubility. Soluble 1 in 90 of water, 1 in 25 of ethanol, 1 in 250 of ether, and 1 in 6 of chloroform.

PHYSOSTIGMINE SULPHATE

A white deliquescent microcrystalline powder. M.p. 144° to 148°.

Solubility. Soluble 1 in less than 1 of water, 1 in less than 1 of ethanol, and 1 in 1200 of ether; soluble in chloroform.

Extraction. Physostigmine is extracted by organic solvents from aqueous alkaline solutions.

Chromatography. PAPER: system P1—Rf 0·43 (location under ultraviolet light, dark blue fluorescence; location reagents: *iodoplatinate spray*, strong reaction; *ninhydrin spray*, purple).

THIN-LAYER: system T1—Rf 0·55 (location reagent *potassium permanganate spray*, positive reaction).

GAS: system G2/225—retention time 0·20 (0·38; 0·61) relative to codeine; system G4—retention time 0·29 relative to codeine.

Colour Tests. MICRO: ammonium molybdate test—grey-green (*sensitivity:* 1·0 μg); ammonium vanadate test—yellow-brown (*sensitivity:* 1·0 μg); Vitali's test—yellow/green/purple—thorough heating is essential (*sensitivity:* 1·0 μg).

Crystal Tests. MICRO: *gold bromide–hydrochloric acid solution*—dark serrated needles (*sensitivity:* 1 in 3000); *lead iodide solution*—serrated blades (*sensitivity:* 1 in 400).

Ultraviolet Absorption Spectrum. Physostigmine in 0·2N sulphuric acid, maxima at 246 mμ (E1%, 1 cm 390) and 302 mμ (E1%, 1 cm 96).

Infra-red Absorption Spectrum. Physostigmine (base). Potassium bromide disk. The principal peaks are: A 1200 or 1243 or 1495 or 1724 (p. 756).

Metabolism. Physostigmine is readily absorbed from the gastro-intestinal tract, the mucous membranes, and the sites of subcutaneous injections. In the body it is hydrolysed at the ester linkage by cholinesterases, and a subcutaneous dose is largely destroyed in 2 hours. Little is excreted in the urine.

Toxicity. Death from physostigmine poisoning may occur within half to two hours from the first onset of symptoms. The skin becomes ashen-grey in colour. Fatalities have occurred following 6 mg of physostigmine orally and 1·2 mg intravenously.

The ingestion of 6 calabar beans by a child has proved fatal.

PHYSOSTIGMINE *N*-OXIDE

Anticholinesterase

Synonyms: Eseridine; Eserine Aminoxide.

Proprietary Name: As the salicylate, it is an ingredient of Geneserine.

N-Oxide of physostigmine

$C_{15}H_{21}N_3O_3 = 291{\cdot}4$

Physostigmine *N*-oxide melts at 129°.

Solubility. Almost insoluble in water; soluble in ethanol, ether, and chloroform.

Extraction. Physostigmine *N*-oxide is extracted by organic solvents from aqueous alkaline solutions.

Chromatography. PAPER: system P1—Rf 0·55 (location under ultraviolet light, weak absorption; location reagent *iodoplatinate spray*, weak reaction); system RP1a—Rf 0·97 (location reagent *iodoplatinate spray*, positive reaction); system RP1b—Rf 0·73 (location as for RP1a).

THIN-LAYER: system T1—Rf 0·31 (location reagent *potassium permanganate spray*, positive reaction).

Colour Tests. MICRO: ammonium molybdate test—pale blue (*sensitivity:* 1·0 μg); Vitali's test—yellow/yellow/yellow (*sensitivity:* 1·0 μg).

Crystal Tests. MICRO: *gold bromide–hydrochloric acid solution*—serrated blades (*sensitivity:* 1 in 200); *picric acid*—rosettes of rods (*sensitivity:* 1 in 400).

Ultraviolet Absorption Spectrum. Physostigmine *N*-oxide in 0·1N sulphuric acid, maxima at 241 mμ (E1%, 1 cm 411) and 300 mμ (E1%, 1 cm 126).

PHYTOMENADIONE

Vitamin

Synonyms: Phylloquinone; Phytonadione; Vitamin K_1.

Proprietary Names: Aquamephyton; Konakion; Mephyton; Mono-Kay.

2-Methyl-3-phytyl-1,4-naphthaquinone

$C_{31}H_{46}O_2 = 450{\cdot}7$

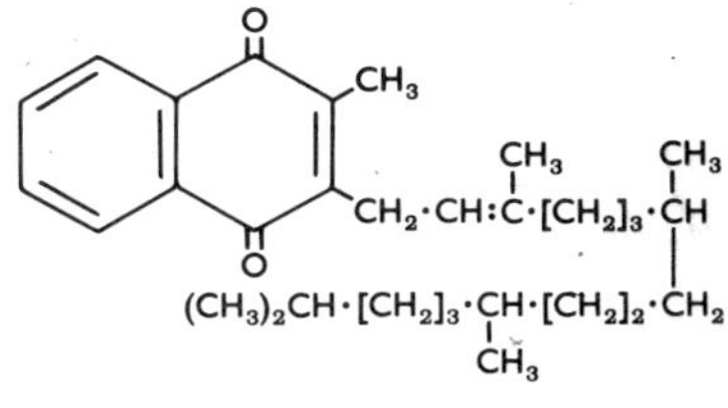

A clear deep-yellow oil which is stable in air but decomposes on exposure to light. Refractive index 1·5255 to 1·5285.

Solubility. Insoluble in water; soluble 1 in 70 of ethanol but more soluble in dehydrated ethanol; freely soluble in ether and chloroform.

Extraction. Phytomenadione is extracted by organic solvents from aqueous acid solutions.

Colour Test. To 0·05 ml, add 10 ml of methanol and 1 ml of a 20% solution of potassium hydroxide in methanol—green; warm gently → purple → reddish-brown.

Ultraviolet Absorption Spectrum. Phytomenadione in trimethylpentane (iso-octane), maxima at 245 mμ (E1%, 1 cm 398), 249 mμ (E1%, 1 cm

420), 263 mμ (E1%, 1 cm 385), 271 mμ (E1%, 1 cm 390), and 327 mμ (E1%, 1 cm 69).

Quantitative Estimation. A colorimetric method of determination in serum, plasma, and urine is described by Kofler (1945).

Metabolism. Phytomenadione is known to be rapidly metabolised *in vivo*, probably by reduction to the corresponding dihydroxy-derivative.
Phytomenadione is a naturally occurring vitamin K which maintains a normal level of prothrombin in the blood-plasma. The average daily human requirement is not known with certainty.

Dose. Up to 20 mg by mouth; up to 50 mg by slow intravenous infusion.

Toxicity. Intravenous injections have caused serious toxic reactions with at least one fatality; they should be given very slowly.

PICROTOXIN *Central Stimulant*

Synonym: Cocculin.

An active principle from the seeds of *Anamirta cocculus* (=*A. paniculata*) (Menispermaceae). The fruits of *A. cocculus* are sometimes known as 'fish berries' or 'Levant berries'.

$C_{30}H_{34}O_{13} = 602{\cdot}6$

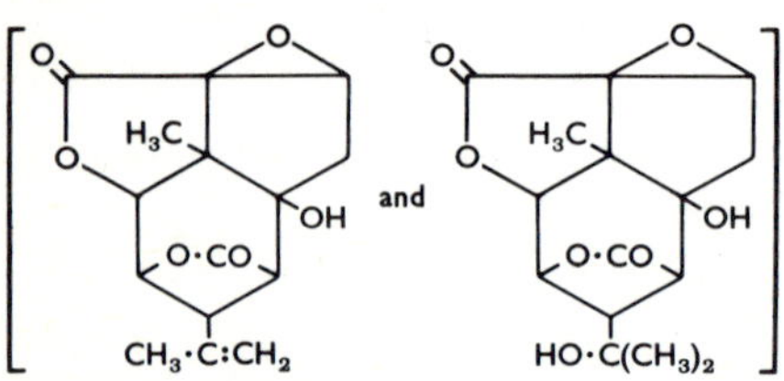

A white crystalline powder which is affected by light. M.p. 199° to 202°.
Solubility. Soluble 1 in 350 of water, 1 in 35 of boiling water, 1 in 16 of ethanol, and 1 in 3 of boiling ethanol; sparingly soluble in ether and chloroform; more readily soluble in dilute acids and alkalis than in water.

Extraction. Picrotoxin is extracted by organic solvents from aqueous acid or alkaline solutions.

Colour Tests. Dissolve in *sulphuric acid*—golden-yellow → reddish-brown, slowly. Add 1 drop of fuming nitric acid to the material—blue-green, discharged by excess acid.

Ultraviolet Absorption Spectrum. Picrotoxin in ethanol, maxima at 253 mμ, 258 mμ, and 264 mμ.

Infra-red Absorption Spectrum. Potassium bromide disk. The principal peaks are: A 1780, B 1123, C 990 (p. 756).

Metabolism. Picrotoxin is readily absorbed upon injection. It disappears rapidly from the blood and tissues; after 2 hours none is detectable although its stimulant effects may endure longer.

Toxicity. Picrotoxin is highly toxic; as little as 20 mg may produce severe poisoning.
LD50 (intraperitoneal): in mice 4·5 mg/kg.

PILOCARPINE *Cholinergic*

An alkaloid obtained from jaborandi, the leaflets of *Pilocarpus microphyllus* (Rutaceae) and other species of *Pilocarpus*.

$C_{11}H_{16}N_2O_2 = 208{\cdot}3$

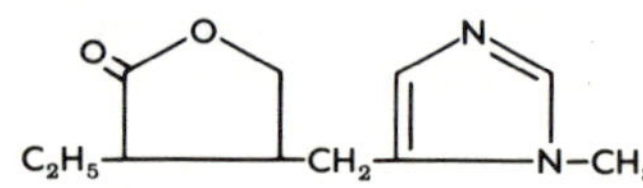

A colourless oil or crystals. M.p. 34°.
Solubility. Soluble in water, ethanol, ether, and chloroform.

PILOCARPINE HYDROCHLORIDE
A white hygroscopic crystalline powder affected by light. M.p. 200° to 205°.
Solubility. Soluble 1 in 0·3 of water, 1 in 3 of ethanol, and 1 in 360 of chloroform; insoluble in ether.

PILOCARPINE NITRATE
Colourless crystals or a white crystalline powder. M.p. 174° to 178°.
Solubility. Soluble 1 in 8 of water and 1 in 160 of ethanol; almost insoluble in ether and chloroform.

Extraction. Pilocarpine is extracted by organic solvents from aqueous alkaline solutions.

Chromatography. PAPER: system P1—Rf 0·10 (location reagents: *iodoplatinate spray*, strong reaction; *bromocresol green spray*, weak reaction); system RP1a—Rf 0·96 (location reagent *iodoplatinate spray*, positive reaction); system RP1b—Rf 0·95 (location as for RP1a).

THIN-LAYER: system T1—Rf 0·60 (location reagent *acidified iodoplatinate spray*, positive reaction).

GAS: system G2/225—retention time 0·36 relative to codeine; system G6—retention time 0·73 relative to codeine.

Crystal Tests. MICRO: *gold bromide solution*—feathery rosettes (*sensitivity:* 1 in 1500); *platinic chloride solution*—plates in clusters (*sensitivity:* 1 in 1500).

Ultraviolet Absorption Spectrum. Pilocarpine in 0·2N sulphuric acid, maximum at 215 mμ (E1%, 1 cm 250).

Infra-red Absorption Spectrum. Pilocarpine (base). Capillary film between potassium bromide windows. The principal peaks are: A 1752, B 1168, C 660 or 1104 (p. 756).

Toxicity. The estimated minimum lethal dose in man is 60 mg. Death is usually due to central respiratory paralysis or to pulmonary oedema and may occur within a few hours.

PIMINODINE *Narcotic Analgesic*

Synonyms: Anopridine; Win 14098.

Ethyl 1-(3-anilinopropyl)-4-phenylpiperidine-4-carboxylate

$C_{23}H_{30}N_2O_2 = 366{\cdot}5$

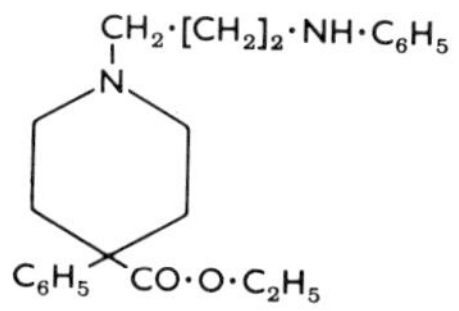

PIMINODINE ESYLATE

Synonym: Piminodine Ethanesulphonate.

Proprietary Name: Alvodine.

A white crystalline powder.

Solubility. Slightly soluble in water and ethanol.

Extraction. Piminodine is extracted by organic solvents from aqueous alkaline solutions.

Chromatography. PAPER: system P1—Rf 0·83 (location under ultraviolet light, dark blue fluorescence; location reagents: *iodoplatinate spray*, strong reaction; *bromocresol green spray*, weak reaction).

THIN-LAYER: system T1—Rf 0·67 (location reagents: *acidified iodoplatinate spray*, positive reaction; *potassium permanganate spray*, positive reaction); system T7—Rf 0·99 (location reagent *iodoplatinate spray*, positive reaction); system T8—Rf 0·73 (location as for T7).

Colour Tests. MICRO: sulphuric acid–formaldehyde test—dull orange (*sensitivity:* 1·0 µg); Vitali's test—orange/yellow/orange (*sensitivity:* 0·1 µg).

Crystal Tests. MICRO: *potassium chromate solution*—bunches of blades (*sensitivity:* 1 in 1000); *potassium iodide solution*—small rosettes of blades (*sensitivity:* 1 in 1000).

Ultraviolet Absorption Spectrum. Piminodine esylate in ethanol:water (1:1), maxima at 245 mµ and 270 mµ; minimum at 223 mµ: in 0·1N hydrochloric acid, maxima at 247 mµ, 253 mµ, 257 mµ, and 263 mµ; minima at 245 mµ, 249 mµ, 252 mµ, and 255 mµ; in 0·1N sodium hydroxide, maximum at 289 mµ; minima at 223 mµ and 271 mµ.

Dose. Up to 50 mg by mouth; up to 20 mg subcutaneously or intramuscularly.

Toxicity. The estimated minimum lethal dose in man is 500 mg. Piminodine possesses marked addiction-producing properties.

LD50 (subcutaneous): in mice 228 mg/kg.

PIPAMAZINE *Anti-emetic*

Synonym: SC 9387.

Proprietary Name: Mornidine.

10 - [3 - (4 - Carbamoylpiperidino)propyl] - 2 - chlorophenothiazine

$C_{21}H_{24}ClN_3OS = 402{\cdot}0$

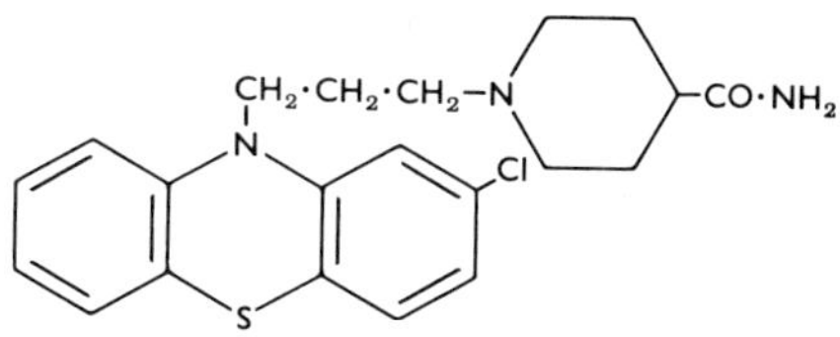

A white crystalline powder. M.p. about 140°.

Solubility. Soluble 1 in 500 of water, 1 in 60 of ethanol, 1 in 200 of ether, and 1 in 5 of chloroform.

Screening Test. *FPN reagent* with urine—purple (see p. 10).

Extraction. Pipamazine is extracted by organic solvents from aqueous alkaline solutions.

Chromatography. PAPER: system P1—Rf 0·50 (location under ultraviolet light, blue fluorescence; location reagent *iodoplatinate spray*, strong reaction); system RP1a—Rf 0·36 (location under ultraviolet light, blue fluorescence; location reagent *iodoplatinate spray*, positive reaction); system RP1b—Rf 0·03 (location as for RP1a).

THIN-LAYER: system T1—Rf 0·62 (location reagent *acidified iodoplatinate spray*, positive reaction); system T6—Rf 0·83 (the spot may be converted on the plate to the sulphoxide, Rf 0·53; location of both spots under ultraviolet light).

Colour Tests. MICRO: sulphuric acid–formaldehyde test—purple (*sensitivity:* 0·1 µg); ammonium molybdate test—purple (*sensitivity:* 0·1 µg); ammonium vanadate test—green → purple (*sensitivity:* 0·1 µg); Vitali's test—purple → yellow/yellow/yellow (*sensitivity:* 0·1 µg).

Ultraviolet Absorption Spectrum. Pipamazine in 0·01N hydrochloric acid, maximum at 255 mµ (E1%, 1cm 800).

Infra-red Absorption Spectrum. Potassium bromide disk. The principal peaks are: A 1644, B 1455, C 747 (p. 757).

Dose. Up to 30 mg daily.

PIPAMPERONE *Tranquilliser*

Synonyms: Floropipamide; R 3345.

Proprietary Names: Dipiperone; Propitan.

1 - [3 - (4 - Fluorobenzoyl)propyl] - 4 - piperidinopiperidine-4-carboxamide

$C_{21}H_{30}FN_3O_2 = 375{\cdot}5$

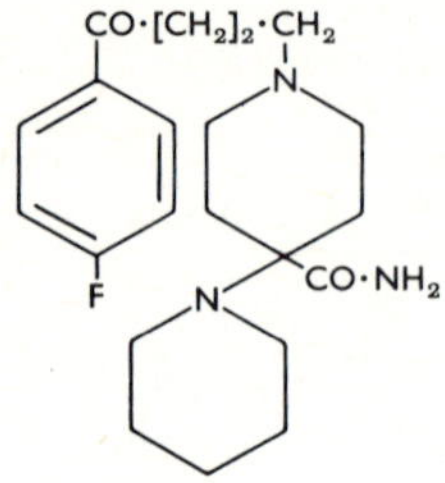

Extraction. Pipamperone is extracted by organic solvents from aqueous alkaline solutions.

Chromatography. PAPER: system P1—Rf 0·18 (location under ultraviolet light, blue fluorescence; location reagents: *iodoplatinate spray*, strong reaction; *bromocresol green spray*, weak reaction; *potassium permanganate spray*, weak reaction).

THIN-LAYER: system T1—Rf 0·53 (location reagent *potassium permanganate spray*, positive reaction).

Crystal Tests. MICRO: *gold bromide–hydrochloric acid solution*—bunches of blades or dense rosettes (*sensitivity:* 1 in 1000); *platinic bromide solution*—dense rosettes (*sensitivity:* 1 in 1000).

Ultraviolet Absorption Spectrum. Pipamperone in 0·1N sulphuric acid, maximum at 248·5 mμ (E1%, 1cm 207·5).

Dose. Up to 600 mg daily.

PIPAZETHATE *Antitussive*

Synonyms: LG 254; Piperestazine.

2-(2-Piperidinoethoxy)ethyl 10-thia-1,9-diazaanthracene-9-carboxylate

$C_{21}H_{25}N_3O_3S = 399{\cdot}5$

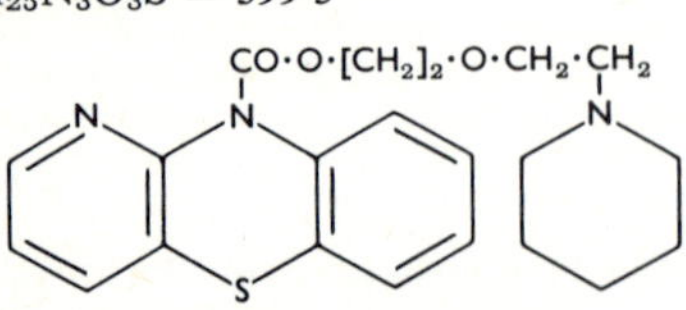

PIPAZETHATE HYDROCHLORIDE

Proprietary Names: Lenopect; Selvigon; Theratuss.

A white crystalline powder. M.p. about 162°.

Solubility. Very soluble in water; soluble in ethanol.

Extraction. Pipazethate is extracted by organic solvents from aqueous alkaline solutions.

Chromatography. PAPER: system P1—Rf 0·54 (location under ultraviolet light, pale yellow fluorescence; location reagent *iodoplatinate spray*, strong reaction).

THIN-LAYER: system T1—Rf 0·40 (location reagent *acidified iodoplatinate spray*, positive reaction).

GAS: system G2/225—retention time 1·70 relative to diphenhydramine.

Colour Test. MICRO: Vitali's test— -/-/yellow (*sensitivity:* 1·0 μg).

Crystal Tests. MICRO: *lead iodide solution*—rods, sometimes in rosettes (*sensitivity:* 1 in 200); *platinic chloride solution*—dense rosettes (*sensitivity:* 1 in 100).

Ultraviolet Absorption Spectrum. Pipazethate in 0·1N sulphuric acid, maximum at 253 mμ (E1%, 1cm 215) and inflexions at about 267 mμ (E1%, 1cm 154) and about 295 mμ (E1%, 1cm 76); pipazethate hydrochloride in methanol, maxima at about 226 mμ, about 254 mμ, and about 273 mμ (E1%, 1cm about 110).

Infra-red Absorption Spectrum. Pipazethate (base). Potassium bromide disk. The principal peaks are: A 1717, B 1225, C 1416 (p. 757).

Dose. Up to 160 mg daily.

PIPENZOLATE BROMIDE *Parasympatholytic*

Synonyms: JB 323; Pipenzolate Methobromide.

Proprietary Name: Piptal.

3 - Benziloyloxy - 1 - ethyl - 1 - methylpiperidinium bromide

$C_{22}H_{28}BrNO_3 = 434{\cdot}4$

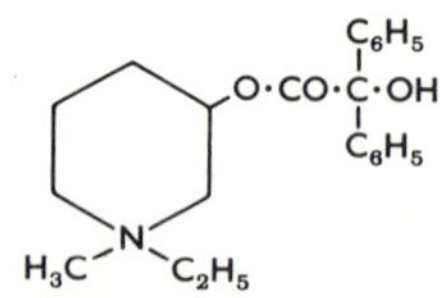

A white crystalline powder. M.p. 179° to 180°.

Solubility. Freely soluble in water.

Extraction. Pipenzolate bromide is a quaternary ammonium compound (see p. 29).

Chromatography. PAPER: system P1—Rf 0·49 (location under ultraviolet light, absorption; location reagent *iodoplatinate spray*, strong reaction); system RP1a—Rf 0·92 (location reagent *iodoplatinate spray*, positive reaction); system RP1b—Rf 0·88 (location as for RP1a).

THIN-LAYER: system T1—Rf 0·04 (location reagent *acidified iodoplatinate spray*, positive reaction).

Colour Tests. MICRO: the following tests are performed on pipenzolate nitrate—see under Colour Tests, p. 134: sulphuric acid–formaldehyde test—orange → green → blue (*sensitivity:* 0·1 μg); ammonium molybdate test—orange → green → blue (*sensitivity:* 0·05 μg); ammonium vanadate test—orange → green (*sensitivity:* 0·05 μg).

Ultraviolet Absorption Spectrum. Pipenzolate bromide in 0·1N sulphuric acid, maxima at

252 mμ (E 1%, 1 cm 9·6), 258 mμ (E 1%, 1 cm 11·1), and about 262 mμ (E 1%, 1 cm 9), and an inflexion at 267·5 mμ (E 1%, 1 cm 5·8).

Infra-red Absorption Spectrum. Potassium bromide disk. The principal peaks are: A 1726, B 698, C 1220 (p. 757).

Dose. Up to 25 mg daily.

Toxicity. The lethal dose in man is probably in the range 10 to 100 mg/kg.

PIPERAZINE *Anthelmintic*

Synonyms: Diethylenediamine; Hexahydropyrazine; Piperazidine.

$C_4H_{10}N_2 = 86·1$

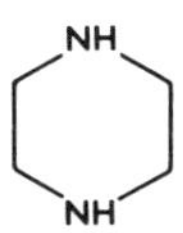

Piperazine melts at 106°.

Solubility. Soluble in water and ethanol; insoluble in ether.

PIPERAZINE HYDRATE

Synonym: Piperazine Hexahydrate.

Proprietary Names: It is an ingredient of Bryrel, Oxyzin, Pipergran, and Urillon.

$C_4H_{10}N_2, 6H_2O = 194·2$

Colourless deliquescent crystals. M.p. 43° to 45°. B.p. 125° to 130°.

Solubility. Soluble 1 in 3 of water and 1 in 1 of ethanol; insoluble in ether.

PIPERAZINE ADIPATE

Proprietary Names: Antivermin; Entacyl; Entazin; Vermicompren.

A white crystalline powder. M.p. about 250°, with decomposition.

Solubility. Soluble 1 in 18 of water; insoluble in ethanol.

PIPERAZINE CALCIUMEDETATE

Synonym: Piperazine Calcium Edathamil.

Proprietary Name: Perin.

Solubility. Soluble in water; very slightly soluble in ethanol and chloroform; almost insoluble in ether.

PIPERAZINE CITRATE

Synonym: Hydrous Triperazine Dicitrate.

Proprietary Names: Antepar (elixir); Helmezine (elixir); Minox; Multifuge; Oxucide; Pipizan.

A fine white granular powder. M.p. about 190°, after drying at 105°.

Solubility. Soluble 1 in 1·5 of water; very slightly soluble in ethanol and ether.

PIPERAZINE PHOSPHATE

Proprietary Names: Antepar (tablets); Helmezine (tablets). It is an ingredient of Pripsen.

A white crystalline powder.

Solubility. Soluble 1 in 60 of water; insoluble in ethanol.

Chromatography. PAPER: system P1—Rf 0·00 (location reagent *iodoplatinate spray*, white).

THIN-LAYER: system T1—Rf 0·03 (location reagent *acidified iodoplatinate spray*, positive reaction).

Colour Test. Add a drop of an aqueous solution to a drop of a dilute aqueous solution of sodium nitroprusside, followed by a drop of acetaldehyde—deep inky-blue.

Crystal Tests. MICRO: *picrolonic acid*—small curved blades (*sensitivity:* 1 in 1000); *platinic chloride solution*—small rectangular plates (*sensitivity:* 1 in 1000).

Infra-red Absorption Spectrum. Piperazine citrate. Potassium bromide disk. The principal peaks are: A 1592, B 1393, C 1442 (p. 757).

Quantitative Estimation. Piperazine in urine may be estimated colorimetrically with 1,2-naphthoquinone-4-sulphonic acid (Rogers, 1958).

Metabolism. Piperazine and its salts are readily absorbed from the gastro-intestinal tract. Some of the drug is metabolised, the remainder is excreted in the urine. No significant difference is observed between the rates of excretion of the adipate, citrate, and phosphate.

Dose. The equivalent of up to 4 g of piperazine hydrate, as a single dose.

Toxicity. Toxic effects during piperazine therapy are rare and are usually due to accumulation after large doses; they disappear rapidly when treatment is discontinued. Children have recovered after doses of 6, 9, and 12 g although these doses had caused symptoms of toxicity. Combes *et al.* (1956) have reported the death of a man who was under treatment with piperazine for threadworm infestation; he had an underlying renal disease and failed to excrete the drug in the urine.

PIPERIDOLATE *Parasympatholytic*

1-Ethylpiperid-3-yl diphenylacetate

$C_{21}H_{25}NO_2 = 323·4$

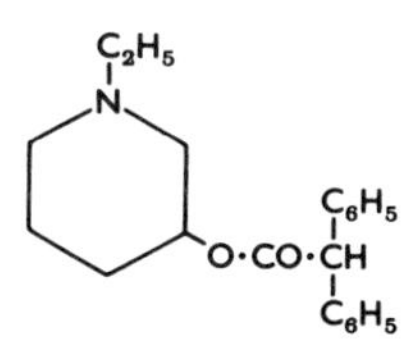

Piperidolate is a liquid. B.p. 191° to 192° at 0·18 mm Hg.

PIPERIDOLATE HYDROCHLORIDE

Synonym: JB 305.

Proprietary Name: Dactil.

A white crystalline powder. M.p. 195° to 196°.

Solubility. Soluble in water.

Extraction. Piperidolate is extracted by organic solvents from aqueous alkaline solutions.

Chromatography. PAPER: system P1—Rf 0·76 (location reagents: *iodoplatinate spray*, strong reaction; *bromocresol green spray*, weak reaction); system RP1a—Rf 0·14 (location reagent *iodoplatinate spray*, positive reaction); system RP1b—Rf 0·00 (location as for RP1a).

THIN-LAYER: system T1—Rf 0·66 (location reagent *acidified iodoplatinate spray*, positive reaction).

GAS: system G2/225—retention time 0·90 relative to codeine.

Colour Tests. MICRO: sulphuric acid–formaldehyde test—faint orange (*sensitivity:* 1·0 μg); ammonium vanadate test—olive (*sensitivity:* 1·0 μg); Vitali's test— -/-/blue (*sensitivity:* 0·5 μg).

Crystal Test. MICRO: *lead iodide solution*—rosettes of plates (*sensitivity:* 1 in 400).

Ultraviolet Absorption Spectrum. Piperidolate in 0·1N sulphuric acid, maxima at 252 mμ (E1%, 1cm 14), 258 mμ (E1%, 1cm 15), and 264 mμ (E1%, 1cm 12).

Dose. Up to 200 mg daily.

Toxicity. The lethal dose in man is probably in the range 10 to 100 mg/kg.

PIPEROCAINE *Local Anaesthetic*

3-(2-Methylpiperidino)propyl benzoate

$C_{16}H_{23}NO_2 = 261·4$

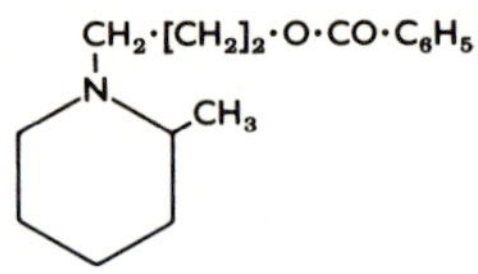

PIPEROCAINE HYDROCHLORIDE

Proprietary Names: Metycaine; Neothesin(e).

A white crystalline powder. M.p. 172° to 175°.

Solubility. Soluble 1 in 1·5 of water and 1 in 4·5 of ethanol; almost insoluble in ether; soluble in chloroform.

Extraction. Piperocaine is extracted by organic solvents from aqueous alkaline solutions.

Chromatography. PAPER: system P1—Rf 0·68 (location under ultraviolet light, absorption; location reagents: *iodoplatinate spray*, strong reaction; *bromocresol green spray*, weak reaction); system RP1a—Rf 0·79 (location under ultraviolet light, absorption; location reagent *iodoplatinate spray*, positive reaction); system RP1b—Rf 0·05 (location as for RP1a).

THIN-LAYER: system T1—Rf 0·55 (location reagent *acidified iodoplatinate spray*, positive reaction).

Crystal Tests. MICRO: *lead iodide solution*—small irregular needles (*sensitivity:* 1 in 1500); *picric acid*—rosettes of blades, best viewed under polarised light (*sensitivity:* 1 in 3000).

Ultraviolet Absorption Spectrum. Piperocaine in 0·1N sulphuric acid, maxima at 232 mμ (E1%, 1cm 627) and 275 mμ (E1%, 1cm 50); piperocaine hydrochloride in 0·01N hydrochloric acid, maximum at 274 mμ (E1%, 1cm about 365).

Infra-red Absorption Spectrum. Piperocaine hydrochloride. Potassium bromide disk. The principal peaks are: A 1278 or 1703, B 711 (p. 757).

Metabolism. Piperocaine undergoes hydrolysis in the plasma; it is reported to be hydrolysed six times faster than procaine.

Toxicity. The maximum amount stated to be safe by injection or topical application is 750 mg. When administered subcutaneously its action and toxicity are similar to those of procaine but when given intravenously it is more toxic.

LD50 (intravenous): in rats 20 mg/kg.

CASE EXAMPLE. A woman died 1 hour after receiving 20 ml of a 1·5% solution of piperocaine for caudal anaesthesia. The spinal fluid contained a total of 135 mg% of piperocaine (Blanke, 1960).

PIPEROXAN *Anti-adrenergic*

Synonyms: Benzodioxane; Compound 933 F; Fourneau 933.

2-Piperidinomethyl-1,4-benzodioxan

$C_{14}H_{19}NO_2 = 233·3$

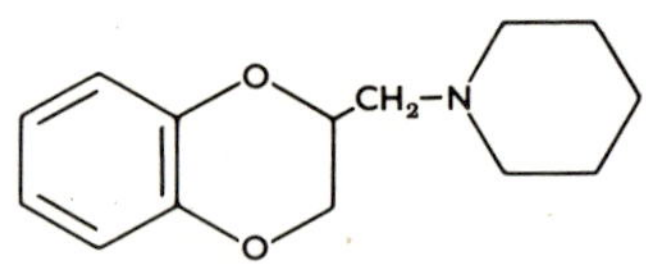

PIPEROXAN HYDROCHLORIDE

Proprietary Name: Benodaine.

A white crystalline powder. M.p. 232° to 237°.

Solubility. Soluble 1 in 3·5 of water and 1 in 12 of ethanol; almost insoluble in ether; soluble in chloroform.

Extraction. Piperoxan is extracted by organic solvents from aqueous alkaline solutions.

Chromatography. PAPER: system P1—Rf 0·62 (location reagents: *iodoplatinate spray*, strong reaction; *bromocresol green spray*, weak reaction); system RP1a—Rf 0·45 (location reagent *iodoplatinate spray*, positive reaction); system RP1b—Rf 0·00 (location as for RP1a).

THIN-LAYER: system T1—Rf 0·65 (location reagent *acidified iodoplatinate spray*, positive reaction).

GAS: system G2/225—retention time 0·98 relative to diphenhydramine; system G4—retention time 0·96 relative to diphenhydramine.

Colour Tests. MICRO: sulphuric acid–formaldehyde test—deep purple (*sensitivity:* 0·1 μg); ammonium molybdate test—blue-green (*sensitivity:* 0·1 μg); ammonium vanadate test—green (*sensitivity:* 0·1 μg); Vitali's test— -/-/faint red (*sensitivity:* 0·1 μg).

Crystal Tests. MICRO: *lead iodide solution*—masses of small irregular needles, often in sheaves (*sensitivity:* 1 in 400); *potassium permanganate solution*—bunches of elongated plates (*sensitivity:* 1 in 400).

Ultraviolet Absorption Spectrum. Piperoxan in

0·1N sulphuric acid, maximum at 274 mμ (E1%, 1 cm 89·5), and inflexion at 279 mμ.

Dose. Up to 20 mg intravenously.

PIPETHANATE *Tranquilliser*

Synonyms: Pentamethate; Piperilate.

2-Piperidinoethyl benzilate

$C_{21}H_{25}NO_3 = 339{\cdot}4$

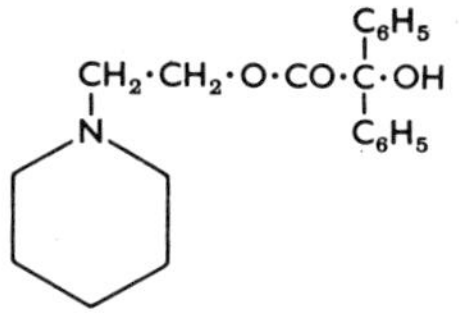

PIPETHANATE HYDROCHLORIDE

Proprietary Name: Sycotrol.

Extraction. Pipethanate is extracted by organic solvents from aqueous alkaline solutions.

Chromatography. PAPER: system P1—Rf 0·71 (location reagents: *iodoplatinate spray*, strong reaction; *bromocresol green spray*, weak reaction).

THIN-LAYER: system T1—Rf 0·68 (location reagent *acidified iodoplatinate spray*, positive reaction).

GAS: system G2/225—retention time 1·30 relative to codeine.

Colour Tests. MICRO: sulphuric acid–formaldehyde test—yellow→green→blue (*sensitivity:* 1·0 μg); ammonium molybdate test—orange (*sensitivity:* 1·0 μg).

Crystal Tests. MICRO: *platinic bromide solution*—fernlike crystals, best viewed under polarised light (*sensitivity:* 1 in 1000); *zinc chloride solution*—rosettes of rods, forming overnight (*sensitivity:* 1 in 200).

Ultraviolet Absorption Spectrum. Pipethanate in 0·1N sulphuric acid, maxima at 252 mμ (E1%, 1 cm 11·2), 258 mμ (E1%, 1 cm 13·3), and 262 mμ (E1%, 1 cm 10·7), and inflexions at about 264 mμ (E1%, 1 cm 10·7) and about 268 mμ (E1%, 1 cm 7·2).

Dose. Up to 18 mg daily.

PIPRADROL *Central Stimulant*

αα-Diphenyl-α-piperid-2-ylmethanol

$C_{18}H_{21}NO = 267{\cdot}4$

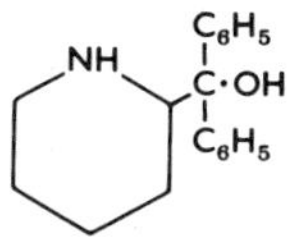

PIPRADROL HYDROCHLORIDE

Synonym: Pipradrol Chloride.

Proprietary Names: Alertol; Gerodyl; Leptidrol; Meratran.

Colourless crystals or a white crystalline powder. M.p. about 295°, with decomposition.

Solubility. Soluble 1 in 30 of water, 1 in 35 of ethanol, and 1 in 1000 of chloroform; almost insoluble in ether.

Extraction. Pipradrol is extracted by organic solvents from aqueous alkaline solutions.

Chromatography. PAPER: system P1—Rf 0·70 (location reagents: *iodoplatinate spray*, weak reaction; *bromocresol green spray*, weak reaction; *ninhydrin spray*, blue).

THIN-LAYER: system T1—Rf 0·61 (location reagent *acidified iodoplatinate spray*, positive reaction).

GAS: system G2/225—retention time 0·51 relative to codeine.

Colour Tests. MICRO: sulphuric acid–formaldehyde test—yellow-orange (*sensitivity:* 0·5 μg); ammonium molybdate test—orange (*sensitivity:* 0·5 μg).

Crystal Tests. MICRO: *gold chloride solution*—clusters of rods (*sensitivity:* 1 in 200); *potassium permanganate solution*—bunches of irregular crystals (*sensitivity:* 1 in 200).

Ultraviolet Absorption Spectrum. Pipradrol in 0·1 N sulphuric acid, maxima at 252·5 mμ (E1%, 1 cm 14·5) and 258 mμ (E1%, 1 cm 17), and an inflexion at about 263 mμ.

Infra-red Absorption Spectrum. Pipradrol hydrochloride. Potassium bromide disk. The principal peaks are: A 701 or 740 or 1448 (p. 757).

Metabolism. Pipradrol is stated to be rapidly absorbed after oral administration and to be excreted in the urine as metabolites which have not been identified.

Dose. Up to 6 mg daily.

PIRITRAMIDE *Narcotic Analgesic*

Synonyms: Pirinitramide; R 3365.

Proprietary Names: Dipidolor; Piridolan.

1 - (3 - Cyano - 3,3 - diphenylpropyl) - 4 - piperidinopiperidine-4-carboxyamide

$C_{27}H_{34}N_4O = 430{\cdot}6$

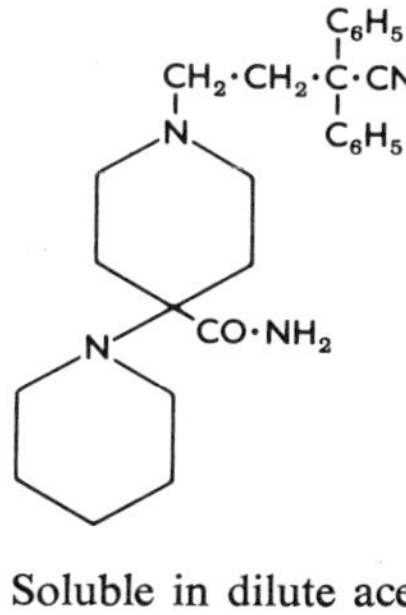

Solubility. Soluble in dilute acetic acid.

Extraction. Piritramide is extracted by organic solvents from aqueous alkaline solutions.

Chromatography. PAPER: system P1—Rf 0·38 (location reagents: *iodoplatinate spray*, strong reaction; *bromocresol green spray*, weak reaction); system RP1a—Rf 0·10 (location reagent *iodoplatinate spray*, positive reaction); system RP1b—Rf 0·00 (location as for RP1a).

THIN-LAYER: system T1—Rf 0·21 (location reagent *acidified iodoplatinate spray*, positive reaction).

Crystal Tests. MICRO: *potassium iodide solution*—rosettes (*sensitivity:* 1 in 1000); *sodium carbonate solution*—rosettes or bunches of plates (*sensitivity:* 1 in 1000).

Toxicity. LD50 (oral): in mice less than 320 and in rats 320 mg/kg.

PLASMOCIDE *Antimalarial*

Synonyms: F 710; Fourneau 710; Rhodoquine; SN 3115.

8 - (3 - Diethylaminopropylamino) - 6 - methoxyquinoline methylenebis-salicylate

$C_{17}H_{25}N_3O, 2C_{15}H_{12}O_6 = 863{\cdot}9$

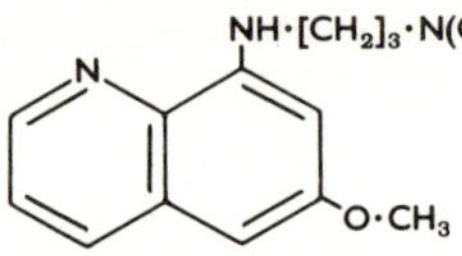

An orange-yellow powder. M.p. 160° to 162°.

Solubility. Insoluble in water; slightly soluble in ethanol.

Extraction. Plasmocide is extracted by organic solvents from aqueous alkaline solutions.

Chromatography. PAPER: system P1—Rf 0·51 (location under ultraviolet light, orange fluorescence; location reagents: *iodoplatinate spray*, strong reaction; *bromocresol green spray*, weak reaction).

THIN-LAYER: system T1—Rf 0·35 (location reagent *acidified iodoplatinate spray*, positive reaction).

Colour Tests. MICRO: sulphuric acid–formaldehyde test—orange (*sensitivity:* 0·25 μg); ammonium molybdate test—pale blue (*sensitivity:* 1·0 μg); ammonium vanadate test—purple→orange (*sensitivity:* 0·5 μg); Vitali's test—yellow/brown/yellow-brown (*sensitivity:* 0·1 μg).

Crystal Tests. MICRO: *picric acid*—rosettes of plates (*sensitivity:* 1 in 400); *potassium mercuric iodide solution*—rods (*sensitivity:* 1 in 1000).

Dose. Up to 60 mg daily.

POLDINE METHYLSULPHATE *Parasympatholytic*

Synonyms: IS 499; Poldine Methosulphate.
Proprietary Names: Nactate; Nacton.

2 - Benziloyloxymethyl - 1,1 - dimethylpyrrolidinium methyl sulphate

$C_{22}H_{29}NO_7S = 451{\cdot}5$

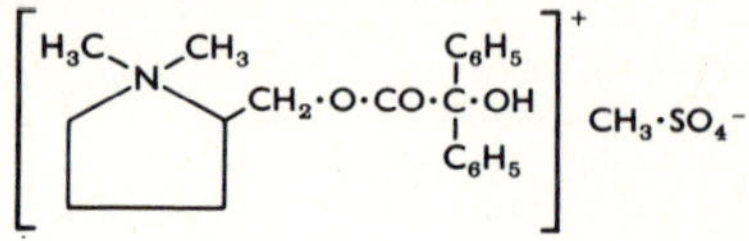

A white crystalline powder. M.p. 137° to 142°.

Solubility. Soluble 1 in 1 of water, 1 in 20 of ethanol, and 1 in 1000 of chloroform.

Extraction. Poldine is a quaternary ammonium compound (see p. 29).

Chromatography. PAPER: system P1—Rf 0·46 (location under ultraviolet light, absorption; location reagent *iodoplatinate spray*, strong reaction).

THIN-LAYER: system T1—Rf 0·02 (location reagent *acidified iodoplatinate spray*, positive reaction).

Colour Tests. MICRO: sulphuric acid–formaldehyde test—orange→green→blue (*sensitivity:* 0·25 μg); ammonium molybdate test—orange→blue (*sensitivity:* 0·05 μg); ammonium vanadate test—orange→green→dull purple (*sensitivity:* 0·05 μg).

Crystal Tests. MICRO: *gold chloride solution*—masses of blades, best viewed under polarised light (*sensitivity:* 1 in 1000); *lead iodide solution*—small feathery rosettes or sheaves of plates (*sensitivity:* 1 in 1000).

Ultraviolet Absorption Spectrum. Poldine in water, maxima at 252 mμ (E1%, 1 cm 9·6), 258 mμ (E1%, 1 cm 11·0); inflexions at 262 mμ, 264 mμ, and 268 mμ; in 0·1N sulphuric acid, maxima at 252 mμ (E1%, 1 cm 11·8), 258 mμ (E1%, 1 cm 13·8) and about 262 mμ (E1%, 1 cm 11·4), and an inflexion at about 268 mμ (E1%, 1 cm 7·4).

Quantitative Estimation. Poldine may be estimated by coupling with methyl orange and determining the resulting complex spectrophotometrically (Langley *et al.*, 1963).

Metabolism. Following repeated daily oral dosage, 70% of poldine methylsulphate or its metabolites is excreted in the faeces (Langley *et al.*, 1966).

Dose. Up to 24 mg daily.

Toxicity. The lethal dose in man is probably in the range 10 to 100 mg/kg.

POLYTHIAZIDE *Diuretic*

Synonym: P 2525.
Proprietary Names: Nephril; Renese.

6 - Chloro - 3,4 - dihydro - 2 - methyl - 7 -

sulphamoyl-3-(2,2,2-trifluoroethylthiomethyl)-2*H*-benzo-1,2,4-thiadiazine 1,1-dioxide
$C_{11}H_{13}ClF_3N_3O_4S_3 = 439{\cdot}9$

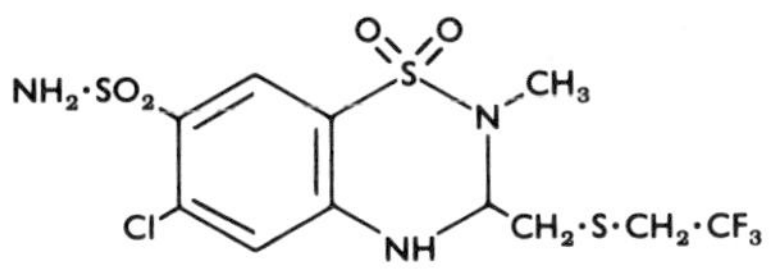

A white crystalline powder. M.p. 209°.
Solubility. Practically insoluble in water and chloroform.

Extraction. Polythiazide may be isolated in the A2 fraction (see p. 27). It may be distinguished from the barbiturates by chromatography (see below) and by the presence of additional ultraviolet maxima in the region 270 to 330 mμ.

Chromatography. PAPER: system P16—Rf 0·88 (location under ultraviolet light, absorption; location reagent *sodium naphthaquinone spray*, strong reaction); system RP1b—Rf 0·05 (location as for P16).

Ultraviolet Absorption Spectrum. Polythiazide in distilled water made alkaline to pH 10 with 2N ammonium hydroxide, maxima at 264 mμ (E1%, 1 cm 460) and 315 mμ (E1%, 1 cm 80); in distilled water made acid to pH 2 with *sulphuric acid*, maxima at 270 mμ (E1%, 1 cm 550) and 310 mμ (E1%, 1 cm 135). These spectra may be confused with those of methyclothiazide.

Metabolism. Polythiazide has a much greater potency and duration of action than chlorothiazide (p. 253). The diuretic action is initiated within about 2 hours and may last for up to 48 hours.

Dose. Usually up to 8 mg daily; max. in 24 hours, 12 mg.

PRALIDOXIME CHLORIDE

Cholinesterase Reactivator

Synonyms: 2-FMPOCl; 2-PAM Chloride; 2-PAMCl; 2-Pyridine Aldoxime Chloride.

2-Hydroxyiminomethyl-1-methylpyridinium chloride
$C_7H_9ClN_2O = 172{\cdot}6$

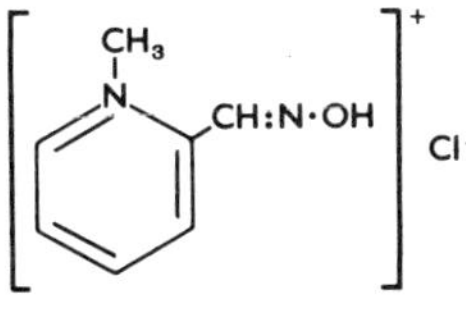

A light yellow crystalline powder. M.p. 220° to 222°, with decomposition.
Solubility. Soluble 1 in 2 of water and 1 in 100 of ethanol.

PRALIDOXIME IODIDE
Synonyms: 2-FMPOI; PAM; P-2-AM; 2-PAMI; 2-PAM Iodide; 2-Pyridine Aldoxime Iodide.

A white to yellow crystalline powder. M.p. 212° to 216°, with decomposition.
Solubility. Soluble 1 in 20 of water; almost insoluble in chloroform and ether. Aqueous solutions are yellowish and unstable.

PRALIDOXIME MESYLATE
Synonyms: 2-FMPOMS; 2-PAMM; P2S; Pralidoxime Methanesulphonate; 2-Pyridine Aldoxime Mesylate; RP 7676.
Proprietary Name: Contrathion.

A colourless or white, crystalline or granular powder.
Solubility. Soluble 1 in 2 of water and 1 in 12 of ethanol; almost insoluble in ether and chloroform.

Extraction. Pralidoxime salts are quaternary ammonium compounds (see p. 29).

Chromatography. PAPER: system P1—Rf 0·10 (location under ultraviolet light, weak absorption; location reagent *iodoplatinate spray*, strong reaction).

THIN-LAYER: system T1—Rf 0·05 (location reagent *acidified iodoplatinate spray*, positive reaction).

Crystal Tests. MICRO: *gold bromide–hydrochloric acid solution*—very small plates or needles (*sensitivity:* 1 in 1000); *potassium bismuth iodide solution*—bunches of rods or prisms (*sensitivity:* 1 in 1000).

Ultraviolet Absorption Spectrum. Pralidoxime chloride in 0·1N hydrochloric acid, maxima at about 242 mμ and about 292 mμ; minimum at about 262 mμ; in 0·1N sodium hydroxide, inflexion at about 280 mμ and maximum at about 332 mμ; minimum at about 250 mμ.

Quantitative Estimation. Pralidoxime in plasma, urine, and faeces may be estimated spectrophotometrically (Drug Standards, *J. pharm. Sci.*, 1965, **54**, 1508).

Metabolism. Pralidoxime is rapidly excreted in the urine, 80% being eliminated within 2 to 3 hours. It does not readily enter the central nervous system.
Pralidoxime reactivates cholinesterase when the activity of the enzyme is depressed and in this way it indirectly reduces an accumulation of acetylcholine. It is not equally antagonistic to all anticholinesterases. It has been reported to be effective in poisoning by some organophosphorus pesticides including malathion and parathion, but it appears to be relatively ineffective against diazinon and dimethoate and against carbamate pesticides and carbamate cholinesterase inhibitors such as neostigmine and pyridostigmine.
Quinby (1964) gives a clinical evaluation of 35 cases of organophosphorus poisoning treated with atropine and pralidoxime chloride or iodide.

Dose. The usual initial dose is 1 g by slow intravenous injection. This dose may be doubled or repeated.

Toxicity. LD50 (oral): in mice 4·1 g/kg of the chloride.

PRAMOXINE *Local Anaesthetic*

Synonym: Pramocaine.

4-[3-(*p*-Butoxyphenoxy)propyl]morpholine

$C_{17}H_{27}NO_3$ = 293·4

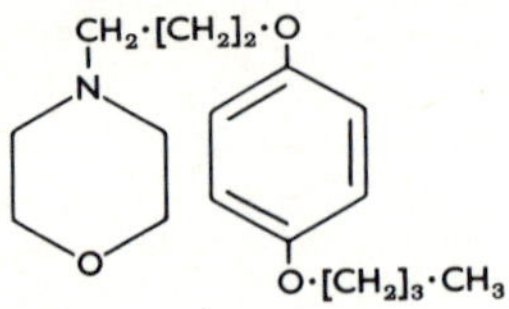

Pramoxine has a boiling point of 196° at 6 mm Hg.

PRAMOXINE HYDROCHLORIDE

Proprietary Names: Tronothane. It is an ingredient of Anugesic.

A white crystalline powder. M.p. 169° to 172°.

Solubility. Freely soluble in water and ethanol; very slightly soluble in ether; soluble 1 in 35 of chloroform.

Extraction. Pramoxine is extracted by organic solvents from aqueous alkaline solutions.

Chromatography. PAPER: system P1—Rf 0·61 (location reagent *iodoplatinate spray*, strong reaction); system RP1a—Rf 0·06 (location under ultraviolet light, absorption; location reagent *iodoplatinate spray*, positive reaction); system RP1b—Rf 0·00 (location as for RP1a).

THIN-LAYER: system T1—Rf 0·67 (location reagent *acidified iodoplatinate spray*, positive reaction).

GAS: system G2/225—retention time 0·73 relative to codeine; system G4—retention time 0·43 relative to codeine.

Colour Tests. MICRO: sulphuric acid-formaldehyde test—yellow→green (*sensitivity:* 0·25 μg); ammonium molybdate test—green (*sensitivity:* 0·25 μg); Vitali's test—yellow/pale brown/pale brown (*sensitivity:* 1·0 μg).

Crystal Tests. MICRO: *picrolonic acid*—bunches of needles, forming overnight (*sensitivity:* 1 in 400); *potassium tri-iodide solution* (*3*)—oily plates, best viewed under polarised light (*sensitivity:* 1 in 400).

Ultraviolet Absorption Spectrum. Pramoxine in 0·1N hydrochloric acid, maxima at 224 mμ and 286 mμ.

Use. It is used topically as a 1% solution, cream, or jelly.

Toxicity. The maximum amount safe for topical application is stated to be 200 mg or 20 ml of a 1% solution.

PREDNISOLONE *Corticosteroid*

Synonyms: 1,2-Dehydrohydrocortisone; Deltadehydrohydrocortisone; Deltahydrocortisone; Metacortandralone.

Proprietary Names: Codelcortone; Dacortin; Delta-Cortef; Deltacortril; Delta-Genacort; Deltastab; Di-Andreson-F; Hostacortin-H; Hydeltra; Marsolone; PreCortisyl; Prenolone; Sterane; Sterolone.

11β,17α,21-Trihydroxypregna-1,4-diene-3,20-dione

$C_{21}H_{28}O_5$ = 360·5

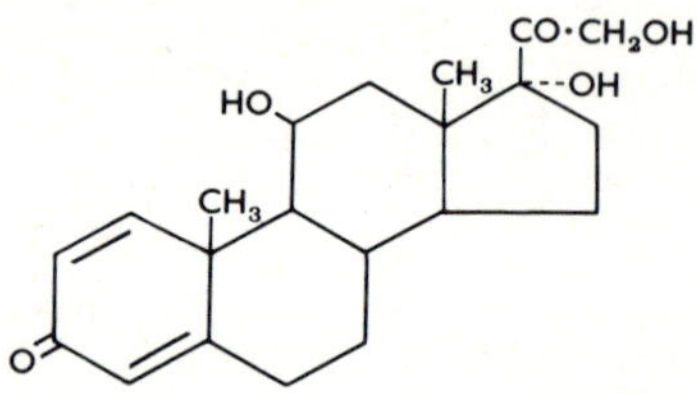

A white crystalline hygroscopic powder. M.p. about 229°, with decomposition. Specific rotation of a 1% solution in dioxan, +96° to +102°.

Solubility. Soluble 1 in 1300 of water, 1 in 35 of ethanol, and 1 in 180 of chloroform.

PREDNISOLONE ACETATE

21-Acetoxy-11β,17α-dihydroxypregna-1,4-diene-3,20-dione.

Proprietary Names: Deltacortril Intramuscular; Delta-Ef-Cortelan; Deltastab Injection; PreCortisyl Injection; Prednelan.

A white crystalline powder. M.p. about 240°. Specific rotation of a 1% solution in dioxan, +112° to +119°.

Solubility. Almost insoluble in water; soluble 1 in 135 of ethanol and 1 in 150 of chloroform.

PREDNISOLONE BUTYLACETATE

11β,17α - Dihydroxy - 21 - t - butylacetoxypregna - 1,4 - diene-3,20-dione.

Proprietary Names: Codelcortone-TBA; Hydeltra-TBA.

A white free-flowing powder.

Solubility. Almost insoluble in water; slightly soluble in chloroform.

PREDNISOLONE PIVALATE

11β,17α-Dihydroxy-21-pivaloyloxypregna-1,4-diene-3,20-dione.

Synonym: Prednisolone Trimethylacetate.

Proprietary Name: Ultracortenol.

A white crystalline powder. M.p. about 229°. Specific rotation of a 1% solution in dioxan, +104° to +112°.

Solubility. Almost insoluble in water; soluble 1 in 150 of ethanol and 1 in 16 of chloroform.

PREDNISOLONE SODIUM PHOSPHATE

Synonym: Prednisolone 21-(Disodium Phosphate).

Proprietary Names: Codelsol Injection; Hydeltrasol; Prednesol; Predsol.

A white hygroscopic crystalline powder.

Solubility. Soluble 1 in 3 of water, 1 in 1000 of ethanol, and 1 in 13 of methanol; insoluble in chloroform.

Extraction. Prednisolone is extracted from neutral solutions with freshly distilled ethyl acetate.

Chromatography. PAPER, for prednisolone: system P13—Rf 0·15 (location reagent *DPST solution*, violet on yellow); for prednisolone acetate: system P14—Rf 0·49 (location as for P13); for prednisolone pivalate: system P14—Rf 0·89 (location as for P13).

THIN-LAYER, for prednisolone: system T19—Rf 0·83 (location reagent *DPST spray*); for prednisolone acetate: system T18—Rf 0·53 (location reagent *DPST spray*); for prednisolone pivalate: system T18—Rf 1·10 (location reagent *DPST spray*).

Colour Test. Dissolve 0·2 mg in 1 ml of *sulphuric acid*—wine-red; after standing for 1 minute the solution exhibits a deep yellow fluorescence in ultraviolet light.

Ultraviolet Absorption Spectrum. Prednisolone in ethanol, maxima at about 240 mμ (E1%, 1 cm 400 to 430) and 263 mμ (E1%, 1 cm 453 to 487); prednisolone acetate in ethanol, maxima at about 240 mμ (E1%, 1 cm 360 to 380) and 263 mμ (E1%, 1 cm 408 to 431); prednisolone pivalate in ethanol, maximum at about 240 mμ (E1%, 1 cm 337); prednisolone sodium phosphate in water, maximum at about 247 mμ (E1%, 1 cm about 312).

Infra-red Absorption Spectrum. Prednisolone. Potassium bromide disk. The principal peaks are: A 1650, B 1610, C 1701 (p. 758).

Metabolism. Prednisolone is a synthetic glucocorticoid which is used as an anti-inflammatory and anti-allergic agent. It appears to be interconvertible with prednisone in man and small amounts of 20β-dihydroprednisolone, 20β-dihydroprednisone, and hydrocortisone have been detected in the urine.
Studies in the horse (Moss and Rylance, 1967) indicate that after oral administration or intramuscular injection less than 10% of the administered prednisolone appears in the urine in the free form; similar amounts of prednisone, 20β-dihydroprednisolone, and 20β-dihydroprednisone are also found, but less hydrocortisone is present. Normally the excretion of prednisolone and its metabolites is complete 3 days after administration.

Dose. Usually up to 100 mg daily.

PREDNISONE *Corticosteroid*

Synonyms: 1,2-Dehydrocortisone; Deltacortisone; Deltadehydrocortisone; Metacortandracin.
Proprietary Names: DeCortisyl; Deltacortone; Deltasone; Deltra; Di-Adreson; Hostacortin; Marsone; Meticorten; Paracort.

17α,21 - Dihydroxypregna - 1,4 - diene - 3,11,20-trione
$C_{21}H_{26}O_5 = 358{\cdot}4$

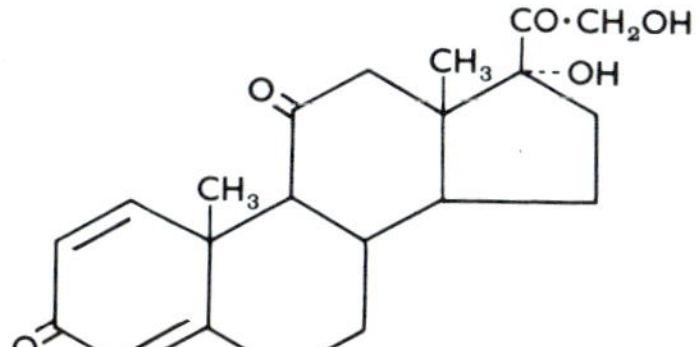

A white crystalline powder. M.p. about 230°, with decomposition. Specific rotation of a 1% solution in dioxan, +167° to +175°.
Solubility. Almost insoluble in water; soluble 1 in 190 of ethanol and 1 in 200 of chloroform.

PREDNISONE ACETATE

Proprietary Name: Delta-Cortelan.

A white crystalline powder. M.p. about 240°, with decomposition. Specific rotation of a 1% solution in dioxan, +183° to +190°.
Solubility. Almost insoluble in water; soluble 1 in 120 of ethanol and 1 in 6 of chloroform.

Extraction. Prednisone is extracted from neutral solutions with freshly distilled ethyl acetate.

Chromatography. PAPER, for prednisone: system P13—Rf 0·55 (location reagent *DPST solution*, violet on yellow); for prednisone acetate: system P14—Rf 0·74 (location as for P13).
THIN-LAYER, for prednisone: system T19—Rf 1·21 (location reagent *DPST spray*); for prednisone acetate: system T18—Rf 0·79 (location reagent *DPST spray*).

Colour Test. Dissolve 0·2 mg in 1 ml of *sulphuric acid*—yellow; after standing for 5 minutes the solution exhibits a pale green fluorescence in ultraviolet light.

Ultraviolet Absorption Spectrum. Prednisone in ethanol, maximum at 240 mμ (E1%, 1 cm 430); prednisone acetate in ethanol, maximum at 240 mμ (E1%, 1 cm 360 to 400).

Infra-red Absorption Spectrum. Prednisone. Potassium bromide disk. The principal peaks are: A 1668, B 1707, C 912 (p. 758).

Metabolism. Prednisone is a synthetic glucocorticoid which is used both as an anti-inflammatory and an anti-allergic agent. It appears to be interconvertible with prednisolone in man and studies in the horse (Moss and Rylance, 1967) indicate that its metabolic pattern is very similar to that of prednisolone.

Dose. Usually up to 100 mg daily.

PRENYLAMINE *Coronary Vasodilator*

Synonym: B 436.

N-(3,3-Diphenylpropyl)-α-methylphenethylamine
$C_{24}H_{27}N = 329{\cdot}5$

$$C_6H_5{\cdot}CH_2{\cdot}\underset{}{\overset{CH_3}{\overset{|}{C}}}H{\cdot}NH{\cdot}[CH_2]_2{\cdot}\overset{C_6H_5}{\overset{|}{C}}H{\cdot}C_6H_5$$

Prenylamine melts at 36·5° to 37·5°.

PRENYLAMINE LACTATE

Synonym: Hoechst 12512.
Proprietary Names: Corontin; Falicor; Segontin; Synadrin.

Prenylamine lactate melts at 140° to 142°.
Solubility. Soluble 1 in 200 of water; freely soluble in ethanol and chloroform; slightly soluble in ether.

Extraction. Prenylamine is extracted by organic solvents from aqueous alkaline solutions.

Chromatography. PAPER: system P1—Rf 0·91 (location under ultraviolet light, absorption;

location reagents: *iodoplatinate spray*, weak reaction; *bromocresol green spray*, weak reaction).

THIN-LAYER: system T1—Rf 0·71 (location reagent *acidified iodoplatinate spray*, positive reaction).

GAS: system G2/225—retention time 1·7 relative to codeine; system G4—retention time 0·89 relative to codeine.

Colour Tests. MICRO: sulphuric acid–formaldehyde test—dull red (*sensitivity:* 1·0 μg); ammonium vanadate test—dull green (*sensitivity:* 1·0 μg); Vitali's test— -/-/grey (*sensitivity:* 1·0 μg).

Crystal Tests. MICRO: *picrolonic acid*—leaflike plates, best viewed under polarised light (*sensitivity:* 1 in 1000); *trinitrobenzoic acid solution*—leaflike plates, best viewed under polarised light (*sensitivity:* 1 in 1000).

Dose. Up to 90 mg daily.

Toxicity. LD50 (oral): in mice 0·2 and in rats 1 g/kg.

PRILOCAINE *Local Anaesthetic*

Synonyms: L 67; Propitocaine.

α-Propylaminopropio-*o*-toluidide

$C_{13}H_{20}N_2O$ = 220·3

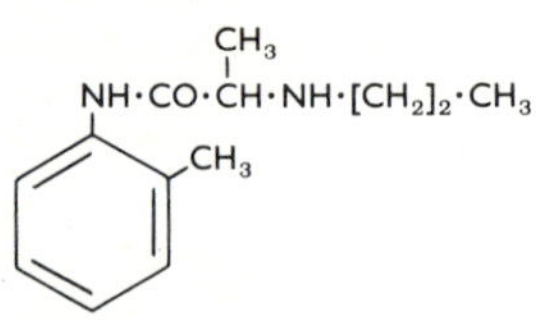

A white crystalline powder. M.p. 36° to 38°. B.p. 156° to 158° at 1·0 mm Hg.

Solubility. Freely soluble in ethanol, ether, and chloroform.

PRILOCAINE HYDROCHLORIDE

Proprietary Name: Citanest.

A white crystalline powder. M.p. 167° to 168°.

Solubility. Readily soluble in water; soluble in ethanol; insoluble in ether.

Extraction. Prilocaine is extracted by organic solvents from aqueous alkaline solutions.

Chromatography. PAPER: system P1—Rf 0·75 (location under ultraviolet light, strong absorption; location reagents: *iodoplatinate spray*, strong reaction; *bromocresol green spray*, weak reaction); system RP1a—Rf 0·66 (location under ultraviolet light, absorption); system RP1b—Rf 0·06 (location as for RP1a).

THIN-LAYER: system T1—Rf 0·65 (location reagent *iodine–carbon tetrachloride spray*, positive reaction).

Colour Test. MICRO: ammonium vanadate test—purple, fading (*sensitivity:* 0·25 μg).

Crystal Test. MICRO: *trinitrobenzoic acid solution*—dense rosettes or rosettes of rods (*sensitivity:* 1 in 400).

Ultraviolet Absorption Spectrum. Prilocaine in 0·1N sulphuric acid, inflexion at 225 mμ (E1%, 1 cm 240).

Infra-red Absorption Spectrum. Prilocaine hydrochloride. Potassium bromide disk. The principal peaks are: A 1700, B 764 or 1540, C 1464 (p. 758).

Metabolism. Following the intramuscular injection of ^{14}C-labelled prilocaine in rats, the organs were found to contain levels decreasing in the following order: lung, kidney, spleen, brain, heart, liver, and blood. Only small amounts of unchanged prilocaine were excreted in the urine and none was detected in the faeces. Two metabolites of prilocaine were identified, *o*-toluidine and *N*-propylaniline (Akerman *et al.*, 1966).

Dose. The maximum adult dose is 400 mg, and 600 mg for solutions containing adrenaline.

Toxicity. At a dosage of 600 mg the formation of methaemoglobin has been observed.

LD50 (intravenous): in rabbits 18 mg/kg.

PRIMAQUINE *Antimalarial*

Synonyms: Primachin; SN 13272.

8 - (4 - Amino - 1 - methylbutylamino) - 6 - methoxyquinoline

$C_{15}H_{21}N_3O$ = 259·4

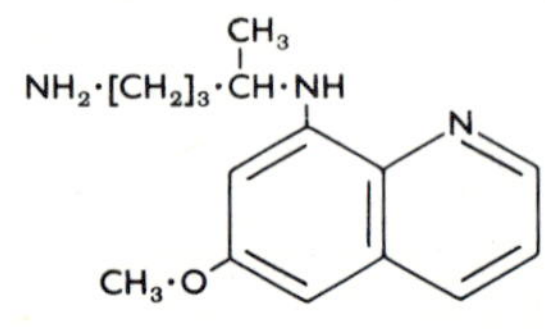

A viscous liquid. B.p. 175° to 179° at 0·2 mm Hg.

Solubility. Moderately soluble in water.

PRIMAQUINE PHOSPHATE

An orange-red crystalline powder. M.p. about 200°.

Solubility. Soluble 1 in 16 of water; insoluble in ethanol, ether, and chloroform.

Extraction. Primaquine is extracted by organic solvents from aqueous alkaline solutions.

Chromatography. PAPER: system P1—Rf 0·45 (location under ultraviolet light, orange fluorescence; location reagent *iodoplatinate spray*, strong reaction).

THIN-LAYER: system T1—Rf 0·20, streaking (location reagent *acidified iodoplatinate spray*, positive reaction).

Colour Tests. Dissolve 10 mg in 5 ml of water and add 1 ml of a 5% solution of ceric ammonium sulphate in dilute nitric acid—deep violet (distinction from chloroquine).

MICRO: sulphuric acid–formaldehyde test—

orange (*sensitivity:* 0·25 μg); ammonium molybdate test—pale blue (*sensitivity:* 1·0 μg); ammonium vanadate test—purple→orange (*sensitivity:* 0·5 μg); Vitali's test—dull green/yellow/orange (*sensitivity:* 0·1 μg).

Crystal Tests. MICRO: *picric acid*—rosettes of curved needles or dense rosettes (*sensitivity:* 1 in 1000); *styphnic acid*—rosettes of rods (*sensitivity:* 1 in 1000).

Ultraviolet Absorption Spectrum. Primaquine in 0·1N sulphuric acid, maxima at 223 mμ (E1%, 1 cm 905), 261 mμ (E1%, 1 cm 585), 282 mμ (E1%, 1 cm 618), 334 mμ (E1%, 1 cm 67), and 406 mμ (E1%, 1 cm 46); primaquine phosphate in 0·01N hydrochloric acid, maxima at 265 mμ (E1%, 1 cm 990) and 282 mμ (E1%, 1 cm about 980).

Infra-red Absorption Spectrum. Primaquine phosphate. Potassium bromide disk. The principal peaks are: A 1611, B 815 or 1595, C 1230 or 1572 (p. 758).

Metabolism. Primaquine is metabolised by 2 general reactions, namely oxidation to a quinone which is an active antimalarial and by *N*-dealkylation. Quinone formation occurs by oxidation of the 5,6-diol formed by hydroxylation at position 5 and *O*-demethylation at position 6—see under The Metabolism of Drugs, p. 161.

Dose. 15 mg (base) daily.

Toxicity. In therapeutic doses primaquine is less toxic than pamaquin. Nevertheless, methaemoglobinaemia and haemolytic anaemia may occur.

PRIMIDONE *Anticonvulsant*

Synonyms: Hexamidine; Primaclone.
Proprietary Names: Lepsiral; Mylepsine; Mysoline.

5-Ethylhexahydro-4,6-dioxo-5-phenylpyrimidine
$C_{12}H_{14}N_2O_2 = 218{\cdot}3$

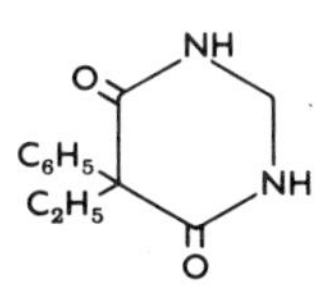

A white crystalline powder. M.p. 279° to 281°.

Solubility. Soluble 1 in 2000 of water and 1 in 170 of ethanol; almost insoluble in ether and chloroform.

Screening Tests. For 2 tests which may be used to detect primidone—see Screening Tests 1 and 2 under Barbiturates, p. 208.

Extraction. Primidone is very insoluble in water but traces may be isolated in the A2 fraction (see p. 27); alternatively it may be oxidised to phenobarbitone (p. 486) and extracted as such.

Chromatography. GAS: system G2/225—retention time 0·65 relative to codeine.

Ultraviolet Absorption Spectrum. Primidone in ethanol, maxima at 251 mμ (E1%, 1 cm 5·4), 258 mμ (E1%, 1 cm 6·0), and 264 mμ (E1%, 1 cm 4·4).

Metabolism. Primidone is an analogue of phenobarbitone in which the oxygen at position 2 of the barbiturate ring is replaced by hydrogen.
Following a dose of 1 g daily in man 15% has been found to be oxidised to phenobarbitone, resulting in blood-levels of phenobarbitone in the therapeutic range; it appears that the action of primidone is due to this metabolic conversion to phenobarbitone (Bogan and Smith, 1968). The phenobarbitone is excreted partly unchanged and partly as its metabolite, *p*-hydroxyphenobarbitone. Fission of the pyrimidine ring may also occur.

Dose. Usually 250 mg daily, gradually increasing as necessary to a maximum of 2 g daily.

Toxicity. The estimated minimum lethal dose in man is 5 g. Serious toxic reactions are rare but cases of megaloblastic anaemia have been reported.

CASE EXAMPLE. A man died 35 hours after taking 32·5 g of primidone (130 tablets); gastric lavage 6 hours after ingestion was of no avail. Post-mortem analysis for phenobarbitone: blood, 9·3 mg%; brain, 7·5 mg%; liver, 27·5 mg%; and urine, 6·7 mg%. About 15% of the primidone was converted to phenobarbitone in the body (Bogan *et al.*, 1965).

PROBARBITAL *Barbiturate*

5-Ethyl-5-isopropylbarbituric acid
$C_9H_{14}N_2O_3 = 198{\cdot}2$

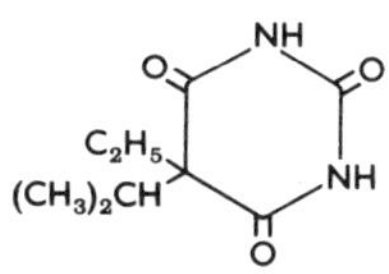

PROBARBITAL SODIUM
Synonym: Ethypropymalnatrium.
Proprietary Name: Ipral Sodium.

A white hygroscopic powder.

Solubility. Very soluble in water; slightly soluble in ethanol; insoluble in ether and chloroform. Aqueous solutions slowly decompose.

Screening Tests. See under Barbiturates, p. 208.

Extraction. Probarbital may be isolated in the A2 fraction (see p. 27).

Chromatography. PAPER: system P2—Rf 0·08 relative to amylobarbitone (location under ultraviolet light, dark spot).

THIN-LAYER: system T10—Rf 0·24 (location reagents: *mercurous nitrate spray*, black; *Zwikker's reagent spray*, pink).

GAS: system G1/180—retention time 0·44 relative to diphenhydramine; system G7—retention time 1·1 relative to barbitone.

Ultraviolet Absorption Spectrum. Probarbital

is a 5,5-derivative—see Screening Test 3 under Barbiturates, p. 208.

Quantitative Estimation. See under Barbiturates, p. 208.

Dose. 250 mg.

Toxicity. The estimated minimum lethal dose is 2 g. It is an intermediate-acting barbiturate —see p. 207.

PROBENECID *Uricosuric Agent*

Proprietary Names: Benemid(e); Probecid; Uricosid. It is an ingredient of Colbenemid.

p-(Dipropylsulphamoyl)benzoic acid
$C_{13}H_{19}NO_4S = 285{\cdot}4$

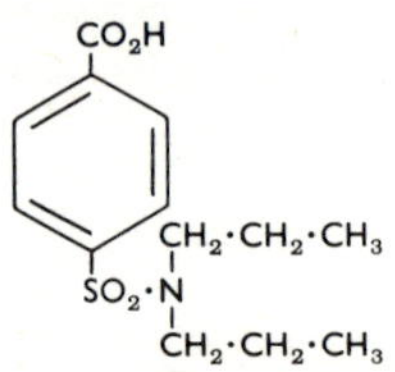

A white crystalline powder. M.p. 198° to 200°.
Solubility. Insoluble in water; soluble 1 in 25 of ethanol.

Extraction. Probenecid is extracted by organic solvents from aqueous acid solutions.

Ultraviolet Absorption Spectrum. Probenecid in ethanol, maxima at 225 mμ and 248 mμ (E 1%, 1 cm 330).

Metabolism. Probenecid is readily absorbed from the gastro-intestinal tract, peak plasma levels being reached in 2 to 4 hours and measurable concentrations persisting for 48 hours. It is only slowly metabolised and excreted, less than 5% of unchanged drug being excreted in the urine in 24 hours. A small amount of probenecid glucuronide appears in the urine; the fate of the remainder has not yet been determined.
Probenecid acts by inhibiting tubular resorption. In the treatment of gout this results in a lowering of the elevated uric acid levels in the plasma and in the slow depletion of urate deposits in the tissues; during treatment, the urine is kept alkaline in order to prevent the precipitation of urates.
Probenecid also reduces the tubular excretion of penicillin, causing an increase in plasma levels, but it has no specific effect on the excretion of other antibiotics. It has also been used to increase the concentrations of aminosalicylates in the plasma, producing a 15 to 50% increase in plasma levels.

Dose. Up to 2 g daily.

Toxicity. Probenecid is relatively non-toxic, side-effects are rare with doses under 1 g. In massive overdosage it causes stimulation of the central nervous system, with convulsions and death from respiratory failure. Recovery has occurred after the ingestion of 47 g.

PROCAINAMIDE *Myocardial Depressant*

Synonym: Procaine Amide.

p-Amino-*N*-(2-diethylaminoethyl)benzamide
$C_{13}H_{21}N_3O = 235{\cdot}3$

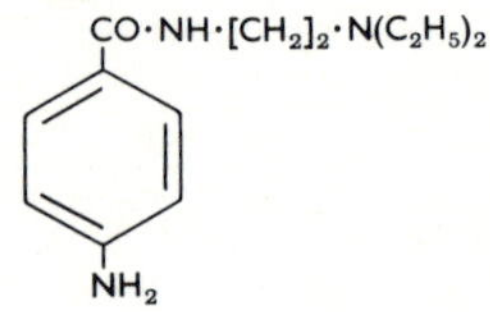

PROCAINAMIDE HYDROCHLORIDE
Proprietary Names: Novocamid; Pronestyl Hydrochloride.
A white hygroscopic crystalline powder. M.p. 165° to 169°.
Solubility. Soluble 1 in 0·25 of water, 1 in 2 of ethanol, and 1 in 140 of chloroform; almost insoluble in ether.

PROCAINAMIDE SULPHATE
A white crystalline powder.
Solubility. Soluble 1 in 0·7 of water and 1 in 200 of ethanol; insoluble in ether and chloroform.

Extraction. It is extracted by organic solvents from aqueous alkaline solutions.

Chromatography. PAPER: system P1—Rf 0·19 (location under ultraviolet light, blue fluorescence; location reagents: *iodoplatinate spray*, strong reaction; *bromocresol green spray*, strong reaction); system RP1a—Rf 0·92 (location under ultraviolet light, blue fluorescence; location reagent *iodoplatinate spray*, positive reaction); system RP1b—Rf 0·90 (location as for RP1a).
THIN-LAYER: system T1—Rf 0·45 (location reagent *acidified iodoplatinate spray*, positive reaction).
GAS: system G2/225—retention time 0·63 relative to codeine.

Colour Tests. MICRO: diazotisation test—red; Vitali's test— -/yellow-brown/yellow (*sensitivity:* 1·0 μg).

Crystal Tests. MICRO: *platinic chloride solution* —rosettes of plates (*sensitivity:* 1 in 200); *potassium bismuth iodide solution*—rhomboidal plates (*sensitivity:* 1 in 3000).

Ultraviolet Absorption Spectrum. Procainamide in 0·02N sodium hydroxide, maximum at 275 mμ (E 1%, 1 cm 693); in 0·1N sulphuric acid, maximum at 224 mμ (E 1%, 1 cm 466) and an inflexion at about 270 mμ.

Infra-red Absorption Spectrum. Procainamide hydrochloride. Potassium bromide disk. The principal peaks are: A 1519 or 1599, B 1632 (p. 758).

Metabolism. Between 50 and 60% of a dose of procainamide is excreted unchanged in the urine in 24 hours; 2 to 10% is metabolised by hydrolysis to *p*-aminobenzoic acid which is recovered in the urine in both the free and conjugated forms.

Procainamide is rapidly and almost completely absorbed from the gastro-intestinal tract. After oral administration peak plasma levels are reached in 15 to 60 minutes. The drug is slowly hydrolysed, so plasma levels decline by only 10 to 15% per hour. Procainamide is well distributed and levels in most tissues are greater than in the plasma.

Dose. Up to 1·5 g.

Toxicity. As little as 200 mg intravenously has caused death, due either to hypersensitivity or to too rapid injection.

PROCAINE *Local Anaesthetic*

2-Diethylaminoethyl *p*-aminobenzoate

$C_{13}H_{20}N_2O_2 = 236{\cdot}3$

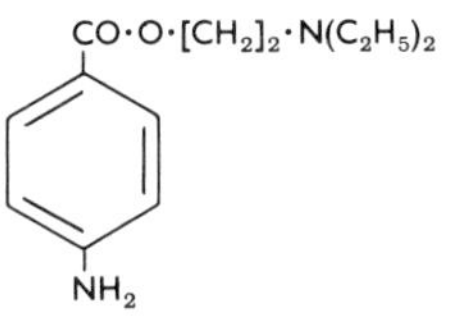

PROCAINE HYDROCHLORIDE

Synonyms: Allocaine; Ethocaine Hydrochloride; Syncaine.

Proprietary Names: Genocaine; Kerocaine; Neocaine; Novocain(e); Novutox; Planocaine.

A white crystalline powder. M.p. 154° to 156°.

Solubility. Soluble 1 in 1 of water, 1 in 15 of ethanol, and 1 in 30 of dehydrated ethanol; almost insoluble in ether; slightly soluble in chloroform.

Extraction. Procaine is extracted by organic solvents from aqueous alkaline solutions.

Chromatography. PAPER: system P1—Rf 0·31 (location under ultraviolet light, blue fluorescence; location reagents: *iodoplatinate spray*, strong reaction; *bromocresol green spray*, strong reaction); system RP1a—Rf 0·89 (location under ultraviolet light, blue fluorescence; location reagent *iodoplatinate spray*, positive reaction); system RP1b—Rf 0·27 (location as for RP1a).

THIN-LAYER: system T1—Rf 0·61 (location reagent *acidified iodoplatinate spray*, positive reaction).

GAS: system G1/180—retention time 1·81 relative to diphenhydramine; system G2/225—retention time 1·63 relative to diphenhydramine; system G3—retention time 3·30 relative to diphenhydramine; system G4—retention time 0·46 relative to codeine; system G6—retention time 0·36 relative to codeine.

Colour Tests. MICRO: diazotisation test—red-orange; Vitali's test— -/yellow/orange (*sensitivity:* 1·0 μg).

Crystal Tests. MICRO: *gold bromide solution*—plates and needles (*sensitivity:* 1 in 1500); *platinic iodide solution*—bunches of prisms (*sensitivity:* 1 in 1500).

Ultraviolet Absorption Spectrum. Procaine in 0·2 N sulphuric acid, maxima at 228 mμ (E1%, 1 cm 450), 272 mμ (E1%, 1 cm 60), and 279 mμ (E1%, 1 cm 60); minima at 258 mμ and 274 mμ: procaine hydrochloride in water, maximum at 290 mμ (E1%, 1 cm 680).

Infra-red Absorption Spectrum. Procaine hydrochloride. Potassium bromide disk. The principal peaks are: A 1274 or 1690, B 1605 (p. 758).

Quantitative Estimation. Procaine and its 2 main metabolites, *p*-aminobenzoic acid and diethylaminoethanol, may be estimated in plasma and urine by the methods described by Brodie *et al.* (1948).

Metabolism. Procaine is very unstable in the body. It is rapidly hydrolysed in the plasma by procaine esterase to *p*-aminobenzoic acid (p. 186) and diethylaminoethanol. Only 2% of a dose administered intravenously is excreted unchanged in the following 24 hours; 90% is excreted as *p*-aminobenzoic acid which is partly free and partly conjugated; of the diethylaminoethanol liberated only about 33% is excreted unchanged—presumably the remainder is metabolised.

Procaine is used chiefly by injection; it is useless for surface application because of its poor penetration of intact mucous membranes.

Toxicity. Although procaine is one of the least toxic of the local anaesthetics it sometimes causes systemic effects in hypersensitive patients and deaths have been reported from the injection of as little as 10 mg. The maximum safe amount by injection in man is stated to be 1 g. Poisoning in piglets following the intramuscular injection of a procaine penicillin preparation was shown to be due to the procaine moiety (Bálintffy and Kovács, 1955).

LD50 (oral): in mice 900 mg/kg.

PROCARBAZINE *Antineoplastic*

Synonyms: Ibenzmethyzin; NSC 77213; Ro 4-6467.

N-*p*-Isopropylcarbamoylbenzyl-*N'*-methylhydrazine

$C_{12}H_{19}N_3O = 221{\cdot}3$

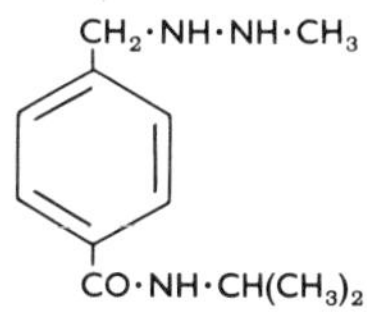

PROCARBAZINE HYDROCHLORIDE

Proprietary Name: Natulan.

Extraction. Procarbazine is extracted by organic solvents from aqueous alkaline solutions.

Chromatography. PAPER: system P1—Rf 0·48 (location under ultraviolet light, strong absorption; location reagents: *iodoplatinate spray*, white; *bromocresol green spray*, weak reaction).

THIN-LAYER: system T1—Rf 0·55 (location reagent *potassium permanganate spray*, positive reaction).

Colour Test. MICRO: ammonium molybdate test—(blue) blue (*sensitivity:* 0·1 μg).

Ultraviolet Absorption Spectrum. Procarbazine in 0·1N sulphuric acid, maximum at 232 mμ (E1%, 1cm 497).

Dose. Up to 300 mg daily.

PROCHLORPERAZINE *Tranquilliser*

Synonym: Prochlorpemazine.
Proprietary Name: Témentil.

2-Chloro-10-[3-(4-methylpiperazin-1-yl)propyl] phenothiazine
$C_{20}H_{24}ClN_3S = 374{\cdot}0$

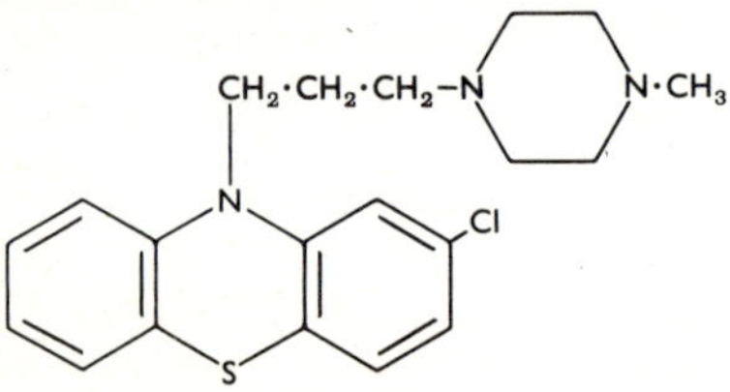

A clear pale yellow viscous liquid, sensitive to light.
Solubility. Very slightly soluble in water; freely soluble in ethanol, ether, and chloroform.

PROCHLORPERAZINE EDISYLATE

Synonym: Prochlorperazine Ethanedisulphonate.
Proprietary Name: Compazine (injection and syrup).

A white crystalline powder.
Solubility. Soluble 1 in 2 of water and 1 in 1500 of ethanol; insoluble in ether and chloroform.

PROCHLORPERAZINE MALEATE

Synonyms: Prochlorperazine Dihydrogen Maleate; Prochlorperazine Dimaleate.
Proprietary Names: Compazine (capsules and tablets); Nipodal (suppositories and tablets); Stemetil (suppositories and tablets).

A white crystalline powder. M.p. 198° to 203°.
Solubility. Almost insoluble in water and ethanol; insoluble in ether; slightly soluble in warm chloroform.

PROCHLORPERAZINE MESYLATE

Synonyms: Prochlorperazine Dimethanesulphonate; Prochlorperazine Methanesulphonate.
Proprietary Name: Stemetil (injection and syrup).

A white powder. M.p. about 242°.
Solubility. Soluble 1 in less than 0·5 of water and 1 in 40 of ethanol; insoluble in ether; slightly soluble in chloroform.

Screening Test. *FPN reagent* with urine—red-purple (see p. 10).

Extraction. Prochlorperazine is extracted by organic solvents from aqueous alkaline solutions; hydrolysis of biological material is required in order to improve the yield.

Chromatography. PAPER: system P1—Rf 0·25 (location under ultraviolet light, blue fluorescence; location reagents: *iodoplatinate spray*, weak reaction; *bromocresol green spray*, weak reaction).

THIN-LAYER: system T1—Rf 0·45 (location reagent *acidified iodoplatinate spray*, positive reaction); system T3—Rf 0·70 (location reagents: *iodoplatinate spray*, positive reaction; *sulphuric acid–ethanol spray*, reddish-pink); system T4—Rf 0·27 (location as for T3); system T5—Rf 0·32 (location as for T3).

Colour Tests. MICRO: sulphuric acid–formaldehyde test—purple (*sensitivity:* 0·1 μg); ammonium molybdate test—blue → purple (*sensitivity:* 0·1 μg); ammonium vanadate test—brown → purple (*sensitivity:* 0·1 μg); Vitali's test—purple → faint yellow/faint yellow/faint yellow (*sensitivity:* 0·5 μg).

Crystal Tests. MICRO: *gold bromide–hydrochloric acid solution*—needles (*sensitivity:* 1 in 1000); *picric acid*—smudge rosettes (*sensitivity:* 1 in 1000).

Ultraviolet Absorption Spectrum. Prochlorperazine in ethanol, maximum at 258 mμ (E1%, 1cm 997): prochlorperazine maleate in ethanol: water (1:1), maxima at 257 mμ (E1%, 1cm 760) and 312 mμ (E1%, 1cm 100); minima at 225 mμ and 280 mμ.

Metabolism. Phillips and Miya (1964), studying prochlorperazine in rats, have shown that about 35% of the administered dose is excreted in the faeces in 24 hours. Unchanged prochlorperazine and its metabolites are detected in the urine but they do not represent a substantial portion of the dose administered. Upon repeated dosage, prochlorperazine reaches peak levels in the tissues 2 hours after administration.

Dose. As an anti-emetic, up to 30 mg daily; in psychiatric states, up to 100 mg daily.

Toxicity. Prochlorperazine is a more potent tranquilliser than chlorpromazine (p. 256). Extrapyramidal symptoms similar to parkinsonism may occur at high dosage levels. Fatal liver damage has been reported and blood dyscrasias may occur.
The acute lethal dose of the phenothiazine tranquillisers in man is stated to be in the range 15 to 150 mg/kg.

PROCYCLIDINE *Parasympatholytic*

1-Cyclohexyl-1-phenyl-3-(pyrrolidin-1-yl)-propan-1-ol
$C_{19}H_{29}NO = 287{\cdot}4$

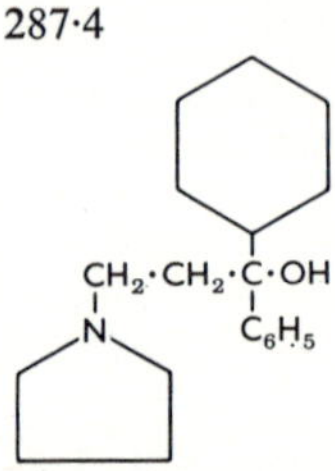

PROCYCLIDINE HYDROCHLORIDE

Proprietary Name: Kemadrin.

A white crystalline powder. M.p. 225° to 227°.
Solubility. Soluble 1 in 40 of water and 1 in 15 of ethanol; insoluble in ether.

Extraction. Procyclidine is extracted by organic solvents from aqueous alkaline solutions.

Chromatography. PAPER: system P1—Rf 0·84 (location reagents: *iodoplatinate spray*, strong reaction; *bromocresol green spray*, weak reaction); system RP1a—Rf 0·53 (location reagent *iodoplatinate spray*, positive reaction); system RP1b—Rf 0·04 (location as for RP1a).

THIN-LAYER: system T1—Rf 0·50 (location reagent *acidified iodoplatinate spray*, positive reaction).

GAS: system G2/225—retention time 0·53 relative to codeine.

Colour Tests. MICRO: sulphuric acid–formaldehyde test—faint purple (*sensitivity:* 1·0 μg); ammonium molybdate test—(blue) grey (*sensitivity:* 0·5 μg); ammonium vanadate test—(grey) black (*sensitivity:* 0·25 μg).

Crystal Tests. MICRO: *picrolonic acid*—clusters of branching needles and oily plates, best viewed under polarised light (*sensitivity:* 1 in 1000); *sodium carbonate solution*—curving needles (*sensitivity:* 1 in 1000).

Ultraviolet Absorption Spectrum. Procyclidine in 0·1N sulphuric acid, maxima at 252 mμ (E1%, 1 cm 5), 258 mμ (E1%, 1 cm 6·5), and 264 mμ (E1%, 1 cm 5).

Infra-red Absorption Spectrum. Procyclidine hydrochloride. Potassium bromide disk. The principal peaks are: A 696, B 1447, C 755 (p. 759).

Dose. Up to 30 mg daily.

Toxicity. The lethal dose in man is probably in the range 10 to 100 mg/kg.

LD50 (oral): in mice 385 mg/kg.

CASE EXAMPLE. In a case of suicide due to the ingestion of procyclidine, fluphenazine, and (unspecified) barbiturates, the procyclidine levels were: duodenum fluid, 2·2 mg%; stomach contents, 27·5 mg; urine, 1·0 mg%; the barbiturate levels were: blood, 3·6 mg%; liver blood, 104 mg%; stomach contents, 1·92 g; urine, 17·6 mg%. The blood also contained 0·4 mg% of fluphenazine (Koumides, 1967).

PROFLAVINE HEMISULPHATE *Antiseptic*

Synonyms: Neutral Proflavine Sulphate; Proflavine.
Proprietary Name: Pancridine.

3,6-Diaminoacridine sulphate dihydrate
$(C_{13}H_{11}N_3)_2,H_2SO_4,2H_2O$ = 552·6

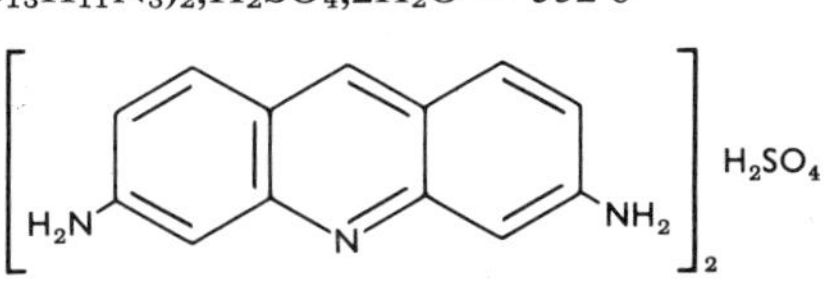

An orange to red, hygroscopic, crystalline powder.
Solubility. Soluble 1 in 300 of water and very soluble in boiling water; very slightly soluble in ethanol; insoluble in ether and chloroform.

Extraction. Proflavine is extracted by organic solvents from aqueous alkaline solutions.

Chromatography. PAPER: system P1—Rf 0·25 (location under ultraviolet light, yellow fluorescence; location reagent *iodoplatinate spray*, strong reaction).

THIN-LAYER: system T1—Rf 0·16 (location by diazotisation followed by *alkaline betanaphthol spray*).

Colour Tests. MICRO: sulphuric acid–formaldehyde test—(orange) pale yellow → orange (*sensitivity:* 0·5 μg); ammonium molybdate test—(orange) very pale yellow (*sensitivity:* 1·0 μg); ammonium vanadate test—(orange) olive (*sensitivity:* 0·5 μg); Vitali's test—–/orange-brown/yellow-brown (*sensitivity:* 1·0 μg).

Crystal Tests. MICRO: *styphnic acid*—small needles (*sensitivity:* 1 in 100); *trinitrobenzoic acid solution*—curving needles or plates (*sensitivity:* 1 in 400).

Ultraviolet Absorption Spectrum. Proflavine hemisulphate in ethanol, maxima at 261 mμ (E1%, 1 cm 1440) and 458 mμ (E1%, 1 cm 1214) and inflexions at about 280 mμ and 296 mμ.

PROGESTERONE *Progestational Steroid*

Synonyms: Luteal Hormone; Luteine; Pregnenedione; Progestin.
Proprietary Names: Corlutone; Gestone; Glanducorpin; Lipo-Lutin; Luteosid; Lutocyclin; Lutoform; Lutogyl; Lutren; Proluton; Syngesterone.

Pregn-4-ene-3,20-dione
$C_{21}H_{30}O_2$ = 314·5

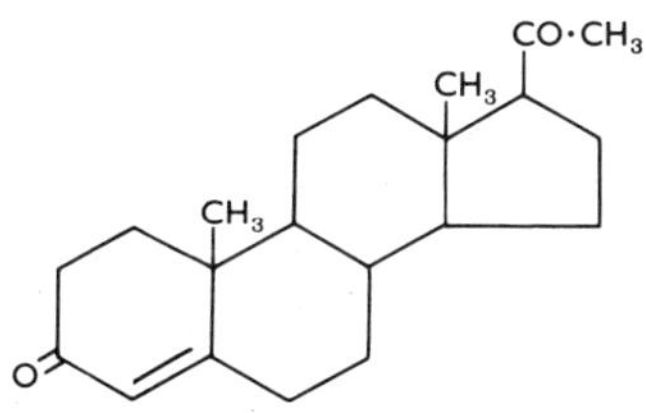

A white crystalline powder. M.p. 128° to 131°, but it may occur with a lower melting-point, about 121°. Specific rotation of a 1% solution in dehydrated ethanol, +186° to +196°.
Solubility. Insoluble in water; soluble 1 in 8 of ethanol, 1 in 16 of ether, and 1 in 0·33 of chloroform.

Extraction. Progesterone is extracted from neutral solutions with freshly distilled ethyl acetate.

Chromatography. THIN-LAYER: thin-layer chromatography on starch-bound silica gel layers involving several solvent systems is described for the separation of progesterone and other steroids by Smith and Foell (1962).

GAS: methods of gas chromatographic determination of progesterone are described by Van Der Molen and Groen (1965) and Lurie *et al.* (1966).

Crystal Test. MICRO: *potassium tri-iodide solution (3)*—rosettes of hairlike crystals.

Ultraviolet Absorption Spectrum. Progesterone in ethanol, maximum at about 240 mμ (E1%, 1 cm 540).

Infra-red Absorption Spectrum. Potassium bromide disk. The principal peaks are: A 1659, B 1691, C 1358 or 1615 (p. 759).

Metabolism. Progesterone is the naturally occurring progestogenic hormone secreted by the corpus luteum. It acts only on tissues which have been previously subjected to the actions of oestrogens. It is essentially concerned with the maintenance of pregnancy. In the adrenal glands progesterone serves as a biosynthetic precursor of hydrocortisone and in the testes as a precursor of testosterone.

Dose. Up to 60 mg daily, intramuscularly.

PROGUANIL *Antimalarial*

Synonyms: Chloriguane; Chloroguanide; Proguanide; RP 3359; SN 12837.

N^1-*p*-Chlorophenyl-N^5-isopropyldiguanide

$C_{11}H_{16}ClN_5 = 253{\cdot}7$

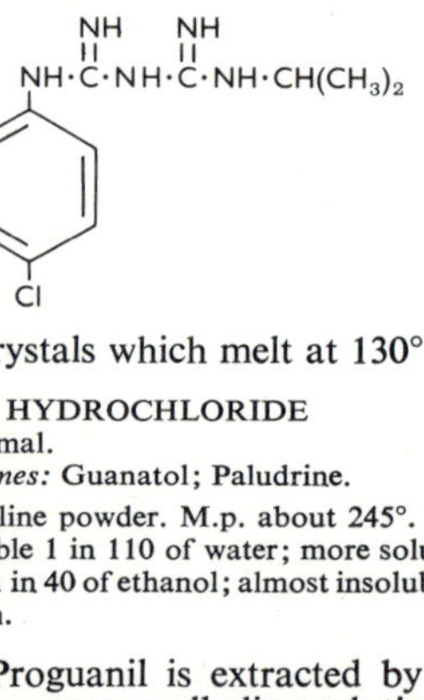

Colourless crystals which melt at 130° to 131°.

PROGUANIL HYDROCHLORIDE

Synonym: Bigumal.

Proprietary Names: Guanatol; Paludrine.

A white crystalline powder. M.p. about 245°.

Solubility. Soluble 1 in 110 of water; more soluble in hot water; soluble 1 in 40 of ethanol; almost insoluble in ether and chloroform.

Extraction. Proguanil is extracted by organic solvents from aqueous alkaline solutions.

Chromatography. PAPER: system P1—Rf 0·78 (location under ultraviolet light, strong absorption; location reagent *iodoplatinate spray*, strong reaction); system RP1a—Rf 0·76 (location under ultraviolet light, absorption; location reagent *iodoplatinate spray*, positive reaction); system RP1b—Rf 0·66 (location under ultraviolet light, absorption).

THIN-LAYER: system T1—Rf 0·30, streaking (location reagent *acidified iodoplatinate spray*, positive reaction).

Colour Test. To 10 ml of a saturated solution of proguanil hydrochloride add 1 drop of 10% copper sulphate solution and 2·5 ml of *dilute ammonia solution* and shake well; add 5 ml of benzene and shake again—benzene layer is purplish-red.

Crystal Tests. MICRO: *gold bromide–hydrochloric acid solution*—long plates (*sensitivity:* 1 in 400); *picrolonic acid*—short rods, some in rosettes, best viewed under polarised light (*sensitivity:* 1 in 400).

Ultraviolet Absorption Spectrum. Proguanil in methanol, maximum at 258 mμ (E1%, 1 cm 715); in 0·1N sulphuric acid, maximum at 247 mμ (E1%, 1 cm 387).

Infra-red Absorption Spectrum. Proguanil hydrochloride. Potassium bromide disk. The principal peaks are: A 1534, B 1492 or 1635, C 1575 (p. 759).

Metabolism. Proguanil is rapidly absorbed from the gastro-intestinal tract. Up to 60% is excreted unchanged in the urine and about 30% as an active metabolite, cycloguanil, p. 274, which is formed by a cyclisation reaction. This metabolite is thought to be mainly responsible for the antimalarial activity of the drug.

Dose. Up to 300 mg daily.

Toxicity. In normal therapeutic doses proguanil rarely provokes toxic symptoms. Large doses may cause vomiting, abdominal pain, and diarrhoea. Recovery has followed the ingestion of as much as 14·5 g.

LD50 (oral): in mice 23 mg/kg.

PROHEPTAZINE *Narcotic*

Synonyms: Dimepheprimine; Wy 757.

Propyl 1,3-dimethyl-4-phenyl-1-azacycloheptane-4-carboxylate

$C_{17}H_{25}NO_2 = 275{\cdot}4$

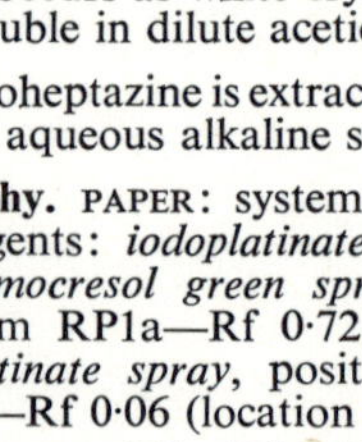

Proheptazine occurs as white crystals.

Solubility. Soluble in dilute acetic acid.

Extraction. Proheptazine is extracted by organic solvents from aqueous alkaline solutions.

Chromatography. PAPER: system P1—Rf 0·56 (location reagents: *iodoplatinate spray*, weak reaction; *bromocresol green spray*, weak reaction); system RP1a—Rf 0·72 (location reagent *iodoplatinate spray*, positive reaction); system RP1b—Rf 0·06 (location as for RP1a).

THIN-LAYER: system T1—Rf 0·40 (location reagent *acidified iodoplatinate spray*, positive reaction).

GAS: system G2/225—retention time 0·48 (1·18; 1·27) relative to diphenhydramine; system G4—retention time 0·46 relative to diphenhydramine.

Colour Tests. MICRO: sulphuric acid–formaldehyde test—dull orange (*sensitivity:* 0·25 μg); ammonium molybdate test—blue-grey → green (*sensitivity:* 0·25 μg); ammonium vanadate test—greyish-purple, fading (*sensitivity:* 0·25 μg).

Crystal Tests. MICRO: *potassium chromate solution*—bunches of plates (*sensitivity:* 1 in 100); *potassium iodide solution*—stout rods or prisms, often in rosettes (*sensitivity:* 1 in 200).

PROLINTANE *Central Stimulant*

Synonym: SP 732.

1-(1-Benzylbutyl)pyrrolidine

$C_{15}H_{23}N = 217·4$

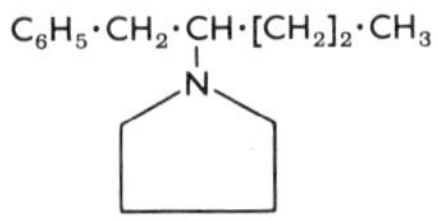

PROLINTANE HYDROCHLORIDE

Proprietary Names: It is an ingredient of Katovit and Villescon.

A white powder. M.p. 132° to 134°.

Solubility. Freely soluble in water, ethanol, and chloroform; insoluble in ether.

Extraction. Prolintane is extracted by organic solvents from aqueous alkaline solutions.

Chromatography. PAPER: system P1—Rf 0·76 (location under ultraviolet light, absorption; location reagents: *iodoplatinate spray*, strong reaction; *bromocresol green spray*, strong reaction).

THIN-LAYER: system T1—Rf 0·48 (location reagents: *acidified iodoplatinate spray*, positive reaction; *potassium permanganate spray*, positive reaction).

GAS: system G2/120—retention time 3·4 relative to ephedrine.

Colour Test. MICRO: sulphuric acid–formaldehyde test—orange → brown (*sensitivity:* 0·1 μg).

Crystal Tests. MICRO: *gold chloride solution*—blades or small crystals in chains (*sensitivity:* 1 in 1000); *lead iodide solution*—masses of needles (*sensitivity:* 1 in 400).

Ultraviolet Absorption Spectrum. Prolintane in 0·1N sulphuric acid, maxima at about 248 mμ (E1%, 1cm 5·1), 252 mμ (E1%, 1cm 6·9), 258 mμ (E1%, 1cm 8·5), and 264 mμ (E1%, 1cm 6·5), and inflexions at about 242 mμ and about 267·5 mμ.

Dose. Up to 40 mg daily.

Toxicity. LD50 (oral): in mice 257 mg/kg.

PROMAZINE *Tranquilliser*

10-(3-Dimethylaminopropyl)phenothiazine

$C_{17}H_{20}N_2S = 284·4$

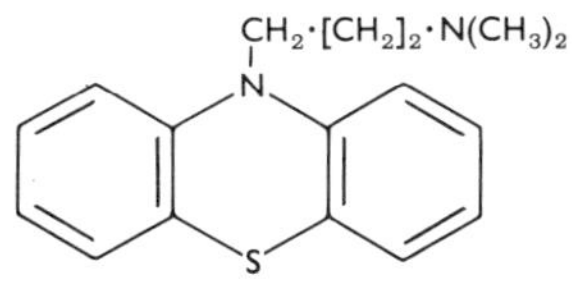

An oily liquid. B.p. 203° to 210° at 0·3 mm Hg.

PROMAZINE HYDROCHLORIDE

Proprietary Names: Prazine; Protactyl; Sparine; Verophen.

A white, slightly hygroscopic, crystalline powder. M.p. 177° to 181°.

Solubility. Soluble 1 in 1 of water, 1 in 2 of ethanol, and 1 in 2 of chloroform; almost insoluble in ether.

Screening Test. *FPN reagent* with urine—orange (see p. 10).

Extraction. Promazine is extracted by organic solvents from aqueous alkaline solutions; hydrolysis of biological material is required in order to improve the yield.

Chromatography. PAPER: system P1—Rf 0·58 (location under ultraviolet light, pale blue fluorescence; location reagents: *iodoplatinate spray*, strong reaction; *bromocresol green spray*, weak reaction); system RP1a—Rf 0·33 (location under ultraviolet light, blue fluorescence; location reagent *iodoplatinate spray*, positive reaction); system RP1b—Rf 0·02 (location as for RP1a).

THIN-LAYER: system T1—Rf 0·42 (location reagent *acidified iodoplatinate spray*, positive reaction); system T3—Rf 0·62 (location reagents: *iodoplatinate spray*, positive reaction; *sulphuric acid–ethanol spray*, positive reaction); system T6—Rf 0·51 (the spot may be converted on the plate to the sulphoxide, Rf 0·37; location of both spots under ultraviolet light).

GAS: system G1/250—retention time 0·89 relative to codeine; system G2/225—retention time 0·86 relative to codeine; system G3—retention time 4·85 relative to diphenhydramine; system G4—retention time 0·6 relative to codeine.

Colour Tests. MICRO: sulphuric acid–formaldehyde test—purple (*sensitivity:* 0·5 μg); ammonium molybdate test—dull green → purple (*sensitivity:* 0·1 μg); ammonium vanadate test—green → purple (*sensitivity:* 0·1 μg); Vitali's test — purple → yellow/yellow/yellow (*sensitivity:* 0·25 μg).

Crystal Tests. MICRO: *gold chloride solution*—rods (*sensitivity:* 1 in 400); *potassium permanganate solution*—branching needles (*sensitivity:* 1 in 400).

Ultraviolet Absorption Spectrum. Promazine in 0·1N sulphuric acid, maxima at 252 mμ (E1%, 1cm 1122) and 300 mμ (E1%, 1cm 130).

Promazine hydrochloride in water, maxima at 251 mμ (E1%, 1cm 910) and 301 mμ: in ethanol:water (1:1), maxima at 253 mμ (E1%, 1cm 930) and 303 mμ (E1%, 1cm 130); minima at 221 mμ and 275 mμ.

Infra-red Absorption Spectrum. Promazine hydrochloride. Potassium bromide disk. The principal peaks are: A 1462, B 748, C 1245 (p. 759).

Metabolism. Promazine is metabolised mainly by sulphoxide formation; some dealkylation may also occur.

Dose. Up to 1 g daily.

Toxicity. Epileptic fits are provoked more often than with other phenothiazines. Fatal agranulocytosis and fatal liver damage have occurred. The acute lethal dose of the phenothiazine tranquillisers in man is stated to be in the range 15 to 150 mg/kg.

CASE EXAMPLES. A 48-year-old woman died after receiving a total of 31·7 g of promazine hydrochloride in 48 days. Examination post mortem showed pulmonary oedema, atelectasis, acute ulcerative colitis, fatty changes in the liver, and agranulocytosis (Woodward and Solomon, 1956).

A man became deeply unconscious after a dose of 1·25 g—he recovered (Hindle and Negus, 1960).

PROMETHAZINE *Antihistamine*

10-(2-Dimethylaminopropyl)phenothiazine

$C_{17}H_{20}N_2S = 284{\cdot}4$

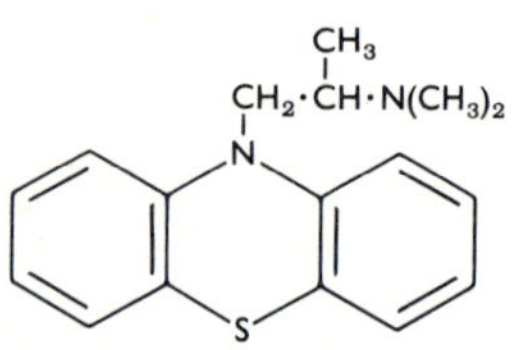

Crystals which melt at 60°. B.p. 190° to 192° at 3 mm Hg.

PROMETHAZINE HYDROCHLORIDE

Synonyms: Diprazine; Proazamine Chloride.

Proprietary Names: Fargan; Phenergan; Prothazin(e).

A white powder which is somewhat unstable in air. M.p. 221° to 225°.

Solubility. Soluble 1 in 0·6 of water, 1 in 9 of ethanol, and 1 in 2 of chloroform; almost insoluble in ether.

PROMETHAZINE THEOCLATE

Synonym: Promethazine 8-Chlorotheophyllinate.

Proprietary Name: Avomine.

A white powder.

Solubility. Very slightly soluble in water; soluble 1 in 70 of ethanol and 1 in 2·5 of chloroform; insoluble in ether.

Screening Test. *FPN reagent* with urine—pink-purple (see p. 10).

Extraction. Promethazine is extracted by organic solvents from aqueous alkaline solutions; hydrolysis of biological material is required in order to improve the yield.

Chromatography. PAPER: system P1—Rf 0·65 (location under ultraviolet light, pale green fluorescence; location reagents: *iodoplatinate spray*, strong reaction; *bromocresol green spray*, weak reaction); system RP1a—Rf 0·23 (location reagent *iodoplatinate spray*, positive reaction); system RP1b—Rf 0·02 (location as for RP1a).

THIN-LAYER: system T1—Rf 0·48 (location reagent *acidified iodoplatinate spray*, positive reaction); system T3—Rf 0·70 (location reagents: *iodoplatinate spray*, positive reaction; *sulphuric acid–ethanol spray*, positive reaction); system T6—Rf 0·66 (the spot may be converted on the plate to the sulphoxide, Rf 0·38; location of both spots under ultraviolet light).

GAS: system G2/225—retention time 0·75 relative to codeine; system G4—retention time 0·46 relative to codeine.

Colour Tests. MICRO: sulphuric acid–formaldehyde test—purple (*sensitivity:* 0·1 μg); ammonium molybdate test—black-violet → purple (*sensitivity:* 0·1 μg); ammonium vanadate test—green → purple (*sensitivity:* 0·1 μg); Vitali's test—purple → yellow/yellow/yellow (*sensitivity:* 1·0 μg).

Crystal Tests. MICRO: *gold cyanide solution*—plates and rods (*sensitivity:* 1 in 1000); *platinic bromide solution*—very small dense rosettes (*sensitivity:* 1 in 1000).

Ultraviolet Absorption Spectrum. Promethazine in ethanol:water (1:1), maxima at 252 mμ (E1%, 1cm 880) and 301 mμ (E1%, 1cm 110); in 0·01N hydrochloric acid, maxima at 249 mμ (E1%, 1cm 1026) and about 300 mμ.

Infra-red Absorption Spectrum. Promethazine hydrochloride. Potassium bromide disk. The principal peaks are: A 757 or 1459, B 1222 (p. 759).

Metabolism. Promethazine sulphoxide is the major metabolite of promethazine found in the urine of subjects given 50 mg of promethazine 8 to 10 hours before the urine collection. A little of the unchanged drug is also found. Small amounts of the sulphoxide are readily identifiable in the urine of the subjects for 10 to 14 days after ingestion of a single 50-mg dose (Cochin and Daly, 1963b).

Dose. Usually up to 50 mg daily; up to 400 mg daily has been given to control parkinsonian symptoms.

Toxicity. Jaundice, agranulocytosis, and photosensitivity reactions have been reported following the use of promethazine. The lethal dose is estimated to be 200 mg/kg orally.

LD50 (oral): in mice 575 mg/kg.

CASE EXAMPLE. A 60-year-old woman was murdered whilst under the influence of drugs. Post-mortem levels of promethazine: brain, 0·33 mg%; liver, 0·33 mg%; intestinal contents, 0·17 mg%; stomach contents, 0·16 mg%. The drug could not be detected in the blood (Heyndrickx *et al.*, 1965).

PROPAMIDINE *Antibacterial*

1,3-Di(4-amidinophenoxy)propane

$C_{17}H_{20}N_4O_2 = 312{\cdot}4$

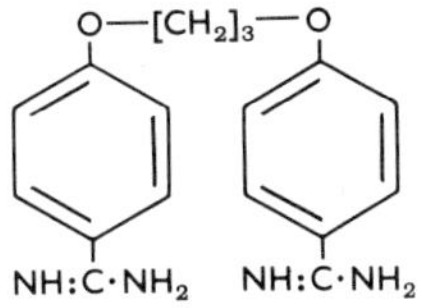

PROPAMIDINE ISETHIONATE

Proprietary Name: Brolene.

A white granular powder. M.p. 235°.

Solubility. Soluble 1 in 4 of water, 1 in 50 of ethanol (90%), and 1 in 300 of absolute ethanol; almost insoluble in ether and chloroform.

Extraction. Propamidine is extracted by organic solvents from aqueous alkaline solutions.

Chromatography. PAPER: system P1—Rf 0·08 (location under ultraviolet light, blue fluorescence; location reagents: *iodoplatinate spray*, strong reaction; *bromocresol green spray*, strong reaction); system RPla—Rf 0·83 (location under ultraviolet light, blue fluorescence; location reagent *iodoplatinate spray*, positive reaction); system RP1b—Rf 0·82 (location as for RP1a). THIN-LAYER: system T1—Rf 0·04 (location reagent *acidified iodoplatinate spray*, positive reaction).

Crystal Tests. MICRO: *mercuric chloride solution*—bunches of fine needles (*sensitivity:* 1 in 1000); *potassium chromate solution*—small hairlike needles (*sensitivity:* 1 in 1000).

Ultraviolet Absorption Spectrum. Propamidine in ethanol, maximum at 267 mμ (E1%, 1 cm 1224).

Use. Propamidine is used in the form of a cream containing 0·15% and an ophthalmic solution containing 0·1%.

PROPANIDID *Anaesthetic*

Synonym: FBA 1420.

Proprietary Name: Epontol.

Propyl 4-diethylcarbamoylmethoxy-3-methoxyphenylacetate

$C_{18}H_{27}NO_5 = 337{\cdot}4$

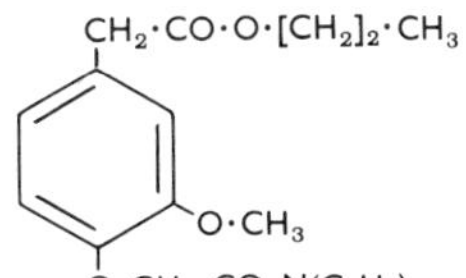

A pale yellow oil. B.p. about 210°.

Solubility. Insoluble in water; soluble in ethanol and chloroform.

Chromatography. PAPER: system P1—Rf 0·97 (location under ultraviolet light, weak absorption; location reagent *iodoplatinate spray*, yellow). THIN-LAYER: system T1—Rf 0·73 (location reagent *Dragendorff spray*, positive reaction).

Colour Test. MICRO: Vitali's test— -/-/bright purple (*sensitivity:* 0·1 μg).

Crystal Test. MICRO: *lead iodide solution*—dense rosettes, forming overnight (*sensitivity:* 1 in 200).

Ultraviolet Absorption Spectrum. Propanidid in ethanol, maximum at about 288 mμ (E1%, 1 cm about 82); minimum at about 255 mμ.

Metabolism. Propanidid is metabolised in the liver, blood-stream, and kidneys mainly by hydrolysis of the ester bond. Some metabolism may occur through demethylation or splitting of the acid amide bond.

Propanidid is a short-acting anaesthetic; recovery begins within 4 minutes and is complete in 12 minutes.

Dose. Up to 10 mg/kg.

PROPANOL *Industrial Solvent*

Synonyms: n-Propanol; Propyl Alcohol; n-Propyl Alcohol.

Propan-1-ol

$CH_3{\cdot}CH_2{\cdot}CH_2OH = 60{\cdot}10$

A clear colourless inflammable liquid. B.p. 97° to 98°. Refractive index 1·386.

Solubility. Miscible with water, ethanol, ether, and chloroform.

Extraction. Propanol is volatile and may be isolated by distillation (see p. 18).

Chromatography. GAS: system G8/100—retention time 3·50 relative to ethanol; system G8/160—retention time 2·30 relative to ethanol.

Colour Test. *Acidified potassium dichromate solution*—green, on warming.

Metabolism. Propanol is readily oxidised *in vivo* through propionaldehyde and propionic acid to carbon dioxide. Less than 1% is conjugated with glucuronic acid.

Toxicity. Propanol is more toxic than isopropanol (p. 385).

LD50 (oral): in rats 1·8 g/kg.

PROPANTHELINE BROMIDE *Parasympatholytic*

Synonym: Propantheline Methobromide.

Proprietary Name: Pro-Banthine.

2-Di-isopropylaminoethyl xanthen-9-carboxylate methobromide

$C_{23}H_{30}BrNO_3 = 448{\cdot}4$

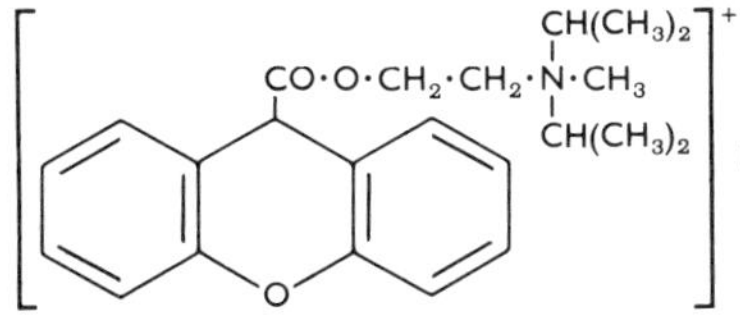

A white powder. M.p. 157° to 162°.

Solubility. Very soluble in water, ethanol, and chloroform; almost insoluble in ether.

Extraction. Propantheline bromide is a quaternary ammonium compound (see p. 29).

Chromatography. PAPER: system P1—Rf 0·54 (location under ultraviolet light, pale green fluorescence; location reagent *iodoplatinate spray*, strong reaction); system RP1a—Rf 0·74 (location under ultraviolet light, pale blue fluorescence; location reagent *iodoplatinate spray*, positive reaction); system RP1b—Rf 0·66 (location as for RP1a).

THIN-LAYER: system T1—Rf 0·04 (location reagent *acidified iodoplatinate spray*, positive reaction).

Colour Tests. MICRO: the following tests are performed on the nitrate (see p. 134): sulphuric acid–formaldehyde test—orange (*sensitivity:* 0·5 μg); ammonium molybdate test—green → yellow (*sensitivity:* 0·025 μg); ammonium vanadate test—orange (*sensitivity:* 0·025 μg); Vitali's test—yellow/–/green (*sensitivity:* 0·5 μg).

Crystal Tests. MICRO: *lead iodide solution*—small dense rosettes, forming overnight (*sensitivity:* 1 in 400); *potassium tri-iodide solution* (*1*)—small oily plates (*sensitivity:* 1 in 1000).

Ultraviolet Absorption Spectrum. Propantheline bromide in 0·1N sulphuric acid, maxima at 243 mμ (E1%, 1 cm 103) and 281 mμ (E1%, 1 cm 52).

Infra-red Absorption Spectrum. Potassium bromide disk. The principal peaks are: A 1260 or 1719, B 1484 (p. 759).

Dose. Up to 150 mg daily.

Toxicity. The lethal dose in man is probably in the range 10 to 100 mg/kg.

PROPERIDINE *Narcotic Analgesic*

Synonyms: Gevelina; Ipropethidine; Isopedine.

Isopropyl 1 - methyl - 4 - phenylpiperidine - 4 - carboxylate

$C_{16}H_{23}NO_2 = 261{\cdot}4$

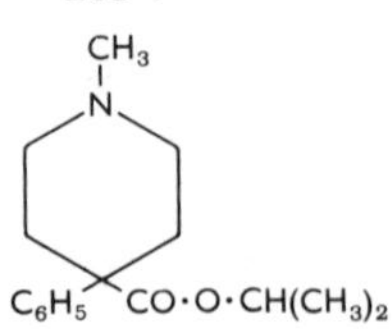

PROPERIDINE HYDROCHLORIDE

Synonym: NU 896.

Proprietary Name: Dolisina B.

Extraction. Properidine is extracted by organic solvents from aqueous alkaline solutions.

Chromatography. PAPER: system P1—Rf 0·50 (location reagents: *iodoplatinate spray*, weak reaction; *bromocresol green spray*, weak reaction); system RP1a—Rf 0·61 (location reagent *iodoplatinate spray*, positive reaction); system RP1b—Rf 0·00 (location as for RP1a).

THIN-LAYER: system T1—Rf 0·53 (location reagent *acidified iodoplatinate spray*, positive reaction).

GAS: system G2/225—retention time 0·75 relative to diphenhydramine; system G4—retention time 0·65 relative to diphenhydramine.

Colour Test. MICRO: sulphuric acid–formaldehyde test—dull orange (*sensitivity:* 1·0 μg).

Crystal Tests. MICRO: *lead iodide solution*—masses of blades, some serrated (*sensitivity:* 1 in 1500); *potassium permanganate solution*—plates, often large and serrated (*sensitivity:* 1 in 1000).

Ultraviolet Absorption Spectrum. Properidine in 0·1N sulphuric acid, maxima at 251 mμ (E1%, 1 cm 7), 257 mμ (E1%, 1 cm 8), and 263 mμ (E1%, 1 cm 6·6).

PROPIOMAZINE *Tranquilliser*

Synonyms: CB 1678; Wy 1359.

10 - (2 - Dimethylaminopropyl) - 2 - propionylphenothiazine

$C_{20}H_{24}N_2OS = 340{\cdot}5$

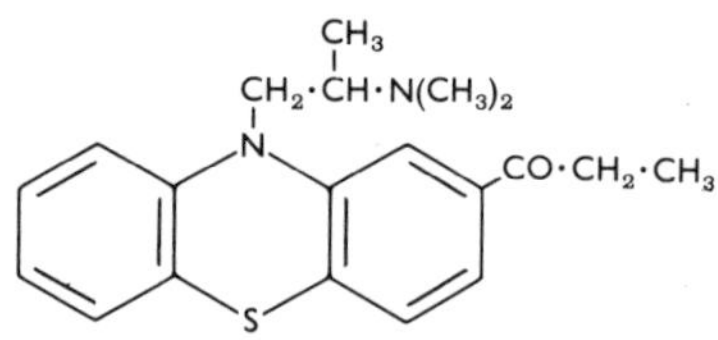

PROPIOMAZINE HYDROCHLORIDE

Proprietary Name: Largon Hydrochloride.

A yellow crystalline powder.

Solubility. Soluble in water; slightly soluble in ethanol.

PROPIOMAZINE MALEATE

Synonym: Propiomazine Hydrogen Maleate.

Proprietary Names: Dorevan; Indorm; Propavan.

A yellow microcrystalline powder.

Solubility. Soluble 1 in 500 of water, 1 in 60 of ethanol, and 1 in 140 of dehydrated ethanol.

Screening Test. *FPN reagent* with urine—faintly red (see p. 10).

Extraction. Propiomazine is extracted by organic solvents from aqueous alkaline solutions; hydrolysis of biological material is necessary in order to improve the yield.

Chromatography. PAPER: system P1—Rf 0·77 (location under ultraviolet light, yellow fluorescence; location reagents: *iodoplatinate spray*, strong reaction; *bromocresol green spray*, weak reaction); system RP1a—Rf 0·07 (location under ultraviolet light, yellow fluorescence; location reagent *iodoplatinate spray*, positive reaction); system RP1b—Rf 0·04 (location as for RP1a).

THIN-LAYER: system T1—Rf 0·61 (location reagent *acidified iodoplatinate spray*, positive reaction); system T6—Rf 0·77 (the spot may be converted on the plate to the sulphoxide, Rf 0·54; location of both spots under ultraviolet light).

GAS: system G2/225—retention time 2·7 relative to codeine; system G4—retention time 2·3 relative to codeine.

Colour Tests. MICRO: sulphuric acid–formaldehyde test—red-purple (*sensitivity:* 0·1 μg); ammonium molybdate test—purple (*sensitivity:* 0·1 μg); ammonium vanadate test—purple (*sensitivity:* 0·1 μg); Vitali's test—purple → yellow/pale yellow/yellow (*sensitivity:* 1·0 μg).

Crystal Test. MICRO: *gold bromide solution*—needles, forming overnight (*sensitivity:* 1 in 400).

Ultraviolet Absorption Spectrum. Propiomazine in 0·01N sulphuric acid, maximum at 241 mμ.

Dose. Up to 40 mg (maleate) by mouth; up to 30 mg (hydrochloride) intramuscularly.

Toxicity. The acute lethal dose of the phenothiazine tranquillisers in man is stated to be in the range 15 to 150 mg/kg.

PROPOXYCAINE *Local Anaesthetic*

2-Diethylaminoethyl 4-amino-2-propoxybenzoate

$C_{16}H_{26}N_2O_3 = 294{\cdot}4$

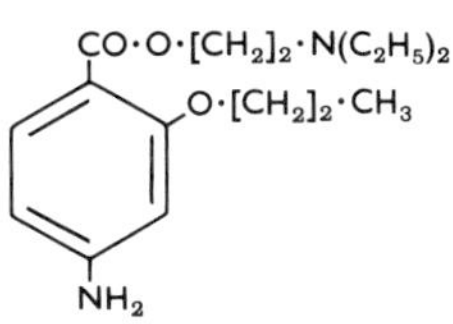

PROPOXYCAINE HYDROCHLORIDE
Proprietary Names: Blockaine; Ravocaine.

A white crystalline powder which discolours if exposed for long to light and air. M.p. 146° to 151°.
Solubility. Very soluble in water; slightly soluble in ethanol and chloroform; almost insoluble in ether.

Extraction. Propoxycaine is extracted by organic solvents from aqueous alkaline solutions.

Chromatography. PAPER: system P1—Rf 0·52 (location under ultraviolet light, blue fluorescence; location reagent *iodoplatinate spray*, strong reaction); system RP1a—Rf 0·83 (location reagent *iodoplatinate spray*, positive reaction); system RP1b—Rf 0·08 (location as for RP1a).

THIN-LAYER: system T1—Rf 0·59 (location reagent *acidified iodoplatinate spray*, positive reaction).

GAS: system G2/225—retention time 0·88 relative to codeine.

Colour Tests. MICRO: ammonium vanadate test—light brown (*sensitivity:* 1·0 μg); diazotisation test—red (*sensitivity:* 0·1 μg); Vitali's test—–/light brown/light brown (*sensitivity:* 1·0 μg).

Crystal Tests. MICRO: *gold bromide–hydrochloric acid solution*—bunches of small serrated plates (*sensitivity:* 1 in 1000); *platinic chloride solution*—bunches of blades, some dense rosettes (*sensitivity:* 1 in 400).

Ultraviolet Absorption Spectrum. Propoxycaine in 0·01N sulphuric acid, maxima at 235 mμ (E1%, 1cm 270) and 298 mμ (E1%, 1cm 189).

Use. Propoxycaine is used in dentistry to prolong and deepen the anaesthesia produced by procaine, 0·4% being added to a 2% solution of procaine hydrochloride.

Toxicity. Propoxycaine is said to be 8 to 10 times more toxic than procaine. The maximum amount stated to be safe by injection is 100 mg.

PROPRANOLOL *Cardiac Depressant*

Synonyms: AY 64043; ICI 45520.

1-Isopropylamino-3-(naphth-1-yloxy)propan-2-ol

$C_{16}H_{21}NO_2 = 259{\cdot}4$

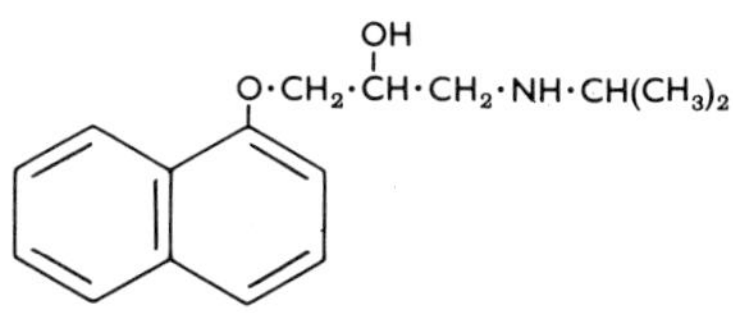

Propranolol melts at 94° to 96°.

PROPRANOLOL HYDROCHLORIDE
Proprietary Names: Dociton; Inderal.

A white crystalline powder. M.p. 163° to 164°.
Solubility. Soluble in water and ethanol; insoluble in ether; slightly soluble in chloroform.

Extraction. Propranolol is extracted by organic solvents from aqueous alkaline solutions.

Chromatography. PAPER: system P1—Rf 0·69 (location under ultraviolet light, blue fluorescence; location reagents: *iodoplatinate spray*, strong reaction; *bromocresol green spray*, weak reaction); system RP1a—Rf 0·73 (location under ultraviolet light, blue fluorescence); system RP1b—Rf 0·20 (location as for RP1a).

THIN-LAYER: system T1—Rf 0·53 (location reagent *acidified iodoplatinate spray*, positive reaction).

GAS: system G2/225—retention time 0·53 relative to codeine.

Colour Tests. MICRO: sulphuric acid–formaldehyde test—green (*sensitivity:* 0·1 μg); ammonium molybdate test—brown → green (*sensitivity:* 0·1 μg); ammonium vanadate test—deep green (*sensitivity:* 0·1 μg); Vitali's test—deep purple → green/yellow/orange (*sensitivity:* 0·1 μg).

Crystal Tests. MICRO: *gold bromide solution*—blades and plates (*sensitivity:* 1 in 1000);

styphnic acid—sheaves of needles (*sensitivity:* 1 in 1000).

Ultraviolet Absorption Spectrum. Propranolol in 0·1N sulphuric acid, inflexions at about 228 mμ and about 282 mμ and maxima at 288·5 mμ (E1%, 1cm 220), 305 mμ (E1%, 1cm 131), and 319·5 mμ (E1%, 1cm 71): propranolol hydrochloride in water, maxima at about 217 mμ (E1%, 1cm 1350) and about 293 mμ (E1%, 1cm about 220); minimum at about 250 mμ.

Metabolism. Propranolol has been shown by Bond (1967) to be metabolised by 2 main routes, viz. by hydroxylation to the 4′-hydroxy-derivative, followed by glucuronide conjugation, and side-chain oxidation to 2-hydroxy-3-(1′-naphthyloxy)propionic acid. Small amounts of these metabolites plus small amounts of unchanged propranolol and its glucuronide conjugate may be found in human urine.

Dose. Usually up to 120 mg daily; up to 400 mg daily has been given.

PROPYLHEXEDRINE *Sympathomimetic*

Proprietary Name: Benzedrex.

2-Cyclohexyl-*N*,1-dimethylethylamine

$C_{10}H_{21}N = 155{\cdot}3$

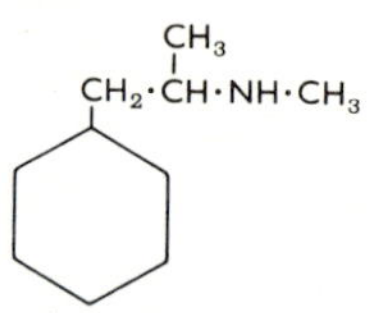

A clear colourless liquid which volatilises at room temperature and absorbs carbon dioxide from the air. B.p. about 204°.

Solubility. Very slightly soluble in water; miscible with ethanol, ether, and chloroform.

PROPYLHEXEDRINE HYDROCHLORIDE

Proprietary Names: Eventin; Obesin.

A crystalline solid. M.p. 138° to 140°.

Solubility. Soluble in water, ethanol, and chloroform; slightly soluble in ether.

Extraction. Propylhexedrine is extracted by organic solvents from aqueous alkaline solutions; it is volatile and may also be isolated by distillation (see p. 18).

Chromatography. PAPER: system P1—Rf 0·63 (location reagents: *iodoplatinate spray*, strong reaction; *bromocresol green spray*, strong reaction).

THIN-LAYER: system T1—Rf 0·26 (location reagent *acidified iodoplatinate spray*, positive reaction).

GAS: system G2/120—retention time 0·34 relative to ephedrine.

Crystal Tests. MICRO: *platinic bromide solution*—bunches of irregular blades (*sensitivity:* 1 in 200); *trinitrobenzoic acid solution*—curved branching needles (*sensitivity:* 1 in 200).

Dose. Up to 100 mg (hydrochloride) daily.

Toxicity. Polster (1965) reports that a 3-year-old boy recovered within 5 days of accidentally ingesting 375 mg of propylhexedrine.

PROTHIONAMIDE *Tuberculostatic*

Synonyms: TH 1321; 2-Propylisonicotinthioamide.
Proprietary Name: Trevintix.

2-Propylpyridine-4-carbothionamide

$C_9H_{12}N_2S = 180{\cdot}3$

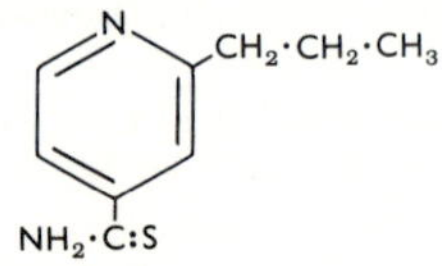

A yellow microcrystalline powder. M.p. 138° to 142°.

Solubility. Almost insoluble in water; soluble in ethanol, acetone, and methanol; slightly soluble in ether and chloroform.

Extraction. Prothionamide is extracted by organic solvents from aqueous alkaline solutions.

Chromatography. PAPER: system P1—Rf 0·88 (location under ultraviolet light, strong absorption; location reagents: *iodoplatinate spray*, white; *bromocresol green spray*, weak reaction); system RP1a—Rf 0·19 (location under ultraviolet light, absorption; location reagent *iodoplatinate spray*, positive reaction); system RP1b—Rf 0·17 (location as for RP1a).

THIN-LAYER: system T1—Rf 0·55, streaking (location reagent *acidified iodoplatinate spray*, positive reaction).

Colour Test. MICRO: ammonium molybdate test—faint blue (*sensitivity:* 1·0 μg).

Crystal Tests. MICRO: *sodium carbonate solution*—strings of plates (*sensitivity:* 1 in 200); *picrolonic acid*—irregular rosettes (*sensitivity:* 1 in 200).

Ultraviolet Absorption Spectrum. Prothionamide in methanol, maximum at 290 mμ; minimum at 255 mμ; in 0·1N sodium hydroxide, maximum at 278 mμ; in 0·1N sulphuric acid, maxima at 234 mμ (E1%, 1cm 414) and 275 mμ (E1%, 1cm 331), and an inflexion at about 315 mμ (E1%, 1cm 156).

Infra-red Absorption Spectrum. Potassium bromide disk. The principal peaks are: A 1398 or 1420, B 833, C 1592 (p. 760).

Dose. Up to 1 g daily.

PROTHIPENDYL *Tranquilliser*

Synonyms: D 206; Phrenotropin.

9 - (3 - Dimethylaminopropyl) - 10 - thia - 1,9 - diaza-anthracene
$C_{16}H_{19}N_3S = 285{\cdot}4$

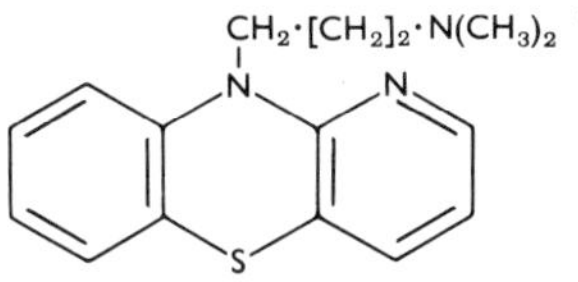

PROTHIPENDYL HYDROCHLORIDE
Proprietary Names: Azacon; Dominal; Timovan; Tolnate.

A crystalline powder. M.p. 108° to 112°.
Solubility. Readily soluble in water; insoluble in ether.

Extraction. Prothipendyl is extracted by organic solvents from aqueous alkaline solutions.

Chromatography. PAPER: system P1—Rf 0·55 (location under ultraviolet light, pale yellow fluorescence; location reagents: *iodoplatinate spray*, strong reaction; *bromocresol green spray*, weak reaction); system RP1a—Rf 0·50 (location reagent *iodoplatinate spray*, positive reaction); system RP1b—Rf 0·04 (location as for RP1a).

THIN-LAYER: system T1—Rf 0·23, streaking (location reagent *acidified iodoplatinate spray*, positive reaction); system T6—Rf 0·69 (the spot may be converted on the plate to the sulphoxide, Rf 0·48; location of both spots under ultraviolet light).

GAS: system G2/225—retention time 0·98 relative to codeine; system G4—retention time 0·53 relative to codeine.

Colour Tests. MICRO: sulphuric acid–formaldehyde test—orange (*sensitivity:* 0·25 μg); ammonium molybdate test—purple-brown (*sensitivity:* 0·1 μg); Vitali's test—yellow flash/–/– (*sensitivity:* 0·5 μg).

Crystal Tests. MICRO: *ammonium thiocyanate solution*—large wedges, best viewed under polarised light (*sensitivity:* 1 in 200); *lead iodide solution*—small needles (*sensitivity:* 1 in 1000).

Ultraviolet Absorption Spectrum. Prothipendyl in 0·1N sodium hydroxide, maximum at 249 mμ (E 1%, 1 cm 907); in 0·1N sulphuric acid, maximum at 242 mμ (E 1%, 1 cm 829).

Infra-red Absorption Spectrum. Prothipendyl hydrochloride. Potassium bromide disk. The principal peaks are: A 1413, B 749 or 1447, C 1488 (p. 760).

Dose. Usually up to 120 mg daily; up to 960 mg daily has been given in severe psychoses.

Toxicity. The lethal dose in man is stated to be between 100 and 500 mg/kg.

PROTOKYLOL *Sympathomimetic*

Synonyms: JB 251; Protochylol.

1 - (3,4 - Dihydroxyphenyl) - 2 - (α - methyl - 3, 4-methylenedioxyphenethylamino)ethanol
$C_{18}H_{21}NO_5 = 331{\cdot}4$

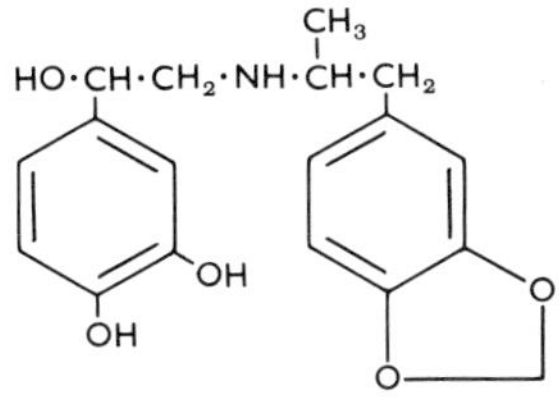

PROTOKYLOL HYDROCHLORIDE
Proprietary Name: Caytine.

A white crystalline powder.
Solubility. Soluble in water.

Extraction. Protokylol is extracted by organic solvents from aqueous ammoniacal solutions.

Chromatography. PAPER: system P1—Rf 0·51 (location under ultraviolet light, absorption; location reagents: *bromocresol green spray*, weak reaction; *potassium permanganate spray*, strong reaction).

THIN-LAYER: system T1—Rf 0·63 (location reagent *potassium permanganate spray*, positive reaction).

Colour Tests. MICRO: sulphuric acid–formaldehyde test—grey-green (*sensitivity:* 0·1 μg); ammonium molybdate test—(yellow) dark grey → brown (*sensitivity:* 0·1 μg); ammonium vanadate test—(grey) yellow → brown (*sensitivity:* 0·5 μg); Vitali's test—faint yellow/yellow/red (*sensitivity:* 0·5 μg).

Ultraviolet Absorption Spectrum. Protokylol in 0·1N sulphuric acid, maxima at 227 mμ (E 1%, 1 cm 222) and 281·5 mμ (E 1%, 1 cm 168).

Dose. Up to 16 mg daily.

PROTOVERATRINE A *Antihypertensive*

Proprietary Name: Protalba.

An alkaloid obtained from *Veratrum album* (Liliaceae).
Protoverine 3 - (+) - 2 - hydroxy - 2 - methyl - butyrate 6,7-diacetate 15-(−)-2-methylbutyrate
$C_{41}H_{63}NO_{14} = 793{\cdot}96$

White crystals. M.p. 259° to 262°; or 302° to 304°, with decomposition.
Solubility. Insoluble in water; soluble in hot ethanol and chloroform.

PROTOVERATRINE B

Synonym: Neoprotoveratrine.

Protoverine 3 - (+) - 2,3 - dihydroxy - 2 - methylbutyrate 6,7-diacetate 15-(−)-2-methylbutyrate
$C_{41}H_{63}NO_{15} = 809{\cdot}96$

White crystals. M.p. 254° to 255°; or 285° to 290°, with decomposition.
Solubility. Insoluble in water; soluble in hot ethanol and chloroform.

PROTOVERATRINES A and B
Proprietary Names: Puroverine; Veralba.

A mixture of protoveratrines A and B.
A white crystalline sternutatory powder. M.p. 256° to 262°, with decomposition.
Solubility. Almost insoluble in water; very slightly soluble in ether; readily soluble in chloroform.

PROTOVERATRINE A and B MALEATES
Proprietary Name: Provell.

A white crystalline powder. M.p. 210° to 222°, with decomposition.
Solubility. Readily soluble in water, ethanol, and chloroform; almost insoluble in ether.

Chromatography. PAPER, for protoveratrine A: system P1—Rf 0·82 (location reagents: *iodoplatinate spray*, weak reaction; *bromocresol green spray*, weak reaction); for protoveratrine B: system P1—Rf 0·66 (location reagents: *iodoplatinate spray*, weak reaction; *bromocresol green spray*, weak reaction).
THIN-LAYER, for protoveratrine A: system T1—Rf 0·72 (location reagent *iodine–carbon tetrachloride spray*, positive reaction); for protoveratrine B: system T1—Rf 0·70 (location reagents: *acidified iodoplatinate spray*, positive reaction; *iodine–carbon tetrachloride spray*, positive reaction; *potassium permanganate spray*, positive reaction).

Crystal Tests. MICRO, for protoveratrine A: *disodium methyl arsonate solution*—dense rosettes (*sensitivity:* 1 in 200); *sodium carbonate solution*—oily rosettes (*sensitivity:* 1 in 400); for protoveratine B: *disodium methyl arsonate solution*—dense rosettes (*sensitivity:* 1 in 200); *picric acid*—oily dendrites (*sensitivity:* 1 in 100).

Dose. Up to 6 mg daily by mouth.

Toxicity. Protoveratrine A is more active than protoveratrine B, but with both alkaloids the margin between the effective antihypertensive dose and the emetic dose is very narrow. Large doses produce respiratory depression which may be followed by bronchiolar constriction and respiratory arrest. With overdosage by mouth, vomiting is so prompt that death is very rare.

PROTRIPTYLINE *Antidepressant*

Synonym: MK 240.

5 - (3 - Methylaminopropyl) - 5*H* - dibenzo[*a*,*d*] cycloheptene
$C_{19}H_{21}N = 263{\cdot}4$

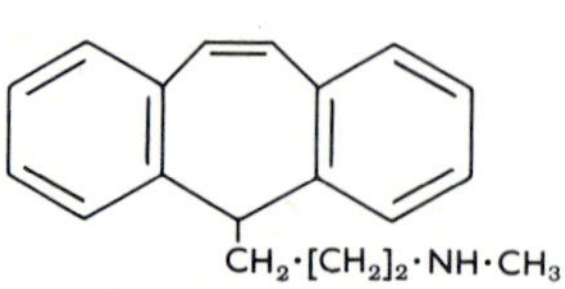

PROTRIPTYLINE HYDROCHLORIDE
Proprietary Names: Concordin; Triptil Hydrochloride; Vivactil Hydrochloride.

A white crystalline solid.
Solubility. Freely soluble in water.

Extraction. Protriptyline is extracted by organic solvents from aqueous alkaline solutions.

Chromatography. PAPER: system P1—Rf 0·70 (location under ultraviolet light, deep blue fluorescence; location reagents: *iodoplatinate spray*, weak reaction; *Marquis reagent*, dull green).
THIN-LAYER: system T1—Rf 0·23 (location reagent *acidified iodoplatinate spray*, positive reaction).
GAS: system G2/225—retention time 0·7 relative to codeine.

Colour Tests. MICRO: sulphuric acid–formaldehyde test—dull green (*sensitivity:* 0·1 μg); ammonium molybdate test—black-purple (*sensitivity:* 0·1 μg); ammonium vanadate test—purple-brown (*sensitivity:* 0·1 μg); Vitali's test—faint yellow/faint yellow/brown (*sensitivity:* 0·1 μg).

Crystal Test. MICRO: *gold cyanide solution*—bunches of plates, forming overnight (*sensitivity:* 1 in 200).

Infra-red Absorption Spectrum. Protriptyline hydrochloride. Potassium bromide disk. The principal peaks are: A 753 or 799, B 772 or 1470 (p. 760).

Metabolism. Protriptyline is well absorbed from the gastro-intestinal tract and is rapidly taken up by a variety of tissues. It appears to undergo extensive metabolism, only low levels being found in the plasma after administration. Only a small amount of unchanged protriptyline is excreted in the urine of the dog and rabbit. Preliminary studies indicate that protriptyline is demethylated to a significant extent, probably in the liver.

Dose. Up to 60 mg daily.

Toxicity. LD50 (oral): in mice 269 mg/kg.

PROXYMETACAINE *Local Anaesthetic*

Synonym: Proparacaine.

2 - Diethylaminoethyl 3 - amino - 4 - propoxy - benzoate
$C_{16}H_{26}N_2O_3 = 294{\cdot}4$

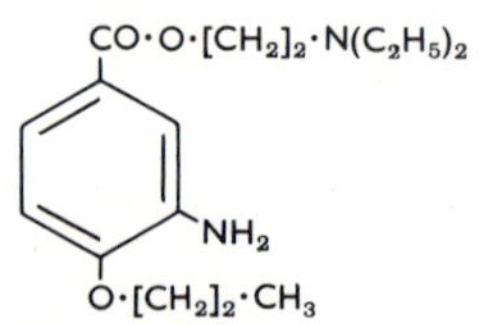

PROXYMETACAINE HYDROCHLORIDE
Proprietary Name: Ophthaine.

A white crystalline powder which discolours on heating or exposure to air.
Solubility. Soluble in water and warm ethanol.

Extraction. Proxymetacaine is extracted by organic solvents from aqueous alkaline solutions.

Chromatography. PAPER: system P1—Rf 0·52

(location under ultraviolet light, blue fluorescence; location reagents: *iodoplatinate spray*, weak reaction; *potassium permanganate spray*, strong reaction).

THIN-LAYER: system T1—Rf 0·59 (location reagents: *acidified iodoplatinate spray*, positive reaction; p-*dimethylaminobenzaldehyde spray*, yellow).

Colour Tests. MICRO: diazotisation test—red (*sensitivity:* 0·1 μg); Vitali's test— –/yellow/dull purple (*sensitivity:* 1·0 μg).

Crystal Tests. MICRO: *lead chloride solution*—needles (*sensitivity:* 1 in 400); *platinic bromide solution*—small rosettes or bunches of needles (*sensitivity:* 1 in 1000).

Use. Proxymetacaine is employed in ophthalmology, usually as eye-drops containing 0·5%.

PROXYPHYLLINE *Xanthine Derivative*

Synonym: Proxiphylline.
Proprietary Names: Brontyl; Purophyllin; Theon. It is an ingredient of Theonyl Tablets.

7-(2-Hydroxypropyl)-1,3-dimethylxanthine
$C_{10}H_{14}N_4O_3$ = 238·2

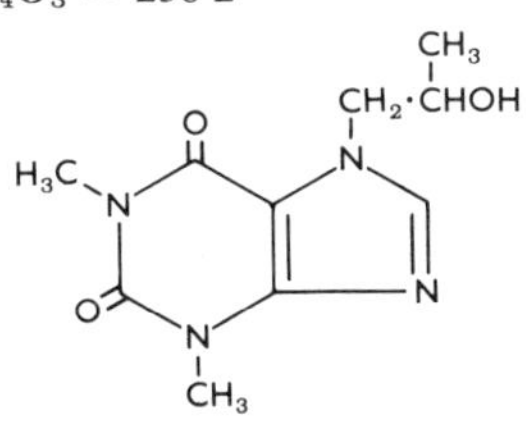

Solubility. Soluble 1 in 1 of water and 1 in 14 of dehydrated ethanol.

Extraction. Proxyphylline is extracted by organic solvents from aqueous alkaline solutions.

Chromatography. PAPER: system P1—Rf 0·73 (location under ultraviolet light, dark blue fluorescence; location by the Clarke-Kalayci test, reddish-purple); system RP1a—Rf 0·83 (location under ultraviolet light, absorption); system RP1b—Rf 0·80 (location as for RP1a).

THIN-LAYER: system T1—Rf 0·59 (location reagent *potassium permanganate spray*, positive reaction).

Colour Test. Amalic acid test—purple (see p. 127).

Crystal Test. MICRO: *gold bromide–hydrochloric acid solution*—small four-pointed stars (*sensitivity:* 1 in 200).

Ultraviolet Absorption Spectrum. Proxyphylline in 0·1N sulphuric acid, inflexion at about 230 mμ (E1%, 1 cm 227) and maximum at 273 mμ (E1%, 1 cm 373).

Infra-red Absorption Spectrum. Proxyphylline (base). Potassium bromide disk. The principal peaks are: A 1656, B 1690, C 750 (p. 760).

Dose. Up to 2 g daily.

PSEUDOEPHEDRINE *Sympathomimetic*

*Synonyms: d-ψ-*Ephedrine; *d*-Isoephedrine.

(+)-2-Methylamino-1-phenylpropan-1-ol
$C_{10}H_{15}NO$ = 165·2

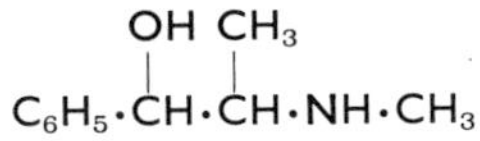

An alkaloid found together with ephedrine in various species of *Ephedra* (Ephedraceae). It is a stereoisomer of ephedrine (p. 327).

Rhombic tablets. M.p. 118° to 119°.
Solubility. Sparingly soluble in water; soluble in ethanol and ether.

PSEUDOEPHEDRINE HYDROCHLORIDE

Proprietary Names: Sudafed. It is an ingredient of Actifed, Benazma, and Emprazil.

A white crystalline powder. M.p. 183° to 186°.
Solubility. Soluble 1 in 1·6 of water, 1 in 4 of ethanol, and 1 in 60 of chloroform.

Extraction. Pseudoephedrine is extracted by organic solvents from aqueous alkaline solutions.

Chromatography. PAPER: system P1—Rf 0·39 (location under ultraviolet light, absorption; location reagents: *iodoplatinate spray*, weak reaction; *bromocresol green spray*, weak reaction); system RP1a—Rf 0·86 (location under ultraviolet light, absorption); system RP1b—Rf 0·85 (location as for RP1a).

THIN-LAYER: system T1—Rf 0·30 (location reagent *potassium permanganate spray*, positive reaction).

GAS: system G2/120—retention time 1·0 relative to ephedrine.

Colour Test. Chen's test—purple.

Ultraviolet Absorption Spectrum. Pseudoephedrine hydrochloride in water, maxima at 250·5 mμ (E1%, 1 cm 7·5), 256·5 mμ (E1%, 1 cm 9·9), and 262·5 mμ (E1%, 1 cm 7·9); minima at 227 mμ, 252·5 mμ, and 259 mμ.

Infra-red Absorption Spectrum. Pseudoephedrine hydrochloride. Potassium bromide disk. The principal peaks are: A 700, B 761 or 1031, C 1000 or 1459 (p. 760).

Dose. Usually up to 180 mg daily.

Toxicity. Ingestion of one 60-mg tablet has caused severe toxic effects.
LD50 (intraperitoneal): in mice 235 mg/kg.

PSEUDOMORPHINE

Synonym: Oxydimorphine.

$C_{34}H_{36}N_2O_6,3H_2O$ = 622·7

White crystals. M.p. 327°, with decomposition.
Solubility. Insoluble in water, ethanol, and ether; soluble in dilute hydrochloric acid, dilute acetic acid, and pyridine.

Extraction. Pseudomorphine is extracted by organic solvents from aqueous alkaline solutions.

Chromatography. PAPER: system P1—Rf 0·02 (location under ultraviolet light, blue fluorescence; location reagent *iodoplatinate spray*, strong reaction); system RP1a—Rf, tailing (location under ultraviolet light, blue fluorescence); system RP1b—Rf, tailing (location as for RP1a).

THIN-LAYER: system T1—Rf 0·13, streaking (location reagent *acidified iodoplatinate spray*, positive reaction).

GAS: system G2/225—retention time 3·0 relative to codeine.

Colour Tests. MICRO: sulphuric acid–formaldehyde test—green (*sensitivity:* 0·1 μg); ammonium molybdate test—purple → blue (*sensitivity:* 0·1 μg); Vitali's test—orange/yellow/brown (*sensitivity:* 1·0 μg).

Crystal Tests. MICRO: *platinic chloride solution*—small rods or tablets (*sensitivity:* 1 in 1000); *potassium iodide solution*—petal-shaped crystals (*sensitivity:* 1 in 1000).

Ultraviolet Absorption Spectrum. Pseudomorphine in 0·1N sulphuric acid, maxima at 231 mμ (E1%, 1cm 308) and 261 mμ (E1%, 1cm 200).

NOTE. Pseudomorphine may be found as an oxidation product of morphine in decomposed viscera.

PSILOCIN *Hallucinogen*

Synonym: 4-Hydroxydimethyltryptamine.

An indole alkaloid obtained from the mushroom, *Psilocybe mexicana* (Agaricaceae).

3-(2-Dimethylaminoethyl)-4-hydroxyindole

$C_{12}H_{16}N_2O = 204{\cdot}3$

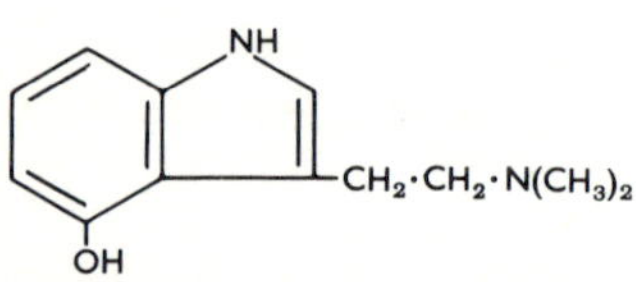

White crystals. M.p. 173° to 176°.

Solubility. Soluble in ethanol and dilute acetic acid.

Extraction. Psilocin is extracted by organic solvents from aqueous ammoniacal solutions.

Chromatography. PAPER: system P1—Rf 0·31 (location under ultraviolet light, absorption; location reagents: *iodoplatinate spray*, strong reaction; *bromocresol green spray*, weak reaction).

THIN-LAYER: system T1—Rf 0·34 (location reagent p-*dimethylaminobenzaldehyde spray*, faint blue).

Colour Tests. MICRO: sulphuric acid–formaldehyde test—greenish-brown (*sensitivity:* 0·25 μg); ammonium molybdate test—greenish-blue → yellow (*sensitivity:* 0·1 μg); Vitali's test—green → brown / brown / red-brown (*sensitivity:* 0·25 μg).

Crystal Tests. MICRO: *gold cyanide solution*—branching needles, best viewed under polarised light (*sensitivity:* 1 in 100); *trinitrobenzoic acid solution*—bunches of needles (*sensitivity:* 1 in 100).

Ultraviolet Absorption Spectrum. Psilocin in 0·01N hydrochloric acid, maxima at 222 mμ, 268 mμ, 285 mμ, and 294 mμ.

Metabolism. Psilocin is less stable than psilocybin which is converted to psilocin in the body. It is thought to be the active hallucinogen.

Dose. 6 to 10 mg of psilocin is sufficient to produce a hallucinogenic syndrome similar to that produced by lysergide.

PSILOCYBIN *Hallucinogen*

Synonym: 4-Phosphoryloxy-*NN*-dimethyltryptamine.
Proprietary Name: Indocybin.

The main indole alkaloid present in the mushroom, *Psilocybe mexicana* (Agaricaceae).

3 - (2 - Dimethylaminoethyl)indol - 4 - yl dihydrogen phosphate

$C_{12}H_{17}N_2O_4P = 284{\cdot}3$

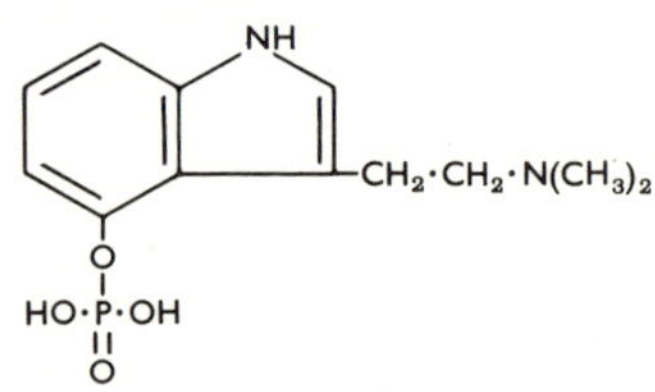

White crystals. M.p. 185° to 195°, with decomposition.

Solubility. Soluble in dilute acetic acid.

Extraction. Psilocybin is extracted by methanol from dry material.

Chromatography. PAPER: system P1—Rf 0·06 (location under ultraviolet light, dark blue fluorescence; location reagents: *iodine vapour*, weak reaction; *Marquis reagent*, faint orange).

THIN-LAYER: system T1—Rf 0·05 (location reagent p-*dimethylaminobenzaldehyde spray*, grey-purple).

Colour Tests. MICRO: sulphuric acid–formaldehyde test—dull orange (*sensitivity:* 0·5 μg); ammonium molybdate test—grey-blue → green → yellow (*sensitivity:* 0·5 μg).

Ultraviolet Absorption Spectrum. Psilocybin in methanol, maxima at 267 mμ and 290 mμ; minima at 242 mμ and 287 mμ.

Metabolism. Psilocybin is rapidly converted in the body by dephosphorylation to psilocin which appears to be the psychoactive compound. After distribution in the body the highest concentration is found in the liver and kidneys.

Up to 11% of a dose is excreted in the urine as unchanged psilocin and 20% as a glucuronic acid derivative; 3·5% is demethylated and degraded to indole acid derivatives. Some 15 to 20% of the dose is found in the bile.

Dose. Doses of 6 to 15 mg may produce a hallucinogenic syndrome similar to that of lysergide.

PULEGIUM OIL *Essential Oil*

Synonym: Pennyroyal Oil.

An oil obtained by distillation from fresh pennyroyal herb, *Mentha pulegium* (Labiatae); it contains not less than 85% of pulegone ($C_{10}H_{16}O$ = 152·2).

A yellow to greenish-yellow oil with an aromatic mint-like odour. Refractive index 1·482 to 1·487.

Solubility. Slightly soluble in water; soluble 1 in 3 of ethanol (70%); soluble in ether and chloroform.

Extraction. Pulegium oil is volatile and may be isolated by distillation (see p. 18).

Colour Tests. Mix a drop with a drop of *sulphuric acid*—orange; mix a drop with a drop of *fuming nitric acid*—deep yellow.

Metabolism. Pulegone has been shown in rabbits to be reduced first to pulegol and then to menthol; both these compounds may be excreted as glucuronides.

Toxicity. The effect of the oil on any particular person is unpredictable; a teaspoonful has caused convulsions and 15 ml of pennyroyal essence (about 1 in 10 of the oil) has produced coma.

CASE EXAMPLE. A healthy woman, aged 24, in the third month of pregnancy, took pulegium oil (dose unknown). The drug produced abortion, vaginal bleeding, haemolytic anaemia, and acute tubular necrosis of the kidney, with death from uraemia on the 14th day (Vallance, 1955).

PUTRESCINE *Putrefactive Base*

Synonym: Tetramethylenediamine.

Butane-1,4-diamine

$H_2N \cdot [CH_2]_4 \cdot NH_2$ = 88·2

Crystals with a strong odour. M.p. 27° to 28°. B.p. 158° to 159°.

Solubility. Very soluble in water.

Extraction. Putrescine is very soluble in water and is not usually found in toxicological extracts. If it is present in large quantities it may be extracted by chloroform.

Chromatography. PAPER: system P1—Rf 0·00 (location reagents: *iodoplatinate spray*, white; *bromocresol green spray*, weak reaction).

THIN-LAYER: system T1—Rf 0·02 (location reagent *acidified iodoplatinate spray*, positive reaction).

Crystal Tests. MICRO: *picric acid*—needles (*sensitivity:* 1 in 1000); *platinic iodide solution*—small rectagular plates (*sensitvity:* 1 in 1000).

Metabolism. Putrescine is formed during putrefaction by bacterial decarboxylation of lysine in the gastro-intestinal tract. It may be deaminated to yield ammonia and an aldehyde.

PYRAZINAMIDE *Tuberculostatic*

Synonym: Pyrazinoic Acid Amide.

Proprietary Names: Aldinamide; Tebrazide; Zinamide.

Pyrazinecarboxyamide

$C_5H_5N_3O$ = 123·1

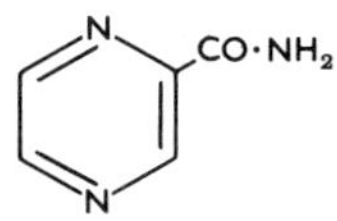

A white crystalline powder. M.p. 188° to 191°.

Solubility. Soluble 1 in 60 of water and 1 in 110 of ethanol; soluble in ether and chloroform.

Extraction. Pyrazinamide is extracted by organic solvents from aqueous acid or alkaline solutions.

Chromatography. PAPER: system P1—Rf 0·56 (location under ultraviolet light, strong absorption; location reagents: *iodoplatinate spray*, white; *potassium permanganate spray*, weak reaction); system RP1a—Rf 0·83 (location under ultraviolet light, absorption); system RP1b—Rf 0·80 (location as for RP1a).

THIN-LAYER: system T1—Rf 0·63 (location reagent *iodine–carbon tetrachloride spray*, positive reaction).

Crystal Tests. MICRO: *mercuric chloride solution*—needles, some curving (*sensitivity:* 1 in 1000); *platinic chloride solution*—grains, best viewed under polarised light (*sensitivity:* 1 in 1000).

Ultraviolet Absorption Spectrum. Pyrazinamide in water, maxima at 268 mμ (E1%, 1 cm 1310) and 310 mμ (E1%, 1 cm 110); in 0·1N sulphuric acid, maxima at 269 mμ (E1%, 1 cm 652) and 312 mμ (E1%, 1 cm 43) and an inflexion at 275 mμ.

Dose. Up to 3 g daily.

Toxicity. Liver damage appears in about 15% of patients taking the maximum dose and jaundice occurs in 2 to 3%.

PYRIDOSTIGMINE BROMIDE *Anticholinesterase*

Proprietary Name: Mestinon.

3 - Dimethylcarbamoyloxy - 1 - methylpyridinium bromide

$C_9H_{13}BrN_2O_2$ = 261·1

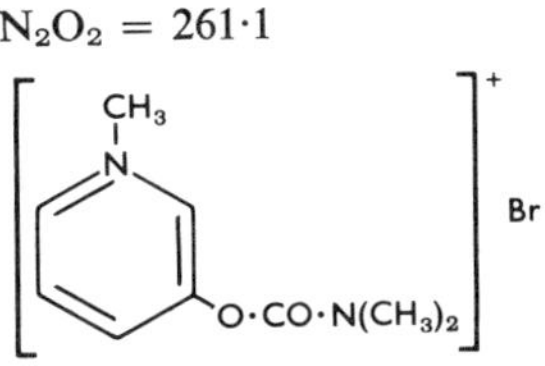

A white deliquescent crystalline powder. M.p. 153° to 156°.

Solubility. Soluble 1 in less than 1 of water, 1 in less than 1 of ethanol, and 1 in 1 of chloroform; almost insoluble in ether.

Extraction. Pyridostigmine bromide is a quaternary ammonium compound (see p. 29).

Chromatography. PAPER: system P1—Rf 0·12 (location under ultraviolet light, strong absorption; location reagent *iodoplatinate spray*, strong reaction).

THIN-LAYER: system T1—Rf 0·04 (location reagent *acidified iodoplatinate spray*, positive reaction).

Crystal Tests. MICRO: *gold bromide solution*—curved branching needles (*sensitivity:* 1 in 400); *gold bromide-hydrochloric acid solution*—rosettes or bunches of serrated plates (*sensitivity:* 1 in 400).

Ultraviolet Absorption Spectrum. Pyridostigmine bromide in water, maximum at 269 mμ (E1%, 1 cm 265); in 0·1N sulphuric acid, maximum at 269 mμ (E1%, 1 cm 180).

Infra-red Absorption Spectrum. Potassium bromide disk. The principal peaks are: A 1728, B 1156, C 1249 (p. 760).

Metabolism. Hydrolysis may occur at the ester linkage.

Dose. Up to 240 mg by mouth; up to 5 mg by injection.

Toxicity. The toxic effects of overdosage usually result from the cholinergic action of pyridostigmine—intestinal cramps, diarrhoea, sweating, miosis, hypotension, bradycardia, fasciculation, bromide rash, and vomiting (A.M.A. Council on Drugs, 1962). The estimated minimum lethal dose in man is 100 mg by mouth.

PYRIDOXINE *Vitamin*

Synonyms: Adermine; Pyridoxol; Vitamin B_6.

3 - Hydroxy - 4,5 - di(hydroxymethyl) - 2 - methylpyridine

$C_8H_{11}NO_3 = 169{\cdot}2$

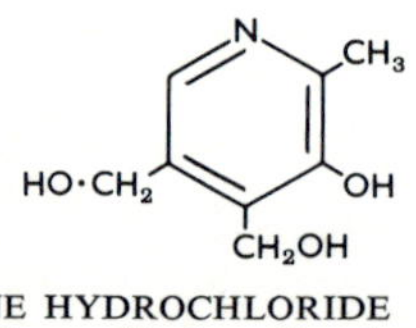

PYRIDOXINE HYDROCHLORIDE

Proprietary Names: Beadox; Benadon; Hexa-Betalin; Hexavibox; Hexobion; Pyrivel.

A white crystalline powder which is slowly affected by sunlight. M.p. about 206°, with decomposition.

Solubility. Soluble 1 in 5 of water and 1 in 100 of ethanol; insoluble in ether and chloroform.

Extraction. Pyridoxine is extracted by organic solvents from aqueous alkaline solutions.

Chromatography. PAPER: system P1—Rf 0·18 (location under ultraviolet light, blue fluorescence; location reagents: *iodoplatinate spray*, white; *bromocresol green spray*, strong reaction); system RP1a—Rf 0·90 (location under ultraviolet light, blue fluorescence); system RP1b—Rf 0·86 (location as for RP1a).

THIN-LAYER: system T1—Rf 0·59 (location reagent *potassium permanganate spray*, positive reaction).

Colour Tests. MICRO: ammonium molybdate test—faint blue (*sensitivity:* 0·25 μg); ammonium vanadate test—blue → grey-green (*sensitivity:* 0·25 μg).

Crystal Tests. MICRO: *platinic iodide solution*—small rectangular crystals (*sensitivity:* 1 in 1000); *potassium bismuth iodide solution*—bunches of plates or blades (*sensitivity:* 1 in 200).

Ultraviolet Absorption Spectrum. Pyridoxine hydrochloride in solution at pH 7, maxima at 254 mμ (E1%, 1 cm about 219) and 324 mμ (E1%, 1 cm 426); in 0·1N hydrochloric acid, maximum at 291 mμ (E1%, 1 cm about 523).

Infra-red Absorption Spectrum. Pyridoxine hydrochloride. Potassium bromide disk. The principal peaks are: A 1536, B 1273, C 1207 (p. 761).

Metabolism. Pyridoxine, pyridoxal, and pyridoxamine, which occur in foodstuffs, are collectively known as vitamin B_6. In the body all three are converted to pyridoxal phosphate which is the coenzyme for amino-acid decarboxylase and for transaminase.

Although, owing to the wide distribution of vitamin B_6 in nature, clinical deficiency symptoms are seldom observed, there is little doubt that pyridoxine is essential in human nutrition. As a nutritional supplement it is usually employed in conjunction with other vitamins of the B group. For adults, the daily requirement of pyridoxine is probably about 2 mg and this amount is present in most normal diets.

Dose. Up to 150 mg daily.

Toxicity. LD50 (oral): in rats 5·5 g/kg.

PYRIMETHAMINE *Antimalarial*

Synonyms: BW 50-63; RP 4753.

Proprietary Names: Daraprim (tablets); Malocide. It is an ingredient of Daraclor.

2,4 - Diamino - 5 - *p* - chlorophenyl - 6 - ethyl - pyrimidine

$C_{12}H_{13}ClN_4 = 248{\cdot}7$

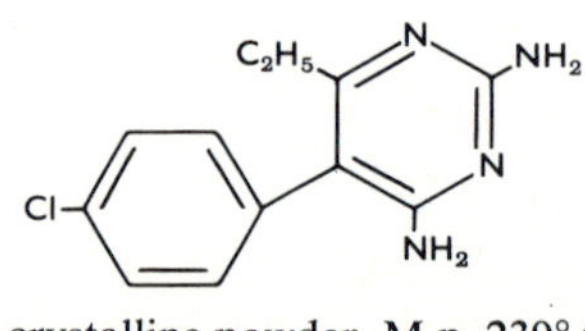

A white crystalline powder. M.p. 239° to 242°.

Solubility. Insoluble in water; soluble 1 in 200 of ethanol and 1 in 125 of chloroform.

PYRIMETHAMINE SULPHATE
Proprietary Name: Daraprim (elixir).

Solubility. Sparingly soluble in cold water; soluble in hot water.

Extraction. Pyrimethamine is extracted by organic solvents from aqueous alkaline solutions.

Chromatography. PAPER: system P1—Rf 0·42 (location under ultraviolet light, blue fluorescence; location reagent *iodoplatinate spray*, weak reaction); system RP1a—Rf 0·42 (location under ultraviolet light, blue fluorescence); system RP1b—Rf 0·08 (location as for RP1a).
THIN-LAYER: system T1—Rf 0·68 (location reagent *acidified iodoplatinate spray*, positive reaction).

Crystal Tests. MICRO: *gold bromide–hydrochloric acid solution*—serrated needles (*sensitivity:* 1 in 1000); *potassium chromate solution*—irregular blades (*sensitivity:* 1 in 1000).

Ultraviolet Absorption Spectrum. Pyrimethamine in ethanol, maximum at 287 mμ (E 1%, 1 cm 365); in 0·005 N hydrochloric acid, maximum at 272 mμ (E 1%, 1 cm 320).

Infra-red Absorption Spectrum. Pyrimethamine (base). Potassium bromide disk. The principal peaks are: A 1445 or 1575 or 1628 (p. 761).

Metabolism. Pyrimethamine affects the nucleoprotein metabolism of the malarial parasites by interference in the folic-folinic acid systems and its action is exerted mainly at the time when the nucleus divides. It has little effect upon immature schizonts in the red corpuscles and therefore it is slow to control a malarial attack; its chief value is as a suppressant.
It has been observed that about 1 mg still remains in the body 30 days after a single dose of 100 mg. It is excreted in the milk of nursing mothers. Several metabolites of pyrimethamine appear in the urine; little is known of their structure or antimalarial activity.

Dose. Up to 50 mg weekly, as a suppressant of malaria.

Toxicity. In a dosage of 25 mg once weekly, pyrimethamine is unlikely to give rise to toxic effects but doses of 25 mg once daily over a prolonged period may cause depression of haemopoiesis due to the interference of the drug in the metabolism of folic acid.
Very large doses of pyrimethamine cause vomiting, convulsions, and collapse. Children have died following the ingestion of 400 mg, 750 mg, and over 1 g of pyrimethamine.

PYRITHIDIUM BROMIDE

Trypanocide (Veterinary)

Proprietary Name: Prothidium.

3 - Amino - 8 - (2 - amino - 6 - methylpyrimidin - 4 - ylamino) - 6 - *p* - aminophenylphenanthridine 5,1′-dimethobromide

$C_{26}H_{27}Br_2N_7$ = 597·4

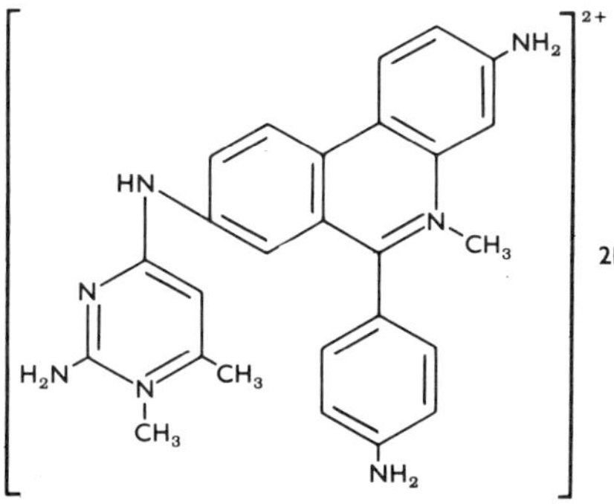

A brick-red to reddish-purple hygroscopic powder.
Solubility. Soluble 1 in 200 of water.

Extraction. Pyrithidium bromide is a quaternary ammonium compound (see p. 29).

Chromatography. PAPER: system P1—Rf 0·00 (location under ultraviolet light, orange fluorescence; location reagents: *iodoplatinate spray*, weak reaction; *potassium permanganate spray*, weak reaction).
THIN-LAYER: system T1—Rf 0·01 (location under ultraviolet light, yellow fluorescence; location reagents: *acidified iodoplatinate spray*, positive reaction; *iodine–carbon tetrachloride spray*, positive reaction).

Crystal Tests. MICRO: *gold cyanide solution*—masses of small oily needles (*sensitivity:* 1 in 1000); *trinitrobenzoic acid solution*—dense or gelatinous rosettes (*sensitivity:* 1 in 200).

Ultraviolet Absorption Spectrum. Pyrithidium bromide in 2N sulphuric acid, maxima at 255 mμ (E 1%, 1 cm 400) and 313 mμ (E 1%, 1 cm 860).

Infra-red Absorption Spectrum. Potassium bromide disk. The principal peaks are: A 1615 or 1642, B 1489, C 1515 (p. 793).

Dose. Cattle, usually 2 mg/kg intramuscularly or subcutaneously.

Toxicity. Doses of 5 mg/kg have occasionally caused death in cattle following loss of weight and liver damage.

PYRROBUTAMINE

Antihistamine

1 - (4 - *p* - Chlorophenyl - 3 - phenylbut - 2 - enyl)pyrrolidine
$C_{20}H_{22}ClN$ = 311·9

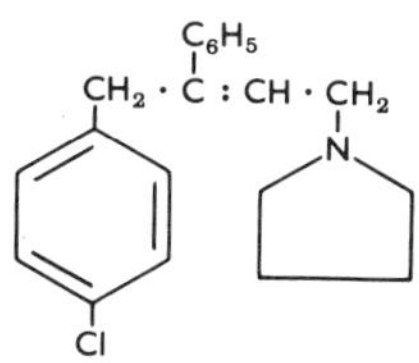

PYRROBUTAMINE PHOSPHATE
Proprietary Names: Proladyl; Pyronil. It is an ingredient of Co-Pyronil.

A white crystalline powder. M.p. 127° to 131°.
Solubility. Soluble in water; slightly soluble in ethanol; practically insoluble in ether and chloroform.

Extraction. Pyrrobutamine is extracted by organic solvents from aqueous alkaline solutions.

Chromatography. PAPER: system P1—Rf 0·84 (location under ultraviolet light, strong absorption; location reagents: *iodoplatinate spray*, strong reaction; *bromocresol green spray*, weak reaction); system RP1a—Rf 0·11 (location under ultraviolet light, absorption; location reagent *iodoplatinate spray*, positive reaction); system RP1b—Rf 0·04 (location as for RP1a).
THIN-LAYER: system T1—Rf 0·49 (location reagent *acidified iodoplatinate spray*, positive reaction); system T3—Rf 0·84 (location reagent *iodoplatinate spray*, positive reaction).
GAS: system G2/225—retention time 1·14 relative to codeine; system G4—retention time 1·2 relative to codeine.

Colour Tests. MICRO: sulphuric acid–formaldehyde test—grey-purple (*sensitivity:* 0·5 µg); ammonium molybdate test—blue → yellow (*sensitivity:* 0·1 µg); ammonium vanadate test—purple (*sensitivity:* 0·5 µg).

Crystal Tests. MICRO: *potassium iodide solution*—irregular blades (*sensitivity:* 1 in 1000); *potassium tri-iodide solution* (*2*)—branching needles (*sensitivity:* 1 in 1000).

Ultraviolet Absorption Spectrum. Pyrrobutamine in 0·1N sulphuric acid, maximum at 227 mµ (E1%, 1 cm 232) and an inflexion at 240 mµ; pyrrobutamine phosphate in 0·1N hydrochloric acid, maximum at about 226 mµ.

Infra-red Absorption Spectrum. Pyrrobutamine (base). Potassium bromide disk. The principal peaks are: A 989 or 1009, B 1080 (p. 761).

Dose. Up to 45 mg daily.

Toxicity. The estimated lethal dose in man is 25 to 250 mg/kg.

QUINALBARBITONE *Barbiturate*

Synonyms: Meballymal; Secobarbital.
Proprietary Name: Seconal.

5-Allyl-5-(1-methylbutyl)barbituric acid
$C_{12}H_{18}N_2O_3 = 238{\cdot}3$

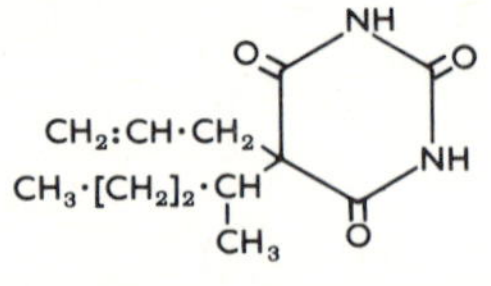

A white amorphous powder. M.p. 100°.
Solubility. Slightly soluble in water; very soluble in ethanol and ether; soluble in solutions of alkali hydroxides.

QUINALBARBITONE SODIUM
Synonyms: Meballymalnatrium; Secobarbital Sodium; Soluble Secobarbital.
Proprietary Names: Evronal Sodium; Imesonal; Quinalspan; Seconal Sodium.

A white hygroscopic powder.
Solubility. Soluble 1 in 3 of water and 1 in 5 of ethanol; almost insoluble in ether.

Screening Tests. See under Barbiturates, p. 208.

Extraction. Quinalbarbitone may be isolated in the A2 fraction (see p. 27).

Chromatography. PAPER: system P2—Rf 1·40, relative to amylobarbitone (location under ultraviolet light, dark spot); system P3—Rf 0·13 (location reagent *silver nitrate spray*, white); system P4—Rf 0·56 (location as for P3); system P5—Rf 1·00 (location under ultraviolet light after exposure to ammonia, absorption); system RP1b—Rf 0·12 (location under ultraviolet light after exposure to ammonia; location reagent *potassium permanganate spray*, yellow on pink).
THIN-LAYER: system T10—Rf 0·44 (location reagents: *mercurous nitrate spray*, black; *potassium permanganate spray*, yellow-brown on purple; *Zwikker's reagent spray*, pink); system T11—Rf 0·46 (location reagents: *mercurous nitrate spray*, white on grey; *potassium permanganate spray*, yellow on purple); system T12—Rf 0·64 (location as for T11); system T13—Rf 0·54 (location as for T11).
GAS: system G1/180—retention time 0·87 relative to diphenhydramine; system G3—retention time 2·40 relative to diphenhydramine; system G5—retention time 3·02 relative to barbitone; system G7—retention time 2·30 relative to barbitone.

Colour Test. Zwikker's test—violet-blue.

Ultraviolet Absorption Spectrum. Quinalbarbitone is a 5,5-derivative—see Screening Test 3 under Barbiturates, p. 208.

Infra-red Absorption Spectrum. Quinalbarbitone sodium. Potassium bromide disk. The principal peaks are: A 1559, B 1648, C 1690 (p. 761).

Quantitative Estimation. See under Barbiturates, p. 208.
A method for the spectrophotometric determination of quinalbarbitone in the presence of amylobarbitone has been described by Moy and Wetherell (1967).

Metabolism. Quinalbarbitone is a short-acting barbiturate—see under Barbiturates, p. 207.
Only a small amount of ingested quinalbarbitone is excreted unchanged in the urine. The remainder is excreted as 5-allyl-5-(1-hydroxy-1-methylbutyl)barbituric acid, 5-(1-methylbutyl)barbituric acid, and 5-(2,3-dihydroxypropyl)-5-(1-methylbutyl)barbituric acid (Waddell, 1963; Cochin and Daly, 1963; Niyogi *et al.*, 1965). 5-Allyl-5-(3-hydroxy-1-methylbutyl)barbituric acid and 5-allyl-5-(4-carboxy-1-methylbutyl)barbituric acid have also been recovered from the urine—see under The Metabolism of Drugs, p. 156.

About 37% of the quinalbarbitone in blood post mortem appears to be protein-bound (Turner, 1964b).

Dose. Up to 400 mg.

Toxicity. The estimated minimum lethal dose in man is 2 g.

CASE EXAMPLE. A 33-year-old woman, found unconscious 9 hours after taking an overdose of quinalbarbitone, died 85 hours later. Post-mortem levels of the barbiturate were: blood, 0·07 mg%; brain, 0·15 mg%; fat, 0·40 mg%; heart, 0·12 mg%; kidney, 4·6 mg%; liver, 0·25 mg%; muscle, 0·20 mg%; stomach contents, 0·13 mg% (Niyogi *et al.*, 1965).

QUINAPYRAMINE CHLORIDE

Trypanocide (*Veterinary*)

Proprietary Name: Antrycide.

4 - Amino - 6 - (2′ - amino - 6′ - methylpyrimid - 4′ - ylamino) - 2 - methylquinoline 1,1′ - di - methochloride dihydrate

$C_{17}H_{22}Cl_2N_6,2H_2O = 417·3$

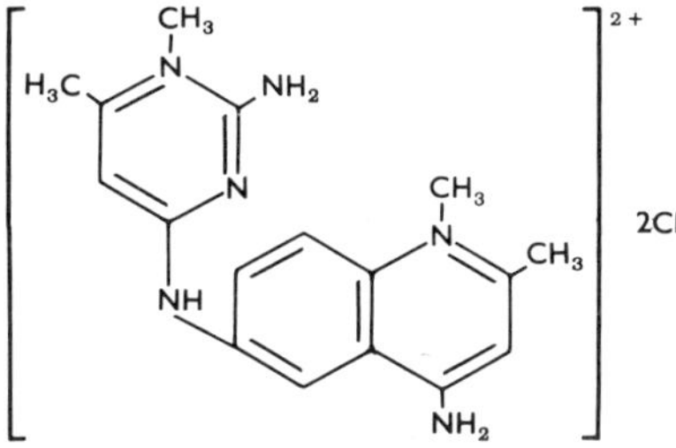

A white crystalline powder. M.p. 310°, with decomposition.

Solubility. Soluble 1 in 850 of water and 1 in 50 of boiling water; almost insoluble in ethanol, ether, and chloroform.

QUINAPYRAMINE SULPHATE

The 1,1′-dimetho(methylsulphate) salt of quinapyramine

A white crystalline powder. M.p. 266°, with decomposition.

Solubility. Soluble 1 in 2 of water; almost insoluble in ethanol, ether, and chloroform.

Extraction. The quinapyramine salts are quaternary ammonium compounds (see p. 29).

Chromatography. PAPER: system P1—Rf 0·01 (location under ultraviolet light, bright blue fluorescence; location reagent *iodoplatinate spray*, strong reaction).

THIN-LAYER: system T1—Rf 0·02 (location reagent *acidified iodoplatinate spray*, positive reaction).

Colour Test. MICRO: Vitali's test—blue-grey/yellow/orange (*sensitivity:* 1·0 μg).

Crystal Tests. MICRO: *platinic chloride solution*—small rosettes of plates (*sensitivity:* 1 in 1000); *potassium iodide solution*—hairlike needles (*sensitivity:* 1 in 1000).

Ultraviolet Absorption Spectrum. Quinapyramine sulphate in 0·1N sulphuric acid, maxima at 248 mμ (E1%, 1cm 415), 296·5 mμ (E1%, 1cm 771), 325 mμ (E1%, 1cm 288), and about 348 mμ (E1%, 1cm 218).

Metabolism. The 1,1′-dimethochloride dihydrate salt is absorbed very much more slowly than the 1,1′-dimetho(methylsulphate) so the two salts are commonly used prophylactically as 'pro-salt R.F.', a mixture of 4 parts of the chloride to 3 of the sulphate. Rapid absorption of the sulphate gives an initial high blood-level which is maintained by slow release from the chloride depot at the injection site.

Dose. 4·4 mg/kg subcutaneously.

Toxicity. Overdosage causes tremors, incoordination, increase in respiration and heart rate, and dementia. Acute inflammation of the gastro-intestinal tract and nephrosis have been found post mortem.

QUINIDINE

Myocardial Depressant

Synonyms: Chinidinum; Quinidina.

An alkaloid obtained from the bark of various species of *Cinchona* (Rubiaceae). It is a stereoisomer of quinine. Commercial samples may contain 20 to 30% of hydroquinidine (p. 372).

$C_{20}H_{24}N_2O_2,2H_2O = 360·5$

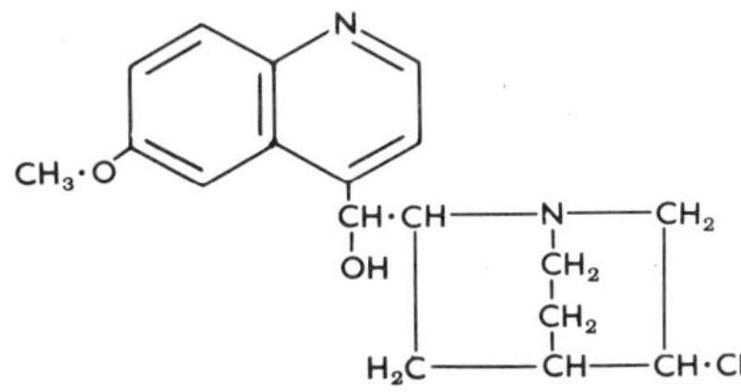

A white amorphous or crystalline powder. Specific rotation of a 1% solution in 0·1N sulphuric acid, not less than +320°.

Solubility. Soluble 1 in 2000 of water, 1 in 750 of boiling water, 1 in 17 of ethanol, and 1 in 70 of ether; the anhydrous alkaloid is soluble 1 in 1·6 of chloroform.

QUINIDINE GLUCONATE

Proprietary Name: Quinaglute.

A white powder.

Solubility. Freely soluble in water; slightly soluble in ethanol.

QUINIDINE SULPHATE

Proprietary Names: Kinidin; Quinicardine; Quinidate.

White needle-like crystals which darken on exposure to light.

Solubility. Soluble 1 in 80 of water, 1 in 15 of boiling water, 1 in 10 of ethanol, and 1 in 15 of chloroform; insoluble in ether.

Extraction. Quinidine is extracted by organic solvents from aqueous alkaline solutions.

Chromatography. PAPER: system P1—Rf 0·48 (location under ultraviolet light, bright blue fluorescence; location reagents: *iodoplatinate spray*, strong reaction; *bromocresol green spray*, weak reaction); system RP1a—Rf 0·71 (location under ultraviolet light, blue fluorescence; location reagent *iodoplatinate spray*, positive reaction); system RP1b—Rf 0·11 (location as for RP1a).

THIN-LAYER: system T1—Rf 0·55 (location reagent *acidified iodoplatinate spray*, positive reaction).

GAS: system G1/250—retention time 2·44 relative to codeine.

Colour Test. Thalleioquin test—green.

Crystal Tests. MICRO: *potassium iodide solution*—irregular crystals, often triangular (*sensitivity:* 1 in 3000); *sodium carbonate solution*—dense rosettes, forming overnight (*sensitivity:* 1 in 1000).

Ultraviolet Absorption Spectrum. Quinidine in ethanol, maxima at 236 mμ (E1%, 1 cm 1110), 278 mμ (E1%, 1 cm 132), and 332 mμ (E1%, 1 cm 163).

Infra-red Absorption Spectrum. Quinidine (base). Potassium bromide disk. The principal peaks are: A 1258, B 1514, C 1040 or 1619 (p. 761).

Metabolism. Quinidine is metabolised by hydroxylation at the 2-position of the quinuclidine nucleus and to a smaller extent at the 2′-position of the quinoline ring—see under The Metabolism of Drugs, p. 161. It is also excreted to some extent in the unchanged form. Oxidation at the 2′-position may result in a loss of activity.

Dose. Up to 3 g daily.

Toxicity. Idiosyncrasy is not uncommon; each patient should receive a test dose before treatment. Quinidine is cumulative in action and overdosage may be fatal; death may follow a dose as low as 300 mg.

LD50 (oral): in mice about 590 mg/kg (of sulphate).

CASE EXAMPLES. Out of 611 case reports of atrial fibrillation treated with quinidine, 20 were recorded as sudden deaths from quinidine shock (Thomson, 1956).

After direct current conversion of her atrial fibrillation, a 45-year-old woman was given two 300-mg doses of quinidine; 10 hours after the first dose she became unconscious and died (Halmos, 1965).

A young woman ingested a fatal quantity of quinidine. Post-mortem analyses: kidneys, 17 mg%; liver, 146 mg%; spleen, 58 mg%; stomach contents, 68 mg; urine, 1144 mg% (Jackson, 1967).

QUININE *Antimalarial*

Synonyms: Chininum; Quinina.

The chief alkaloid of various species of *Cinchona* (Rubiaceae). It is a stereo-isomer of quinidine, and normally exists as the trihydrate.

$C_{20}H_{24}N_2O_2, 3H_2O = 378{\cdot}5$

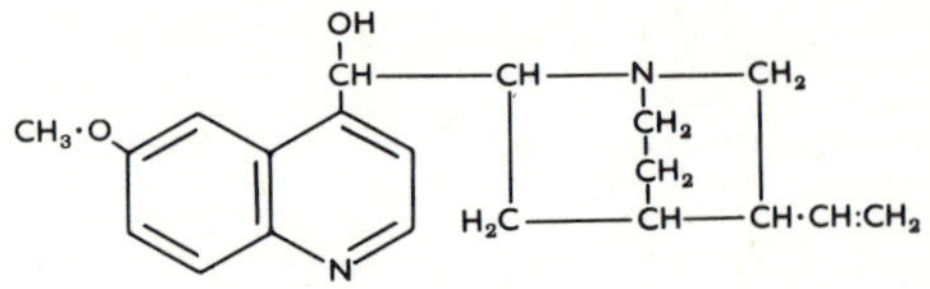

A white, granular, slightly efflorescent, microcrystalline powder. M.p. of the anhydrous substance, about 174°. Specific rotation of a 1% solution in 0·2N sulphuric acid, −266° to −277°.

Solubility. Slightly soluble in water; soluble 1 in 1 of ethanol, 1 in 4 of ether saturated with water, and 1 in 3 of chloroform.

QUININE BISULPHATE

Synonyms: Neutral Quinine Sulphate; Quinine Acid Sulphate.

A white efflorescent crystalline powder which darkens on exposure to light. Specific rotation of a 3% solution in 0·1N hydrochloric acid, about −210°.

Solubility. Soluble 1 in 8 of water, 1 in 1 of boiling water, 1 in 50 of ethanol, and 1 in 625 of chloroform.

QUININE DIHYDROBROMIDE.

Synonyms: Neutral Quinine Hydrobromide; Quinine Acid Hydrobromide.

White crystals or powder.

Solubility. Soluble 1 in 7 of water; very soluble in ethanol; insoluble in ether.

QUININE DIHYDROCHLORIDE

Synonyms: Neutral Quinine Hydrochloride; Quinine Acid Hydrochloride.

Proprietary Name: It is an ingredient of Coryzin.

A white powder. Specific rotation of a 3% solution in 0·1N hydrochloric acid, about −225°.

Solubility. Soluble 1 in 0·5 of water, 1 in 14 of ethanol, and 1 in 7 of chloroform; almost insoluble in ether.

QUININE ETHYL CARBONATE

Synonym: Euquinina.

White masses of silky crystals which darken on exposure to light.

Solubility. Slightly soluble in water; soluble 1 in 2 of ethanol, 1 in 10 of ether, and 1 in 1 of chloroform.

QUININE HYDROBROMIDE

Synonym: Basic Quinine Hydrobromide.

White silky efflorescent crystals which darken on exposure to light.

Solubility. Soluble 1 in 55 of water, 1 in 1 of boiling water, 1 in 0·7 of ethanol, and 1 in 1 of chloroform; slightly soluble in ether.

QUININE HYDROCHLORIDE

Synonyms: Basic Quinine Hydrochloride; Quinine Hydrochlorate; Quininium Chloride.

Colourless or white, needle-like crystals which effloresce in warm air and become yellowish on exposure to light. Specific rotation of a 3% solution in 0·1N hydrochloric acid, about −245°.

Solubility. Soluble 1 in 23 of water, 1 in less than 1 of ethanol, and 1 in 2 of chloroform; very slightly soluble in ether.

QUININE PHOSPHATE
Fine white needles or crystalline powder.
Solubility. Soluble 1 in about 600 of water, 1 in about 200 of ethanol, and 1 in 60 of boiling ethanol.

QUININE SALICYLATE
White crystals or a crystalline powder which becomes pink on keeping.
Solubility. Very slightly soluble in water; soluble 1 in 24 of ethanol, 1 in 160 of ether, and 1 in 25 of chloroform.

QUININE SULPHATE
Synonyms: Basic Quinine Sulphate; Quininium Sulphate.
White needle-like crystals which become brown on exposure to light. Specific rotation of a 3% solution in 0·1N hydrochloric acid, about −240°.
Solubility. Soluble 1 in 810 of water, 1 in 35 of boiling water, 1 in 95 of ethanol, and 1 in 10 of boiling ethanol; slightly soluble in ether and chloroform.

QUININE TANNATE
A pale yellow or yellowish-white amorphous powder.
Solubility. Slightly soluble in cold water; soluble 1 in 30 of boiling water and 1 in 3 of ethanol.

Extraction. Quinine is extracted by organic solvents from aqueous alkaline solutions.

Chromatography. PAPER: system P1—Rf 0·46 (location under ultraviolet light, bright blue fluorescence; location reagents: *iodoplatinate spray*, strong reaction; *bromocresol green spray*, weak reaction); system RP1a—Rf 0·71 (location under ultraviolet light, blue fluorescence; location reagent *iodoplatinate spray*, positive reaction); system RP1b—Rf 0·11 (location as for RP1a).

THIN-LAYER: system T1—Rf 0·52 (location under ultraviolet light, blue fluorescence; location reagent *acidified iodoplatinate spray*, positive reaction).

GAS: system G1/250—retention time 2·44 relative to codeine; system G6—retention time 2·81 relative to codeine.

Colour Test. Thalleioquin test—green.

Crystal Tests. MICRO: *platinic iodide solution*—curved serrated needles, forming overnight (*sensitivity:* 1 in 1500); *sodium phosphate solution*—needles (*sensitivity:* 1 in 1000).

Ultraviolet Absorption Spectrum. Quinine in ethanol, maxima at 236 mμ (E1%, 1cm 1110), 278 mμ (E1%, 1cm 133), and 332 mμ (E1%, 1cm 163); in 0·1N sulphuric acid, maxima at 250 mμ (E1%, 1cm 1005), 316 mμ (E1%, 1cm 154), and 346 mμ (E1%, 1cm 188).

Infra-red Absorption Spectrum. Quinine (base). Potassium bromide disk. The principal peaks are: A 1235, B 1510, C 1030 or 1619 (p. 761).

Metabolism. Quinine is metabolised by hydroxylation at the 2-position of the quinuclidine nucleus and to a smaller extent at the 2′-position of the quinoline ring—see under The Metabolism of Drugs, p. 161. It is also excreted to some extent in the unchanged form. Oxidation in the 2′-position may result in a loss of activity.

Dose. Therapeutic, 1·8 g daily for 4 days; as a suppressive, up to 600 mg daily.

Toxicity. Many cases of poisoning have been due to the use of quinine in attempts to procure abortion. The average fatal dose is 8 g although larger doses have been survived; 4 g usually causes untoward effects. Death, which usually occurs in coma from respiratory failure, may result in a few hours or may be delayed for one or two days.
In 3 non-fatal cases of quinine poisoning the following serum levels were determined on admission to hospital: 0·73 mg%; 1·01 mg%; and 0·675 mg%; 24 hours later the levels in the first 2 cases had dropped to 0·37 mg% (Tompsett, 1966).

CASE EXAMPLES. Fatal quinine poisoning occurred in 3 females, 2 aged 18 years and 1 aged 16 years. The post-mortem levels were: (i) intestines, 280 mg%; kidneys, 30 mg%; liver, 150 mg%; spleen, 60 mg%. (ii) blood, 1·1 mg%; kidneys, 9·6 mg%; liver, 3·9 mg%; spleen, 8·7 mg%. (iii) kidneys, 41 mg%; liver, 15 mg%; stomach contents, 82 mg; urine, 86 mg%; vomit, 168 mg (Walker, 1964).
A 22-year-old woman died 7 hours after taking quinine, probably about 15 g. Autopsy showed no cause of death or indication of poisoning. References to 10 other fatal cases are given where the estimated doses ranged from 0·4 to 16 g and the times of survival varied from 10 minutes after taking 16 g to 12 days after taking 1·5 g (Corby *et al.*, 1963).
An 18-year-old girl took 3·84 g of quinine sulphate in an attempt to abort a suspected pregnancy. On admission to hospital 2 hours later a plasma quinine level of 0·92 mg% was found. Peritoneal dialysis was instituted and by the following day the plasma quinine level was 0·525 mg%. In the first 19 hours a total of 1·632 g of quinine was recovered from the urine and dialysate, i.e. 42·5% of the ingested dose, 10·8% of the amount recovered being found in the dialysate (Markham *et al.*, 1967).

QUINURONIUM SULPHATE

Antiprotozoal (Veterinary)

Synonyms: Acaprin; Acapron; Quinolyl Urea.
Proprietary Names: Babesan; Pirevan.

NN′-Diquinol-6-ylurea 1,1′-dimetho(methyl sulphate)

$C_{23}H_{26}N_4O_9S_2 = 566·6$

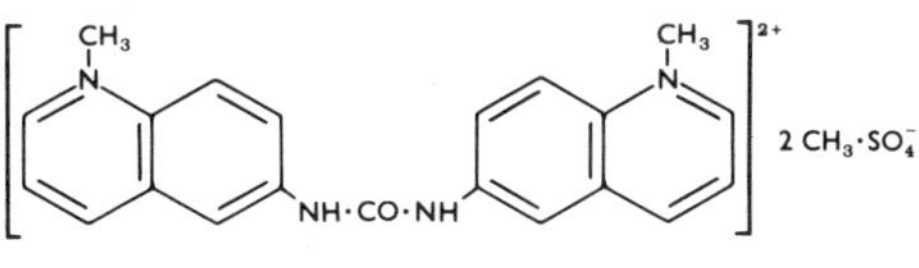

A white crystalline powder. Aqueous solutions may decompose on heating. M.p. 235°, with decomposition.
Solubility. Very soluble in water; very slightly soluble in ethanol, ether, and chloroform.

Extraction. Quinuronium sulphate is a quaternary ammonium compound (see p. 29).

Chromatography. PAPER: system P1—Rf 0·00 (location under ultraviolet light, blue fluorescence; location reagents: *iodoplatinate spray*, strong reaction; *bromocresol green spray*, weak reaction; *potassium permanganate spray*, strong reaction).

THIN-LAYER: system T1—Rf 0·00 (location reagent *acidified iodoplatinate spray*, positive reaction).

Colour Test. MICRO: Vitali's test — (yellow)-/pale yellow/orange (*sensitivity:* 0·5 μg).

Crystal Tests. MICRO: *potassium chromate solution*—bunches or rosettes of small needles (*sensitivity:* 1 in 3000); *zinc chloride solution*—bunches or rosettes of small needles (*sensitivity:* 1 in 3000).

Infra-red Absorption Spectrum. Potassium bromide disk. The principal peaks are: A 1210, B 1248, C 1276 or 1572 (p. 762).

Dose. 0·25 mg/kg in dogs and up to 1 mg/kg for horses and cattle, subcutaneously.

Toxicity. The margin between the toxic dose and the therapeutic dose in animals is very small. An overdose may cause a precipitate fall in blood-pressure which can be fatal if not treated immediately by adrenaline or atropine.

RACEMETHORPHAN *Narcotic*

Synonym: Ro 1-5470.

(±)-3-Methoxy-*N*-methylmorphinan

$C_{18}H_{25}NO = 271{\cdot}4$

A white crystalline powder.

NOTE. For a microcrystalline method of differentiation of racemethorphan from dextromethorphan (p. 289) and levomethorphan (p. 390) see Microcrystal Tests, p. 140.

Extraction. Racemethorphan is extracted by organic solvents from aqueous alkaline solutions.

Chromatography. PAPER: system P1—Rf 0·50 (location reagents: *iodoplatinate spray*, strong reaction; *bromocresol green spray*, weak reaction); system RP1a—Rf 0·78 (location reagent *iodoplatinate spray*, positive reaction); system RP1b—Rf 0·00 (location as for RP1a). THIN-LAYER: system T1—Rf 0·25 (location reagent *acidified iodoplatinate spray*, positive reaction).

GAS: system G2/225—retention time 0·50 relative to codeine.

Colour Test. MICRO: ammonium molybdate test —blue → green (*sensitivity:* 0·25 μg).

Crystal Tests. MICRO: *styphnic acid*—rosettes of plates and needles, forming overnight (*sensitivity:* 1 in 400); *trinitrobenzoic acid solution*—rosettes of crystals (*sensitivity:* 1 in 400).

Ultraviolet Absorption Spectrum. Racemethorphan in ethanol, maxima at 220 to 221 mμ, 281 mμ, and 289 mμ; in 0·1N sulphuric acid, maximum at 277 mμ (E1%, 1cm 71) and an inflexion at 283 mμ (E1%, 1cm 66).

RACEMORAMIDE *Narcotic Analgesic*

Synonyms: NIH 7421; R 610; SKF 5137.

Proprietary Name: Eupharma.

(±) - 1 - (3 - Methyl - 4 - morpholino - 2,2 - diphenylbutyryl)pyrrolidine

$C_{25}H_{32}N_2O_2 = 392{\cdot}5$

A white crystalline powder.

NOTE. For a microcrystalline method of differentiation of racemoramide from dextromoramide (p. 290) and levomoramide (p. 391) see Microcrystal Tests, p. 140.

Extraction. Racemoramide is extracted by organic solvents from aqueous alkaline solutions.

Chromatography. PAPER: system P1—Rf 0·61 (location reagent *iodoplatinate spray*, weak reaction); system RP1a—Rf 0·11 (location reagent *iodoplatinate spray*, positive reaction); system RP1b—Rf 0·00 (location as for RP1a). THIN-LAYER system T1—Rf 0·70 (location reagent *acidified iodoplatinate spray*, positive reaction).

GAS: system G2/225—retention time 4·70 relative to codeine.

Crystal Tests. MICRO: *gold chloride solution*—oily needles, some serrated, forming overnight (*sensitivity:* 1 in 1000); *picrolonic acid*—rosettes of branching rods, sometimes dense (*sensitivity:* 1 in 1000).

Ultraviolet Absorption Spectrum. Racemoramide in 0·1N sulphuric acid, maxima at 253·5 mμ (E1%, 1cm 9·2), 258·5 mμ (E1%, 1cm 10) and 264 mμ (E1%, 1cm 8·5), and minor inflexions at about 267 mμ and about 270 mμ.

Dose. Up to 20 mg.

RACEMORPHAN *Narcotic*

(±)-3-Hydroxy-*N*-methylmorphinan

$C_{17}H_{23}NO = 257{\cdot}4$

A white powder. Soluble in dilute acetic acid.

NOTE. For a microcrystalline method of differentiation of racemorphan from dextrorphan (p. 291) and levorphanol (p. 391) see Microcrystal Tests, p. 140.

Extraction. Racemorphan is extracted by organic solvents from aqueous ammoniacal solutions.

Chromatography. PAPER: system P1—Rf 0·59 (location reagents: *iodoplatinate spray*, strong reaction; *bromocresol green spray*, weak reaction); system RP1a—Rf 0·94 (location reagent *iodoplatinate spray*, positive reaction); system RP1b—Rf 0·08 (location as for RP1a). THIN-LAYER: system T1—Rf 0·26 (location reagent *acidified iodoplatinate spray*, positive reaction).

GAS: system G2/225—retention time 0·63 relative to codeine.

Colour Tests. MICRO: ammonium molybdate test—blue → green (*sensitivity:* 0·25 μg); Vitali's test—yellow/yellow/orange (*sensitivity:* 0·25 μg).

Crystal Tests. MICRO: *disodium methyl arsonate*

solution—rosettes of prisms (*sensitivity:* 1 in 400); *sodium carbonate solution*—plates or rods in bunches (*sensitivity:* 1 in 400).

Ultraviolet Absorption Spectrum. Racemorphan in 0·2N sulphuric acid, maximum at 279 mμ (E1%, 1cm 50); in 0·1N sulphuric acid, maximum at 278·5 mμ (E1%, 1cm 81·5) and an inflexion at 284 mμ (E1%, 1cm 75).

RACEPHEDRINE *Sympathomimetic*

Synonyms: dl-Ephedrine; Racemic Ephredine.

(±)-2-Methylamino-1-phenylpropan-1-ol

$C_{10}H_{15}NO = 165{\cdot}2$

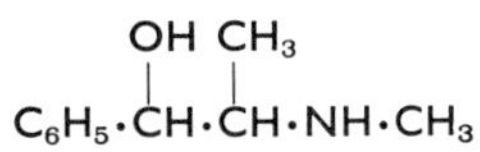

Racephedrine occurs as crystals. M.p. 79°.

Solubility. Soluble in water, ethanol, ether, and chloroform.

RACEPHEDRINE HYDROCHLORIDE

Proprietary Name: Ephetonin.

Fine white crystals or powder, affected by light. M.p. 187° to 188°.

Solubility. Soluble 1 in 4 of water and 1 in 25 of ethanol; insoluble in ether.

Extraction. Racephedrine is extracted by organic solvents from aqueous alkaline solutions.

Chromatography. PAPER: system P1—Rf 0·48 (location under ultraviolet light, absorption; location reagents: *iodoplatinate spray*, weak reaction; *bromocresol green spray*, weak reaction).

THIN-LAYER: system T1—Rf 0·28 (location reagent *potassium permanganate spray*, positive reaction).

Crystal Test. MICRO: *potassium bismuth iodide solution*—plates, jagged or irregular (*sensitivity:* 1 in 1000).

Dose. Up to 300 mg daily.

RESCINNAMINE *Antihypertensive/Tranquilliser*

Proprietary Names: Anaprel; Moderil; Rescisan.

Methyl 18-(3,4,5-trimethoxycinnamoyl)reserpate

$C_{35}H_{42}N_2O_9 = 634{\cdot}7$

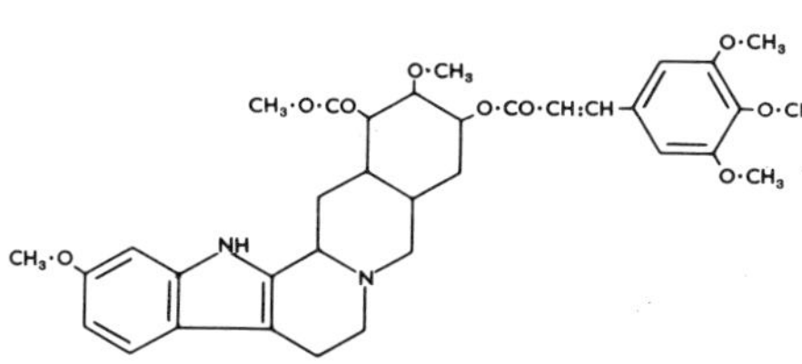

An alkaloid obtained from the roots of certain species of *Rauwolfia* (Apocynaceae), mainly *R. serpentina* and *R. vomitoria*, or by synthesis.

A white crystalline powder which darkens slowly on exposure to light but more rapidly when in solution. M.p. 238°.

Solubility. Almost insoluble in water; slightly soluble in ethanol; soluble in chloroform and acetic acid.

Extraction. Rescinnamine is extracted by organic solvents from aqueous alkaline solutions.

Chromatography. PAPER: system P1—Rf 0·72 (location under ultraviolet light, blue fluorescence; location reagents: *iodoplatinate spray*, weak reaction; *bromocresol green spray*, weak reaction).

THIN-LAYER: system T1—Rf 0·77 (location reagent *potassium permanganate spray*, positive reaction).

Colour Tests. MICRO: sulphuric acid–formaldehyde test—grey-green (*sensitivity:* 0·1 μg); ammonium molybdate test—greenish-blue (*sensitivity:* 0·1 μg); ammonium vanadate test—brown (*sensitivity:* 0·5 μg); Vitali's test—red-brown/yellow-brown/brown (*sensitivity:* 0·25 μg).

Crystal Test. MICRO: *sodium carbonate solution*—large rosettes or irregular crystals (*sensitivity:* 1 in 200).

Ultraviolet Absorption Spectrum. Rescinnamine in *borate buffer solution*, maxima at 228 mμ (E1%, 1cm 777) and 301 mμ (E1%, 1cm 380).

Dose. Up to 12 mg daily.

Toxicity. Rescinnamine has a relatively low toxicity but even in minimum therapeutic doses it may give rise to a number of side-effects. In the main, the side-effects are transient and quickly clear up on reduction of dosage or discontinuation of treatment.

Tolerance to rescinnamine does not develop and it does not appear to be habit-forming.

RESERPINE *Antihypertensive/Tranquilliser*

Proprietary Names: Bioserpine; Eskaserp; Quiescin; Rau-sed; Reserpoid; Sandril; Serpasil; Serpiloid.

Methyl 18-(3,4,5-trimethoxybenzoyl)reserpate

$C_{33}H_{40}N_2O_9 = 608{\cdot}7$

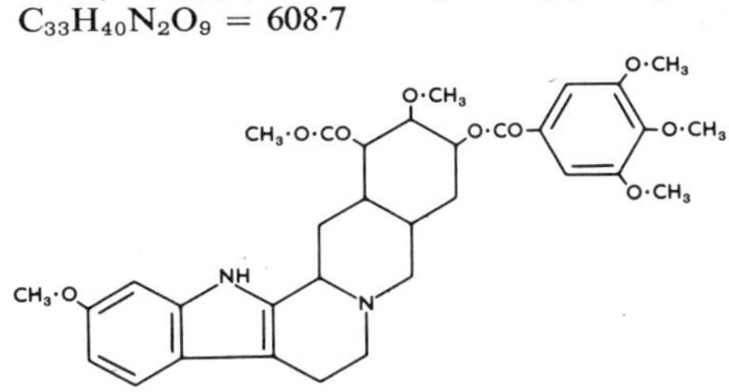

An alkaloid obtained from the roots of certain species of *Rauwolfia* (Apocynaceae), mainly *R. serpentina* and *R. vomitoria*, or by synthesis.

White crystals, or crystalline powder which darkens slowly on exposure to light. M.p. about 270°, with decomposition.

Solubility. Almost insoluble in water and ether; soluble 1 in 2000 of ethanol and 1 in 6 of chloroform.

Extraction. Reserpine is extracted by organic solvents from aqueous alkaline solutions.

Chromatography. PAPER: system P1—Rf 0·78 (location under ultraviolet light, pale green fluorescence; location reagents: *iodoplatinate spray*, weak reaction; *bromocresol green spray*, weak reaction).

THIN-LAYER: system T1—Rf 0·77 (location reagent *potassium permanganate spray*, positive reaction).

Colour Tests. MICRO: sulphuric acid–formaldehyde test—grey-green → brown (*sensitivity:* 0·1 μg); ammonium molybdate test—blue (*sensitivity:* 0·1 μg); ammonium vanadate test —green (*sensitivity:* 0·1 μg); Vitali's test—purple flash → orange/orange/brown (*sensitivity:* 1·0 μg).

Crystal Tests. MICRO: *potassium cyanide solution* —small rosettes (*sensitivity:* 1 in 1000); *ammonium thiocyanate solution*—plates (*sensitivity:* 1 in 1000).

Ultraviolet Absorption Spectrum. Reserpine in ethanol, maxima at 267 mμ (E1%, 1 cm 239) and 294 mμ (E1%, 1 cm 150).

Infra-red Absorption Spectrum. Potassium bromide disk. The principal peaks are: A 1120 or 1220, B 1330 (p. 762).

Quantitative Estimation. Reserpine may be estimated by spectrofluorimetry (Jakovljevic *et al.*, 1962). Reserpine, ajmaline, and yohimbine may be separated by thin-layer chromatography and determined by spectrophotometry or spectrofluorimetry (Wullen and Stainer, 1967).

Metabolism. The most likely possibilities for metabolic breakdown of reserpine would be hydrolysis of the ester linkage and *O*-demethylation—see under The Metabolism of Drugs, p. 163.

The metabolites of reserpine include trimethoxybenzoic acid, methyl reserpate, reserpic acid, syringomethyl reserpate, syringic acid, and carbon dioxide.

After oral administration to rats, 22% appears in the urine and 45% in the faeces as methyl reserpate; the same dose given parenterally results in a urinary level of methyl reserpate of less than 1%. Only small amounts of methyl reserpate are found in the excreta and tissues in other animals. After intravenous injection, reserpine appears to be rapidly removed from the blood-stream (Domino, 1962).

Dose. Up to 5 mg daily.

Toxicity. High dosage may occasionally cause a parkinsonian-like syndrome and severe depression which may lead to suicide. In the main, the side-effects are transient and quickly clear up on reduction of dosage or discontinuation of treatment.

Tolerance to reserpine does not develop and it does not appear to be habit-forming.

LD50 (oral): in mice 390 mg/kg.

RIBOFLAVINE *Vitamin*

Synonyms: Lactoflavin; Vitamin B_2; Vitamin G.
Proprietary Names: Beflavin; Beflavit; Flavaxin; Ribovel.

6,7-Dimethyl-9-(D-1-ribityl)isoalloxazine

$C_{17}H_{20}N_4O_6 = 376{\cdot}4$

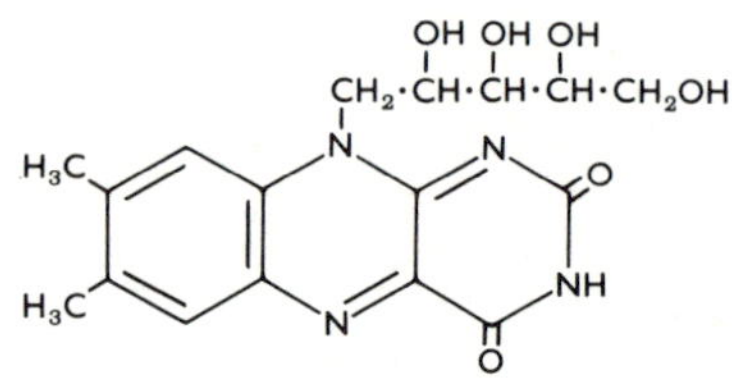

An orange-yellow crystalline powder. M.p. about 280°, with decomposition. Solutions deteriorate on exposure to light.

Solubility. Slightly soluble in water; sparingly soluble in ethanol; insoluble in ether and chloroform.

Colour Test. Dissolve 1 mg in 100 ml of water; the solution is greenish-yellow when viewed by transmitted light and shows an intense yellowish-green fluorescence which disappears on adding mineral acids, alkalis, and reducing agents such as sodium dithionite.

Ultraviolet Absorption Spectrum. Riboflavine in water, maxima at 222 mμ (E1%, 1 cm 942), 267 mμ (E1%, 1 cm 873), 371·5 mμ (E1%, 1 cm 277), and 445 mμ (E1%, 1 cm 324).

Infra-red Absorption Spectrum. Potassium bromide disk. The principal peaks are: A 1544, B 1575, C 1641 (p. 762).

Metabolism. Riboflavine is a component of the flavoprotein enzymes which form part of an enzyme system for the transference of hydrogen. The flavoproteins are necessary for the oxidation of carbohydrates, amino-acids, aldehydes, and other products of metabolism.

Before it can be utilised, riboflavine must be phosphorylated, the process occurring in the intestinal wall, liver, and red blood-cells.

The exact role of riboflavine in human nutrition is unknown but it probably plays a part in the nutrition of the eye, the formation of red blood-cells, and protein metabolism. It is absorbed from the intestinal mucosa, stored chiefly in the liver and kidneys and excreted in the urine. For normal health, an adult requires about 1·5 to 3 mg of riboflavine daily and a child 0·6 to 2 mg.

Dose. Up to 10 mg daily.

ROLITETRACYCLINE *Antibiotic*

Synonyms: PMT; Pyrrolidinomethyltetracycline.
Proprietary Names: Reverin; Syntetrex; Syntetrin; Syntodecin; Velacycline.

4 - Dimethylamino - 1,4,4a,5,5a,6,11,12a - octahydro - 3,6,10,12,12a - pentahydroxy - 6 - methyl - 1,11 - dioxo - *N* - pyrrolidin - 1′ - ylmethylnaphthacene-2-carboxyamide

$C_{27}H_{33}N_3O_8 = 527{\cdot}6$

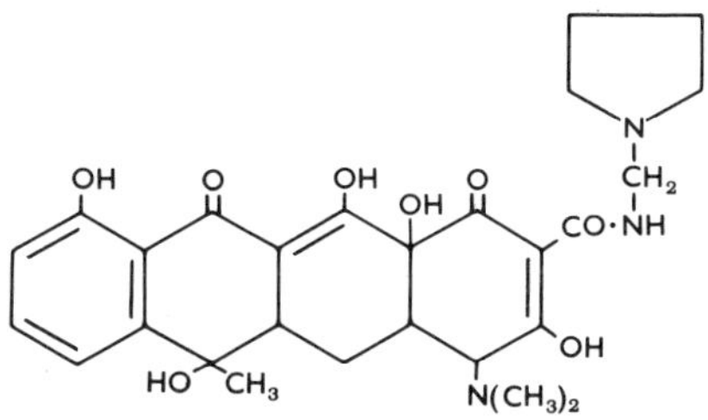

Fine, light yellow, acicular crystals.
Solubility. Soluble 1 in less than 1 of water.

Extraction. Rolitetracycline is extracted by organic solvents from aqueous alkaline solutions.

Chromatography. THIN-LAYER: system T1—Rf 0·05, streaking (location under ultraviolet light, orange fluorescence; location reagent *potassium permanganate spray*, positive reaction).

Colour Tests. MICRO: sulphuric acid–formaldehyde test—dull orange (*sensitivity:* 0·25 μg); ammonium molybdate test—black-purple (*sensitivity:* 0·25 μg); ammonium vanadate test—purple → red → orange (*sensitivity:* 0·25 μg); sulphuric acid test—purple → yellow; Vitali's test—yellow/yellow/brown (*sensitivity:* 1·0 μg).

Crystal Test. MICRO: *mercuric chloride solution*—dense rosettes (*sensitivity:* 1 in 1000).

Dose. Up to 1·4 g daily by injection.

Toxicity. Liver damage may occur; this is more likely after intravenous than after intramuscular administration.

ROTENONE *Pesticide*

(−) - 2 - Isopropenyl - 8,9 - dimethoxy - 6 - oxo - 1,2,6,6a,12,12a - hexahydrofuro[2, 3 - *h*][1]benzopyrano-[3,4-*b*][1]benzopyran

$C_{23}H_{22}O_6 = 394{\cdot}4$

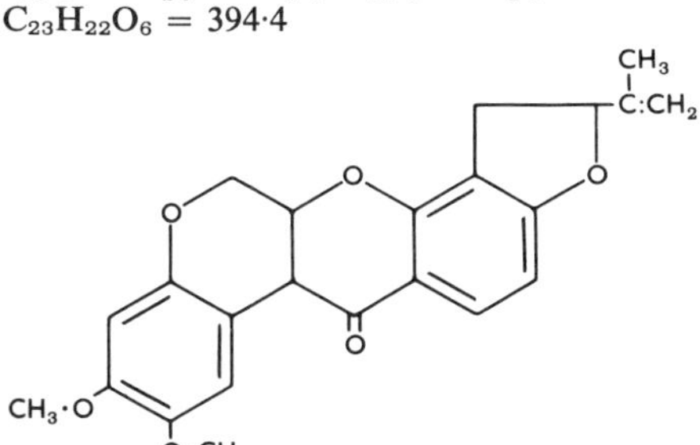

Rotenone is the principal active constituent of derris, the dried rhizome and roots of *Derris elliptica*, *D. malaccensis*, and other species of *Derris* (Leguminosae), which contains not less than 3%.

A white crystalline powder which decomposes on exposure to light and air. M.p. about 163°. A dimorphic form melts at 181°.

Solubility. Almost insoluble in water; soluble 1 in 300 of ethanol, 1 in 200 of ether, and 1 in 3 of chloroform. Solutions in organic solvents are laevorotatory.

Extraction. Rotenone is extracted by organic solvents from aqueous acid solutions.

Ultraviolet Absorption Spectrum. Rotenone in 0·1N sulphuric acid, maxima at 235 mμ (E1%, 1 cm 480) and 292 mμ (E1%, 1 cm 550).

Quantitative Estimation. Rotenone may be determined colorimetrically (Joint Committee of the Pharmaceutical Society and the Society for Analytical Chemistry on Methods of Assay of Crude Drugs, 1961).

Toxicity. The estimated oral lethal dose in man is 200 g.
LD50 (oral): in rats 133 mg/kg.

STP *Hallucinogen*

Synonyms: 2,5-Dimethoxy-4-methylamphetamine; DOM.

α-Methyl-2,5-dimethoxy-4-methylphenethylamine

$C_{12}H_{19}NO_2 = 209{\cdot}3$

Melting-points of 59° and 69·5° have been reported.
Solubility. Insoluble in water; soluble in chloroform.

STP HYDROCHLORIDE

A white powder. M.p. 190°.
Solubility. Soluble in water.

Extraction. STP is extracted by organic solvents from aqueous ammoniacal solutions.

Chromatography. PAPER: system P1—Rf 0·57 (location under ultraviolet light, absorption; location reagents: *bromocresol green spray*, weak reaction; *Marquis reagent*, yellow).

THIN-LAYER: system T1—Rf 0·51 (location reagent *potassium permanganate spray*, positive reaction).

Colour Tests. MICRO: sulphuric acid–formaldehyde test—yellow (*sensitivity:* 0·1 μg); ammonium molybdate test—yellow (*sensitivity:* 0·25 μg); Vitali's test— –/–/purple-brown (*sensitivity:* 0·1 μg).

Crystal Tests. MICRO: *gold bromide solution*—long irregular curving needles (*sensitivity:* 1 in 400); *picrolonic acid*—rosettes of fine branching needles (*sensitivity:* 1 in 1000).

Ultraviolet Absorption Spectrum. STP in dilute

hydrochloric acid, maxima at 214 mμ, about 225 mμ, and 288 mμ; minimum at 252 mμ.

NOTE. In doses of less than 3 mg, pure STP produces a mild euphoria; doses greater than 3 mg may cause pronounced hallucinogenic effects which last about 8 hours (Synder *et al.*, 1967).
The abuse of STP as a hallucinogenic agent has been reported in several countries. It has been used principally in the form of capsules containing about 10 mg. It appears that the preparations so used often contain an atropine-like drug in addition to STP (Solursh and Clement, 1968).

SACCHARIN *Sweetening Agent*

Synonyms: Benzosulphimide; Garantose; Gluside.

o-Benzoicsulphimide

$C_7H_5NO_3S = 183{\cdot}2$

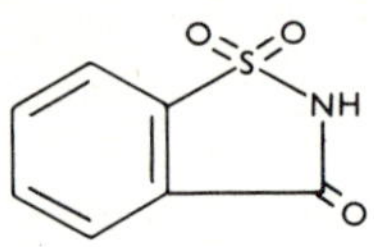

A white crystalline powder. M.p. 226° to 230°.
Solubility. Soluble 1 in 290 of water, 1 in 25 of boiling water, and 1 in 30 of ethanol; slightly soluble in ether and chloroform.

SACCHARIN CALCIUM
White crystals or crystalline powder.
Solubility. Soluble 1 in 1·5 of water.

SACCHARIN SODIUM
Synonyms: Soluble Gluside; Soluble Saccharin.
Proprietary Names: Hermesetas; Limmisax; Saxin.
A white crystalline powder which effloresces in dry air.
Solubility. Soluble 1 in 1·5 of water and 1 in 50 of ethanol.

Colour Tests. Heat a little dry material with an excess of resorcinol in *sulphuric acid* to just below boiling—green; cool the solution, dilute, and make alkaline with sodium hydroxide—green fluorescence. Melt with a little dry potassium hydroxide in a tube for about half a minute, cool, dissolve in water and make just acid, pH 4 to 5—salicylic acid (p. 539) may be identified in the solution.

Ultraviolet Absorption Spectrum. Saccharin in 0·01N sodium hydroxide, maxima at 234·5 mμ (E1%, 1cm 351) and 268 mμ (E1%, 1cm 89) and an inflexion at 284 mμ; saccharin sodium in water, maximum at 267·5 mμ (E1%, 1cm 69); minimum at 244·5 mμ.

Infra-red Absorption Spectrum. Saccharin. Potassium bromide disk. The principal peaks are: A 1334 or 1705, B 1170 (p. 762).

Metabolism. Saccharin is rapidly absorbed from the gastro-intestinal tract and excreted unchanged, mostly in the urine, within 24 hours.

Toxicity. 5 g has caused nausea, vomiting, and diarrhoea. Injection may cause local thrombophlebitis.

SALICYLAMIDE *Analgesic and Antipyretic*

Synonym: Salamid.
Proprietary Names: Salicim; Salimed; Salrin. It is an ingredient of Arthripax, Delimon, and Mephosol.

o-Hydroxybenzamide

$C_7H_7NO_2 = 137{\cdot}1$

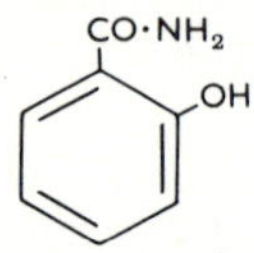

A white crystalline powder. M.p. 139° to 142°.
Solubility. Soluble 1 in 500 of water; more soluble in hot water; soluble 1 in 15 of ethanol, 1 in 35 of ether, and 1 in 100 of chloroform.

Screening Test. *Ferric chloride solution* with urine—blue-violet, after hydrolysis (indicative of a salicylate—see p. 8).

Extraction. Salicylamide is extracted by ether from acidified urine but cannot be extracted from the ether into aqueous bicarbonate. It is, however, extracted into 3% sodium hydroxide solution, from which it cannot be re-extracted by ether until the aqueous phase is acidified. Thus, salicylamide accompanies the barbiturates in extraction, not salicylic acid (Stevens, 1965).

Chromatography. PAPER: system P12—Rf 0·45 (location under ultraviolet light, bright blue fluorescence; location reagent *ferric chloride spray*, violet); system RP1b—Rf 0·87 (location reagent *bromine–starch–potassium iodide*).
GAS: system G5—retention time 1·04 relative to barbitone.

Colour Test. *Trinder's reagent*—purple.

Ultraviolet Absorption Spectrum. Salicylamide in ethanol, maxima at 235 mμ (E1%, 1cm 543) and 302 mμ (E1%, 1cm 295); in 0·1N sodium hydroxide, maxima at 242 mμ (E1%, 1cm 536) and 328 mμ (E1%, 1cm 435).

Quantitative Estimation. Salicylamide may be estimated as salicylic acid by the spectrophotometric methods of Trinder (1954) and Stevenson (1960)—see under Salicylic Acid, p. 539.

Metabolism. Salicylamide is metabolised in man mainly by the formation of glucuronide and sulphate conjugates. Three metabolites have been found in the urine: a glucuronide conjugate of salicylamide, a sulphate conjugate of salicylamide, and a glucuronide conjugate of gentisamide. Peak serum levels are reached some time between ½ and 1 hour after oral administration.

Dose. Usually up to 1 g; in acute rheumatism, up to 12 g daily.

Toxicity. LD50 (oral): in mice 1·4 and in rats 1·2 g/kg.

SALICYLIC ACID *Antimicrobial*

o-Hydroxybenzoic acid

$C_7H_6O_3 = 138{\cdot}1$

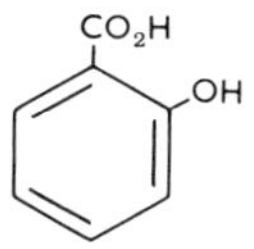

A white crystalline powder. M.p. 158·5° to 161°.

Solubility. Soluble 1 in 550 of water, 1 in 15 of boiling water, 1 in 4 of ethanol, 1 in 3 of ether, and 1 in 55 of chloroform.

CHOLINE SALICYLATE

Proprietary Names: Actasal; Arthropan. It is the main ingredient of Cholisate.

A white crystalline, very hygroscopic powder. M.p. about 50°.

Solubility. Very soluble in water and ethanol; insoluble in ether.

SODIUM SALICYLATE

Colourless crystals, crystalline flakes, or white powder.

Solubility. Soluble 1 in 1 of water and 1 in 11 of ethanol; insoluble in chloroform and ether. Concentrated aqueous solutions are liable to deposit crystals of the hexahydrate on standing.

Screening Test. *Ferric chloride solution* with urine—blue-violet (see p. 8).

Extraction. Salicylic acid may be isolated in the A1 fraction (see p. 27).

Chromatography. PAPER: system P12—Rf 0·52 (location under ultraviolet light, moderate blue fluorescence; location reagent *ferric chloride spray*, violet); system RP1a—Rf 0·90 (location reagent *bromine–starch–potassium iodide*).

THIN-LAYER: system T17—Rf 0·57, approximately (location under ultraviolet light, absorption).

GAS: system G5—retention time 0·54 relative to barbitone.

Colour Tests. *Trinder's reagent*—purple. McNally's test—red.

NOTE. Neither *m*- nor *p*-hydroxybenzoic acid give positive reactions with McNally's test, but all 3 acids (*o*-, *m*-, and *p*-) give a yellow colour with *Liebermann's reagent.*

Ultraviolet Absorption Spectrum. Salicylic acid in 0·5N sodium hydroxide, maximum at 300 mμ (E1%, 1 cm 260); in 0·1N sulphuric acid, maximum at 302 mμ (E1%, 1 cm 259).

Infra-red Absorption Spectrum. Salicylic acid. Potassium bromide disk. The principal peaks are: A 758, B 1446, C 1288 or 1657 (p. 762).

Quantitative Estimation. Salicylates in blood, plasma, cerebrospinal fluid, and urine may be estimated spectrophotometrically or colorimetrically following the addition of *Trinder's reagent* (Trinder, 1954); salicylic acid and acetylsalicylic acid in blood, serum, or plasma may be estimated directly by spectrophotometry after extraction into 0·4% malonic acid in butyl ether (Stevenson, 1960).

Metabolism. A large proportion of salicylic acid is excreted unchanged but conjugation with glycine and glucuronic acid occurs, yielding salicyluric acid, *o*-hydroxybenzoyl glucuronide, and *o*-carboxyphenylglucuronide. Hydroxylation to yield gentisic acid, 2,3-dihydroxybenzoic acid, and 2,3,5-trihydroxybenzoic acid may also occur.

Salicylic acid is rapidly absorbed and distributed throughout the whole body. It has been detected in brain tissues, eyes, and milk. It may take several days to eliminate salicylate after a single dose.

Use. Salicylic acid is applied externally in dusting-powders, lotions, and ointments for the treatment of chronic ulcers, dandruff, eczema, psoriasis, and parasitic skin diseases. Sodium salicylate may be given in a dosage of up to 16 g daily in the treatment of acute rheumatism. Choline salicylate has been used for the same purposes as aspirin in similar doses.

Toxicity. The estimated lethal dose in man is in the range 5 to 15 g. A serum salicylate level above 30 mg% is indicative of poisoning. Levels as high as 25 mg% may be found in arthritic patients who are taking large doses. LD50 (oral): in rats 1·5 to 2 g/kg.

SALOL

Synonym: Phenyl Salicylate.

Phenyl *o*-hydroxybenzoate

$C_{13}H_{10}O_3 = 214{\cdot}2$

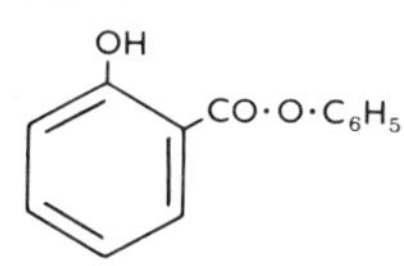

Colourless crystals or white crystalline powder. M.p. 42° to 43·5°. B.p. 173° at 12 mm Hg.

Solubility. Soluble 1 in 7000 of water, 1 in 9 of ethanol, 3 in 1 of ether, and 3 in 1 of chloroform.

Screening Test. *Ferric chloride solution* with an ethanolic solution of salol—blue-violet (see p. 8).

Extraction. Salol is extracted by organic solvents from aqueous acid or alkaline solutions.

Ultraviolet Absorption Spectrum. Salol in ethanol, maxima at 242 mμ (E1%, 1 cm 664) and 310 mμ (E1%, 1 cm 248).

Quantitative Estimation. Salol may be estimated as salicylic acid by the spectrophotometric methods of Trinder (1954) and Stevenson (1960)—see under Salicylic Acid.

Dose. Doses of up to 6 g daily have been given but salol is rarely used therapeutically.

Toxicity. It was formerly used as an intestinal antiseptic, but effective doses are toxic owing to the liberation of phenol in the intestines.

SANTONIN *Anthelmintic*

Synonym: Santolactone.

A lactone which may be obtained from santonica, the unexpanded flowerheads of *Artemisia cina* (Compositae) and other *Artemisia* spp.

$C_{15}H_{18}O_3$ = 246·3

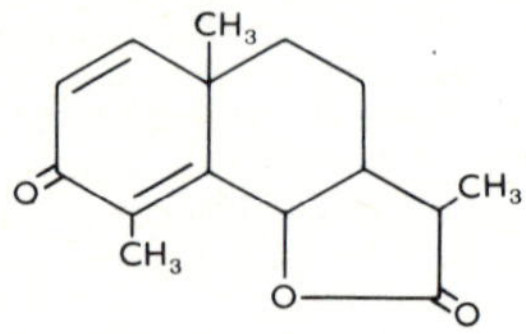

A white crystalline powder which becomes yellow on exposure to sunlight. M.p. 171° to 174°. Specific rotation of a 1% solution in ethanol, −172° to −176°.

Solubility. Almost insoluble in water; soluble 1 in 50 of ethanol, 1 in 140 of ether, and 1 in 2 of chloroform.

Extraction. Santonin is extracted by organic solvents from aqueous acid or alkaline solutions.

Chromatography. GAS: system G2/225—retention time 0·55 relative to codeine.

Colour Test. 10 mg warmed in 1 ml of a 10% ethanolic potassium hydroxide solution—violet-red.

Ultraviolet Absorption Spectrum. Santonin in ethanol: water (1:1), maximum at 245 mμ (E1%, 1cm 450).

Metabolism. An oxidation product of absorbed santonin colours acid urine bright yellow or orange and alkaline urine purplish-red.

Dose. Up to 200 mg daily for 3 days; maximum single and daily dose 300 mg.

Toxicity. Santonin is efficacious only when given in potentially toxic doses and it has now been largely superseded by other less toxic anthelmintics. Poisoning chiefly affects vision; large doses may give rise to epileptiform convulsions followed by coma. Death may be caused by respiratory failure. In children, 60 mg has produced serious poisoning, and two such doses have been fatal.

SECBUTOBARBITONE *Barbiturate*

Synonyms: Butabarbital (distinguish from Butobarbitone); Secbutabarbital; Secumalum.

5-Ethyl-5-s-butylbarbituric acid

$C_{10}H_{16}N_2O_3$ = 212·3

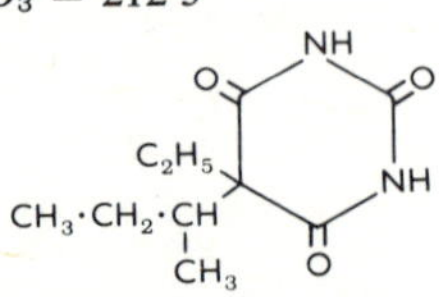

SECBUTOBARBITONE SODIUM

Proprietary Names: Bubartal Sodium; Butak; Butazem; Butisol Sodium; Insolat; Mebutal.

A white powder.

Solubility. Soluble 1 in 2 of water and 1 in 7 of ethanol; almost insoluble in ether.

Screening Tests. See under Barbiturates, p. 208.

Extraction. Secbutobarbitone may be isolated in the A2 fraction (see p. 27).

Chromatography. PAPER: system P2—Rf 0·52, relative to amylobarbitone (location under ultraviolet light, dark spot).

THIN-LAYER: system T11—Rf 0·49 (location reagent *mercurous nitrate spray*, white on grey); system T12—Rf 0·52 (location as for T11); system T13—Rf 0·62 (location as for T11).

GAS: system G5—retention time 1·94 relative to barbitone; system G7—retention time 1·7 relative to barbitone.

Colour Test. Zwikker's test—violet-blue.

Ultraviolet Absorption Spectrum. Secbutobarbitone is a 5,5-derivative—see Screening Test 3 under Barbiturates, p. 208.

Quantitative Estimation. See under Barbiturates, p. 208.

Metabolism. Secbutobarbitone is an intermediate-acting barbiturate—see under Barbiturates, p. 207.

It is rapidly metabolised, probably in the liver. About a third of a dose is excreted as a γ-oxidation product, 5-ethyl-5-(2′-carboxy-1′-methylethyl)barbituric acid—see under The Metabolism of Drugs, p. 157. It is excreted unchanged in the urine only when excessive doses are given.

Dose. Up to 200 mg as a hypnotic.

Toxicity. The estimated minimum lethal dose in man is 2 g.

SEROTONIN

Synonyms: Enteramine; 5-HT; 5-Hydroxytryptamine.

3-(2-Aminoethyl)-5-hydroxyindole

$C_{10}H_{12}N_2O$ = 176·2

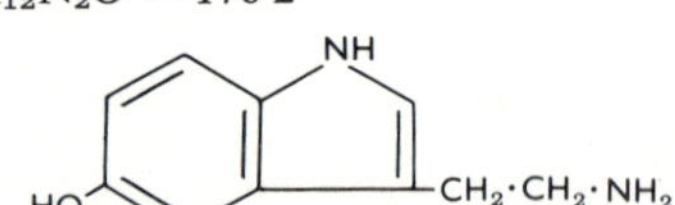

White crystals.

Solubility. Soluble in water.

Chromatography. PAPER: system P1—Rf 0·12 (location under ultraviolet light, white fluorescence; location reagents: *iodoplatinate spray*, white; *ninhydrin spray*, grey-blue).

THIN-LAYER: system T1—Rf 0·25 (location reagent *potassium permanganate spray*, positive reaction).

Colour Tests. MICRO: sulphuric acid–formaldehyde test—brown, appearing slowly (*sensitivity:* 1·0 μg); ammonium molybdate test—blue→green (*sensitivity:* 0·25 μg); Vitali's test—grey-green/brown/brown (*sensitivity:* 0·25 μg).

Crystal Tests. MICRO: *gold bromide–hydrochloric acid solution*—small plates, forming overnight (*sensitivity:* 1 in 100); *styphnic acid*—oily dendrites, forming overnight (*sensitivity:* 1 in 100).

Ultraviolet Absorption Spectrum. Serotonin in 0·1N hydrochloric acid, maximum at 275 mμ and inflexion at about 295 mμ.

Infra-red Absorption Spectrum. Potassium bromide disk. The principal peaks are: A 1084, B 1548 or 1747 (p. 762).

Quantitative Estimation. Curzon (1955) describes a rapid paper chromatographic test for the detection of serotonin and 5-hydroxyindolylacetic acid in urine.

Metabolism. Serotonin is widely distributed in the body. It has been suggested that it has a physiological function in the central nervous system and is involved in the transmission of nervous impulses as well as in the control of the tone of the viscera.
Serotonin arises from the hydroxylation and subsequent decarboxylation of tryptophan. It is metabolised chiefly by oxidative deamination to 5-hydroxyindolylacetic acid; *N*-methylation in the side-chain may also occur.

SOLANIDINE *Alkaloid*

Synonym: Solatubine.

$C_{27}H_{43}NO$ = 397·6

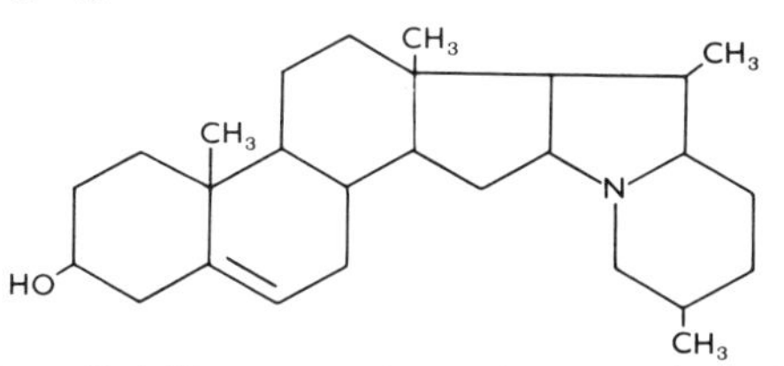

An alkaloid present in various species of *Solanum* (Solanaceae). It is the aglycone of solanine.
A white crystalline powder. M.p. 218° to 219°, with decomposition.
Solubility. Almost insoluble in water and ether; slightly soluble in ethanol; freely soluble in chloroform; soluble in dilute acids.

Extraction. Solanidine is extracted by organic solvents from aqueous alkaline solutions.

Chromatography. PAPER: system P1—Rf 0·90 (location reagents: *iodoplatinate spray*, weak reaction; *bromocresol green spray*, weak reaction).
THIN-LAYER: system T1—Rf 0·68 (location reagent *iodine–carbon tetrachloride spray*, positive reaction).

Colour Tests. MICRO: sulphuric acid–formaldehyde test—purple (*sensitivity:* 0·25 μg); ammonium molybdate test—yellow→olive→purple (*sensitivity:* 0·25 μg); ammonium vanadate test—orange→purple→blue (*sensitivity:* 0·25 μg); paraformaldehyde-phosphoric acid test—steel-blue.

SOLANINE *Alkaloid*

Synonym: Solatunine.

$C_{45}H_{73}NO_{15}$ = 868·1

A glycosidal alkaloid present in various species of *Solanum* (Solanaceae). Solanine is stated to be a mixture of 3 alkaloids which differ in the sugar moiety combined with the aglycone solanidine (q.v.) (Prelog and Jeger, 1960).
A white crystalline powder which decomposes at about 285°.
Solubility. Insoluble in water, ether, and chloroform; soluble in hot ethanol, dilute acids, and amyl alcohol.

Extraction. Solanine may be extracted by amyl alcohol from alkaline solutions.

Chromatography. PAPER: system P1—Rf 0·15 (location reagent *iodoplatinate spray*, weak reaction).
THIN-LAYER: system T1—Rf 0·52 (location reagents: *iodine–carbon tetrachloride spray*, positive reaction; *Marquis reagent*, positive reaction).

Colour Tests. MICRO: sulphuric acid–formaldehyde test—yellow→purple (*sensitivity:* 0·25 μg); ammonium molybdate test—yellow→olive→purple (*sensitivity:* 0·25 μg); ammonium vanadate test—orange→purple→blue (*sensitivity:* 0·25 μg); paraformaldehyde–phosphoric acid test—steel-blue.

Crystal Test. MICRO: *styphnic acid*—oily dendrites (*sensitivity:* 1 in 100).

Toxicity. Solanine exerts a direct irritant effect on the mucous membranes of the gastro-intestinal tract and, on absorption into the blood-stream, causes haemolysis of the red cells.
The berries, particularly the unripe berries, of Woody Nightshade (*Solanum dulcamara*) and of Black Nightshade (*Solanum nigrum*) have caused poisoning when eaten by children; the quantity of toxic alkaloids present varies considerably with conditions of soil and climate.
Green and sprouting potatoes may contain large quantities of solanine and can be dangerous. Poisoning of farm stock, particularly pigs, from eating green potato haulms or meal made from sprouting potatoes has been recorded on numerous occasions.
CASE EXAMPLES. A 9-year-old girl who had eaten the berries of woody nightshade (*Solanum dulcamara*) showed severe toxic symptoms including abdominal pain, thirst, vomiting, and dyspnoea. Her condition deteriorated and she died 2 days later. The liver contained about 21 mg of solanine (Alexander *et al.*, 1948).
For a report of solanine poisoning from eating potato shoots and for references to previous cases of solanine poisoning and details of previously published figures of the solanine content of potatoes see Willimott (1933).

Solanine poisoning in 4 persons who ate baked unpeeled potatoes. A 5th person who ate the pulp but not the skin of the potatoes was not affected. Potatoes from the same batch were found to contain 50 mg% of solanine. The average content of solanine in potatoes is about 8 mg% and the toxic dose for man is about 20 to 25 mg. The solanine content is higher in and immediately beneath the skin of the potato than in the flesh itself (Wilson, 1959).

SPARTEINE *Oxytocic*

Synonyms: Lupinidine; *l*-Sparteine.

(−)-Sparteine

$C_{15}H_{26}N_2 = 234{\cdot}4$

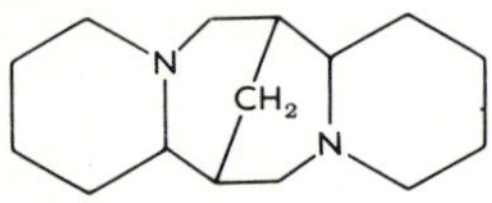

An alkaloid obtained from scoparium, the dried tops of broom, *Sarothamnus scoparius* (Leguminosae). A viscous oily liquid. B.p. 173° at 8 mm Hg.

Solubility. Soluble 1 in 325 of water; very soluble in ethanol, ether, and chloroform.

SPARTEINE SULPHATE

Proprietary Names: Spartocin; Tocine; Tocosamine.

Colourless crystals or white crystalline granules which decompose at 136°.

Solubility. Soluble 1 in 0·5 of water and 1 in 5 of ethanol; insoluble in ether and chloroform.

Extraction. Sparteine is extracted by organic solvents from aqueous alkaline solutions; it may also be isolated by distillation (see p. 18).

Chromatography. PAPER: system P1—Rf 0·13 (location reagents: *iodoplatinate spray*, strong reaction; *bromocresol green spray*, weak reaction); system RP1a—Rf 0·93 (location reagent *iodoplatinate spray*, positive reaction); system RP1b—Rf 0·82 (location as for RP1a).

THIN-LAYER: system T1—Rf 0·04 (location reagent *acidified iodoplatinate spray*, positive reaction).

GAS: system G6—retention time 0·20 relative to codeine.

Crystal Tests. MICRO: *gold chloride solution*—small irregular blades (*sensitivity:* 1 in 3000); *potassium cadmium iodide solution*—long plates (*sensitivity:* 1 in 1500).

Ultraviolet Absorption Spectrum. Sparteine in ethanol, maximum at 214 mμ (E1%, 1 cm 3·7).

Infra-red Absorption Spectrum. Sparteine sulphate. Potassium bromide disk. The principal peaks are: A 1118, B 1421 or 1447 (p. 763).

Dose. As an oxytocic agent, usually 150 mg intramuscularly.

SPIRAMYCIN *Antibiotic*

Synonyms: IC 5902; NSC 64393.

Proprietary Names: Rovamycin; Selectomycin.

A mixture of spiramycin I, $C_{45}H_{78}N_2O_{15} = 887{\cdot}1$ (about 63%), spiramycin II, $C_{47}H_{80}N_2O_{16} = 929{\cdot}2$ (about 24%), and spiramycin III, $C_{48}H_{82}N_2O_{16} = 943{\cdot}2$ (about 13%), produced by the growth of *Streptomyces ambofaciens*.

A white amorphous powder.

Solubility. Soluble 1 in 50 of water; very soluble in ethanol and chloroform.

Extraction. Spiramycin is extracted by organic solvents from aqueous alkaline solutions.

Chromatography. PAPER: system P1—Rf 0·23 (location under ultraviolet light, absorption; location reagents: *iodoplatinate spray*, strong reaction; *bromocresol green spray*, weak reaction); system RP1a—Rf 0·21 (location under ultraviolet light, absorption); system RP1b—Rf 0·00 (location as for RP1a).

THIN-LAYER: system T1—Rf 0·42 (location reagent *potassium permanganate spray*, positive reaction).

Colour Tests. MICRO: sulphuric acid–formaldehyde test—dull orange (*sensitivity:* 1·0 μg); ammonium molybdate test—grey-brown (*sensitivity:* 1·0 μg); ammonium vanadate test—orange-brown (*sensitivity:* 1·0 μg); Vitali's test—faint red/–/– (*sensitivity:* 1·0 μg).

Metabolism. Spiramycin is readily absorbed from the gastro-intestinal tract after oral administration and is widely distributed in the tissues. An oral dose of 12·5 mg/kg produces blood-levels of approximately 0·1 mg% after 1 hour. Peak blood-levels are maintained for 4 to 6 hours after a single dose and the drug may be detectable in the blood after 24 hours. Spiramycin is slowly eliminated; substantial amounts are excreted in the bile and about 10% in the urine. High concentrations appear in human milk.

Dose. Up to 5 g daily.

Toxicity. LD50 (intravenous): in mice 110 mg/kg.

SPIRONOLACTONE *Diuretic*

Synonyms: SC 9420; Spirolactone.

Proprietary Name: Aldactone-A.

7α - Acetylthio - 17β - hydroxy - 3 - oxo - 17α - pregn-4-ene-21-carboxylic acid γ-lactone

$C_{24}H_{32}O_4S = 416{\cdot}6$

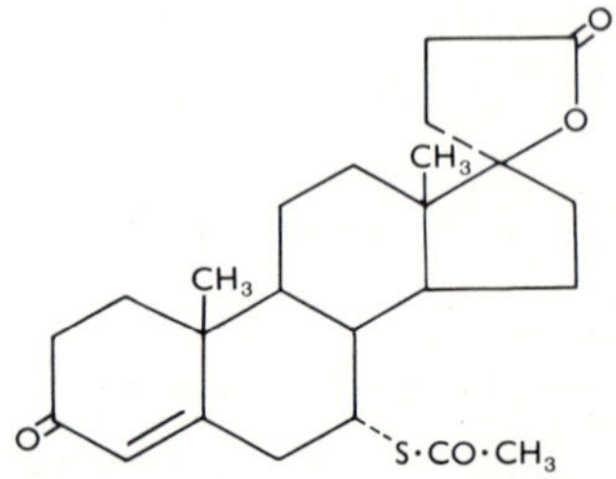

A buff powder. M.p. about 205°. Specific rotation of a 1% solution in dioxan, −47·5° to −52·5°.

Solubility. Soluble 1 in 400 of water, 1 in 80 of ethanol, 1 in 100 of ether, and 1 in 3 of chloroform.

Extraction. Spironolactone is extracted from neutral solutions with chloroform.

Colour Test. Shake 10 mg with 2 ml of 50% v/v sulphuric acid—orange solution with intense yellowish-green fluorescence; heat the solution gently—deep red and hydrogen sulphide is evolved.

Ultraviolet Absorption Spectrum. Spironolactone in methanol, maximum at about 238 mμ (E1%, 1 cm 470).

Quantitative Estimation. A method of paper chromatographic separation and subsequent spectrofluorimetric determination of spironolactone and its major metabolite is described by Gochman and Gantt (1962).

Metabolism. Spironolactone is a competitive inhibitor of the naturally occurring hormone aldosterone, which promotes retention of sodium and excretion of potassium by the distal renal tubules. It thus increases sodium and reduces potassium excretion.

Upon oral administration the dethioacetylated metabolite appears rapidly in the plasma, attaining peak levels after 4 to 6 hours. Significant amounts remain in the circulation for longer than 24 hours (Gochman and Gantt, 1962). Seven metabolites of spironolactone have been detected in the urine (Zicha *et al.*, 1964).

Dose. Up to 200 mg daily.

STILBAMIDINE *Antiprotozoal*

Synonym: M&B 744.

4,4′-Diamidinostilbene

$C_{16}H_{16}N_4 = 264{\cdot}3$

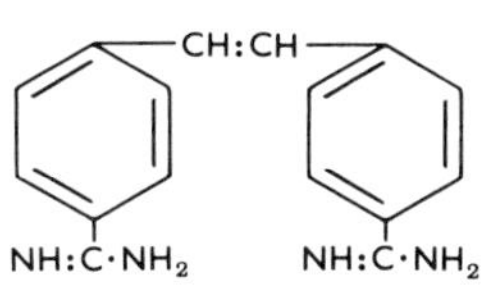

STILBAMIDINE ISETHIONATE

A white crystalline powder which decomposes on exposure to light and darkens when heated above 250°. M.p. 325° to 335°, with decomposition.

Solubility. Freely soluble in water; slightly soluble in ethanol.

Extraction. Stilbamidine is extracted by organic solvents from aqueous alkaline solutions.

Chromatography. PAPER: system P1—Rf 0·02 (location under ultraviolet light, bright blue fluorescence; location reagents: *iodoplatinate spray*, strong reaction; *bromocresol green spray*, weak reaction); system RP1a—Rf tailing (location under ultraviolet light, blue fluorescence; location reagent *iodoplatinate spray*, positive reaction); system RP1b—Rf tailing (location as for RP1a).

THIN-LAYER: system T1—Rf 0·04 (location reagent *acidified iodoplatinate spray*, positive reaction).

Colour Test. MICRO: ammonium molybdate test—pale blue (*sensitivity:* 1·0 μg).

Crystal Tests. MICRO: *potassium iodide solution*—small rods or needles (*sensitivity:* 1 in 1000); *zinc chloride solution*—small rods (*sensitivity:* 1 in 100).

Dose. 3 to 5 mg/kg, on alternate days, by intravenous injection, has been given.

Toxicity. Stilbamidine sometimes causes hypoglycaemia and, if administered intravenously, it may produce sudden hypotension. A serious late reaction is a neuropathy which may not develop until 2 to 5 months after a course of treatment.

STILBOESTROL *Oestrogen*

Synonyms: Diethylstilbestrol; Stilbol.

Proprietary Names: Cyren A; Oestromon; Pabestrol; Stilbetin. It is an ingredient of many proprietary preparations—see Extra Pharmacopoeia (Martindale), 25th Edn, pp. 1312–3.

3,4-Di(*p*-hydroxyphenyl)hex-3-ene

$C_{18}H_{20}O_2 = 268{\cdot}4$

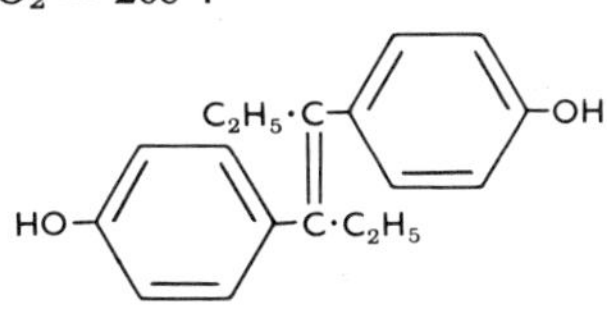

A white crystalline powder. M.p. about 172°.

Solubility. Very slightly soluble in water; soluble 1 in 5 of ethanol, 1 in 3 of ether, and 1 in 200 of chloroform.

STILBOESTROL DIPHOSPHATE

Disodium dihydrogen 3,4-di(*p*-phosphonyloxyphenyl)hex-3-ene

Proprietary Names: Honvan; Stilphostrol.

A white crystalline powder.

Solubility. Sparingly soluble in water.

STILBOESTROL DIPROPIONATE

3,4-Di-*p*-propionyloxyphenylhex-3-ene

Proprietary Names: Cyren B; Syntestrin.

A white crystalline powder. M.p. 104° to 106°.

Solubility. Slightly soluble in water; soluble 1 in 100 of ethanol and 1 in 6 of ether; soluble in chloroform.

Extraction. Stilboestrol is extracted from neutral solutions with freshly distilled ethyl acetate.

Chromatography. PAPER: system P15—Rf 0·85 (location reagents: *diazotised* p-*nitroaniline spray*, brown; *Pauly's reagent*, yellow).

GAS: system G2/225—retention time 0·78 relative to codeine.

Colour Test. Dissolve about 0·5 mg in 0·2 ml of glacial acetic acid, add 1 ml of phosphoric acid, and heat on a water-bath for 3 minutes—deep yellow, disappearing on dilution with 3 ml of glacial acetic acid. (This test distinguishes stilboestrol from dienoestrol (p. 300), which produces a magenta colour.)

Ultraviolet Absorption Spectrum. Stilboestrol in 0·1N sodium hydroxide, maximum at 259 mμ (E1%, 1cm 764).

Infra-red Absorption Spectrum. Stilboestrol. Potassium bromide disk. The principal peaks are: A 1198, B 1515, C 1165 (p. 763).

Metabolism. Stilboestrol is a synthetic oestrogen which is not a steroid but has actions similar to those of oestradiol. It is readily absorbed from the gastro-intestinal tract.

Dose. In carcinoma, up to 150 mg daily may be given; for menopausal disorders, up to 1 mg daily.

STREPTOMYCIN *Antibiotic/Tuberculostatic*

2, 4-Diguanidino-3,5,6-trihydroxycyclohexyl-5-deoxy-2-*O*-(2-deoxy-2-methylamino-α-L-glucopyranosyl)-3-formyl-β-L-lyxopentanofuranoside

$C_{21}H_{39}N_7O_{12} = 581{\cdot}6$

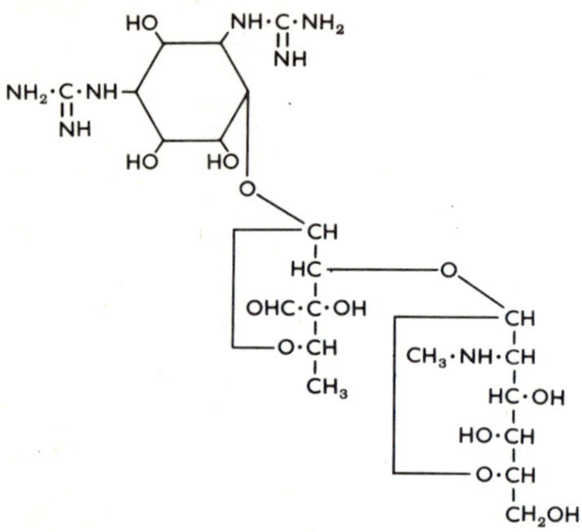

STREPTOMYCIN HYDROCHLORIDE

A hygroscopic white powder or granules.

Solubility. Very soluble in water; almost insoluble in ethanol, ether, and chloroform.

STREPTOMYCIN SULPHATE

Proprietary Names: Strepolin; Streptaquaine.

A white hygroscopic powder or granules.

Solubility. Very soluble in water; almost insoluble in ethanol, ether, and chloroform.

Chromatography. PAPER: system P1—Rf 0·00 (location reagents: *bromine–starch–potassium iodide*, weak reaction; *iodine vapour*, weak reaction).

THIN-LAYER: system T1—Rf 0·00 (location reagent *potassium permanganate spray*, positive reaction).

Colour Test. Boil a small quantity of streptomycin sulphate with 1N sodium hydroxide, add a slight excess of *hydrochloric acid* and a few drops of *ferric chloride solution*—brilliant violet.

Ultraviolet Absorption Spectrum. Streptomycin in 0·2N sulphuric acid, maximum at 280 mμ (E1%, 1cm 0·2).

Metabolism. Streptomycin is not appreciably absorbed or inactivated in the gastro-intestinal tract and most of a dose administered by mouth is excreted unchanged in the faeces.

After intramuscular injection, maximum blood-levels are reached in 1 or 2 hours but the time taken and the level attained, which may be as high as 5 mg%, vary considerably. A minimum effective serum level is stated to be about 0·7 mg%. After the intramuscular injection of 1 g of streptomycin, therapeutic serum levels may persist for 6 to 8 hours or longer and significant amounts may still be present after 24 hours. Maximum concentration in the blood is obtained within a few minutes of intravenous injection but declines more rapidly than after intramuscular injection.

The rate of excretion varies in different individuals and the concentration of streptomycin in the urine is often very high; as much as 70% of a parenterally administered dose may be excreted in the urine in 24 hours. Significant amounts are excreted in the bile and smaller amounts in milk, saliva, sweat, and tears.

Streptomycin diffuses rapidly into most body tissues and is present in the extracellular fluids. It is not absorbed through intact skin.

Dose. Up to 1·5 g daily by mouth; usually up to 1 g daily intramuscularly.

Toxicity. The most serious toxic effect is damage to the eighth cranial nerve, causing deafness which may be permanent. Liver and kidney damage have occurred after large doses.

STROPHANTHIN-K *Cardiac Glycoside*

Synonyms: Kombé Strophanthin; K-Strophanthin; Strophanthin; Strophanthoside-K.

A mixture of glycosides from the seeds of *Strophanthus kombé* (Apocynaceae) adjusted to possess 40% of the activity of anhydrous ouabain (p. 457).

A white crystalline powder which is affected by light.

Solubility. Moderately soluble in water and ethanol; less soluble in dehydrated ethanol; almost insoluble in ether and chloroform.

Extraction. Strophanthin-K is extracted with chloroform from acid solutions; it may also be isolated by continuous extraction under reduced pressure with ethanol (see p. 29).

Colour Test. Dissolve strophanthin-K in a cold mixture of *sulphuric acid* and water (4:1)—emerald green, immediately (distinction from ouabain, p. 457).

Infra-red Absorption Spectrum. Potassium bromide disk. The principal peaks are: A 1071, B 1035, C 1733 (p. 763).

Metabolism. Strophanthin-K is poorly absorbed from the gastro-intestinal tract; it is thought that it is destroyed there to a considerable extent. It is usually administered intravenously and becomes effective within 5 to 15 minutes, the effect lasting about 24 hours.

Dose. Up to 1 mg intravenously or intramuscularly.

Toxicity. Strophanthin-K has an action on the heart similar to that of digitalis but it is absorbed more rapidly and is less cumulative.

CASE EXAMPLE. Too rapid injection of strophanthin-K—0·125 mg in each injection—caused the deaths, within 10 minutes of treatment, of 3 women with cardiac insufficiency (Laves, 1960).

STRYCHNINE *Central Stimulant*

An alkaloid obtained from the seeds of *Strychnos nux-vomica* (Loganiaceae) and other *Strychnos* spp.

$C_{21}H_{22}N_2O_2$ = 334·4

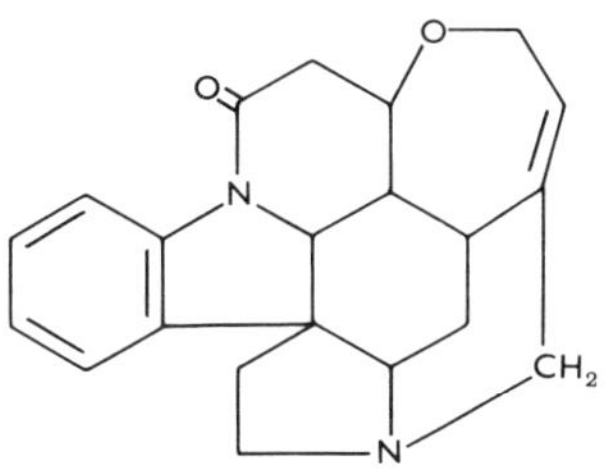

A white crystalline powder. M.p. 268°.

Solubility. Soluble 1 in 7000 of water, 1 in 250 of ethanol, 1 in 5500 of ether, and 1 in 6 of chloroform.

STRYCHNINE HYDROCHLORIDE
A white efflorescent crystalline powder.
Solubility. Soluble 1 in 40 of water and 1 in 85 of ethanol; insoluble in ether.

STRYCHNINE NITRATE.
A white crystalline powder.
Solubility. Soluble 1 in 50 of water, 1 in 150 of ethanol, and 1 in 110 of chloroform; insoluble in ether.

STRYCHNINE PHOSPHATE
A white powder.
Solubility. Soluble 1 in 30 of water and more soluble in hot water; slightly soluble in ethanol.

STRYCHNINE SULPHATE
A white crystalline powder which effloresces in dry air. Melts when anhydrous at about 200°, with decomposition.
Solubility. Soluble 1 in 50 of water and 1 in 135 of ethanol; insoluble in ether; slightly soluble in chloroform.

Extraction. Strychnine is extracted by organic solvents from aqueous alkaline solutions.

Chromatography. PAPER: system P1—Rf 0·30 (location under ultraviolet light, strong absorption; location reagent *iodoplatinate spray*, strong reaction).

THIN-LAYER: system T1—Rf 0·22 (location reagent *acidified iodoplatinate spray*, positive reaction).

GAS: system G1/250—retention time 4·83 relative to codeine.

Colour Tests. MICRO: ammonium vanadate test —blue→purple→red (*sensitivity:* 0·05 μg); Vitali's test— -/-/orange (*sensitivity:* 0·5 μg).

Crystal Tests. MICRO: *platinic chloride solution* —small plates (*sensitivity:* 1 in 1000); *potassium mercuric iodide solution*—wedge-shaped crystals, sometimes curved.

Ultraviolet Absorption Spectrum. Strychnine in ethanol, maximum at 255 mμ (E 1%, 1 cm 377); in 0·1N sulphuric acid, maximum at 255 mμ (E 1%, 1 cm 315).

Infra-red Absorption Spectrum. Strychnine (base). Potassium bromide disk. The principal peaks are: A 1664, B 764 or 1392, C 1480 (p. 763).

Quantitative Estimation. Bogan *et al.* (1966) describe a method of extraction from blood, urine, and tissues, followed by spectrophotometric estimation.

Metabolism. Strychnine is absorbed rapidly from the gastro-intestinal tract, through mucous membranes and intact skin, and upon injection. It leaves the blood-stream rapidly; 50% enters the tissues in 5 minutes. Up to 80% of a dose is rapidly oxidised, mainly by the liver. The remainder is slowly excreted in the urine. The action of strychnine may therefore be cumulative.

Strychnine is very stable and may be found in cadavers exhumed many years after death.

Dose. Up to 8 mg has been administered as a 'tonic'.

Toxicity. For adults the fatal dose is between 60 and 100 mg although, with adequate treatment, the patient may recover after ingesting 250 mg or more. Death is due to medullary paralysis following convulsive seizures which may occur within 10 to 15 minutes of each other.

Fatalities have arisen through the accidental ingestion of overdoses of various preparations containing strychnine, in particular Easton's Syrup and Easton's Tablets; the syrup contains 0·025% of strychnine; each tablet formerly contained 0·5 or 1 mg but the amounts have now been reduced (*B.P.C.* 1968) to 0·05 and 0·1 mg. When strychnine is taken in coated tablets, the toxic symptoms are much longer in appearing than when it is taken in solution.

When strychnine is injected, the toxic symptoms appear almost at once and death follows rapidly.

The toxic dose for horses is about 200 to 300 mg; for dogs and cats 5 to 20 mg (0·75 mg/kg).

CASE EXAMPLES. A 2-year-old girl swallowed an unknown quantity of strychnine, was promptly given an emetic, became unconscious and jerky but recovered following the administration of phenobarbitone sodium and mephenesin. Blood, urine, and stomach contents showed the presence of strychnine (Jacoby and Boyle, 1956).

An 18-year-old boy ingested approximately 6 oz of rat poison containing 0·2% of strychnine; he recovered within a few hours after being treated by gastric lavage and intravenous infusion of mephenesin (Swissman and Jacoby, 1964).

A young boy died about 8½ hours after being forced to swallow some strychnine powder. Prior to death a strychnine level of 0·7 mg% was found in the urine. At post-mortem examination the following levels of strychnine were found: brain, 0·047 mg%; kidney, 0·007 mg%; spinal cord, 0·18 mg%; urine, 0·77 mg% (Bogan *et al.*, 1966).

STYRAMATE *Muscle Relaxant*

Proprietary Name: Sinaxar.

β-Hydroxyphenethyl carbamate

$C_9H_{11}NO_3 = 181{\cdot}2$

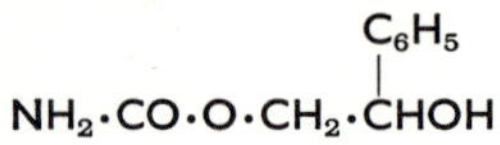

A crystalline powder. M.p. 108° to 110°.

Solubility. Sparingly soluble in water; soluble in ethanol, ether, and chloroform.

Screening Test. See under Screening Tests, p. 13.

Extraction. Styramate is extracted by organic solvents from aqueous acid or alkaline solutions.

Chromatography. PAPER: system P6—Rf 0·76 (location under ultraviolet light, absorption; location reagent *furfural–hydrochloric acid spray*, positive reaction); system P7—Rf 0·78 (location as for P6); system RP1b—Rf 0·73 (location as for P6).

THIN-LAYER: system T1—Rf 0·74 (location reagent p-*dimethylaminobenzaldehyde spray*, positive reaction).

GAS: system G5—retention time 1·88 (1·3; 0·54) relative to barbitone.

Ultraviolet Absorption Spectrum. Styramate in 0·1 N sulphuric acid, maxima at about 247 mμ (E1%, 1 cm 6·4), 251 mμ (E1%, 1 cm 8·6), 257 mμ (E1%, 1 cm 10·9), and 263 mμ (E1%, 1 cm 8·4).

Infra-red Absorption Spectrum. Potassium bromide disk. The principal peaks are: A 1660, B 1059, C 1425 (p. 763).

Dose. Up to 1·6 g daily.

SUCCINYLSULPHATHIAZOLE *Sulphonamide*

Synonyms: Succinylsulfathiazole; Sulfasuccithiazol.

Proprietary Names: Sulfasuxidine. It is an ingredient of Cremomycin, Cremostrep, Cremosuxidine, Kaovax, Neovax, and Sulfadigesin.

2 - [*p* - (3 - Carboxypropionamido)benzenesul - phonamido]thiazole monohydrate

$C_{13}H_{13}N_3O_5S_2,H_2O = 373{\cdot}4$

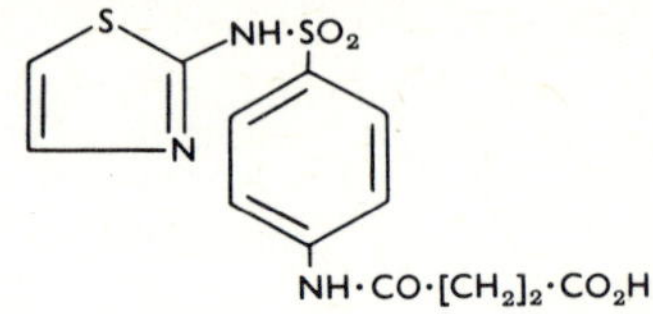

A white crystalline powder which darkens on exposure to light. M.p. about 190°, with decomposition.

Solubility. Soluble 1 in 5000 of water, 1 in 150 of boiling water, and 1 in 200 of ethanol; insoluble in ether and chloroform; soluble in aqueous solutions of alkali hydroxides.

Extraction. Succinylsulphathiazole may be extracted by ether from aqueous acid solutions; addition of an equal volume of acetone to the aqueous phase prior to extraction greatly increases the yield.

Chromatography. THIN-LAYER: system T23—Rf 0·43 (location under ultraviolet light, faintly blue fluorescence; location reagent *bromocresol purple spray*, blue or purple on yellow).

Colour Test. Copper sulphate test—grey-green.

Ultraviolet Absorption Spectrum. Succinylsulphathiazole in ethanol, maxima at 258 mμ (E1%, 1 cm 577) and 287 mμ (E1%, 1 cm 612).

Metabolism. Succinylsulphathiazole is poorly absorbed from the gastro-intestinal tract, consequently it is used for its local bacteriostatic action in the gastro-intestinal tract. It is hydrolysed in the large intestine to sulphathiazole, which is believed to be the bacteriostatically active substance.

The blood concentration of sulphathiazole following usual doses does not exceed 4 mg% and only about 5% is excreted in the urine. The concentration of sulphathiazole in the faeces reaches 80 to 200 mg%.

Dose. Up to 20 g daily.

Toxicity. Toxic effects following therapeutic doses are usually very slight owing to the low concentration in the blood and tissues.

LD50 (intraperitoneal): in mice 5·7 to 7·5 g/kg.

SULPHACETAMIDE *Sulphonamide*

Synonyms: Acetosulfaminum; Sulfacetamide; *N*-Sulfanilylacetamide.

Proprietary Names: Sulamyd; Urosulfon.

N-*p*-Aminobenzenesulphonylacetamide

$C_8H_{10}N_2O_3S = 214{\cdot}2$

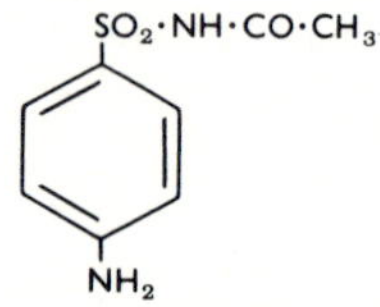

A white crystalline powder. M.p. 181° to 184°.

Solubility. Soluble 1 in 150 of water and 1 in 15 of ethanol; slightly soluble in ether; very slightly soluble in chloroform; soluble in mineral acids and in alkali hydroxides and carbonates.

SULPHACETAMIDE SODIUM
Synonym: Sulfacylum Solubile.
Proprietary Names: Albucid; Bleph; Ocusol; Steramide Sodium; Vasosulf.

A white microcrystalline powder which slowly darkens on exposure to light. In moist air it absorbs carbon dioxide and becomes less soluble. M.p. about 183°.
Solubility. Soluble 1 in 1·5 of water; sparingly soluble in ethanol; almost insoluble in ether and chloroform.

Extraction. Sulphacetamide may be extracted by ether from aqueous acid solutions; addition of an equal volume of acetone to the aqueous phase prior to extraction greatly increases the yield.

Chromatography. PAPER: system P1—Rf 0·81 (location under ultraviolet light, absorption; location by diazotisation followed by *alkaline betanaphthol spray*).
THIN-LAYER: system T1—Rf 0·70 (location by diazotisation followed by *alkaline betanaphthol spray*); system T22—Rf 0·42 (location by diazotisation followed by N-*1-naphthylethylenediamine spray*, reddish-purple).

Colour Test. Copper sulphate test—pale blue.

Crystal Test. MICRO: *gold bromide solution*—burrs or branching needles, forming overnight (*sensitivity:* 1 in 100).

Infra-red Absorption Spectrum. Sulphacetamide sodium. Potassium bromide disk. The principal peaks are: A 1145, B 1264, C 1552 (p. 763).

Quantitative Estimation. Bratton and Marshall (1939) describe a colorimetric method for the quantitative determination of diazotised sulphonamides in biological fluids and tissues.

Metabolism. Sulphacetamide is used for the treatment of urinary tract infections. It is more soluble in water than other sulphonamides and is readily absorbed from the gastro-intestinal tract and rapidly excreted in the urine, largely unchanged. A maximum blood-level of 3·7 mg% is reached 3 hours after a single dose of 4 g; after 72 hours it is not detectable in blood. The average blood-level at a dosage of 1 g four times daily by mouth was found to be 4 to 5 mg% of free sulphacetamide.
Sulphacetamide sodium is used mainly by local application in infections or injuries of the eyes. The 30% solution, which is not irritating to mucous membranes, is rapidly absorbed by ocular tissues; it is claimed that concentrations as high as 800 mg% are attained within 15 minutes after application to the cornea.

Dose. Up to 4 g daily.

Toxicity. Toxic effects following therapeutic doses are usually mild and occur infrequently. The incidence of crystalluria is low due to the high solubility of sulphacetamide even in acid urine.

LD50 (oral) of the base: in mice 16·5 g/kg; of the sodium salt: in mice 10 g/kg.

SULPHADIAZINE *Sulphonamide*

Synonym: Sulfadiazine.
Proprietary Names: Adiazine; Microsulfon. It is the active ingredient of Cremodiazine.

2-(*p*-Aminobenzenesulphonamido)pyrimidine
$C_{10}H_{10}N_4O_2S = 250{\cdot}3$

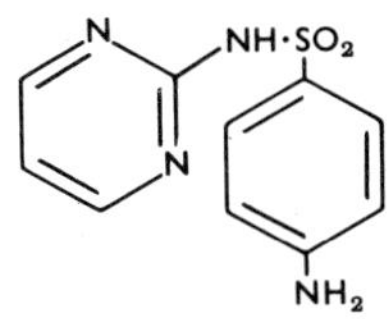

A white crystalline powder which slowly darkens on exposure to light. M.p. about 255°, with decomposition.
Solubility. Soluble 1 in 13,000 of water and 1 in 60 of boiling water; sparingly soluble in ethanol; almost insoluble in ether and chloroform; soluble in dilute mineral acids and aqueous solutions of alkali hydroxides and carbonates.

SULPHADIAZINE SODIUM
Synonym: Soluble Sulphadiazine.

A white powder which slowly darkens on exposure to light. On prolonged exposure to humid air it absorbs carbon dioxide, liberating sulphadiazine and becoming only partly soluble in water.
Solubility. Soluble 1 in 2 of water; slightly soluble in ethanol; almost insoluble in ether and chloroform.

Extraction. Sulphadiazine may be extracted by ether from aqueous acid solutions; addition of an equal volume of acetone to the aqueous phase prior to extraction greatly increases the yield.

Chromatography. PAPER: system P1—Rf 0·75 (location under ultraviolet light, absorption; location by diazotisation followed by *alkaline betanaphthol spray*).
THIN-LAYER: system T1—Rf 0·64 (location by diazotisation followed by *alkaline betanaphthol spray*); system T22—Rf 0·47 (location by diazotisation followed by N-*1-naphthylethylenediamine spray*, reddish-purple).

Colour Test. Copper sulphate test—purple-brown.

Crystal Tests. MICRO: *potassium tri-iodide solution (1)*—rosettes of blades or needles (*sensitivity:* 1 in 100); *sodium phosphate solution*—rosettes of rods or needles (*sensitivity:* 1 in 100).

Ultraviolet Absorption Spectrum. Sulphadiazine in ethanol, maximum at 270 mμ (E1%, 1 cm 844).

Infra-red Absorption Spectrum. Sulphadiazine

(base). Potassium bromide disk. The principal peaks are: A 1150, B 1577, C 1323 (p. 764).

Quantitative Estimation. Bratton and Marshall (1939) describe a colorimetric method for the quantitative determination of diazotised sulphonamides in biological fluids and tissues.

Metabolism. Sulphadiazine is well absorbed from the gastro-intestinal tract in spite of the fact that it is practically insoluble in water. A single dose, even when it is large, will not produce a peak blood-level for several hours but an effective blood-level may be maintained with an average dose of 1 g every 4 hours. At a blood-level of about 10 mg%, about half the sulphadiazine is bound to plasma protein. Sulphadiazine is excreted slowly in the urine, from 15 to 40% being acetylated; approximately 50% of a single oral dose is eliminated within 24 hours and 60 to 85% within 48 to 72 hours. About 75% of an intravenously administered dose is excreted within 24 hours. Normal doses produce bactericidal levels in the urine.

Dose. Up to 4 g daily.

Toxicity. Sulphadiazine therapy rarely leads to serious toxic effects. It is generally well tolerated; the urine should be kept alkaline to prevent crystallisation during excretion.

SULPHADIMETHOXINE *Sulphonamide*

Synonym: Sulfadimethoxine.
Proprietary Names: Madribon; Madriquid; Sulfoplan.

4-(*p*-Aminobenzenesulphonamido)-2,6-dimethoxypyrimidine

$C_{12}H_{14}N_4O_4S = 310{\cdot}3$

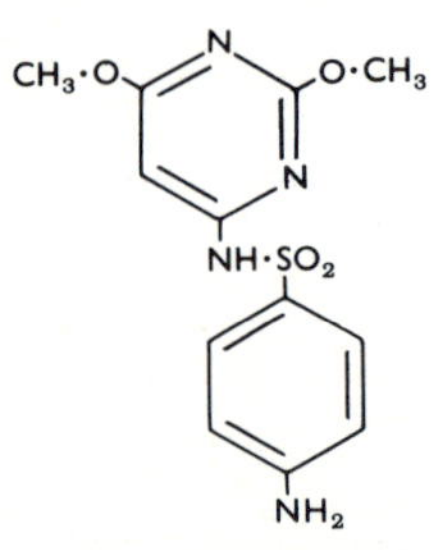

A white crystalline powder. M.p. 198° to 204°.
Solubility. Almost insoluble in water; soluble 1 in 200 of ethanol; slightly soluble in ether and chloroform; soluble in dilute mineral acids and in solutions of alkali hydroxides and carbonates.

Extraction. Sulphadimethoxine may be extracted by ether from aqueous acid solutions; addition of an equal volume of acetone to the aqueous phase prior to extraction greatly increases the yield.

Chromatography. PAPER: system P1—Rf 0·86 (location under ultraviolet light, absorption; location by diazotisation followed by *alkaline betanaphthol spray*).

THIN-LAYER: system T1—Rf 0·65 (location by diazotisation followed by *alkaline betanaphthol spray*).

Colour Test. Copper sulphate test—yellow-green.

Crystal Tests. MICRO: *potassium bismuth iodide solution*—serrated blades (*sensitivity:* 1 in 100); *sodium carbonate solution*—blades, best viewed under polarised light (*sensitivity:* 1 in 100).

Ultraviolet Absorption Spectrum. Sulphadimethoxine in 0·001N sodium hydroxide, maximum at 269 mμ (E1%, 1 cm 840).

Quantitative Estimation. Bratton and Marshall (1939) describe a colorimetric method for the quantitative determination of diazotised sulphonamides in biological fluids and tissues.

Metabolism. Sulphadimethoxine is a long-acting sulphonamide, being rapidly absorbed and slowly excreted. After a single dose of 2 g by mouth, a maximum blood-level is reached in 4 to 6 hours and at least half of this is still detectable after 24 hours. About 10% is present in the acetylated form and a little is present as the glucuronide. About 95% is bound to the plasma protein. Diffusion into the cerebrospinal fluid is poor.
Sulphadimethoxine is slowly excreted by the kidneys, since tubular resorption takes place. About 5% is excreted as sulphadimethoxine, 15% as the acetylated form, and the remainder as the glucuronide, a very soluble but bacteriologically inactive derivative.

Dose. Usually up to 2 g initially, followed by 500 mg daily.

Toxicity. The toxic effects of sulphadimethoxine are similar to those of other long-acting sulphonamides—see under Sulphamethoxypyridazine, p. 553.

SULPHADIMIDINE *Sulphonamide*

Synonyms: Sulfadimerazine; Sulfadimezine; Sulfadimidine; Sulfamethazine; Sulphadimethylpyrimidine.

NOTE. Sulphadimethylpyrimidine has been used as a synonym for both sulphadimidine and sulphasomidine; the 2 compounds are isomeric.

Proprietary Names: S-mez; Sulphamezathine. It is an ingredient of Orastrep and Sulpenin V.

2 - (*p* - Aminobenzenesulphonamido) - 4,6 - dimethylpyrimidine

$C_{12}H_{14}N_4O_2S = 278{\cdot}3$

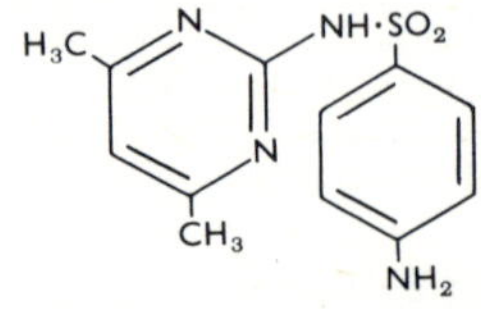

A white crystalline powder which may darken on exposure to light. M.p. 197° to 199°.
Solubility. Almost insoluble in water; soluble

1 in 120 of ethanol, 1 in 2500 of ether, and 1 in 600 of chloroform; soluble in dilute mineral acids and in aqueous solutions of alkali hydroxides and carbonates.

SULPHADIMIDINE SODIUM
Synonym: Soluble Sulfamethazine.
Proprietary Name: Sulphamezathine Sodium.

A white hygroscopic powder which slowly darkens on exposure to light. On prolonged exposure to moist air it absorbs carbon dioxide and becomes less soluble.
Solubility. Soluble 1 in 2·5 of water and 1 in 60 of ethanol.

Extraction. Sulphadimidine may be extracted by ether from aqueous acid solutions; addition of an equal volume of acetone to the aqueous phase prior to extraction greatly increases the yield.

Chromatography. PAPER: system P1—Rf 0·79 (location under ultraviolet light, weak absorption; location by diazotisation followed by *alkaline betanaphthol spray*).

THIN-LAYER: system T1—Rf 0·62 (location by diazotisation followed by *alkaline betanaphthol spray*).

Colour Test. Copper sulphate test—green → red-brown.

Crystal Tests. MICRO: *platinic bromide solution* —bunches of blades (*sensitivity:* 1 in 100); *potassium tri-iodide solution* (*1*)—dense rosettes or rosettes of plates (*sensitivity:* 1 in 100).

Ultraviolet Absorption Spectrum. Sulphadimidine in water, maxima at 240 mμ (E 1%, 1 cm 600) and 272 mμ (E 1%, 1 cm 660).

Quantitative Estimation. Bratton and Marshall (1939) describe a colorimetric method for the quantitative determination of diazotised sulphonamides in biological fluids and tissues.

Metabolism. Sulphadimidine is rapidly absorbed from the gastro-intestinal tract so that with regular dosage by mouth the blood concentration can be maintained at 5 to 10 mg%. Sulphadimidine is highly acetylated, about 30% in the blood and at least 60% in the urine being in the form of the acetyl derivative. It is firmly bound to plasma proteins and is therefore excreted slowly.

Dose. Up to 6 g daily by mouth; up to 2 g of the sodium salt by injection.

Toxicity. Sulphadimidine in therapeutic doses rarely causes serious toxic effects. The acetylated form of the drug is very soluble, even in acid urine, hence it is less likely to give rise to anuria and haematuria than sulphadiazine or sulphathiazole. Total doses of about 30 g, given over periods of 5 to 11 days, have produced thrombocytopenia and haemolytic anaemia in children.

SULPHAETHIDOLE *Sulphonamide*

Synonyms: Aethazolum; Ethazol; SETD; Sulphaethylthiadiazole.
Proprietary Names: Sethadil; Sul-Spansion; Sul-Spantab.

2 - *p* - Aminobenzenesulphonamido - 5 - ethyl - 1,3,4-thiadiazole
$C_{10}H_{12}N_4O_2S_2 = 284{\cdot}4$

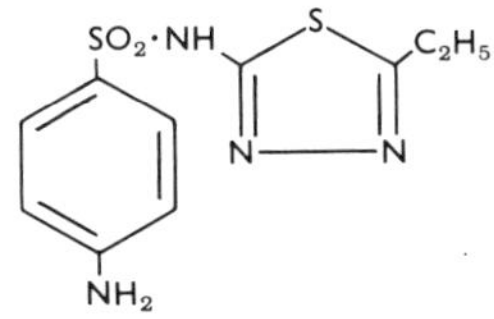

A white crystalline powder.
Solubility. Almost insoluble in water and ether; slightly soluble in ethanol; soluble in dilute mineral acids and in solutions of alkali hydroxides.

Extraction. Sulphaethidole may be extracted by ether from aqueous acid solutions; addition of an equal volume of acetone to the aqueous phase prior to extraction greatly increases the yield.

Chromatography. PAPER: system P1—Rf 0·88 (location under ultraviolet light, absorption; location by diazotisation followed by *alkaline betanaphthol spray*).

THIN-LAYER: system T1—Rf 0·67 (location by diazotisation followed by *alkaline betanaphthol spray*).

Colour Test. Copper sulphate test—bright green.

Crystal Tests. MICRO: *platinic bromide solution* —fine needles (*sensitivity:* 1 in 100); *potassium tri-iodide solution* (*3*)—small blades, best viewed under polarised light (*sensitivity:* 1 in 100).

Quantitative Estimation. Bratton and Marshall (1939) describe a colorimetric method for the quantitative determination of diazotised sulphonamides in biological fluids and tissues.

Metabolism. Sulphaethidole is readily absorbed from the gastro-intestinal tract. Only a small proportion is acetylated; about 90 to 95% appears in the blood and urine in the free form. Both sulphaethidole and its conjugated forms are soluble in urine, thus minimising the risk of crystalluria and renal toxicity.

Dose. Up to 1·95 g every 12 hours.

SULPHAFURAZOLE *Sulphonamide*

Synonyms: NU 445; Sulfisoxazole.
Proprietary Name: Gantrisin (tablets).

5 - (*p* - Aminobenzenesulphonamido) - 3,4 - dimethylisoxazole
$C_{11}H_{13}N_3O_3S = 267{\cdot}3$

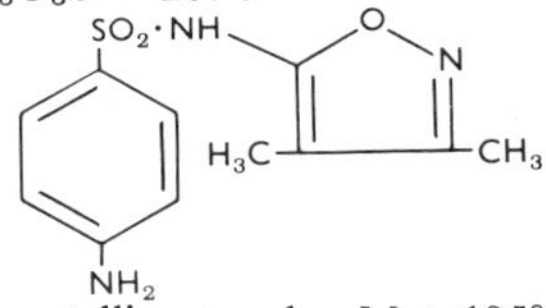

A white crystalline powder. M.p. 195° to 198°.

Solubility. Soluble 1 in 7000 of water, 1 in 50 of ethanol, 1 in 800 of ether, and 1 in 1000 of chloroform; freely soluble in dilute hydrochloric acid.

ACETYL SULPHAFURAZOLE
Proprietary Name: Gantrisin (suspension).

A white crystalline powder. M.p. 192° to 195°.
Solubility. Almost insoluble in water; slightly soluble in ethanol; sparingly soluble in chloroform.

SULPHAFURAZOLE DIETHANOLAMINE
Proprietary Name: Gantrisin (injection).

A slightly yellowish crystalline powder.
Solubility. Very soluble in water; soluble in ethanol; almost insoluble in ether; very slightly soluble in chloroform.

Extraction. Sulphafurazole may be extracted by ether from aqueous acid solutions; addition of an equal volume of acetone to the aqueous phase prior to extraction greatly increases the yield.

Chromatography. PAPER: system P1—Rf 0·88 (location under ultraviolet light, absorption; location by diazotisation followed by *alkaline betanaphthol spray*).

THIN-LAYER: system T1—Rf 0·65 (location by diazotisation followed by *alkaline betanaphthol spray*).

Colour Test. Copper sulphate test—pale green.

Crystal Tests. MICRO: *lead iodide solution*—rectangular plates (*sensitivity:* 1 in 100); *picrolonic acid*—irregular prisms, best viewed under polarised light (*sensitivity:* 1 in 100).

Ultraviolet Absorption Spectrum. Sulphafurazole in 0·01 N hydrochloric acid, maximum at 268 mμ (E1%, 1 cm 480); in 0·01 N sodium hydroxide, maximum at 253 mμ (E1%, 1 cm 780).

Quantitative Estimation. Bratton and Marshall (1939) describe a colorimetric method for the quantitative determination of diazotised sulphonamides in biological fluids and tissues.

Metabolism. Sulphafurazole is rapidly absorbed and excreted, about 95% of a single dose appearing in the urine in 24 hours. The concentration in the cerebrospinal fluid reaches about one-third of that in the blood.
Owing to its relatively high solubility, even in acid urine, it is especially useful in the treatment of infections of the urinary tract.

Dose. Up to 6 g (base) daily.

Toxicity. With therapeutic doses the usual mild toxic sulphonamide reactions may occur but the relatively high solubility of sulphafurazole in urine renders crystalluria unlikely.

SULPHAGUANIDINE *Sulphonamide*

Synonyms: Sulfamidinum; Sulfaguanidine; Sulgin.
Proprietary Names: Guanicil; Resulfon; Ruocid. It is an ingredient of Guanimycin and Ivax.

N - *p* - Aminobenzenesulphonylguanidine monohydrate

$C_7H_{10}N_4O_2S,H_2O = 232{\cdot}3$

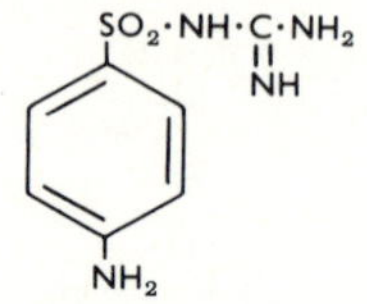

A white crystalline powder which slowly darkens on exposure to light. M.p. 190° to 192·5°.
Solubility. Soluble 1 in 1000 of water, 1 in 10 of boiling water, and 1 in 250 of ethanol; almost insoluble in ether; freely soluble in dilute mineral acids.

Extraction. Sulphaguanidine may be extracted by ether from aqueous acid solutions; addition of an equal volume of acetone to the aqueous phase prior to extraction greatly increases the yield.

Chromatography. PAPER: system P1—Rf 0·32 (location under ultraviolet light, absorption; location by diazotisation followed by *alkaline betanaphthol spray*).

THIN-LAYER: system T1—Rf 0·65 (location by diazotisation followed by *alkaline betanaphthol spray*).

Colour Test. Copper sulphate test—blue.

Crystal Test. MICRO: *picrolonic acid*—dense rosettes, or rosettes of curved needles (*sensitivity:* 1 in 100).

Ultraviolet Absorption Spectrum. Sulphaguanidine in water, maximum at 259 mμ (E1%, 1 cm 635); in ethanol, maximum at 264 mμ (E1%, 1 cm 800).

Infra-red Absorption Spectrum. Potassium bromide disk. The principal peaks are: A 1129 or 1620, B 1230 or 1537 (p. 764).

Quantitative Estimation. Bratton and Marshall (1939) describe a colorimetric method for the quantitative determination of diazotised sulphonamides in biological fluids and tissues.

Metabolism. Sulphaguanidine is not readily absorbed from the gastro-intestinal tract and it has therefore been employed in the treatment of local intestinal infections. The portion which is absorbed is mainly acetylated.

Dose. Up to 20 g daily.

SULPHAMERAZINE *Sulphonamide*

Synonyms: Sulfamerazine; Sulfamethyldiazine; Sulfamethylpyrimidine.

2 - (*p* - Aminobenzenesulphonamido) - 4 - methylpyrimidine

$C_{11}H_{12}N_4O_2S$ = 264·3

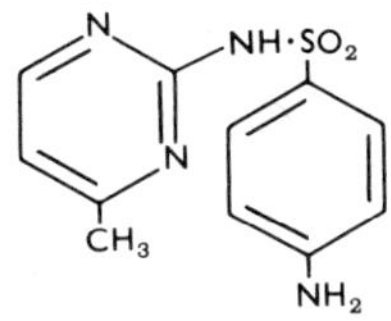

A white crystalline powder. M.p. 234° to 238°.

Solubility. Soluble 1 in 6250 of water at 20°, 1 in 3300 of water at 37°, 1 in 300 of boiling water, and 1 in 300 of ethanol; very slightly soluble in ether and chloroform; soluble in dilute mineral acids and in solutions of alkali hydroxides.

SULPHAMERAZINE SODIUM

Synonym: Soluble Sulphamerazine.

A white powder which slowly darkens on exposure to light. In moist air it absorbs carbon dioxide and becomes less soluble.

Solubility. Soluble 1 in 3·5 of water; slightly soluble in ethanol; almost insoluble in ether and chloroform.

Extraction. Sulphamerazine may be extracted by ether from aqueous acid solutions; addition of an equal volume of acetone to the aqueous phase prior to extraction greatly increases the yield.

Chromatography. PAPER: system P1—Rf 0·71 (location under ultraviolet light, absorption; location by diazotisation followed by *alkaline betanaphthol spray*).

THIN-LAYER: system T1—Rf 0·65 (location by diazotisation followed by *alkaline betanaphthol spray*); system T22—Rf 0·57 (location by diazotisation followed by N-*1-naphthylethylenediamine spray*, reddish-purple).

Colour Test. Copper sulphate test—green → dark brown.

Crystal Tests. MICRO: *gold chloride solution*—dense rosettes (*sensitivity:* 1 in 100); *potassium bismuth iodide solution*—irregular crystals or bunches of prisms (*sensitivity:* 1 in 100).

Ultraviolet Absorption Spectrum. Sulphamerazine in water, maxima at 244 mμ (E1%, 1 cm 875) and 257 mμ (E1%, 1 cm 822); in ethanol, maximum at 271 mμ (E1%, 1 cm 835).

Infra-red Absorption Spectrum. Sulphamerazine. Potassium bromide disk. The principal peaks are: A 1143, B 1592, C 1559 (p. 764).

Quantitative Estimation. Bratton and Marshall (1939) describe a colorimetric method for the quantitative determination of diazotised sulphonamides in biological fluids and tissues.

Metabolism. Sulphamerazine is rapidly and completely absorbed from the gastro-intestinal tract. It is more slowly excreted than sulphadiazine; thus it is possible to have an effective concentration in the blood with smaller doses than are required with sulphadiazine. About 50% of the drug is excreted in the urine in the acetylated form.

Dose. Up to 4·5 g daily.

Toxicity. Sulphamerazine in therapeutic doses has caused haematuria and persistent albuminuria in children, especially in those aged less than 6 years, even when fluid intake has been normal.

CASE EXAMPLE. A 2-year-old girl died after receiving 12½ tablets (about 6 g) of sulphamerazine in 84 hours. At post-mortem examination, death was found to be due to uraemia, cerebral oedema, acute tubular nephritis due to sulphonamide crystallisation in the renal tract, and bilateral otitis media (*Pharm. J.*, ii/1950, 221).

SULPHAMETHIZOLE *Sulphonamide*

Synonyms: Sulfamethizole; Sulfamethylthiadiazole.

Proprietary Names: Lucosil; Rufol; Sulfametin; Sulfurine; Thiosulfil; Urolucosil; Utrasul.

NOTE. Sulfametin is also the U.S. Adopted Name for Sulphamethoxydiazine (p. 552).

2 - (*p* - Aminobenzenesulphonamido) - 5 - methyl - 1,3,4 - thiadiazole

$C_9H_{10}N_4O_2S_2$ = 270·3

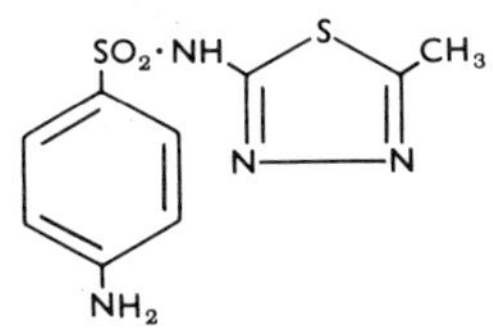

A white crystalline powder. M.p. 208° to 211°.

Solubility. Soluble 1 in 3000 of water, 1 in 60 of boiling water, 1 in 25 of ethanol, 1 in 4000 of ether, and 1 in 1700 of chloroform; soluble in dilute mineral acids and in solutions of alkali hydroxides.

Extraction. Sulphamethizole may be extracted by ether from aqueous acid solutions; addition of an equal volume of acetone to the aqueous phase prior to extraction greatly increases the yield.

Chromatography. PAPER: system P1—Rf 0·84 (location under ultraviolet light, absorption; location by diazotisation followed by *alkaline betanaphthol spray*).

THIN-LAYER: system T1—Rf 0·65 (location by diazotisation followed by *alkaline betanaphthol spray*).

Colour Test. Copper sulphate test—green.

Crystal Tests. MICRO: *picrolonic acid*—small leaflike plates (*sensitivity:* 1 in 100); *potassium tri-iodide solution* (*3*)—small plates and rods, often in rosettes (*sensitivity:* 1 in 100).

Quantitative Estimation. Bratton and Marshall (1939) describe a colorimetric method for the quantitative determination of diazotised sulphonamides in biological fluids and tissues.

Metabolism. Sulphamethizole is rapidly absorbed from the gastro-intestinal tract. In 5 hours about 60% is excreted and in 15 hours practically all is eliminated. Only 5 to 7% appears in the urine in the acetylated form.

Dose. Up to 1·2 g daily.

Toxicity. Sulphamethizole in therapeutic doses is well tolerated and the risk of crystalluria is slight.

SULPHAMETHOXAZOLE *Sulphonamide*

Synonyms: Ro 4-2130; Sulfamethoxazole.
Proprietary Name: Gantanol.

3-*p*-Aminobenzenesulphonamido-5-methylisoxazole

$C_{10}H_{11}N_3O_3S = 253{\cdot}3$

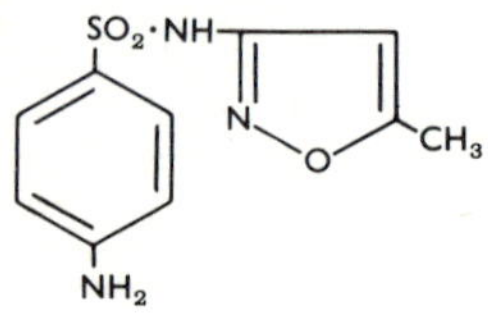

A white crystalline powder.

Solubility. Very slightly soluble in water; almost insoluble in ether and chloroform.

Extraction. Sulphamethoxazole may be extracted by ether from aqueous acid solutions; addition of an equal volume of acetone to the aqueous phase prior to extraction greatly increases the yield.

Chromatography. PAPER: system P1—Rf 0·90 (location under ultraviolet light, absorption; location by diazotisation followed by *alkaline betanaphthol spray*).

THIN-LAYER: system T1—Rf 0·65 (location by diazotisation followed by *alkaline betanaphthol spray*).

Colour Test. Copper sulphate test—green.

Crystal Tests. MICRO: *lead iodide solution*—small irregular crystals and small rods (*sensitivity:* 1 in 100); *sodium phosphate solution*—small irregular rods (*sensitivity:* 1 in 100).

Quantitative Estimation. Bratton and Marshall (1939) describe a colorimetric method for the quantitative determination of diazotised sulphonamides in biological fluids and tissues.

Metabolism. Sulphamethoxazole closely resembles sulphafurazole (p. 549) chemically but its rates of absorption and excretion are slower. Following a 2-g dose, a peak level is reached in the blood within 4 to 6 hours and about 25% is eliminated in the urine within 8 hours, about 60% of this being acetylated.

Dose. Up to 3 g daily.

Toxicity. When sulphamethoxazole is administered therapeutically, special precautions must be taken against crystalluria since the acetyl derivative of sulphamethoxazole is relatively insoluble.

LD50 (oral): in mice 3·2 g/kg.

SULPHAMETHOXYDIAZINE

Sulphonamide

Synonyms: AHR 857; Sulfametin; Sulfametorinum; Sulfametoxydiazine.
Proprietary Names: Bayrena; Durenat(e); Kirocid; Kiron; Sulla.

NOTE. Sulfametin is also a proprietary name for sulphamethizole (p. 551).

2-*p*-Aminobenzenesulphonamido-5-methoxypyrimidine

$C_{11}H_{12}N_4O_3S = 280{\cdot}3$

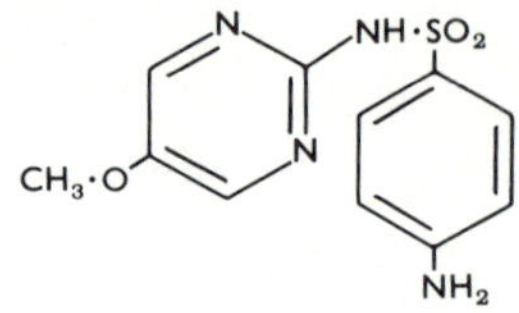

A white crystalline powder. M.p. 209° to 213°.

Solubility. Almost insoluble in water, ether, and chloroform; slightly soluble in ethanol and dilute hydrochloric acid; freely soluble in aqueous solutions of alkali hydroxides and carbonates.

Extraction. Sulphamethoxydiazine may be extracted by ether from aqueous acid solutions; addition of an equal volume of acetone to the aqueous phase prior to extraction greatly increases the yield.

Chromatography. PAPER: system P1—Rf 0·78 (location under ultraviolet light, absorption; location by diazotisation followed by *alkaline betanaphthol spray*).

THIN-LAYER: system T1—Rf 0·60 (location by diazotisation followed by *alkaline betanaphthol spray*).

Colour Test. Copper sulphate test—purple-brown.

Crystal Tests. MICRO: *gold chloride solution*—bunches of rectangular plates, best viewed under polarised light (*sensitivity:* 1 in 100); *potassium tri-iodide solution* (*1*)—very small rhomboids.

Quantitative Estimation. Bratton and Marshall (1939) describe a colorimetric method for the quantitative determination of diazotised sulphonamides in biological fluids and tissues.

Metabolism. Sulphamethoxydiazine is a long-acting sulphonamide which is rapidly absorbed but slowly excreted. After a single dose by mouth, a maximum blood-level is reached in about 4 hours, and 48 hours after a dose of 1 g, serum-levels are still half their original level. About 10% is present in the acetylated form and about 75 to 80% is bound to the serum protein. Levels in the cerebrospinal fluid reach about one-third of those in the blood.

Sulphamethoxydiazine is slowly excreted in the urine, resorption taking place. About 50% is excreted unchanged, 20% in the acetylated form and the remainder as other metabolites, one of which is the glucuronide conjugate.

Dose. Usually up to 2 g initially, followed by 500 mg daily.

Toxicity. The toxic effects of sulphamethoxydiazine are similar to those of other long-acting sulphonamides—see under Sulphamethoxypyridazine, below.

SULPHAMETHOXYPYRIDAZINE

Sulphonamide

Synonyms: CT 879; RP 7522; Sulfamethoxypyridazine; SMP.

Proprietary Names: Durox; Kynex; Lederkyn; Longamid; Midicel; Midikel; Minikel; Sulfadurazin; Sultirène.

3 - (*p* - Aminobenzenesulphonamido) - 6 - methoxypyridazine

$C_{11}H_{12}N_4O_3S = 280{\cdot}3$

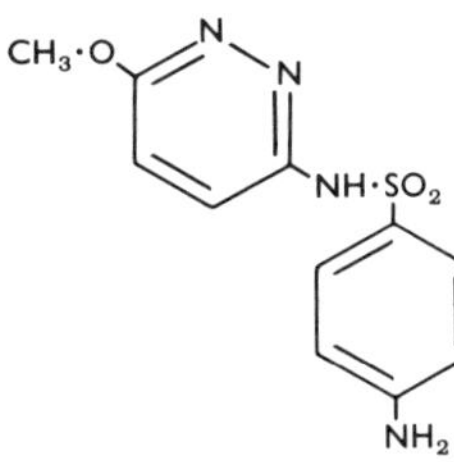

A white crystalline powder which slowly darkens on exposure to light. M.p. 180° to 183°.

Solubility. Very slightly soluble in water; sparingly soluble in ethanol; almost insoluble in chloroform; freely soluble in dilute mineral acids and in solutions of alkali hydroxides.

ACETYL SULPHAMETHOXYPYRIDAZINE

3 - (N^1 - Acetyl - *p* - aminobenzenesulphonamido) - 6 - methoxypyridazine.

Synonyms: Lederkyn Acetyl (suspension); Midicel (suspension).

Crystals which melt at 186° to 187°, with decomposition.

Solubility. Very soluble in water.

Extraction. Sulphamethoxypyridazine may be extracted by ether from aqueous acid solutions; addition of an equal volume of acetone to the aqueous phase prior to extraction greatly increases the yield.

Chromatography. PAPER: system P1—Rf 0·80 (location under ultraviolet light, absorption; location by diazotisation followed by *alkaline betanaphthol spray*).

THIN-LAYER: system T1—Rf 0·65 (location by diazotisation followed by *alkaline betanaphthol spray*).

Colour Test. Copper sulphate test—greenish-brown.

Crystal Tests. MICRO: *potassium bismuth iodide solution*—very small dense rosettes (*sensitivity:* 1 in 100); *potassium tri-iodide solution* (*1*)—small rhomboids, sometimes in rosettes (*sensitivity:* 1 in 100).

Ultraviolet Absorption Spectrum. Sulphamethoxypyridazine in ethanol, maximum at 267 mμ (E1%, 1 cm 800).

Infra-red Absorption Spectrum. Sulphamethoxypyridazine. Potassium bromide disk. The principal peaks are: A 1152 or 1475 or 1485 (p. 764).

Quantitative Estimation. Bratton and Marshall (1939) describe a colorimetric method for the quantitative determination of diazotised sulphonamides in biological fluids and tissues.

Metabolism. Sulphamethoxypyridazine is a long-acting sulphonamide which is rapidly absorbed and slowly excreted. After a single oral dose of 4 g, maximum blood-levels of 11 to 18 mg% are reached in 5 hours. On the first day a quarter of the dose is excreted and on the second day a further 20%, but sulphamethoxypyridazine is detectable in the serum even after 4 days. The rate of excretion is higher in alkaline urine. About 85% is bound to the plasma protein. The level in the cerebrospinal fluid is about 5 to 10% of that in the plasma. Twenty to 30% of the total dose is excreted in the urine in 24 hours, of which about 50% is unchanged and 50% is acetylated.

Dose. Usually up to 2 g initially, followed by 500 mg daily.

Toxicity. Sulphamethoxypyridazine and the other long-acting sulphonamides are more strongly bound to proteins and more slowly excreted than sulphonamides with a short duration of action. The concentration in the plasma must be higher to achieve the same therapeutic effect as that given by the short-acting sulphonamides, and the possibility of toxicity is thereby increased.

Patients treated with long-acting sulphonamides may develop a severe form of erythema multiforme, associated with widespread lesions of the skin and mucous membranes, termed the Stevens-Johnson syndrome (erythema multiforme gravis; erythema multiforme exudativum) which may be fatal in about 25% of cases.

CASE EXAMPLES. Sulphamethoxypyridazine was considered to have caused the death of 3 elderly patients who developed acute interstitial myocarditis after being treated with the drug (Blanchard and Mertens, 1958).

A 67-year-old woman, treated with sulphamethoxypyridazine after an operation developed mental confusion, urinary frequency, and a temperature of 104°F; she also had severe aplastic anaemia. She died, despite blood transfusions (Holsinger *et al.*, 1958).

After treatment with 500 mg of sulphamethoxypyridazine daily for 10 days, a man of 34 died from thrombocytopenic purpura (Janovsky, 1960).

For reports of the occurrence of the Stevens-Johnson syndrome, particularly in children, associated with sulphamethoxypyridazine therapy see Extra Pharmacopoeia (Martindale), 25th Edn, p. 1394.

SULPHANILAMIDE

Sulphonamide

Synonyms: Streptocidum Album; Sulfanilamide; Sulfaminum.

Proprietary Names: Prontosil Album; Streptocide. It is an ingredient of Rhinamid.

p-Aminobenzenesulphonamide
$C_6H_8N_2O_2S = 172{\cdot}2$

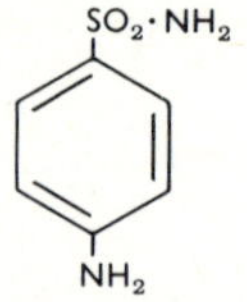

A white crystalline powder. On heating the dry powder it becomes violet-blue and eventually aniline and ammonia are produced. M.p. 164·5° to 166·5°.

Solubility. Soluble 1 in 250 of water at 15·5°, 1 in 170 at 20°, 1 in 2 of boiling water, and 1 in 37 of ethanol; almost insoluble in ether and chloroform; soluble in solutions of alkali hydroxides.

Extraction. Sulphanilamide may be extracted by ether from aqueous acid solutions; addition of an equal volume of acetone to the aqueous phase prior to extraction greatly increases the yield.

Chromatography. PAPER: system P1—Rf 0·49 (location by diazotisation followed by *alkaline betanaphthol spray*).

THIN-LAYER: system T1—Rf 0·67 (location by diazotisation followed by *alkaline betanaphthol spray*); system T22—Rf 0·53 (location by diazotisation followed by N-*1-naphthylethylenediamine spray*, reddish-purple).

Colour Test. Copper sulphate test—blue.

Crystal Test. MICRO: *potassium chromate solution*—dense rosettes (*sensitivity:* 1 in 100).

Ultraviolet Absorption Spectrum. Sulphanilamide in ethanol, maximum at 263 mμ (E1%, 1 cm 1106); in 0·1N sodium hydroxide, maximum at 254 mμ (E1%, 1 cm 1402).

Infra-red Absorption Spectrum. Potassium bromide disk. The principal peaks are: A 1144, B 1593, C 1312 or 1624 (p. 764).

Quantitative Estimation. Bratton and Marshall (1939) describe a colorimetric method for the quantitative determination of diazotised sulphonamides in biological fluids and tissues.

Metabolism. Sulphanilamide is metabolised by acetylation; usually up to 50% of a dose is acetylated.

Dose. Up to 9 g daily has been given.

Toxicity. LD50 (oral): in mice 3·7 to 4·2 and in rats 3·9 to 10 g/kg.

SULPHAPHENAZOLE *Sulphonamide*

Synonyms: C 17922; Sulphophenylpyrazol.
Proprietary Names: Microsulf; Orisul(f); Sulfabid.

5 - *p* - Aminobenzenesulphonamido - 1 - phenylpyrazole
$C_{15}H_{14}N_4O_2S = 314{\cdot}4$

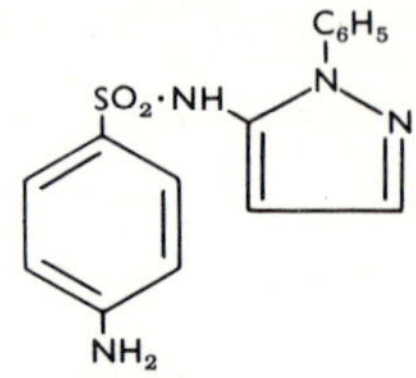

A white crystalline powder. M.p. 179° to 183°. When heated, the powder becomes brown; when further heated, it produces yellow fumes and an odour of sulphur dioxide.

Solubility. Almost insoluble in water, ethanol, ether, and chloroform; soluble in mineral acids and in solutions of alkali hydroxides.

Extraction. Sulphaphenazole may be extracted by ether from aqueous acid solutions; addition of an equal volume of acetone to the aqueous phase prior to extraction greatly increases the yield.

Chromatography. PAPER: system P1—Rf 0·93 (location under ultraviolet light, absorption; location by diazotisation followed by *alkaline betanaphthol spray*).

THIN-LAYER: system T1—Rf 0·69 (location by diazotisation followed by *alkaline betanaphthol spray*).

Colour Test. Copper sulphate test—grey-blue.

Crystal Tests. MICRO: *lead iodide solution*—short rods (*sensitivity:* 1 in 100); *sodium phosphate solution*—prisms (*sensitivity:* 1 in 100).

Ultraviolet Absorption Spectrum. Sulphaphenazole in methanol, maximum at 267 mμ (E1%, 1 cm 654).

Infra-red Absorption Spectrum. Potassium bromide disk. The principal peaks are: A 1148, B 1313 or 1507, C 1592 (p. 764).

Quantitative Estimation. Bratton and Marshall (1939) describe a colorimetric method for the quantitative determination of diazotised sulphonamides in biological fluids and tissues.

Metabolism. Sulphaphenazole is rapidly excreted and slowly absorbed. After a single dose, peak blood concentrations are attained in 3 to 4 hours and they are maintained for about 12 hours, although sulphaphenazole is still detectable in the serum after 36 hours.

Dose. Up to 3 g daily for two days, followed by 1 g daily for a few days.

Toxicity. Since sulphaphenazole has a fairly long duration of action it may produce toxic effects similar to those caused by sulphamethoxypyridazine (p. 553).

SULPHAPYRIDINE *Sulphonamide*

Synonym: Sulfapyridine.
Proprietary Name: M & B 693.

2-(*p*-Aminobenzenesulphonamido)pyridine

$C_{11}H_{11}N_3O_2S = 249{\cdot}3$

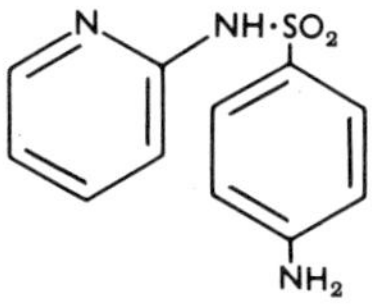

A white crystalline powder which slowly darkens on exposure to light. M.p. 191° to 193°.

Solubility. Soluble 1 in 3000 of water, 1 in 100 of boiling water, and 1 in 400 of ethanol; almost insoluble in ether and chloroform; soluble in dilute mineral acids and aqueous solutions of alkaline hydroxides.

SULPHAPYRIDINE SODIUM

Synonym: Soluble Sulphapyridine.
Proprietary Name: M & B 693 Soluble.

A white crystalline powder. On exposure to air, it slowly absorbs carbon dioxide, liberating sulphapyridine and becoming incompletely soluble in water.

Solubility. Soluble 1 in 3 of water and 1 in 10 of ethanol.

Extraction. Sulphapyridine may be extracted by ether from aqueous acid solutions; addition of an equal volume of acetone to the aqueous phase prior to extraction greatly increases the yield.

Chromatography. PAPER: system P1—Rf 0·66 (location under ultraviolet light, blue fluorescence; location by diazotisation followed by *alkaline betanaphthol spray*).

THIN-LAYER: system T1—Rf 0·67 (location by diazotisation followed by *alkaline betanaphthol spray*).

Colour Test. Copper sulphate test—green → brownish-green.

Crystal Tests. MICRO: *gold chloride solution*—clumps of small irregular crystals (*sensitivity:* 1 in 100); *platinic bromide solution*—rosettes of blades (*sensitivity:* 1 in 100).

Ultraviolet Absorption Spectrum. Sulphapyridine in water, maxima at 244 mμ (E1%, 1 cm 620) and 261 mμ (E1%, 1 cm 680); in ethanol, maximum at 270 mμ (E1%, 1 cm 857).

Metabolism. Sulphapyridine is metabolised mainly by acetylation but hydroxylation at position 5 of the pyridine ring may occur; the hydroxy-derivative is excreted in urine as its glucuronide conjugate.

Dose. Up to 4 g daily.

Toxicity. As for Sulphathiazole, p. 557.

LD50 (oral): in mice 15 g/kg (base); in mice 27 mg/kg (sodium salt).

SULPHAQUINOXALINE

Sulphonamide (Veterinary)

Proprietary Names: Embazin; Sulfacox.

2-(*p*-Aminobenzenesulphonamido)quinoxaline

$C_{14}H_{12}N_4O_2S = 300{\cdot}3$

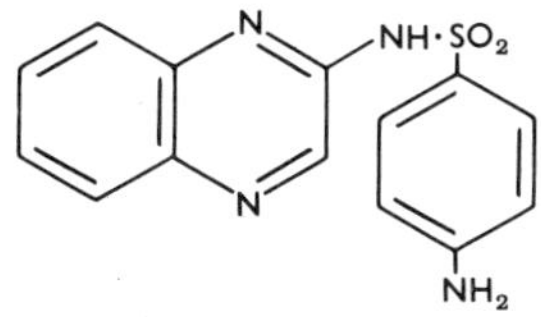

A yellow powder. M.p. 250°, with decomposition.

Solubility. Insoluble in water; very slightly soluble in ethanol; almost insoluble in ether; soluble in dilute mineral acids and in solutions of alkalis.

Extraction. Sulphaquinoxaline may be extracted by ether from aqueous acid solutions; addition of an equal volume of acetone to the aqueous phase prior to extraction greatly improves the yield.

Chromatography. PAPER: system P1—Rf 0·45, streaking (location by diazotisation followed by *alkaline betanaphthol spray*).

THIN-LAYER: system T1—Rf 0·71 (location by diazotisation followed by *alkaline betanaphthol spray*).

Colour Test. Copper sulphate test—yellow-green.

Ultraviolet Absorption Spectrum. Sulphaquinoxaline in 0·01N sodium hydroxide, maximum at 252 mμ (E1%, 1 cm 1100).

Use. Sulphaquinoxaline is mainly employed in the treatment of caecal coccidiosis in poultry; it is administered in the feed or in the drinking water.

Toxicity. The lethal oral dose in mice is 15 g/kg.

SULPHASALAZINE *Sulphonamide*

Synonyms: Salazosulfapyridine; Salicylazosulphapyridine.
Proprietary Names: Azulfidine; Salazopyrin.

4 - Hydroxy - 4′ - (pyrid - 2 - ylsulphamoyl) azobenzene-3-carboxylic acid

$C_{18}H_{14}N_4O_5S = 398{\cdot}4$

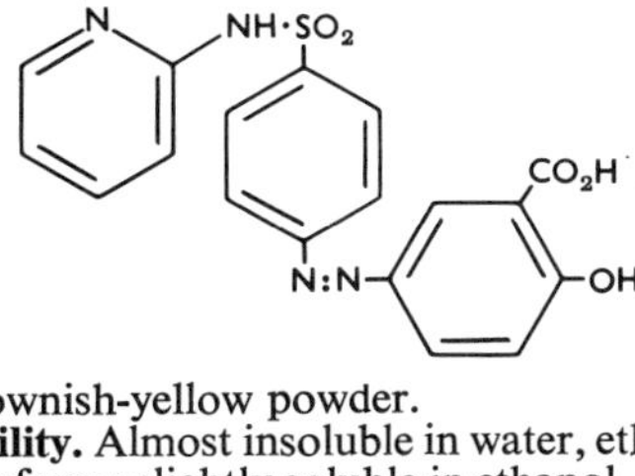

A brownish-yellow powder.

Solubility. Almost insoluble in water, ether, and chloroform; slightly soluble in ethanol.

Extraction. Sulphasalazine may be extracted

by ether from aqueous acid solutions; addition of an equal volume of acetone to the aqueous phase prior to extraction greatly increases the yield.

Chromatography. PAPER: system P1—Rf 0·83, visible orange spot.

THIN-LAYER: system T1—Rf 0·66, visible orange spot.

Colour Test. Copper sulphate test—orange-brown.

Dose. Up to 9 g daily.

Toxicity. Blood dyscrasias involving fatal agranulocytosis have occurred following sulphasalazine therapy.

SULPHASOMIDINE *Sulphonamide*

Synonyms: Sulfa-isodimerazine; Sulfaisodimidine; Sulfasomidine; Sulfisomidine.

NOTE. Sulphadimethylpyrimidine has been used as a synonym for both sulphasomidine and sulphadimidine; the 2 compounds are isomeric.

Proprietary Names: Aristamid; Elkosin.

4-(*p*-Aminobenzenesulphonamido)-2,6-dimethylpyrimidine

$C_{12}H_{14}N_4O_2S = 278{\cdot}3$

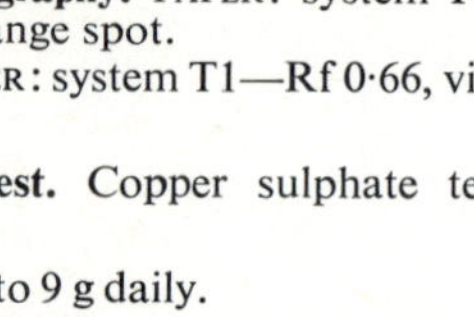

A white crystalline powder which slowly darkens on exposure to light. M.p. about 240°, with decomposition.

Solubility. Slightly soluble in water; soluble 1 in 60 of boiling water; slightly soluble in ethanol; very slightly soluble in ether and chloroform; readily soluble in dilute mineral acids and in solutions of alkali hydroxides.

Extraction. Sulphasomidine may be extracted by ether from aqueous acid solutions; addition of an equal volume of acetone to the aqueous phase prior to extraction greatly increases the yield.

Chromatography. PAPER: system P1—Rf 0·67 (location under ultraviolet light, yellow fluorescence; location by diazotisation followed by *alkaline betanaphthol spray*).

THIN-LAYER: system T1—Rf 0·64 (location by diazotisation followed by *alkaline betanaphthol spray*).

Colour Test. Copper sulphate test—green.

Crystal Tests. MICRO: *platinic bromide solution*—dense rosettes (*sensitivity:* 1 in 100); *potassium bismuth iodide solution*—bundles of rhomboids (*sensitivity:* 1 in 100).

Infra-red Absorption Spectrum. Potassium bromide disk. The principal peaks are: A 1125 or 1480, B 1138 or 1260 (p. 765).

Quantitative Estimation. Bratton and Marshall (1939) describe a colorimetric method for the quantitative determination of diazotised sulphonamides in biological fluids and tissues.

Metabolism. Sulphasomidine is rapidly absorbed and excreted; its relatively high solubility makes it useful in the treatment of urinary tract infections. It is only slightly acetylated in the body.

Dose. Up to 6 g daily.

Toxicity. Toxic effects following therapeutic doses are rare, owing to the relatively high solubility of the drug in urine.

SULPHASOMIZOLE *Sulphonamide*

Synonyms: M & B 4438; Sulfasomizole; TH 2132.

Proprietary Names: Amidozol; Bidizole.

5-(*p*-Aminobenzenesulphonamido)-3-methylisothiazole

$C_{10}H_{11}N_3O_2S_2 = 269{\cdot}3$

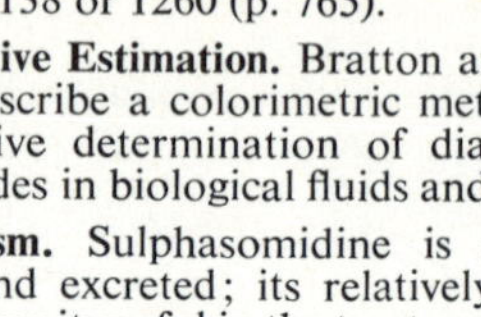

A white powder.

Solubility. Soluble 1 in 2000 of water; almost insoluble in ether and chloroform.

Extraction. Sulphasomizole may be extracted by ether from aqueous acid solutions; addition of an equal volume of acetone to the aqueous phase prior to extraction greatly increases the yield.

Chromatography. PAPER: system P1—Rf 0·93 (location under ultraviolet light, absorption; location by diazotisation followed by *alkaline betanaphthol spray*).

THIN-LAYER: system T1—Rf 0·66 (location by diazotisation followed by *alkaline betanaphthol spray*).

Colour Test. Copper sulphate test—brown.

Crystal Tests. MICRO: *lead iodide solution*—needles (*sensitivity:* 1 in 100); *sodium phosphate solution*—needles and plates (*sensitivity:* 1 in 100).

Ultraviolet Absorption Spectrum. Sulphasomizole in 0·1N hydrochloric acid, maxima at 245 mμ and 301 mμ; in 0·1N sodium hydroxide, maxima at 257 mμ and 280 mμ.

Quantitative Estimation. Bratton and Marshall (1939) describe a colorimetric method for the quantitative determination of diazotised sulphonamides in biological fluids and tissues.

Metabolism. Sulphasomizole is rapidly absorbed and fairly slowly excreted.

After an oral dose of 30 mg/kg, 5 patients excreted an average of 60% of the total dose in urine in the succeeding 24 hours. Of the total drug excreted, 62% was unchanged sulphasomizole, 37% consisted of the *N*-4-acetylated metabolite, and 0·7% was identified as a *N*-4-glucuronide which is thought to be an artefact, not a true metabolite. There was also a trace of *N*-4-sulphosulphasomizole (Bridges and Williams, 1963).

Dose. Up to 1 g daily.

Toxicity. Since sulphasomizole has a fairly long duration of action it may produce toxic effects similar to those caused by sulphamethoxypyridazine (p. 553).

SULPHATHIAZOLE *Sulphonamide*

Synonyms: Norsulfazol; Sulfanilamidothiazolum; Sulfathiazole; Sulfonazolum.
Proprietary Names: Cibazol; Eleudron; Sulfex; Thiazamide.

2-(*p*-Aminobenzenesulphonamido)thiazole
$C_9H_9N_3O_2S_2$ = 255·3

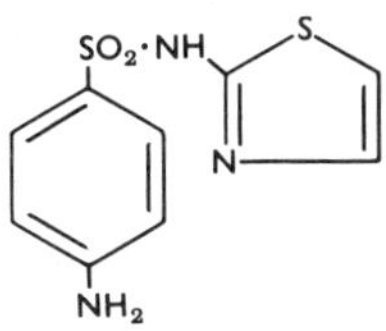

A white crystalline powder which slowly darkens on exposure to light. M.p. 200° to 203°.
Solubility. Soluble 1 in 2500 of water, 1 in 40 of boiling water, and 1 in 200 of ethanol; almost insoluble in ether and chloroform; soluble in dilute mineral acids and in solutions of alkali hydroxides and carbonates.

SULPHATHIAZOLE SODIUM

Synonym: Soluble Sulphathiazole.

A white crystalline powder which slowly darkens on exposure to light; on exposure to moist air it absorbs carbon dioxide, liberating sulphathiazole, and becomes incompletely soluble.
Solubility. Soluble 1 in 3 of water and 1 in 20 of ethanol.

Extraction. Sulphathiazole may be extracted by ether from aqueous acid solutions; addition of an equal volume of acetone to the aqueous phase prior to extraction greatly increases the yield.

Chromatography. PAPER: system P1—Rf 0·69 (location under ultraviolet light, absorption; location by diazotisation followed by *alkaline betanaphthol spray*).
THIN-LAYER: system T1—Rf 0·66 (location by diazotisation followed by *alkaline betanaphthol spray*); system T22—Rf 0·50 (location by diazotisation followed by N-*1-naphthylethylenediamine spray*, reddish-purple).

Colour Test. Copper sulphate test—purple-brown.

Crystal Tests. MICRO: *gold bromide solution*—feathery needles (*sensitivity:* 1 in 100); *potassium tri-iodide solution* (*1*)—large irregular crystals (*sensitivity:* 1 in 100).

Ultraviolet Absorption Spectrum. Sulphathiazole in water, maxima at 258 mμ (E 1%, 1 cm 452) and 284 mμ (E 1%, 1 cm 549).

Quantitative Estimation. Bratton and Marshall (1939) describe a colorimetric method for the quantitative determination of diazotised sulphonamides in biological fluids and tissues.

Metabolism. Sulphathiazole is rapidly absorbed when given by mouth and the peak blood concentration, 5 to 10 mg%, is attained in about 4 to 6 hours. A single dose is almost completely excreted in 24 hours, partly in the form of an insoluble acetyl derivative.

Dose. Up to 6 g daily.

Toxicity. Toxic effects following therapeutic doses of sulphathiazole are common; excretion of the insoluble acetyl derivative may cause blocking of the renal tubules leading to anuria or haematuria.
LD50 (oral): in mice 4·5 g/kg.

SULPHINPYRAZONE *Uricosuric*

Synonyms: G 28315; Sulfinpyrazone; Sulphoxyphenylpyrazolidine.
Proprietary Name: Anturan(e).

4 - (2 - Benzenesulphinylethyl) - 3,5 - dioxo - 1, 2-diphenylpyrazolidine
$C_{23}H_{20}N_2O_3S$ = 404·5

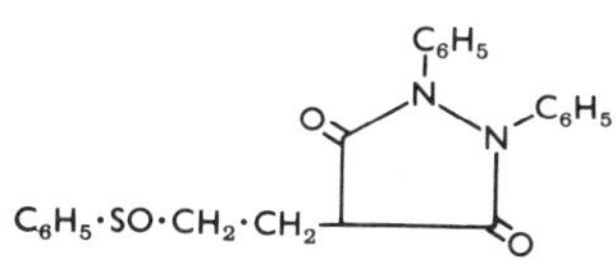

A white crystalline powder. M.p. 131° to 135°.
Solubility. Slightly soluble in water; soluble 1 in 40 of ethanol, 1 in 750 of ether, and 1 in 2 of chloroform.

Colour Test. *Liebermann's reagent*—orange.

Ultraviolet Absorption Spectrum. Sulphinpyrazone in 0·01N sodium hydroxide, maximum at 260 mμ (E 1%, 1 cm about 560).

Metabolism. Sulphinpyrazone is an analogue of phenylbutazone and has a much stronger uricosuric effect but much weaker analgesic and anti-inflammatory properties. Its action is limited almost exclusively to enhancing urate excretion through the kidneys, probably by blocking tubular resorption of urate.
Sulphinpyrazone is rapidly and completely absorbed from the gastro-intestinal tract and its uricosuric effect may last for 10 hours.
About 50% of an orally administered dose is excreted in the urine in 24 hours. Most of the drug is excreted unchanged but metabolism to the *p*-hydroxy-derivative may occur.

Dose. Up to 600 mg daily.

Toxicity. The acute fatal dose is stated to be in the region of 5 to 30 g.
LD50 (intravenous): in mice 240 mg/kg.

SULPHONAL *Hypnotic*

Synonym: Sulphonmethane.

2,2-Di(ethylsulphonyl)propane
$C_7H_{16}O_4S_2 = 228{\cdot}3$

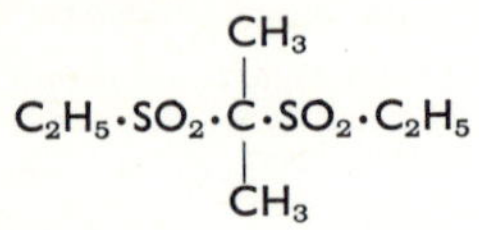

A white powder. M.p. 125° to 127°.

Solubility. Soluble 1 in 450 of water, 1 in 15 of boiling water, 1 in 80 of ethanol, 1 in 90 of ether, and 1 in 3 of chloroform.

Chromatography. GAS: system G2/225—retention time 0·35 relative to diphenhydramine; system G4—retention time 1·15 relative to diphenhydramine.

Colour Test. Heat with a few drops of *sulphuric acid* containing a trace of phenol—green.

Metabolism. Sulphonal is largely metabolised by oxidation of the sulphone groups to unknown metabolites, possibly sulphonic acids. It is excreted very slowly and successive doses may have a dangerous cumulative effect.

Dose. Up to 1·2 g.

Toxicity. A single dose of 2 to 30 g may cause acute fatal poisoning but recovery has followed very much larger doses. The effects caused by accumulation of sulphonal makes it one of the most dangerous of the hypnotics. It may lead to the destruction of haemoglobin in the blood, with the appearance of haematoporphyrins in the urine, which acquires a cherry-red colour and reduces Fehling's solution.

SULPHORMETHOXINE *Sulphonamide*

Synonyms: Ro 4-4393; Sulphorthodimethoxine.
Proprietary Name: Fanasil.

4-*p*-Aminobenzenesulphonamido-5,6-dimethoxypyrimidine
$C_{12}H_{14}N_4O_4S = 310{\cdot}3$

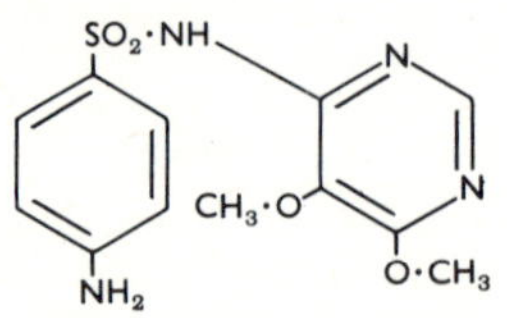

Solubility. Almost insoluble in ether and chloroform.

Extraction. Sulphormethoxine may be extracted by ether from aqueous acid solutions; addition of an equal volume of acetone to the aqueous phase prior to extraction greatly increases the yield.

Chromatography. PAPER: system P1—Rf 0·86 (location under ultraviolet light, strong absorption; location by diazotisation followed by *alkaline betanaphthol spray*).
THIN-LAYER: system T1—Rf 0·67 (location by diazotisation followed by *alkaline betanaphthol spray*).

Colour Test. Copper sulphate test—pale green.

Crystal Tests. MICRO: *lead iodide solution*—bunches of irregular crystals (*sensitivity:* 1 in 100); *potassium bismuth iodide solution*—rosettes of plates (*sensitivity:* 1 in 100).

Quantitative Estimation. Bratton and Marshall (1939) describe a colorimetric method for the quantitative determination of diazotised sulphonamides in biological fluids and tissues.

Metabolism. Sulphormethoxine is a long-acting sulphonamide. It gives a high and early blood concentration and is excreted very slowly.
Studies in children (Vest, 1966) have shown that after a single dose of 25 mg/kg, the blood concentration falls from an initial value of 8 to 12 mg% to 2 to 6 mg% over a period of 7 days. The percentage of acetylated metabolites in the serum is usually below 10% of the total concentration and that of the glucuronide conjugates is even less. In the urine, 16 to 46% of the administered dose is recovered in one week, 30% being in the free form, 60% being acetylated, and the rest being conjugated with glucuronic acid.

Dose. Up to 1 g as a single dose, once weekly.

Toxicity. The toxic effects of sulphormethoxine are similar to those of other long-acting sulphonamides—see under Sulphamethoxypyridazine, p. 553.

SULTHIAME *Anticonvulsant*

Synonyms: Riker 594; Sultiame.
Proprietary Name: Ospolot.

Tetrahydro-2-*p*-sulphamoylphenyl-2*H*-1,2-thiazine 1,1-dioxide
$C_{10}H_{14}N_2O_4S_2 = 290{\cdot}4$

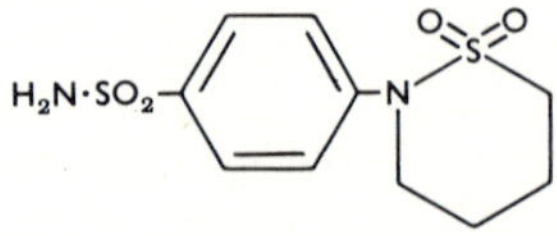

A colourless crystalline powder. M.p. 185° to 187°.

Solubility. Soluble 1 in 2000 of water, 1 in 350 of ethanol, 1 in 500 of ether, and 1 in 700 of chloroform.

Extraction. Sulthiame is extracted by ethyl acetate from aqueous acid solutions.

Chromatography. PAPER: system P12—Rf 0·55 (location under ultraviolet light, absorption; location reagent p-*dimethylaminobenzaldehyde* *spray*, followed by exposure to ammonia vapour, yellow spot).

Metabolism. In animal studies over 80% of sulthiame was excreted in the urine (Friebel and Sommer, 1960).

Dose. Up to 600 mg daily.

Toxicity. The most frequently reported toxic effects due to sulthiame therapy are ataxia, anorexia, and lethargy; tachypnoea and dyspnoea provoked by metabolic acidosis occur frequently, especially in children.

CASE EXAMPLE. A youth swallowed 4 g of sulthiame in a suicide attempt; 6 hours later poisoning symptoms included vomiting, ataxia, and hyperpnoea; about 15 hours later, after a rise in the urinary pH to 9·4, about 20% of a urine sample crystallised on cooling. The crystals were pure sulthiame. The high pH probably prevented renal damage (Rockley, 1965).

SUXAMETHONIUM CHLORIDE

Muscle Relaxant

Synonyms: Choline Chloride Succinate; Succinylcholine Chloride.

Proprietary Names: Anectine; Lysthenon; Midarine; Pantolax; Quelicin Chloride; Scoline; Sucostrin Chloride.

2-Dimethylaminoethyl succinate dimethochloride dihydrate

$C_{14}H_{30}Cl_2N_2O_4, 2H_2O = 397{\cdot}3$

A white powder. M.p. about 160°.

Solubility. Soluble 1 in 1 of water and 1 in 350 of ethanol; insoluble in ether; slightly soluble in chloroform.

SUXAMETHONIUM BROMIDE

Proprietary Name: Brevidil M.

A white powder. M.p. about 225°.

Solubility. Soluble 1 in 0·3 of water and 1 in 5 of ethanol; insoluble in ether and chloroform.

SUXAMETHONIUM IODIDE

Proprietary Name: Celocurin.

A white, slightly hygroscopic, crystalline powder. M.p. 243° to 245°.

Solubility. Soluble in water; slightly soluble in ethanol; insoluble in ether.

Extraction. The suxamethonium salts are quaternary ammonium compounds (see p. 29).

Chromatography. PAPER: system P1—Rf 0·00 (location reagent *iodoplatinate spray*, strong reaction); system RP1a—Rf 1·00 (location reagent *iodoplatinate spray*, positive reaction); system RP1b—Rf 1·00 (location as for RP1a). THIN-LAYER: system T1—Rf 0·01 (location reagent *acidified iodoplatinate spray*, positive reaction).

Crystal Tests. MICRO: *potassium cadmium iodide solution*—long needles (*sensitivity:* 1 in 1000); *potassium permanganate solution*—irregular blades and needles (*sensitivity:* 1 in 1000).

Infra-red Absorption Spectrum. Suxamethonium chloride. Potassium bromide disk. The principal peaks are: A 1724, B 1148, C 1308 (p. 765).

Metabolism. Suxamethonium salts are slowly and incompletely absorbed from the gastro-intestinal tract. Suxamethonium chloride is hydrolysed relatively rapidly by plasma cholinesterase to its acid and alcohol components, succinic acid and choline being formed. Normally, less than 3% of an intravenous dose is excreted unchanged in the urine.

Dose. Usually up to 40 mg (base) intravenously.

Toxicity. Prolonged apnoea occurs in patients with low serum pseudocholinesterase levels.

CASE EXAMPLES. Two reports of death of newborn babies immediately after an injection of suxamethonium chloride in mistake for distilled water (*Pharm. J.*, ii/1965, 412; ibid., ii/1966, 254).

SUXETHONIUM BROMIDE

Muscle Relaxant

Proprietary Name: Brevidil E.

2-Dimethylaminoethyl succinate diethobromide

$C_{16}H_{34}Br_2N_2O_4 = 478{\cdot}3$

A white, slightly hydroscopic, crystalline powder. M.p. 158°.

Solubility. Readily soluble in water.

Extraction. Suxethonium bromide is a quaternary ammonium compound (see p. 29).

Chromatography. PAPER: system P1—Rf 0·00 (location reagent *iodoplatinate spray*, strong reaction); system RP1a—Rf 1·00 (location reagent *iodoplatinate spray*, positive reaction); system RP1b—Rf 1·00 (location as for RP1a). THIN-LAYER: system T1—Rf 0·01 (location reagent *acidified iodoplatinate spray*, positive reaction).

Crystal Tests. MICRO: *platinic chloride solution*—bunches of prisms (*sensitivity:* 1 in 1000); *potassium permanganate solution*—coarse needles (*sensitivity:* 1 in 100).

Metabolism. Suxethonium bromide is hydrolysed rapidly to succinic acid and choline. The rate of hydrolysis is about 1½ times that of suxamethonium, hence it has a shorter duration of action than the latter.

Dose. Up to 100 mg (base) intravenously.

SYROSINGOPINE

Antihypertensive

Synonyms: Methyl Carbethoxysyringoyl Reserpate; SU 3118.

Proprietary Names: Isotense; Raunova; Singoserp.

Methyl 18-(4-ethoxycarbonyl-3,5-dimethoxybenzoyl)reserpate

$C_{35}H_{42}N_2O_{11} = 666{\cdot}7$

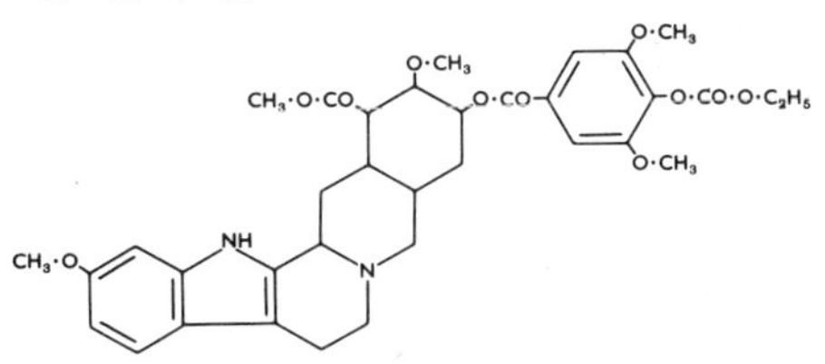

A white crystalline powder which is affected by light. M.p. 220° to 225°.

Solubility. Almost insoluble in water; slightly soluble in ether; soluble 1 in about 4 of chloroform; soluble in dilute acetic acid.

Extraction. Syrosingopine is extracted by organic solvents from aqueous alkaline solutions.

Chromatography. PAPER: system P1—Rf 0·81 (location under ultraviolet light, pale green fluorescence; location reagents: *iodoplatinate spray*, weak reaction; *bromocresol green spray*, weak reaction; *potassium permanganate spray*, strong reaction).

THIN-LAYER: system T1—Rf 0·78 (location reagent *potassium permanganate spray*, positive reaction).

Colour Tests. MICRO: sulphuric acid–formaldehyde test—pale brown (*sensitivity:* 1·0 μg); ammonium molybdate test—blue → green (*sensitivity:* 1·0 μg); ammonium vanadate test—greenish-brown (*sensitivity:* 1·0 μg); Vitali's test—pale yellow/pale yellow/brown (*sensitivity:* 1·0 μg).

Ultraviolet Absorption Spectrum. Syrosingopine in methanol, maxima at 258 mμ and 298 mμ.

Dose. Up to 6 mg daily has been given.

TACRINE *Narcotic Antagonist*

Synonym: Tetrahydroaminacrine.

5-Amino-1,2,3,4-tetrahydroacridine

$C_{13}H_{14}N_2 = 198{\cdot}3$

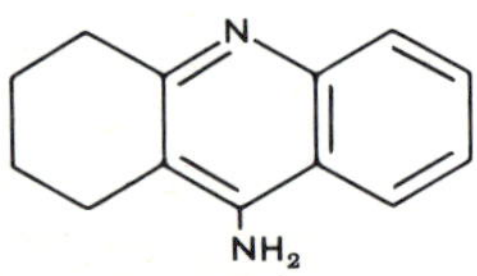

TACRINE HYDROCHLORIDE

Proprietary Names: Romotal; THA.

A pale yellow crystalline powder.

Solubility. Readily soluble in water.

Extraction. Tacrine is extracted by organic solvents from aqueous alkaline solutions.

Chromatography. PAPER: system P1—Rf 0·60 (location under ultraviolet light, blue fluorescence; location reagents: *iodoplatinate spray*, strong reaction; *bromocresol green spray*, weak reaction); system RP1a—Rf 0·64 (location under ultraviolet light, blue fluorescence; location reagent *iodoplatinate spray*, positive reaction); system RP1b—Rf 0·41 (location as for RP1a).

THIN-LAYER: system T1—Rf 0·43 (location reagent *acidified iodoplatinate spray*, positive reaction).

GAS: system G2/225—retention time 0·55 relative to codeine.

Crystal Tests. MICRO: *mercuric chloride solution*—small needles (*sensitivity:* 1 in 1500); *potassium permanganate solution*—stout needles (*sensitivity:* 1 in 1000).

Ultraviolet Absorption Spectrum. Tacrine in 0·1N sulphuric acid, maxima at 240 mμ (E1%, 1cm 1554), 323·5 mμ (E1%, 1cm 385), and 336 mμ (E1%, 1cm 340), and an inflexion at about 301 mμ (E1%, 1cm 174).

Quantitative Estimation. Tacrine and its metabolites in urine may be estimated by spectrophotometry (Kaul, 1962).

Metabolism. Following the oral and intramuscular administration of tacrine to human subjects, a lower percentage of the administered dose was excreted by those who received the drug orally.

At least 4 metabolites have been separated from rat urine and 2 of these correspond to 2 metabolites which have been isolated from the urine of human subjects receiving intramuscular tacrine plus morphine. These 2 metabolites have ultraviolet absorption spectra showing a close resemblance to that of tacrine which seems to indicate that the ring system of the tacrine molecule remains almost unchanged. However, one of these metabolites possesses a cyclic carbonyl group which might arise through an oxidative deamination of tacrine (Kaul, 1962).

Dose. Up to 60 mg by mouth or intravenously.

TALBUTAL *Barbiturate*

Synonym: Butalbital.

NOTE. The synonym Butalbital is also applied to allylbarbituric acid (p. 179).

Proprietary Name: Lotusate.

5-Allyl-5-s-butylbarbituric acid

$C_{11}H_{16}N_2O_3 = 224{\cdot}3$

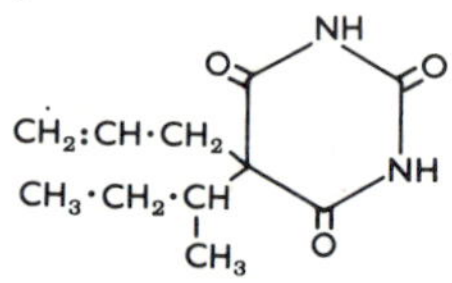

A white crystalline powder.

Solubility. Almost insoluble in water; soluble in ethanol, ether, and chloroform.

Screening Tests. See under Barbiturates, p. 208.

Extraction. Talbutal may be isolated in the A2 fraction (see p. 27).

Chromatography. PAPER: system RP1b—Rf 0·24 (location under ultraviolet light after exposure to ammonia; location reagent *potassium permanganate spray*, yellow on pink).

GAS: system G5—retention time 1·31 relative to barbitone; system G7—retention time 1·90 relative to barbitone.

Ultraviolet Absorption Spectrum. Talbutal is a 5,5-derivative—see Screening Test 3 under Barbiturates, p. 208.

Quantitative Estimation. See under Barbiturates, p. 208.

Dose. Usually 120 mg as a hypnotic.

Toxicity. It is an intermediate-acting barbiturate—see p. 207. The estimated minimum lethal dose in man is 2 g.

TECLOTHIAZIDE *Diuretic*

Synonym: Tetrachlormethiazide.

6 - Chloro - 3,4 - dihydro - 7 - sulphamoyl - 3 - trichloromethyl - 2*H* - benzo - 1,2,4 - thiadiazine 1,1-dioxide

$C_8H_7Cl_4N_3O_4S_2 = 415{\cdot}1$

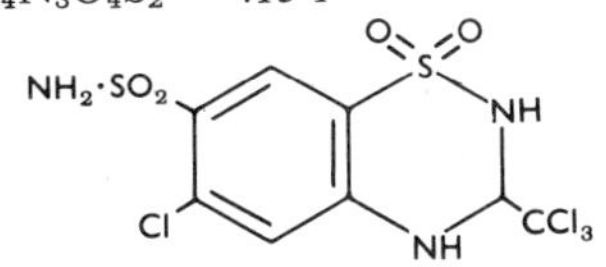

Teclothiazide melts at 230°, with decomposition.

TECLOTHIAZIDE POTASSIUM

Proprietary Names: Dépléil; Deplet. It is an ingredient of Hydeplet.

A white crystalline powder.

Solubility. Soluble in water; insoluble in most organic solvents.

Extraction. Teclothiazide may be isolated in the A2 fraction (see p. 27); it is distinguished from the barbiturates by chromatography (see below) and by the presence of additional ultraviolet maxima in the region 270 to 330 mμ.

Chromatography. PAPER: system P16—Rf 0·72 (location under ultraviolet light, absorption; location reagent *sodium naphthaquinone spray*, strong reaction); system RP1b—Rf 0·21 (location as for P16).

Ultraviolet Absorption Spectrum. Teclothiazide in water made alkaline to pH 10 with 2N ammonium hydroxide, maxima at 270 mμ (E 1%, 1 cm 350) and 315 mμ (E 1%, 1 cm 80).

Dose. Up to 220 mg daily.

TESTOSTERONE *Androgen*

Proprietary Names: Androlin; Andronage; Androteston; Andrusol; Malestrone (Injection); Mertestate; Neo-Hombreol F; Oreton Suspension; Synandrol F; Testandrone; Testoral Sublings; Testosteroid; Testrone; Testryl.

17β-Hydroxyandrost-4-en-3-one

$C_{19}H_{28}O_2 = 288{\cdot}4$

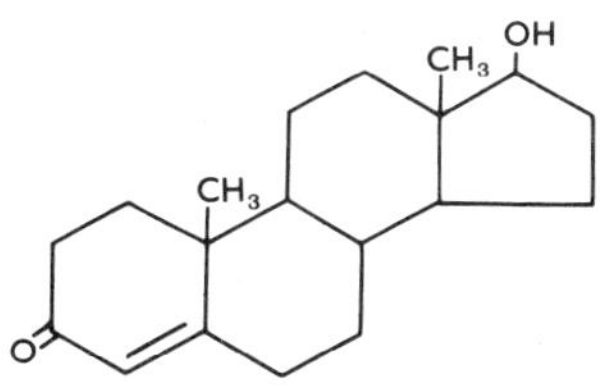

A white crystalline powder. M.p. 152° to 156°. Specific rotation of a 1% solution in ethanol, +106° to +112°.

Solubility. Almost insoluble in water; soluble 1 in 5 of ethanol, 1 in 100 of ether, and 1 in 2 of chloroform.

TESTOSTERONE ACETATE

17β-Acetoxyandrost-4-en-3-one.

Proprietary Name: Acéto-Sterandryl.

White crystals.

Solubility. Insoluble in water; soluble in dehydrated ethanol; very soluble in chloroform.

TESTOSTERONE CYPIONATE

17β-(3-Cyclopentylpropionyloxy)androst-4-en-3-one.

Synonym: Testosterone Cyclopentylpropionate.

Proprietary Names: Depo-Testosterone; Depovirin; Pertestis Depositum.

A white crystalline powder. M.p. 98° to 104°.

Solubility. Insoluble in water; freely soluble in ethanol, ether, and chloroform.

TESTOSTERONE ENANTHATE

17β-Heptanoyloxyandrost-4-en-3-one.

Synonyms: Testosterone Heptanoate; Testosterone Oenanthate.

Proprietary Names: Androtardyl; Delatestryl; Primoteston-Depot; Testoviron-Depot.

A white crystalline powder which should be stored at a temperature below 30°. M.p. 34° to 39°. Specific rotation of a 2% solution in dioxan, +77° to +82°.

Solubility. Insoluble in water; soluble 1 in 0·3 of ethanol and 1 in 0·3 of ether; soluble in chloroform.

TESTOSTERONE PHENYLPROPIONATE

17β-(β-Phenylpropionyloxy)androst-4-en-3-one.

Proprietary Name: Tes. P. P.

A white crystalline powder. M.p. 114° to 117°. Specific rotation of a 1% solution in dioxan, +86° to +91°.

Solubility. Almost insoluble in water; soluble 1 in 40 of ethanol.

TESTOSTERONE PROPIONATE

17β-Propionyloxyandrost-4-en-3-one.

Proprietary Names: Andronate; Andrusol(P); Neo-Hombreol; Oreton (injection); Pantestin (injection); Perandren (injection); Sterandryl; Testosid (injection); Testoviron; Virormone (injection).

A white crystalline powder. M.p. 119° to 122°. Specific rotation of a 1% solution in dioxan, +83° to +90°.

Solubility. Almost insoluble in water; soluble 1 in 6 of ethanol; soluble in ether and chloroform.

Extraction. Testosterone is extracted from neutral solutions with freshly distilled ethyl acetate.

Ultraviolet Absorption Spectrum. Testosterone in ethanol, maximum at 240 mμ (E 1%, 1 cm 560); testosterone phenylpropionate and testosterone propionate in ethanol, maximum at about 240 mμ (E 1%, 1 cm 395).

Infra-red Absorption Spectrum. Testosterone. Potassium bromide disk. The principal peaks are: A 1650, B 1051 or 1061, C 872 or 1225 (p. 765).

Quantitative Estimation. Brownie *et al.* (1964) describe a gas chromatographic method for the determination of testosterone in peripheral blood.

Metabolism. Testosterone is the androgenic hormone formed in the testes. It controls the development and maintenance of the male sex organs and the male secondary sex characteristics. It is metabolised, chiefly in the liver, to androstane-3α,17β-diol, androsterone, and etiocholanolone. These metabolites are excreted in the urine.

Dose. Varies according to the type of preparation used and the condition treated; usually administered intramuscularly or by implantation.

Toxicity. Testosterone and other androgens give rise to side-effects which can be related to their androgenic or anabolic activities. Large and repeated doses in early puberty may cause closure of the epiphyses and stop linear growth. In women, the inhibitory action of testosterone on the activity of the anterior pituitary results in the suppression of ovarian activity and menstruation. In men, large doses suppress spermatogenesis and cause degenerative changes in the seminiferous tubules.

TETRACHLOROETHANE *Industrial Solvent*

Synonym: Acetylene Tetrachloride.
Proprietary Names: Bonoform; Cellon.

1,1,2,2-Tetrachloroethane
$Cl_2{\cdot}CH{\cdot}CH{\cdot}Cl_2 = 167{\cdot}9$

A colourless, mobile, non-flammable, corrosive, heavy liquid. B.p. 146°. Refractive index at 25°, 1·4918.
Solubility. Almost insoluble in water; miscible with ethanol, ether, and chloroform.

Extraction. Tetrachloroethane is volatile and may be isolated by distillation (see p. 18).

Chromatography. GAS: system G8/160—retention time 14·0 relative to n-propanol.

Metabolism. Tetrachloroethane is absorbed fairly rapidly from the lungs. It is metabolised and eliminated rather slowly and tends to remain unchanged in various tissues.
During a 4-hour period following exposure only 19·6% of the amount absorbed was exhaled. Seventeen hours after exposure the brain, heart, liver, lungs, kidneys, and fat all contained amounts ranging from 4·7 to 63·3 mg%.
It has been suggested that tetrachloroethane is metabolised by hydrolysis followed by oxidation to yield oxalic acid. Oxalic acid may contribute to the high toxicity of tetrachloroethane. It seems to have been established that its metabolism is not a process of dehydrochlorination eventually yielding trichloroacetic acid, since this has not been found as an excretion product.

Toxicity. Tetrachloroethane is one of the most poisonous of the chlorinated hydrocarbons. Inhalation or ingestion has a narcotic effect and causes degenerative changes in the liver. The lethal dose is about 3 ml and the maximum permissible atmospheric concentration is 5 p.p.m.

CASE EXAMPLE. A 67-year-old man died at least 8 hours after ingesting tetrachloroethane; 4 ml of tetrachloroethane was recovered from the stomach contents and a positive qualitative test for the presence of tetrachloroethane was given by a blood sample (Lynch, 1967).

TETRACHLOROETHYLENE *Anthelmintic/Solvent*

Synonym: Perchlorethylene.
Proprietary Name: Perchlor.

$Cl_2{\cdot}C{:}C{\cdot}Cl_2 = 165{\cdot}8$

A colourless mobile non-flammable liquid. F.p. −22°. B.p. 119° to 122°.
Solubility. Insoluble in water; soluble in ethanol; miscible with ether and chloroform.

Extraction. Tetrachloroethylene is volatile and may be isolated by distillation (see p. 18).

Colour Test. Tetrachloroethylene may be distinguished from carbon tetrachloride and chloroform by the following test: to 5 ml of tetrachloroethylene in a stoppered cylinder add 5 ml of a saturated solution of bromine in water and shake vigorously at intervals of 15 minutes for 1 hour—bromine colour fades and there is a white turbidity in the lower layer.

Metabolism. In contrast to trichloroethylene, tetrachloroethylene is slowly metabolised by the body, hence its excretion is prolonged. It is partly excreted unchanged through the lungs but is also converted into an unknown water-soluble metabolite.

Dose. Up to 3 ml as a single dose.

Toxicity. Tetrachloroethylene is less toxic than carbon tetrachloride (p. 240). Inhalation of the vapour in concentrations of more than 200 p.p.m. for any length of time may produce dizziness, excessive perspiration, nausea and vomiting, stupor, and loss of consciousness. Kidney and liver damage may occur and some deaths have been reported.
The estimated lethal dose is stated to be 10 g. The maximum permissible concentration in a factory atmosphere is 100 p.p.m.

TETRACYCLINE *Antibiotic*

Proprietary Name: Tetrabon.

4 - Dimethylamino - 1,4,4a,5,5a,6,11,12a - octahydro - 3,6,10,12,12a - pentahydroxy - 6 - methyl - 1,11-dioxonaphthacene-2-carboxyamide
$C_{22}H_{24}N_2O_8 = 444{\cdot}4$

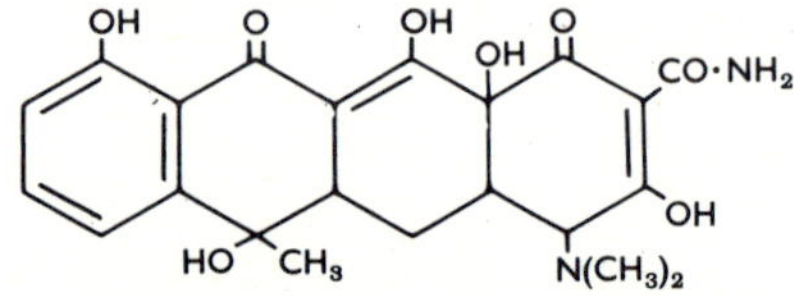

A yellow crystalline powder which darkens on exposure to strong sunlight.
Solubility. Soluble 1 in 2500 of water and 1 in 50 of ethanol; almost insoluble in ether and chloroform; freely soluble in dilute acids and in alkali hydroxide solutions.

TETRACYCLINE HYDROCHLORIDE
Proprietary Names: Achromycin; Ambramycin; Economycin; Hostacycline; Panmycin; Polycycline; Sanclomycin; Steclin; Tetracyn; Totomycin.

A yellow hygroscopic crystalline powder which darkens in moist air on exposure to strong sunlight. M.p. about 214°, with decomposition.
Solubility. Soluble 1 in 10 of water and 1 in 100 of ethanol; almost insoluble in ether and chloroform.

Chromatography. PAPER: system P1—Rf 0·25 (location under ultraviolet light, orange fluorescence; location reagents: *ninhydrin spray*, orange; *potassium permanganate spray*, weak reaction); system RP1a—Rf 0·67 (location under ultraviolet light, yellow fluorescence); system RP1b—Rf 0·74 (location as for RP1a).
A paper chromatographic method of separation of tetracycline derivatives in blood and urine is described by Addison and Clark (1963).

THIN-LAYER: system T1—Rf 0·05, streaking (location under ultraviolet light, orange fluorescence; location reagent *potassium permanganate spray*, positive reaction).
Ascione *et al.* (1967) describe a thin-layer method for the separation of tetracyclines and their derivatives.

Colour Tests. MICRO: sulphuric acid–formaldehyde test—dull orange (*sensitivity:* 0·5 μg); ammonium molybdate test—black-purple (*sensitivity:* 0·5 μg); ammonium vanadate test—purple → red → orange (*sensitivity:* 0·5 μg); sulphuric acid test—purple → yellow; Vitali's test—yellow/yellow/brown (*sensitivity:* 0·5 μg).

Crystal Tests. MICRO: *sodium carbonate solution*—plates, best viewed under polarised light (*sensitivity:* 1·0 μg); *sodium phosphate solution*—rhomboidal plates, best viewed under polarised light (*sensitivity:* 1·0 μg).

Ultraviolet Absorption Spectrum. Tetracycline in water, maximum at 380 mμ (E 1%, 1 cm 365); in 0·1N sulphuric acid, maxima at 270 mμ (E 1%, 1 cm 501) and 356 mμ (E 1%, 1 cm 360).

Infra-red Absorption Spectrum. Tetracycline hydrochloride. Potassium chloride disk. The principal peaks are: A 1612, B 1580, C 1666 (p. 765).

Quantitative Estimation. Kohn (1961) and Silvestrov *et al.* (1963) have described spectrofluorimetric methods of estimating tetracycline in biological fluids.

Metabolism. After oral administration of the hydrochloride or other soluble salts, the tetracyclines are incompletely and irregularly absorbed from the gastro-intestinal tract. Therapeutically effective blood-levels of 0·1 to 0·3 mg% can usually be maintained by the 6-hourly administration of doses of 250 mg.
After absorption the tetracyclines diffuse into body fluids; they are bound in varying degrees to plasma protein. They are slowly excreted in the bile and urine; 20 to 25% of an orally administered dose and 50% of an intravenous dose are excreted in the urine.

Dose. Up to 4 g by mouth daily.

Toxicity. The side-effects of tetracycline hydrochloride are common to all tetracyclines and include nausea, diarrhoea, and symptoms resulting from the overgrowth of non-susceptible organisms. Occasionally, severe and sometimes fatal liver damage has occurred in pregnant women.
The degradation products, epianhydrotetracycline and anhydrotetracycline, which are produced on storage in the presence of heat and moisture, may lead to nausea, vomiting, proteinuria, glycosuria, and acidosis.
LD50 (oral): in mice more than 3 g/kg.
CASE EXAMPLES. Six young pregnant women who developed acute pyelonephritis were given 2·4 to 4 g (average) of tetracycline intravenously daily for 3 to 9 days. Jaundice soon developed, then azotaemia and terminal shock. Examination post mortem showed fine-droplet fatty metamorphosis of all liver lobules but no necrosis (Schultz *et al.*, 1963).

TETRAHYDROZOLINE *Sympathomimetic*

Synonym: Tetryzoline.

2-(1,2,3,4-Tetrahydronaphth-1-yl)-2-imidazoline

$C_{13}H_{16}N_2 = 200{\cdot}3$

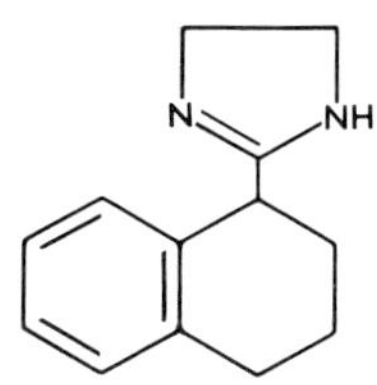

A white crystalline powder.
Solubility. Soluble in water and chloroform.

TETRAHYDROZOLINE HYDROCHLORIDE
Proprietary Names: Tyzanol; Tyzine; Visine.
A white crystalline powder.
Solubility. Freely soluble in water and ethanol; almost insoluble in ether; very slightly soluble in chloroform.

Extraction. Tetrahydrozoline is extracted by organic solvents from aqueous alkaline solutions.

Chromatography. PAPER: system P1—Rf 0·58 (location reagents: *iodoplatinate spray*, strong reaction; *bromocresol green spray*, weak reaction); system RP1a—Rf 1·00 (location reagent *iodoplatinate spray*, positive reaction); system RP1b—Rf 1·00 (location as for RP1a).

THIN-LAYER: system T1—Rf 0·15 (location reagent *acidified iodoplatinate spray*, positive reaction).

GAS: system G2/225—retention time 0·92 relative to diphenhydramine.

Colour Test. MICRO: Vitali's test— –/–/yellow (*sensitivity:* 1·0 μg).

Crystal Tests. MICRO: *gold bromide–hydrochloric*

acid solution—plates and prisms (*sensitivity:* 1 in 400); *lead iodide solution*—rosettes or sheaves of needles (*sensitivity:* 1 in 200).

Ultraviolet Absorption Spectrum. Tetrahydrozoline in 0·1N sulphuric acid, maxima at about 260 mμ (E1%, 1 cm 17·4), 265 mμ (E1%, 1 cm 21·3), and 272 mμ (E1%, 1 cm 19·8); tetrahydrozoline hydrochloride in water, maxima at about 264 mμ and about 271·5 mμ.

Infra-red Absorption Spectrum. Tetrahydrozoline hydrochloride. Potassium bromide disk. The principal peaks are: A 1600, B 742, C 1293 (p. 765).

Use. A 0·1% solution is used as nasal drops or nasal spray; 0·05% as eye-drops.

CASE EXAMPLE. A 1-year-old girl slowly recovered after ingesting about ½ to 1 teaspoonful of eye-drops containing 0·05% of tetrahydrozoline (Mindlin, 1966).

TETRAMISOLE *Anthelmintic (Veterinary)*

Synonyms: ICI 50627; McN-JR 8299; R 8299.

(±) - 2,3,5,6 - Tetrahydro - 6 - phenylimidazo - [2,1-*b*]thiazole

$C_{11}H_{12}N_2S$ = 204·3

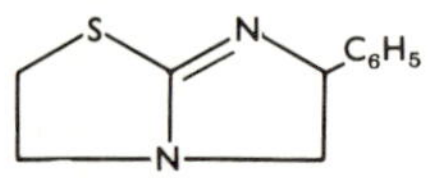

Solubility. Insoluble in water; soluble in chloroform.

TETRAMISOLE HYDROCHLORIDE

Proprietary Name: Nilverm.

A white amorphous powder.

Solubility. Soluble 1 in 6 of water; soluble in ethanol and chloroform.

Extraction. Tetramisole is extracted by organic solvents from aqueous alkaline solutions.

Chromatography. PAPER: system P1—Rf 0·41 (location under ultraviolet light, strong absorption; location reagents: *iodoplatinate spray*, strong reaction; *bromocresol green spray*, weak reaction).

THIN-LAYER: system T1—Rf 0·66 (location reagent *acidified iodoplatinate spray*, positive reaction).

Colour Test. MICRO: ammonium molybdate test—(pale blue) blue (*sensitivity:* 0·1 μg).

Crystal Tests. MICRO: *picrolonic acid*—bunches of blades or plates, best viewed under polarised light (*sensitivity:* 1 in 1000); *platinic chloride solution*—blades, often in crosses (*sensitivity:* 1 in 1000).

THALIDOMIDE *Sedative/Hypnotic*

Synonym: K 17.

Proprietary Names: see list in Extra Pharmacopoeia (Martindale), 25th Edn, p. 311.

α-Phthalimidoglutarimide

$C_{13}H_{10}N_2O_4$ = 258·2

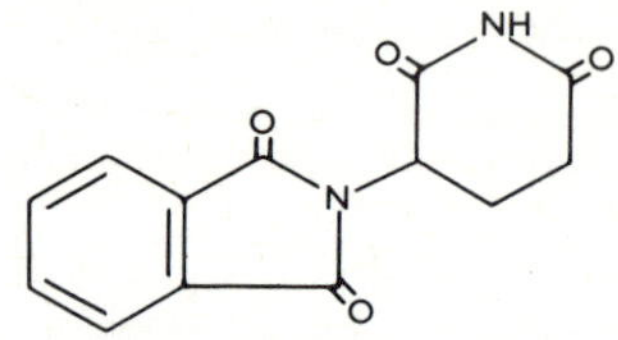

A white crystalline powder. M.p. 269° to 271°.

Solubility. Slightly soluble in water and ethanol; insoluble in ether and chloroform.

Extraction. Thalidomide is extracted by organic solvents from aqueous acid or alkaline solutions.

Chromatography. PAPER: system RP1b—Rf 0·65 (location reagent *bromine–starch–potassium iodide*).

Schumacher *et al.* (1964) describe a 2-dimensional paper chromatographic method of separation of thalidomide and its 12 spontaneous hydrolysis products.

Ultraviolet Absorption Spectrum. Thalidomide in ethanol, maxima at 218 mμ (E1%, 1 cm 2010) and 292·5 mμ; in 0·1N hydrochloric acid, maxima at 220 mμ (E1%, 1 cm 1950) and 299·5 mμ.

Quantitative Estimation. Thalidomide in blood, plasma, or urine may be estimated by spectrophotometry (Green and Benson, 1961).

Metabolism. At physiological pH values, thalidomide is hydrolysed, forming mainly α-(*o*-carboxybenzamido)glutarimide, although many other hydrolysis products are also detectable. Thalidomide reacts with putrescine, spermidine, ethylenediamine, and cadaverine.

After oral administration of thalidomide to pregnant mice, it was found that the thalidomide was distributed in similar concentrations in the brain, liver, lungs, and spleen. After 8 hours, about 70% of the dose administered was accounted for in the faeces, urine, and gastro-intestinal contents. Chromatography of the extracts of the foetal tissue showed that 1½ hours after administration only thalidomide could be detected. However, after 4 and 8 hours, the drug and one of its hydrolysis products, α-(*o*-carboxybenzamido)glutarimide, were present.

Thalidomide has been shown to have immunosuppressive activity. It has recently been tried in the treatment of cancer and of lepra reaction.

Toxicity. In November 1961 it was reported that thalidomide apparently had teratogenic effects when administered to women early in pregnancy and this was soon followed by further reports which implicated thalidomide beyond doubt. Thalidomide was withdrawn from the British market in December 1961.

Other toxic effects due to thalidomide include paraesthesias and peripheral neuritis.

CASE EXAMPLES. See Extra Pharmacopoeia (Martindale), 25th Edn, p. 310.

THEBACON *Narcotic Analgesic*

Synonyms: Acethydrocodone; Acetyldihydrocodeinone; Acétylodéméthylodihydrothébaine; Diacodon; Dihydrocodeinone Enol Acetate.

6 - Acetoxy - 4,5 - epoxy - 3 - methoxy - *N* - methylmorphin - 6 - ene

$C_{20}H_{23}NO_4 = 341{\cdot}4$

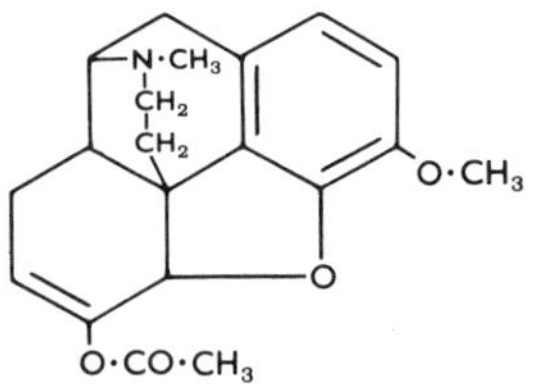

A white powder. M.p. 154°.

Solubility. Insoluble in water; soluble in ethanol, ether, chloroform, and dilute acetic acid.

THEBACON HYDROCHLORIDE

Proprietary Names: Acedicon; Cofadicon; Novocodon; Thebacetyl.

White crystals. M.p. 132° to 135°, with decomposition.

Extraction. Thebacon is extracted by organic solvents from aqueous alkaline solutions.

Chromatography. PAPER: system P1—Rf 0·36 (location under ultraviolet light, strong absorption; location reagent *iodoplatinate spray*, strong reaction); system RP1a—Rf 0·83 (location reagent *iodoplatinate spray*, positive reaction); system RP1b—Rf 0·00 (location under ultraviolet light, absorption; location reagent *iodoplatinate spray*, positive reaction).

THIN-LAYER: system T1—Rf 0·42 (location reagent *acidified iodoplatinate spray*, positive reaction).

GAS: system G2/225—retention time 1·52 relative to codeine.

Colour Tests. MICRO: sulphuric acid–formaldehyde test—yellow→purple (*sensitivity:* 0·25 μg); ammonium molybdate test—green→blue (*sensitivity:* 0·25 μg); Vitali's test—faint yellow/faint yellow/orange (*sensitivity:* 1·0 μg).

Crystal Tests. MICRO: *potassium cadmium iodide solution*—fine dendrites (*sensitivity:* 1 in 1000); *potassium mercuric iodide solution*—feathery rosettes (*sensitivity:* 1 in 1000).

Ultraviolet Absorption Spectrum. Thebacon in 0·1N sulphuric acid, maximum at 281 mμ (E 1%, 1 cm 41·2) and inflexion at 276 mμ.

Dose. Up to 10 mg.

THEBAINE *Narcotic*

Synonym: Paramorphine.

3,6 - Dimethoxy - 4,5 - epoxy - *N* - methyl - morphin-6,8-diene

$C_{19}H_{21}NO_3 = 311{\cdot}4$

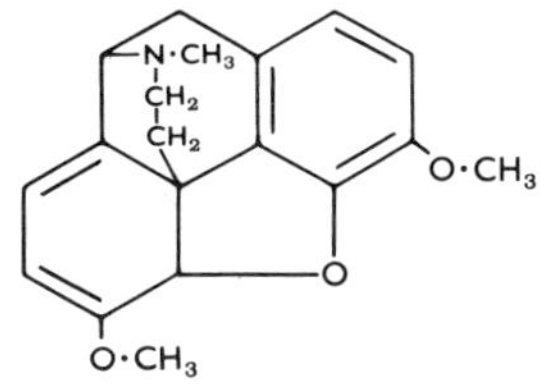

A white powder. M.p. 193°.

Solubility. Soluble 1 in 1500 of water, 1 in 10 of ethanol, 1 in 200 of ether, and 1 in 13 of chloroform; soluble in dilute acetic acid.

THEBAINE HYDROCHLORIDE

White crystals.

Solubility. Soluble 1 in 16 of water.

Extraction. Thebaine is extracted by organic solvents from aqueous alkaline solutions.

Chromatography. PAPER: system P1—Rf 0·32 (location under ultraviolet light, strong absorption; location reagents: *iodoplatinate spray*, strong reaction; *bromocresol green spray*, weak reaction); system RP1a—Rf 0·72 (location under ultraviolet light, absorption; location reagent *iodoplatinate spray*, positive reaction); system RP1b—Rf 0·06 (location as for RP1a).

THIN-LAYER: system T1—Rf 0·41 (location reagent *acidified iodoplatinate spray*, positive reaction).

GAS: system G6—retention time 1·44 relative to codeine.

Colour Tests. MICRO: sulphuric acid–formaldehyde test—red→orange (*sensitivity:* 0·05 μg); ammonium molybdate test—greenish-brown→red-brown (*sensitivity:* 0·1 μg); ammonium vanadate test—orange-brown (*sensitivity:* 0·1 μg); Vitali's test—yellow/yellow/orange (*sensitivity:* 1·0 μg).

Crystal Tests. MICRO: *platinic chloride solution*—dense rosettes (*sensitivity:* 1 in 1500); *sodium carbonate solution*—rosettes of small plates (*sensitivity:* 1 in 3000).

Ultraviolet Absorption Spectrum. Thebaine in 0·1N sulphuric acid, maximum at 283 mμ (E 1%, 1 cm 288).

Infra-red Absorption Spectrum. Thebaine hydrochloride. Potassium bromide disk. The principal peaks are: A 1234, B 1144 or 1605 (p. 793).

Toxicity. Thebaine is much less narcotic than morphine; in large doses and in some species of animals it may produce convulsions similar to those caused by strychnine.

THENALIDINE *Antihistamine*

Synonyms: AS 716; Thenopiperidine.

1-Methyl-4-(*N*-then-2-ylanilino)piperidine
$C_{17}H_{22}N_2S = 286{\cdot}4$

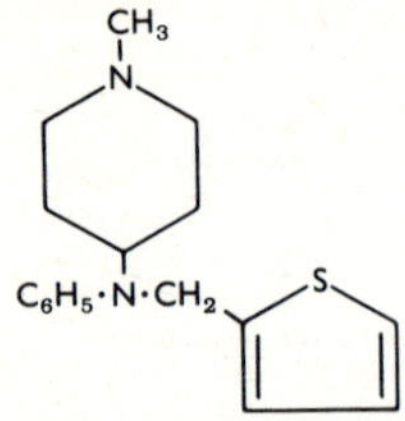

Solubility. Insoluble in water; soluble in chloroform.

THENALIDINE TARTRATE
Proprietary Name: Sandosten.

A white crystalline powder.
Solubility. Soluble in water.

Extraction. Thenalidine is extracted by organic solvents from aqueous alkaline solutions.

Chromatography. PAPER: system P1—Rf 0·60 (location under ultraviolet light, strong absorption; location reagents: *iodoplatinate spray*, strong reaction; *bromocresol green spray*, weak reaction); system RP1a—Rf 0·30 (location under ultraviolet light, absorption; location reagent *iodoplatinate spray*, positive reaction); system RP1b—Rf 0·05 (location as for RP1a). THIN-LAYER: system T1—Rf 0·45 (location reagent *acidified iodoplatinate spray*, positive reaction).

Colour Tests. MICRO: sulphuric acid–formaldehyde test—grey-purple (*sensitivity:* 0·5 μg); ammonium molybdate test—grey (*sensitivity:* 1·0 μg); ammonium vanadate test—orange→brown (*sensitivity:* 0·5 μg); Vitali's test—yellow/yellow/yellow (*sensitivity:* 1·0 μg).

Crystal Tests. MICRO: *picric acid*—branching needles or dense rosettes (*sensitivity:* 1 in 1000); *styphnic acid*—small rosettes (*sensitivity:* 1 in 1000).

Ultraviolet Absorption Spectrum. Thenalidine in 0·1N sulphuric acid, maximum at 234 mμ (E1%, 1 cm 280).

Toxicity. Cases of agranulocytosis following its therapeutic use have been reported.

THENIUM CLOSYLATE

Anthelmintic (Veterinary)

Proprietary Names: It is an ingredient of Ancaris and Bancaris.

Dimethyl(2 - phenoxyethyl)then - 2 - yl - ammonium *p*-chlorobenzenesulphonate
$C_{21}H_{24}ClNO_4S_2 = 454{\cdot}0$

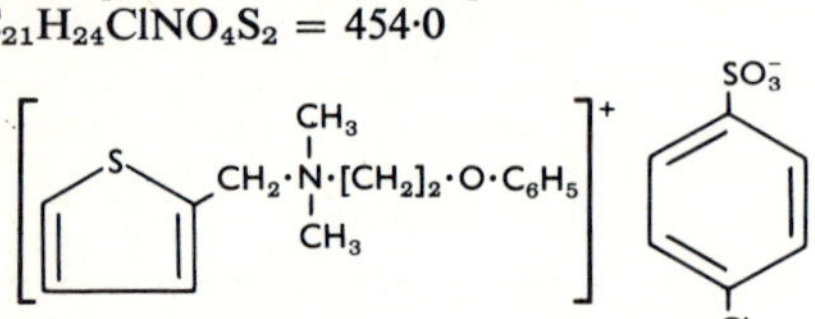

A white crystalline powder. M.p. 156° to 162°.

Solubility. Soluble 1 in 200 of water, 1 in 25 of ethanol, and 1 in 35 of chloroform; readily soluble in hot water, any excess forming an oily layer.

Extraction. Thenium closylate is a quaternary ammonium compound (see p. 29).

Chromatography. PAPER: system P1—Rf 0·61 (location under ultraviolet light, strong absorption; location reagent *iodoplatinate spray*, strong reaction); system RP1a—Rf 0·83 (location under ultraviolet light, absorption; location reagent *iodoplatinate spray*, positive reaction); system RP1b—Rf 0·81 (location as for RP1a).
THIN-LAYER: system T1—Rf 0·02 (location reagent *acidified iodoplatinate spray*, positive reaction).

Colour Tests. MICRO: sulphuric acid–formaldehyde test—purple (*sensitivity:* 0·1 μg); ammonium molybdate test—blue (*sensitivity:* 0·1 μg); ammonium vanadate test—green (*sensitivity:* 0·1 μg); Vitali's test— -/-/yellow-orange (*sensitivity:* 0·1 μg).

Crystal Tests. MICRO: *mercuric chloride solution*—bunches of irregular rhomboids (*sensitivity:* 1 in 1000); *potassium tri-iodide solution* (*1*)—rods (*sensitivity:* 1 in 1000).

Ultraviolet Absorption Spectrum. Thenium closylate in 0·1N sulphuric acid, maxima at 223 mμ (E1%, 1 cm 589), 268 mμ (E1%, 1 cm 46), and 275 mμ (E1%, 1 cm 36) and an inflexion at about 243 mμ (E1%, 1 cm 167).

Dose. For adult dogs: up to 500 mg (base equivalent) in combination with piperazine phosphate as a compound tablet.

THENYLDIAMINE

Antihistamine

Synonym: Win 2848.
Proprietary Name: Thenfadil.

NN - Dimethyl - *N′* - pyrid - 2 - yl - *N′* - then - 3 - yl ethylenediamine
$C_{14}H_{19}N_3S = 261{\cdot}4$

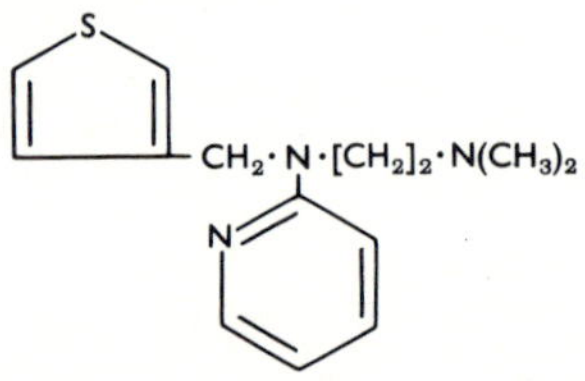

NOTE. Thenyldiamine is an isomer of methapyrilene (p. 410).

Thenyldiamine occurs as a liquid. B.p. 169° to 172° at 1·0 mm Hg.
Solubility. Insoluble in water; soluble in chloroform.

THENYLDIAMINE HYDROCHLORIDE
A white crystalline powder. M.p. 167° to 171°.
Solubility. Soluble 1 in 5 of water, 1 in 5 of ethanol, and 1 in 5 of chloroform; almost insoluble in ether.

Extraction. Thenyldiamine is extracted by organic solvents from aqueous alkaline solutions.

Chromatography. PAPER: system P1—Rf 0·27 (location under ultraviolet light, blue fluorescence; location reagents: *iodoplatinate spray*, strong reaction; *bromocresol green spray*, weak reaction); system RP1a—Rf 0·65 (location under ultraviolet light, blue fluorescence; location reagent *iodoplatinate spray*, positive reaction); system RP1b—Rf 0·07 (location as for RP1a).

THIN-LAYER: system T1—Rf 0·47 (location reagent *acidified iodoplatinate spray*, positive reaction).

Colour Tests. MICRO: sulphuric acid–formaldehyde test—black-purple (*sensitivity:* 0·1 μg); ammonium molybdate test—brown (*sensitivity:* 0·25 μg); ammonium vanadate test—olive (*sensitivity:* 0·1 μg).

Crystal Tests. MICRO: *gold bromide solution*—plates and needles (*sensitivity:* 1 in 1000); *platinic chloride solution*—feathery rosettes (*sensitivity:* 1 in 1000).

Ultraviolet Absorption Spectrum. Thenyldiamine in ethanol, maxima at 244 mμ (E1%, 1 cm 600) and 307 mμ (E1%, 1 cm 120); in 0·1N sulphuric acid, maxima at 239 mμ (E1%, 1 cm 735) and 315 mμ (E1%, 1 cm 319): thenyldiamine hydrochloride in ethanol, maximum at about 246 mμ.

Dose. Up to 180 mg daily.

Toxicity. The estimated acute lethal dose of thenyldiamine is stated to be in the range 25 to 250 mg/kg.

LD50 (oral): in rats 525 mg/kg.

THEOBROMINE *Xanthine Derivative*

Synonyms: Santheose; Teobromina.

An alkaloid contained in the seeds of *Theobroma cacao* (Sterculiaceae).

3,7-Dimethylxanthine

$C_7H_8N_4O_2 = 180{\cdot}2$

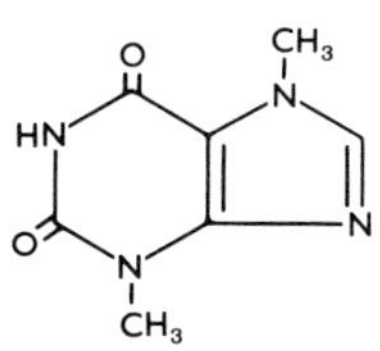

A white crystalline powder which sublimes at about 290°.

Solubility. Soluble 1 in 2000 of water, 1 in 150 of boiling water, 1 in 2500 of ethanol, and 1 in 6000 of chloroform; insoluble in ether.

Extraction. Theobromine may be isolated in the D1 fraction (see p. 27). As it is a weak base, a small amount may be extracted by organic solvents from aqueous acid solutions.

Chromatography. PAPER: system P1—Rf 0·35 (location under ultraviolet light, blue fluorescence; location by the Clarke-Kalayci test, reddish-purple).

GAS: system G6—retention time 1·08 relative to codeine.

Colour Test. Amalic acid test—purple (see p. 127).

Crystal Tests. MICRO: *gold bromide solution*—hairlike needles which are unstable (*sensitivity:* 1 in 3000); *platinic iodide solution*—small rods and plates (*sensitivity:* 1 in 1000).

Ultraviolet Absorption Spectrum. Theobromine in solution at pH 9·4, maximum at 273 mμ (E1%, 1 cm 550).

Infra-red Absorption Spectrum. Potassium bromide disk. The principal peaks are: A 1690, B 1221, C 1550 (p. 765).

Metabolism. Theobromine is well absorbed from the gastro-intestinal tract. It is metabolised by demethylation, mainly to 7-methylxanthine together with some 3-methylxanthine. The 7-methylxanthine derivative is further oxidised to 7-methyluric acid, about 3 to 4% of a 1-g dose being excreted as such.

Dose. Up to 600 mg.

Toxicity. In large doses, theobromine may cause nausea and anorexia. Cocoa meal, which may contain 2·5% of theobromine, has been found to be toxic to pigs.

THEOPHYLLINE *Xanthine Derivative*

Synonyms: Anhydrous Theophylline; Teofilina.

Proprietary Preparations: Theophylline is an ingredient of many proprietary preparations—see Extra Pharmacopoeia (Martindale), 25th Edn, p. 255.

1,3-Dimethylxanthine

$C_7H_8N_4O_2 = 180{\cdot}2$

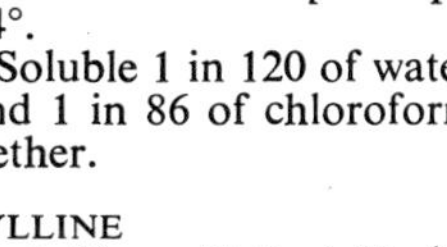

A white crystalline or amorphous powder. M.p. 269° to 274°.

Solubility. Soluble 1 in 120 of water, 1 in 80 of ethanol, and 1 in 86 of chloroform; sparingly soluble in ether.

AMINOPHYLLINE

Synonyms: Euphyllinum; Methaphyllin; Theophyllamin; Theophylline Ethylenediamine.

Proprietary Names: Cardophylin; Delaminoph; Diaphyllin.

Aminophylline is a mixture of theophylline and ethylenediamine, its composition approximately corresponding to the formula $(C_7H_8N_4O_2)_2, C_2H_4(NH_2)_2, 2H_2O = 456{\cdot}5$.

A white powder or granules. Aqueous solutions absorb

carbon dioxide from the air and become turbid due to the precipitation of theophylline.
Solubility. Soluble 1 in 5 of water but additional ethylenediamine or ammonia may be needed to give complete solution; insoluble in ethanol and ether.

CHOLINE THEOPHYLLINATE
Synonyms: Oxtriphylline; Theophylline Cholinate.
Proprietary Name: Choledyl.

A white microcrystalline powder. M.p. 187° to 192°.
Solubility. Soluble 1 in less than 1 of water and 1 in 10 of ethanol; very slightly soluble in ether and chloroform.

THEOPHYLLINE MEGLUMINE
Synonym: Theophylline Methylglucamine.
Proprietary Name: Glucophylline.
A mixture of theophylline hydrate ($C_7H_8N_4O_2$, H_2O) and *N*-methylglucamine ($C_7H_{17}NO_5$) in approximately equimolecular proportions.

A white powder.
Solubility. Freely soluble in water.

THEOPHYLLINE MONOETHANOLAMINE
Proprietary Name: Monotheamin.
A stable compound of anhydrous theophylline 75% and monoethanolamine 25%.

A white crystalline powder.
Solubility. Soluble in water.

THEOPHYLLINE SODIUM GLYCINATE
Synonym: Theophylline Sodium Aminoacetate.
Proprietary Names: Aminomed; Cinaphyl; Dorsaphyllin; Englate; Glynazan; Synophylate; Theoglycinate.
An equilibrium mixture of theophylline sodium ($C_7H_7N_4NaO_2$) and aminoacetic acid ($C_2H_5NO_2$).

A white crystalline powder.
Solubility. Freely soluble in water; very slightly soluble in ethanol; almost insoluble in chloroform.

Extraction. Theophylline may be isolated in the D1 fraction (see p. 27). As it is a weak base, a small amount may be extracted by organic solvents from aqueous acid solutions.

Chromatography. PAPER: system P1—Rf 0·58 (location under ultraviolet light, blue fluorescence; location by the Clarke-Kalayci test, reddish-purple); system RP1a—Rf 0·72 (location under ultraviolet light, absorption); system RP1b—Rf 0·73 (location as for RP1a).

Colour Test. Amalic acid test—purple (see p. 127).

Crystal Tests. MICRO: *gold bromide–hydrochloric acid solution*—needles which are unstable (*sensitivity:* 1 in 400); *mercuric chloride solution*—sheaves of broad needles (*sensitivity:* 1 in 400).

Ultraviolet Absorption Spectrum. Theophylline in 0·1N hydrochloric acid, maximum at 270 mμ (E1%, 1cm 530): aminophylline in 0·1N sodium hydroxide, maximum at 274 mμ (E1%, 1cm 575); in 0·1N sulphuric acid, maximum at 270 mμ (E1%, 1cm 500).

Infra-red Absorption Spectrum. Theophylline. Potassium bromide disk. The principal peaks are: A 1660, B 1700, C 1445 or 1560 (p. 766). Choline theophyllinate. Potassium bromide disk. The principal peaks are: A 1627, B 1676, C 1536 (p. 735).

Metabolism. After the oral ingestion of 750 mg of theophylline in man, 50% of the dose is excreted as 1,3-dimethyluric acid, nearly 20% as 1-methyluric acid, and about 10% unchanged. Theophylline is of low solubility, so that administration of the more soluble derivatives such as aminophylline, choline theophyllinate, and theophylline sodium glycinate is preferred.

Dose. Theophylline, max. single dose 500 mg.

Toxicity. Orally administered theophylline preparations are liable to cause gastric irritation. Toxic reactions occurring after intravenous administration of aminophylline may be fatal. Aminophylline has proved very poisonous to pigs after oral administration.
LD50 (oral): for aminophylline, in mice 540 mg/kg.

THIABENDAZOLE *Anthelmintic*

Synonym: MK 360.
Proprietary Names: Equizole; Mintezol; Thibenzole.

2-(Thiazol-4-yl)benzimidazole
$C_{10}H_7N_3S = 201{\cdot}3$

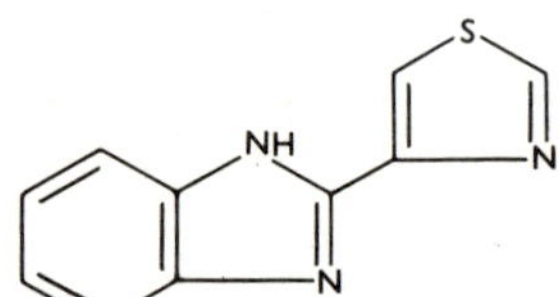

A white powder. M.p. 300°.
Solubility. Almost insoluble in water; soluble 1 in 150 of ethanol and 1 in 300 of chloroform; slightly soluble in ether; soluble in dilute mineral acids.

Extraction. Thiabendazole is extracted by organic solvents from aqueous alkaline solutions.

Chromatography. PAPER: system P1—Rf 0·06 (location under ultraviolet light, absorption; location reagents: *bromocresol green spray*, strong reaction; *potassium permanganate spray*, weak reaction).
THIN-LAYER: system T1—Rf 0·63 (location reagent *acidified iodoplatinate spray*, positive reaction, white).

Crystal Tests. MICRO: *picric acid*—clusters of small plates (*sensitivity:* 1 in 1000); *trinitrobenzoic acid solution*—long plates, best viewed under polarised light (*sensitivity:* 1 in 1000).

Ultraviolet Absorption Spectrum. Thiabendazole in 0·1N hydrochloric acid, maxima at 243 mμ (E1%, 1cm 620) and 302 mμ (E1%, 1cm 1240).

Infra-red Absorption Spectrum. Potassium bromide disk. The principal peaks are: A 1408, B 740, C 906 (p. 766).

Quantitative Estimation. Thiabendazole and its metabolites may be estimated spectrofluorimetrically in biological fluids and tissues (Tocco *et al.*, 1965).

Metabolism. Thiabendazole is metabolised chiefly to 5-hydroxythiabendazole which is excreted in the urine as glucuronide and sulphate conjugates. Thiabendazole is rapidly absorbed from the gastro-intestinal tract and peak plasma levels of 1·3 to 1·8 mg% are found within an hour of ingestion. The drug and its metabolite are excreted rapidly, 87% in the urine and 5% in the faeces within 48 hours. Small amounts of both unchanged thiabendazole and free 5-hydroxythiabendazole may be found in both the plasma and the urine.

Dose. In man, 50 mg/kg in 2 divided doses. In horses and cattle, up to 100 mg/kg.

Toxicity. LD50 (oral): in mice 3·6 and in rats 3·1 g/kg.

THIALBARBITONE *Barbiturate*

Synonyms: Thialbarbital; Thiohexallymal.

5-Allyl-5-cyclohex-2′-enyl-2-thiobarbituric acid

$C_{13}H_{16}N_2O_2S = 264{\cdot}3$

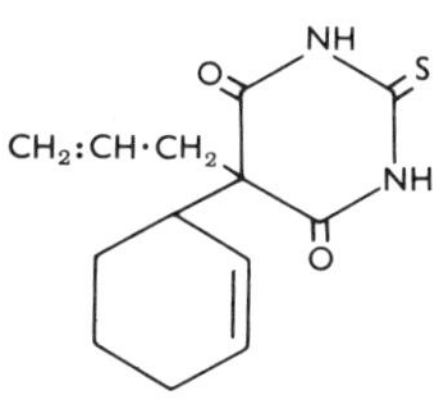

Solubility. Sparingly soluble in water; readily soluble in most organic solvents.

THIALBARBITONE SODIUM

Synonym: Thiohexallymalnatrium.

Proprietary Name: Kemithal Sodium.

A pale yellow hygroscopic powder.

Solubility. Very soluble in water and ethanol; insoluble in ether; slightly soluble in chloroform.

Screening Tests. See under Barbiturates, p. 208.

Extraction. Thialbarbitone may be isolated in the A2 fraction (see p. 27).

Chromatography. PAPER: system P2—Rf 1·80 relative to amylobarbitone (location under ultraviolet light, dark spot); system RP1b—Rf 0·05 (location under ultraviolet light after exposure to ammonia; location reagent *potassium permanganate spray*, yellow on pink).

THIN-LAYER: system T10—Rf 0·69 (location reagents: *mercurous nitrate spray*, black; *potassium permanganate spray*, yellow-brown; *Zwikker's reagent spray*, green).

Ultraviolet Absorption Spectrum. Thialbarbitone is a thiobarbiturate—see Screening Test 3, under Barbiturates, p. 208.

Infra-red Absorption Spectrum. Thialbarbitone sodium. Potassium bromide disk. The principal peaks are: A 1482, B 1685, C 1408 (p. 766).

Quantitative Estimation. See under Barbiturates, p. 208.

Metabolism. Thialbarbitone is a very short-acting barbiturate—see under Barbiturates, p. 207.

Studies in rabbits have shown the presence of thiourea and the thiourea derivative of thialbarbitone in the urine, indicating that hydrolysis of the barbiturate ring had occurred to a minor extent. Desulphuration has also been demonstrated; 2·7% of the corresponding oxybarbiturate and 2% of unchanged drug have been recovered from rabbit urine.

Dose. 0·5 to 1·5 g intravenously, for the induction of anaesthesia.

Toxicity. Thialbarbitone is said to give rise to less respiratory depression than other intravenously administered barbiturates.

THIAMBUTOSINE *Antileprotic*

Synonyms: DPT; Diphenylthiourea; Thiambutoxine; Thiocarbanilide; SU 1906.

Proprietary Name: Ciba 1906.

N-*p*-Butoxyphenyl-*N′*-*p*-dimethylamino-phenylthiourea

$C_{19}H_{25}N_3OS = 343{\cdot}5$

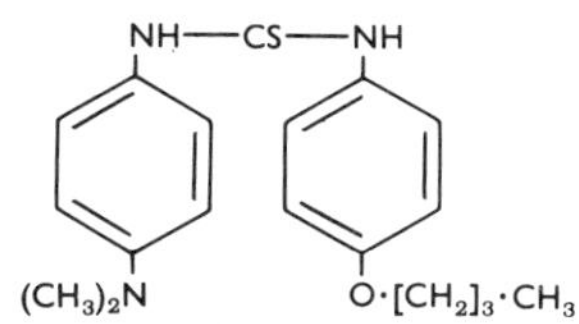

A white crystalline powder. M.p. 123° to 127°.

Solubility. Almost insoluble in water; soluble 1 in 300 of ether and 1 in 1·5 of chloroform.

Extraction. Thiambutosine is extracted by organic solvents from aqueous acid or alkaline solutions.

Chromatography. PAPER: system P1—Rf 0·93 (location under ultraviolet light, strong absorption; location reagent *nitrogen dioxide vapour*, orange).

THIN-LAYER: system T1—Rf 0·71 (location reagent *nitrogen dioxide vapour*, green).

GAS: system G2/225—retention time 0·68 (0·29) relative to diphenhydramine; system G4—retention time 0·76 (0·45; 1·0) relative to diphenhydramine.

Colour Tests. MICRO: ammonium molybdate test—pale blue→yellow-green (*sensitivity:* 1·0 μg); Vitali's test—yellow→blue-green/orange-brown/purple-brown (*sensitivity:* 0·25 μg).

Ultraviolet Absorption Spectrum. Thiambutosine in ethanol, maximum at 270 mμ (E1%, 1 cm 700).

Quantitative Estimation. Thiambutosine and its metabolites in the urine and faeces may be estimated colorimetrically (Ellard and Naylor, 1961).

Metabolism. Upon absorption the butoxy-group of thiambutosine is rapidly metabolised and water-soluble metabolites are formed. Only about 10% of oral doses of thiambutosine of up to 1·5 g are absorbed, and the metabolites are rapidly excreted in the urine. About 75% of the dose is excreted unchanged in the faeces. Intramuscular injections of aqueous suspensions of thiambutosine are absorbed extremely slowly and metabolites can be demonstrated in the urine up to 4 months later. The urinary excretion of thiambutosine and its metabolites does not exceed 41% of the injected dose; it is possible that the drug is incompletely absorbed from the site of injection. Very little faecal excretion is found after injection.

Dose. Up to 3 g daily.

THIAMINE *Vitamin*

Synonym: Aneurine.

3-(4-Amino-2-methylpyrimidin-5-ylmethyl)-5-(2-hydroxyethyl)-4-methylthiazolium chloride

$C_{12}H_{17}ClN_4OS = 300{\cdot}8$

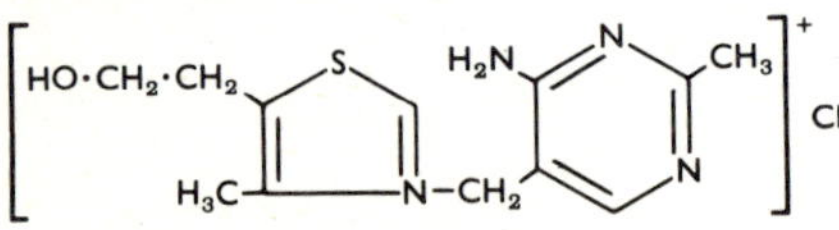

THIAMINE HYDROCHLORIDE

Synonyms: Aneurine Chloride Hydrochloride; Vitamin B_1.
Proprietary Name: Benerva; Betavel.

A white crystalline powder. M.p. about 207°, with darkening and decomposition.
Solubility. Soluble 1 in 1 of water and 1 in 100 of ethanol; almost insoluble in ether.

THIAMINE MONONITRATE

Synonyms: Aneurine Nitrate; Vitamin B_1 Mononitrate.

White crystals or crystalline powder.
Solubility. Soluble 1 in 35 of water; slightly soluble in ethanol and chloroform.

Extraction. Johnson *et al.* (1945) have described a method of extraction of thiamine from urine with an activated cation-exchange resin.

Chromatography. PAPER: system P1—Rf 0·00 (location reagents: *iodoplatinate spray*, strong reaction; *bromocresol green spray*, weak reaction); system RP1a—Rf 0·89 (location under ultraviolet light, absorption; location reagent *iodoplatinate spray*, positive reaction).

THIN-LAYER: system T1—Rf 0·01 (location reagent *acidified iodoplatinate spray*, positive reaction).

Colour Tests. Dissolve about 5 mg of thiamine hydrochloride in a mixture of 1 ml of *lead acetate solution* and 1 ml of 10% sodium hydroxide solution—yellow; after heating on a steam-bath—brown; on standing—a black precipitate of lead sulphide.

MICRO: Vitali's test— –/–/faint yellow (*sensitivity:* 1·0 µg).

Crystal Tests. MICRO: *gold chloride solution*—feathery rosettes (*sensitivity:* 1 in 1000); *platinic chloride solution*—small irregular plates or needles (*sensitivity:* 1 in 1000).

Ultraviolet Absorption Spectrum. Thiamine in ethanol, maxima at 233 mµ (E1%, 1 cm 380) and 267 mµ (E1%, 1 cm 240); in 0·1N sulphuric acid, maximum at 247 mµ (E1%, 1 cm 253) and an inflexion at about 260 mµ.

Metabolism. Thiamine is converted in the body, particularly in the liver, kidneys, and white blood-cells, to its pyrophosphate (co-carboxylase) which acts as the coenzyme of carboxylase, an enzyme essential for the breakdown of pyruvic acid in the body. In cases of thiamine deficiency, pyruvic and lactic acids accumulate in the tissues and this deranges the earlier phases of carbohydrate metabolism.
Thiamine is not stored in the body and is rapidly lost from the tissues during short periods of deficiency, therefore the normal diet must contain an adequate amount of the vitamin. Under normal conditions there is probably little destruction of thiamine in the gastro-intestinal tract, but intestinal disturbances may seriously retard its absorption.

Human Requirements. The optimum daily requirement is believed to be from 1 to 2 mg. The requirement is directly related to the carbohydrate intake and metabolic rate and is increased during periods of active growth or heavy muscular work, during pregnancy and lactation, and in pathological conditions such as fevers and hyperthyroidism, and in other conditions causing increased metabolism and diuresis.

Dose. Therapeutic, up to 100 mg daily; prophylactic, up to 5 mg daily.

Toxicity. When administered orally thiamine is non-toxic even in amounts many times greater than the therapeutic dose. Toxic reactions have been produced by injections of 50 mg and sudden death has been reported following the intravenous injection of 100 mg.
LD50 (oral): in mice 3 g/kg.

THIETHYLPERAZINE *Anti-emetic*

Synonym: GS 95.

2 - Ethylthio - 10 - [3 - (4 - methylpiperazin - 1 - yl)propyl]phenothiazine

$C_{22}H_{29}N_3S_2 = 399{\cdot}6$

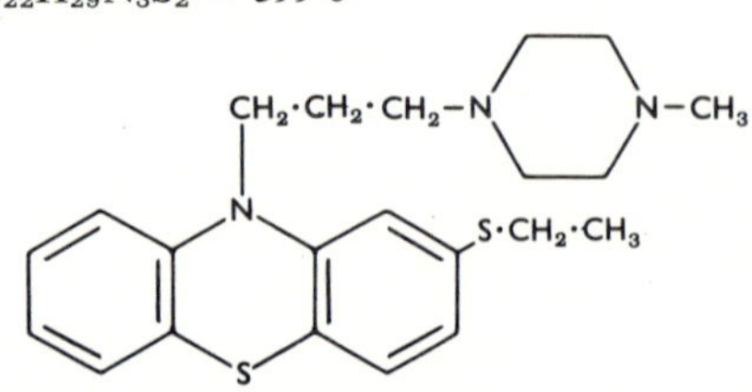

Solubility. Insoluble in water.

THIETHYLPERAZINE MALATE

Proprietary Name: Torecan (injection).

A white crystalline powder. M.p. 139°.
Solubility. Soluble 1 in 50 to 100 of water, 1 in 200 of ethanol, and 1 in less than 200 parts of ether and of chloroform.

THIETHYLPERAZINE MALEATE

Proprietary Name: Torecan (suppositories and tablets).

A yellow crystalline powder. M.p. 183·5°.

Solubility. Soluble 1 in less than 200 parts of water, ether, and chloroform; soluble 1 in 200 of ethanol.

Screening Test. *FPN reagent* with urine—blue (see p. 10).

Extraction. Thiethylperazine is extracted by organic solvents from aqueous alkaline solutions; hydrolysis of biological material is required in order to improve the yield.

Chromatography. PAPER: system P1—Rf 0·40 (location under ultraviolet light, pale green fluorescence; location reagents: *iodoplatinate spray*, strong reaction; *bromocresol green spray*, weak reaction; *FPN spray*, blue).

THIN-LAYER: system T1—Rf 0·48 (location reagent *acidified iodoplatinate spray*, positive reaction); system T6—Rf 0·47 (the spot may be converted on the plate to the sulphoxide, Rf 0·28; location of both spots under ultraviolet light).

Colour Tests. MICRO: sulphuric acid–formaldehyde test—dull red→dull green (*sensitivity:* 0·25 μg); ammonium molybdate test—(blue) blue (*sensitivity:* 0·1 μg); ammonium vanadate test—(green) purple, with excess reagent, or blue, with excess compound (*sensitivity:* 0·5 μg); Vitali's test—blue-green/brown/brown (*sensitivity:* 0·5 μg).

Crystal Test. MICRO: *potassium tri-iodide solution* (2)—rosettes, often shell-like (*sensitivity:* 1 in 1000).

Ultraviolet Absorption Spectrum. Thiethylperazine in ethanol, maxima at 264 mμ (E1%, 1 cm 973) and 316 mμ (E1%, 1 cm 123); in 0·1N sulphuric acid, maxima at 255 mμ (E1%, 1 cm 857) and 307 mμ (E1%, 1 cm 98).

Infra-red Absorption Spectrum. Thiethylperazine maleate. Potassium bromide disk. The principal peaks are: A 1356 or 1462, B 1568 (p. 766).

Dose. Up to 30 mg.

Toxicity. The acute lethal dose in man of the phenothiazine tranquillisers appears to be in the range 15 to 150 mg/kg.

THIOPENTONE *Barbiturate*

Synonyms: Pentothiobarbital; Thiomebumal; Thiopental.

5-Ethyl-5-(1-methylbutyl)-2-thiobarbituric acid

$C_{11}H_{18}N_2O_2S = 242{\cdot}3$

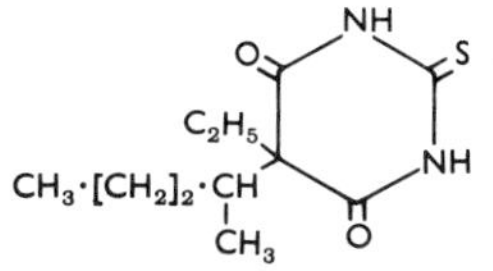

THIOPENTONE SODIUM

Synonyms: Soluble Thiopentobarbital; Thiomebumal-natrium.

Proprietary Names: Intraval Sodium; Nesdonal; Pentothal; Trapanal.

A yellowish-white hygroscopic powder.

Solubility. Soluble 1 in 1·5 of water; partly soluble in ethanol; insoluble in ether.

Screening Tests. See under Barbiturates, p. 208.

Extraction. Thiopentone may be isolated in the A2 fraction (see p. 27).

Chromatography. PAPER: system P2—Rf 1·8 relative to amylobarbitone (location under ultraviolet light, dark spot); system RP1b—Rf 0·03 (location under ultraviolet light after exposure to ammonia; location reagent *potassium permanganate spray*, yellow on pink).

THIN-LAYER: system T10—Rf 0·68 (location reagents: *mercurous nitrate spray*, black; *potassium permanganate spray*, yellow-brown on purple; *Zwikker's reagent spray*, green); system T11—Rf 0·73 (location reagents: *mercurous nitrate spray*, white on grey; *potassium permanganate spray*, yellow on purple); system T12—Rf 0·70 (location as for T11); system T13—Rf 0·94 (location as for T11).

GAS: system G5—retention time 4·8 relative to barbitone; system G7—retention time 2·38 relative to barbitone.

Colour Test. Zwikker's test—violet-blue.

Ultraviolet Absorption Spectrum. Thiopentone is a thiobarbiturate—see Screening Test 3 under Barbiturates, p. 208.

Infra-red Absorption Spectrum. Thiopentone sodium. Potassium bromide disk. The principal peaks are: A 1484, B 1409, C 1688 (p. 766).

Quantitative Estimation. See under Barbiturates, p. 208. Oroszlan and Maengwyn-Davies (1960) describe a spectrophotometric method of determination of thiopentone in blood.

Metabolism. Thiopentone is a very short-acting barbiturate—see under Barbiturates, p. 207. It is administered intravenously for the production of complete anaesthesia of short duration or for the induction of general anaesthesia.

Thiopentone appears to be almost completely metabolised; side-chain ω-oxidation to 5-ethyl-5-(3-carboxy-1-methylpropyl)-2-thiobarbituric acid appears to be a major route of metabolism, although some desulphuration to pentobarbitone also occurs. After the administration of 2- to 4-g doses in man, only about 0·3% is excreted unchanged in the urine over 48 hours and 10 to 25% is excreted as the carboxylic acid. Ring fission has been reported to occur in animals. The brain has been shown to take up thiopentone very rapidly upon injection, a peak level of 10% of the dose being reached within 1 minute. Very little is concentrated in the fat during the first 20 minutes after injection.

Dose. 100 to 500 mg intravenously; 40 mg/kg to a maximum dose of 2 g, by rectal injection.

Toxicity. The chief danger arising during

anaesthesia with thiopentone sodium is respiratory depression. Extravasation may cause tissue necrosis.

CASE EXAMPLES. Campbell (1960) reports 11 fatalities in the immediate post-operative period after thiopentone administration. He gives tissue and fluid thiopentone levels in the 11 cases.

A 29-year-old physician committed suicide by injecting 2 g of thiopentone intravenously; thiopentone was not found in the blood or urine (Frýdl, 1967).

THIOPROPAZATE *Tranquilliser*

10 - {3 - [4 - (2 - Acetoxyethyl)piperazin - 1 - yl]propyl}-2-chlorophenothiazine

$C_{23}H_{28}ClN_3O_2S = 446{\cdot}0$

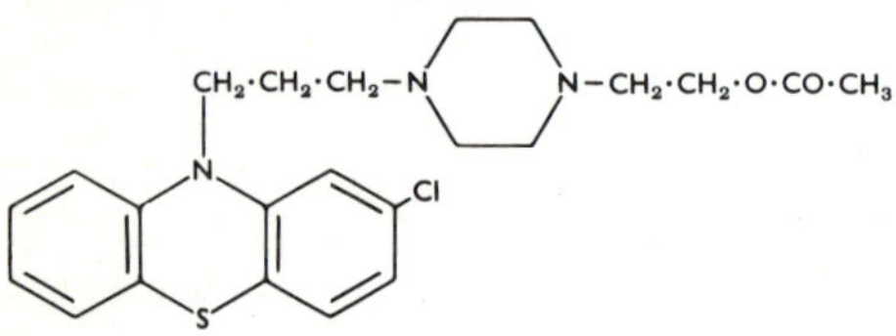

Thiopropazate has a boiling-point between 214° and 218° at 0·1 mm Hg.

Solubility. Insoluble in water; soluble in ether and chloroform.

THIOPROPAZATE HYDROCHLORIDE

Proprietary Names: Dartal; Dartalan.

An almost white crystalline powder. M.p. about 230°, with decomposition.

Solubility. Soluble 1 in 4 of water and 1 in 130 of ethanol; insoluble in ether; very slightly soluble in chloroform.

Screening Test. *FPN reagent* with urine—red (see p. 10).

Extraction. Thiopropazate is extracted by organic solvents from aqueous alkaline solutions; hydrolysis of biological material is required in order to improve the yield.

Chromatography. PAPER: system P1—Rf 0·53 (location under ultraviolet light, pale blue fluorescence; location reagents: *iodoplatinate spray*, strong reaction; *FPN spray*, purple); system RP1a—Rf 0·67 (location under ultraviolet light, blue fluorescence; location reagent *iodoplatinate spray*, positive reaction); system RP1b—Rf 0·03 (location as for RP1a).

THIN-LAYER: system T1—Rf 0·67 (location reagent *acidified iodoplatinate spray*, positive reaction); system T3—Rf 0·97 (location reagents: *iodoplatinate spray*, positive reaction; *sulphuric acid–ethanol spray*, green); system T4—Rf 0·67 (location as for T3); system T6—Rf 0·77 (the spot may be converted on the plate to the sulphoxide, Rf 0·25; location of both spots under ultraviolet light).

Colour Tests. MICRO: sulphuric acid–formaldehyde test—purple (*sensitivity:* 0·5 μg); ammonium molybdate test—deep purple (*sensitivity:* 0·5 μg); ammonium vanadate test—purple (*sensitivity:* 0·5 μg); Vitali's test—purple→yellow/yellow/yellow (*sensitivity:* 0·5 μg).

Crystal Test. MICRO: *picric acid*—masses of small crystals, forming overnight, best viewed under polarised light (*sensitivity:* 1 in 400).

Ultraviolet Absorption Spectrum. Thiopropazate in 0·01N hydrochloric acid, maxima at 256 mμ (E 1%, 1 cm 707) and 305 mμ (E 1%, 1 cm 93).

Infra-red Absorption Spectrum. Thiopropazate hydrochloride. Potassium bromide disk. The principal peaks are: A 1222 or 1462, B 1728 (p. 766).

Dose. Usually 15 to 30 mg initially; max. in 24 hours 100 mg.

Toxicity. The acute lethal dose in man of the phenothiazine tranquillisers appears to be in the range 15 to 150 mg/kg, although severe symptoms have occurred with doses of less than 1 mg/kg.

LD50 (oral): in mice 279 mg/kg.

THIOPROPERAZINE *Tranquilliser*

Synonym: RP 7843.

NN - Dimethyl - 10 - [3 - (4 - methylpiperazin - 1 - yl)propyl]phenothiazine - 2 - sulphonamide

$C_{22}H_{30}N_4O_2S_2 = 446{\cdot}6$

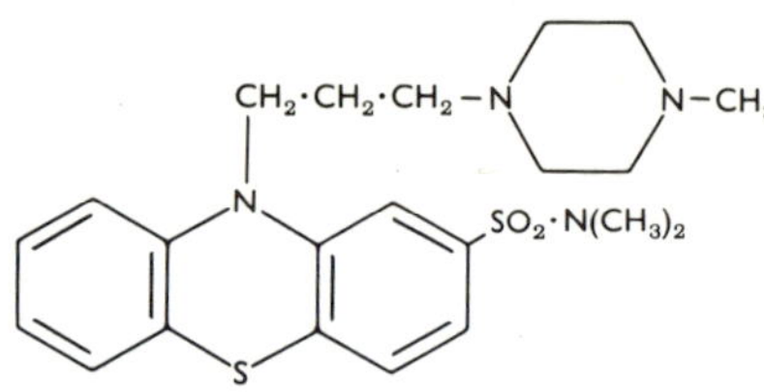

Solubility. Insoluble in water.

THIOPROPERAZINE MESYLATE

Synonyms: Thioproperazine Dimethanesulphonate; Thioproperazine Methanesulphonate.

Proprietary Names: Majeptil; Vontil.

A fine white powder which becomes pale yellow on exposure to light.

Solubility. Soluble in water; slightly soluble in ethanol; fairly soluble in boiling ethanol.

Screening Test. *FPN reagent* with urine—red (see p. 10).

Extraction. Thioproperazine is extracted by organic solvents from aqueous alkaline solutions; hydrolysis of biological material is required in order to improve the yield.

Chromatography. PAPER: system P1—Rf 0·20 (location under ultraviolet light, yellow-green fluorescence; location reagents: *iodoplatinate spray*, weak reaction; *FPN spray*, red); system RP1a—Rf 0·16 (location under ultraviolet light, green fluorescence; location reagent *iodoplatinate spray*, positive reaction); system RP1b—Rf 0·08 (location as for RP1a).

THIN-LAYER: system T1—Rf 0·44 (location reagent *acidified iodoplatinate spray*, positive reaction); system T6—Rf 0·43 (the spot may be converted on the plate to the sulphoxide, Rf 0·26; location of both spots under ultraviolet light).

Colour Tests. MICRO: sulphuric acid–formaldehyde test—red (*sensitivity:* 0·25 μg); ammonium molybdate test—dull purple→red (*sensitivity:* 0·25 μg); ammonium vanadate test—brown→green→purple (*sensitivity:* 0·25 μg); Vitali's test—purple→yellow/light brown/orange (*sensitivity:* 1·0 μg).

Crystal Tests. MICRO: *potassium tri-iodide solution* (*1*)—branching needles or shell-like crystals, forming overnight (*sensitivity:* 1 in 400); *sodium carbonate solution*—very small crystals, forming overnight, best viewed under polarised light (*sensitivity:* 1 in 100).

Ultraviolet Absorption Spectrum. Thioproperazine in 0·01N sulphuric acid, maxima at 265 mμ and 315 mμ.

Dose. Usually 15 mg daily, initially; up to 90 mg thrice daily is given in the treatment of acute and chronic schizophrenia.

Toxicity. The acute lethal dose in man of the phenothiazine tranquillisers appears to be in the range 15 to 150 mg/kg.

CASE EXAMPLE. A man aged 21 was given 7·5 mg of thioproperazine mesylate intramuscularly and died within 24 hours. Post-mortem examination indicated an almost selective depression of the respiratory centre by thioproperazine (Annesley and Mant, 1962).

THIORIDAZINE *Tranquilliser*

Synonym: TP 21.

10 - [2 - (1 - Methylpiperid - 2 - yl)ethyl] - 2 - methylthiophenothiazine

$C_{21}H_{26}N_2S_2 = 370·6$

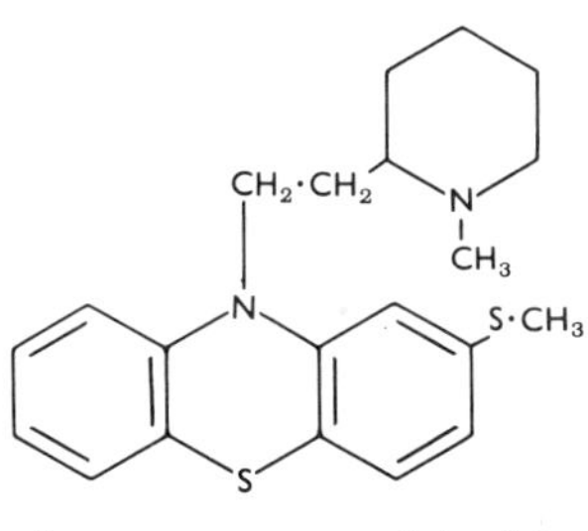

Thioridazine occurs as crystals. M.p. 72° to 74°. B.p. 230° at 0·02 mm Hg.

Solubility. Insoluble in water; soluble in chloroform.

THIORIDAZINE HYDROCHLORIDE

Proprietary Names: Melleretten; Melleril.

A white crystalline powder. M.p. 159° to 163°.

Solubility. Soluble 1 in 9 of water, 1 in 10 of ethanol, and 1 in 1·5 of chloroform; almost insoluble in ether.

Screening Test. *FPN reagent* with urine—blue (see p. 10).

Extraction. Thioridazine is extracted by organic solvents from aqueous alkaline solutions.

Chromatography. PAPER: system P1—Rf 0·76 (location under ultraviolet light yellow-green fluorescence; location reagents *iodoplatinate spray*, strong reaction; *bromocresol green spray*, weak reaction; *FPN spray*, blue); system RP1a—Rf 0·67 (location under ultraviolet light, pale green fluorescence; location reagent *iodoplatinate spray*, positive reaction); system RP1b—Rf 0·05 (location as for RP1a).

THIN-LAYER: system T1—Rf 0·47 (location reagent *acidified iodoplatinate spray*, positive reaction); system T3—Rf 0·97 (location reagents: *iodoplatinate spray*, positive reaction; *sulphuric acid–ethanol spray*, green); system T4—Rf 0·65 (location as for T3); system T6—Rf 0·71 (the spot may be converted on the plate to the sulphoxide, Rf 0·46; location of both spots under ultraviolet light).

Colour Tests. MICRO: sulphuric acid–formaldehyde test—purple-red→blue-green (*sensitivity:* 0·1 μg); ammonium molybdate test—deep blue-green (*sensitivity:* 0·1 μg); ammonium vanadate test—deep blue→purple (*sensitivity:* 0·1 μg); Vitali's test—blue-purple/purple-brown/yellow-brown (*sensitivity:* 0·25 μg).

Crystal Test. MICRO: *gold cyanide solution*—branching needles, forming overnight (*sensitivity:* 1 in 200).

Ultraviolet Absorption Spectrum. Thioridazine in ethanol, maxima at 263 mμ (E1%, 1 cm 1030) and 314 mμ (E1%, 1 cm 124); in 0·1N sulphuric acid, maxima at about 230 mμ (E1%, 1 cm 565), 263 mμ (E1%, 1 cm 1240), and 313 mμ (E1%, 1 cm 141).

Infra-red Absorption Spectrum. Thioridazine hydrochloride. Potassium bromide disk. The principal peaks are: A 1460, B 1402, C 755 (p. 793).

Quantitative Estimation. Thioridazine may be estimated spectrophotometrically after extraction from urine (Neve, 1961; Forrest *et al.*, 1965).

Metabolism. The major excretion product of thioridazine is its sulphoxide derivative. Dealkylation and hydroxylation may also occur and the metabolites are excreted chiefly as glucuronide conjugates in both the urine and the faeces. An average of 10·4% of the dose of thioridazine may be recovered unchanged within 24 hours in the urine, and excretion of the metabolites reaches a peak within 24 hours.

Dose. Up to 600 mg daily, initially, later reduced.

Toxicity. The toxic effects of thioridazine are milder and less frequent than with chlorpromazine; liver damage and blood dyscrasias have been reported. Serum-levels of between 0·24 and 1·18 mg% have been found in non-fatal poisoning cases.

CASE EXAMPLES. A 61-year-old man took twenty 100-mg tablets of thioridazine hydrochloride and died 2 hours later. Post-mortem levels were: blood, 0·18 mg%; liver,

7·8 mg%; stomach contents, 270 mg; thioridazine was not detected in the urine (Curry, 1962).

A 40-year-old woman died 5 days after starting treatment with 1600 mg of thioridazine hydrochloride and 20 mg of trifluoperazine hydrochloride daily. Previously she had been receiving up to 2400 mg of chlorpromazine daily for 5 weeks. Post-mortem blood-levels were: 0·1 mg% of thioridazine and 0·5 mg% of trifluoperazine. It is suggested that these levels are consistent with the therapeutic doses administered (Hollister and Kosek, 1965).

THIOTHIXENE *Tranquilliser*

Synonym: P4657B.
Proprietary Name: Navane.

cis-2-Dimethylsulphamoyl-9-[3-(4-methylpiperazin-1-yl)propylidene]thiaxanthen
$C_{23}H_{29}N_3O_2S_2 = 443·6$

Chromatography. PAPER: system P1—Rf 0·25 (location under ultraviolet light, blue fluorescence; location reagents: *iodoplatinate spray*, strong reaction; *bromocresol green spray*, weak reaction).

THIN-LAYER: system T1—Rf 0·45 (location reagent *acidified iodoplatinate spray*, positive reaction).

Colour Tests. MICRO: sulphuric acid–formaldehyde test—red (*sensitivity:* 0·1 μg); ammonium molybdate test—red (*sensitivity:* 0·1 μg); ammonium vanadate test—red (*sensitivity:* 0·25 μg); Vitali's test—red/–/faint green (*sensitivity:* 0·1 μg).

Ultraviolet Absorption Spectrum. Thiothixene in 0·1N sulphuric acid, maxima at 228 mμ and 308 mμ and an inflexion at 257 mμ.

Metabolism. Studies with ^{35}S-labelled thiothixene in rats and dogs (Hobbs, 1968) show it to be well absorbed from the gastro-intestinal tract, rapidly distributed, and metabolised to a variety of related compounds which are excreted mainly in the bile. The only metabolite tentatively identified is the *N*-demethylated derivative.

THONZYLAMINE *Antihistamine*

Synonym: Histazylamine.

N-(*p*-Methoxybenzyl)-*N'N'*-dimethyl-*N*-(pyrimid-2-yl)ethylenediamine
$C_{16}H_{22}N_4O = 286·4$

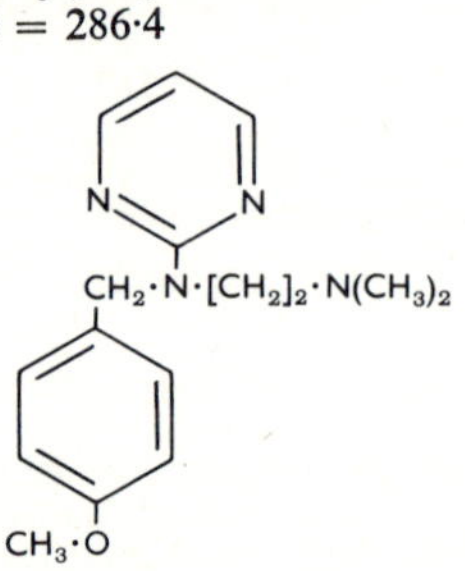

Thonzylamine occurs as an oily liquid.
Solubility. Insoluble in water; soluble in chloroform.

THONZYLAMINE HYDROCHLORIDE
Proprietary Names: Neo-hetramine; Resistab.

A white crystalline powder. M.p. 173° to 176°.
Solubility. Soluble 1 in 1 of water, 1 in 6 of ethanol, and 1 in 4 of chloroform; almost insoluble in ether.

Extraction. Thonzylamine is extracted by organic solvents from aqueous alkaline solutions.

Chromatography. PAPER: system P1—Rf 0·52 (location under ultraviolet light, blue fluorescence; location reagent *iodoplatinate spray*, strong reaction); system RP1a—Rf 0·73 (location under ultraviolet light, blue fluorescence; location reagent *iodoplatinate spray*, positive reaction); system RP1b—Rf 0·05 (location as for RP1a).

THIN-LAYER: system T1—Rf 0·47 (location reagent *acidified iodoplatinate spray*, positive reaction); system T2—Rf 0·59 (location reagent *iodoplatinate spray*, positive reaction); system T3—Rf 0·65 (location as for T2).

GAS: system G1/180—retention time 3·38 relative to diphenhydramine; system G2/225—retention time 0·53 relative to codeine; system G3—retention time 2·42 relative to diphenhydramine; system G4—retention time 0·39 relative to codeine.

Colour Tests. MICRO: ammonium molybdate test—blue-violet (*sensitivity:* 0·25 μg); ammonium vanadate test—red-violet (*sensitivity:* 0·5 μg).

Crystal Tests. MICRO: *gold chloride solution*—serrated needles (*sensitivity:* 1 in 1000); *lead iodide solution*—feathery rosettes (*sensitivity:* 1 in 400).

Ultraviolet Absorption Spectrum. Thonzylamine in 0·1N sodium hydroxide, maxima at 241 mμ (E1%, 1 cm 767), 273 mμ (E1%, 1 cm 90), 279 mμ (E1%, 1 cm 86), and 312 mμ (E1%, 1 cm 90); in 0·1N sulphuric acid, maxima at 235 mμ (E1%, 1 cm 902), 273 mμ (E1%, 1 cm 95), and 313 mμ (E1%, 1 cm 135).

Dose. Up to 400 mg daily.

Toxicity. The estimated acute lethal dose in man is stated to be in the range 25 to 250 mg/kg.

THURFYL NICOTINATE *Peripheral Vasodilator*

Synonym: Nicotafuryl.
Proprietary Name: Trafuril.

Tetrahydrofurfuryl pyridine-3-carboxylate
$C_{11}H_{13}NO_3 = 207·2$

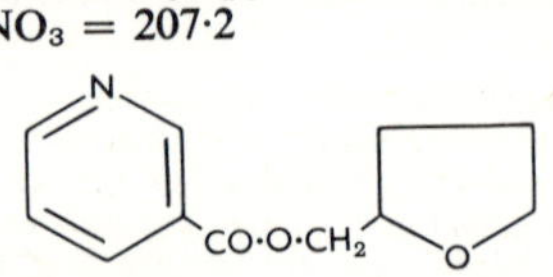

A colourless liquid.
Solubility. Soluble in water and chloroform.

Extraction. Thurfyl nicotinate is extracted by organic solvents from aqueous alkaline solutions.

Chromatography. PAPER: system P1—Rf 0·90 (location under ultraviolet light, strong absorption; location reagent *iodoplatinate spray*, white); system RP1a—Rf 0·33 (location under ultraviolet light, absorption; location reagent *iodoplatinate spray*, positive reaction); system RP1b—Rf 0·20 (location as for RP1a).
THIN-LAYER: system T1—Rf 0·62 (location reagent *acidified iodoplatinate spray*, positive reaction).

Crystal Tests. MICRO: *gold bromide–hydrochloric acid solution*—four-pointed stars (*sensitivity:* 1 in 400); *mercuric chloride solution*—feathery rosettes (*sensitivity:* 1 in 400).

Use. It is used by topical application in creams and ointments.

THYMOXAMINE *Peripheral Vasodilator*

Synonym: Moxisylyte.

4 - (2 - Dimethylaminoethoxy) - 5 - isopropyl - 2-methylphenyl acetate
$C_{16}H_{25}NO_3 = 279·4$

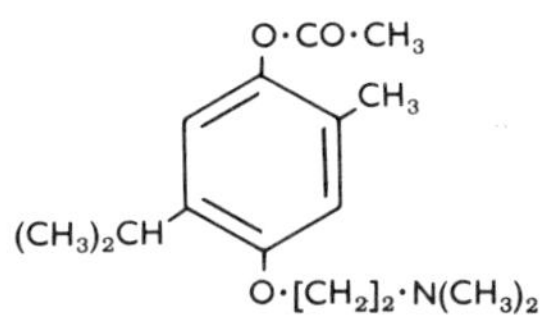

Solubility. Insoluble in water; soluble in chloroform.

THYMOXAMINE HYDROCHLORIDE
Proprietary Name: Opilon.
A white crystalline powder.
Solubility. Soluble in water.

Extraction. Thymoxamine is extracted by organic solvents from aqueous alkaline solutions.

Chromatography. PAPER: system P1—Rf 0·65 (location reagent *iodoplatinate spray*, strong reaction); system RP1a—Rf 0·56 (location reagent *iodoplatinate spray*, positive reaction); system RP1b—Rf 0·02 (location as for RP1a).
THIN-LAYER: system T1—Rf 0·52 (location reagent *acidified iodoplatinate spray*, positive reaction).
GAS: system G2/225—retention time 0·95 relative to diphenhydramine; system G4—retention time 0·90 (0·48) relative to diphenhydramine.

Colour Tests. MICRO: sulphuric acid–formaldehyde test—yellow-brown (*sensitivity:* 1·0 μg); ammonium molybdate test—brown→green→blue (*sensitivity:* 0·1 μg); Vitali's test—brown→yellow/–/faint brown (*sensitivity:* 1·0 μg).

Crystal Tests. MICRO: *lead iodide solution*—small dense rosettes (*sensitivity:* 1 in 1000); *styphnic acid*—bunches of irregular blades (*sensitivity:* 1 in 1000).

Ultraviolet Absorption Spectrum. Thymoxamine in 0·1N sulphuric acid, maximum at 275 mμ (E1%, 1 cm 57) and an inflexion at about 280 mμ (E1%, 1 cm 52).

Metabolism. Thymoxamine produces peripheral vasodilatation less potent than dihydroergotamine but greater than piperoxan.

Dose. Up to 40 mg daily.

TIGLOIDINE *Parasympatholytic*

Synonym: Tiglylpseudotropeine.

ψ-Tropine tiglate
$C_{13}H_{21}NO_2 = 223·3$

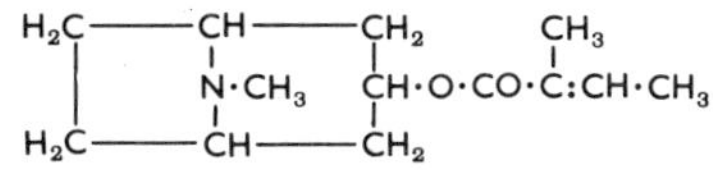

Tigloidine was first isolated from *Duboisia myoporoides* (Solanaceae) but is now synthesised.
A thin syrupy liquid.

TIGLOIDINE HYDROBROMIDE
Proprietary Name: Tiglyssin.
A white crystalline solid.
Solubility. Soluble in water.

Extraction. Tigloidine is extracted by organic solvents from aqueous alkaline solutions.

Chromatography. PAPER: system P1—Rf 0·49 (location under ultraviolet light, absorption; location reagents: *iodoplatinate spray*, strong reaction; *bromocresol green spray*, weak reaction).
THIN-LAYER: system T1—Rf 0·26 (location reagent *acidified iodoplatinate spray*, positive reaction).

Crystal Tests. MICRO: *picric acid*—long plates or segmented needles, best viewed under polarised light (*sensitivity:* 1 in 1500); *potassium mercuric iodide solution*—serrated blades (*sensitivity:* 1 in 1500).

Dose. Up to 2 g daily.

Toxicity. LD50 (intravenous): in small animals 200 to 250 mg/kg.

TOLAZAMIDE *Antidiabetic*

Synonym: U 17835.
Proprietary Names: Diabewas; Tolanase; Tolinase.

N - Hexahydroazepin - 1 - yl - *N′* - toluene - *p* - sulphonylurea
$C_{14}H_{21}N_3O_3S = 311·4$

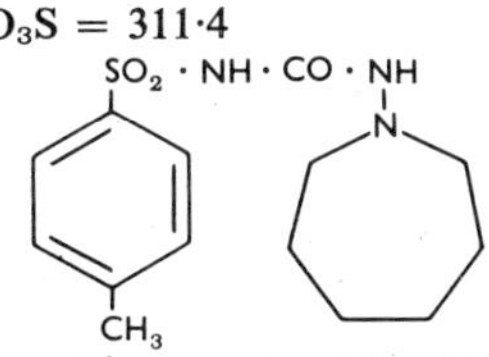

A white crystalline powder. M.p. 170° to 173°.
Solubility. Soluble in ethanol.

Extraction. Tolazamide is extracted by organic solvents from aqueous acid or alkaline solutions.

Ultraviolet Absorption Spectrum. Tolazamide in ethanol, maximum at about 228 mμ; minimum at about 212 mμ.

Quantitative Estimation. Kern (1963) describes a method of extraction of tolazamide from blood followed by nitration of the tolyl moiety, diazotisation, coupling with *N*-1-naphthylethylenediamine, and final spectrophotometric determination.
Tolazamide may be extracted from acidified serum by chloroform and then estimated spectrophotometrically as a complex with bromocresol purple (Forist, 1967).

Metabolism. Tolazamide is absorbed more slowly from the gastro-intestinal tract than are the other sulphonylurea compounds. Peak blood-levels are reached 4 to 8 hours after oral administration of therapeutic doses; tolazamide does not accumulate in the blood. About 85% of a dose is excreted in the urine in the form of metabolites which are more soluble than tolazamide itself.

Dose. Up to 750 mg daily.

Toxicity. LD50 (oral): in rats more than 5 g/kg.

TOLAZOLINE *Peripheral Vasodilator*

Synonym: Benzazoline.

2-Benzyl-2-imidazoline
$C_{10}H_{12}N_2 = 160{\cdot}2$

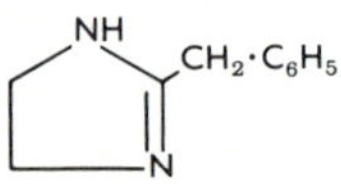

Solubility. Soluble in water and chloroform.

TOLAZOLINE HYDROCHLORIDE

Proprietary Names: Lambral; Priscol; Priscoline; Tolavad; Tolpal; Vasodil; Zoline.

A white crystalline powder. M.p. 172° to 176°.
Solubility. Soluble 1 in 0·5 of water, 1 in 2 of ethanol, and 1 in 2·5 of chloroform; insoluble in ether.

Extraction. Tolazoline is extracted by organic solvents from aqueous alkaline solutions.

Chromatography. PAPER: system P1—Rf 0·40 (location under ultraviolet light, absorption; location reagent *iodoplatinate spray*, strong reaction); system RP1a—Rf 0·96 (location under ultraviolet light, absorption; location reagent *iodoplatinate spray*, positive reaction); system RP1b—Rf 0·92 (location as for RP1a).
THIN-LAYER: system T1—Rf 0·15 (location reagent *acidified iodoplatinate spray*, positive reaction).
GAS: system G2/225—retention time 0·43 relative to diphenhydramine.

Colour Test. MICRO: Vitali's test— –/–/orange (*sensitivity:* 0·1 μg).

Crystal Tests. MICRO: *gold bromide solution*—long branching plates with a few hexagons (*sensitivity:* 1 in 1000); *platinic chloride solution*—irregular prisms (*sensitivity:* 1 in 200).

Ultraviolet Absorption Spectrum. Tolazoline in ethanol, maxima at 257 mμ (E1%, 1cm 15) and 263 mμ (E1%, 1cm 10·5).

Infra-red Absorption Spectrum. Tolazoline (base). Potassium bromide disk. The principal peaks are: A 1608, B 1296, C 721 (p. 767).

Metabolism. Tolazoline is extremely stable *in vivo*; it is concentrated mainly in the liver and kidneys. About 90% of an oral dose is excreted unchanged in 12 hours.

Dose. Up to 75 mg. The maximum safe dose is said to be 100 mg orally or intravenously.

CASE EXAMPLE. About 3 hours after taking 2·5 g of tolazoline hydrochloride a 54-year-old woman died. The following levels were found post mortem: femoral blood, 13 mg%; liver, 10·2 mg%; stomach, traces only (Turner, 1964a).

TOLBUTAMIDE *Antidiabetic*

Synonyms: Butamide; D 860; Tolglybutamide; U 2043.
Proprietary Names: Arcosal; Artosin; Dolipol; Ipoglicone; Mobenol; Orinase; Rastinon; Toluvan.

N-Butyl-*N′*-toluene-*p*-sulphonylurea
$C_{12}H_{18}N_2O_3S = 270{\cdot}4$

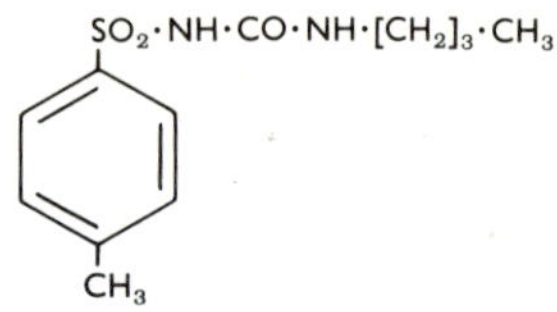

A white crystalline powder. M.p. 126° to 130°.
Solubility. Insoluble in water; soluble 1 in 10 of ethanol; soluble in chloroform.

Extraction. Tolbutamide may be extracted from neutral solutions with chloroform.

Chromatography. PAPER: system P1—Rf 0·96 (location reagent *bromocresol green spray*, weak reaction).
THIN-LAYER: system T1—Rf 0·76 (location reagent *acidified iodoplatinate spray*, positive reaction).

Ultraviolet Absorption Spectrum. Tolbutamide in ethanol, maxima at 228 mμ (E1%, 1cm 500), 257 mμ (E1%, 1cm 22), 262 mμ (E1%, 1cm 26), 267 mμ (E1%, 1cm 25), and 274 mμ (E1%, 1cm 22).

Infra-red Absorption Spectrum. Potassium bromide disk. The principal peaks are: A 1157 or 1658, B 1336 or 1552 (p. 767).

Quantitative Estimation. Kern (1963) describes a method of extraction of tolbutamide from blood followed by nitration of the tolyl moiety, diazotisation, coupling with *N*-1-naphthylethylenediamine, and final spectrophotometric determination.
Nelson *et al.* (1960) describe a method of determination of carboxytolbutamide in urine.

Metabolism. Tolbutamide is an orally active hypoglycaemic agent which reduces the blood-sugar level without affecting glucose tolerance. It probably acts by stimulating insulin secretion. It is excreted more rapidly than chlorpropamide, consequently its duration of action is shorter. Peak hypoglycaemic activity occurs within 4 to 6 hours of oral administration.

Tolbutamide is fairly rapidly metabolised to carboxytolbutamide which is inactive. About 75% of an oral dose can be recovered from the urine of normal subjects as carboxytolbutamide; in diabetic subjects the amount is between 24 and 67%.

Dose. Up to 2 g daily for maintenance; up to 4 g may be given at the start of therapy.

Toxicity. Toxic effects may include skin sensitisation, gastro-intestinal disturbances, weakness, paraesthesias, tinnitus, headache, intolerance to alcohol, and jaundice. Blood dyscrasias have also been reported including agranulocytosis, leucopenia, thrombocytopenia, and eosinophilia.

CASE EXAMPLE. Daily 1-g doses of tolbutamide for 16 months were considered to have caused pancytopenia and subsequent death of a 61-year-old woman (Chapman and Wan Ho Cheung, 1963).

TOLNAFTATE *Antimycotic*

Proprietary Names: Dermoxin; Naphthiomate-T; Tinactin; Tinaderm.

Naphth-2-yl *N*-methyl-*N*-*m*-tolylthiocarbamate

$C_{19}H_{17}NOS = 307·4$

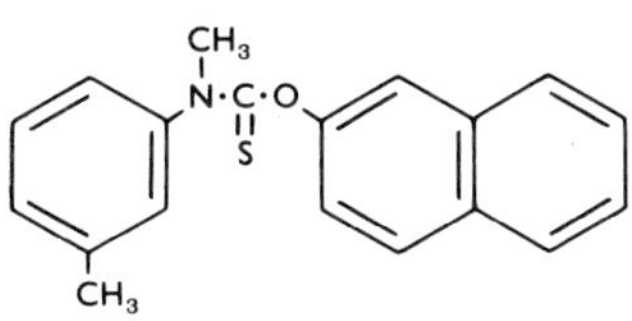

A white crystalline powder. M.p. 110° to 113°.

Solubility. Almost insoluble in water; slightly soluble in ethanol and ether; freely soluble in chloroform.

Extraction. Tolnaftate is extracted by organic solvents from aqueous acid or alkaline solutions.

Colour Tests. MICRO: sulphuric acid–formaldehyde test—blue-green; ammonium vanadate test—brown; Vitali's test—yellow/yellow/red-brown.

Ultraviolet Absorption Spectrum. Tolnaftate in ethanol, maximum at 257 mμ (E1%, 1 cm about 660); minimum at 243 mμ.

Use. Topically as a 1% solution or cream.

TOLONIUM CHLORIDE *Dye/Antiheparin Compound*

Synonyms: C.I. Basic Blue 17; Colour Index No. 52040; Toluidine Blue O.

Proprietary Name: Blutene Chloride.

3 - Amino - 7 - dimethylamino - 2 - methyl - phenazothionium chloride

$C_{15}H_{16}ClN_3S = 305·8$

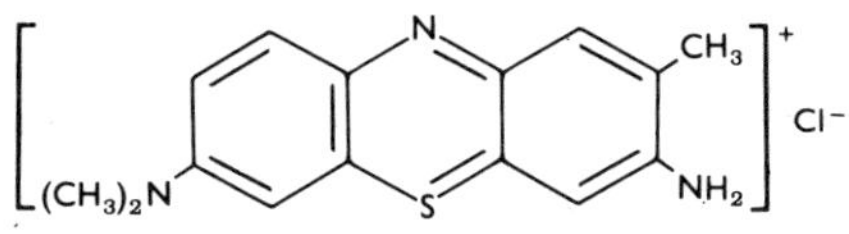

A green crystalline powder with a bronze lustre.

Solubility. Soluble 1 in 20 of water; slightly soluble in ethanol; almost insoluble in ether; very slightly soluble in chloroform.

Extraction. Tolonium chloride is a quaternary ammonium compound (see p. 29).

Chromatography. PAPER: system P1—Rf 0·17, visible blue streak (location under ultraviolet light, red fluorescence).

THIN-LAYER: system T1—Rf 0·01 (location under ultraviolet light, red fluorescence; location reagent *acidified iodoplatinate spray*, positive reaction).

Colour Tests. MICRO: sulphuric acid–formaldehyde test—(blue) green (*sensitivity:* 0·1 μg); ammonium molybdate test—(blue) green (*sensitivity:* 0·1 μg); ammonium vanadate test—(blue) purple → green (*sensitivity:* 0·1 μg); Vitali's test—(blue) blue/blue/dull red (*sensitivity:* 0·5 μg).

Ultraviolet Absorption Spectrum. Tolonium chloride in 0·1N sulphuric acid, maxima at 245 mμ (E1%, 1 cm 276) and 285 mμ (E1%, 1 cm 469).

Action. Tolonium chloride inhibits the anticoagulant effect of heparinoid substances in the blood.

Dose. Up to 300 mg daily.

NOTE. During treatment with tolonium chloride the urine of patients assumes a blue-green colour.

TOLPROPAMINE *Antihistamine*

NN-Dimethyl-3-phenyl-3-*p*-tolylpropylamine

$C_{18}H_{23}N = 253·4$

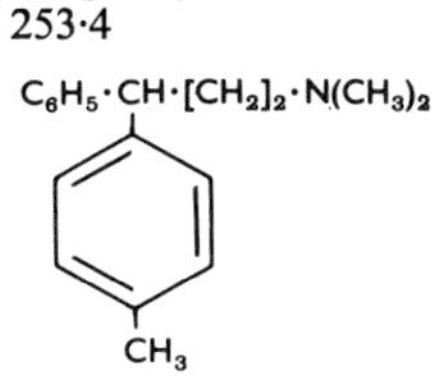

Solubility. Insoluble in water; soluble in chloroform.

TOLPROPAMINE HYDROCHLORIDE

Proprietary Names: It is the active ingredient of Pragman Gelee and Tylagel.

A white crystalline powder.

Solubility. Soluble in water and ethanol; insoluble in ether and chloroform.

Extraction. Tolpropamine is extracted by organic solvents from aqueous alkaline solutions.

Chromatography. PAPER: system P1—Rf 0·70 (location reagents: *iodoplatinate spray*, strong reaction; *bromocresol green spray*, strong reaction); system RP1a—Rf 0·33 (location reagent *iodoplatinate spray*, positive reaction); system RP1b—Rf 0·00 (location as for RP1a). THIN-LAYER: system T1—Rf 0·48 (location reagent *acidified iodoplatinate spray*, positive reaction).

Colour Tests. MICRO: sulphuric acid–formaldehyde test—dull red (*sensitivity:* 0·25 μg); ammonium molybdate test—green→blue (*sensitivity:* 0·5 μg); ammonium vanadate test—brown (*sensitivity:* 0·25 μg); Vitali's test—-/-/faint yellow (*sensitivity:* 1·0 μg).

Crystal Tests. MICRO: *gold bromide solution*—oily blades, best viewed under polarised light (*sensitivity:* 1 in 3000); *styphnic acid*—masses of irregular blades (*sensitivity:* 1 in 3000).

Ultraviolet Absorption Spectrum. Tolpropamine in 0·1N sulphuric acid, maxima at 260 mμ (E1%, 1 cm 27), 264·5 mμ (E1%, 1 cm 27), and 273 mμ (E1%, 1 cm 18) and inflexions at 253 mμ and 267 mμ.

Infra-red Absorption Spectrum. Tolpropamine hydrochloride. Potassium bromide disk. The principal peaks are: A 700 or 727 or 776, B 802 or 1450 or 1480 (p. 767).

Use. By topical application as a jelly containing 1%.

TOLUENE *Industrial Solvent*

Synonym: Toluole.

Methylbenzene

$C_6H_5 \cdot CH_3 = 92 \cdot 14$

A colourless, mobile, highly inflammable liquid which burns with a smoky flame. B.p. 109·5° to 111·5°.

Solubility. Insoluble in water; miscible with ethanol, ether, chloroform, and other organic solvents.

Extraction. Toluene is volatile and may be isolated by distillation (p. 18).

Chromatography. PAPER and THIN-LAYER: Bonnichsen *et al.* (1966) describe a paper system and a thin-layer system, both of which detect the nitration products of toluene, following steam distillation into carbon tetrachloride and subsequent nitration.

GAS: system G8/160—retention time 6·0 relative to n-propanol.

Ultraviolet Absorption Spectrum. Toluene in ethanol, maxima at 249 mμ (E1%, 1 cm 14·4), 253·5 mμ (E1%, 1 cm 18·8), 255·3 mμ (E1%, 1 cm 20), 259·7 mμ (E1%, 1 cm 22·6), 261·6 mμ (E1%, 1 cm 27·5), 264·5 mμ (E1%, 1 cm 18·1), and 268·2 mμ (E1%, 1 cm 25·3).

Quantitative Estimation. Toluene may be estimated in biological fluids and tissues by steam distillation into carbon tetrachloride, nitration, and subsequent spectrophotometric determination (Bonnichsen *et al.*, 1966).

Metabolism. Following inhalation, about 80% of the toluene is oxidised to benzoic acid and 20% is eliminated by the lungs unchanged. The benzoic acid is excreted almost entirely as hippuric acid.

Toxicity. Concentrations exceeding 200 p.p.m. in air are dangerous. Toluene has about the same acute toxicity as benzene but it is a less serious industrial hazard, probably because it is mainly metabolised to the non-toxic hippuric acid and not hydroxylated to phenols.

CASE EXAMPLES. Bonnichsen *et al.* (1966) present detailed case reports, including figures of toluene levels found at post-mortem examination, on 4 probable suicides, 6 accidental poisonings, 2 cases of 'sniffing', and 2 in which the source of the toluene was not known.

TOLYCAINE *Local Anaesthetic*

Methyl 2-diethylaminoacetamido-3-methylbenzoate

$C_{15}H_{22}N_2O_3 = 278 \cdot 4$

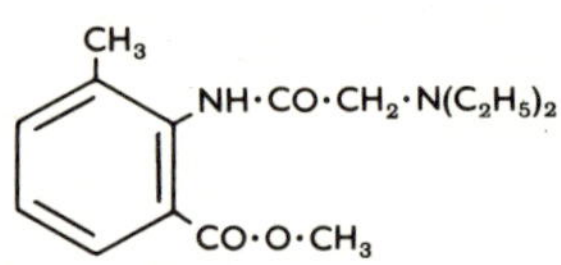

Solubility. Insoluble in water; soluble in chloroform.

TOLYCAINE HYDROCHLORIDE

Proprietary Name: Baycain(e).

A white crystalline powder.

Solubility. Soluble in water.

Extraction. Tolycaine is extracted by organic solvents from aqueous alkaline solutions.

Chromatography. PAPER: system P1—Rf 0·61 (location under ultraviolet light, pale green fluorescence; location reagent *iodoplatinate spray*, weak reaction).

THIN-LAYER: system T1—Rf 0·70 (location under ultraviolet light, green fluorescence; location reagent *acidified iodoplatinate spray*, positive reaction).

Colour Test. MICRO: Vitali's test— -/-/yellow (*sensitivity:* 1·0 μg).

Crystal Tests. MICRO: *gold bromide–hydrochloric acid solution*—long plates, often serrated, best viewed under polarised light (*sensitivity:* 1 in 1000); *potassium mercuric iodide solution*—branching blades and needles (*sensitivity:* 1 in 1000).

Ultraviolet Absorption Spectrum. Tolycaine in water, maximum at 283 mμ (E1%, 1 cm 66).

Use. It is used as a 3% solution with adrenaline and noradrenaline.

TRAMAZOLINE *Sympathomimetic*

2-(5,6,7,8-Tetrahydronaphth-1-ylamino)-2-imidazoline

$C_{13}H_{17}N_3 = 215{\cdot}3$

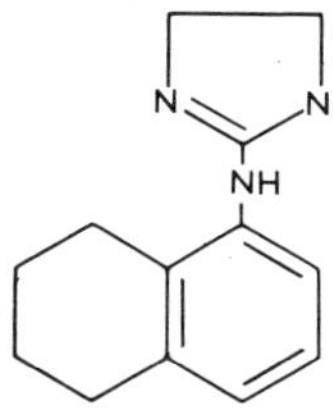

TRAMAZOLINE HYDROCHLORIDE

Proprietary Name: It is an ingredient of Dexa-Rhinaspray.

A white crystalline solid. M.p. 171°.

Solubility. Soluble 1 in 6 of water.

Extraction. Tramazoline is extracted by organic solvents from aqueous alkaline solutions.

Chromatography. PAPER: system P1—Rf 0·70 (location under ultraviolet light, strong absorption; location reagents: *iodoplatinate spray*, strong reaction; *bromocresol green spray*, weak reaction; *potassium permanganate spray*, weak reaction); system RP1a—Rf 0·82 (location under ultraviolet light, absorption; location reagent *iodoplatinate spray*, positive reaction); system RP1b—Rf 0·62 (location as for RP1a).

THIN-LAYER: system T1—Rf 0·21, streaking (location reagent *potassium permanganate spray*, positive reaction).

Colour Tests. MICRO: sulphuric acid–formaldehyde test—red-purple (*sensitivity:* 0·25 μg); ammonium molybdate test—faint grey-blue→yellow (*sensitivity:* 1·0 μg); ammonium vanadate test—brown (*sensitivity:* 1·0 μg); Vitali's test—-/-/bright orange-red (*sensitivity:* 0·1 μg).

Crystal Tests. MICRO: *platinic bromide solution*—dendrites, often curving (*sensitivity:* 1 in 1000); *potassium mercuric iodide solution*—plates, some serrated (*sensitivity:* 1 in 1000).

Use. It is used as a nasal decongestant.

Toxicity. LD50 (oral): in mice 175 mg/kg.

TRANYLCYPROMINE

Antidepressant/Monoamine Oxidase Inhibitor

Synonyms: SKF 385; Transamine.

trans-(±)-2-Phenylcyclopropylamine

$C_9H_{11}N = 133{\cdot}2$

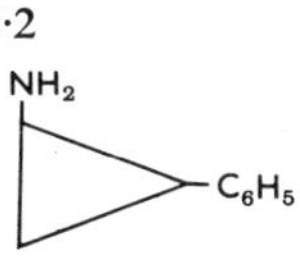

TRANYLCYPROMINE SULPHATE

Proprietary Names: Parnate. It is an ingredient of Partelin and Jatrosom.

A white crystalline powder.

Solubility. Soluble 1 in 20 of water and 1 in 2000 of ether; very slightly soluble in ethanol; insoluble in chloroform.

Extraction. Tranylcypromine is extracted by organic solvents from aqueous alkaline solutions.

Chromatography. PAPER: system P1—Rf 0·45 (location under ultraviolet light, absorption; location reagents: *iodoplatinate spray*, white; *bromocresol green spray*, weak reaction); system RP1a—Rf 0·79 (location under ultraviolet light, absorption); system RP1b—Rf 0·00 (location as for RP1a).

THIN-LAYER: system T1—Rf 0·61 (location reagents: *acidified iodoplatinate spray*, positive reaction; *Marquis reagent*, positive reaction; *ninhydrin spray*, positive reaction).

GAS: system G2/120—retention time 0·45 relative to ephedrine.

Colour Tests. MICRO: sulphuric acid–formaldehyde test—red→brown (*sensitivity:* 0·25 μg); ammonium molybdate test—blue→grey (*sensitivity:* 0·25 μg); ammonium vanadate test—green or purple, depending on the relative concentrations of the test substance and the reagent (*sensitivity:* 0·25 μg); Vitali's test—-/yellow/brown (*sensitivity:* 0·25 μg).

Crystal Tests. MICRO: *platinic chloride solution*—small irregular crystals (*sensitivity:* 1 in 200); *potassium bismuth iodide solution*—plates, often rectangular (*sensitivity:* 1 in 400).

Ultraviolet Absorption Spectrum. Tranylcypromine sulphate in 0·2N sulphuric acid, maxima at 258 mμ (E1%, 1 cm about 14·4), 264 mμ (E1%, 1 cm about 16·2), and 271 mμ (E1%, 1 cm about 11·6).

Infra-red Absorption Spectrum. Tranylcypromine sulphate. Potassium bromide disk. The principal peaks are: A 1120, B 1497, C 690 (p. 767).

Quantitative Estimation. Turner *et al.* (1966) describe a method of spectrofluorimetric determination in urine.

Metabolism. Tranylcypromine is rapidly excreted in the urine.

Dose. Usually 20 mg daily, initially; for the intensive treatment of severe depression up to 60 mg daily has been given.

Toxicity. Fatal hypertensive crises have occurred following low doses. Recovery with the aid of haemodialysis is reported after the ingestion of 350 mg (Matter *et al.*, 1965).

For the toxicity of monoamine oxidase inhibitors see under Phenelzine, p. 482.

LD50 (oral): in mice 32·4 to 38·5 mg/kg.

CASE EXAMPLES. An 18-year-old girl died 6½ hours after admission to hospital, following ingestion of approximately 170 mg of tranylcypromine. Post-mortem examination revealed congestion of the lungs, brain, and kidneys, and blood in the bowels. Microscopic examination showed necrosis of the gastro-intestinal mucosa, cloudy swelling of the liver parenchyma and renal tubules, and haemorrhagic pulmonary oedema (Bell and Scaff, 1963).

Death of a 40-year-old man who consumed cheese while under treatment with chlordiazepoxide and tranylcypromine. Examination post mortem showed extensive pulmonary congestion and haemorrhage, severe liver damage, and brain congestion. Tranylcypromine was found in the following organs: intestines, 0·1 mg%; liver and kidneys, 0·1 mg%; spleen and lungs, 0·1 mg% (Cuthill *et al.*, 1964).

After taking 30 tablets of Parstelin (tranylcypromine 10 mg and trifluoperazine hydrochloride 1 mg in each tablet), a 27-year-old man died. At post-mortem examination a test for trifluoperazine in the urine was negative but tranylcypromine was found in a concentration of 4 mg%. The length of time between ingestion of the tablets and the onset of severe toxic symptoms, over 30 hours, is unusual (MacCaig and Edmondson, 1965).

TRIACETYLOLEANDOMYCIN

Antibiotic

Proprietary Names: Cyclamycin; Evramycin; Olicin; Tao.

The triacetyl ester of oleandomycin

$C_{41}H_{67}NO_{15}$ = 814·0

A white crystalline powder. M.p. 176°, with decomposition.

Solubility. Slightly soluble in water and ether; soluble 1 in 10 of ethanol and 1 in 1 of chloroform.

Extraction. Triacetyloleandomycin is extracted by organic solvents from aqueous alkaline solutions.

Chromatography. PAPER: system P1—Rf 0·75 (location reagents: *iodoplatinate spray*, weak reaction; *iodine vapour*, weak reaction).

THIN-LAYER: system T1—Rf 0·65 (location reagent *acidified iodoplatinate spray*, positive reaction).

Colour Tests. Heat 10 mg with 5 ml of *hydrochloric acid* on a water-bath—greenish-yellow.

MICRO: sulphuric acid–formaldehyde test—faint yellow-brown (*sensitivity:* 1·0 μg); ammonium molybdate test—dull purple, appearing slowly (*sensitivity:* 1·0 μg); ammonium vanadate test—dull purple, appearing slowly (*sensitivity:* 1·0 μg).

Metabolism. Triacetyloleandomycin is not destroyed by the acid of the gastric secretion. After oral administration it is rapidly absorbed from the gastro-intestinal tract and distributed in body tissues. Peak blood concentrations are achieved about 2 hours after a therapeutic dose; effective blood-levels may persist for up to 6 hours and detectable amounts for 12 hours.

It is excreted in the urine and bile; about 20% of a dose can be recovered in active form from the urine.

Dose. Up to the equivalent of 2 g of oleandomycin daily.

TRIAMCINOLONE

Corticosteroid

Synonym: Triamcortisone.

Proprietary Names: Adcortyl; Aristocort; Kenacort; Ledercort.

9α-Fluoro-11β,16α,17α,21-tetrahydroxypregna-1,4-diene-3,20-dione

$C_{21}H_{27}FO_6$ = 394·4

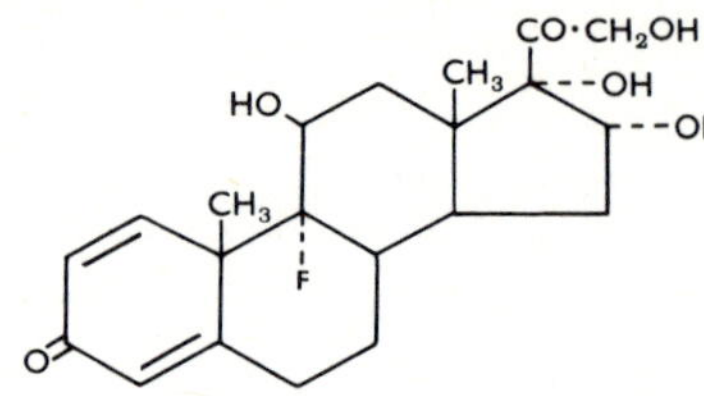

A white crystalline powder. M.p. 264° to 268°.

Solubility. Soluble 1 in 500 of water and 1 in 200 of ethanol; very slightly soluble in ether and chloroform.

TRIAMCINOLONE ACETONIDE

9α - Fluoro - 11β,21 - dihydroxy - 16α,17α - isopropylidenedioxypregna-1,4-diene-3,20-dione.

Proprietary Names: Adcortyl A; Adcortyl E; Kenalog; Ledercort Acetonide.

A white crystalline powder. M.p. 276° to 279°. Specific rotation of a 1% solution in dioxan, +101° to +107°.

Solubility. Very slightly soluble in water; soluble 1 in 150 of ethanol and 1 in 40 of chloroform.

TRIAMCINOLONE DIACETATE

16α,21-Diacetoxy - 9α - fluoro - 11β,17α - dihydroxypregna-1,4-diene-3,20-dione.

Proprietary Names: Aristocort Forte; Kenacort Diacetate; Ledercort Diacetate.

Extraction. Triamcinolone is extracted from neutral solutions with freshly distilled ethyl acetate.

Chromatography. PAPER, for triamcinolone acetonide: system P14—Rf 0·52 (location reagent *DPST solution*, violet on yellow).

THIN-LAYER, for triamcinolone acetonide: system T18—Rf 0·50 (location reagent *DPST spray*); system T19—Rf 1·39 (location reagent *DPST spray*); for triamcinolone: system T19—Rf 0·59 (location reagent *DPST spray*).

Ultraviolet Absorption Spectrum. Triamcinolone in ethanol, maximum at about 238 mμ (E1%, 1 cm 380); triamcinolone acetonide in methanol, maximum at about 238 mμ (E1%, 1 cm 330 to 360).

Metabolism. Triamcinolone is a synthetic glucocorticoid with an anti-inflammatory action similar to that of prednisone.

Upon intravenous injection of 2 mg/kg in dogs, the plasma half-life was found to be nearly 2 hours, the longest half-life in the dog of any corticosteroid. The excretion was equally divided between the urine and the faeces, and about 20% of the unchanged drug was recovered from the urine.

In the rat, triamcinolone has been found to

be deposited primarily in the muscles, liver, intestines, skin, and kidneys.

Dose. Up to 48 mg daily, initially; up to 8 mg for maintenance daily.

TRIAMTERENE *Diuretic*

Synonym: SKF 8542.
Proprietary Names: Dytac; Dyrenium. It is an ingredient of Dytide.

2,4,7-Triamino-6-phenylpteridine
$C_{12}H_{11}N_7 = 253{\cdot}3$

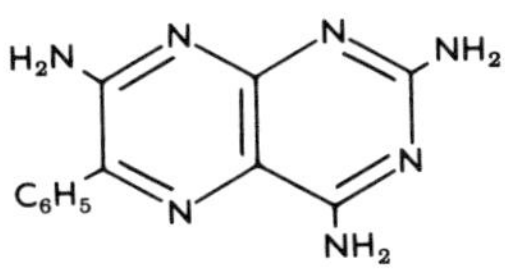

A yellow crystalline powder.
Solubility. Soluble 1 in 1000 of water, 1 in 3000 of ethanol, and 1 in 4000 of chloroform; insoluble in ether.

Chromatography. PAPER: system P1—Rf 0·25 (location under ultraviolet light, bright blue fluorescence; location reagent *iodoplatinate spray*, weak reaction).
THIN-LAYER: system T1—Rf 0·59 (location under ultraviolet light, bright blue fluorescence).

Colour Tests. MICRO: sulphuric acid–formaldehyde test—yellow (*sensitivity:* 1·0 μg); Vitali's test—yellow/yellow/orange-brown (*sensitivity:* 1·0 μg).

Crystal Tests. MICRO: *gold bromide–hydrochloric acid solution*—small needles (*sensitivity:* 1 in 1000); *potassium mercuric iodide solution*—rosettes of needles (*sensitivity:* 1 in 200).

Ultraviolet Absorption Spectrum. Triamterene in an aqueous solution containing 10% v/v of acetic acid, maximum at 360 mμ (E1%, 1 cm 840).

Infra-red Absorption Spectrum. Potassium bromide disk. The principal peaks are: A 1428 or 1572 or 1612 (p. 767).

Metabolism. Triamterene is metabolised chiefly by hydroxylation of the phenyl ring in the *p*-position. The resulting metabolite is excreted as the sulphate conjugate although a little is excreted free. Unchanged triamterene and its conjugate are also excreted. In all, about 30% of an oral dose is recovered in the urine within 24 hours.

Dose. Up to a max. of 300 mg daily.

Toxicity. LD50 (oral): in mice about 300 mg/kg.

TRICHLORMETHIAZIDE *Diuretic*

Synonym: CMR 807.
Proprietary Names: Fluitran; Metahydrin; Naqua.

6 - Chloro - 3 - dichloromethyl - 3,4 - dihydro - 7 - sulphamoyl - 2*H* - benzo - 1,2,4 - thiadiazine 1,1-dioxide
$C_8H_8Cl_3N_3O_4S_2 = 380{\cdot}7$

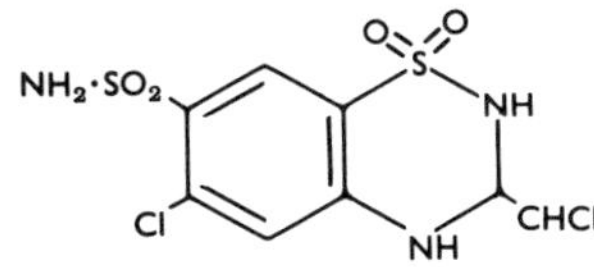

Extraction. Trichlormethiazide may be isolated in the A2 fraction (see p. 27); it is distinguished from the barbiturates by chromatography (see below).

Chromatography. PAPER: system P1—Rf 0·91 (location under ultraviolet light, absorption).
THIN-LAYER: system T1—Rf 0·80 (location reagents: *iodine–carbon tetrachloride spray*, positive reaction; *potassium permanganate spray*, positive reaction).

Metabolism. Trichlormethiazide is a diuretic with a greater potency and duration of action than chlorothiazide (p. 253). Diuresis is initiated within 2 hours of administration, reaches its maximum in about 6 hours and lasts for more than 24 hours. The drug is rapidly absorbed from the gastro-intestinal tract. Studies in dogs have shown that after 5 hours 69% may be recovered from the urine.

Dose. Usually up to 4 mg daily, but some patients may need up to 8 mg.

Toxicity. LD50 (oral): in mice 2·96 and in rats 5·60 g/kg.

TRICHLOROETHANE *Industrial Solvent*

Synonym: Methyl Chloroform.
Proprietary Names: Chlorothene; Genklene. It is the principal ingredient of Thawpit.

1,1,1-Trichloroethane
$Cl_3{\cdot}C{\cdot}CH_3 = 133{\cdot}4$

A colourless liquid. F.p. −32·5° to −32·7°. B.p. 71° to 81°.
Solubility. Insoluble in water; soluble in ethanol, ether, and acetone.

Screening Test. Fujiwara's test—pink or red (see p. 15).

Extraction. Trichloroethane is volatile and may be isolated by distillation (see p. 18).

Chromatography. GAS: system G8/160—retention time 2·30 relative to n-propanol.

Quantitative Estimation. Trichloroethane may be determined in the breath, blood, and tissues by infra-red spectrophotometry or gas chromatography (Stewart and Dodd, 1964; Stewart and Erley, 1965; Stewart *et al.*, 1965; Stewart and Andrews, 1966).

Metabolism. Trichloroethane is rapidly absorbed from the gastro-intestinal tract after ingestion and through the lungs during exposure to its vapour. It is poorly absorbed through the intact skin and, although it may remove the natural greases, it is unlikely that toxic quantities will be absorbed. It is mainly eliminated unchanged via the lungs. A small percentage is metabolised to carbon dioxide and trichloroethanol, the latter appearing in the urine as a glucuronide conjugate.

Use. Trichloroethane is a non-inflammable solvent which effectively dissolves oils, greases, waxes, rubber, and bitumen. It is used for cleaning articles which are contaminated with these materials and as a solvent in adhesives, rubber formulations, grease preparations, polishes, and aerosols, and for waxes including silicones. It is a particularly suitable solvent for dry cleaning operations because it is less toxic than other chlorinated hydrocarbon solvents.

Toxicity. The estimated lethal dose by ingestion is stated to be 2 g. The maximum permissible atmospheric concentration is 500 p.p.m. Blood-levels of 35 to 100 mg% may cause fatal poisoning. Recovery occurred following the ingestion of about 0·6 g/kg—about 42 g (Stewart and Andrews, 1966).

CASE EXAMPLES. A 29-year-old man found dead had a trichloroethane blood-level of 13 mg%. Since no drugs or solvents were found in the stomach contents, the man had presumably inhaled the solvent. A similar case in a young woman who had a history of 'sniffing'; the blood-level was 72 mg% (Hall and Hine, 1966).

TRICHLOROETHYLENE

Anaesthetic/Solvent

Synonym: Trichlorethylene.
Proprietary Names: Chlorylen(e); Gemalgene; Trethylene; Trichlor; Trilene; Westrosol.

1,1,2-Trichloroethylene
$Cl{\cdot}CH{:}CCl_2 = 131{\cdot}4$

A colourless mobile liquid which is slowly decomposed by light in the presence of moisture. The anaesthetic grade contains thymol 0·01% w/w as a preservative and may contain not more than 0·001% w/w of a suitable blue colouring matter. B.p. 86° to 88°.

Solubility. Almost insoluble in water; miscible with ethanol, ether, and chloroform.

Screening Test. Fujiwara's test—pink or red (see p. 15).

Extraction. Trichloroethylene is volatile and may be isolated by distillation (see p. 18).

Chromatography. GAS: system G8/160—retention time 3·10 relative to n-propanol.

Quantitative Estimation. Abrahamsen (1960) describes 2 methods of extraction of trichloroethylene and trichloroacetic acid from serum and urine followed by spectrophotometric estimation based on Fujiwara's test. Feldstein (1965) describes an infra-red spectrophotometric method for the determination of blood-levels. Bonnichsen and Maehly (1966) describe a method of determination in blood, urine, or finely cut tissue, based on Fujiwara's test.

Metabolism. Trichloroethylene is metabolised to chloral hydrate which is in turn metabolised to trichloroethanol and trichloroacetic acid. Trichloroethanol is excreted mainly as the glucuronide conjugate and trichloroacetic acid is excreted very slowly in the urine.

It seems that trichloroethylene or a breakdown product is stored in the tissues from which it is only slowly released so that the concentration of trichloroacetic acid in the serum remains low and decreases only gradually.

After anaesthesia, very small amounts of trichloroethylene have been found in the expired air and in the blood, but only during the first 1 to 2 days.

NOTE. For a review of the literature over 40 years dealing with the pharmacology and toxicology of trichloroethylene and giving over 400 references see Defalque (1961).

Uses. Trichloroethylene resembles chloroform in its effects but it is less potent as an anaesthetic and more potent as an analgesic, and it is less toxic. It is a useful cleansing agent for dirty and greasy wounds. It is used in industry in a less pure form as a solvent for oils and fats, for degreasing metals, and for dry cleaning.

Toxicity. Although less toxic than chloroform, trichloroethylene may produce cardiac irregularities such as atrial or ventricular extrasystoles. It may increase the respiratory rate, inducing short jerky inspirations. It may also give rise to nausea, vomiting, headache, and confusion.

In industry, exposure to high concentrations of trichloroethylene vapour has caused acute poisoning and fatalities have occurred, although temporary unconsciousness is a more common manifestation. Chronic poisoning arising from the industrial use of trichloroethylene may result in ataxia, trigeminal paralysis, optic neuritis, paralysis of the oculomotor nerve, and permanent blindness. In acute cases of poisoning the metabolites of trichloroethylene play a minor role but upon chronic exposure considerable amounts of the metabolites may be excreted in the urine. The maximum permissible atmospheric concentration is 100 p.p.m.

Prolonged contact with trichloroethylene can cause dermatitis, eczema, burns, and conjunctivitis.

Addiction to trichloroethylene vapour has occurred among medical personnel and factory workers.

The lethal dose by ingestion or inhalation is estimated to be 5 ml.

CASE EXAMPLES. A 41-year-old man was in direct contact with trichloroethylene in a dry cleaning establishment for 7 years. At the end of this time his urine was found to contain 20 mg% of trichloroacetic acid. During the following 9 years he was not in direct contact with trichloroethylene but he then drank about 40 ml of the solvent. On admission to hospital several hours later, trichloroacetic acid was found in the urine, 127 mg%, and in the serum, about 15 mg%, and it was present for the following 53 days, but no longer by the 85th day.

A 20-year-old seaman was ill after cleaning, for 2 hours in a cabin, some carpets with 2 litres of Motorin (trichloroethylene with some turpentine). In hospital, about 4 hours later, trichloroacetic acid was found in his urine and serum and was present in both for the next 14 days. The serum concentration reached a maximum, about 14 mg%, nearly 48 hours after inhalation and then decreased very slowly; the maximum urine concentration, attained concomitantly, was about 47 mg% (Abrahamsen, 1960).
With suicidal intent, an adolescent girl swallowed 400 to 500 ml of trichloroethylene and fell into deep coma with depressed respiration. With tracheostomy, glucose infusions, and artificial respiration, she eventually recovered completely (Warembourg *et al.*, 1964).
After inadvertently inhaling trichloroethylene, a man developed acute renal failure and toxic myocarditis. The latter was believed to be related to retention of trichloroethylene or its metabolic products because of the renal failure. The man recovered after peritoneal dialysis (Gutch *et al.*, 1965).
Post-mortem findings in 19 fatal cases of trichloroethylene poisoning ranged as follows: blood, 0·2 to 4·1 mg%; brain, 0·4 to 7·4 mg%; kidneys, 0·4 to 14 mg%; liver, 0·1 to 25 mg%; lungs, 0·1 to 1·5 mg%; stomach contents, 0·9 to 200 mg%; urine, a trace to 9·1 mg%. Of these cases, 8 were due to ingestion and 11 to inhalation (Bonnichsen and Maehly, 1966).
Atmospheric concentrations of trichloroethylene ranged from 0·015 to 0·19 mg% in 30 small Italian dry-cleaning works. The concentration of trichloroacetic acid in the urine of workers in these establishments ranged from a trace to over 7 mg%. Levels of over 20 mg% were found in 22 of the cases and these persons also had the highest incidence of abnormal clinical findings, e.g. moderate hepatomegaly, chronic cholecystitis, asthenia, and contact dermatitis (Brancaccio *et al.*, 1966).
A middle-aged man consumed an unknown amount of trichloroethylene from a 'labelled beer bottle'. He was seriously ill but survived. On admission to hospital the serum trichloroethylene level was 3·3 mg%, and the first 24-hour urine collection contained 3·8 mg% of trichloroethylene (Tompsett, 1967c).

TRICLOBISONIUM CHLORIDE

Antimicrobial

Synonym: Ro 5-0810.
Proprietary Name: Triburon Chloride.

Hexamethylenebis{dimethyl[1-methyl-3-(2,2,6-trimethylcyclohexyl)propyl]ammonium chloride}

$C_{36}H_{74}Cl_2N_2$ = 605·9

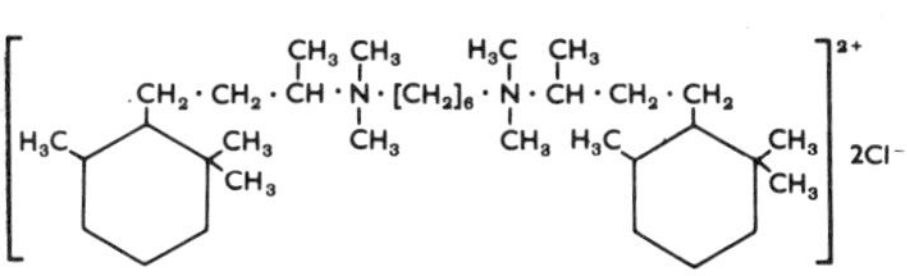

A white hygroscopic crystalline powder. M.p. about 243°.
Solubility. Soluble in water, ethanol, and chloroform; insoluble in ether.

Extraction. Triclobisonium chloride is a quaternary ammonium compound (see p. 29).

Chromatography. PAPER: system P1—Rf 0·50 (location reagents: *iodoplatinate spray*, weak reaction; *iodine vapour*, weak reaction).

THIN-LAYER: system T1—Rf 0·01 (location reagent *acidified iodoplatinate spray*, positive reaction).

Colour Test. MICRO: ammonium molybdate test—blue (*sensitivity:* 1·0 μg).

Use. Topically as a 0·1% ointment.

TRICYCLAMOL CHLORIDE

Parasympatholytic

Proprietary Names: Elorine; Lergine; Tricoloid.

(±) - *N* - (3 - Cyclohexyl - 3 - hydroxy - 3 - phenylpropyl)-*N*-methylpyrrolidinium chloride
$C_{20}H_{32}ClNO$ = 337·9

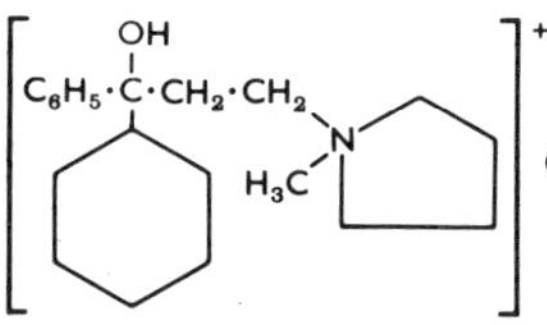

A white crystalline powder. M.p. 165° to 168°.
Solubility. Soluble 1 in 3 of water, 1 in 3 of ethanol, and 1 in 25 of chloroform; insoluble in ether.

Extraction. Tricyclamol chloride is a quaternary ammonium compound (see p. 29).

Chromatography. PAPER: system P1—Rf 0·63 (location reagent *iodoplatinate spray*, strong reaction); system RP1a—Rf 0·89 (location under ultraviolet light, absorption; location reagent *iodoplatinate spray*, positive reaction); system RP1b—Rf 0·74 (location as for RP1a).
THIN-LAYER: system T1—Rf 0·06 (location reagent *acidified iodoplatinate spray*, positive reaction).

Colour Tests. MICRO: sulphuric acid–formaldehyde test—dull purple (*sensitivity:* 1·0 μg); ammonium molybdate test—grey (*sensitivity:* 1·0 μg); ammonium vanadate test—grey-purple (*sensitivity:* 0·25 μg).

Crystal Tests. MICRO: *platinic bromide solution*—rosettes or sheaves of needles (*sensitivity:* 1 in 400); *potassium chromate solution*—small oily rods, sometimes in rosettes (*sensitivity:* 1 in 3000).

Ultraviolet Absorption Spectrum. Tricyclamol chloride in water, maxima at 252 mμ (E1%, 1 cm 4·5), 257 mμ (E1%, 1 cm 5·6), and 263 mμ (E1%, 1 cm 4·2).

Dose. Up to 600 mg daily.

Toxicity. The lethal dose in man is probably in the range 10 to 100 mg/kg.

TRIDIHEXETHYL CHLORIDE

Parasympatholytic

Proprietary Name: Pathilon Chloride.

(3 - Cyclohexyl - 3 - hydroxy - 3 - phenyl - propyl)triethylammonium chloride

$C_{21}H_{36}ClNO = 354·0$

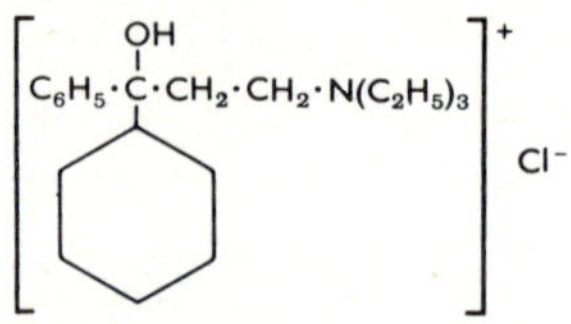

A white crystalline powder. M.p. 198° to 202°.

Solubility. Freely soluble in water and chloroform; almost insoluble in ether.

Extraction. Tridihexethyl chloride is a quaternary ammonium compound (see p. 29).

Chromatography. PAPER: system P1—Rf 0·78 (location reagent *iodoplatinate spray*, strong reaction); system RP1a—Rf 0·89 (location under ultraviolet light, absorption; location reagent *iodoplatinate spray*, positive reaction); system RP1b—Rf 0·74 (location as for RP1a).

THIN-LAYER: system T1—Rf 0·07 (location reagent *acidified iodoplatinate spray*, positive reaction).

Colour Tests. MICRO: sulphuric acid–formaldehyde test—brown-purple (*sensitivity:* 1·0 µg); ammonium molybdate test—black-purple (*sensitivity:* 1·0 µg); ammonium vanadate test—faint purple (*sensitivity:* 1·0 µg).

Crystal Test. MICRO: *potassium chromate solution*—hedgehogs or rosettes of fine needles (*sensitivity:* 1 in 100).

Infra-red Absorption Spectrum. Tridihexethyl chloride. Potassium bromide disk. The principal peaks are: A 717, B 710 or 1492, C 1400 or 1450 (p. 767).

Dose. Usually up to 200 mg by mouth daily.

Toxicity. The lethal dose in man is probably in the range 10 to 100 mg/kg.

TRIFLUOPERAZINE *Tranquilliser*

Synonym: SKF 5019.

10 - [3 - (4 - Methylpiperazin - 1 - yl)propyl] - 2 - trifluoromethylphenothiazine

$C_{21}H_{24}F_3N_3S = 407·5$

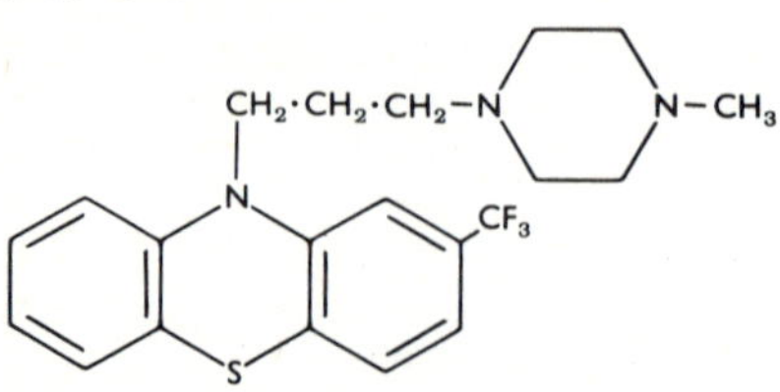

TRIFLUOPERAZINE HYDROCHLORIDE

Proprietary Names: Jatroneural; Stelazine; Terfluzine. It is an ingredient of Amylozine, Parstelin, and Stelabid.

A pale cream-coloured crystalline powder. M.p. about 240°.

Solubility. Soluble 1 in 2 of water; slightly soluble in ethanol; insoluble in ether.

Screening Test. *FPN reagent* with urine—orange (see p. 10).

Extraction. Trifluoperazine is extracted by organic solvents from aqueous alkaline solutions; hydrolysis of biological material is required in order to improve the yield.

Chromatography. PAPER: system P1—Rf 0·34 (location under ultraviolet light, yellow fluorescence; location reagents: *iodoplatinate spray*, strong reaction; *bromocresol green spray*, weak reaction; *FPN spray*, orange); system RP1a—Rf 0·06 (location under ultraviolet light, yellow fluorescence; location reagent *iodoplatinate spray*, positive reaction); system RP1b—Rf 0·03 (location under ultraviolet light, yellow fluorescence; location reagent *iodoplatinate spray*, positive reaction).

THIN-LAYER: system T1—Rf 0·48 (location reagent *acidified iodoplatinate spray*, positive reaction); system T3—Rf 0·69 (location reagents: *iodoplatinate spray*, positive reaction; *sulphuric acid–ethanol spray*, orange); system T4—Rf 0·33 (location as for T3); system T5—Rf 0·40 (location as for T3); system T6—Rf 0·63 (the spot may be converted on the plate to the sulphoxide, Rf 0·41; location of both spots under ultraviolet light).

GAS: system G2/225—retention time 2·28 relative to codeine.

Colour Tests. MICRO: sulphuric acid–formaldehyde test—red-purple (*sensitivity:* 0·5 µg); ammonium molybdate test—red-brown (*sensitivity:* 0·5 µg); ammonium vanadate test—red-brown (*sensitivity:* 0·5 µg); Vitali's test—purple → yellow/yellow/bright yellow (*sensitivity:* 0·5 µg).

Crystal Tests. MICRO: *gold chloride solution*—curved needles (*sensitivity:* 1 in 100); *zinc chloride solution*—needles, forming overnight (*sensitivity:* 1 in 100).

Ultraviolet Absorption Spectrum. Trifluoperazine in 0·01N hydrochloric acid, maximum at 256 mµ (E1%, 1 cm 739).

Infra-red Absorption Spectrum. Trifluoperazine hydrochloride. Potassium bromide disk. The principal peaks are: A 1106, B 1426, C 1316 (p. 768).

Dose. In psychiatric states, up to 30 mg daily by mouth or up to 5 mg daily intramuscularly. As an anti-emetic, up to 6 mg daily by mouth or up to 3 mg daily intramuscularly.

Toxicity. The acute lethal dose of the phenothiazine tranquillisers is stated to be in the range 15 to 150 mg/kg.

TRIMEPERIDINE *Narcotic Analgesic*

Synonym: Trimethylmeperidine.

1,2,5 - Trimethyl - 4 - phenyl - 4 - propionyloxypiperidine

$C_{17}H_{25}NO_2 = 275{\cdot}4$

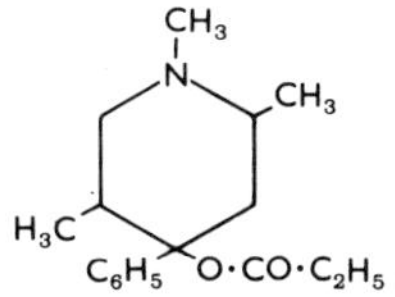

TRIMEPERIDINE HYDROCHLORIDE

Synonym: Promedol.

A white crystalline powder.

Solubility. Soluble in water, ethanol, and chloroform; insoluble in ether.

Extraction. Trimeperidine is extracted by organic solvents from aqueous alkaline solutions; hydrolysis of biological material is required in order to improve the yield.

Chromatography. PAPER: system P1—Rf 0·65 (location reagents: *iodoplatinate spray*, strong reaction; *bromocresol green spray*, weak reaction); system RP1a—Rf 0·70 (location reagent *iodoplatinate spray*, positive reaction); system RP1b—Rf 0·05 (location as for RP1a).

THIN-LAYER: system T1—Rf 0·52 (location reagent *acidified iodoplatinate spray*, positive reaction).

GAS: system G2/225—retention time 0·92 relative to diphenhydramine.

Colour Test. MICRO: sulphuric acid–formaldehyde test—red-purple (*sensitivity:* 0·25 μg).

Crystal Tests. MICRO: *lead iodide solution*—rosettes of needles (*sensitivity:* 1 in 400); *styphnic acid*—fans or bunches of rods, often serrated, forming overnight (*sensitivity:* 1 in 1000).

Ultraviolet Absorption Spectrum. Trimeperidine in 0·1N sulphuric acid, maxima at about 242 mμ (E1%, 1 cm 3·7), about 247 mμ (E1%, 1 cm 4·8), 251 mμ (E1%, 1 cm 6·2), 257 mμ (E1%, 1 cm 7·6), and 263 mμ (E1%, 1 cm 6).

Dose. Max. single 60 mg; max. in 24 hours 120 mg.

Toxicity. When given over a prolonged period, symptoms of tolerance and addiction may develop.

TRIMEPRAZINE *Antihistamine*

Synonym: Alimemazine.

10 - (3 - Dimethylamino - 2 - methylpropyl) - phenothiazine

$C_{18}H_{22}N_2S = 298{\cdot}5$

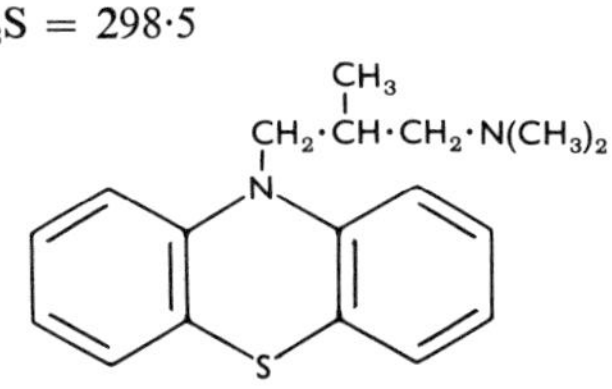

Trimeprazine occurs as crystals. M.p. 68°. B.p. 150° to 175° at 0·3 mm Hg.

TRIMEPRAZINE TARTRATE

Proprietary Names: Panectyl; Repeltin; Temaril; Théralène; Vallergan.

A white powder which darkens on exposure to light. M.p. 159° to 163°.

Solubility. Soluble 1 in 4 of water, 1 in 30 of ethanol, and 1 in 75 of chloroform; very slightly soluble in ether.

Screening Test. *FPN reagent* with urine—orange-red (see p. 10).

Extraction. Trimeprazine is extracted by organic solvents from aqueous alkaline solutions; hydrolysis of biological material is required in order to improve the yield.

Chromatography. PAPER: system P1—Rf 0·70 (location under ultraviolet light, blue fluorescence; location reagents: *iodoplatinate spray*, strong reaction; *FPN spray*, orange-red); system RP1a—Rf 0·29 (location under ultraviolet light, blue fluorescence; location reagent *iodoplatinate spray*, positive reaction); system RP1b—Rf 0·94 (location as for RP1a).

THIN-LAYER: system T1—Rf 0·55 (location reagent *acidified iodoplatinate spray*, positive reaction); system T3—Rf 0·96 (location reagents: *iodoplatinate spray*, positive reaction; *sulphuric acid–ethanol spray*, orange); system T4—Rf 0·64 (location as for T3); system T5—Rf 0·30 (location as for T3); system T6—Rf 0·71 (the spot may be converted on the plate to the sulphoxide, Rf 0·50; location of both spots under ultraviolet light).

GAS: system G2/225—retention time 0·85 relative to codeine; system G4—retention time 0·47 relative to codeine.

Colour Tests. MICRO: sulphuric acid–formaldehyde test—purple (*sensitivity:* 0·5 μg); ammonium molybdate test—purple (*sensitivity:* 0·5 μg); ammonium vanadate test—purple (*sensitivity:* 0·5 μg); Vitali's test—yellow/yellow/yellow (*sensitivity:* 1·0 μg).

Crystal Tests. MICRO: *gold chloride solution*—needles, some serrated (*sensitivity:* 1 in 400); *picrolonic acid*—rosettes of rods (*sensitivity:* 1 in 200).

Ultraviolet Absorption Spectrum. Trimeprazine in 0·01N hydrochloric acid, maxima at 251 mμ (E1%, 1 cm 876) and 302 mμ.

Infra-red Absorption Spectrum. Trimeprazine tartrate. Potassium bromide disk. The principal peaks are: A 1461, B 748, C 1248 (p. 768).

Metabolism. After oral administration of a single 15-mg dose of ^{35}S-labelled trimeprazine, about 70% of the radioactivity was excreted in the urine in 48 hours. Less than 3% of the radioactivity was excreted in the faeces over a period of 4 days (Johnson and Masters, 1962).

Dose. Up to 40 mg daily for relief of pruritus; up to 5 mg/kg for pre-operative medication of children.

Toxicity. Acute poisoning may be associated

with profound depression of the central nervous system. Agranulocytosis may occasionally occur.

TRIMETAPHAN CAMSYLATE

Antihypertensive

Synonyms: Méthioplégium; NU 2222; Trimethaphan Camphorsulphonate.
Proprietary Name: Arfonad.

4,6 - Dibenzyl - 5 - oxo - 1 - thia - 4,6 - diazatricyclo[6,3,0,$0^{3,7}$]undecanium (+)-β-camphorsulphonate

$C_{22}H_{25}N_2OS, C_{10}H_{15}O_4S = 596{\cdot}8$

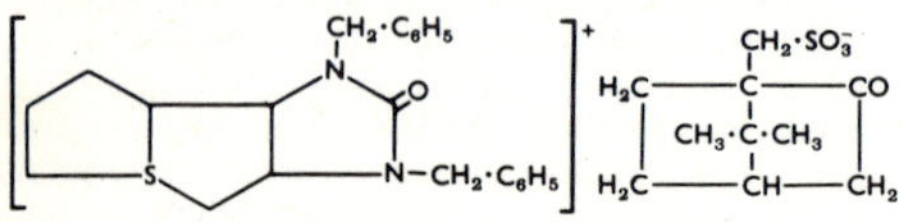

A white crystalline powder. M.p. about 245°, with decomposition.
Solubility. Soluble 1 in 5 of water and 1 in 2 of ethanol; very slightly soluble in ether; soluble in chloroform.

Extraction. Trimetaphan camsylate is a quaternary ammonium compound (see p. 29).

Chromatography. PAPER: system P1—Rf 0·55 (location reagent *iodoplatinate spray*, strong reaction); system RP1a—Rf 0·85 (location under ultraviolet light, absorption; location reagent *iodoplatinate spray*, positive reaction); system RP1b—Rf 0·77 (location as for RP1a).
THIN-LAYER: system T1—Rf 0·02 (location reagent *acidified iodoplatinate spray*, positive reaction).

Colour Test. MICRO: Vitali's test— -/-/orange (*sensitivity:* 1·0 μg).

Crystal Tests. MICRO: *potassium iodide solution*—masses of fine needles (*sensitivity:* 1 in 1000); *potassium permanganate solution*—bunches of branching serrated needles (*sensitivity:* 1 in 1000).

Ultraviolet Absorption Spectrum. Trimetaphan camsylate in water, maxima at 252 mμ (E1%, 1cm about 7·6), 258 mμ (E1%, 1cm about 7·8), and 264 mμ (E1%, 1cm about 5·8).

Infra-red Absorption Spectrum. Potassium bromide disk. The principal peaks are: A 1220 or 1701, B 1184 or 1735 (p. 768).

Uses. Trimetaphan is used for inducing controlled hypotension during surgical procedures. It is administered as a slow intravenous infusion, the usual strength being 1 mg/ml and the dose being determined according to the patient's needs.

TRIMETAZIDINE

Coronary Vasodilator

Synonyms: S 4004; Trimetazine.

1-(2,3,4-Trimethoxybenzyl)piperazine
$C_{14}H_{22}N_2O_3 = 266{\cdot}3$

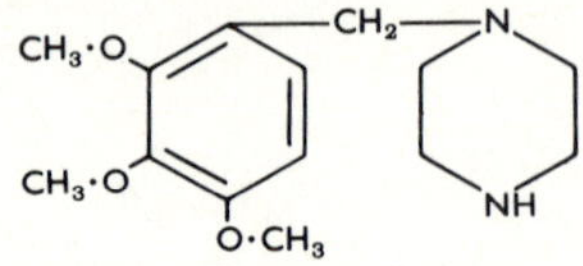

TRIMETAZIDINE HYDROCHLORIDE
Proprietary Name: Vastarel.

A crystalline powder which melts at 222° to 228°.
Solubility. Soluble in water; very slightly soluble in ethanol.

Extraction. Trimetazidine is extracted by organic solvents from aqueous alkaline solutions.

Chromatography. PAPER: system P1—Rf 0·04 (location under ultraviolet light, absorption; location reagents: *iodoplatinate spray*, strong reaction; *bromocresol green spray*, strong reaction); system RP1a—Rf 0·92 (location under ultraviolet light, absorption; location reagent *iodoplatinate spray*, positive reaction); system RP1b—Rf 0·63 (location as for RP1a).
THIN-LAYER: system T1—Rf 0·18 (location reagent *acidified iodoplatinate spray*, positive reaction).

Colour Tests. MICRO: sulphuric acid–formaldehyde test—faint yellow, fading (*sensitivity:* 1·0 μg); ammonium molybdate test—purple-brown (*sensitivity:* 1·0 μg); ammonium vanadate test—purple (*sensitivity:* 1·0 μg); Vitali's test—dull purple/dull purple/faint brown (*sensitivity:* 1·0 μg).

Crystal Tests. MICRO: *platinic bromide solution*—small plates and needles (*sensitivity:* 1 in 1000); *platinic chloride solution*—small needles in bunches (*sensitivity:* 1 in 1000).

Ultraviolet Absorption Spectrum. Trimetazidine in 0·1N sulphuric acid, maxima at 232 mμ (E1%, 1cm 305) and 269 mμ (E1%, 1cm 23), and an inflexion at about 275 mμ.

Dose. Up to 6 mg daily.

Toxicity. LD50 (intravenous): in mice 130 mg/kg.

TRIMETHOPRIM

Antimicrobial

Synonym: Trimethoxyprim.
Proprietary Name: Syraprim.

2,4 - Diamino - 5 - (3,4,5 - trimethoxybenzyl) - pyrimidine
$C_{14}H_{18}N_4O_3 = 290{\cdot}3$

Extraction. Trimethoprim is extracted by

organic solvents from aqueous alkaline solutions.

Chromatography. PAPER: system P1—Rf 0·23 (location under ultraviolet light, strong absorption; location reagents: *iodoplatinate spray*, weak reaction; *bromocresol green spray*, strong reaction).

THIN-LAYER: system T1—Rf 0·50 (location reagent *acidified iodoplatinate spray*, positive reaction).

GAS: system G2/225—retention time 2·07 relative to codeine.

Colour Tests. MICRO: sulphuric acid–formaldehyde test—orange (*sensitivity:* 0·1 μg); ammonium molybdate test—bluish-green (*sensitivity:* 0·1 μg); ammonium vanadate test—yellow-brown (*sensitivity:* 0·5 μg); Vitali's test—purple-red/brown/brown (*sensitivity:* 0·1 μg).

Crystal Tests. MICRO: *ammonium thiocyanate solution*—needles (*sensitivity:* 1 in 400); *potassium iodide solution*—fans of needles (*sensitivity:* 1 in 400).

Ultraviolet Absorption Spectrum. Trimethoprim in 0·1N sulphuric acid, maximum at 271 mμ (E1%, 1 cm 212).

Dose. Up to 800 mg daily has been given.

TRIMETHOXYAMPHETAMINE *Hallucinogen*

Synonym: TMA.

α-Methyl-3,4,5-trimethoxyphenethylamine
$C_{12}H_{19}NO_3 = 225{\cdot}3$

Trimethoxyamphetamine is the α-methyl homologue of mescaline (p. 404). It occurs as an oil.
Solubility. Insoluble in water; soluble in chloroform.

The hydrochloride is soluble in water; m.p. 219° to 220°.

Extraction. Trimethoxyamphetamine is extracted by organic solvents from aqueous alkaline solutions.

Chromatography. PAPER: system P1—Rf 0·41 (location under ultraviolet light, absorption; location reagents: *iodoplatinate spray*, weak reaction; *bromocresol green spray*, weak reaction).

THIN-LAYER: system T1—Rf 0·35 (location reagent *acidified iodoplatinate spray*, positive reaction).

Colour Tests. MICRO: sulphuric acid–formaldehyde test—dull orange (*sensitivity:* 0·25 μg); ammonium molybdate test—blue-green (*sensitivity:* 0·1 μg); Vitali's test—dull red-purple/red/yellow (*sensitivity:* 1·0 μg).

Crystal Tests. MICRO: *gold bromide solution*—bunches of serrated needles (*sensitivity:* 1 in 1000); *picric acid*—branching irregular needles (*sensitivity:* 1 in 1000).

Ultraviolet Absorption Spectrum. In 0·1N sulphuric acid, maximum at 269 mμ.

NOTE. Doses of 0·8 to 2 mg/kg in human volunteers produced fairly vivid hallucinations similar to those produced by mescaline. At higher dosage, 2·8 to 3·5 mg/kg, dramatic and dangerous psychotropic responses occurred; the initial effects, about 2 hours after ingestion, were mescaline-like, but between 3 and 5 hours after ingestion, anger, hostility, and megalomaniac euphoria dominated the subjects' thoughts and conversation and it was thought that provocation of the subjects would have precipitated homicidal violence (Shulgin *et al.*, 1961).

TRIMIPRAMINE *Antidepressant*

Synonyms: IL 6001; RP 7162; Trimeprimine.

5 - (3 - Dimethylamino - 2 - methylpropyl) - 10,11-dihydro-5*H*-dibenz[*b*,*f*]azepine
$C_{20}H_{26}N_2 = 294{\cdot}4$

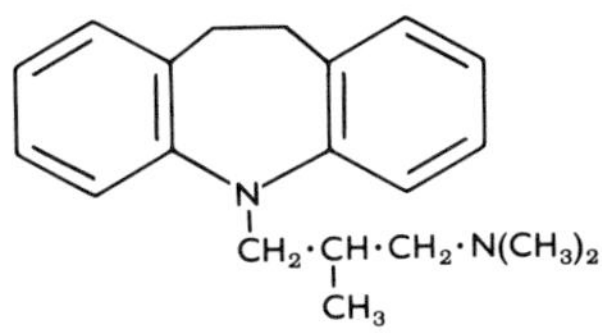

A pale yellowish waxy solid. M.p. about 45°.
Solubility. Insoluble in water; readily soluble in ethanol.

TRIMIPRAMINE MALEATE
Proprietary Name: Surmontil (tablets).

A white crystalline substance. M.p. 142°.
Solubility. Sparingly soluble in water and ethanol; practically insoluble in ether; soluble in chloroform.

TRIMIPRAMINE MESYLATE
Synonym: Trimeprimine Methanesulphonate.
Proprietary Name: Surmontil (injection).

Screening Test. See under Screening Tests, p. 13.

Extraction. Trimipramine is extracted by organic solvents from aqueous alkaline solutions; hydrolysis of biological material is required in order to improve the yield.

Chromatography. PAPER: system P1—Rf 0·73 (location under ultraviolet light, blue fluorescence; location reagents: *iodoplatinate spray*, strong reaction; *bromocresol green spray*, weak reaction).

THIN-LAYER: system T1—Rf 0·58 (location reagent *acidified iodoplatinate spray*, positive reaction).

GAS: system G2/225—retention time 0·64 relative to codeine; system G4—retention time 0·30 (0·15) relative to codeine.

Colour Tests. MICRO: ammonium molybdate test — blue (*sensitivity:* 0·1 μg); ammonium vanadate test—blue (*sensitivity:* 0·1 μg); Vitali's test — deep green/yellow/yellow (*sensitivity:* 0·1 μg).

Crystal Tests. MICRO: *platinic chloride solution*—needles, often serrated (*sensitivity:* 1 in 1000); *trinitrobenzoic acid solution*—dense rosettes (*sensitivity:* 1 in 1000).

Ultraviolet Absorption Spectrum. Trimipramine

in 0·1N sulphuric acid, maximum at 250 mμ (E1%, 1cm 300) and an inflexion at about 268 mμ (E1%, 1 cm 250).

Infra-red Absorption Spectrum. Trimipramine maleate. Potassium bromide disk. The principal peaks are: A 1488, B 1351, C 1580 (p. 768).

Quantitative Estimation. See under Imipramine, p. 379.

Metabolism. Studies in rabbits and dogs have shown that trimipramine is extensively metabolised.

Dose. Usually up to 300 mg daily; as much as 800 mg daily has been given for periods of up to 6 months.

Toxicity. LD50 (oral): in mice 250 mg/kg.

TRIPELENNAMINE *Antihistamine*

N - Benzyl - *N'N'* - dimethyl - *N* - pyrid - 2 - ylethylenediamine

$C_{16}H_{21}N_3 = 255·4$

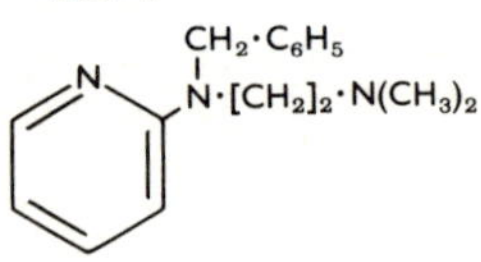

Tripelennamine has a boiling-point between 167° and 172° at 0·1 mm Hg.

TRIPELENNAMINE CITRATE

Proprietary Name: Pyribenzamine Citrate (elixir).

A white crystalline powder. M.p. about 107°.

Solubility. Soluble 1 in about 1 of water; freely soluble in ethanol; very slightly soluble in ether; almost insoluble in chloroform.

TRIPELENNAMINE HYDROCHLORIDE

Proprietary Names: Azaron; Piristina; Pyribenzamine Hydrochloride (tablets).

A white crystalline powder which slowly darkens on exposure to light. M.p. 187° to 192°.

Solubility. Soluble 1 in 1 of water, 1 in 8 of ethanol, and 1 in 4 of chloroform; insoluble in ether.

Extraction. Tripelennamine is extracted by organic solvents from aqueous alkaline solutions.

Chromatography. PAPER: system P1—Rf 0·35 (location under ultraviolet light, bright blue fluorescence; location reagents: *iodoplatinate spray*, strong reaction; *bromocresol green spray*, weak reaction); system RP1a—Rf 0·74 (location under ultraviolet light, blue fluorescence; location reagent *iodoplatinate spray*, positive reaction); system RP1b—Rf 0·57 (location as for RP1a).

THIN-LAYER: system T1—Rf 0·48 (location reagent *acidified iodoplatinate spray*, positive reaction); system T2—Rf 0·62 (location reagent *iodoplatinate spray*, positive reaction); system T3—Rf 0·92 (location as for T2).

GAS: system G1/180—retention time 1·54 relative to diphenhydramine.

Colour Tests. MICRO: sulphuric acid–formaldehyde test—red-brown (*sensitivity:* 0·1 μg); ammonium molybdate test—yellow-brown (*sensitivity:* 0·1 μg); ammonium vanadate test—yellow-brown (*sensitivity:* 0·5 μg).

Crystal Tests. MICRO: *lead iodide solution*—snowflake rosettes or masses of small needles (*sensitivity:* 1 in 1000); *platinic chloride solution*—rosettes of plates (*sensitivity:* 1 in 1000).

Ultraviolet Absorption Spectrum. Tripelennamine in 0·1N sulphuric acid, maxima at 239 mμ (E1%, 1cm 570) and 314 mμ (E1%, 1 cm 320).

Infra-red Absorption Spectrum. Tripelennamine hydrochloride. Potassium bromide disk. The principal peaks are: A 1496, B 1592, C 770 (p. 768).

Metabolism. Tripelennamine is less potent than promethazine (p. 518), has a shorter duration of action, and generally causes less sedation. It seems to be metabolised in the liver. In 24 hours 20% of the dose is excreted in the urine. After ingestion of a single dose of 400 mg, the drug appears in the blood in 2 hours.

Dose. Up to 400 mg daily, by mouth; up to 100 mg daily, by injection.

Toxicity. Following the accidental ingestion of large doses, several cases of coma and convulsions have been reported, but the occurrence of severe central nervous system disturbances is rare. The estimated acute lethal dose in man is between 25 and 250 mg/kg.

TRIPROLIDINE *Antihistamine*

trans - 1 - Pyrid - 2′ - yl - 3 - pyrrolidin - 1″ - yl - 1-*p*-tolylprop-1-ene

$C_{19}H_{22}N_2 = 278·4$

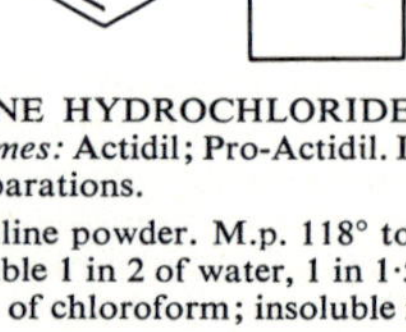

TRIPROLIDINE HYDROCHLORIDE

Proprietary Names: Actidil; Pro-Actidil. It is an ingredient of Actifed preparations.

A white crystalline powder. M.p. 118° to 121°.

Solubility. Soluble 1 in 2 of water, 1 in 1·5 of ethanol, and 1 in less than 1 of chloroform; insoluble in ether.

Extraction. Triprolidine is extracted by organic solvents from aqueous alkaline solutions.

Chromatography. PAPER: system P1—Rf 0·59 (location under ultraviolet light, bright blue fluorescence; location reagents: *iodoplatinate spray*, strong reaction; *bromocresol green spray*, weak reaction); system RP1a—Rf 0·74 (location reagent *iodoplatinate spray*, positive reaction); system RP1b—Rf 0·28 (location as for RP1a).

THIN-LAYER: system T1—Rf 0·43 (location reagent *acidified iodoplatinate spray*, positive reaction); system T2—Rf 0·81 (location reagent *iodoplatinate spray*, positive reaction); system T3—Rf 0·40 (location as for T3).

GAS: system G2/225—retention time 0·69 relative to codeine.

Crystal Tests. MICRO: *picric acid*—rosettes (*sensitivity:* 1 in 1000); *platinic bromide solution*—bunches of blades (*sensitivity:* 1 in 1000).

Ultraviolet Absorption Spectrum. Triprolidine in 0·1N sulphuric acid, maxima at 230 mμ, 276 mμ (E1%, 1cm 276), and 290 mμ.

Infra-red Absorption Spectrum. Triprolidine hydrochloride. Potassium bromide disk. The principal peaks are: A 775, B 1461, C 1421 (p. 768).

Metabolism. Triprolidine is one of the most potent of the antihistamines. Its action is of somewhat shorter duration than that of promethazine (p. 518), persisting for up to 12 hours.

Dose. Up to 15 mg daily.

Toxicity. The estimated acute lethal dose in man is between 25 and 250 mg/kg.

TROPACOCAINE *Local Anaesthetic*

Benzoylpseudotropëine

$C_{15}H_{19}NO_2 = 245{\cdot}3$

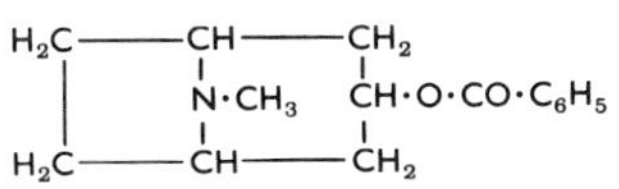

A white crystalline powder. M.p. 49°.

Solubility. Slightly soluble in water; soluble in ethanol, ether, chloroform, and dilute acids.

TROPACOCAINE HYDROCHLORIDE

A white crystalline powder. M.p. 283°, with decomposition.

Solubility. Very soluble in water; less soluble in ethanol; almost insoluble in ether.

Extraction. Tropacocaine is extracted by organic solvents from aqueous alkaline solutions.

Chromatography. PAPER: system P1—Rf 0·51 (location under ultraviolet light, strong absorption; location reagents: *iodoplatinate spray*, strong reaction; *bromocresol green spray*, weak reaction); system RP1a—Rf 0·89 (location under ultraviolet light, absorption; location reagent *iodoplatinate spray*, positive reaction); system RP1b—Rf 0·57 (location as for RP1a).

THIN-LAYER: system T1—Rf 0·35 (location reagent *acidified iodoplatinate spray*, positive reaction).

Crystal Tests. MICRO: *gold chloride solution*—bunches of serrated needles (*sensitivity:* 1 in 3000); *potassium permanganate solution*—irregular plates (*sensitivity:* 1 in 3000).

Ultraviolet Absorption Spectrum. Tropacocaine in ethanol:water (1:1), maxima at 230 mμ (E1%, 1cm 590) and 273 mμ (E1%, 1cm 30).

Dose. Up to 300 mg daily.

Toxicity. Anaesthesia is produced more quickly than with cocaine but is more transitory. The minimum intravenous lethal dose in rats is 20 mg/kg.

TROPICAMIDE *Mydriatic and Cycloplegic*

Synonyms: Bistropamide; Ro 1-7683.

Proprietary Names: Mydriacyl; Mydriaticum.

N-Ethyl-*N*-pyrid-4-ylmethyltropamide

$C_{17}H_{20}N_2O_2 = 284{\cdot}4$

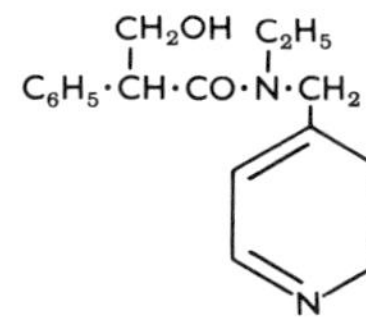

A yellow amorphous powder.

Solubility. Soluble in water and ethanol; insoluble in ether.

Extraction. Tropicamide is extracted by organic solvents from aqueous acid or alkaline solutions.

Chromatography. PAPER: system P1—Rf 0·60 (location under ultraviolet light, blue fluorescence; location reagent *iodoplatinate spray*, weak reaction).

THIN-LAYER: system T1—Rf 0·65 (location reagent *acidified iodoplatinate spray*, positive reaction).

Colour Tests. MICRO: ammonium molybdate test—faint blue (*sensitivity:* 1·0 μg); Vitali's test— -/-/yellow (*sensitivity:* 0·1 μg).

Crystal Tests. MICRO: *picrolonic acid*—rosettes (*sensitivity:* 1 in 1000); *potassium tri-iodide solution (1)*—blades or dense rosettes (*sensitivity:* 1 in 1000).

Ultraviolet Absorption Spectrum. Tropicamide in 0·1N sulphuric acid, maximum at 254 mμ (E1%, 1cm 194).

Use. As eye-drops in 0·5 or 1% solution.

TROPINE

Tropan-3-ol

$C_8H_{15}NO = 141{\cdot}2$

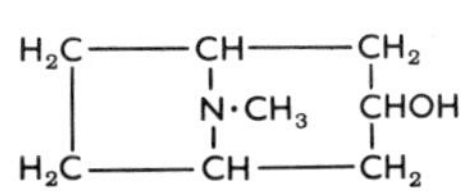

A white powder, which may be obtained by the hydrolysis of atropine. M.p. 63°. B.p. 233°.

Solubility. Soluble in water, ethanol, ether, and chloroform.

Extraction. Tropine is extracted by organic solvents from aqueous acid or alkaline solutions.

Chromatography. PAPER: system P1—Rf 0·05 (location reagents: *iodoplatinate spray*, strong reaction; *bromocresol green spray*, weak reaction).

THIN-LAYER: system T1—Rf 0·40 (location reagent *acidified iodoplatinate spray*, positive reaction).

Crystal Tests. MICRO: *gold bromide solution*—rhomboids (*sensitivity:* 1 in 3000); *picric acid*—needles (*sensitivity:* 1 in 3000).

TROXIDONE *Anticonvulsant*

Synonyms: Trimethadione; Trimethin.
Proprietary Names: Epidione; Tridione.

3,5,5-Trimethyloxazolidine-2,4-dione
$C_6H_9NO_3 = 143{\cdot}1$

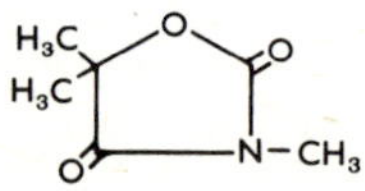

Colourless granular crystals. M.p. 45° to 47°.
Solubility. Soluble 1 in 13 of water and 1 in 2 of ethanol; freely soluble in ether and chloroform.

Extraction. Troxidone is extracted by organic solvents from aqueous acid solutions.

Chromatography. GAS: system G5—retention time 0·12 relative to barbitone.

Ultraviolet Absorption Spectrum. Troxidone in 0·1N sulphuric acid, inflexion at about 226 mμ (E1%, 1 cm 85).

Infra-red Absorption Spectrum. Potassium bromide disk. The principal peaks are: A 1730, B 1802, C 1098 (p. 769).

Metabolism. Troxidone is metabolised chiefly by *N*-demethylation.

Dose. Usually 900 mg daily, initially, increasing up to 1·8 g daily.

Toxicity. Troxidone is highly toxic. The estimated minimum lethal dose in man is 5 g.

TRYPTAMINE *Putrefactive Base*

Synonym: Aminoethylindole.

2-(3-Indolyl)ethylamine
$C_{10}H_{12}N_2 = 160{\cdot}2$

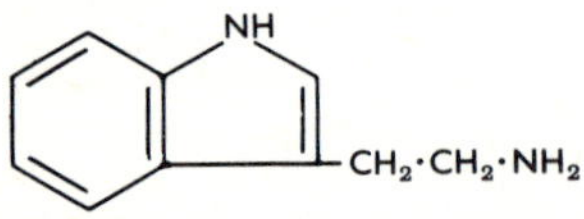

A white crystalline powder. M.p. 116°.

Solubility. Almost insoluble in water, ether, and chloroform; soluble in ethanol.

TRYPTAMINE HYDROCHLORIDE
A white crystalline powder. M.p. 252°.
Solubility. Soluble in water.

Extraction. Tryptamine is extracted by organic solvents from aqueous alkaline solutions.

Chromatography. PAPER: system P1—Rf 0·35 (location under ultraviolet light, blue fluorescence; location reagents: *iodoplatinate spray*, white; *bromocresol green spray*, weak reaction; *potassium permanganate spray*, strong reaction); system RP1a—Rf 0·79 (location under ultraviolet light, blue fluorescence); system RP1b—Rf 0·58 (location as for RP1a).

THIN-LAYER: system T1—Rf 0·27 (location reagent *acidified iodoplatinate spray*, positive reaction).

GAS: system G2/225—retention time 0·78 relative to diphenhydramine.

Colour Tests. MICRO: sulphuric acid–formaldehyde test—dull orange (*sensitivity:* 0·5 μg); ammonium molybdate test—blue → green → yellow (*sensitivity:* 1·0 μg); Vitali's test—yellow/dull yellow/red-brown (*sensitivity:* 1·0 μg).

Crystal Tests. MICRO: *gold cyanide solution*—branching needles (*sensitivity:* 1 in 200); *potassium bismuth iodide solution*—dense rosettes or prisms (*sensitivity:* 1 in 400).

Ultraviolet Absorption Spectrum. Tryptamine in 0·1N sulphuric acid, maxima at about 272·5 mμ (E1%, 1 cm 336), 278 mμ (E1%, 1 cm 349), and 287 mμ (E1%, 1 cm 285).

Metabolism. Tryptamine is formed during putrefaction by bacterial decarboxylation of tryptophan in the gastro-intestinal tract. Reaction with acetaldehyde may occur to form tetrahydroharman; the latter may then be reduced to harman (p. 358).

TUAMINOHEPTANE *Sympathomimetic*

1-Methylhexylamine
$C_7H_{17}N = 115{\cdot}2$

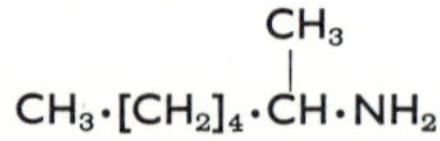

A pale yellow or colourless liquid.
Solubility. Sparingly soluble in water; soluble in ethanol, ether, and chloroform.

TUAMINOHEPTANE SULPHATE
Proprietary Names: Heptédrine; Tuamine Sulphate.

A white powder.
Solubility. Freely soluble in water; soluble in ethanol; sparingly soluble in ether.

Extraction. Tuaminoheptane is extracted by organic solvents from aqueous alkaline solutions; it is volatile and may be isolated by distillation from alkaline solutions (see p. 18).

Chromatography. PAPER: system P1—Rf 0·62

(location reagents: *iodoplatinate spray*, white; *bromocresol green spray*, strong reaction).
THIN-LAYER: system T1—Rf 0·33 (location reagent *acidified iodoplatinate spray*, positive reaction).
GAS: system G2/120—retention time 0·10 relative to ephedrine.

Crystal Tests. MICRO: *platinic bromide solution*—plates, some serrated (*sensitivity:* 1 in 400); *platinic iodide solution*—masses of rods or plates (*sensitivity:* 1 in 1500).

Use. The base is used in inhalers; the sulphate is employed in solutions containing up to 2% as nasal drops or spray.

Toxicity. The estimated minimum lethal dose in young children is stated to be 200 mg orally.

TUBOCURARINE CHLORIDE

Muscle Relaxant

Synonym: d-Tubocurarine Chloride.
Proprietary Names: Curarin; Intocostrin-T; Tubadil; Tubarine.

(+)-Tubocurarine chloride
$C_{38}H_{44}Cl_2N_2O_6,5H_2O = 785{\cdot}8$

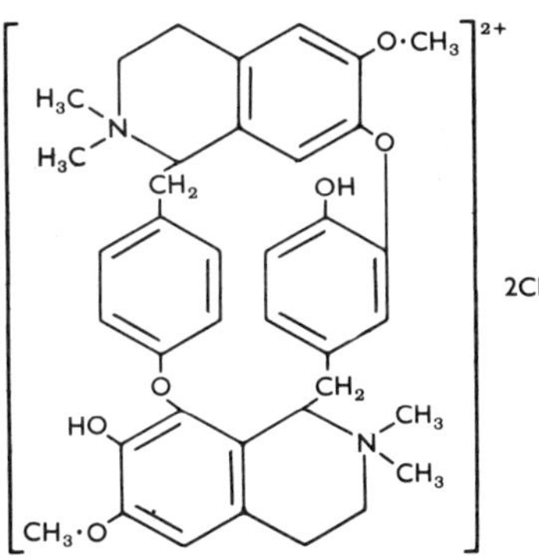

The chloride of an alkaloid, (+)-tubocurarine, which is obtained from the stems of plants of the genus *Chondodendron* (Menispermaceae).
A white microcrystalline powder. M.p. about 270°, with decomposition.
Solubility. Soluble 1 in 20 of water and 1 in 25 of ethanol; almost insoluble in ether and chloroform.

Extraction. Tubocurarine chloride is a quaternary ammonium compound (see p. 29); it is extracted with ethylene dichloride from plasma buffered with a potassium iodide–glycine buffer (Cohen, 1963).

Chromatography. PAPER: system P1—Rf 0·04 (location under ultraviolet light, absorption; location reagent *iodoplatinate spray*, strong reaction); system RP1a—Rf 0·82 (location under ultraviolet light, purple fluorescence; location reagent *iodoplatinate spray*, positive reaction); system RP1b—Rf 0·47 (location as for RP1a).
THIN-LAYER: system T1—Rf 0·00 (location reagent *acidified iodoplatinate spray*, positive reaction).
GAS: system G6—retention time 1·17 relative to codeine.

Colour Tests. MICRO: ammonium molybdate test—deep blue → green → yellow (*sensitivity:* 0·025 μg); ammonium vanadate test—brown (*sensitivity:* 0·1 μg); Vitali's test—purple-brown/brown/orange-brown (*sensitivity:* 0·1 μg).

Crystal Tests. MICRO: *sodium phosphate solution*—very small needles (*sensitivity:* 1 in 200); *zinc chloride solution*—bunches of small plates (*sensitivity:* 1 in 200).

Ultraviolet Absorption Spectrum. Tubocurarine chloride in water, maximum at about 280 mμ (E 1%, 1 cm 148); minimum at 255 mμ.

Infra-red Absorption Spectrum. Potassium bromide disk. The principal peaks are: A 1516, B 1228, C 1120 or 1280 (p. 769).

Quantitative Estimation. Tubocurarine chloride may be estimated spectrofluorimetrically or spectrophotometrically (Cohen, 1963).

Metabolism. Tubocurarine, when given by injection, produces paralysis of voluntary muscle. The action is rapid, the maximum effect being attained within 3 to 5 minutes of intravenous injection.
About 60% of injected tubocurarine is destroyed in the body and 30% is recovered unchanged in the urine. The main site of metabolism is thought to be the liver. Tubocurarine is only slowly and incompletely absorbed from the gastro-intestinal tract.

Dose. Usually 10 to 20 mg intravenously, as an adjuvant to anaesthesia.

Toxicity. Overdosage may produce respiratory paralysis within 7 to 10 minutes.

TYBAMATE

Tranquilliser

Synonym: W 713.
Proprietary Names: Benvil; Solacen.

2 - Butylcarbamoyloxymethyl - 2 - carbamoyl - oxymethylpentane
$C_{13}H_{26}N_2O_4 = 274{\cdot}4$

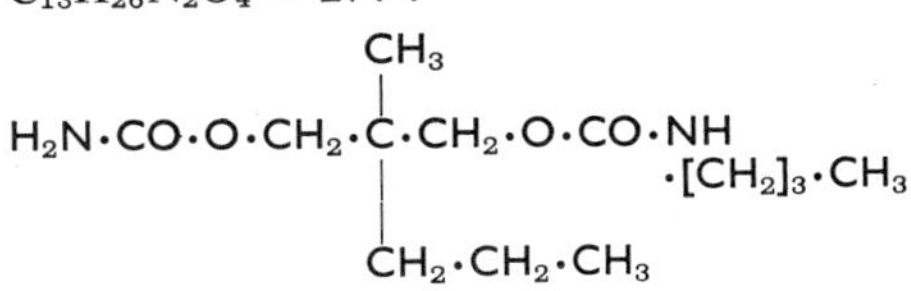

A white crystalline powder. M.p. about 49°.
Solubility. Very slightly soluble in water; very soluble in ethanol; freely soluble in ether.

Extraction. Tybamate is extracted by organic solvents from aqueous acid or alkaline solutions.

Chromatography. THIN-LAYER: system T1—Rf 0·77 (location reagent *iodine–carbon tetrachloride spray*, positive reaction).

GAS: system G5—retention time 6·9 (2·3) relative to barbitone.

Infra-red Absorption Spectrum. Potassium bromide disk. The principal peaks are: A 1695, B 1342, C 1065 or 1250 (p. 769).

Metabolism. Tybamate is a minor tranquilliser chemically related to meprobamate (p. 403). At least 3 metabolites are found in the urine of dogs after oral administration: a hydroxylated derivative, the *N*-dealkylated compound, and a derivative which is both hydroxylated and *N*-dealkylated. Hydroxytybamate is the major metabolite; hydroxymeprobamate is excreted in somewhat smaller amounts. Only traces of meprobamate, glucuronide conjugates, and the unchanged drug are found.

Dose. Up to 2 g daily.

TYMAZOLINE *Vasoconstrictor*

2-(*p*-Mentha-1,3,5-trien-3-yloxymethyl)-2-imidazoline

$C_{14}H_{20}N_2O = 232·3$

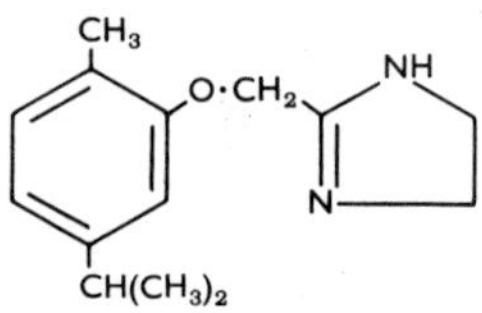

TYMAZOLINE HYDROCHLORIDE

Proprietary Name: Pernazene.

A white powder.

Solubility. Soluble in water.

Extraction. Tymazoline is extracted by organic solvents from aqueous alkaline solutions.

Chromatography. PAPER: system P1—Rf 0·74 (location under ultraviolet light, absorption; location reagents: *iodoplatinate spray*, strong reaction; *bromocresol green spray*, strong reaction); system RP1a—Rf 0·84 (location under ultraviolet light, absorption; location reagent *iodoplatinate spray*, positive reaction); system RP1b—Rf 0·82 (location as for RP1a). THIN-LAYER: system T1—Rf 0·38 (location reagent *acidified iodoplatinate spray*, positive reaction).

Colour Tests. MICRO: sulphuric acid–formaldehyde test—red (*sensitivity:* 0·1 μg); ammonium molybdate test—blue (*sensitivity:* 0·1 μg); ammonium vanadate test—green (*sensitivity:* 1·0 μg); Vitali's test—brown flash/–/faint brown (*sensitivity:* 0·5 μg).

Crystal Tests. MICRO: *ammonium thiocyanate solution*—needles (*sensitivity:* 1 in 1000); *potassium permanganate solution*—small fine needles (*sensitivity:* 1 in 1000).

Infra-red Absorption Spectrum. Tymazoline (base). Potassium bromide disk. The principal peaks are: A 1617, B 1258, C 1279 or 1508 (p. 793).

Use. As a 0·05% nasal spray.

TYRAMINE

Synonym: Tyrosamine.

p-(2-Aminoethyl)phenol

$C_8H_{11}NO = 137·2$

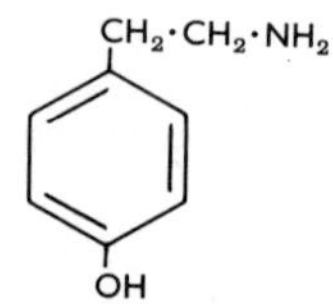

Colourless crystals. M.p. 164° to 165°.

Solubility. Soluble 1 in 95 of water and 1 in 10 of boiling ethanol.

TYRAMINE HYDROCHLORIDE

Crystals which melt at about 270°, with decomposition.

Solubility. Soluble in water.

Extraction. Tyramine is extracted by organic solvents from aqueous ammoniacal solutions; hydrolysis of biological material is required in order to improve the yield.

NOTE. Tyramine is a frequently occurring impurity found together with morphine in the D3 fraction (see p. 27); it may be distinguished from morphine by chromatography and colour and crystal tests (see below and p. 431).

Chromatography. PAPER: system P1—Rf 0·25 (location under ultraviolet light, strong absorption; location reagent *bromocresol green spray*, weak reaction); system RP1a—Rf 0·89 (location under ultraviolet light, absorption); system RP1b—Rf 0·89 (location as for RP1a). THIN-LAYER: system T1—Rf 0·31 (location reagent *potassium permanganate spray*, positive reaction).

Colour Tests. MICRO: sulphuric acid–formaldehyde test—brown → green (*sensitivity:* 0·25 μg); ammonium molybdate test—blue → yellow (*sensitivity:* 1·0 μg); Vitali's test—yellow/yellow/orange (*sensitivity:* 0·25 μg).

Crystal Tests. MICRO: *platinic chloride solution*—long plates (*sensitivity:* 1 in 100); *platinic iodide solution*—bunches of irregular plates (*sensitivity:* 1 in 100).

Ultraviolet Absorption Spectrum. Tyramine in 0·1N hydrochloric acid, maxima at 230 mμ and 275 mμ; minimum at 240 mμ: in 0·1N sodium hydroxide, maxima at 235 mμ and 290 mμ; minimum at 270 mμ.

Metabolism. Tyramine is a normal constituent of human urine, the daily excretion being of the order of 0·2 to 0·5 mg. It is a precursor of several sympathomimetic amines, and it may be found in considerable amounts in cheese, especially Cheddar cheese. It is formed during putrefaction by bacterial decarboxylation of tyrosine.

Use. Tyramine has been used in a test for diagnosing phaeochromocytoma.

URETHANE *Antineoplastic*

Synonyms: Ethylurethane; Urethan.

Ethyl carbamate

$H_2N \cdot CO \cdot O \cdot C_2H_5 = 89{\cdot}10$

Colourless prismatic crystals or leaflets which are volatile at room temperature. M.p. 48° to 50°.

Solubility. Soluble 1 in 1·5 of water, 1 in 1 of ethanol, 1 in 2 of ether, and 1 in 1 of chloroform.

Extraction. Urethane is extracted by organic solvents from aqueous acid or alkaline solutions; it is volatile and may be isolated by distillation (see p. 18).

Chromatography. PAPER: system P6—Rf 0·73 (location reagent *furfural–hydrochloric acid spray*, positive reaction); system P7—Rf 0·89 (location as for P6).

NOTE. Urethane evaporates rapidly therefore chromatograms must be run immediately it is spotted on the paper.

Infra-red Absorption Spectrum. Potassium bromide disk. The principal peaks are: A 1713, B 1340, C 1075 or 1385 (p. 769).

Quantitative Estimation. Boyland and Nery (1964) describe a colorimetric method of determination of urethane and its metabolites in urine.

Metabolism. The cytotoxic action of urethane resembles that of the nitrogen mustards although it is much less potent. Urethane is cumulative in action and dosage must be carefully controlled by frequent blood-counts. It is partly metabolised by *N*-hydroxylation giving rise to the excretion of *N*-hydroxyurethane. The *N*- and *O*-acetyl derivatives are also excreted in the urine. *N*-Hydroxyurethane is also an active cytotoxic agent.

Dose. Up to 6 g daily.

Toxicity. Continuous medication with urethane may give rise to bone-marrow depression, anaemia, neutropenia, and thrombocytopenia.

CASE EXAMPLE. A man died from hepatic failure after being treated for multiple myeloma with 2 to 4 g of urethane daily for 10½ months. Post-mortem examination revealed massive acute centrilobular liver necrosis and marked tubular injury, both attributed to urethane (Flanagan, 1955).

VALETHAMATE BROMIDE *Spasmolytic*

Proprietary Names: Epidosin; Murel.

Diethylmethyl(2-β-methyl-α-phenylvaleryloxyethyl)ammonium bromide

$C_{19}H_{32}BrNO_2 = 386{\cdot}4$

Colourless crystals or white crystalline powder.

Solubility. Soluble in water.

Extraction. Valethamate bromide is a quaternary ammonium compound (see p. 29).

Chromatography. PAPER: system P1—Rf 0·64 (location reagent *iodoplatinate spray*, strong reaction).

THIN-LAYER: system T1—Rf 0·02 (location reagent *acidified iodoplatinate spray*, positive reaction).

Crystal Tests. MICRO: *platinic bromide solution*—oily needles (*sensitivity:* 1 in 1000); *platinic chloride solution*—small needles (*sensitivity:* 1 in 1000).

Ultraviolet Absorption Spectrum. Valethamate bromide in 0·1N sulphuric acid, maxima at 253 mμ (E1%, 1cm 5), 259 mμ (E1%, 1cm 5·4), and 265 mμ (E1%, 1cm 4).

Dose. Up to 80 mg daily.

VANCOMYCIN *Antibiotic*

An amphoteric antimicrobial substance produced by the growth of *Streptomyces orientalis.*

VANCOMYCIN HYDROCHLORIDE

Proprietary Name: Vancocin.

A light brown powder.

Solubility. Soluble 1 in 10 of water and 1 in 700 of ethanol; slightly soluble in ether; almost insoluble in chloroform.

Extraction. Vancomycin is extracted by organic solvents from neutral solutions.

Chromatography. PAPER: system P1—Rf 0·01 (location under ultraviolet light, strong absorption; location reagents: *iodine vapour*, weak reaction; *potassium permanganate spray*, weak reaction).

THIN-LAYER: system T1—Rf 0·22 (location reagent *potassium permanganate spray*, positive reaction).

Colour Tests. MICRO: sulphuric acid–formaldehyde test—pale yellow (*sensitivity:* 1·0 μg); Vitali's test— -/-/yellow (*sensitivity:* 1·0 μg).

Crystal Tests. MICRO: *mercuric chloride solution*—irregular crystals, forming overnight (*sensitivity:* 1 in 1000); *picric acid*—irregular rosettes, forming overnight (*sensitivity:* 1 in 1000).

Ultraviolet Absorption Spectrum. Vancomycin hydrochloride in 0·1N sulphuric acid, maximum at 280·5 mμ (E1%, 1cm 34).

Metabolism. Vancomycin is not absorbed from the gastro-intestinal tract. In order to obtain systemic action, it is administered intravenously. Therapeutically effective blood-levels are maintained by the intravenous injection of 500 mg every 6 hours or 1 g every 12 hours.

Vancomycin diffuses into pleural, ascitic, and synovial effusions but it does not readily penetrate the cerebrospinal fluid. Serum concentrations have been reported to range from 5 to 14 μg/ml following a dosage of 500 mg every 5 hours. It is excreted mainly in the urine; levels as high as 240 mg% have been found one hour after a single injection of 500 mg. The average urinary concentration 6 hours after injection exceeds 30 mg% and is almost 10 mg% after 24 hours.

Dose. Up to 2 g daily, by slow intravenous injection.

Toxicity. Large doses may produce deafness which may be irreversible.
LD50 (intravenous): in mice 400 mg/kg.

VERATRINE

A mixture of alkaloids from sabadilla, the ripe seeds of *Schoenocaulon officinale* (Liliaceae).

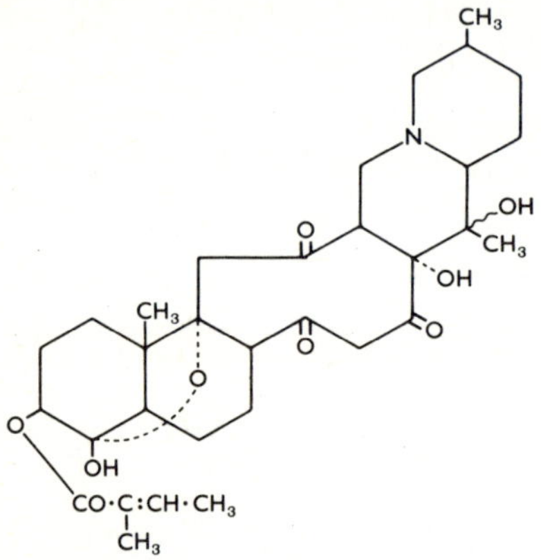

A white powder.

CAUTION. *Veratrine has a violent irritant action on mucous membranes, even in minute doses, and must be handled with great care.*

Solubility. Almost insoluble in water; soluble 1 in 3 of ethanol, 1 in 6 of ether, and 1 in 3 of chloroform.

Extraction. Veratrine is extracted by organic solvents from aqueous alkaline solutions.

Chromatography. PAPER: system P1—Rf 0·68 (location under ultraviolet light, blue fluorescence; location reagent *iodine vapour*, positive reaction); system RP1a—Rf 0·57 (location under ultraviolet light, blue fluorescence); system RP1b—Rf 0·03 (location under ultraviolet light, blue fluorescence; location reagent *iodoplatinate spray*, positive reaction).
THIN-LAYER: system T1—Rf 0·61 (location reagent *iodine vapour*, positive reaction).

Colour Tests. MICRO: sulphuric acid–formaldehyde test—orange (*sensitivity:* 1·0 μg); ammonium vanadate test—yellow → orange → purple-brown (*sensitivity:* 0·25 μg); sulphuric acid test—yellow (orange rim) → pale violet edge → violet (*sensitivity:* 0·025 μg); Vitali's test — –/–/bright purple (*sensitivity:* 0·5 μg).

Ultraviolet Absorption Spectrum. Veratrine in 0·1N sulphuric acid, maxima at 263 mμ (E1%, 1 cm 67) and 293 mμ (E1%, 1 cm 35).

Infra-red Absorption Spectrum. Potassium bromide disk. The principal peaks are: A 1270, B 1085, C 1111 (p. 769).

Toxicity. Veratrine is an intense local irritant and a powerful muscle poison, having a direct stimulating action on all forms of muscle tissue. It causes violent vomiting, purging, intense burning in the mouth and throat, and death in convulsions or consequent upon paralysis.
It was formerly applied externally for its analgesic properties and as a parasiticide, especially for head lice, but even when used in this way there is danger of systemic poisoning from absorption.
LD50 (intraperitoneal): in mice 7·5 to 8·5 mg/kg.

VINBARBITONE *Barbiturate*

Synonyms: Butenemal; Vinbarbital.
Proprietary Names: Delvinal; Diminal.

5 - Ethyl - 5 - (1 - methylbut - 1 - enyl)barbituric acid
$C_{11}H_{16}N_2O_3 = 224{\cdot}3$

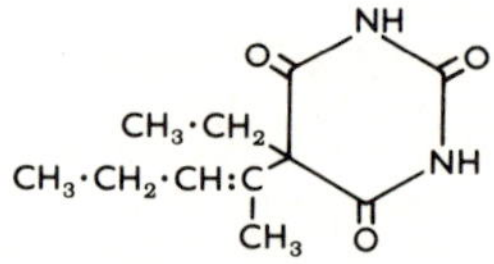

A white powder. M.p. 160° to 163°.
Solubility. Very slightly soluble in water; soluble in ethanol; sparingly soluble in ether.

VINBARBITONE SODIUM
A white hygroscopic powder which absorbs carbon dioxide from moist air, liberating vinbarbitone.
Solubility. Soluble in water and ethanol; slightly soluble in ether and chloroform.

Screening Tests. See under Barbiturates, p. 208.

Extraction. Vinbarbitone may be isolated in the A2 fraction (see p. 27).

Chromatography. PAPER: system P2—Rf 0·21 relative to amylobarbitone (location under ultraviolet light, dark spot).
THIN-LAYER: system T10—Rf 0·28 (location reagents: *mercurous nitrate spray*, black; *potassium permanganate spray*, yellow-brown; *Zwikker's reagent spray*, pink).
GAS: system G5—retention time 2·37 relative to barbitone; system G7—retention time 2·20 relative to barbitone.

Colour Test. Zwikker's test—violet-blue.

Quantitative Estimation. See under Barbiturates, p. 208.

Ultraviolet Absorption Spectrum. Vinbarbitone is a 5,5-derivative—see Screening Test 3 under Barbiturates, p. 208.

Infra-red Absorption Spectrum. Vinbarbitone. Potassium bromide disk. The principal peaks are: A 1370 or 1675 or 1760 (p. 769).

Dose. 30 to 200 mg.

Toxicity. Vinbarbitone is an intermediate-acting barbiturate—see under Barbiturates, p. 207. The estimated minimum lethal dose in man is 2 g.

VINBLASTINE *Antineoplastic*

Synonyms: LE 29060; NSC 49842; Vincaleukoblastine.

$C_{46}H_{58}N_4O_9 = 811{\cdot}0$

An alkaloid extracted from *Vinca rosea* (Apocynaceae).

VINBLASTINE SULPHATE

Proprietary Names: Velban; Velbe.

A white crystalline powder.

Solubility. Soluble in water and methanol; insoluble in ethanol.

Chromatography. PAPER: system RP1a—Rf 0·10 (location under ultraviolet light, purple fluorescence; location reagent *iodoplatinate spray*, positive reaction); system RP1b—Rf 0·00 (location as for RP1a).

Colour Test. MICRO: sulphuric acid–formaldehyde test—wine-red.

Quantitative Estimation. Vinblastine may be estimated spectrophotometrically (Jakovljevic, 1962).

Metabolism. Vinblastine is a cytotoxic agent which is only partially absorbed from the gastro-intestinal tract. It is cleared very rapidly from the blood. Within minutes of intravenous injection, radioactively labelled vinblastine has been detected mostly in the liver. It is excreted primarily in the faeces; less than 5% appears in the urine.

Dose. Initial, 0·1 mg/kg weekly, intravenously.

VIOMYCIN *Antibiotic/Tuberculostatic*

Synonyms: Celiomycin; Florimycin.

Proprietary Names: Viocin; Vionactane.

An antimicrobial polypeptide base produced by certain strains of *Streptomyces griseus* var. *purpureus*.

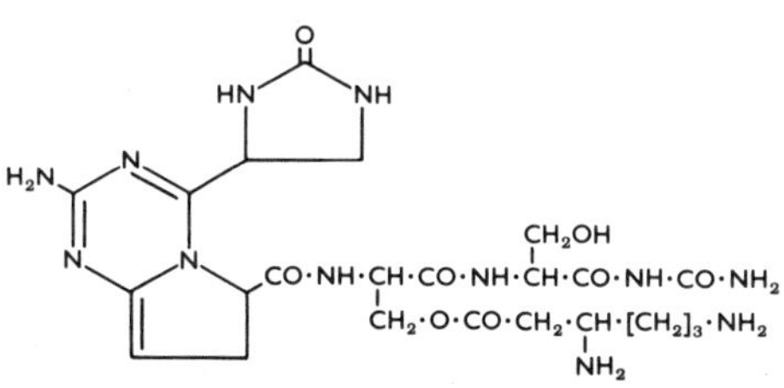

VIOMYCIN SULPHATE

A white, somewhat hygroscopic powder. M.p. 252° (anhydrous) or 280°, with decomposition.

Solubility. Very soluble in water; slightly soluble in ethanol; almost insoluble in ether.

Chromatography. PAPER: system P1—Rf 0·01 (location under ultraviolet light, strong absorption; location reagents: *bromine–starch–potassium iodide*, weak reaction; *potassium permanganate spray*, strong reaction).

THIN-LAYER: system T1—Rf 0·00 (location reagent *potassium permanganate spray*, positive reaction).

Colour Test. MICRO: ammonium molybdate test—faint blue (*sensitivity:* 1·0 μg).

Ultraviolet Absorption Spectrum. Viomycin sulphate in water, maximum at about 268·5 mμ; in 0·1N sulphuric acid, maximum at 269 mμ (E1%, 1 cm 259).

Metabolism. Viomycin is only partially absorbed when given by mouth and therapeutic blood-levels are difficult to attain by this route of administration. It does not readily pass the normal blood-brain barrier or into peritoneal or pleural effusions. It is mainly excreted by the kidneys. Serum concentrations of viomycin have been reported to range from 12 to 45 μg/ml one hour after a dose of 500 mg intramuscularly, falling to about 5 μg/ml after 8 hours.

Dose. Up to 1 mega unit daily, intramuscularly.

Toxicity. LD50 (intravenous): in mice 165 to 240 mg/kg.

VIPRYNIUM EMBONATE *Anthelmintic*

Synonym: Pyrvinium Pamoate.

Proprietary Names: Pamovin; Povan; Vanquin.

6 - Dimethylamino - 2 - [2 - (2,5 - dimethyl - 1 - phenylpyrrol-3-yl)vinyl] - 1 - methylquinolinium 4,4′-methylenedi(3-hydroxy-2-naphthoate)

$C_{75}H_{70}N_6O_6 = 1151{\cdot}4$

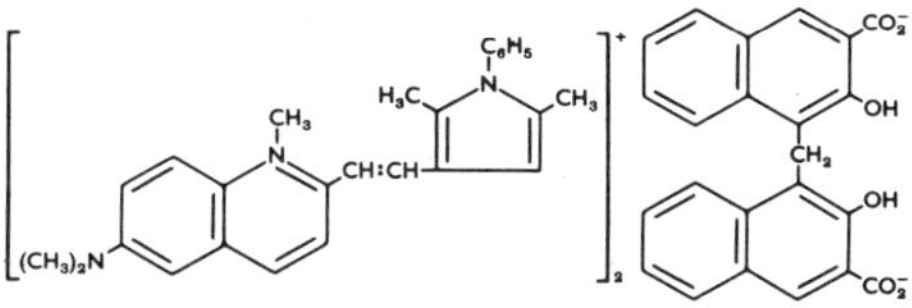

A bright orange or orange-red to almost black crystalline powder. M.p. about 206°, with decomposition.

Solubility. Almost insoluble in water and ether; very slightly soluble in ethanol; soluble 1 in 1000 of chloroform.

Extraction. Viprynium embonate is a quaternary ammonium compound (see p. 29).

Chromatography. PAPER: system P1—Rf 0·64 (location under ultraviolet light, bright orange fluorescence; location reagent *potassium permanganate spray*, weak reaction).

THIN-LAYER: system T1—Rf 0·67 (location reagent *potassium permanganate spray*, weak reaction).

Colour Tests. MICRO: sulphuric acid–formaldehyde test—pale yellow (*sensitivity:* 1·0 μg); ammonium vanadate test—(red) yellow (*sensitivity:* 1·0 μg).

Crystal Tests. MICRO: *picric acid*—bunches of plates (*sensitivity:* 1 in 3000); *trinitrobenzoic acid solution*—plates or tablets (*sensitivity:* 1 in 3000).

Ultraviolet Absorption Spectrum. Viprynium embonate in methoxyethanol, maxima at 239 mμ, 358 mμ, and 508 mμ (E1%, 1cm 785).

Dose. 5 mg/kg (base), as a single dose.

NOTE. Viprynium embonate is an effective anthelmintic in the treatment of threadworm infestation. It stains the stools bright red and will stain clothing if vomiting occurs.

WARFARIN *Anticoagulant/Rodenticide*

3-(α-Acetonylbenzyl)-4-hydroxycoumarin

$C_{19}H_{16}O_4$ = 308·3

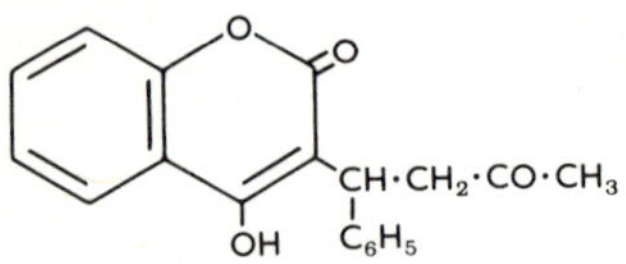

A white felty substance consisting of long well-formed needles. M.p. of the purified compound 159° to 160°; of the technical grade 157°.
Solubility. Almost insoluble in water.

WARFARIN POTASSIUM
Proprietary Name: Athrombin-K.

A white crystalline powder which discolours on exposure to light.
Solubility. Soluble in water and ethanol; very slightly soluble in ether and chloroform.

WARFARIN SODIUM
Proprietary Names (as medicinal anticoagulants): Coumadin; Marevan; Panwarfin; Prothromadin; (as a rodenticide): Dethmor(e).

A white crystalline powder which discolours on exposure to light.
Solubility. Soluble 1 in less than 1 of water and 1 in less than 1 of ethanol; slightly soluble in ether and chloroform.

Extraction. Warfarin is extracted by organic solvents from aqueous acid solutions.

Chromatography. GAS: system G1/180—retention time 0·28 relative to diphenhydramine; system G3—retention time 0·78 relative to diphenhydramine; system G5—retention time 0·78 relative to barbitone.

Colour Test. *Liebermann's reagent*—orange.

Ultraviolet Absorption Spectrum. Warfarin in 0·01N sodium hydroxide, maximum at 308 mμ (E1%, 1cm 462).

Infra-red Absorption Spectrum. Warfarin sodium. Potassium bromide disk. The principal peaks are: A 1517, B 1599, C 1640 (p. 770).

Quantitative Estimation. Warfarin in biological materials may be estimated by spectrophotometry (Wanntorp, 1960; Fishwick and Taylor, 1967).

Metabolism. Warfarin is used medicinally as an anticoagulant. The therapeutic effect takes from 12 to 18 hours to develop and may persist for 5 to 6 days. Following oral doses of 1·5 mg/kg in man, the concentration of the drug in the plasma has been found to be maximal from 2 to 12 hours. Absorption is relatively rapid and complete. No unchanged warfarin is found in the urine but significant amounts of a metabolite are found. The action of warfarin as an anticoagulant is thought to be due to competitive inhibition at the enzyme sites utilised by vitamin K.
Warfarin is an effective rodenticide primarily because it is metabolised and excreted fairly slowly; it therefore accumulates in the animal and gives rise to internal haemorrhages.

Dose. As an anticoagulant, up to 50 mg initially; subsequent doses adjusted according to the prothrombin activity of the blood.

Toxicity. Single doses of warfarin, unless very large, do not usually exert a lethal action; in man, doses above 100 mg may be dangerous. Rats may survive single doses of 50 mg/kg, but they are killed by repeated dosing for 5 days with 1 mg/kg. Sheep and cattle will tolerate single doses of up to 50 mg/kg.
Since 1960, 3 apparently independent outbreaks of resistance to warfarin in rats have been reported; the resistance has been shown to be heritable and to be dependent on a single dominant autosomal gene (Greaves and Ayres, 1967).

CASE EXAMPLES. A naval recruit attempted suicide by taking 1 cartonful (567 mg of warfarin) of rat poison concentrate over 6 days. Two days later he had kidney and abdominal pain, vomited and had periodic nose bleeding. Two days later still, in hospital, laboratory findings revealed a prothrombin time of 4 minutes 6 seconds (control time 15 seconds), a coagulation time of 35 minutes, and a clotting time of 9 minutes. He recovered after blood transfusion and vitamin K therapy (Holmes and Love, 1952).
Widespread haemorrhages seen post mortem in 4 greyhounds who suddenly died when racing indicated poisoning due to warfarin. It was concluded that the biscuit meal fed to the dogs had been slightly but continuously contaminated by the excreta of rats and mice that had been consuming warfarin from 2 baiting points close to the stored sacks of biscuit meal (Bowden *et al.*, 1960).

XENYSALATE *Dermatological Agent*

Synonym: Biphenamine.

2-Diethylaminoethyl 2-hydroxy-3-phenylbenzoate

$C_{19}H_{23}NO_3$ = 313·4

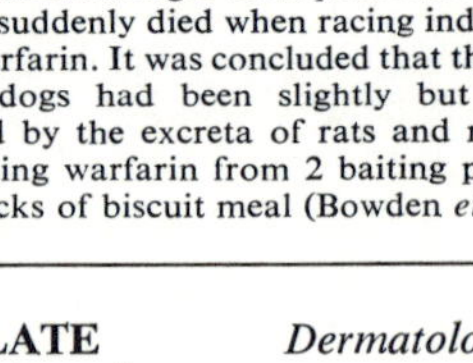

White crystals.
Solubility. Soluble in water.

XENYSALATE HYDROCHLORIDE
Proprietary Names: It is an ingredient of Sebaclen and Alvinine Shampoo.

Extraction. Xenysalate is extracted by organic solvents from aqueous alkaline solutions.

Chromatography. PAPER: system P1—Rf 0·74 (location under ultraviolet light, pale yellow-green fluorescence; location reagents: *iodoplatinate spray*, strong reaction; *bromocresol green spray*, strong reaction); system RP1a—Rf 0·05 (location under ultraviolet light, green fluorescence; location reagent *iodoplatinate spray*, positive reaction); system RP1b—Rf 0·07 (location under ultraviolet light, green fluorescence).
THIN-LAYER: system T1—Rf 0·62 (location reagent *acidified iodoplatinate spray*, positive reaction).
GAS: system G2/225—retention time 1·20 relative to codeine.

Colour Tests. MICRO: sulphuric acid–formaldehyde test—olive-green (*sensitivity:* 0·25 μg); ammonium molybdate test—blue (*sensitivity:* 0·1 μg); ammonium vanadate test—green (*sensitivity:* 0·1 μg); Vitali's test— –/faint yellow/bright yellow (*sensitivity:* 0·1 μg).

Crystal Tests. MICRO: *gold bromide solution*—rods and needles, forming overnight (*sensitivity:* 1 in 3000); *platinic chloride solution*—irregular rosettes (*sensitivity:* 1 in 1000).

Ultraviolet Absorption Spectrum. Xenysalate in 0·1N sulphuric acid, maxima at 231 mμ (E1%, 1cm 892) and 319 mμ (E1%, 1cm 179).

Use. It is used in shampoos for the control of seborrhoeic dermatitis and dandruff.

XYLENE *Solvent*

Synonym: Xylol(e).

A mixture of *o*-, *m*-, and *p*-dimethylbenzene in which the *m*-isomer predominates.
C_8H_{10} = 106·2

A clear, colourless, mobile, inflammable liquid. B.p. 138° to 142°.
Solubility. Insoluble in water; miscible with ethanol, ether, and other organic solvents.

Extraction. Xylene is extracted by organic solvents from aqueous acid solutions; it may be isolated by distillation (see p. 18).

Chromatography. PAPER and THIN-LAYER: Bonnichsen *et al.* (1966) describe a paper system and a thin-layer system, both of which detect the nitration products of xylene, following steam distillation into carbon tetrachloride and subsequent nitration.
GAS: system G8/160—retention time 13·9 relative to n-propanol.

Quantitative Estimation. Xylene may be estimated in biological fluids and tissues by steam distillation into carbon tetrachloride, nitration, and subsequent spectrophotometric determination at 570 mμ (Bonnichsen *et al.*, 1966).

Metabolism. Xylene and its isomers are largely metabolised in man to the relatively non-toxic toluic acids. In rabbits, the main metabolite of the *o*-isomer is *o*-toluic acid, which is partly excreted as such and partly as the glucuronide conjugate. Hydroxylation may also occur. The *m*- and *p*-isomers are more highly oxidised to the corresponding toluic acids than is the *o*-isomer, and they are excreted almost entirely as glycine conjugates.

Toxicity. Xylene has about the same toxic potency as toluene. The maximum permissible atmospheric concentration is 200 p.p.m. The minimum oral lethal dose in rats is 4 g/kg.

CASE EXAMPLES. Three probable suicide cases are described in which liquids containing xylene were ingested. The following post-mortem xylene levels were measured: blood, 0·3 mg% and 2 mg%; liver, 0·07 mg% and 0·1 mg%; stomach contents, 6 mg% and 73 mg%.
A 17-month-old child swallowed an unknown quantity of a preparation containing about 3·7% of xylene and died 4 days later; 3 mg% of xylene was found in the kidneys post mortem (Bonnichsen *et al.*, 1966).

XYLOMETAZOLINE *Vasoconstrictor*

2 - (2,6 - Dimethyl - 4 - t - butylbenzyl) - 2 - imidazoline
$C_{16}H_{24}N_2$ = 244·4

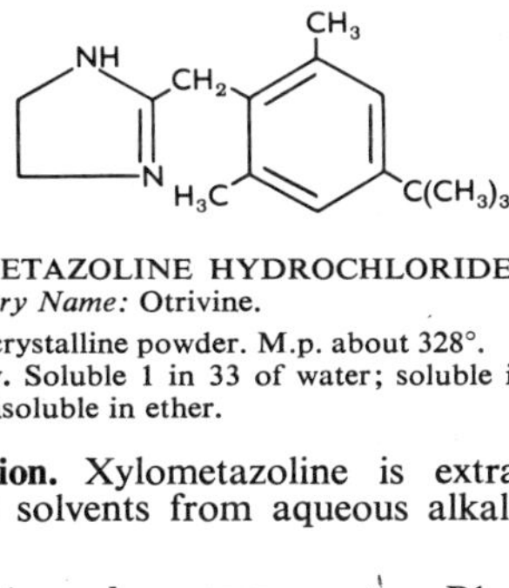

XYLOMETAZOLINE HYDROCHLORIDE
Proprietary Name: Otrivine.

A white crystalline powder. M.p. about 328°.
Solubility. Soluble 1 in 33 of water; soluble in ethanol; almost insoluble in ether.

Extraction. Xylometazoline is extracted by organic solvents from aqueous alkaline solutions.

Chromatography. PAPER: system P1—Rf 0·75 (location reagents: *iodoplatinate spray*, strong reaction; *bromocresol green spray*, strong reaction); system RP1a—Rf 0·79 (location reagent *iodoplatinate spray*, positive reaction).
THIN-LAYER: system T1—Rf 0·13 (location reagent *acidified iodoplatinate spray*, positive reaction).
GAS: system G2/225—retention time 1·35 relative to diphenhydramine.

Colour Tests. MICRO: sulphuric acid–formaldehyde test—dull orange (*sensitivity:* 1·0 μg); ammonium molybdate test—faint grey (*sensitivity:* 1·0 μg); ammonium vanadate test—faint red (*sensitivity:* 1·0 μg).

Crystal Tests. MICRO: *gold bromide–hydrochloric acid solution*—fernlike crystals and plates (*sensitivity:* 1 in 3000); *potassium permanganate solution*—long plates (*sensitivity:* 1 in 1000).

Ultraviolet Absorption Spectrum. Xylometazoline in 0·1N sulphuric acid, maximum at 266 mμ (E1%, 1cm 9), and inflexions at 271 mμ (E1%, 1cm 8) and 275 mμ (E1%, 1cm 6).

Infra-red Absorption Spectrum. Xylometazoline hydrochloride. Potassium bromide disk. The principal peaks are: A 1602, B 1253, C 1298 (p. 770).

Use. It is used in 0·05 to 0·1% solution for the relief of nasal congestion.

YOHIMBINE *Alkaloid*

Synonyms: Aphrodine; Corynine; Quebrachine.

$C_{21}H_{26}N_2O_3 = 354·5$

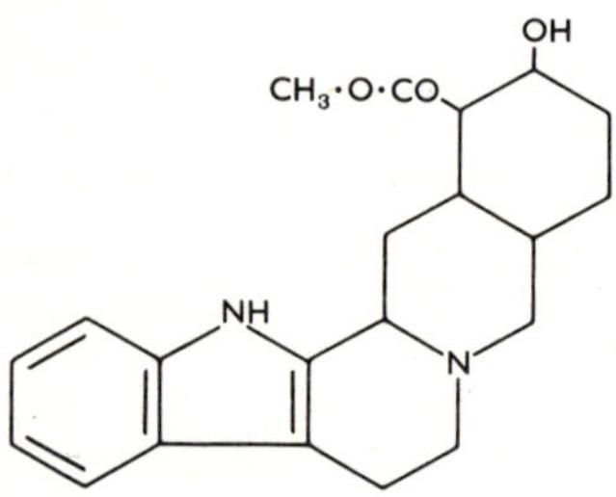

The principal alkaloid of the bark of the yohimbe tree, *Pausinystalia yohimbe* (=*Corynanthe yohimbi*) (Rubiaceae).

Glistening needles. M.p. 234°.

Solubility. Very slightly soluble in water; soluble in ethanol and chloroform; sparingly soluble in ether.

YOHIMBINE HYDROCHLORIDE

Proprietary Names: Yobinol; it is an ingredient of Potensan.

A white crystalline powder. M.p. 302°, with decomposition.

Solubility. Soluble 1 in 100 of water; more soluble in hot water and ethanol.

Extraction. Yohimbine is extracted by organic solvents from aqueous alkaline solutions.

Chromatography. PAPER: system P1—Rf 0·54 (location under ultraviolet light, pale blue fluorescence; location reagents: *iodoplatinate spray*, weak reaction; *bromocresol green spray*, weak reaction); system RP1a—Rf 0·64 (location under ultraviolet light, blue fluorescence); system RP1b—Rf 0·07 (location as for RP1a). THIN-LAYER: system T1—Rf 0·55 (location reagent *acidified iodoplatinate spray*, positive reaction). GAS: system G6—retention time 0·38 relative to codeine.

Colour Tests. MICRO: ammonium molybdate test—blue, slowly → green (*sensitivity:* 0·025 μg); ammonium vanadate test—blue → green, fading (*sensitivity:* 0·1 μg); Vitali's test—yellow/yellow/violet (*sensitivity:* 0·1 μg).

Crystal Tests. MICRO: *potassium cyanide solution*—rosettes of rods (*sensitivity:* 1 in 1500); *sodium carbonate solution*—rosettes of rods or dense rosettes (*sensitivity:* 1 in 1500).

Ultraviolet Absorption Spectrum. Yohimbine in 0·1N sulphuric acid, maxima at 220 mμ (E1% 1cm 1064), 272 mμ (E1%, 1cm 208), about 278 mμ (E1%, 1cm 204), and 287·5 mμ (E1%, 1cm 153).

Infra-red Absorption Spectrum. Yohimbine hydrochloride. Potassium bromide disk. The principal peaks are: A 1705, B 741, C 1160 or 1197 or 1436 (p. 770).

Quantitative Estimation. See under Reserpine, p. 536.

Dose. It has been given in doses of up to 10 mg thrice daily for its alleged aphrodisiac properties but convincing evidence of such an effect is lacking.

Addenda

It should be noted that the analytical data in the following additional monographs are not recorded in the analytical indexes in Part 3.

BROMHEXINE *Bronchial Mucolytic*

Synonym: Na 274.

Proprietary Name: Bisolvon is the hydrochloride.

N-(2-Amino-3,5-dibromobenzyl)-*N*-cyclohexylmethylamine

$C_{14}H_{20}Br_2N_2 = 376{\cdot}1$

Solubility. Insoluble in water; soluble in chloroform.

The hydrochloride is very slightly soluble in water, slightly soluble in ethanol, and practically insoluble in chloroform, and melts at 233° to 242°.

Chromatography. PAPER: system P1—Rf 0·87 (location under ultraviolet light, absorption; location reagent *iodoplatinate spray*, strong reaction).

THIN-LAYER: system T1—Rf 0·75 (location reagent *acidified iodoplatinate spray*, positive reaction).

Ultraviolet Absorption Spectrum. Bromhexine in 0·1N sulphuric acid, maximum at 311 mμ (E1%, 1 cm 71).

DIETHYLAMINOETHYL DIPHENYLPROPIONATE *Parasympatholytic*

Proprietary Names: Spasmadryl (hydrochloride). The hydrochloride is an ingredient of Sedalby Tablets.

2-Diethylaminoethyl αβ-diphenylpropionate

$C_{21}H_{27}NO_2 = 325{\cdot}5$

The hydrochloride is very soluble in water, soluble in ethanol, and sparingly soluble in ether, and melts at 111° to 112°.

Chromatography. PAPER: system P1—Rf 0·80 (location under ultraviolet light, pale yellow fluorescence; location reagent *iodoplatinate spray*, strong reaction).

THIN-LAYER: system T1—Rf 0·64 (location reagent *acidified iodoplatinate spray*, positive reaction).

Colour Test. MICRO: Vitali's test— –/–/purple (*sensitivity:* 0·1 μg).

Ultraviolet Absorption Spectrum. Diethylaminoethyl diphenylpropionate in 0·1N sulphuric acid, maxima at 252 mμ (E1%, 1 cm 3·9), 258 mμ (E1%, 1 cm 4·3), and 264·5 mμ (E1%, 1 cm 3·2).

FAMPROFAZONE *Analgesic and Antipyretic*

Proprietary Name: An ingredient of Gevodin.

4 - Isopropyl - 1 - methyl - 5 - [*N* - methyl - *N* - (α - methylphenethyl)aminomethyl] - 3 - oxo - 2 - phenylpyrazoline

$C_{24}H_{31}N_3O = 377{\cdot}5$

A white powder.

Solubility. Insoluble in water; soluble in ethanol and chloroform.

Chromatography. PAPER: system P1—Rf 0·94 (location under ultraviolet light, strong absorption; location reagent *iodoplatinate spray*, strong reaction).

THIN-LAYER: system T1—Rf 0·80 (location reagent *acidified iodoplatinate spray*, positive reaction).

Ultraviolet Absorption Spectrum. Famprofazone in 0·1N sulphuric acid, maxima at about 243 mμ (E1%, 1 cm 202) and 278 mμ (E1%, 1 cm 253).

IMINODIMETHYLPHENYLTHIAZOLIDINE *Sympathomimetic*

Proprietary Name: Priatan preparations contain either the thiocyanate or the theophyllin-7-ylacetate salt.

(−)-2-Imino-3,4-dimethyl-5-phenylthiazolidine

$C_{11}H_{14}N_2S = 206{\cdot}3$

Solubility. Insoluble in water; soluble in chloroform.

Chromatography. PAPER: system P1—Rf 0·62 (location under ultraviolet light, absorption; location reagent *iodoplatinate spray*, weak reaction).

THIN-LAYER: system T1—Rf 0·48 (location reagent *acidified iodoplatinate spray*, positive reaction).

Colour Test. MICRO: ammonium vanadate test —(green) orange (*sensitivity:* 0·1 μg).

IPRINDOLE *Antidepressant*

Synonyms: Pramindole; Wy 3263.

Proprietary Name: Prondol is the hydrochloride.

5-[3-(Dimethylamino)propyl]-6,7,8,9,10,11-hexahydro-5*H*-cyclo-oct[*b*]indole

$C_{19}H_{28}N_2 = 284{\cdot}4$

The hydrochloride is soluble in water, ethanol, and chloroform, and melts at 142° to 147°.

Chromatography. PAPER: system P1—Rf 0·76 (location under ultraviolet light, pale blue fluorescence; location reagent *iodoplatinate spray*, strong reaction).

THIN-LAYER: system T1—Rf 0·41 (location reagent *acidified iodoplatinate spray*, positive reaction).

Colour Test. MICRO: ammonium molybdate test —blue (*sensitivity:* 0·1 μg).

Ultraviolet Absorption Spectrum. Iprindole in 0·1N sulphuric acid, maxima at 286 mμ (E1%, 1 cm 209) and about 293 mμ (E1%, 1 cm 202).

PIMOZIDE

Tranquilliser

Synonym: R 6238.

1-{1-[4,4-Di(*p*-fluorophenyl)butyl]piperid-4-yl}-2-oxobenzimidazoline
$C_{28}H_{29}F_2N_3O = 461{\cdot}6$

A white powder.
Solubility. Insoluble in water and ethanol; soluble in chloroform and dilute acetic acid.

Chromatography. PAPER: system P1—Rf 0·94 (location reagent *iodoplatinate spray*, weak reaction).

THIN-LAYER: system T1—Rf 0·78 (location reagent *acidified iodoplatinate spray*, positive reaction).

Colour Tests. MICRO: sulphuric acid–formaldehyde test—dull purple (*sensitivity:* 1·0 μg); ammonium vanadate test—purple flash (*sensitivity:* 0·1 μg); Vitali's test— –/–/yellow (*sensitivity:* 0·5 μg).

Ultraviolet Absorption Spectrum. Pimozide in ethanol, maxima at 268 mμ (E1%, 1cm 97), 274 mμ (E1%, 1cm 134), and 283 mμ (E1%, 1cm 153).

PROPYPHENAZONE

Analgesic

Synonyms: Isopropylantipyrine; Isopropylphenazone; Propylantipyrine; Propylphenazone.
Proprietary Names: An ingredient of Gevodin and Saridone.

4-Isopropyl-1,5-dimethyl-3-oxo-2-phenylpyrazoline
$C_{14}H_{18}N_2O = 230{\cdot}3$

A white powder.
Solubility. Insoluble in water; soluble in ethanol.

Chromatography. PAPER: system P1—Rf 0·96 (location under ultraviolet light, strong absorption; location reagent *potassium permanganate spray*, weak reaction).

THIN-LAYER: system T1—Rf 0·71 (location reagent *potassium permanganate spray*, positive reaction).

Ultraviolet Absorption Spectrum. Propyphenazone in ethanol, maxima at 248 mμ (E1%, 1cm 483) and 277 mμ (E1%, 1cm 493).

PROQUAMEZINE

Antispasmodic (Veterinary)

Synonyms: Aminopromazine; Tetrameprozine.
Proprietary Names: Lispamol and Myspamol as the fumarate.

10 - [2,3 - Di(dimethylamino)propyl]phenothiazine
$C_{19}H_{25}N_3S = 327{\cdot}5$

The fumarate is soluble 1 in 11 of water and 1 in 200 of ethanol, and melts at 166° to 170°, with decomposition.

Chromatography. PAPER: system P1—Rf 0·30 (location under ultraviolet light, yellow-green fluorescence; location reagent *iodoplatinate spray*, strong reaction).

THIN-LAYER: system T1—Rf 0·43 (location reagent *acidified iodoplatinate spray*, positive reaction).

Colour Tests. MICRO: sulphuric acid–formaldehyde test—bright purple (*sensitivity:* 0·1 μg); ammonium molybdate test—blue-purple (*sensitivity:* 0·1 μg); ammonium vanadate test—orange→purple (*sensitivity:* 0·5 μg); Vitali's test—yellow/red/dull purple (*sensitivity:* 0·5 μg).

Ultraviolet Absorption Spectrum. Proquamezine in 0·1N sulphuric acid, maxima at about 250 mμ and about 297 mμ.

TRIFLUPERIDOL

Tranquilliser

Synonym: R 2498.
Proprietary Name: Triperidol.

p-Fluoro-*γ*-[4-hydroxy-4-(*α*,*α*,*α*-trifluoro-*m*-tolyl)piperidino]butyrophenone
$C_{22}H_{23}F_4NO_2 = 409{\cdot}4$

Chromatography. PAPER: system P1—Rf 0·93 (location under ultraviolet light, strong absorption; location reagent *iodoplatinate spray*, strong reaction).

THIN-LAYER: system T1—Rf 0·73 (location reagent *Dragendorff spray*, positive reaction).

Ultraviolet Absorption Spectrum. Trifluperidol in 0·1N sulphuric acid, maximum at 248 mμ (E1%, 1cm 302).

PART 3

Indexes to Analytical Data

Melting-points

d = 'with decomposition'

°C	
8·4	Formic Acid, p. 349
>11	Paraldehyde, p. 466
>14·8	Acetic Acid, p. 171
18·4	Dimethyl Sulphoxide, p. 310
23–25	Nikethamide, p. 443
24	Amylmetacresol, p. 195
27–28	Menthol, p. 400
	Putrescine, p. 527
28–32	Monosulfiram, p. 430
30–32	Menthol, p. 400
33–34	Myrophine, p. 433
33–35	Fluoroacetic Acid, p. 348
33–37	Ephedrine, Anhydrous, p. 327
34	Pilocarpine, p. 500
34–39	Testosterone Enanthate, p. 561
35	Nandrolone Decanoate, p. 435
35–36	Mescaline, p. 404
36–37	Prenylamine, p. 509
36–38	Prilocaine, p. 510
38–39	Benzydamine, p. 217
38–40	Phenoxybenzamine, p. 489
39	Methyl Nicotinate, p. 419
>40	Phenol, p. 487
40–41	Ephedrine, p. 327
41–46	Amethocaine, p. 184
42	Parachlorophenol, p. 466
42–43	Salol, p. 539
42–44	Menthol, p. 400
43–44	Amolanone, p. 191
43–45	Piperazine Hydrate, p. 503
43–47	Cannabidiolic Acid, p. 236
45	Trimipramine, p. 587
45–47	Troxidone, p. 590
46	Ethosuximide, p. 338
48–50	Urethane, p. 593
49	Diethylcarbamazine, p. 301
	Tropacocaine, p. 589
	Tybamate, p. 591
50	Choline Salicylate, p. 539
50–52	Metyrapone, p. 429
50–56	Methsuximide, p. 418
50–58	Chloral Hydrate, p. 245
51	Benactyzine, p. 209
51–52	Dimethoate, p. 309
53–54	Paradichlorobenzene, p. 466
53–56	Methylpentynol Carbamate, p. 425
56–58	Emylcamate, p. 326
57–59	Butyl Aminobenzoate, p. 232
57–60	Leptazol, p. 389
58–60	Cetalkonium Chloride, p. 243
59	Hyoscine (monohydrate), p. 376
	STP, p. 537
60	Promethazine, p. 518
60–62	Apoatropine, p. 198
61	Erythrityl Tetranitrate, p. 329
62–65	Butylated Hydroxyanisole, p. 232
63	Tropine, p. 589
63–65	Cinchocaine, p. 262
64–66	Naepaine, p. 433
64–67	Dichloralphenazone, p. 296
65	Isobutyl Aminobenzoate, p. 381
66	Lucanthone, p. 394
66–67	Cannabidiol, p. 236
66–68	Hexylresorcinol, p. 364
66–69	Lignocaine, p. 392
68	Fluanisone, p. 346
	Trimeprazine, p. 585
68–69	Isometheptene Hydrochloride, p. 383
68–70	Dioxaphetyl Butyrate, p. 313
69	STP, p. 537
>69	Butylated Hydroxytoluene, p. 233
69–70	Disulfiram, p. 319
69–71	Diphenyl, p. 316
69–72	Phensuximide, p. 491
70–73	Mephenesin, p. 401
72–74	Thioridazine, p. 573
73–74	Azinphos-methyl, p. 205
74	Emetine, p. 325
74–75	Methyl Phenidate, p. 419
74–77	Methyprylone, p. 426
75	Phenadoxone, p. 478
75–76	Cannabinol, p. 236
76	Hydroxyquinoline, p. 375
76–79	Lignocaine Hydrochloride, p. 392
>77	Chlorbutol, p. 246
77–78	Norpseudoephedrine, p. 450
77–83	Cetylpyridinium Chloride, p. 244
78	Butylchloral Hydrate, p. 233
79	Racephedrine, p. 535
80	Anileridine, p. 197
	Naphthalene, p. 436
80–85	Lysergide, p. 395
83–84	Fentanyl, p. 345
	Histamine, p. 364
84–88	Cholecalciferol, p. 260
85–86	Bretylium Tosylate, p. 224
85–88	Glutethimide, p. 353
86	Benzoylecgonine (hydrated), p. 215
	Dinitro-orthocresol, p. 312
87–88	Chloroquine, p. 252
88–91	Benzocaine, p. 214
89	Anileridine, p. 197
	Chloramphenicol Palmitate, p. 246
	Methoxychlor, p. 417
89–91	Hydroxychloroquine, p. 374
90	Aldrin (technical), p. 177
	Ethotoin, p. 338
90–95	Carbetapentane Citrate, p. 238
90–96	Cycrimine, p. 277

m.p.	Substance
168	Hydrocortisone Hydrogen Succinate, p. 370
	Naphazoline Nitrate, p. 435
168d	Edrophonium Chloride, p. 324
	Phenindamine Tartrate, p. 484
168–169	Chlortetracycline, p. 259
	Dimethylthiambutene Hydrochloride, p. 310
168–172	Diphenhydramine Hydrochloride, p. 315
169	Amydricaine Hydrochloride, p. 194
	Hydroquinidine, p. 372
169–171	Hydrocortisone Sodium Succinate, p. 370
169–172	Paracetamol, p. 465
	Pramoxine Hydrochloride, p. 508
170	Diamorphine, p. 292
170d	Bephenium Hydroxynaphthoate, p. 219
	Norbutrine Hydrochloride, p. 447
170–171	Hydroquinone, p. 373
	Narceine, p. 436
170–172	Dimenoxadole, p. 307
170–173	Isoniazid, p. 383
	Methacholine Chloride, p. 407
	Tolazamide, p. 575
170–174	Imipramine Hydrochloride, p. 379
171	Tramazoline Hydrochloride, p. 579
171d	Methoserpidine, p. 415
171–174	Cyclobarbitone, p. 274
	Santonin, p. 540
171–174d	Pecazine Hydrochloride, p. 470
171–177	Methanthelinium Bromide, p. 409
172	Dipyrone, p. 318
	Halopyramine Hydrochloride, p. 357
	Heptabarbitone, p. 359
	Stilboestrol, p. 543
172d	Methylergometrine, p. 424
172–173	Hydrallazine, p. 367
172–174	Allobarbitone, p. 179
	Dicyclomine Hydrochloride, p. 299
	Methylamphetamine Hydrochloride, p. 421
172–175	Arecoline Hydrobromide, p. 201
	Piperocaine Hydrochloride, p. 504
172–176	Tolazoline Hydrochloride, p. 576
172–177	Nicomorphine Hydrochloride, p. 439
173	Hydroquinine, p. 372
173–174	Fluopromazine Hydrochloride, p. 347
173–176	Chloroprocaine Hydrochloride, p. 251
	Psilocin, p. 526
173–176	Thonzylamine Hydrochloride, p. 574
174	Phenmetrazine Hydrochloride, p. 486
	Phenylephrine, p. 493
	Quinine (anhydrous), p. 532
174–176	Noscapine, p. 451
174–177	Buformin Hydrochloride, p. 226
	Phenobarbitone, p. 486
174–178	Dichlorophen, p. 297
	Metaraminol Tartrate, p. 406
	Pilocarpine Nitrate, p. 500
174–179	Camphor, p. 235
175	Amisometradine, p. 189
	Cyclamic Acid, p. 273
	Norethynodrel, p. 448
	Phentolamine, p. 492
175–176	Dicyclomine Hydrochloride, p. 323
175–177	Naepaine Hydrochloride, p. 433
	Normethadone Hydrochloride, p. 449
175–178	Hydroxyquinoline Sulphate, p. 375
	Oestradiol, p. 453
176	Levallorphan Tartrate, p. 390
176d	Triacetyloleandomycin, p. 580
176–178	Isometheptene, p. 383
177d	Phenglutarimide Hydrochloride, p. 483
177–179	Amylocaine Hydrochloride, p. 196
177–181	Benactyzine Hydrochloride, p. 209
	Phentolamine Mesylate, p. 492
	Promazine Hydrochloride, p. 517
178	Brucine (anhydrous), p. 225
	Gelsemine, p. 353
178–181	Aminopentamide Sulphate, p. 188
	Methylphenobarbitone, p. 425
179	Ethyl Biscoumacetate, p. 338
179–180	Pipenzolate Bromide, p. 502
179–183	Sulphaphenazole, p. 554
>180	Lobeline Hydrochloride, p. 393
180d	Clioquinol, p. 265
180–181	Phenazocine, p. 479
180–182	Levallorphan, p. 390
180–183	Sulphamethoxypyridazine, p. 553
181	Rotenone, p. 537
181–184	Metabutethamine Hydrochloride, p. 405
	Sulphacetamide, p. 546
182–184	Ethinyloestradiol, p. 335
	Heteronium Bromide, p. 360
	Hexylcaine Hydrochloride, p. 363
183	Sulphacetamide Sodium, p. 547
	Thiethylperazine Maleate, p. 571
183–184	Aminopentamide, p. 187
	Dextromoramide, p. 290

M.p.	Substance
200d	Strychnine Sulphate (anhydrous), p. 545
>200	Endrin, p. 326
	Hyoscyamine Sulphate, p. 378
>200d	Lymecycline, p. 394
200–203	Sulphathiazole, p. 557
200–204	Amicarbalide Isethionate, p. 185
200–205	Pilocarpine Hydrochloride, p. 500
200–210	Hexocyclium Methylsulphate, p. 363
200–215	Di-iodohydroxyquinoline, p. 306
201–206	Norethisterone, p. 447
201–208	Isoxsuprine Hydrochloride, p. 386
202	Ethambutol Hydrochloride, p. 332
204	Acetorphine Hydrochloride, p. 172
204–208	Guanoxan Sulphate, p. 356
205	Ecgonine (dry), p. 324
	Orciprenaline Sulphate, p. 456
	Spironolactone, p. 542
205d	Methacycline Hydrochloride, p. 408
205–206	Oxazepam, p. 458
206	Diphenylpyraline Hydrochloride, p. 317
206d	Furaltadone, p. 351
	Pentolinium Tartrate, p. 474
	Pyridoxine Hydrochloride, p. 528
	Viprynium Embonate, p. 595
207d	Thiamine Hydrochloride, p. 570
207–209	Guanoclor Sulphate, p. 356
208	Amodiaquine, p. 190
	Nalorphine, p. 434
208d	Frusemide, p. 350
208–209	Bamipine Hydrochloride, p. 206
208–211	Sulphamethizole, p. 551
209	Fludrocortisone Acetate, p. 346
	Polythiazide, p. 506
209–213	Sulphamethoxydiazine, p. 552
209–220	Ambutonium Bromide, p. 183
210	Bialamicol Hydrochloride, p. 222
210d	Carbachol, p. 237
	Chlortetracycline Hydrochloride, p. 259
	Cinchonidine, p. 262
210–211d	Opipramol Hydrochloride, p. 455
210–222d	Protoveratrine A and B Maleates, p. 524
211	Bethanechol Chloride, p. 221
	Coniine Hydrobromide, p. 270
212d	Adrenaline, p. 175
	Hydrastinine Hydrochloride, p. 368
	Isothipendyl Hydrochloride, p. 385
212–214d	Ergotamine, p. 328
212–215	Azamethonium Bromide, p. 204
212–216	Lachesine Chloride, p. 387
	Methoxamine Hydrochloride, p. 417
	Phenacemide, p. 477
212–216d	Pralidoxime Iodide, p. 507
212–218d	Chlordiazepoxide Hydrochloride, p. 248
213–214	Alphacetylmethadol Hydrochloride, p. 181
214d	Hydrocortisone, p. 370
	Tetracycline Hydrochloride, p. 562
214–215	Etorphine, p. 341
214–216d	Cyproheptadine Hydrochloride, p. 278
214–217d	Homatropine Hydrobromide, p. 365
214–218	Desipramine Hydrochloride, p. 285
215–218	Chloroquine Phosphate, p. 252
215–225	Papaverine Hydrochloride, p. 464
216	Methyclothiazide, p. 419
216–218	Cantharidin, p. 236
217d	Diminazene Aceturate, p. 312
	Noradrenaline, p. 445
217–220	Ephedrine Hydrochloride, p. 327
217–221	Acetyldigitoxin, p. 173
	Doxapram Hydrochloride, p. 322
217–224d	Cortisone, p. 270
218	Nortriptyline Hydrochloride, p. 451
218–219d	Solanidine, p. 541
218–220	Alphaprodine Hydrochloride, p. 182
	Oxycodone, p. 460
218–224	Griseofulvin, p. 355
219	Bethanechol Chloride, p. 221
219–220	Trimethoxyamphetamine Hydrochloride, p. 587
220	Cyclothiazide, p. 277
220d	Chlorthalidone, p. 259
	Hydrocortisone Acetate, p. 370
220–222d	Pralidoxime Chloride, p. 507
220–225	Syrosingopine, p. 559
220–235	Deslanoside, p. 286
221–225	Promethazine Hydrochloride, p. 518
222–223	Atropine Methobromide, p. 203
222–228	Hyoscine Methobromide, p. 377
	Trimetazidine Hydrochloride, p. 586
223–226	Buphenine Hydrochloride, p. 227
224d	Meclozine Hydrochloride, p. 398
224–225d	Phenadoxone Hydrochloride, p. 478
224–226	Nitrazepam, p. 443
225	Fludrocortisone Acetate, p. 346

Paper Chromatographic Data

SYSTEM P1 (p. 34)—Rf Values and Location Data

Rf	*Compound*	*Ultraviolet Light*	*Primary Location Reagent*
0·00	Cadaverine, p. 233	white fluorescence	*iodoplatinate spray*
	Dihydrostreptomycin, p. 306	—	*bromine–starch–potassium iodide*
	Framycetin, p. 350	—	*bromine–starch–potassium iodide*
	Gallamine, p. 352	—	*iodoplatinate spray*
	Hexamethonium Bromide, p. 361	—	*iodoplatinate spray*
	Histamine, p. 364	—	*iodoplatinate spray*
	Kanamycin, p. 386	—	*bromine–starch–potassium iodide*
	Lymecycline (methylenelysine moiety), p. 394	—	*ninhydrin spray*
	Neomycin, p. 437	—	*bromine–starch–potassium iodide*
	Paraquat, p. 468	strong absorption	*iodoplatinate spray*
	Pentolinium Tartrate, p. 474	—	*iodoplatinate spray*
	Pethidine, p. 476	—	*Dragendorff spray*
	Piperazine, p. 503	—	*iodoplatinate spray*
	Putrescine, p. 527	—	*iodoplatinate spray*
	Pyrithidium Bromide, p. 529	orange fluorescence	*iodoplatinate spray*
	Quinuronium Sulphate, p. 533	blue fluorescence	*iodoplatinate spray*
	Streptomycin, p. 544	—	*bromine–starch–potassium iodide*
	Suxamethonium Salts, p. 559	—	*iodoplatinate spray*
	Suxethonium Bromide, p. 559	—	*iodoplatinate spray*
	Thiamine, p. 570	—	*iodoplatinate spray*
0·01	Diquat, p. 319	pale green fluorescence with an absorbing centre	*iodoplatinate spray*
	Quinapyramine Salts, p. 531	bright blue fluorescence	*iodoplatinate spray*
	Vancomycin, p. 593	strong absorption	*iodine vapour*
	Viomycin, p. 595	strong absorption	*potassium permanganate spray*
0·02	Azamethonium Bromide, p. 204	absorption	*iodoplatinate spray*
	Cycloserine, p. 276	absorption	*iodoplatinate spray*
	Diminazene, p. 312	orange fluorescence	*iodoplatinate spray*
	Mebezonium Iodide, p. 397	—	*iodoplatinate spray*
	Pholcodine, p. 496	strong absorption	*iodoplatinate spray*
	Pseudomorphine, p. 525	blue fluorescence	*iodoplatinate spray*
	Stilbamidine, p. 543	bright blue fluorescence	*iodoplatinate spray*
0·03	Amicarbalide, p. 185	blue fluorescence	*iodoplatinate spray*
	Amprolium Hydrochloride, p. 193	pale blue fluorescence	*iodoplatinate spray*
	Carbachol, p. 237	—	*iodoplatinate spray*
	Cytisine, p. 279	blue fluorescence	*iodoplatinate spray*
	Distigmine Bromide, p. 319	strong absorption	*bromocresol green spray*

Rf	*Compound*	*Ultraviolet Light*	*Primary Location Reagent*
0·03	Ecgonine, p. 324	—	*iodoplatinate spray*
	Guanethidine, p. 356	—	*iodoplatinate spray*
0·04	Acetylcholine, p. 173	—	*iodoplatinate spray*
	Decamethonium Iodide, p. 280	—	*iodoplatinate spray*
	Noradrenaline, p. 445	absorption	*potassium permanganate spray*
	Pemoline, p. 470	absorption	*bromine–starch–potassium iodide*
	Phenamidine, p. 478	blue fluorescence	*bromocresol green spray*
	Trimetazidine, p. 586	absorption	*iodoplatinate spray*
	Tubocurarine Chloride, p. 591	absorption	*iodoplatinate spray*
0·05	Bethanechol Chloride, p. 221	—	*iodoplatinate spray*
	Cephaloridine, p. 243	absorption	*iodoplatinate spray*
	Choline, p. 261	—	*iodoplatinate spray*
	Ethambutol, p. 332	—	*bromocresol green spray*
	Tropine, p. 589	—	*iodoplatinate spray*
0·06	Adrenaline, p. 175	absorption	*potassium permanganate spray*
	Chlorisondamine Chloride, p. 249	—	*iodoplatinate spray*
	Psilocybin, p. 526	dark blue fluorescence	*iodine vapour*
	Thiabendazole, p. 568	absorption	*bromocresol green spray*
0·07	Dimethyltubocurarine Salts, p. 311	strong absorption	*iodoplatinate spray*
	Metformin, p. 407	strong absorption	*iodoplatinate spray*
	Methyldopa, p. 423	absorption	*ninhydrin spray*
	Nicotine, p. 440	strong absorption	*iodoplatinate spray*
0·08	Ambazone, p. 182	brown fluorescence	*potassium permanganate spray*
	Ametazole, p. 184	—	*iodoplatinate spray*
	Furaltadone, p. 351	green fluorescence	*iodoplatinate spray*
	Hydromorphinol, p. 371	absorption	*iodoplatinate spray*
	Paraphenylenediamine, p. 467	absorption	*iodoplatinate spray*
	Propamidine, p. 519	blue fluorescence	*iodoplatinate spray*
0·09	Oxymorphone, p. 461	dark blue fluorescence	*iodoplatinate spray*
0·10	Ambenonium Chloride, p. 183	absorption	*iodoplatinate spray*
	Methacholine Bromide, p. 407	—	*iodoplatinate spray*
	Pilocarpine, p. 500	—	*iodoplatinate spray*
	Pralidoxime Chloride, p. 507	weak absorption	*iodoplatinate spray*
0·11	Adrenalone, p. 176	pale blue fluorescence	*potassium permanganate spray*
	Cephaëline, p. 242	blue fluorescence	*iodoplatinate spray*
	Dehydroemetine, p. 280	—	*iodoplatinate spray*
	Lysergamide, p. 395	blue fluorescence	*iodoplatinate spray*
	Normetanephrine, p. 449	absorption	*bromocresol green spray*

Rf	*Compound*	*Ultraviolet Light*	*Primary Location Reagent*
0·12	Clamoxyquin, p. 264	pale yellow fluorescence	*iodoplatinate spray*
	Dopamine, p. 321	strong absorption	*potassium permanganate spray*
	Hydrallazine, p. 367	absorption	*iodoplatinate spray*
	Hydroxychloroquine, p. 374	blue fluorescence	*iodoplatinate spray*
	Normorphine, p. 450	strong absorption	*iodoplatinate spray*
	Pyridostigmine Bromide, p. 528	strong absorption	*iodoplatinate spray*
	Serotonin, p. 540	white fluorescence	*iodoplatinate spray*
0·13	Dibromopropamidine, p. 295	strong absorption	*iodoplatinate spray*
	Sparteine, p. 542	—	*iodoplatinate spray*
0·14	Alcuronium Chloride, p. 177	absorption	*iodoplatinate spray*
	Etamiphylline, p. 331	absorption	*iodoplatinate spray*
	Hydrastinine, p. 368	bright blue fluorescence	*iodoplatinate spray*
	Morphine, p. 431	strong absorption	*iodoplatinate spray*
	Morphine *N*-Oxide, p. 432	strong absorption	*iodoplatinate spray*
0·15	Arecoline, p. 201	absorption	*iodoplatinate spray*
	Hydromorphone, p. 371	strong absorption	*iodoplatinate spray*
	Metanephrine, p. 406	strong absorption	*bromocresol green spray*
	Oxedrine, p. 459	strong absorption	*bromocresol green spray*
	Solanine, p. 541	—	*iodoplatinate spray*
0·16	Amopyroquine, p. 191	pale yellow fluorescence	*iodoplatinate spray*
	Bufotenine, p. 227	white fluorescence	*iodoplatinate spray*
	Codeine, p. 268	strong absorption	*iodoplatinate spray*
	Dihydromorphine, p. 305	strong absorption	*iodoplatinate spray*
	Nicotinyl Alcohol, p. 442	strong absorption	*iodoplatinate spray*
	Oxycodone, p. 460	strong absorption	*iodoplatinate spray*
0·17	Brucine, p. 226	—	*iodoplatinate spray*
	Pentamidine, p. 472	dark blue fluorescence	*iodoplatinate spray*
	Tolonium Chloride, p. 577	red fluorescence	visible blue streak—without reagent
0·18	Azacosterol, p. 204	—	*iodoplatinate spray*
	Ethylnoradrenaline, p. 340	absorption	*bromocresol green spray*
	Laudexium Methylsulphate, p. 388	blue fluorescence	*iodoplatinate spray*
	Lincomycin, p. 393	—	*iodoplatinate spray*
	Neopine, p. 438	strong absorption	*iodoplatinate spray*
	Norcodeine, p. 447	absorption	*iodoplatinate spray*
	Pipamperone, p. 502	blue fluorescence	*iodoplatinate spray*
	Pyridoxine, p. 528	blue fluorescence	*iodoplatinate spray*
0·19	Amodiaquine, p. 190	yellow fluorescence	*iodoplatinate spray*
	Chloroquine, p. 252	blue fluorescence	*iodoplatinate spray*
	Codeine *N*-Oxide, p. 269	strong absorption	*iodoplatinate spray*
	Cotarnine, p. 271	green fluorescence	*iodoplatinate spray*
	Emetine, p. 325	—	*iodoplatinate spray*
	Lysergic Acid, p. 395	blue fluorescence	*iodoplatinate spray*
	Procainamide, p. 512	blue fluorescence	*iodoplatinate spray*

Rf	*Compound*	*Ultraviolet Light*	*Primary Location Reagent*
0·20	Dihydrocodeine, p. 304	strong absorption	*iodoplatinate spray*
	Homatropine Methobromide, p. 366	absorption	*iodoplatinate spray*
	Hyoscine Methonitrate, p. 378	—	*iodoplatinate spray*
	Neostigmine Bromide, p. 438	absorption	*iodoplatinate spray*
	Opipramol, p. 455	yellow fluorescence	*iodoplatinate spray*
	Thioproperazine, p. 572	yellow-green fluorescence	*iodoplatinate spray*
0·21	Buformin, p. 226	absorption	*iodoplatinate spray*
	Diaveridine, p. 293	white fluorescence	*iodoplatinate spray*
0·22	Anileridine, p. 197	pale green fluorescence	*iodoplatinate spray*
	Hydrocodone, p. 369	strong absorption	*iodoplatinate spray*
	Isoprenaline, p. 384	blue fluorescence	*bromocresol green spray*
	Morpheridine, p. 431	—	*iodoplatinate spray*
0·23	Acetophenazine, p. 172	yellow fluorescence	*iodoplatinate spray*
	Acriflavine, p. 175	yellow-green fluorescence	*iodoplatinate spray*
	Hordenine, p. 367	absorption	*iodoplatinate spray*
	Hyoscine, p. 376	absorption	*iodoplatinate spray*
	Perphenazine, p. 475	blue fluorescence	*iodoplatinate spray*
	Spiramycin, p. 542	absorption	*iodoplatinate spray*
	Trimethoprim, p. 587	strong absorption	*bromocresol green spray*
0·24	Metopon, p. 429	strong absorption	*iodoplatinate spray*
	Oxytetracycline Dihydrate, p. 463	orange fluorescence	*bromine–starch–potassium iodide*
	Phenylephrine, p. 493	strong absorption	*bromocresol green spray*
0·25	Atropine Methobromide, p. 203	absorption	*iodoplatinate spray*
	Atropine Methonitrate, p. 203	absorption	*iodoplatinate spray*
	Berberine, p. 219	faint yellow fluorescence	*iodoplatinate spray*
	Cycloguanil, p. 275	weak absorption	—
	Edrophonium Chloride, p. 324	absorption	*iodoplatinate spray*
	Ergometrine, p. 328	bright blue fluorescence	p-*dimethylaminobenzaldehyde spray*
	Lymecycline (tetracycline moiety), p. 394	orange fluorescence	*bromocresol green spray*
	Mescaline, p. 404	absorption	*iodoplatinate spray*
	Methyldihydromorphine, p. 422	absorption	*iodoplatinate spray*
	Nicomorphine, p. 439	absorption	*iodoplatinate spray*
	Phenformin, p. 483	strong absorption	*bromocresol green spray*
	Prochlorperazine, p. 514	blue fluorescence	*iodoplatinate spray*
	Proflavine Hemisulphate, p. 515	yellow fluorescence	*iodoplatinate spray*
	Tetracycline, p. 563	orange fluorescence	*ninhydrin spray*
	Thiothixene, p. 574	blue fluorescence	*iodoplatinate spray*
	Triamterene, p. 581	bright blue fluorescence	*iodoplatinate spray*
	Tyramine, p. 592	strong absorption	*bromocresol green spray*
0·26	Carphenazine, p. 242	yellow fluorescence	*iodoplatinate spray*
	Orciprenaline, p. 455	absorption	*iodoplatinate spray*

Rf	*Compound*	*Ultraviolet Light*	*Primary Location Reagent*
0·27	Dequalinium Chloride, p. 284	bright blue fluorescence	*iodoplatinate spray*
	Mepacrine, p. 400	green fluorescence	*iodoplatinate spray*
	Pheniramine, p. 485	dark blue fluorescence	*iodoplatinate spray*
	Thenyldiamine, p. 566	blue fluorescence	*iodoplatinate spray*
0·28	Acepifylline, p. 169	weak absorption	Clarke-Kalayci test
	Chlorhexidine, p. 249	strong absorption	*iodoplatinate spray*
	Diamthazole, p. 293	absorption	*iodoplatinate spray*
	Diethylcarbamazine, p. 301	—	*iodoplatinate spray*
0·29	Demecolcine, p. 281	pale yellow fluorescence	—
	Desferrioxamine, p. 285	—	*potassium permanganate spray*
	6–Monoacetylmorphine, p. 430	absorption	*iodoplatinate spray*
0·30	Butaperazine, p. 229	yellow fluorescence	*potassium permanganate spray*
	Doxylamine, p. 322	blue fluorescence	*iodoplatinate spray*
	Homatropine, p. 365	absorption	*iodoplatinate spray*
	Nalorphine, p. 434	absorption	*iodoplatinate spray*
	Norbutrine, p. 447	absorption	*potassium permanganate spray*
	Strychnine, p. 545	strong absorption	*iodoplatinate spray*
0·30, tailing	Betaprodine, p. 221	—	*iodoplatinate spray*
0·31	Metaraminol, p. 406	strong absorption	p-*dimethylaminobenzaldehyde spray*
	Nicocodine, p. 439	absorption	*iodoplatinate spray*
	Procaine, p. 513	blue fluorescence	*iodoplatinate spray*
	Psilocin, p. 526	absorption	*iodoplatinate spray*
0·32	Demethylchlortetracycline, p. 281	orange fluorescence	*Dragendorff spray*
	Dipyrone, p. 318	absorption	*potassium permanganate spray*
	Isoniazid, p. 383	absorption	*iodoplatinate spray*
	Mepyramine, p. 403	bright blue fluorescence	*iodoplatinate spray*
	Methapyrilene, p. 410	bright blue fluorescence	*iodoplatinate spray*
	Sulphaguanidine, p. 550	absorption	diazotisation followed by *alkaline betanaphthol spray*
	Thebaine, p. 565	strong absorption	*iodoplatinate spray*
0·33	Apomorphine, p. 199	blue fluorescence	*iodoplatinate spray*
	Diamorphine, p. 292	—	*iodoplatinate spray*
	Norharman, p. 448	bright blue fluorescence	*iodoplatinate spray*
0·34	Acetyldihydrocodeine, p. 174	strong absorption	*iodoplatinate spray*
	Clopenthixol, p. 266	dark blue fluorescence	*iodoplatinate spray*
	Phenethylamine, p. 482	absorption	*iodoplatinate spray*
	Trifluoperazine, p. 584	yellow fluorescence	*iodoplatinate spray*
0·35	Desomorphine, p. 286	absorption	*iodoplatinate spray*
	Ethylmorphine, p. 340	dark blue fluorescence	*iodoplatinate spray*
	Metabutethamine, p. 405	bright blue fluorescence	*iodoplatinate spray*
	Methacycline, p. 408	orange fluorescence	*ninhydrin spray*
	Phenglutarimide, p. 483	absorption	*iodoplatinate spray*

Rf	*Compound*	*Ultraviolet Light*	*Primary Location Reagent*
0·35	Theobromine, p. 567	blue fluorescence	Clarke-Kalayci test
	Tripelennamine, p. 588	bright blue fluorescence	*iodoplatinate spray*
	Tryptamine, p. 590	blue fluorescence	*iodoplatinate spray*
0·36	Dihydrallazine, p. 304	blue fluorescent streak	*iodoplatinate spray*
	Fluphenazine, p. 348	yellow fluorescence	*iodoplatinate spray*
	Hydroxyamphetamine, p. 373	absorption	*potassium permanganate spray*
	Thebacon, p. 565	strong absorption	*iodoplatinate spray*
0·37	Atropine, p. 202	absorption	*iodoplatinate spray*
	Chlortetracycline, p. 259	orange fluorescence	*iodine vapour*
	Dithiazanine Iodide, p. 320	red fluorescence	*iodoplatinate spray*
	Harmine, p. 359	bright blue fluorescence	*iodoplatinate spray*
	Hyoscyamine, p. 378	absorption	*iodoplatinate spray*
	Norpseudoephedrine, p. 450	weak absorption	*bromocresol green spray*
	Phanquone, p. 476	yellow fluorescence	*Dragendorff spray*
0·38	Cocaine, p. 267	strong absorption	*iodoplatinate spray*
	Dimethindene, p. 307	white fluorescence	*iodoplatinate spray*
	Dimethyltryptamine, p. 311	blue fluorescence	*iodoplatinate spray*
	Guanoxan, p. 356	absorption	*bromocresol green spray*
	Hexocyclium Methylsulphate, p. 363	—	*iodoplatinate spray*
	Hydrastine, p. 368	blue fluorescence	*iodoplatinate spray*
	Meclofenoxate, p. 398	absorption	*iodoplatinate spray*
	Phenelzine Sulphate, p. 482	weak absorption	*iodoplatinate spray*
	Pholedrine, p. 497	absorption	*iodoplatinate spray*
	Piritramide, p. 505	—	*iodoplatinate spray*
0·39	Harmaline, p. 358	green fluorescence	*iodoplatinate spray*
	Homidium Bromide, p. 366	bright orange fluorescence	*iodoplatinate spray*
	Isoetharine, p. 382	absorption	*bromocresol green spray*
	Pseudoephedrine, p. 525	absorption	*iodoplatinate spray*
0·40	Amydricaine, p. 194	dark blue fluorescence	*iodoplatinate spray*
	Atropine *N*-Oxide, p. 203	—	*iodoplatinate spray*
	Benzoylecgonine, p. 215	absorption	*iodoplatinate spray*
	Benzylmorphine, p. 218	absorption	*iodoplatinate spray*
	Gelsemine, p. 353	strong absorption	*iodoplatinate spray*
	Methyldopate, p. 423	absorption	*ninhydrin spray*
	Methylergometrine, p. 424	bright blue fluorescence	p-*dimethylaminobenzaldehyde spray*
	Noscapine, p. 451	bright blue fluorescence	*iodoplatinate spray*
	Thiethylperazine, p. 570	pale green fluorescence	*iodoplatinate spray*
	Tolazoline, p. 576	absorption	*iodoplatinate spray*
0·41	Aminohippuric Acid, p. 187	blue fluorescence	diazotisation followed by *alkaline betanaphthol spray*
	Cinchonidine, p. 262	blue fluorescence	*iodoplatinate spray*
	Tetramisole, p. 564	strong absorption	*iodoplatinate spray*
	Trimethoxyamphetamine, p. 587	absorption	*iodoplatinate spray*
0·42	Harman, p. 358	blue fluorescence	*iodoplatinate spray*
	Pyrimethamine, p. 528	blue fluorescence	*iodoplatinate spray*

Rf	*Compound*	*Ultraviolet Light*	*Primary Location Reagent*
0·43	Ambutonium Bromide, p. 183	weak absorption	*iodoplatinate spray*
	Debrisoquine, p. 279	—	*iodoplatinate spray*
	Methoxamine, p. 417	absorption	*diazotised* p-*nitroaniline–sodium hydroxide spray*
	Physostigmine, p. 498	dark blue fluorescence	*iodoplatinate spray*
0·44	Bretylium Tosylate, p. 224	absorption	*iodoplatinate spray*
	Heteronium Bromide, p. 360	strong absorption	*iodoplatinate spray*
	Lachesine Chloride, p. 387	absorption	*iodoplatinate spray*
	Methyldesorphine, p. 422	—	*iodoplatinate spray*
	Pempidine, p. 471	—	*iodoplatinate spray*
	Phenylpropanolamine, p. 494	absorption	*bromocresol green spray*
0·45	Amiphenazole, p. 188	absorption	*iodoplatinate spray*
	Brompheniramine, p. 225	absorption	*iodoplatinate spray*
	Chloroprocaine, p. 251	strong absorption	*iodoplatinate spray*
	Chlorpheniramine, p. 254	blue fluorescence	*iodoplatinate spray*
	Dexbrompheniramine, p. 288	strong absorption	*iodoplatinate spray*
	Dexchlorpheniramine, p. 289	blue fluorescence	*iodoplatinate spray*
	Ephedrine, p. 327	absorption	*iodoplatinate spray*
	Eucatropine, p. 342	absorption	*iodoplatinate spray*
	Halopyramine, p. 358	blue fluorescence	*iodoplatinate spray*
	Mepenzolate Bromide, p. 401	absorption	*iodoplatinate spray*
	Methysergide, p. 427	blue fluorescence	*iodoplatinate spray*
	Metoclopramide, p. 428	blue fluorescence	*iodoplatinate spray*
	Primaquine, p. 510	orange fluorescence	*iodoplatinate spray*
	Tranylcypromine, p. 579	absorption	*iodoplatinate spray*
0·45, streaking	Sulphaquinoxaline, p. 555	—	diazotisation followed by *alkaline betanaphthol spray*
0·46	Carbinoxamine, p. 239	blue fluorescence	*iodoplatinate spray*
	Diphenylpyraline, p. 317	absorption	*iodoplatinate spray*
	Methylephedrine, p. 423	absorption	*bromocresol green spray*
	Narceine, p. 436	strong absorption	*iodoplatinate spray*
	Poldine Methylsulphate, p. 506	absorption	*iodoplatinate spray*
	Quinine, p. 532	bright blue fluorescence	*iodoplatinate spray*
0·47	Aminopentamide, p. 187	weak absorption	*iodoplatinate spray*
	Bamifylline, p. 206	strong absorption	*iodoplatinate spray*
	Cinchonine, p. 263	bright blue fluorescence	*iodoplatinate spray*
	Dibenzepin, p. 295	pale yellow fluorescence	*iodoplatinate spray*
	Diprophylline, p. 317	dark blue fluorescence	Clarke-Kalayci test
	Lysergide, p. 395	blue fluorescence	*iodoplatinate spray*
	Nicotinamide, p. 440	strong absorption	*iodoplatinate spray*
0·48	Amethocaine, p. 184	blue fluorescence	*iodoplatinate spray*
	Ethacridine, p. 331	pale green fluorescence	*iodoplatinate spray*
	Hydroquinine, p. 372	bright blue fluorescence	*iodoplatinate spray*
	Hydroxypethidine, p. 375	absorption	*iodoplatinate spray*
	Metazocine, p. 407	absorption	*iodoplatinate spray*
	Phendimetrazine, p. 481	—	*iodoplatinate spray*
	Procarbazine, p. 513	strong absorption	*iodoplatinate spray*

Rf	*Compound*	*Ultraviolet Light*	*Primary Location Reagent*
0·48	Quinidine, p. 531	bright blue fluorescence	*iodoplatinate spray*
	Racephedrine, p. 535	absorption	*iodoplatinate spray*
0·49	Papaverine, p. 464	pale yellow-green fluorescence	*iodoplatinate spray*
	Phenmetrazine, p. 486	—	*iodoplatinate spray*
	Pipenzolate Bromide, p. 502	absorption	*iodoplatinate spray*
	Sulphanilamide, p. 553	—	diazotisation followed by *alkaline betanaphthol spray*
	Tigloidine, p. 575	absorption	*iodoplatinate spray*
0·50	Glycopyrronium Bromide, p. 355	—	*iodoplatinate spray*
	Ketobemidone, p. 387	absorption	*iodoplatinate spray*
	Methoxyamphetamine, p. 417	absorption	*bromocresol green spray*
	Pipamazine, p. 501	blue fluorescence	*iodoplatinate spray*
	Properidine, p. 520	—	*iodoplatinate spray*
	Racemethorphan, p. 534	—	*iodoplatinate spray*
	Triclobisonium Chloride, p. 583	—	*iodoplatinate spray*
0·51	Amphetamine, p. 192	—	*iodoplatinate spray*
	Apoatropine, p. 198	absorption	*iodoplatinate spray*
	Butethamine, p. 230	blue fluorescence	*iodoplatinate spray*
	Dexamphetamine, p. 287	—	*iodoplatinate spray*
	Levamphetamine, p. 390	—	*iodoplatinate spray*
	Naphazoline, p. 435	pale blue fluorescence	*iodoplatinate spray*
	Phenisonone, p. 485	pale blue fluorescence	*bromocresol green spray*
	Phenylpropylmethylamine, p. 495	absorption	*iodoplatinate spray*
	Plasmocide, p. 506	orange fluorescence	*iodoplatinate spray*
	Protokylol, p. 523	absorption	*potassium permanganate spray*
	Tropacocaine, p. 589	strong absorption	*iodoplatinate spray*
0·52	Benzilonium Bromide, p. 214	—	*iodoplatinate spray*
	Ethoheptazine, p. 336	—	*iodoplatinate spray*
	Methyridine, p. 427	absorption	*iodoplatinate spray*
	Phenyramidol, p. 495	blue fluorescence	*iodoplatinate spray*
	Propoxycaine, p. 521	blue fluorescence	*iodoplatinate spray*
	Proxymetacaine, p. 524	blue fluorescence	*potassium permanganate spray*
	Thonzylamine, p. 574	blue fluorescence	*iodoplatinate spray*
0·53	Clidinium Bromide, p. 265	—	*iodoplatinate spray*
	Dimefline, p. 306	dark blue fluorescence	*iodoplatinate spray*
	Fenethylline, p. 343	strong absorption	*iodoplatinate spray*
	Hydroquinidine, p. 372	bright blue fluorescence	*iodoplatinate spray*
	Methanthelinium Bromide, p. 409	pale blue fluorescence	*iodoplatinate spray*
	Thiopropazate, p. 572	pale blue fluorescence	*iodoplatinate spray*
0·54	Chloropyrilene, p. 251	bright blue fluorescence	*iodoplatinate spray*
	Dimethoxanate, p. 309	yellow-green fluorescence	*iodoplatinate spray*
	Etoxeridine, p. 341	absorption	*iodoplatinate spray*
	Pipazethate, p. 502	pale yellow fluorescence	*iodoplatinate spray*
	Propantheline Bromide, p. 519	pale green fluorescence	*iodoplatinate spray*
	Yohimbine, p. 598	pale blue fluorescence	*iodoplatinate spray*

Rf	*Compound*	*Ultraviolet Light*	*Primary Location Reagent*
0·55	Acepromazine, p. 169	yellow fluorescence	*iodoplatinate spray*
	Cyclizine, p. 273	absorption	*iodoplatinate spray*
	Isopropamide Iodide, p. 384	—	*iodoplatinate spray*
	Ketamine, p. 387	absorption	*iodoplatinate spray*
	Mebhydrolin, p. 397	blue fluorescence	*iodoplatinate spray*
	Nicotinic Acid, p. 441	absorption	*iodoplatinate spray*
	Pargyline, p. 469	absorption	*iodoplatinate spray*
	Physostigmine *N*-Oxide, p. 499	weak absorption	*iodoplatinate spray*
	Prothipendyl, p. 522	pale yellow fluorescence	*iodoplatinate spray*
	Trimetaphan Camsylate, p. 586	—	*iodoplatinate spray*
0·56	Bibenzonium Bromide, p. 222	—	*iodoplatinate spray*
	Coniine, p. 270	—	*iodoplatinate spray*
	Etafedrine, p. 330	—	*iodoplatinate spray*
	Guanoclor, p. 356	—	*iodoplatinate spray*
	Methylamphetamine, p. 420	absorption	*iodoplatinate spray*
	Octatropine Methylbromide, p. 452	—	*iodoplatinate spray*
	Proheptazine, p. 516	—	*iodoplatinate spray*
	Pyrazinamide, p. 527	strong absorption	*iodoplatinate spray*
0·57	Oxypertine, p. 461	blue fluorescence	*iodoplatinate spray*
	STP, p. 537	absorption	*Marquis reagent*
0·58	Alphaprodine, p. 182	—	*iodoplatinate spray*
	Aminacrine, p. 185	bright blue fluorescence	*iodoplatinate spray*
	Benzydamine, p. 217	blue fluorescence	*iodoplatinate spray*
	Bufylline, p. 227	strong absorption	—
	Dibutoline Sulphate, p. 296	—	*iodoplatinate spray*
	Diethylpropion, p. 301	strong absorption	*iodoplatinate spray*
	Homochlorcyclizine, p. 366	absorption	*iodoplatinate spray*
	Imolamine, p. 380	absorption	*iodoplatinate spray*
	Isothipendyl, p. 385	pale green fluorescence	*iodoplatinate spray*
	Methoxyphenamine, p. 418	absorption	*iodoplatinate spray*
	Methylaminoheptane, p. 420	—	*bromocresol green spray*
	Penthienate Methobromide, p. 473	strong absorption	*iodoplatinate spray*
	Promazine, p. 517	pale blue fluorescence	*iodoplatinate spray*
	Tetrahydrozoline, p. 563	—	*iodoplatinate spray*
	Theophylline, p. 567	blue fluorescence	Clarke-Kalayci test
0·59	Droperidol, p. 323	strong absorption	*iodoplatinate spray*
	Pericyazine, p. 475	pale green fluorescence	*iodoplatinate spray*
	Racemorphan, p. 534	—	*iodoplatinate spray*
	Triprolidine, p. 588	bright blue fluorescence	*iodoplatinate spray*
0·60	Amylocaine, p. 196	absorption	*iodoplatinate spray*
	Azacyclonol, p. 204	—	*iodoplatinate spray*
	Bamethan, p. 206	absorption	—
	Benzquinamide, p. 216	white fluorescence	*iodoplatinate spray*
	Cyclopentolate, p. 276	—	*iodoplatinate spray*
	Dextromethorphan, p. 289	—	*iodoplatinate spray*
	Dextrorphan, p. 291	—	*iodoplatinate spray*

Rf	*Compound*	*Ultraviolet Light*	*Primary Location Reagent*
0·60	Dimethylthiambutene, p. 310	strong absorption	*iodoplatinate spray*
	Diphemanil Methylsulphate, p. 314	strong absorption	*iodoplatinate spray*
	Doxapram, p. 322	—	*iodoplatinate spray*
	Levomethorphan, p. 390	—	*iodoplatinate spray*
	Levorphanol, p. 391	—	*iodoplatinate spray*
	Methylhexaneamine, p. 424	—	*bromocresol green spray*
	Norlevorphanol, p. 449	absorption	*iodoplatinate spray*
	Oleandomycin, p. 455	—	*iodoplatinate spray*
	Phenazopyridine, p. 480	red-brown fluorescence	visible red spot—without reagent
	Phenelzine, p. 482	—	*iodoplatinate spray*
	Phentermine, p. 491	absorption	*bromocresol green spray*
	Tacrine, p. 560	blue fluorescence	*iodoplatinate spray*
	Thenalidine, p. 565	strong absorption	*iodoplatinate spray*
	Tropicamide, p. 589	blue fluorescence	*iodoplatinate spray*
0·61	Amprotropine, p. 194	—	*iodoplatinate spray*
	Aniline, p. 197	—	diazotisation followed by *alkaline betanaphthol spray*
	Betameprodine, p. 220	—	*iodoplatinate spray*
	Dextromoramide, p. 290	—	*iodoplatinate spray*
	Levomoramide, p. 391	—	*iodoplatinate spray*
	Pramoxine, p. 508	—	*iodoplatinate spray*
	Racemoramide, p. 534	—	*iodoplatinate spray*
	Thenium Closylate, p. 566	strong absorption	*iodoplatinate spray*
	Tolycaine, p. 578	pale green fluorescence	*iodoplatinate spray*
0·62	Aconitine, p. 174	absorption	*iodoplatinate spray*
	Amidopyrine, p. 185	dark blue fluorescence	*iodoplatinate spray*
	Bethanidine, p. 222	absorption	*iodoplatinate spray*
	Dimenoxadole, p. 307	absorption	*iodoplatinate spray*
	Diphenhydramine, p. 315	absorption	*iodoplatinate spray*
	Leucinocaine, p. 389	blue fluorescence	*iodoplatinate spray*
	Lignocaine, p. 392	strong absorption	*iodoplatinate spray*
	Mephentermine, p. 401	absorption	*iodoplatinate spray*
	Mepivacaine, p. 402	absorption	*iodoplatinate spray*
	Methoxypromazine, p. 418	blue fluorescence	*iodoplatinate spray*
	Oxyphenonium Bromide, p. 463	—	*iodoplatinate spray*
	Phenyltoloxamine, p. 495	—	*iodoplatinate spray*
	Piperoxan, p. 504	—	*iodoplatinate spray*
	Tuaminoheptane, p. 590	—	*iodoplatinate spray*
0·63	Bamipine, p. 206	absorption	*iodoplatinate spray*
	Chlophedianol, p. 244	absorption	*iodoplatinate spray*
	Cyprenorphine, p. 278	absorption	*iodoplatinate spray*
	Dihydroergotamine, p. 305	pale green fluorescence	p-*dimethylaminobenzaldehyde spray*
	Dimethothiazine, p. 309	pale green fluorescence	*iodoplatinate spray*
	Etorphine, p. 341	absorption	*iodoplatinate spray*
	Imipramine, p. 379	dark blue fluorescence	*iodoplatinate spray*
	Methyl Phenidate, p. 419	—	*iodoplatinate spray*
	Phenindamine, p. 484	pale green fluorescence	*iodoplatinate spray*
	Propylhexedrine, p. 522	—	*iodoplatinate spray*
	Tricyclamol Chloride, p. 583	—	*iodoplatinate spray*

Rf	*Compound*	*Ultraviolet Light*	*Primary Location Reagent*
0·64	Azapetine, p. 205	blue fluorescence	*iodoplatinate spray*
	Benactyzine, p. 209	absorption	*iodoplatinate spray*
	Cyclopentamine, p. 275	—	*iodoplatinate spray*
	Hydroxyquinoline, p. 375	pale yellow fluorescence	*iodoplatinate spray*
	Mecamylamine, p. 397	blue fluorescence	*iodoplatinate spray*
	Methdilazine, p. 412	blue fluorescence	*iodoplatinate spray*
	Valethamate Bromide, p. 593	—	*iodoplatinate spray*
	Viprynium Embonate, p. 595	bright orange fluorescence	*potassium permanganate spray*
0·65	Aletamine, p. 178	—	*iodoplatinate spray*
	Caffeine, p. 234	deep blue fluorescence	Clarke-Kalayci test
	Chlorphentermine, p. 255	—	*iodoplatinate spray*
	Chlorproguanil, p. 256	strong absorption	*iodoplatinate spray*
	Desipramine, p. 285	dark blue fluorescence	*iodoplatinate spray*
	Dioxyline, p. 313	yellow fluorescence	*iodoplatinate spray*
	Ergotamine, p. 328	blue fluorescence	p-*dimethylaminobenzaldehyde spray*
	Methotrimeprazine, p. 416	blue fluorescence	*iodoplatinate spray*
	Promethazine, p. 518	pale green fluorescence	*iodoplatinate spray*
	Thymoxamine, p. 575	—	*iodoplatinate spray*
	Trimeperidine, p. 584	—	*iodoplatinate spray*
0·66	Bephenium Hydroxynaphthoate, p. 219	yellow fluorescence	*iodoplatinate spray*
	Methixene, p. 414	absorption	*iodoplatinate spray*
	Naepaine, p. 434	blue fluorescence	*iodoplatinate spray*
	Protoveratrine B, p. 523	—	*iodoplatinate spray*
	Sulphapyridine, p. 555	blue fluorescence	diazotisation followed by *alkaline betanaphthol spray*
0·67	Clorprenaline, p. 267	—	*bromocresol green spray*
	Diethylthiambutene, p. 302	strong absorption	*iodoplatinate spray*
	Hydroxyzine, p. 376	absorption	*iodoplatinate spray*
	Methaphenilene, p. 410	strong absorption	*iodoplatinate spray*
	Normethadone, p. 449	—	*iodoplatinate spray*
	Orphenadrine, p. 456	—	*iodoplatinate spray*
	Pamaquin, p. 464	orange fluorescence	*iodoplatinate spray*
	Sulphasomidine, p. 556	yellow fluorescence	diazotisation followed by *alkaline betanaphthol spray*
0·68	Acetorphine, p. 172	absorption	*iodoplatinate spray*
	Chlorpromazine, p. 256	blue fluorescence	*iodoplatinate spray*
	Clonitazene, p. 266	strong absorption	*iodoplatinate spray*
	Fenpipramide, p. 344	—	*iodoplatinate spray*
	Metofoline, p. 428	—	*iodoplatinate spray*
	Pentaquin, p. 472	orange fluorescence	*iodoplatinate spray*
	Phenampromide, p. 479	—	*iodoplatinate spray*
	Phenomorphan, p. 488	—	*iodoplatinate spray*
	Piperocaine, p. 504	absorption	*iodoplatinate spray*
	Veratrine, p. 594	blue fluorescence	*iodine vapour*
0·69	Bromodiphenhydramine, p. 224	absorption	*iodoplatinate spray*
	Phenoxypropazine, p. 490	absorption	*iodoplatinate spray*
	Propranolol, p. 521	blue fluorescence	*iodoplatinate spray*
	Sulphathiazole, p. 557	absorption	diazotisation followed by *alkaline betanaphthol spray*

Rf	Compound	Ultraviolet Light	Primary Location Reagent
0·70	Denatonium Benzoate, p. 282	—	*iodoplatinate spray*
	Dimethisoquin, p. 308	bright blue fluorescence	*iodoplatinate spray*
	Furethidine, p. 351	—	*iodoplatinate spray*
	Isometheptene, p. 383	—	*iodoplatinate spray*
	Oxybuprocaine, p. 459	blue fluorescence	*iodoplatinate spray*
	Pipradrol, p. 505	—	*iodoplatinate spray*
	Protriptyline, p. 524	deep blue fluorescence	*iodoplatinate spray*
	Tolpropamine, p. 577	—	*iodoplatinate spray*
	Tramazoline, p. 579	strong absorption	*iodoplatinate spray*
	Trimeprazine, p. 585	blue fluorescence	*iodoplatinate spray*
0·71	Cetrimide, p. 244	—	*iodoplatinate spray*
	Clothiapine, p. 267	strong absorption	*iodoplatinate spray*
	Ethylmethylthiambutene, p. 339	absorption	*iodoplatinate spray*
	Pipethanate, p. 505	—	*iodoplatinate spray*
	Sulphamerazine, p. 550	absorption	diazotisation followed by *alkaline betanaphthol spray*
0·72	Amolanone, p. 191	absorption	*iodoplatinate spray*
	Butethamate, p. 230	—	*iodoplatinate spray*
	Caramiphen, p. 237	—	*iodoplatinate spray*
	Deserpidine, p. 284	pale blue fluorescence	*iodoplatinate spray*
	Ethionamide, p. 335	absorption	*iodoplatinate spray*
	Ethopropazine, p. 337	yellow fluorescence	*iodoplatinate spray*
	Etonitazene, p. 341	absorption	*iodoplatinate spray*
	Fluopromazine, p. 347	yellow fluorescence	*iodoplatinate spray*
	Lucanthone, p. 394	orange fluorescence	*iodoplatinate spray*
	Methimazole, p. 413	absorption	*iodoplatinate spray*
	Oxyphencyclimine, p. 462	—	*iodoplatinate spray*
	Pecazine, p. 470	pale blue fluorescence	*iodoplatinate spray*
	Rescinnamine, p. 535	blue fluorescence	*iodoplatinate spray*
0·73	Isomethadone, p. 382	—	*iodoplatinate spray*
	Levallorphan, p. 390	—	*iodoplatinate spray*
	Methoserpidine, p. 415	white fluorescence	*iodoplatinate spray*
	Nifenazone, p. 442	strong absorption	*iodoplatinate spray*
	Proxyphylline, p. 525	dark blue fluorescence	Clarke-Kalayci test
	Trimipramine, p. 587	blue fluorescence	*iodoplatinate spray*
0·74	Adiphenine, p. 175	—	*iodoplatinate spray*
	Alphamethadol, p. 181	absorption	*iodoplatinate spray*
	Antazoline, p. 198	absorption	*iodoplatinate spray*
	Chlorcyclizine, p. 247	absorption	*iodoplatinate spray*
	Dipyridamole, p. 318	bright yellow fluorescence	*iodoplatinate spray*
	Histapyrrodine, p. 365	dark blue fluorescence	*iodoplatinate spray*
	Methadone, p. 408	absorption	*iodoplatinate spray*
	Nortriptyline, p. 451	absorption	*iodoplatinate spray*
	Phentolamine, p. 492	strong absorption	*iodoplatinate spray*
	Tymazoline, p. 592	absorption	*iodoplatinate spray*
	Xenysalate, p. 596	yellow-green fluorescence	*iodoplatinate spray*
0·75	Allylprodine, p. 180	—	*iodoplatinate spray*
	Alphacetylmethadol, p. 180	absorption	*iodoplatinate spray*
	Alphameprodine, p. 181	—	*iodoplatinate spray*
	Benzamine, p. 210	absorption	*iodoplatinate spray*
	Benzphetamine, p. 215	absorption	*iodoplatinate spray*
	Butoxamine, p. 231	—	*bromocresol green spray*

Rf	*Compound*	*Ultraviolet Light*	*Primary Location Reagent*
0·75	Cetoxime, p. 243	strong absorption	*iodine vapour*
	Chlorphenoxamine, p. 255	—	*iodoplatinate spray*
	Chlorprothixene, p. 258	dark blue fluorescence	*iodoplatinate spray*
	Dextropropoxyphene, p. 290	—	*iodoplatinate spray*
	Diethazine, p. 300	yellow fluorescence	*iodoplatinate spray*
	Dioxaphetyl Butyrate, p. 313	absorption	*iodoplatinate spray*
	Iproniazid, p. 381	absorption	*iodoplatinate spray*
	Levopropoxyphene, p. 391	—	*iodoplatinate spray*
	Metyrapone, p. 429	strong absorption	*iodoplatinate spray*
	Prilocaine, p. 510	strong absorption	*iodoplatinate spray*
	Sulphadiazine, p. 547	absorption	diazotisation followed by *alkaline betanaphthol spray*
	Triacetyloleandomycin, p. 580	—	*iodoplatinate spray*
	Xylometazoline, p. 597	—	*iodoplatinate spray*
0·76	Benzethonium Chloride, p. 213	—	*iodoplatinate spray*
	Benztropine, p. 216	—	*iodoplatinate spray*
	Carbetapentane, p. 238	—	*iodoplatinate spray*
	Diampromide, p. 292	—	*iodoplatinate spray*
	Oxymetazoline, p. 460	absorption	*iodoplatinate spray*
	Piperidolate, p. 503	—	*iodoplatinate spray*
	Prolintane, p. 517	absorption	*iodoplatinate spray*
	Thioridazine, p. 573	yellow-green fluorescence	*iodoplatinate spray*
0·77	Amitriptyline, p. 189	absorption	*iodoplatinate spray*
	Clemizole, p. 264	dark blue fluorescence	*iodoplatinate spray*
	Cyproheptadine, p. 278	blue fluorescence	*iodoplatinate spray*
	Diphenidol, p. 316	—	*iodoplatinate spray*
	Octaverine, p. 453	green fluorescence	*iodoplatinate spray*
	Phenadoxone, p. 478	—	*iodoplatinate spray*
	Propiomazine, p. 520	yellow fluorescence	*iodoplatinate spray*
0·78	Butacaine, p. 228	blue fluorescence	*iodoplatinate spray*
	Butanilicaine, p. 229	—	*iodoplatinate spray*
	Butriptyline, p. 231	—	*iodoplatinate spray*
	Cinchocaine, p. 262	blue fluorescence	*iodoplatinate spray*
	Dyclonine, p. 323	absorption	*iodoplatinate spray*
	Nialamide, p. 439	absorption	*iodoplatinate spray*
	Proguanil, p. 516	strong absorption	*iodoplatinate spray*
	Reserpine, p. 535	pale green fluorescence	*iodoplatinate spray*
	Sulphamethoxydiazine, p. 552	absorption	diazotisation followed by *alkaline betanaphthol spray*
	Tridihexethyl Chloride, p. 583	—	*iodoplatinate spray*
0·79	Ajmaline, p. 177	blue fluorescence	*iodoplatinate spray*
	Cetylpyridinium Chloride, p. 244	absorption	*iodoplatinate spray*
	Embramine, p. 324	absorption	*iodoplatinate spray*
	Ethomoxane, p. 337	—	*iodoplatinate spray*
	Fencamfamin, p. 343	—	*iodoplatinate spray*
	Isoxsuprine, p. 386	absorption	*iodoplatinate spray*
	Noracymethadol, p. 445	—	*bromocresol green spray*
	Orthocaine, p. 456	blue fluorescence	*iodoplatinate spray*
	Sulphadimidine, p. 549	weak absorption	diazotisation followed by *alkaline betanaphthol spray*

Rf	*Compound*	*Ultraviolet Light*	*Primary Location Reagent*
0·80	Aminosalicylic Acid, p. 188	blue fluorescence	diazotisation followed by *alkaline betanaphthol spray*
	Buphenine, p. 227	—	*Marquis reagent*
	Dihydroergotoxine Mesylate, p. 305	green fluorescence	p-*dimethylaminobenzaldehyde spray*
	Domiphen Bromide, p. 321	absorption	*iodoplatinate spray*
	Fluanisone, p. 346	strong absorption	*iodoplatinate spray*
	Metronidazole, p. 429	strong absorption	*iodoplatinate spray*
	Pentazocine, p. 473	—	*bromocresol green spray*
	Phencyclidine, p. 481	—	*iodoplatinate spray*
	Sulphamethoxypyridazine, p. 553	absorption	diazotisation followed by *alkaline betanaphthol spray*
0·81	Hexylcaine, p. 363	absorption	*iodoplatinate spray*
	Sulphacetamide, p. 546	absorption	diazotisation followed by *alkaline betanaphthol spray*
	Syrosingopine, p. 559	pale green fluorescence	*iodoplatinate spray*
0·82	Chlordiazepoxide, p. 248	strong absorption	*iodoplatinate spray*
	Ergotoxine, p. 329	blue fluorescence	p-*dimethylaminobenzaldehyde spray*
	Fenfluramine, p. 344	absorption	*iodoplatinate spray*
	Fenpiprane, p. 345	absorption	*iodoplatinate spray*
	Lobeline, p. 393	strong absorption	*iodoplatinate spray*
	Oxeladin, p. 459	—	*iodoplatinate spray*
	Protoveratrine A, p. 523	—	*iodoplatinate spray*
0·83	Aminobenzoic Acid, p. 186	blue fluorescence	diazotisation followed by *alkaline betanaphthol spray*
	Colchicine, p. 269	yellow fluorescence	—
	Cycrimine, p. 277	—	*iodoplatinate spray*
	Myrophine, p. 433	absorption	*iodoplatinate spray*
	Piminodine, p. 501	dark blue fluorescence	*iodoplatinate spray*
	Sulphasalazine, p. 555	—	visible orange spot—without reagent
0·84	Amisometradine, p. 189	absorption	*iodine vapour*
	Captodiame, p. 236	strong absorption	*iodoplatinate spray*
	Carbamazepine, p. 238	blue fluorescence	*potassium permanganate spray*
	Dicyclomine, p. 299	—	*iodoplatinate spray*
	Haloperidol, p. 357	strong absorption	*iodoplatinate spray*
	Levophenacylmorphan, p. 391	absorption	*iodoplatinate spray*
	Procyclidine, p. 514	—	*iodoplatinate spray*
	Pyrrobutamine, p. 529	strong absorption	*iodoplatinate spray*
	Sulphamethizole, p. 551	absorption	diazotisation followed by *alkaline betanaphthol spray*
0·85	Benzhexol, p. 213	—	*iodoplatinate spray*
	Bupivacaine, p. 228	—	*iodoplatinate spray*
	Chlorthalidone, p. 259	absorption	—
	Diperodon, p. 314	strong absorption	*iodoplatinate spray*
	Dipipanone, p. 317	absorption	*iodoplatinate spray*
	Leptazol, p. 389	—	*iodoplatinate spray*

Rf	*Compound*	*Ultraviolet Light*	*Primary Location Reagent*
0·86	Alverine, p. 182	—	*iodoplatinate spray*
	Fentanyl, p. 345	—	*iodoplatinate spray*
	Nikethamide, p. 443	strong absorption	*iodoplatinate spray*
	Phenazocine, p. 479	—	*iodoplatinate spray*
	Sulphadimethoxine, p. 548	absorption	diazotisation followed by *alkaline betanaphthol spray*
	Sulphormethoxine, p. 558	strong absorption	diazotisation followed by *alkaline betanaphthol spray*
0·87	Biperiden, p. 223	—	*iodoplatinate spray*
	Cyclomethycaine, p. 275	blue fluorescence	*iodoplatinate spray*
	Norbormide, p. 446	bright blue fluorescence	*iodoplatinate spray*
	Oxethazaine, p. 459	—	*iodoplatinate spray*
	Phenazone, p. 480	strong absorption	*iodoplatinate spray*
0·88	Clomiphene, p. 265	absorption	*iodoplatinate spray*
	Prothionamide, p. 522	strong absorption	*iodoplatinate spray*
	Sulphaethidole, p. 549	absorption	diazotisation followed by *alkaline betanaphthol spray*
	Sulphafurazole, p. 549	absorption	diazotisation followed by *alkaline betanaphthol spray*
0·89	Diazepam, p. 294	—	*iodoplatinate spray*
	Mephenesin Carbamate, p. 401	—	*Marquis reagent*
0·90	Acinitrazole, p. 174	absorption	*potassium permanganate spray*
	Benzocaine, p. 214	blue fluorescence	diazotisation followed by *alkaline betanaphthol spray*
	Bisacodyl, p. 223	absorption	*iodoplatinate spray*
	Carbimazole, p. 238	absorption	*iodoplatinate spray*
	Cinnarizine, p. 263	—	*iodoplatinate spray*
	Diphenoxylate, p. 316	—	*iodoplatinate spray*
	Erythromycin, p. 330	—	*iodoplatinate spray*
	Etymide, p. 342	—	*iodoplatinate spray*
	Hexetidine, p. 361	—	*iodoplatinate spray*
	Phenelzine, p. 482	strong absorption	*iodoplatinate spray*
	Phenoperidine, p. 488	—	*iodoplatinate spray*
	Solanidine, p. 541	—	*iodoplatinate spray*
	Sulphamethoxazole, p. 552	absorption	diazotisation followed by *alkaline betanaphthol spray*
	Thurfyl Nicotinate, p. 574	strong absorption	*iodoplatinate spray*
0·91	Benzethidine, p. 212	—	*iodoplatinate spray*
	Benzyl Nicotinate, p. 218	absorption	*iodoplatinate spray*
	Butyl Aminobenzoate, p. 232	strong absorption	*diazotised* p-*nitroaniline–sodium hydroxide spray*
	Prenylamine, p. 509	absorption	*iodoplatinate spray*
	Trichlormethiazide, p. 581	absorption	—
0·92	Cetalkonium Chloride, p. 243	—	*iodoplatinate spray*

Rf	*Compound*	*Ultraviolet Light*	*Primary Location Reagent*
0·92	Cyclothiazide, p. 277	absorption	*potassium permanganate spray*
	Meclozine, p. 398	—	*bromocresol green spray*
	Nitrazepam, p. 443	strong absorption	—
	Phenoxybenzamine, p. 489	—	*iodoplatinate spray*
0·93	Carbromal, p. 240	absorption	*bromine–starch–potassium iodide*
	Chlormethiazole, p. 250	absorption	*iodoplatinate spray*
	Chlorzoxazone, p. 260	absorption	—
	Cropropamide, p. 272	strong absorption	*potassium permanganate spray*
	Crotethamide, p. 272	strong absorption	*potassium permanganate spray*
	Ethinamate, p. 334	—	*iodine vapour*
	Ethosuximide, p. 338	—	*bromine–starch–potassium iodide*
	Glutethimide, p. 353	—	*bromine–starch–potassium iodide*
	Hyoscine Butylbromide, p. 377	—	*iodoplatinate spray*
	Sulphaphenazole, p. 554	absorption	diazotisation followed by *alkaline betanaphthol spray*
	Sulphasomizole, p. 556	absorption	diazotisation followed by *alkaline betanaphthol spray*
	Thiambutosine, p. 569	strong absorption	*nitrogen dioxide vapour*
0·94	Buclizine, p. 226	—	*iodoplatinate spray*
	Isocarboxazid, p. 382	strong absorption	*iodoplatinate spray*
	Methaqualone, p. 411	strong absorption	*iodine vapour*
	Methsuximide, p. 418	absorption	*iodine vapour*
	Methyprylone, p. 426	—	*bromine–starch–potassium iodide*
	Pheneturide, p. 483	absorption	*iodine vapour*
0·95	Carbutamide, p. 241	—	diazotisation followed by *alkaline betanaphthol spray*
	Chloramphenicol, p. 246	strong absorption	—
	Monosulfiram, p. 430	absorption	*iodoplatinate spray*
0·96	Chlorpropamide, p. 258	absorption	*ninhydrin spray*
	Isobutyl Aminobenzoate, p. 381	blue fluorescence	diazotisation followed by *alkaline betanaphthol spray*
	Oxyphenbutazone, p. 462	strong absorption	p-*dimethylaminobenzaldehyde spray*
	Phenylbutazone, p. 492	absorption	*potassium permanganate spray*
	Tolbutamide, p. 576	—	*bromocresol green spray*
0·97	Fenimide, p. 344	—	*bromine–starch–potassium iodide*
	Propanidid, p. 519	weak absorption	*iodoplatinate spray*

SYSTEM P2 (p. 34)—Rf Values Relative to Amylobarbitone

Rf	*Compound*
0·06	Barbitone, p. 207
	Phenylmethylbarbituric Acid, p. 494
0·08	Probarbital, p. 511
0·09	Allobarbitone, p. 179
	Phenobarbitone, p. 486
0·21	Vinbarbitone, p. 594
0·24	Cyclobarbitone, p. 274
0·29	Ibomal, p. 378
0·40	Allylbarbituric Acid, p. 179
0·52	Butobarbitone, p. 231
	Secbutobarbitone, p. 540
0·58	Heptabarbitone, p. 359
0·72	Nealbarbitone, p. 437
1·00	Amylobarbitone, p. 195
1·16	Pentobarbitone, p. 473
1·35	Metharbitone, p. 412
1·40	Quinalbarbitone, p. 530
1·68	Methohexitone, p. 415
1·80	Thialbarbitone, p. 569
	Thiopentone, p. 571
2·00	Methylphenobarbitone, p. 425
2·40	Hexobarbitone, p. 362

SYSTEM P3 (p. 35)—Rf Values

Rf	*Compound*
0·06	Barbitone, p. 207
0·07	Phenobarbitone, p. 486
0·13	Quinalbarbitone, p. 530
0·15	Allobarbitone, p. 179
0·18	Cyclobarbitone, p. 274
0·19	Aprobarbitone, p. 200
0·24	Butobarbitone, p. 231
0·31	Amylobarbitone, p. 195
0·41	Pentobarbitone, p. 473
0·63	Methylphenobarbitone, p. 425
0·77	Hexobarbitone, p. 362

SYSTEM P4 (p. 36)—Rf Values

Rf	*Compound*
0·06	Phenobarbitone, p. 486
0·09	Barbitone, p. 207
0·12	Allobarbitone, p. 179
0·23	Cyclobarbitone, p. 274
0·29	Aprobarbitone, p. 200
0·35	Butobarbitone, p. 231
0·46	Amylobarbitone, p. 195
0·56	Quinalbarbitone, p. 530
0·64	Pentobarbitone, p. 473
0·85	Hexobarbitone, p. 362
0·90	Methylphenobarbitone, p. 425

SYSTEM P5 (p. 36)—Rf Values Relative to Quinalbarbitone

Rf	*Compound*
0·07	Barbitone, p. 207
0·10	Phenobarbitone, p. 486
0·22	Cyclobarbitone, p. 274
0·39	Butobarbitone, p. 231
0·66	Amylobarbitone, p. 195
0·70	Pentobarbitone, p. 473
1·00	Quinalbarbitone, p. 530
2·35	Hexobarbitone, p. 362

SYSTEM P6 (p. 37)—Rf Values

Rf	*Compound*
0·00	Carbachol, p. 237
0·73	Urethane, p. 593
0·76	Styramate, p. 546
0·83	Mephenesin Carbamate, p. 401
0·86	Meprobamate, p. 403
0·88	Methylpentynol Carbamate, p. 425
0·93	Ethinamate, p. 334

SYSTEM P7 (p. 37)—Rf Values

Rf	*Compound*
0·51	Ethinamate, p. 334
0·64	Mephenesin Carbamate, p. 401
0·71	Meprobamate, p. 403
0·72	Methylpentynol Carbamate, p. 425
0·78	Styramate, p. 546
0·82	Carbachol, p. 237
0·89	Urethane, p. 593

SYSTEM P8 (p. 38)—Rf Values

Rf	*Compound*
0·60	Salicylic Acid, p. 539
0·75	Ethyl Biscoumacetate, p. 338
0·76	Dicoumarol, p. 298
0·77	Phenindione, p. 484
0·88	Nicoumalone, p. 442

SYSTEM P9 (p. 38)—Rf Values

Rf	*Compound*
0·04	Phenindione, p. 484
0·05	Salicylic Acid, p. 539
0·23	Ethyl Biscoumacetate, p. 338
0·28	Nicoumalone, p. 442
0·31	Dicoumarol, p. 298

SYSTEM P10 (p. 38)—Rf Values

Rf	*Compound*
0·80	Nicoumalone, p. 442
0·82	Salicylic Acid, p. 539
0·96	Dicoumarol, p. 298
0·96	Ethyl Biscoumacetate, p. 338
	Phenindione, p. 484

SYSTEM P11 (p. 39)—Rf Values

Rf	*Compound*
0·56	Diazinon, p. 294
0·71	Parathion, p. 468
0·90	Malathion, p. 396

SYSTEM P12 (p. 39)—Rf Values

Rf	*Compound*
0·15	Salicyluric Acid, p. 202
0·19	Aminosalicylic Acid, p. 188
0·32	Gentisic Acid, p. 202
0·45	Salicylamide, p. 538
0·52	Aspirin, p. 202
0·52	Salicylic Acid, p. 539
0·55	Sulthiame, p. 558
0·80	Mefenamic Acid, p. 399

SYSTEM P13 (p. 40)—Rf Values

Rf	*Compound*
0·15	Prednisolone, p. 508
0·16	Betamethasone, p. 220
0·21	Dexamethasone, p. 287
0·26	Hydrocortisone, p. 370
0·55	Prednisone, p. 509
0·62	Cortisone, p. 270

SYSTEM P14 (p. 40)—Rf Values

Rf	*Compound*
0·40	Fluocinolone Acetonide, p. 346
0·44	Betamethasone Acetate
0·45	Fludrocortisone Acetate, p. 346
0·49	Prednisolone Acetate, p. 508
0·52	Triamcinolone Acetonide, p. 580
0·59	Hydrocortisone Acetate, p. 370
0·60	Dexamethasone Acetate, p. 287
0·74	Prednisone Acetate, p. 509
0·80	Cortisone Acetate, p. 271
0·86	Betamethasone 17-Valerate, p. 220
0·89	Betamethasone 21-Valerate, p. 220
	Prednisolone Pivalate, p. 508

SYSTEM P15 (p. 41)—Rf Values

Rf	*Compound*
0·85	Dienoestrol, p. 300
	Hexoestrol, p. 363
0·85	Stilboestrol, p. 543

SYSTEM P16 (p. 41)—Rf Values

Rf	*Compound*
0·05	Chlorothiazide, p. 253
0·08	Hydrochlorothiazide, p. 368
0·22	Bendrofluazide, p. 210
0·36	Benzthiazide, p. 216
0·62	Hydroflumethiazide, p. 370
0·72	Teclothiazide, p. 561
0·73	Methyclothiazide, p. 419
0·75	Frusemide, p. 350
0·80	Cyclopenthiazide, p. 276
0·88	Polythiazide, p. 506

SYSTEM RP1a (p. 41)—Rf Values

Rf	*Compound*
0·00	Diphenoxylate, p. 316
	Meclozine, p. 398
	Myrophine, p. 433
	Phenadoxone, p. 478
0·02	Chlorcyclizine, p. 247
0·04	Clemizole, p. 264
	Isobutyl Aminobenzoate, p. 381
	Oxethazaine, p. 459
	Oxyphenbutazone, p. 462
0·05	Xenysalate, p. 596
0·06	Methaqualone, p. 411
	Octaverine, p. 452
	Phenylbutazone, p. 492
	Pramoxine, p. 508
	Trifluoperazine, p. 584
0·07	Dicyclomine, p. 299
	Dioxyline, p. 313
	Propiomazine, p. 520
0·08	Cetoxime, p. 243
	Papaverine, p. 464
0·10	Cyclothiazide, p. 277
	Levophenacylmorphan, p. 391
	Piritramide, p. 505
	Vinblastine, p. 595
0·11	Ethacridine, p. 331
	Pyrrobutamine, p. 529
	Racemoramide, p. 534
0·12	Dimethindene, p. 307
	Fluopromazine, p. 347
0·13	Dipyridamole, p. 318
	Fluphenazine, p. 348
	Glutethimide, p. 353
	Levomoramide, p. 391
	Methotrimeprazine, p. 416
0·14	Ethopropazine, p. 337
	Piperidolate, p. 503
0·16	Diperodon, p. 314
	Dipipanone, p. 317
	Phenprobamate, p. 491
	Thioproperazine, p. 572
0·17	Benzphetamine, p. 215
	Isocarboxazid, p. 382
0·18	Pheneturide, p. 483
0·19	Diampromide, p. 292
	Perphenazine, p. 475
	Prothionamide, p. 522
0·20	Azapetine, p. 205
	Chlorpromazine, p. 256
	Cyproheptadine, p. 278
	Phenoperidine, p. 488
0·21	Hydrastine, p. 368
	Spiramycin, p. 542
0·22	Diethylthiambutene, p. 302
0·23	Diethazine, p. 300
	Promethazine, p. 518
0·25	Dextropropoxyphene, p. 290
	Doxapram, p. 322
0·26	Diazepam, p. 294
0·27	Berberine, p. 219
	Fentanyl, p. 345
	Methimazole, p. 413
	Methixene, p. 414
0·28	Ethylmethylthiambutene, p. 339
	Hydroxyzine, p. 376
0·29	Benzhexol, p. 213
	Carbamazepine, p. 238
	Trimeprazine, p. 585
0·30	Cinchocaine, p. 262
	Homidium Bromide, p. 366
	Thenalidine, p. 565
0·31	Bromodiphenhydramine, p. 224
	Norharman, p. 448
	Pecazine, p. 470
0·32	Adiphenine, p. 175
	Amitriptyline, p. 189
	Domiphen Bromide, p. 321
	Embramine, p. 324
0·33	Promazine, p. 517
	Thurfyl Nicotinate, p. 574
	Tolpropamine, p. 577
0·35	Caramiphen, p. 237
0·36	Pipamazine, p. 501
0·37	Phenindamine, p. 484

Rf	*Compound*
0·38	Cycrimine, p. 277 Metyrapone, p. 429
0·39, 0·66	Acinitrazole, p. 174
0·40	Cropropamide, p. 272 Dimethylthiambutene, p. 310
0·41	Bamipine, p. 206
0·42	Oxeladin, p. 459 Pyrimethamine, p. 528
0·43	Ambazone, p. 182 Butacaine, p. 228 Chlophedianol, p. 244 Ethionamide, p. 335 Histapyrrodine, p. 365
0·44	Imipramine, p. 379
0·45	Aminacrine, p. 185 Piperoxan, p. 504
0·46	Methysergide, p. 427
0·47	Cyclizine, p. 273 Opipramol, p. 455
0·48	Leucinocaine, p. 389
0·50	Diphenylpyraline, p. 317 Harman, p. 358 Prothipendyl, p. 522
0·52	Diethylpropion, p. 301 Orthocaine, p. 456
0·53	Hydroxypethidine, p. 375 Ketobemidone, p. 387 Phencyclidine, p. 481 Procyclidine, p. 514
0·54	Acepromazine, p. 169
0·55	Apomorphine, p. 199 Nortriptyline, p. 450 Phenazocine, p. 479
0·56	Allylprodine, p. 180 Amethocaine, p. 184 Benzylmorphine, p. 218 Lysergic Acid, p. 395 Nicomorphine, p. 439 Thymoxamine, p. 575
0·57	Alphameprodine, p. 181 Veratrine, p. 594
0·58	Halopyramine, p. 357
0·59	Methadone, p. 408
0·60	Amodiaquine, p. 190 Betameprodine, p. 220
0·61	Dimethoxanate, p. 309 Haloperidol, p. 357 Pentaquin, p. 472 Properidine, p. 520

Rf	*Compound*
0·64	Ethomoxane, p. 337 Lignocaine, p. 392 Tacrine, p. 560 Yohimbine, p. 598
0·65	Nikethamide, p. 443 Thenyldiamine, p. 566
0·66	Nicocodine, p. 439 Prilocaine, p. 510
0·66, 0·39	Acinitrazole, p. 174
0·67	Dextromoramide, p. 290 Hydroquinine, p. 372 Isoxsuprine, p. 386 Tetracycline, p. 562 Thiopropazate, p. 572 Thioridazine, p. 573
0·68	Amidopyrine, p. 185 Hydroquinidine, p. 372
0·69	Imolamine, p. 380
0·70	Chloroquine, p. 252 Cinchonidine, p. 262 Desipramine, p. 285 Diphenhydramine, p. 315 Trimeperidine, p. 584
0·71	Laudexium Methylsulphate, p. 388 Mepyramine, p. 403 Methapyrilene, p. 410 Orphenadrine, p. 456 Quinidine, p. 531 Quinine, p. 532
0·72	Azacosterol, p. 204 Benztropine, p. 216 Cinchonine, p. 263 Proheptazine, p. 516 Thebaine, p. 565 Theophylline, p. 567
0·73	Bufylline, p. 227 Carbetapentane, p. 238 Propranolol, p. 521 Thonzylamine, p. 574
0·74	Levallorphan, p. 390 Propantheline Bromide, p. 519 Tripelennamine, p. 588 Triprolidine, p. 588
0·75	Amiphenazole, p. 188 Buphenine, p. 227
0·76	Levomethorphan, p. 390 Morpheridine, p. 430 Proguanil, p. 516
0·77	Brucine, p. 225 Dextromethorphan, p. 289 Doxylamine, p. 322 Methanthelinium Bromide, p. 409 Metoclopramide, p. 428

Rf	*Compound*
0·96	Pilocarpine, p. 500
	Tolazoline, p. 576
0·97	Physostigmine *N*-Oxide, p. 499
0·98	Atropine Methobromide, p. 203
	Atropine Methonitrate, p. 203
0·99	Decamethonium Iodide, p. 280
	Dimethisoquin, p. 308
	Nicotine, p. 440
1·00	Azamethonium Bromide, p. 204
	Distigmine Bromide, p. 319
	Hexamethonium Bromide, p. 361
	Hordenine, p. 367
	Neostigmine Bromide, p. 438
	Suxamethonium Chloride, p. 559
	Suxethonium Bromide, p. 559
	Tetrahydrozoline, p. 563
Tailing	Acetophenazine, p. 172
	Amicarbalide, p. 185
	Amopyroquine, p. 191
	Chlorproguanil, p. 256
	Gallamine, p. 352
	Pentamidine, p. 472
	Pseudomorphine, p. 525
	Stilbamidine, p. 543

SYSTEM RP1b (p. 42)—**Rf Values**

Rf	*Compound*
0·00	Acetophenazine, p. 172
	Adiphenine, p. 175
	Allylprodine, p. 180
	Alphameprodine, p. 181
	Alverine, p. 182
	Amethocaine, p. 184
	Amitriptyline, p. 189
	Amodiaquine, p. 190
	Amydricaine, p. 194
	Azacosterol, p. 204
	Azapetine, p. 205
	Bamipine, p. 206
	Benzethidine, p. 212
	Benzhexol, p. 213
	Benzphetamine, p. 215
	Benzylmorphine, p. 218
	Betameprodine, p. 220
	Bromodiphenhydramine, p. 224
	Butacaine, p. 228
	Caramiphen, p. 237
	Chlorcyclizine, p. 247
	Cinchocaine, p. 262
	Clemizole, p. 264
	Cyclizine, p. 273
	Cyproheptadine, p. 278
	Denatonium Benzoate, p. 282
	Diethylpropion, p. 301
	Dimethisoquin, p. 308
	Diperodon, p. 314
	Diphenhydramine, p. 315
	Diphenoxylate, p. 316
	Dipipanone, p. 317
	Doxapram, p. 322
	Embramine, p. 324
	Ethomoxane, p. 337
	Fencamfamin, p. 343
	Fentanyl, p. 345
	Haloperidol, p. 357
	Homatropine, p. 365
	Hydroxyzine, p. 376
	Imipramine, p. 379
	Isopropamide Iodide, p. 384
	Levomoramide, p. 391
	Levophenacylmorphan, p. 391
	Meclozine, p. 398
	Methadone, p. 408
	Methimazole, p. 413
	Methixene, p. 414
	Myrophine, p. 433
	Nicomorphine, p. 439
	Normethadone, p. 449
	Octaverine, p. 452
	Orphenadrine, p. 456
	Oxeladin, p. 459
	Oxethazaine, p. 459
	Papaverine, p. 464
	Pecazine, p. 470
	Perphenazine, p. 475
	Phenadoxone, p. 478
	Phenazocine, p. 479
	Phencyclidine, p. 481
	Phenindamine, p. 484
	Phenoperidine, p. 488
	Piperidolate, p. 503
	Piperoxan, p. 504
	Piritramide, p. 505
	Pramoxine, p. 508
	Properidine, p. 520
	Racemethorphan, p. 534
	Racemoramide, p. 534
	Spiramycin, p. 542
	Thebacon, p. 565
	Tolpropamine, p. 577
	Tranylcypromine, p. 579
	Vinblastine, p. 595
0·02	Chlorpromazine, p. 256
	Dioxyline, p. 313
	Histapyrrodine, p. 365
	Promazine, p. 517
	Promethazine, p. 518
	Thymoxamine, p. 575
0·03	Methohexitone, p. 415
	Pethidine, p. 476
	Pipamazine, p. 501
	Thiopentone, p. 571
	Thiopropazate, p. 572
	Trifluoperazine, p. 584
	Veratrine, p. 594
0·04	Betaprodine, p. 221
	Butyl Aminobenzoate, p. 232

Rf	*Compound*
0·04	Dextromethorphan, p. 289
	Diethazine, p. 300
	Dimethindene, p. 307
	Dimethoxanate, p. 309
	Diphenylpyraline, p. 317
	Halopyramine, p. 357
	Isobutyl Aminobenzoate, p. 381
	Lignocaine, p. 392
	Methaqualone, p. 411
	Methotrimeprazine, p. 416
	Nortriptyline, p. 450
	Opipramol, p. 455
	Procyclidine, p. 514
	Propiomazine, p. 520
	Prothipendyl, p. 522
	Pyrrobutamine, p. 529
0·05	Buphenine, p. 227
	Ethopropazine, p. 337
	Imolamine, p. 380
	Mepyramine, p. 403
	Methapyrilene, p. 410
	Piperocaine, p. 504
	Polythiazide, p. 506
	Thenalidine, p. 565
	Thialbarbitone, p. 569
	Thioridazine, p. 573
	Thonzylamine, p. 574
	Trimeperidine, p. 584
0·06	Amopyroquine, p. 191
	Cyclopenthiazide, p. 276
	Desipramine, p. 285
	Dextromoramide, p. 290
	Diethylthiambutene, p. 302
	Etoxeridine, p. 341
	Hydroflumethiazide, p. 370
	Isoxsuprine, p. 386
	Levallorphan, p. 390
	Nicocodine, p. 439
	Oxycodone, p. 460
	Phenampromide, p. 479
	Prilocaine, p. 510
	Proheptazine, p. 516
	Thebaine, p. 565
0·07	Acepromazine, p. 169
	Dipyridamole, p. 318
	Emetine, p. 325
	Fluopromazine, p. 347
	Fluphenazine, p. 348
	Hydrastine, p. 368
	Thenyldiamine, p. 566
	Xenysalate, p. 596
	Yohimbine, p. 598
0·08	Benztropine, p. 216
	Carbetapentane, p. 238
	Dimethylthiambutene, p. 310
	Ethylmethylthiambutene, p. 339
	Norharman, p. 448
	Pentaquin, p. 472
	Propoxycaine, p. 521
	Pyrimethamine, p. 528
	Racemorphan, p. 534
	Thioproperazine, p. 572

Rf	*Compound*
0·09	Harman, p. 358
	Leucinocaine, p. 389
	Levomethorphan, p. 390
0·10	Acetyldihydrocodeine, p. 174
	Carbinoxamine, p. 239
	Cinchonine, p. 263
0·11	Apomorphine, p. 199
	Phenprobamate, p. 491
	Quinidine, p. 531
	Quinine, p. 532
0·12	Diamorphine, p. 292
	Ethylmorphine, p. 340
	Hydroquinine, p. 372
	Mepivacaine, p. 402
	Quinalbarbitone, p. 530
0·13	Ethacridine, p. 331
	Glutethimide, p. 353
	Hydrocodone, p. 369
	Hydroquinidine, p. 372
	Hydroxypethidine, p. 375
	Morpheridine, p. 430
0·14	Chloroquine, p. 252
	Hexobarbitone, p. 362
0·15	Amylobarbitone, p. 195
	Carbromal, p. 240
	Domiphen Bromide, p. 321
	Pentazocine, p. 473
	Pheneturide, p. 483
0·16	Methysergide, p. 427
	Pentobarbitone, p. 473
0·17	Doxylamine, p. 322
	Ethoheptazine, p. 336
	Frusemide, p. 350
	Prothionamide, p. 522
0·18	Heptabarbitone, p. 359
0·20	Cinchonidine, p. 262
	Cyclobarbitone, p. 274
	Isocarboxazid, p. 382
	Methyclothiazide, p. 419
	Pheniramine, p. 485
	Propranolol, p. 521
	Thurfyl Nicotinate, p. 574
0·21	Teclothiazide, p. 561
0·22	Codeine, p. 268
	Desomorphine, p. 286
0·24	Aprobarbitone, p. 200
	Butethamine, p. 230
	Talbutal, p. 560
0·26	Ethinamate, p. 334
0·27	Butobarbitone, p. 231
	Procaine, p. 513
0·28	Ambazone, p. 182
	Metyrapone, 429
	Triprolidine, p. 588

Rf	*Compound*
0·29	Phenyramidol, p. 495 Pholcodine, p. 496
0·30	Carbamazepine, p. 238 Cropropamide, p. 272 Hydroxychloroquine, p. 374
0·31	Chlorproguanil, p. 256 Homidium Bromide, p. 366
0·33	Oxymorphone, p. 461
0·34	Amiphenazole, p. 188
0·35	Apronal, p. 200 Berberine, p. 219 Dihydrocodeine, p. 304 Phenacetin, p. 477
0·36	Metoclopramide, p. 428 Nalorphine, 434
0·38	Aminacrine, p. 185
0·39	Ethionamide, p. 335 Nicotine, p. 440
0·41	Tacrine, p. 560
0·43	Phenylbutazone, p. 492
0·46	Mephenesin, p. 401
0·47	Brucine, p. 225 Tubocurarine Chloride, p. 591
0·48	Phenobarbitone, p. 486
0·49	Levorphanol, p. 391
0·50	Crotethamide, p. 272
0·51	Allobarbitone, p. 179
0·52	Antazoline, p. 198
0·53	Amidopyrine, p. 185
0·54	Orthocaine, p. 456
0·55	Methyprylone, p. 426
0·56	Benzthiazide, p. 216 Phentolamine, p. 492
0·57	Acetylcholine, p. 173 Hyoscine, p. 376 Tripelennamine, p. 588 Tropacocaine, p. 589
0·58	Hordenine, p. 367 Laudexium Methylsulphate, p. 388 Oxyphenbutazone, p. 462 Tryptamine, p. 590
0·60	Bemegride, p. 209
0·61	Lysergic Acid, p. 395
0·62	Hydrochlorothiazide, p. 368 Tramazoline, p. 579
0·63	Trimetazidine, p. 586
0·64	Bendrofluazide, p. 210 Meprobamate, p. 403
0·65	Thalidomide, p. 564
0·66	Neostigmine Bromide, p. 438 Proguanil, p. 516 Propantheline Bromide, p. 519
0·68	Nikethamide, p. 443
0·70	Barbitone, p. 207
0·72	Pentamidine, p. 472
0·73	Physostigmine *N*-Oxide, p. 499 Styramate, p. 546 Theophylline, p. 567
0·74	Caffeine, p. 234 Diphemanil Methylsulphate, p. 314 Tetracycline, p. 562 Tricyclamol Chloride, p. 583 Tridihexethyl Chloride, p. 583
0·75	Amisometradine, p. 189 Bufylline, p. 227 Chlorothiazide, p. 253 Methanthelinium Bromide, p. 409
0·76	Hexocyclium Methylsulphate, p. 363 Naphazoline, p. 435 Oxyphenonium Bromide, p. 463
0·77	Nialamide, p. 439 Trimetaphan Camsylate, p. 586
0·79	Iproniazid, p. 381 Nicotinamide, p. 440 Phenamidine, p. 478 Phenazone, p. 480
0·80	Paracetamol, p. 465 Proxyphylline, p. 525 Pyrazinamide, p. 527
0·81	Metronidazole, p. 429 Morphine, p. 431 Nicotinyl Alcohol, p. 442 Thenium Closylate, p. 566
0·82	Guanethidine, p. 356 Hydromorphone, p. 371 Normorphine, p. 450 Propamidine, p. 519 Sparteine, p. 542 Tymazoline, p. 592
0·84	Bephenium Hydroxynaphthoate, p. 219 Bibenzonium Bromide, p. 222 Glycopyrronium Bromide, p. 355

Rf	*Compound*
0·85	Ambutonium Bromide, p. 183
	Clidinium Bromide, p. 265
	Pseudoephedrine, p. 525
0·86	Ambenonium Chloride, p. 183
	Pyridoxine, p. 528
0·87	Ametazole, p. 184
	Hydrastinine, p. 368
	Nicotinic Acid, p. 441
	Salicylamide, p. 538
0·88	Amprolium Hydrochloride, p. 193
	Dihydromorphine, p. 305
	Orciprenaline, p. 455
	Oxymetazoline, p. 460
	Pipenzolate Bromide, p. 502
0·89	Tyramine, p. 592
0·90	Benzilonium Bromide, p. 214
	Cotarnine, p. 271
	Mepenzolate Bromide, p. 401
	Procainamide, p. 512
0·92	Tolazoline, p. 576
0·93	Homatropine Methobromide, p. 365

Rf	*Compound*
0·93	Hyoscine Methonitrate, p. 378
	Paraquat, p. 468
	Penthienate Methobromide, p. 473
	Phenisonone, p. 485
0·94	Edrophonium Chloride, p. 324
	Mescaline, p. 404
	Phenformin, p. 483
	Trimeprazine, p. 585
0·95	Atropine Methobromide, p. 203
	Atropine Methonitrate, p. 203
	Metformin, p. 407
	Pilocarpine, p. 500
0·96	Decamethonium Iodide, p. 280
	Distigmine Bromide, p. 319
1·00	Azamethonium Bromide, p. 204
	Hexamethonium Bromide, p. 361
	Pentolinium Tartrate, p. 474
	Suxamethonium Chloride, p. 559
	Suxethonium Bromide, p. 559
	Tetrahydrozoline, p. 563
Tailing	Amicarbilide, p. 185
	Gallamine, p. 352
	Pseudomorphine, p. 525
	Stilbamidine, p. 543

Thin-layer Chromatographic Data

SYSTEM T1 (p. 46)—Rf Values and Location Reagents

Rf	*Compound*	*Primary Location Reagent*
0·00	Azamethonium Bromide, p. 204	*acidified iodoplatinate spray*
	Decamethonium Iodide, p. 280	*acidified iodoplatinate spray*
	Dimethyltubocurarine Bromide, p. 311	*acidified iodoplatinate spray*
	Diquat, p. 319	*acidified iodoplatinate spray*
	Distigmine Bromide, p. 319	*acidified iodoplatinate spray*
	Framycetin, p. 350	*potassium permanganate spray*
	Gallamine, p. 352	*acidified iodoplatinate spray*
	Hexamethonium Bromide, p. 361	*acidified iodoplatinate spray*
	Hydrastinine, p. 368	*acidified iodoplatinate spray*
	Mebezonium Iodide, p. 397	*acidified iodoplatinate spray*
	Neomycin, p. 437	*potassium permanganate spray*
	Paraquat, p. 468	*acidified iodoplatinate spray*
	Pentolinium Tartrate, p. 474	*acidified iodoplatinate spray*
	Quinuronium Sulphate, p. 533	*acidified iodoplatinate spray*
	Streptomycin, p. 544	*potassium permanganate spray*
	Tubocurarine Chloride, p. 591	*acidified iodoplatinate spray*
	Viomycin, p. 595	*potassium permanganate spray*
0·01	Alcuronium Chloride, p. 177	*potassium permanganate spray*
	Bretylium Tosylate, p. 224	*acidified iodoplatinate spray*
	Carbachol, p. 237	*acidified iodoplatinate spray*
	Chlorisondamine Chloride, p. 249	*acidified iodoplatinate spray*
	Dibromopropamidine, p. 295	*acidified iodoplatinate spray*
	Dihydrostreptomycin, p. 306	*potassium permanganate spray*
	Hexylcaine, p. 363	*acidified iodoplatinate spray*
	Kanamycin, p. 386	*potassium permanganate spray*
	Laudexium Methylsulphate, p. 388	*acidified iodoplatinate spray*
	Mepenzolate Bromide, p. 401	*acidified iodoplatinate spray*
	Pyrithidium Bromide, p. 529	*acidified iodoplatinate spray*
	Suxamethonium Chloride, p. 559	*acidified iodoplatinate spray*
	Suxethonium Bromide, p. 559	*acidified iodoplatinate spray*
	Thiamine, p. 570	*acidified iodoplatinate spray*
	Tolonium Chloride, p. 577	*acidified iodoplatinate spray*
	Triclobisonium Chloride, p. 583	*acidified iodoplatinate spray*
0·02	Acetylcholine, p. 173	*acidified iodoplatinate spray*
	Ambenonium Chloride, p. 183	*acidified iodoplatinate spray*
	Amprolium Hydrochloride, p. 193	*acidified iodoplatinate spray*
	Atropine Methobromide, p. 203	*acidified iodoplatinate spray*
	Atropine Methonitrate, p. 203	*acidified iodoplatinate spray*
	Bethanechol Chloride, p. 221	*acidified iodoplatinate spray*
	Bibenzonium Bromide, p. 222	*acidified iodoplatinate spray*
	Cadaverine, p. 233	*acidified iodoplatinate spray*
	Cetrimide, p. 244	*acidified iodoplatinate spray*
	Choline, p. 261	*acidified iodoplatinate spray*
	Clamoxyquin, p. 264	*acidified iodoplatinate spray*
	Clidinium Bromide, p. 265	*acidified iodoplatinate spray*
	Cotarnine, p. 271	*acidified iodoplatinate spray*
	Dibutoline Sulphate, p. 296	*acidified iodoplatinate spray*
	Diphemanil Methylsulphate, p. 314	*acidified iodoplatinate spray*
	Hexocyclium Methylsulphate, p. 363	*acidified iodoplatinate spray*
	Homatropine Methobromide, p. 365	*acidified iodoplatinate spray*
	Hyoscine Methobromide, p. 377	*acidified iodoplatinate spray*
	Hyoscine Methonitrate, p. 378	*acidified iodoplatinate spray*
	Lachesine Chloride, p. 387	*acidified iodoplatinate spray*
	Methacholine Bromide, p. 407	*acidified iodoplatinate spray*

Rf	*Compound*	*Primary Location Reagent*
0·02	Methanthelinium Bromide, p. 409	*acidified iodoplatinate spray*
	Neostigmine Bromide, p. 438	*acidified iodoplatinate spray*
	Octatropine Methylbromide, p. 452	*acidified iodoplatinate spray*
	Penthienate Methobromide, p. 473	*acidified iodoplatinate spray*
	Poldine Methylsulphate, p. 506	*acidified iodoplatinate spray*
	Putrescine, p. 527	*acidified iodoplatinate spray*
	Quinapyramine Chloride, p. 531	*acidified iodoplatinate spray*
	Thenium Closylate, p. 566	*acidified iodoplatinate spray*
	Trimetaphan Camsylate, p. 586	*acidified iodoplatinate spray*
	Valethamate Bromide, p. 593	*acidified iodoplatinate spray*
0·03	Ambutonium Bromide, p. 183	*acidified iodoplatinate spray*
	Benzethonium Chloride, p. 213	*acidified iodoplatinate spray*
	Benzilonium Bromide, p. 214	*acidified iodoplatinate spray*
	Dequalinium Chloride, p. 284	*acidified iodoplatinate spray*
	Glycopyrronium Bromide, p. 355	*acidified iodoplatinate spray*
	Heteronium Bromide, p. 360	*acidified iodoplatinate spray*
	Oxyphencyclimine, p. 462	*acidified iodoplatinate spray*
	Oxyphenonium Bromide, p. 463	*acidified iodoplatinate spray*
	Piperazine, p. 503	*acidified iodoplatinate spray*
0·04	Acepifylline, p. 169	*strongly acid iodoplatinate spray*
	Diminazene, p. 312	*acidified iodoplatinate spray*
	Pipenzolate Bromide, p. 502	*acidified iodoplatinate spray*
	Propamidine, p. 519	*acidified iodoplatinate spray*
	Propantheline Bromide, p. 519	*acidified iodoplatinate spray*
	Pyridostigmine Bromide, p. 527	*acidified iodoplatinate spray*
	Sparteine, p. 542	*acidified iodoplatinate spray*
	Stilbamidine, p. 543	*acidified iodoplatinate spray*
0·04, streaking	Phenamidine, p. 478	*acidified iodoplatinate spray*
0·05	Domiphen Bromide, p. 321	*acidified iodoplatinate spray*
	Guanethidine, p. 356	*acidified iodoplatinate spray*
	Isopropamide Iodide, p. 384	*acidified iodoplatinate spray*
	Pralidoxime Chloride, p. 507	*acidified iodoplatinate spray*
	Psilocybin, p. 526	p-*dimethylaminobenzaldehyde spray*
0·05, streaking	Amicarbalide, p. 185	*acidified iodoplatinate spray*
	Chlortetracycline, p. 259	*potassium permanganate spray*
	Demethylchlortetracycline, p. 281	*potassium permanganate spray*
	Lymecycline, p. 394	*potassium permanganate spray*
	Methacycline, p. 408	*potassium permanganate spray*
	Oxytetracycline Dihydrate, p. 463	*potassium permanganate spray*
	Rolitetracycline, p. 537	*potassium permanganate spray*
	Tetracycline, p. 562	*potassium permanganate spray*
0·06	Tricyclamol Chloride, p. 583	*acidified iodoplatinate spray*
0·07	Acriflavine, p. 175	ultraviolet light—yellow-green fluorescence
	Berberine, p. 219	*acidified iodoplatinate spray*
	Edrophonium Chloride, p. 324	*acidified iodoplatinate spray*
	Tridihexethyl Chloride, p. 583	*acidified iodoplatinate spray*
0·08, streaking	Desferrioxamine, p. 285	*potassium permanganate spray*
0·09	Metformin, p. 407	*acidified iodoplatinate spray*

Rf	*Compound*	*Primary Location Reagent*
0·10	Denatonium Benzoate, p. 282	*acidified iodoplatinate spray*
0·11	Bethanidine, p. 222	*Dragendorff spray*
0·12	Azacosterol, p. 204	*acidified iodoplatinate spray*
	Benztropine, p. 216	*acidified iodoplatinate spray*
	Brucine, p. 225	*acidified iodoplatinate spray*
0·12, streaking	Cetalkonium Chloride, p. 243	*acidified iodoplatinate spray*
	Norlevorphanol, p. 449	*acidified iodoplatinate spray*
	Oxethazaine, p. 459	*acidified iodoplatinate spray*
0·13	Histamine, p. 364	*acidified iodoplatinate spray*
	Naphazoline, p. 435	*acidified iodoplatinate spray*
	Xylometazoline, p. 597	*acidified iodoplatinate spray*
0·13, streaking	Pseudomorphine, p. 525	*acidified iodoplatinate spray*
0·14, streaking	Oxymetazoline, p. 460	*acidified iodoplatinate spray*
0·15	Azacyclonol, p. 204	*acidified iodoplatinate spray*
	Homatropine, p. 365	*acidified iodoplatinate spray*
	Tetrahydrozoline, p. 563	*acidified iodoplatinate spray*
	Tolazoline, p. 576	*acidified iodoplatinate spray*
0·15, streaking	Cycloserine, p. 276	*acidified iodoplatinate spray*
	Levophenacylmorphan, p. 391	*acidified iodoplatinate spray*
0·16	Proflavine Hemisulphate, p. 515	diazotisation followed by *alkaline betanaphthol spray*
0·17	Ecgonine, p. 324	*acidified iodoplatinate spray*
	Normorphine, p. 450	*acidified iodoplatinate spray*
	Pempidine, p. 471	*acidified iodoplatinate spray*
0·18	Apoatropine, p. 198	*acidified iodoplatinate spray*
	Atropine, p. 202	*acidified iodoplatinate spray*
	Hyoscyamine, p. 378	*acidified iodoplatinate spray*
	Trimetazidine, p. 586	*acidified iodoplatinate spray*
0·18, streaking	Adrenaline, p. 175	*potassium permanganate spray*
	Cyclopentamine, p. 275	*potassium permanganate spray*
	Dopamine, p. 321	*potassium permanganate spray*
0·19	Meclofenoxate, p. 398	*potassium permanganate spray*
0·20	Cetylpyridinium Chloride, p. 244	*acidified iodoplatinate spray*
	Ethambutol, p. 332	*potassium permanganate spray*
	Pentaquin, p. 472	*diazotised* p-*nitroaniline–sodium hydroxide spray*
0·20, streaking	Debrisoquine, p. 279	*acidified iodoplatinate spray*
	Primaquine, p. 510	*acidified iodoplatinate spray*

Rf	*Compound*	*Primary Location Reagent*
0·21	Atropine *N*-Oxide, p. 203	*acidified iodoplatinate spray*
	Benzoylecgonine, p. 215	*acidified iodoplatinate spray*
	Metanephrine, p. 406	*potassium permanganate spray*
	Metazocine, p. 407	*acidified iodoplatinate spray*
	Piritramide, p. 505	*acidified iodoplatinate spray*
0·21, streaking	Tramazoline, p. 579	*potassium permanganate spray*
0·22	Acriflavine, p. 175	ultraviolet light—yellow-green fluorescence
	Mescaline, p. 404	*acidified iodoplatinate spray*
	Oxedrine, p. 458	*potassium permanganate spray*
	Pamaquin, p. 464	*diazotised* p-*nitroaniline–sodium hydroxide spray*
	Strychnine, p. 545	*acidified iodoplatinate spray*
	Vancomycin, p. 593	*potassium permanganate spray*
0·22, streaking	Mecamylamine, p. 397	*iodine vapour*
	Phanquone, p. 476	*acidified iodoplatinate spray*
0·23	Antazoline, p. 198	*acidified iodoplatinate spray*
	Codeine *N*-Oxide, p. 269	*acidified iodoplatinate spray*
	Dihydromorphine, p. 305	*acidified iodoplatinate spray*
	Morphine *N*-Oxide, p. 432	*acidified iodoplatinate spray*
	Noradrenaline, p. 445	*potassium permanganate spray*
	Protriptyline, p. 524	*acidified iodoplatinate spray*
0·23, streaking	Prothipendyl, p. 522	*acidified iodoplatinate spray*
0·24	Ametazole, p. 184	*potassium permanganate spray*
	Desipramine, p. 285	*acidified iodoplatinate spray*
	Dextromethorphan, p. 289	*acidified iodoplatinate spray*
	Dextrorphan, p. 291	*acidified iodoplatinate spray*
	Hydromorphone, p. 371	*acidified iodoplatinate spray*
	Isometheptene, p. 383	*potassium permanganate spray*
	Levomethorphan, p. 390	*acidified iodoplatinate spray*
	Levorphanol, p. 391	*acidified iodoplatinate spray*
	Mephentermine, p. 401	*acidified iodoplatinate spray*
	Methoxyphenamine, p. 418	*acidified iodoplatinate spray*
	Pholedrine, p. 497	*potassium permanganate spray*
0·24, streaking	Cyclizine, p. 273	*acidified iodoplatinate spray*
	Isoetharine, p. 382	*potassium permanganate spray*
0·25	Dihydrocodeine, p. 304	*acidified iodoplatinate spray*
	Ethoheptazine, p. 336	*potassium permanganate spray*
	Hydroxyamphetamine, p. 373	*potassium permanganate spray*
	Metopon, p. 428	*acidified iodoplatinate spray*
	Racemethorphan, p. 534	*acidified iodoplatinate spray*
	Serotonin, p. 540	*potassium permanganate spray*
0·26	Acetyldihydrocodeine, p. 174	*acidified iodoplatinate spray*
	Coniine, p. 270	*acidified iodoplatinate spray*
	Propylhexedrine, p. 522	*acidified iodoplatinate spray*
	Racemorphan, p. 534	*acidified iodoplatinate spray*
	Tigloidine, p. 575	*acidified iodoplatinate spray*
0·26, streaking	Methyldopa, p. 422	*potassium permanganate spray*

Rf	*Compound*	*Primary Location Reagent*
0·27	Hydrocodone, p. 369	*acidified iodoplatinate spray*
	Methdilazine, p. 412	*acidified iodoplatinate spray*
	Pholcodine, p. 496	*acidified iodoplatinate spray*
	Tryptamine, p. 590	*acidified iodoplatinate spray*
0·28	Acriflavine, p. 175	ultraviolet light—yellow-green fluorescence
	Ephedrine, p. 327	*potassium permanganate spray*
	Homochlorcyclizine, p. 366	*acidified iodoplatinate spray*
	Methotrimeprazine, p. 416	*acidified iodoplatinate spray*
	Methylamphetamine, p. 420	*acidified iodoplatinate spray*
	Methyldihydromorphine, p. 422	*acidified iodoplatinate spray*
	Nortriptyline, p. 450	*acidified iodoplatinate spray*
	Phenylephrine, p. 493	*potassium permanganate spray*
	Racephedrine, p. 535	*potassium permanganate spray*
0·29	Desomorphine, p. 286	*acidified iodoplatinate spray*
	Phentolamine, p. 492	*acidified iodoplatinate spray*
0·30	Aminopentamide, p. 187	*acidified iodoplatinate spray*
	Phenylpropylmethylamine, p. 495	*potassium permanganate spray*
	Pseudoephedrine, p. 525	*potassium permanganate spray*
0·30, streaking	Phenisonone, p. 485	*potassium permanganate spray*
	Proguanil, p. 516	*acidified iodoplatinate spray*
0·31	Chloroquine, p. 252	*acidified iodoplatinate spray*
	Physostigmine *N*-Oxide, p. 499	*potassium permanganate spray*
	Tyramine, p. 592	*potassium permanganate spray*
0·32	Bufotenine, p. 227	p-*dimethylaminobenzaldehyde spray*
	Cytisine, p. 279	*acidified iodoplatinate spray*
	Dexchlorpheniramine, p. 289	*acidified iodoplatinate spray*
	Hordenine, p. 367	*potassium permanganate spray*
	Methylephedrine, p. 423	*acidified iodoplatinate spray*
	Neopine, p. 438	*acidified iodoplatinate spray*
	Pheniramine, p. 485	*acidified iodoplatinate spray*
0·32, streaking	Hydroxyquinoline, p. 375	*acidified iodoplatinate spray*
0·33	Chlorhexidine, p. 249	*strongly acid iodoplatinate spray*
	Dexbrompheniramine, p. 288	*acidified iodoplatinate spray*
	Narceine, p. 436	*acidified iodoplatinate spray*
	Normetanephrine, p. 449	*potassium permanganate spray*
	Tuaminoheptane, p. 590	*acidified iodoplatinate spray*
0·33, streaking	Isoprenaline, p. 384	*potassium permanganate spray*
	Phenethylamine, p. 482	*acidified iodoplatinate spray*
0·34	Brompheniramine, p. 225	*acidified iodoplatinate spray*
	Dimethyltryptamine, p. 311	*acidified iodoplatinate spray*
	Morphine, p. 431	*acidified iodoplatinate spray*
	Psilocin, p. 526	p-*dimethylaminobenzaldehyde spray*
0·35	Codeine, p. 268	*acidified iodoplatinate spray*
	Methyldesorphine, p. 422	*acidified iodoplatinate spray*
	Plasmocide, p. 506	*acidified iodoplatinate spray*
	Trimethoxyamphetamine, p. 587	*acidified iodoplatinate spray*
	Tropacocaine, p. 589	*acidified iodoplatinate spray*

Rf	*Compound*	*Primary Location Reagent*
0·36	Dehydroemetine, p. 280	*acidified iodoplatinate spray*
	Dimethindene, p. 307	*acidified iodoplatinate spray*
	Dimethoxanate, p. 309	*acidified iodoplatinate spray*
	Ethylmorphine, p. 340	*acidified iodoplatinate spray*
	Mepacrine, p. 400	*acidified iodoplatinate spray*
	Nicocodine, p. 439	*acidified iodoplatinate spray*
	Nicomorphine, p. 439	*acidified iodoplatinate spray*
0·37	Benzylmorphine, p. 218	*acidified iodoplatinate spray*
	Methadone, p. 408	*acidified iodoplatinate spray*
0·38	Carbinoxamine, p. 239	*acidified iodoplatinate spray*
	Chlorpheniramine, p. 254	*acidified iodoplatinate spray*
	Etafedrine, p. 330	*potassium permanganate spray*
	Harmaline, p. 358	*acidified iodoplatinate spray*
	Phenglutarimide, p. 483	*acidified iodoplatinate spray*
	Tymazoline, p. 592	*acidified iodoplatinate spray*
0·39	Methoxypromazine, p. 418	*acidified iodoplatinate spray*
0·40	Acepromazine, p. 169	*acidified iodoplatinate spray*
	Benzydamine, p. 217	*acidified iodoplatinate spray*
	Methoxyamphetamine, p. 417	*acidified iodoplatinate spray*
	Metoclopramide, p. 428	*acidified iodoplatinate spray*
	Pipazethate, p. 502	*acidified iodoplatinate spray*
	Proheptazine, p. 516	*acidified iodoplatinate spray*
	Tropine, p. 589	*acidified iodoplatinate spray*
0·41	Amydricaine, p. 194	*acidified iodoplatinate spray*
	Diphenylpyraline, p. 317	*acidified iodoplatinate spray*
	Thebaine, p. 565	*acidified iodoplatinate spray*
0·42	Diampromide, p. 292	*acidified iodoplatinate spray*
	Hydroquinine, p. 372	*acidified iodoplatinate spray*
	Hydroxychloroquine, p. 374	*acidified iodoplatinate spray*
	Ketobemidone, p. 387	*acidified iodoplatinate spray*
	Promazine, p. 517	*acidified iodoplatinate spray*
	Spiramycin, p. 542	*potassium permanganate spray*
	Thebacon, p. 565	*acidified iodoplatinate spray*
0·43	Doxylamine, p. 322	*acidified iodoplatinate spray*
	Imipramine, p. 379	*acidified iodoplatinate spray*
	Tacrine, p. 560	*acidified iodoplatinate spray*
	Triprolidine, p. 588	*acidified iodoplatinate spray*
0·43, streaking	Guanoxan, p. 356	*potassium permanganate spray*
0·44	Hydroquinidine, p. 372	*acidified iodoplatinate spray*
	6–Monoacetylmorphine, p. 430	*acidified iodoplatinate spray*
	Thioproperazine, p. 572	*acidified iodoplatinate spray*
0·45	Alphaprodine, p. 182	*acidified iodoplatinate spray*
	Amopyroquine, p. 191	*acidified iodoplatinate spray*
	Diamorphine, p. 292	*acidified iodoplatinate spray*
	Eucatropine, p. 342	*acidified iodoplatinate spray*
	Oleandomycin, p. 455	*potassium permanganate spray*
	Oxeladin, p. 459	*acidified iodoplatinate spray*
	Procainamide, p. 512	*acidified iodoplatinate spray*
	Prochlorperazine, p. 514	*acidified iodoplatinate spray*
	Thenalidine, p. 565	*acidified iodoplatinate spray*
	Thiothixene, p. 574	*acidified iodoplatinate spray*

Rf	*Compound*	*Primary Location Reagent*
0·46	Bamipine, p. 206	*acidified iodoplatinate spray*
	Carbetapentane, p. 238	*acidified iodoplatinate spray*
	Furaltadone, p. 351	*acidified iodoplatinate spray*
	Normethadone, p. 449	*acidified iodoplatinate spray*
0·47	Hydroxypethidine, p. 375	*potassium permanganate spray*
	Metaraminol, p. 406	*potassium permanganate spray*
	Thenyldiamine, p. 566	*acidified iodoplatinate spray*
	Thioridazine, p. 573	*acidified iodoplatinate spray*
	Thonzylamine, p. 574	*acidified iodoplatinate spray*
0·48	Amphetamine, p. 192	*potassium permanganate spray*
	Butaperazine, p. 229	*potassium permanganate spray*
	Cinchonine, p. 263	*acidified iodoplatinate spray*
	Dexamphetamine, p. 287	*potassium permanganate spray*
	Diethylcarbamazine, p. 301	*Dragendorff spray*
	Halopyramine, p. 357	*acidified iodoplatinate spray*
	Hydrallazine, p. 367	*acidified iodoplatinate spray*
	Hydromorphinol, p. 371	*acidified iodoplatinate spray*
	Isothipendyl, p. 385	*acidified iodoplatinate spray*
	Methapyrilene, p. 410	*acidified iodoplatinate spray*
	Methixene, p. 414	*acidified iodoplatinate spray*
	Nialamide, p. 439	*acidified iodoplatinate spray*
	Norpseudoephedrine, p. 450	*potassium permanganate spray*
	Pethidine, p. 476	*acidified iodoplatinate spray*
	Phenelzine Sulphate, p. 482	*acidified iodoplatinate spray*
	Prolintane, p. 517	*acidified iodoplatinate spray*
	Promethazine, p. 518	*acidified iodoplatinate spray*
	Thiethylperazine, p. 570	*acidified iodoplatinate spray*
	Tolpropamine, p. 577	*acidified iodoplatinate spray*
	Trifluoperazine, p. 584	*acidified iodoplatinate spray*
	Tripelennamine, p. 588	*acidified iodoplatinate spray*
0·48, streaking	Ethylnoradrenaline, p. 340	*potassium permanganate spray*
	Guanoclor, p. 356	*acidified iodoplatinate spray*
0·49	Amitriptyline, p. 189	*acidified iodoplatinate spray*
	Bromodiphenhydramine, p. 224	*acidified iodoplatinate spray*
	Chlorpromazine, p. 256	*acidified iodoplatinate spray*
	Etamiphylline, p. 331	*acidified iodoplatinate spray*
	Gelsemine, p. 353	*acidified iodoplatinate spray*
	Mepyramine, p. 403	*acidified iodoplatinate spray*
	Pyrrobutamine, p. 529	*acidified iodoplatinate spray*
0·50	Chlorphenoxamine, p. 255	*acidified iodoplatinate spray*
	Cyproheptadine, p. 278	*acidified iodoplatinate spray*
	Diamthazole, p. 293	*acidified iodoplatinate spray*
	Fenfluramine, p. 344	*acidified iodoplatinate spray*
	Oxymorphone, p. 461	*acidified iodoplatinate spray*
	Phendimetrazine, p. 481	*acidified iodoplatinate spray*
	Phenmetrazine, p. 486	*potassium permanganate spray*
	Phenyltoloxamine, p. 495	*acidified iodoplatinate spray*
	Procyclidine, p. 514	*acidified iodoplatinate spray*
	Trimethoprim, p. 586	*acidified iodoplatinate spray*
0·50, streaking	Alphameprodine, p. 181	*acidified iodoplatinate spray*
	Droperidol, p. 323	*acidified iodoplatinate spray*
0·51	Acetophenazine, p. 172	*acidified iodoplatinate spray*
	Cephaëline, p. 242	*acidified iodoplatinate spray*
	Cinchonidine, p. 262	*acidified iodoplatinate spray*

Rf	*Compound*	*Primary Location Reagent*
0·51	Diphenhydramine, p. 315	*acidified iodoplatinate spray*
	Isoniazid, p. 383	*acidified iodoplatinate spray*
	Noracymethadol, p. 445	*acidified iodoplatinate spray*
	Orphenadrine, p. 456	*acidified iodoplatinate spray*
	STP, p. 537	*potassium permanganate spray*
0·52	Dibenzepin, p. 295	*acidified iodoplatinate spray*
	Emetine, p. 325	*acidified iodoplatinate spray*
	Myrophine, p. 433	*acidified iodoplatinate spray*
	Pecazine, p. 470	*acidified iodoplatinate spray*
	Phenoxypropazine, p. 490	*acidified iodoplatinate spray*
	Phenylpropanolamine, p. 494	*potassium permanganate spray*
	Quinine, p. 532	*acidified iodoplatinate spray*
	Solanine, p. 541	*iodine–carbon tetrachloride spray*
	Thymoxamine, p. 575	*acidified iodoplatinate spray*
	Trimeperidine, p. 584	*acidified iodoplatinate spray*
0·53	Arecoline, p. 201	*potassium permanganate spray*
	Carphenazine, p. 242	*acidified iodoplatinate spray*
	Chloropyrilene, p. 252	*acidified iodoplatinate spray*
	Cyclomethycaine, p. 275	*acidified iodoplatinate spray*
	Fluopromazine, p. 347	*acidified iodoplatinate spray*
	Lucanthone, p. 394	*acidified iodoplatinate spray*
	Methaphenilene, p. 410	*acidified iodoplatinate spray*
	Opipramol, p. 455	*acidified iodoplatinate spray*
	Oxycodone, p. 460	*acidified iodoplatinate spray*
	Pipamperone, p. 501	*potassium permanganate spray*
	Properidine, p. 520	*acidified iodoplatinate spray*
	Propranolol, p. 521	*acidified iodoplatinate spray*
0·54	Aminacrine, p. 185	*acidified iodoplatinate spray*
	Chlophedianol, p. 244	*acidified iodoplatinate spray*
	Chlorphentermine, p. 255	*acidified iodoplatinate spray*
	Dimethothiazine, p. 309	*acidified iodoplatinate spray*
	Embramine, p. 324	*acidified iodoplatinate spray*
	Hyoscine, p. 376	*acidified iodoplatinate spray*
0·54, streaking	Nicotinamide, p. 440	*iodine vapour*
0·55	Aminohippuric Acid, p. 187	p-*dimethylaminobenzaldehyde spray*
	Chlorprothixene, p. 258	*acidified iodoplatinate spray*
	Dimethylthiambutene, p. 310	*acidified iodoplatinate spray*
	Homidium Bromide, p. 366	*potassium permanganate spray*
	Lobeline, p. 393	*acidified iodoplatinate spray*
	Methoxamine, p. 417	*potassium permanganate spray*
	Phenformin, p. 483	*Marquis reagent*
	Physostigmine, p. 498	*potassium permanganate spray*
	Piperocaine, p. 504	*acidified iodoplatinate spray*
	Procarbazine, p. 513	*potassium permanganate spray*
	Quinidine, p. 531	*acidified iodoplatinate spray*
	Trimeprazine, p. 585	*acidified iodoplatinate spray*
	Yohimbine, p. 598	*acidified iodoplatinate spray*
0·55, streaking	Prothionamide, p. 522	*acidified iodoplatinate spray*
0·56	Demecolcine, p. 281	p-*dimethylaminobenzaldehyde spray*
	Dimefline, p. 306	*acidified iodoplatinate spray*
	Dimethisoquin, p. 308	*acidified iodoplatinate spray*
	Fenethylline, p. 343	*acidified iodoplatinate spray*
	Fenpipramide, p. 344	*acidified iodoplatinate spray*

Rf	*Compound*	*Primary Location Reagent*
0·56	Imolamine, p. 380	*acidified iodoplatinate spray*
	Morpheridine, p. 430	*acidified iodoplatinate spray*
	Orciprenaline, p. 455	*potassium permanganate spray*
	Phentermine, p. 491	*acidified iodoplatinate spray*
0·57	Alphamethadol, p. 181	*acidified iodoplatinate spray*
	Amethocaine, p. 184	*acidified iodoplatinate spray*
	Apomorphine, p. 199	*acidified iodoplatinate spray*
	Benzamine, p. 210	*acidified iodoplatinate spray*
	Chlorcyclizine, p. 247	*acidified iodoplatinate spray*
	Dyclonine, p. 323	*acidified iodoplatinate spray*
	Metofoline, p. 428	*acidified iodoplatinate spray*
	Nicotine, p. 440	*acidified iodoplatinate spray*
	Nifenazone, p. 442	*potassium permanganate spray*
	Norbutrine, p. 447	*potassium permanganate spray*
	Phenindamine, p. 484	*acidified iodoplatinate spray*
0·58	Alverine, p. 182	*potassium permanganate spray*
	Aminobenzoic Acid, p. 186	p-*dimethylaminobenzaldehyde spray*
	Bamethan, p. 206	*potassium permanganate spray*
	Chlorproguanil, p. 256	*potassium permanganate spray*
	Clopenthixol, p. 266	*acidified iodoplatinate spray*
	Diaveridine, p. 293	*acidified iodoplatinate spray*
	Diphenidol, p. 316	*acidified iodoplatinate spray*
	Ethylmethylthiambutene, p. 339	*acidified iodoplatinate spray*
	Lysergic Acid, p. 395	p-*dimethylaminobenzaldehyde spray*
	Mebhydrolin, p. 397	*acidified iodoplatinate spray*
	Methyprylone, p. 426	*potassium permanganate spray*
	Nicotinic Acid, p. 441	*iodine vapour*
	Perphenazine, p. 475	*acidified iodoplatinate spray*
	Trimipramine, p. 587	*acidified iodoplatinate spray*
0·59	Alphacetylmethadol, p. 180	*acidified iodoplatinate spray*
	Clomiphene, p. 265	*acidified iodoplatinate spray*
	Fluphenazine, p. 348	*acidified iodoplatinate spray*
	Phencylidine, p. 481	*acidified iodoplatinate spray*
	Propoxycaine, p. 521	*acidified iodoplatinate spray*
	Proxymetacaine, p. 524	*acidified iodoplatinate spray*
	Proxyphylline, p. 525	*potassium permanganate spray*
	Pyridoxine, p. 528	*potassium permanganate spray*
	Triamterene, p. 581	ultraviolet light—bright blue fluorescence
0·60	Benactyzine, p. 209	*acidified iodoplatinate spray*
	Butethamine, p. 230	*acidified iodoplatinate spray*
	Butoxamine, p. 231	*potassium permanganate spray*
	Chloroprocaine, p. 251	*acidified iodoplatinate spray*
	Clothiapine, p. 267	*acidified iodoplatinate spray*
	Cocaine, p. 267	*acidified iodoplatinate spray*
	Dimenoxadole, p. 307	*acidified iodoplatinate spray*
	Dipyrone, p. 318	*acidified iodoplatinate spray*
	Ethacridine, p. 331	diazotisation followed by *alkaline betanaphthol spray*
	Fencamfamin, p. 343	*acidified iodoplatinate spray*
	Histapyrrodine, p. 365	*acidified iodoplatinate spray*
	Lysergamide, p. 395	p-*dimethylaminobenzaldehyde spray*
	Metabutethamine, p. 405	*acidified iodoplatinate spray*
	Methyl Phenidate, p. 419	*acidified iodoplatinate spray*
	Pentazocine, p. 473	*acidified iodoplatinate spray*
	Pilocarpine, p. 500	*acidified iodoplatinate spray*
	Sulphamethoxydiazine, p. 552	diazotisation followed by *alkaline betanaphthol spray*

Rf	*Compound*	*Primary Location Reagent*
0·60, streaking	Dipipanone, p. 317	*acidified iodoplatinate spray*
0·61	Adiphenine, p. 175	*acidified iodoplatinate spray*
	Amodiaquine, p. 190	*acidified iodoplatinate spray*
	Betaprodine, p. 221	*acidified iodoplatinate spray*
	Butriptyline, p. 231	*acidified iodoplatinate spray*
	Diethazine, p. 300	*acidified iodoplatinate spray*
	Diprophylline, p. 317	*potassium permanganate spray*
	Fenpiprane, p. 345	*acidified iodoplatinate spray*
	Hydrastine, p. 368	*acidified iodoplatinate spray*
	Isomethadone, p. 382	*acidified iodoplatinate spray*
	Paraphenylenediamine, p. 467	*acidified iodoplatinate spray*
	Pericyazine, p. 475	*acidified iodoplatinate spray*
	Pipradrol, p. 505	*acidified iodoplatinate spray*
	Procaine, p. 513	*acidified iodoplatinate spray*
	Propiomazine, p. 520	*acidified iodoplatinate spray*
	Tranylcypromine, p. 579	*acidified iodoplatinate spray*
	Veratrine, p. 594	*iodine vapour*
0·62	Acriflavine, p. 175	ultraviolet light—yellow-green fluorescence
	Ajmaline, p. 177	*potassium permanganate spray*
	Biperiden, p. 223	*acidified iodoplatinate spray*
	Colchicine, p. 269	p-*dimethylaminobenzaldehyde spray*
	Leucinocaine, p. 389	*acidified iodoplatinate spray*
	Nalorphine, p. 434	*acidified iodoplatinate spray*
	Noscapine, p. 451	*acidified iodoplatinate spray*
	Pipamazine, p. 501	*acidified iodoplatinate spray*
	Sulphadimidine, p. 548	diazotisation followed by *alkaline betanaphthol spray*
	Thurfyl Nicotinate, p. 574	*acidified iodoplatinate spray*
	Xenysalate, p. 596	*acidified iodoplatinate spray*
0·63	Aletamine, p. 178	*acidified iodoplatinate spray*
	Butethamate, p. 230	*acidified iodoplatinate spray*
	Caffeine, p. 234	*strongly acid iodoplatinate spray*
	Cinchocaine, p. 262	*acidified iodoplatinate spray*
	Clorprenaline, p. 267	*potassium permanganate spray*
	Diethylthiambutene, p. 302	*acidified iodoplatinate spray*
	Dihydroergotamine, p. 305	p-*dimethylaminobenzaldehyde spray*
	Ethopropazine, p. 337	*acidified iodoplatinate spray*
	Levallorphan, p. 390	*acidified iodoplatinate spray*
	Naepaine, p. 433	*acidified iodoplatinate spray*
	Oxybuprocaine, p. 459	*acidified iodoplatinate spray*
	Protokylol, p. 523	*potassium permanganate spray*
	Pyrazinamide, p. 527	*iodine–carbon tetrachloride spray*
	Thiabendazole, p. 568	*acidified iodoplatinate spray*
0·64	Betameprodine, p. 220	*acidified iodoplatinate spray*
	Etoxeridine, p. 341	*acidified iodoplatinate spray*
	Iproniazid, p. 381	*potassium permanganate spray*
	Leptazol, p. 389	*acidified iodoplatinate spray*
	Metronidazole, p. 429	*potassium permanganate spray*
	Pemoline, p. 470	*potassium permanganate spray*
	Sulphadiazine, p. 547	diazotisation followed by *alkaline betanaphthol spray*
	Sulphasomidine, p. 556	diazotisation followed by *alkaline betanaphthol spray*
0·65	Cycrimine, p. 277	*acidified iodoplatinate spray*
	Ethomoxane, p. 337	*acidified iodoplatinate spray*

Rf	*Compound*	*Primary Location Reagent*
0·65	Methyldopate, p. 423	*potassium permanganate spray*
	Methyridine, p. 427	*acidified iodoplatinate spray*
	Metyrapone, p. 429	*acidified iodoplatinate spray*
	Nicotinyl Alcohol, p. 442	*iodine–carbon tetrachloride spray*
	Phenazone, p. 480	*acidified iodoplatinate spray*
	Piperoxan, p. 504	*acidified iodoplatinate spray*
	Prilocaine, p. 510	*iodine–carbon tetrachloride spray*
	Sulphadimethoxine, p. 548	diazotisation followed by *alkaline betanaphthol spray*
	Sulphafurazole, p. 549	diazotisation followed by *alkaline betanaphthol spray*
	Sulphaguanidine, p. 550	diazotisation followed by *alkaline betanaphthol spray*
	Sulphamerazine, p. 550	diazotisation followed by *alkaline betanaphthol spray*
	Sulphamethizole, p. 551	diazotisation followed by *alkaline betanaphthol spray*
	Sulphamethoxazole, p. 552	diazotisation followed by *alkaline betanaphthol spray*
	Sulphamethoxypyridazine, p. 553	diazotisation followed by *alkaline betanaphthol spray*
	Triacetyloleandomycin, p. 580	*acidified iodoplatinate spray*
	Tropicamide, p. 589	*acidified iodoplatinate spray*
0·66	Ambazone, p. 182	*potassium permanganate spray*
	Amidopyrine, p. 185	*acidified iodoplatinate spray*
	Amylocaine, p. 196	*acidified iodoplatinate spray*
	Captodiame, p. 236	*acidified iodoplatinate spray*
	Caramiphen, p. 237	*acidified iodoplatinate spray*
	Dextropropoxyphene, p. 290	*acidified iodoplatinate spray*
	Dicyclomine, p. 299	*acidified iodoplatinate spray*
	Furethidine, p. 351	*acidified iodoplatinate spray*
	Hydroxyzine, p. 376	*acidified iodoplatinate spray*
	Lysergide, p. 395	p-*dimethylaminobenzaldehyde spray*
	Methysergide, p. 427	p-*dimethylaminobenzaldehyde spray*
	Papaverine, p. 464	*acidified iodoplatinate spray*
	Phenazocine, p. 479	*acidified iodoplatinate spray*
	Piperidolate, p. 503	*acidified iodoplatinate spray*
	Sulphasalazine, p. 555	no reagent—visible orange spot
	Sulphasomizole, p. 556	diazotisation followed by *alkaline betanaphthol spray*
	Sulphathiazole, p. 557	diazotisation followed by *alkaline betanaphthol spray*
	Tetramisole, p. 564	*acidified iodoplatinate spray*
0·67	Butacaine, p. 228	*acidified iodoplatinate spray*
	Chlordiazepoxide, p. 248	*acidified iodoplatinate spray*
	Ergometrine, p. 328	p-*dimethylaminobenzaldehyde spray*
	Ethionamide, p. 335	*acidified iodoplatinate spray*
	Lincomycin, p. 393	*potassium permanganate spray*
	Methimazole, p. 413	*acidified iodoplatinate spray*
	Nikethamide, p. 443	*iodine vapour*
	Pentamidine, p. 472	*acidified iodoplatinate spray*
	Piminodine, p. 501	*acidified iodoplatinate spray*
	Pramoxine, p. 508	*acidified iodoplatinate spray*
	Sulphaethidole, p. 549	diazotisation followed by *alkaline betanaphthol spray*
	Sulphanilamide, p. 553	diazotisation followed by *alkaline betanaphthol spray*
	Sulphapyridine, p. 555	diazotisation followed by *alkaline betanaphthol spray*
	Sulphormethoxine, p. 558	diazotisation followed by *alkaline betanaphthol spray*

Rf	*Compound*	*Primary Location Reagent*
0·67	Thiopropazate, p. 572	*acidified iodoplatinate spray*
	Viprynium Embonate, p. 595	*potassium permanganate spray*
0·68	Amisometradine, p. 189	*potassium permanganate spray*
	Bamifylline, p. 206	*acidified iodoplatinate spray*
	Benzhexol, p. 213	*acidified iodoplatinate spray*
	Buphenine, p. 227	*potassium permanganate spray*
	Doxapram, p. 322	*acidified iodoplatinate spray*
	Ergotamine, p. 328	p-*dimethylaminobenzaldehyde spray*
	Harmine, p. 359	*acidified iodoplatinate spray*
	Norharman, p. 448	*acidified iodoplatinate spray*
	Pipethanate, p. 505	*acidified iodoplatinate spray*
	Pyrimethamine, p. 528	*acidified iodoplatinate spray*
	Solanidine, p. 541	*iodine–carbon tetrachloride spray*
0·69	Benzquinamide, p. 216	*acidified iodoplatinate spray*
	Deptropine, p. 283	*potassium permanganate spray*
	Dioxyline, p. 313	*acidified iodoplatinate spray*
	Haloperidol, p. 357	*acidified iodoplatinate spray*
	Sulphaphenazole, p. 554	diazotisation followed by *alkaline betanaphthol spray*
0·70	Aminosalicylic Acid, p. 188	p-*dimethylaminobenzaldehyde spray*
	Benzyl Nicotinate, p. 218	*potassium permanganate spray*
	Bisacodyl, p. 223	*acidified iodoplatinate spray*
	Butanilicaine, p. 229	*acidified iodoplatinate spray*
	Clonitazene, p. 266	*acidified iodoplatinate spray*
	Dextromoramide, p. 290	*acidified iodoplatinate spray*
	Ethosuximide, p. 338	*iodine vapour*
	Etonitazene, p. 341	*acidified iodoplatinate spray*
	Harman, p. 358	*acidified iodoplatinate spray*
	Hexetidine, p. 361	*acidified iodoplatinate spray*
	Levomoramide, p. 391	*acidified iodoplatinate spray*
	Mepivacaine, p. 402	*acidified iodoplatinate spray*
	Methaqualone, p. 411	*acidified iodoplatinate spray*
	Methocarbamol, p. 414	*strongly acid iodoplatinate spray*
	Methylergometrine, p. 424	p-*dimethylaminobenzaldehyde spray*
	Pargyline, p. 469	*acidified iodoplatinate spray*
	Phenazopyridine, p. 480	*potassium permanganate spray*
	Protoveratrine B, p. 523	*acidified iodoplatinate spray*
	Racemoramide, p. 534	*acidified iodoplatinate spray*
	Sulphacetamide, p. 546	diazotisation followed by *alkaline betanaphthol spray*
	Tolycaine, p. 578	*acidified iodoplatinate spray*
0·71	Aconitine, p. 174	*acidified iodoplatinate spray*
	Amiphenazole, p. 188	*acidified iodoplatinate spray*
	Amolanone, p. 191	*acidified iodoplatinate spray*
	Amprotropine, p. 194	*acidified iodoplatinate spray*
	Bupivacaine, p. 228	*acidified iodoplatinate spray*
	Diethylpropion, p. 301	*acidified iodoplatinate spray*
	Dihydroergotoxine Mesylate, p. 305	p-*dimethylaminobenzaldehyde spray*
	Fentanyl, p. 345	*acidified iodoplatinate spray*
	Lignocaine, p. 392	*acidified iodoplatinate spray*
	Orthocaine, p. 456	p-*dimethylaminobenzaldehyde spray*
	Prenylamine, p. 509	*acidified iodoplatinate spray*
	Sulphaquinoxaline, p. 555	diazotisation followed by *alkaline betanaphthol spray*
	Thiambutosine, p. 569	*nitrogen dioxide vapour*

Rf	*Compound*	*Primary Location Reagent*
0·72	Acetorphine, p. 172	*acidified iodoplatinate spray*
	Aniline, p. 197	p-*dimethylaminobenzaldehyde spray*
	Azapetine, p. 205	*acidified iodoplatinate spray*
	Carbimazole, p. 238	*acidified iodoplatinate spray*
	Chlormethiazole, p. 250	*acidified iodoplatinate spray*
	Chlorpropamide, p. 257	*potassium permanganate spray*
	Cinnarizine, p. 263	*acidified iodoplatinate spray*
	Clemizole, p. 264	*acidified iodoplatinate spray*
	Cropropamide, p. 272	*potassium permanganate spray*
	Dioxaphetyl Butyrate, p. 313	*acidified iodoplatinate spray*
	Diperodon, p. 314	*acidified iodoplatinate spray*
	Dipyridamole, p. 318	*acidified iodoplatinate spray*
	Embutramide, p. 325	*potassium permanganate spray*
	Etorphine, p. 341	*acidified iodoplatinate spray*
	Etymide, p. 342	*acidified iodoplatinate spray*
	Isocarboxazid, p. 382	*potassium permanganate spray*
	Ketamine, p. 387	*acidified iodoplatinate spray*
	Norbormide, p. 446	*acidified iodoplatinate spray*
	Phenomorphan, p. 488	*acidified iodoplatinate spray*
	Phenyramidol, p. 495	*potassium permanganate spray*
	Protoveratrine A, p. 523	*iodine–carbon tetrachloride spray*
0·73	Anileridine, p. 197	*acidified iodoplatinate spray*
	Benzethidine, p. 212	*acidified iodoplatinate spray*
	Benzocaine, p. 214	p-*dimethylaminobenzaldehyde spray*
	Benzphetamine, p. 215	*acidified iodoplatinate spray*
	Carbamazepine, p. 238	*potassium permanganate spray*
	Cephaloridine, p. 243	*potassium permanganate spray*
	Crotethamide, p. 272	*potassium permanganate spray*
	Ergotoxine, p. 329	p-*dimethylaminobenzaldehyde spray*
	Fluanisone, p. 346	*potassium permanganate spray*
	Oxypertine, p. 461	*acidified iodoplatinate spray*
	Phenampromide, p. 479	*acidified iodoplatinate spray*
	Propanidid, p. 519	*Dragendorff spray*
0·74	Hydroxyphenamate, p. 375	p-*dimethylaminobenzaldehyde spray*
	Isoxsuprine, p. 386	*potassium permanganate spray*
	Nitrazepam, p. 443	*Dragendorff spray*
	Styramate, p. 546	p-*dimethylaminobenzaldehyde spray*
0·75	Cetoxime, p. 243	*potassium permanganate spray*
	Cyprenorphine, p. 278	*acidified iodoplatinate spray*
	Deserpidine, p. 284	*acidified iodoplatinate spray*
	Diazepam, p. 294	*Dragendorff spray*
	Fenimide, p. 344	*strongly acid iodoplatinate spray*
	Glutethimide, p. 353	*strongly acid iodoplatinate spray*
	Monosulfiram, p. 430	*acidified iodoplatinate spray*
	Octaverine, p. 452	*potassium permanganate spray*
	Phenoperidine, p. 488	*acidified iodoplatinate spray*
	Phenprobamate, p. 491	*strongly acid iodoplatinate spray*
	Phensuximide, p. 491	*iodine–carbon tetrachloride spray*
0·76	Ethinamate, p. 334	*furfural–hydrochloric acid spray*
	Methsuximide, p. 418	*iodine–carbon tetrachloride spray*
	Pheneturide, p. 483	*iodine–carbon tetrachloride spray*
	Phenoxybenzamine, p. 489	*acidified iodoplatinate spray*
	Tolbutamide, p. 576	*acidified iodoplatinate spray*

Rf	*Compound*	*Primary Location Reagent*
0·77	Bephenium Hydroxynaphthoate, p. 219	*potassium permanganate spray*
	Cyclothiazide, p. 277	*potassium permanganate spray*
	Isobutyl Aminobenzoate, p. 381	diazotisation followed by *alkaline betanaphthol spray*
	Mephenesin, p. 401	*Marquis reagent*
	Methoserpidine, p. 415	*acidified iodoplatinate spray*
	Oxyphenbutazone, p. 462	*potassium permanganate spray*
	Phenadoxone, p. 478	*acidified iodoplatinate spray*
	Rescinnamine, p. 535	*potassium permanganate spray*
	Reserpine, p. 535	*potassium permanganate spray*
	Tybamate, p. 591	*iodine–carbon tetrachloride spray*
0·78	Carbutamide, p. 241	diazotisation followed by *alkaline betanaphthol spray*
	Syrosingopine, p. 559	*potassium permanganate spray*
0·79	Diphenoxylate, p. 316	*acidified iodoplatinate spray*
	Hyoscine Butylbromide, p. 377	*acidified iodoplatinate spray*
	Phenylbutazone, p. 492	*potassium permanganate spray*
0·80	Acinitrazole, p. 174	*potassium permanganate spray*
	Meclozine, p. 398	*acidified iodoplatinate spray*
	Trichlormethiazide, p. 581	*iodine–carbon tetrachloride spray*

SYSTEM T2 (p. 46)—Rf Values

Rf	*Compound*
0·38	Antazoline, p. 198
0·48	Brompheniramine, p. 225
0·49	Chlorcyclizine, p. 247
0·52	Chlorpheniramine, p. 254
0·53	Diphenhydramine, p. 315
0·56	Mepyramine, p. 403
	Methapyrilene, p. 410
0·59	Thonzylamine, p. 574
0·60	Doxylamine, p. 322
0·62	Tripelennamine, p. 588
0·63	Bromodiphenhydramine, p. 224
	Carbinoxamine, p. 239
	Pheniramine, p. 485
0·65	Phenindamine, p. 484
0·66	Chloropyrilene, p. 251
0·70	Chlordiazepoxide, p. 248
0·81	Triprolidine, p. 588
0·84	Hydroxyzine, p. 376

SYSTEM T3 (p. 47)—Rf Values

Rf	*Compound*
0·10	Chlordiazepoxide, p. 248
0·27	Hydroxyzine, p. 376
0·31	Antazoline, p. 198
0·33	Carbinoxamine, p. 239
0·34	Fluphenazine, p. 348
0·36	Perphenazine, p. 475
0·40	Chlorpheniramine, p. 254
	Methdilazine, p. 412
	Triprolidine, p. 588
0·42	Brompheniramine, p. 225
0·52	Doxylamine, p. 322
0·62	Promazine, p. 517
0·65	Thonzylamine, p. 574
0·68	Pheniramine, p. 485
0·69	Trifluoperazine, p. 584
0·70	Chloropyrilene, p. 251
	Prochlorperazine, p. 514
	Promethazine, p. 518
0·74	Amitriptyline, p. 189
	Methoxypromazine, p. 418
0·80	Chlorprothixene, p. 258
0·82	Mepyramine, p. 403
0·83	Methapyrilene, p. 410
0·84	Pyrrobutamine, p. 529
0·86	Bromodiphenhydramine, p. 224
	Imipramine, p. 379
0·90	Chlorcyclizine, p. 247
	Phenindamine, p. 484
0·91	Diphenhydramine, p. 315
0·92	Tripelennamine, p. 588
0·94	Chlorpromazine, p. 256
0·95	Fluopromazine, p. 347
0·96	Trimeprazine, p. 585
0·97	Thiopropazate, p. 572
	Thioridazine, p. 573

SYSTEM T4 (p. 48)—Rf Values

Rf	*Compound*
0·27	Prochlorperazine, p. 514
0·33	Trifluoperazine, p. 584
0·38	Promazine, p. 517
0·38, tailing	Doxylamine, p. 322
	Pheniramine, p. 485
0·40, tailing	Carbinoxamine, p. 239
0·41, tailing	Chlorpheniramine, p. 254
0·43, tailing	Mepyramine, p. 403
0·44	Perphenazine, p. 475
0·47, tailing	Brompheniramine, p. 225
0·48, tailing	Tripelennamine, p. 588
	Triprolidine, p. 588
0·52, tailing	Methapyrilene, p. 410
0·56, tailing	Chloropyrilene, p. 251
0·57	Pecazine, p. 470
	Thonzylamine, p. 574
0·58	Fluphenazine, p. 348
	Methoxypromazine, p. 418
0·59	Promethazine, p. 518
0·61	Diphenhydramine, p. 315
	Methdilazine, p. 412
0·64	Trimeprazine, p. 585
0·65	Amitriptyline, p. 189
	Thioridazine, p. 573
0·67	Chlordiazepoxide, p. 248
	Phenindamine, p. 484
	Thiopropazate, p. 572
0·68	Chlorcyclizine, p. 247
0·70	Chlorpromazine, p. 256
	Hydroxyzine, p. 376
0·72	Antazoline, p. 198
	Pipamazine, p. 501
0·73	Chlorprothixene, p. 258
0·77	Imipramine, p. 379
0·79	Fluopromazine, p. 347
0·80	Bromodiphenhydramine, p. 224
0·82	Pyrrobutamine, p. 529

SYSTEM T5 (p. 48)—Rf Values

Rf	*Compound*
0·16	Brompheniramine, p. 225
	Methdilazine, p. 412
0·17	Carbinoxamine, p. 239
	Doxylamine, p. 322
0·19	Pheniramine, p. 485
0·20	Chlorpheniramine, p. 254
	Thioridazine, p. 573
0·22	Promethazine, p. 518
0·23	Tripelennamine, p. 588
0·24	Methoxypromazine, p. 418
0·25	Diphenhydramine, p. 315
0·26	Triprolidine, p. 588
0·27	Mepyramine, p. 403
0·29	Chloropyrilene, p. 251
	Imipramine, p. 379
	Pecazine, p. 470
0·30	Chlorpromazine, p. 256
	Methapyrilene, p. 410
	Trimeprazine, p. 585
0·32	Prochlorperazine, p. 514
	Pyrrobutamine, p. 529
	Thonzylamine, p. 574
0·33	Bromodiphenhydramine, p. 224
0·37	Promazine, p. 517
0·39	Amitriptyline, p. 189
0·40	Antazoline, p. 198
	Chlorcyclizine, p. 247
	Fluopromazine, p. 347
	Trifluoperazine, p. 584
0·46	Chlorprothixene, p. 258
0·48	Perphenazine, p. 475
	Phenindamine, p. 484
0·56	Pipamazine, p. 501
0·62	Hydroxyzine, p. 376
0·68	Fluphenazine, p. 348
0·70	Thiopropazate, p. 572
0·73	Chlordiazepoxide, p. 248

SYSTEM T6[a] (p. 49)—Rf Values

Rf	*Compound*
0·43	Thioproperazine, p. 572
0·47	Thiethylperazine, p. 570
0·51	Promazine, p. 517
0·55	Prochlorperazine, p. 514
0·56	Dimethoxanate, p. 309
0·58	Acepromazine, p. 169
0·62	Chlorpromazine, p. 256
0·63	Trifluoperazine, p. 584
0·64	Isothipendyl, p. 385
	Methdilazine, p. 412
0·65	Perphenazine, p. 475
0·66	Chlorprothixene, p. 258
	Promethazine, p. 518
0·67	Methoxypromazine, p. 418
0·69	Acetophenazine, p. 172
	Diethazine, p. 300
	Fluopromazine, p. 347
	Phenothiazine, p. 489
	Prothipendyl, p. 522
0·70	Ethopropazine, p. 337
0·71	Carphenazine, p. 242
	Thioridazine, p. 573
	Trimeprazine, p. 585
0·75	Fluphenazine, p. 348
0·77	Propiomazine, p. 520
	Thiopropazate, p. 572
0·83	Pipamazine, p. 501

SYSTEM T6[b] (p. 49)—Rf Values

Rf	*Compound*
0·15	Prochlorperazine, p. 514
0·16	Acetophenazine, p. 172
	Carphenazine, p. 242
0·25	Thiopropazate, p. 572
0·26	Thioproperazine, p. 572
0·28	Thiethylperazine, p. 570
0·35	Methoxypromazine, p. 418
0·37	Phenothiazine, p. 489
	Promazine, p. 517
0·38	Promethazine, p. 518
0·39	Acepromazine, p. 169
0·41	Dimethoxanate, p. 309
	Isothipendyl, p. 385
	Trifluoperazine, p. 584
0·43	Methdilazine, p. 412
0·44	Diethazine, p. 300
0·45	Chlorprothixene, p. 258
	Perphenazine, p. 475
0·46	Thioridazine, p. 573
0·47	Ethopropazine, p. 337
0·48	Chlorpromazine, p. 256
	Prothipendyl, p. 522
0·50	Fluopromazine, p. 347
	Trimeprazine, p. 585
0·53	Pipamazine, p. 501
0·54	Propiomazine, p. 520
0·59	Fluphenazine, p. 348

SYSTEM T7 (p. 50)—Rf Values

Rf	*Compound*
0·04	Normorphine, p. 450
0·10	Dihydromorphine, p. 305
0·11	Morphine, p. 431
0·13	Norcodeine, p. 447
0·17	Hydromorphone, p. 371
0·35	Nalorphine, p. 434
0·39	Codeine, p. 268
0·41	Hydrocodone, p. 369
0·46	Ethylmorphine, p. 340
0·47	Ketobemidone, p. 387
0·64	6-Monoacetylmorphine, p. 430
0·76	Diamorphine, p. 292
0·80	Dextrorphan, p. 291
	Levorphanol, p. 391
0·91	Levomethorphan, p. 390
0·93	Alphaprodine, p. 182
0·97	Dextropropoxyphene, p. 290
	Pethidine, p. 476
	Phenazocine, p. 479
0·98	Levallorphan, p. 390
0·99	Methadone, p. 408
	Piminodine, p. 501

SYSTEM T8 (p. 51)—Rf Values

Rf	*Compound*
0·21	Dihydromorphine, p. 305
	Hydromorphone, p. 371
0·25	Ethylmorphine, p. 340
	Hydrocodone, p. 369
0·27	Morphine, p. 431
0·29	Codeine, p. 268
0·35	Diamorphine, p. 292
0·39	Ketobemidone, p. 387
0·40	Alphaprodine, p. 182
	6-Monoacetylmorphine, p. 430
0·41	Pethidine, p. 476
0·43	Levomethorphan, p. 390
0·47	Dextrorphan, p. 291
	Levorphanol, p. 391
0·48	Normorphine, p. 450
0·50	Norcodeine, p. 447
0·55	Nalorphine, p. 434
0·59	Methadone, p. 408
0·68	Dextropropoxyphene, p. 290
0·70	Levallorphan, p. 390
0·73	Piminodine, p. 501
0·87	Phenazocine, p. 479

SYSTEM T9[i] (p. 51)—Rf Values

Rf	*Compound*
0·05	Lysergic Acid, p. 395
0·18	Ergometrine Maleate, p. 328
0·35	Dihydroergotamine, p. 305
0·45	Ergotoxine, p. 329
0·52	Ergotamine Tartrate, p. 328
0·60	Lysergide, p. 395
0·69	Ergotoxine, p. 329
0·71	Ergocristine, p. 329
0·81	Ergotoxine, p. 329

SYSTEM T9[ii] (p. 51)—Rf Values

Rf	*Compound*
0·19	Ergometrine Maleate, p. 328
0·23	Methylergometrine, p. 424
0·35	Methysergide, p. 427
0·45	Dihydroergotamine, p. 305
0·51	Ergotamine Tartrate, p. 328
0·61	Lysergide, p. 395

SYSTEM T9[iii] (p. 51)—Rf Values

Rf	*Compound*
0·01	Lysergic Acid, p. 395
0·18	Lysergamide, p. 395
0·23	Ergometrine Maleate, p. 328
0·30	Methylergometrine, p. 424
0·49	Methysergide, p. 427
0·56	Dihydroergotamine, p. 305
0·58	Ergotamine Tartrate, p. 328
0·63	Lysergide, p. 395
0·78	Ergotoxine, p. 329

SYSTEM T10 (p. 52)—Rf Values

Rf	*Compound*
0·12	Phenylmethylbarbituric Acid, p. 494
0·20	Phenytoin, p. 496
0·22	Barbitone, p. 207
0·24	Phenobarbitone, p. 486
	Probarbital, p. 511
0·26	Bromvaletone, p. 225
0·27	Allobarbitone, p. 179
0·28	Butallylonal, p. 229
	Vinbarbitone, p. 594
0·30	Aprobarbitone, p. 200
0·31	Heptabarbitone, p. 359
0·32	Cyclobarbitone, p. 274
0·33	Amylobarbitone, p. 195
0·33	Butobarbitone, p. 231
	Pentobarbitone, p. 473
0·36	Allylbarbituric Acid, p. 179
0·38	Nealbarbitone, p. 437
0·39	Bemegride, p. 209
0·44	Quinalbarbitone, p. 530
0·50	Carbromal, p. 240
	Hexobarbitone, p. 362
0·52	Glutethimide, p. 353
0·55	Metharbitone, p. 412
0·59	Methylphenobarbitone, p. 425
0·67	Methohexitone, p. 415
0·68	Thiopentone, p. 571
0·69	Thialbarbitone, p. 569

SYSTEM T11 (p. 52)—Rf Values

Rf	*Compound*
0·32	Ethchlorvynol, p. 333
0·36	Phenobarbitone, p. 486
0·38	Barbitone, p. 207
0·40	Pentobarbitone, p. 473
0·42	Amylobarbitone, p. 195
0·43	Allobarbitone, p. 179
0·46	Quinalbarbitone, p. 530
0·48	Allylbarbituric Acid, p. 179
0·49	Hexobarbitone, p. 362
0·49	Secbutobarbitone, p. 540
0·53	Metharbitone, p. 412
0·54	Glutethimide, p. 353
0·55	Cyclobarbitone, p. 274
0·65	Ethinamate, p. 334
0·73	Thiopentone, p. 571
0·75	Methohexitone, p. 415
0·81	Methyprylone, p. 426
0·85	Methylphenobarbitone, p. 425

SYSTEM T12 (p. 53)—Rf Values

Rf	*Compound*
0·26	Phenobarbitone, p. 486
0·38	Cyclobarbitone, p. 274
0·40	Barbitone, p. 207
0·45	Methyprylone, p. 426
0·48	Allobarbitone, p. 179
0·49	Pentobarbitone, p. 473
0·50	Allylbarbituric Acid, p. 179
0·52	Amylobarbitone, p. 195
	Secbutobarbitone, p. 540
0·54	Quinalbarbitone, p. 530
0·55	Ethinamate, p. 334
0·58	Hexobarbitone, p. 362
0·60	Methylphenobarbitone, p. 425
0·66	Metharbitone, p. 412
0·70	Thiopentone, p. 571
0·78	Methohexitone, p. 415
0·95	Ethchlorvynol, p. 333
0·99	Glutethimide, p. 353

SYSTEM T13 (p. 54)—Rf Values

Rf	*Compound*
0·50	Barbitone, p. 207
	Methyprylone, p. 426
	Phenobarbitone, p. 486
0·55	Allobarbitone, p. 179
0·57	Pentobarbitone, p. 473
0·60	Amylobarbitone, p. 195
0·62	Secbutobarbitone, p. 540
0·64	Quinalbarbitone, p. 530
0·67	Allylbarbituric Acid, p. 179
0·68	Cyclobarbitone, p. 274
0·77	Hexobarbitone, p. 362
0·80	Glutethimide, p. 353
0·81	Ethinamate, p. 334
0·85	Metharbitone, p. 412
0·92	Methohexitone, p. 415
0·94	Thiopentone, p. 571
0·95	Ethchlorvynol, p. 333
0·98	Methylphenobarbitone, p. 425

SYSTEM T14 (p. 54)—Rf Values

Rf	*Compound*
0·09	Ouabain, p. 457
0·27	Deslanoside, p. 286
0·36	Lanatoside C, p. 388
0·62	Digoxin, p. 303
0·72	Digitoxin, p. 302
0·82	Acetyldigitoxin, p. 173

SYSTEM T15 (p. 54)—Rf Values

Rf	*Compound*
0·14	Azinphos-methyl, p. 205
0·29	Malathion, p. 396
0·50	Diazinon, p. 294

SYSTEM T16 (p. 55)—Rf Values

Rf	*Compound*
0·03	Dimethoate, p. 309
0·19	Demeton-S, p. 282
0·38	Diazinon, p. 294
0·40	Azinphos-methyl, p. 205
0·45	Malathion, p. 396
0·60	Demeton-O, p. 282

SYSTEM T17 (p. 55)—Rf Values

Rf	*Compound*
0·19	Salicyluric Acid, p. 202
0·34	Gentisic Acid, p. 202
0·50	Aspirin, p. 201
0·57	Salicylic Acid, p. 539

SYSTEM T18 (p. 56)—Rf Values

Rf	*Compound*
0·19	Hydrocortisone, p. 370
0·26	Betamethasone, p. 220
0·50	Triamcinolone Acetonide, p. 580
0·53	Fluocinolone Acetonide, p. 346
	Prednisolone Acetate, p. 508
0·66	Hydrocortisone Acetate, p. 370
0·71	Betamethasone 17-Valerate, p. 220
0·79	Dexamethasone Acetate, p. 287
	Prednisone Acetate, p. 509
0·87	Fludrocortisone Acetate, p. 346
1·10	Prednisolone Pivalate, p. 508
1·92	Deoxycortone Acetate, p. 283
2·22	Deoxycortone Pivalate, p. 283

SYSTEM T19 (p. 56)—Rf Values

Rf	*Compound*
0·18	Hydrocortisone Hydrogen Succinate, p. 370
0·59	Triamcinolone, p. 580
0·83	Prednisolone, p. 508
1·00	Betamethasone, p. 220
1·00	Dexamethasone, p. 287
1·21	Prednisone, p. 509
1·39	Triamcinolone Acetonide, p. 580
1·40	Fluocinolone Acetonide, p. 346
1·88	Cortisone Acetate, p. 271

SYSTEM T20 (p. 56)—Rf Values

Rf	*Compound*
0·07	Oestriol, p. 454
0·37	Oestradiol, p. 453
0·58	Oestrone, p. 454

SYSTEM T21a (p. 57)—Rf Values

Rf	*Compound*
0·30	Cholesterol, p. 261
0·32	Cholecalciferol, p. 260
0·33	Calciferol, p. 234

SYSTEM T21b (p. 57)—Rf Values

Rf	*Compound*
0·41	Cholesterol, p. 261
0·44	Calciferol, p. 234
0·44	Cholecalciferol, p. 260

SYSTEM T21c (p. 57)—Rf Values

Rf	*Compound*
0·15	Calciferol, p. 234
0·15	Cholecalciferol, p. 260

SYSTEM T22 (p. 57)—Rf Values

Rf	*Compound*
0·42	Sulphacetamide, p. 546
0·47	Sulphadiazine, p. 547
0·50	Sulphathiazole, p. 557
0·53	Sulphanilamide, p. 553
0·57	Sulphamerazine, p. 550
0·64	Sulphadimidine, p. 548
0·66	Sulphaquinoxaline, p. 555

SYSTEM T23 (p. 58)—Rf Values

Rf	*Compound*
0·43	Succinylsulphathiazole, p. 546
0·51	Phthalylsulphacetamide, p. 497
0·61	Phthalylsulphathiazole, p. 498

Gas Chromatographic Data

SYSTEM G1/180 (p. 82)—**Retention Time Relative to Diphenhydramine**

RRT	*Compound*
0·28	Warfarin, p. 596
0·37	Barbitone, p. 207
0·40	Methyprylone, p. 426
0·44	Probarbital, p. 511
0·60	Phenacetin, p. 477
0·69	Amylobarbitone, p. 195
	Pethidine, p. 476
0·73	Pentobarbitone, p. 473
0·74	Hydroxyphenamate, p. 375
0·83	Pheniramine, p. 485
0·87	Caffeine, p. 234
	Quinalbarbitone, p. 530
1·00	Glutethimide, p. 353
1·01	Meprobamate, p. 403
1·03	Lignocaine, p. 392
1·20	Methylphenobarbitone, p. 425
1·54	Tripelennamine, p. 588
1·56	Chlorpheniramine, p. 254
	Methapyrilene, p. 410
1·80	Phenobarbitone, p. 486
1·81	Procaine, p. 513
2·78	Methadone, p. 408
2·82	Bromodiphenhydramine, p. 224
3·17	Dextropropoxyphene, p. 290
3·22	Atropine, p. 202
3·38	Thonzylamine, p. 574
3·56	Chlorcyclizine, p. 247
3·95	Amethocaine, p. 184
6·00	Dicophane, p. 297

SYSTEM G1/250 (p. 82)—**Retention Time Relative to Codeine**

RRT	*Compound*
0·72	Chlorcyclizine, p. 247
0·89	Antazoline, p. 198
	Chlordiazepoxide, p. 248
	Hyoscine, p. 376
	Promazine, p. 517
1·05	Phenytoin, p. 496
1·11	Ethylmorphine, p. 340
1·22	Chlorpromazine, p. 256
1·28	Morphine, p. 431
1·44	Chloroquine, p. 252
1·55	Cinchonidine, p. 262
	Cinchonine, p. 263
1·67	Diamorphine, p. 292
1·72	Cinchocaine, p. 262
2·44	Anileridine, p. 197
	Quinidine, p. 531
	Quinine, p. 532
3·44	Meclozine, p. 398
4·83	Strychnine, p. 545

SYSTEM G2/120 (p. 82)—**Retention Time Relative to Ephedrine**

RRT	*Compound*
0·10	Tuaminoheptane, p. 590
0·21	Cyclopentamine, p. 275
	Isometheptene, p. 383
0·28	Amphetamine, p. 192
0·33	Phentermine, p. 491
0·34	Propylhexedrine, p. 522
0·40	Methylamphetamine, p. 420
0·43	Pargyline, p. 469
0·45	Tranylcypromine, p. 579
0·46	Fenfluramine, p. 344
0·51	Mephentermine, p. 401
0·62	Aletamine, p. 178
0·77	Chlorphentermine, p. 255
0·82	Norpseudoephedrine, p. 450
0·84	Nicotine, p. 440
0·91	Methoxyphenamine, p. 418
1·00	Pseudoephedrine, p. 525
1·13	Methylephedrine, p. 423
1·25	Phenmetrazine, p. 486
1·40	Phendimetrazine, p. 481
1·50	Etafedrine, p. 330
	Phenoxypropazine, p. 490
1·60	Diethylpropion, p. 301
1·90	Leptazol, p. 389
	Nikethamide, p. 443
3·40	Prolintane, p. 517
3·70	Fencamfamin, p. 343
5·50	Methyl Phenidate, p. 419
8·80	Benzphetamine, p. 215

SYSTEM G2/225 (p. 82)—Retention Time Relative to Codeine

RRT	*Compound*
0·20 (0·38; 0·61)	Physostigmine, p. 498
0·21	Diphenhydramine, p. 315
0·36	Homatropine, p. 365
	Naphazoline, p. 435
	Pilocarpine, p. 500
0·37	Bufotenine, p. 227
	Eucatropine, p. 342
0·38	Phenothiazine, p. 489
0·40	Ketobemidone, p. 387
0·45	Carbinoxamine, p. 239
0·49 (0·44)	Norbormide, p. 446
0·50	Dextromethorphan, p. 289
	Quinuronium Sulphate, p. 533
	Racemethorphan, p. 534
0·51	Methaqualone, p. 411
	Pipradrol, p. 505
0·53	Oxypertine, p. 461
	Procyclidine, p. 514
	Propranolol, p. 521
	Thonzylamine, p. 574
0·54	Phenindamine, p. 484
0·55	Methadone, p. 408
	Santonin, p. 540
	Tacrine, p. 560
0·56	Butriptyline, p. 231
	Dieldrin, p. 299
0·56, tailing	Dopamine, p. 321
0·57	Embramine, p. 324
0·58	Amitriptyline, p. 189
	Chloroprocaine, p. 251
0·60	Oxymetazoline, p. 460
0·61	Fluopromazine, p. 347
0·63	Nortriptyline, p. 450
	Procainamide, p. 512
	Racemorphan, p. 534
0·64	Trimipramine, p. 587
0·64, tailing	Mefenamic Acid, p. 399
0·65	Levorphanol, p. 391
	Mepyramine, p. 403
	Primidone, p. 511
0·66	Amolanone, p. 191
0·67	Chlorcyclizine, p. 247
	Harmine, p. 359
0·68	Desipramine, p. 285
	Phenoxybenzamine, p. 489
0·69	Triprolidine, p. 588
0·70	Azacyclonol, p. 204
	Levomethorphan, p. 390
	Protriptyline, p. 524
0·73	Pramoxine, p. 508
0·74	Benzhexol, p. 213
0·75	Dimethindene, p. 307
	Imipramine, p. 379
	Pentazocine, p. 473
	Promethazine, p. 518
0·76	Isothipendyl, p. 385
0·78	Desomorphine, p. 286
	Stilboestrol, p. 543
0·79	Biperiden, p. 223
	Bupivacaine, p. 228
0·81	Carbamazepine, p. 238
	Methyldesorphine, p. 422
0·82	Dicophane, p. 297
0·84	Hyoscine, p. 376
0·85	Etoxeridine, p. 341
	Trimeprazine, p. 585
0·86	Promazine, p. 517
0·88	Propoxycaine, p. 521
0·90	Oxazepam, p. 458
	Piperidolate, p. 503
0·91, tailing	Buphenine, p. 227
0·92	Benztropine, p. 216
0·94	Cyproheptadine, p. 278
0·95	Levallorphan, p. 390
0·98	Prothipendyl, p. 522
1·00	Dihydrocodeine, p. 304
	Ethopropazine, p. 337
	Methyldihydromorphine, p. 422
	Metopon, p. 428
1·00 (1·25)	Phenylbutazone, p. 492
1·04	Diethazine, p. 300
1·10	Ethylmorphine, p. 340
1·14	Pyrrobutamine, p. 529
1·15	Morphine, p. 431
1·16	Diazepam, p. 294
	Hydrocodone, p. 369
1·17	Oxycodone, p. 460
1·20	Dihydromorphine, p. 305
	Xenysalate, p. 596
1·22	Methdilazine, p. 412
1·26	Mebhydrolin, p. 397
1·27	Acetyldihydrocodeine, p. 174
1·28	Dibenzepin, p. 295
1·29	Hydromorphone, p. 371
1·30	Pipethanate, p. 505
1·35	Dipipanone, p. 317
	Phenyramidol, p. 495
1·38	Chlorpromazine, p. 256
1·39	Androsterone, p. 196
1·40	Methixene, p. 414
1·43	Chlorprothixene, p. 258
1·45	6-Monoacetylmorphine, p. 430
1·46	Chlordiazepoxide, p. 248
1·52	Thebacon, p. 565
1·54	Morpheridine, p. 430
1·56	Methotrimeprazine, p. 416
1·58	Pecazine, p. 470
1·60	Oxymorphone, p. 461
	Phenadoxone, p. 478
1·70	Pentaquin, p. 472
	Prenylamine, p. 509

RRT	*Compound*
1·76	Nalorphine, p. 434
1·93	Deptropine, p. 283
2·04	Methyltestosterone, p. 426
2·07	Trimethoprim, p. 586
2·08	Diamorphine, p. 292
2·15	Phenazocine, p. 479
2·25	Clemizole, p. 264
2·28	Trifluoperazine, p. 584
2·44	Acepromazine, p. 169
2·53	Benzethidine, p. 212
2·62	Cinchocaine, p. 262
2·65	Fentanyl, p. 345
2·66	Gallamine, p. 352
2·70	Propiomazine, p. 520
2·76	Captodiame, p. 236
2·94	Nitrazepam, p. 443
3·00	Pseudomorphine, p. 525
3·24	Hexachlorophane, p. 360
3·26	Hydroquinidine, p. 372
3·50	Papaverine, p. 464
3·60	Hydroxyzine, p. 376
4·20	Doxapram, p. 322
4·70	Racemoramide, p. 534
4·86	Dextromoramide, p. 290
5·98	Benzylmorphine, p. 218
6·90	Cinnarizine, p. 263
6·95	Cholesterol, p. 261
16·00	Buclizine, p. 226

SYSTEM G2/225 (p. 82)—Retention Time Relative to Diphenhydramine

RRT	*Compound*
0·24	Chlorphentermine, p. 255
0·25	Ephedrine, p. 327
0·32	Phendimetrazine, p. 481
0·33	Etafedrine, p. 330
	Pheneturide, p. 483
0·35	Sulphonal, p. 558
0·35, 2·91	Chlormezanone, p. 250
0·40	Phenprobamate, p. 491
0·43	Methimazole, p. 413
	Tolazoline, p. 576
0·44	Metronidazole, p. 429
0·48 (1·18; 1·27)	Proheptazine, p. 516
0·50	Nifenazone, p. 442
0·58	Mescaline, p. 404
0·61	Carbimazole, p. 238
0·63	Hydroxyphenamate, p. 375
0·63 (1·27), (2·71)	Dextropropoxyphene, p. 290
0·65	Dicyclomine, p. 299
0·68 (0·29)	Thiambutosine, p. 569
0·69	Chlorzoxazone, p. 260
0·70	Methoxamine, p. 417
0·74	Dimethyltryptamine, p. 311
0·75	Butethamate, p. 230
	Meclofenoxate, p. 398
	Properidine, p. 520
0·77	Chlorpropamide, p. 257
0·78	Pethidine, p. 476
	Tryptamine, p. 590
0·84	Alphaprodine, p. 182
	Betaprodine, p. 221
0·87	Pheniramine, p. 485
0·92	Betameprodine, p. 220
	Tetrahydrozoline, p. 563
	Trimeperidine, p. 584
0·95	Thymoxamine, p. 575
0·98	Piperoxan, p. 504
1·00	Alphameprodine, p. 181
	Ethoheptazine, p. 336
	Ketamine, p. 387
	Lignocaine, p. 392
1·00, tailing	Lachesine Chloride, p. 387
1·10	Dimethylthiambutene, p. 310
	Doxylamine, p. 322
1·28	Orphenadrine, p. 456
1·30	Azapetine, p. 205
	Ethylmethylthiambutene, p. 339
	Methaphenilene, p. 410
	Phencyclidine, p. 481
	Phenyltoloxamine, p. 495
1·35	Xylometazoline, p. 597
1·40	Caramiphen, p. 237
	Hexylcaine, p. 363
1·50	Ethomoxane, p. 337
1·53	Dexchlorpheniramine, p. 289
1·60	Diethylthiambutene, p. 302
1·63	Procaine, p. 513
1·65	Butanilicaine, p. 229
1·66	Cyclopentolate, p. 276
1·70	Amprotropine, p. 194
	Eucatropine, p. 342
	Pipazethate, p. 502
1·75	Apoatropine, p. 198
	Hydroxypethidine, p. 375
1·77	Cyclizine, p. 273
1·80	Butethamine, p. 230
	Chloropyrilene, p. 251
1·90	Chlorphenoxamine, p. 255
	Mepivacaine, p. 402
2·00	Chlophedianol, p. 244
	Dexbrompheniramine, p. 288
2·05	Diphenylpyraline, p. 317
2·10	Carbinoxamine, p. 239
2·20 (1·90)	Methyl Phenidate, p. 419
2·55	Alphamethadol, p. 181

RRT	*Compound*	*RRT*	*Compound*
2·65	Butriptyline, p. 231	3·13	Chlorcyclizine, p. 247
2·70	Alphacetylmethadol, p. 181	3·50	Isothipendyl, p. 385
	Chloroprocaine, p. 251	3·76	Carbamazepine, p. 238
2·91, 0·35	Chlormezanone, p. 250	3·80	Antazoline, p. 198
3·04	Amethocaine, p. 184	4·65	Codeine, p. 268

SYSTEM G3 (p. 82)—Retention Time Relative to Diphenhydramine

RRT	*Compound*	*RRT*	*Compound*
0·57	Hydroxyphenamate, p. 375	2·42	Thonzylamine, p. 574
0·78	Warfarin, p. 596	3·00	Amidopyrine, p. 185
0·92	Dextropropoxyphene, p. 290	3·30	Glutethimide, p. 353
	Pheniramine, p. 485		Procaine, p. 513
1·20	Barbitone, p. 207	3·80	Atropine, p. 202
1·40	Methyprylone, p. 426	3·90	Lignocaine, p. 392
1·57	Phenacetin, p. 477	4·70	Phenobarbitone, p. 486
1·90	Caffeine, p. 234	4·80	Chlordiazepoxide, p. 248
2·00	Amylobarbitone, p. 195	4·85	Promazine, p. 517
2·07	Pentobarbitone, p. 473	5·06	Amethocaine, p. 184
2·10	Benzhexol, p. 213	6·10	Phenazone, p. 480
2·30	Chlorcyclizine, p. 247	6·60	Antazoline, p. 198
2·40	Quinalbarbitone, p. 530	10·70	Hyoscine, p. 376

SYSTEM G4 (p. 83)—Retention Time Relative to Codeine

RRT	*Compound*	*RRT*	*Compound*
0·10	Diphenhydramine, p. 315	0·66	Desomorphine, p. 286
0·22	Dextromethorphan, p. 289	0·69	Amethocaine, p. 184
0·27	Embramine, p. 324	0·72	Ethopropazine, p. 337
	Eucatropine, p. 342	0·75	Bupivacaine, p. 228
0·29	Amitriptyline, p. 189	0·81	Chlorprothixene, p. 258
	Physostigmine, p. 498	0·89	Prenylamine, p. 509
0·30	Phenindamine, p. 484	0·90	Pheniramine, p. 485
0·30 (0·15)	Trimipramine, p. 587	0·95	Dihydrocodeine, p. 304
0·35	Biperiden, p. 223	0·96	Phenadoxone, p. 478
	Metronidazole, p. 429	1·00	Ethylmorphine, p. 340
0·39	Homatropine, p. 365	1·05	Etoxeridine, p. 341
	Thonzylamine, p. 574	1·08	Oxazepam, p. 458
0·42	Benztropine, p. 216	1·10	Methotrimeprazine, p. 416
0·43	Amolanone, p. 191		Pecazine, p. 470
	Pramoxine, p. 508	1·20	Pyrrobutamine, p. 529
0·44	Fluopromazine, p. 347	1·28	Ketobemidone, p. 387
0·46	Procaine, p. 513	1·34	Dibenzepin, p. 295
	Promethazine, p. 518	1·39	Hyoscine, p. 376
0·47	Butanilicaine, p. 229	1·60	Hydroxyzine, p. 376
	Dimethindene, p. 307	1·70	Androsterone, p. 196
	Trimeprazine, p. 585		Benzethidine, p. 212
0·53	Isothipendyl, p. 386	1·77	Diazepam, p. 294
	Methaqualone, p. 411	2·05	Oxycodone, p. 460
	Prothipendyl, p. 522	2·08	Chlordiazepoxide, p. 248
0·55	Dipipanone, p. 317	2·30	Propiomazine, p. 520
0·56	Hydroxypethidine, p. 375	3·00	Cholesterol, p. 261
0·60	Diethazine, p. 300	3·30	Methyltestosterone, p. 426
	Promazine, p. 517	5·80	Doxapram, p. 322

SYSTEM G4 (p. 83)—Retention Time Relative to Diphenhydramine

RRT	*Compound*
0·30	Chlorphentermine, p. 255
0·40	Betameprodine, p. 220
0·41	Betaprodine, p. 221
0·46	Proheptazine, p. 516
0·48	Alphameprodine, p. 181
0·50	Hydroxyphenamate, p. 375
0·58	Butethamate, p. 230
0·60	Dextropropoxyphene, p. 290
0·65	Properidine, p. 520
0·74	Dimethylthiambutene, p. 310
0·75	Diethylthiambutene, p. 302
0·76 (0·45; 1·0)	Thiambutosine, p. 569
0·80	Ethylmethylthiambutene, p. 339
0·84	Phencyclidine, p. 481
0·85	Benzphetamine, p. 215
0·90 (0·48)	Thymoxamine, p. 575
0·91	Alphaprodine, p. 182
0·93	Dicyclomine, p. 299
0·96	Piperoxan, p. 504
1·00	Pheneturide, p. 483
1·07	Ethoheptazine, p. 336
1·15	Sulphonal, p. 558
1·17	Caramiphen, p. 237
1·20	Antazoline, p. 198
1·30	Meclofenoxate, p. 398
1·40	Doxylamine, p. 322
1·50, tailing	Lachesine Chloride, p. 387
1·60	Cyclizine, p. 273
1·70	Ketamine, p. 387
1·80	Ethomoxane, p. 337
1·89	Chlorphenoxamine, p. 255
2·00	Dexchlorpheniramine, p. 289
	Dimethyltryptamine, p. 311
2·10	Diphenylpyraline, p. 317
2·18	Apoatropine, p. 198
2·20	Alphacetylmethadol, p. 180
	Butriptyline, p. 231
2·25	Oxypertine, p. 461
2·30	Lignocaine, p. 392
2·40	Amprotropine, p. 194
2·44	Alphamethadol, p. 181
2·50	Dexbrompheniramine, p. 288
2·56	Benzhexol, p. 213
2·66	Captodiame, p. 236
2·92	Chlophedianol, p. 244
2·95	Chloropyrilene, p. 251
3·20	Chlorcyclizine, p. 247
9·60	Codeine, p. 268

SYSTEM G5 (p. 83)—Retention Time Relative to Barbitone

RRT	*Compound*
0·10	Camphor, p. 235
0·12	Phenol, p. 487
	Troxidone, p. 590
0·14	Butylchoral Hydrate, p. 233
0·16	Chlorbutol, p. 246
0·17	Paramethadione, p. 467
0·21	Paradichlorobenzene, p. 466
0·22	Acetylcarbromal, p. 172
0·23	Coniine, p. 270
0·25	Phenelzine, p. 482
0·28	Ethosuximide, p. 338
0·31	Carbromal, p. 240
	Nicotinyl Alcohol, p. 442
0·32	Benzoic Acid, p. 214
	Menthol, p. 400
0·36	Aspirin, p. 201
0·37	Apronal, p. 200
0·45	Naphthalene, p. 436
0·49	Ethinamate, p. 334
0·54	Salicylic Acid, p. 539
0·62	Bemegride, p. 209
0·69	Alphamethadol, p. 181
0·71	Nicotine, p. 440
0·78	Warfarin, p. 596
0·98	Hydroxyquinoline, p. 375
1·00	Phendimetrazine, p. 481
1·04	Salicylamide, p. 538
1·09 (2·18)	Methyridine, p. 427
1·30	Methyprylone, p. 426
	Phenprobamate, p. 491
1·31	Talbutal, p. 560
1·36	Phentermine, p. 491
1·40 (3·80)	Mephenesin, p. 401
1·47	Allobarbitone, p. 179
1·48	Benzocaine, p. 214
1·62	Aprobarbitone, p. 200
1·84	Butobarbitone, p. 231
1·88 (1·3; 0·54)	Styramate, p. 546
1·94	Secbutobarbitone, p. 540
2·14	Amylobarbitone, p. 195
2·30	Dinitro-orthocresol, p. 312
	Meprobamate, p. 403
	Methohexitone, p. 415
	Phenacetin, p. 477
2·35	Nealbarbitone, p. 437
2·37	Vinbarbitone, p. 594
2·40	Paracetamol, p. 465
2·50	Hydroxyphenamate, p. 375
2·55	Pentobarbitone, p. 473
2·92	Chlorpropamide, p. 257
3·02	Quinalbarbitone, p. 530

RRT	Compound	RRT	Compound
3·49	Carisoprodol, p. 241	5·15	Phenazone, p. 480
4·05	Hexobarbitone, p. 362	5·60	Phenylmethylbarbituric Acid, p. 494
4·38	Caffeine, p. 234	6·90	Phenobarbitone, p. 486
4·50	Glutethimide, p. 353	6·90 (2·30)	Tybamate, p. 591
4·60	Methylphenobarbitone, p. 425	7·20	Cyclobarbitone, p. 274
4·80	Thiopentone, p. 571	10·50	Heptabarbitone, p. 359
5·10	Ibomal, p. 378		

SYSTEM G5 (p. 83)—Retention Time Relative to Phenobarbitone

RRT	Compound	RRT	Compound
0·14	Barbitone, p. 207	0·31	Amylobarbitone, p. 195
0·21	Allobarbitone, p. 179		

SYSTEM G6 (p. 83)—Retention Time Relative to Codeine

RRT	Compound	RRT	Compound
0·08	Nicotine, p. 440	1·15	Colchicine, p. 269
0·18	Pethidine, p. 476	1·17	Tubocurarine Chloride, p. 591
0·20	Sparteine, p. 542	1·18	Hydrastine, p. 368
0·21	Mescaline, p. 404		Hydrocodone, p. 369
0·22	Caffeine, p. 234	1·21	Emetine, p. 325
0·23	Cotarnine, p. 271		Ethylmorphine, p. 340
0·36	Procaine, p. 513		Morphine, p. 431
0·38	Yohimbine, p. 598	1·28	Apomorphine, p. 199
0·41	Berberine, p. 219	1·39	Diamorphine, p. 292
0·44	Homatropine, p. 365	1·44	Thebaine, p. 565
0·49	Methadone, p. 408	1·45	Cinchonidine, p. 262
0·57	Cocaine, p. 267		Cinchonine, p. 263
0·59	Atropine, p. 202	1·47	Hydromorphone, p. 371
	Hyoscyamine, p. 378	1·85	Nalorphine, p. 434
0·73	Pilocarpine, p. 500	2·12	Cinchocaine, p. 262
0·84	Hyoscine, p. 376	2·81	Gelsemine, p. 353
1·08	Aconitine, p. 174		Quinine, p. 532
	Theobromine, p. 567	3·17	Papaverine, p. 464

SYSTEM G7 (p. 83)—Retention Time Relative to Barbitone

RRT	Compound	RRT	Compound
0·76	Metharbitone, p. 412	2·09	Pentobarbitone, p. 473
1·10	Probarbital, p. 511	2·20	Vinbarbitone, p. 594
1·30	Allobarbitone, p. 179	2·30	Quinalbarbitone, p. 530
1·47	Allylbarbituric Acid, p. 179	2·38	Thiopentone, p. 571
1·54	Aprobarbitone, p. 200	2·90	Hexobarbitone, p. 362
1·60	Butobarbitone, p. 231	3·30	Methylphenobarbitone, p. 425
1·70	Secbutobarbitone, p. 540	4·40	Hydroxyamylobarbitone, p. 195
1·90	Talbutal, p. 560	4·80	Phenobarbitone, p. 486
2·00	Amylobarbitone, p. 195	5·00	Cyclobarbitone, p. 274

SYSTEM G8/100 (p. 83)—Retention Time Relative to n-Propanol

RRT	Compound	RRT	Compound
0·10	Methanol, p. 409	0·62	Isopropanol, p. 385
0·28	Ethanol, p. 332	1·03	Ether, p. 334
0·59	Acetone, p.171		

SYSTEM G8/160 (p. 83)—**Retention Time Relative to n-Propanol**

RRT	*Compound*	*RRT*	*Compound*
0·22	Methanol, p. 409	2·80	Acetaldehyde, p. 169
0·44	Ethanol, p. 332		Paraldehyde, p. 466
0·70	Acetone, p. 171	2·90	Benzene, p. 211
0·76	Isopropanol, p. 385	3·10	Trichloroethylene, p. 582
0·98	Ether, p. 334	5·10	Amyl Alcohol, p. 194
1·45	Chloroform, p. 250	6·00	Toluene, p. 578
1·62	Halothane, p. 358	13·90	Xylene, p. 597
2·30	Trichloroethane, p. 581	14·00	Tetrachloroethane, p. 562

The Marquis Test

Colours given with the sulphuric acid–formaldehyde test

The colours given in the following lists are those obtained by the microtechnique described on page 133 with a 1% solution of the pure substance. They have been listed in the order of the spectrum—purple/violet, blue, green, yellow, orange, red—preceded by black and followed by brown and grey. Under each prime colour the recorded colour or colours for each substance are arranged in two main classes:

(1) single colours, e.g. red, orange-red, red-orange, red-brown, etc.

(2) colour changes, e.g. yellow→red, orange→red, purple-red→blue-green, etc.

As with the prime colours, the compound terms are arranged in spectral order, the first colour taking precedence over the subsequent colour or colours of the term. The colour given in any test depends on the quantity of material used and on its purity, and may be described differently by different individuals. To allow for this, the following lists must be used in as wide a sense as possible. For example, if the test material gives a colour which the operator regards as red, he should look up the compounds listed under red. If this produces no satisfactory result, i.e. no compound whose chromatographic and spectrophotometric data correspond with those of the unknown, he should then look in the list of qualified colours, e.g. red-orange, purple-red. If this fails, he should realise that he may have missed some evanescent colour and turn to the list of colour changes, e.g. orange→red, yellow-green→red. Similarly, excess of material or presence of impurity will sometimes produce a colour change not shown in the table, and what the operator records as brown→purple may be listed here under the latter heading only.

Black

BLACK-PURPLE	Methapyrilene, p. 410	Thenyldiamine, p. 566
BLUE-BLACK	Allylprodine, p. 180	
PURPLE→BLACK	Apomorphine, p. 199	
YELLOW→PURPLE→BLACK	Ethylmorphine, p. 340	
BLACK-PURPLE→GREEN	Dextropropoxyphene, p. 290	

Purple/Violet

Acetyldihydrocodeine, p. 174
Ajmaline, p. 177
Bisacodyl, p. 223
Butriptyline, p. 231
Captodiame, p. 236
Chloropyrilene, p. 251
Chlorpromazine, p. 256
Codeine, p. 268
Desomorphine, p. 286
Diamorphine, p. 292
Diethylthiambutene, p. 302
Dihydrocodeine, p. 304
Dimethoxanate, p. 309
Doxylamine, p. 322
Ethopropazine, p. 337
Guanoxan, p. 356
Hexocyclium, p. 363
Hydromorphinol, p. 371
Laudexium, p. 388
Mepyramine, p. 403
Methaphenilene, p. 410
Methoxypromazine, p. 418
Methyldesorphine, p. 422
Methyldihydromorphine, p. 422
Metopon, p. 428
6-Monoacetylmorphine, p. 430
Morphine, p. 431
Nalorphine, p. 434
Normorphine, p. 450
Pecazine, p. 470
Penthienate, p. 473
Perphenazine, p. 475
Phenoxybenzamine, p. 489
Phenyltoloxamine, p. 495
Pholcodine, p. 496
Pipamazine, p. 501
Piperoxan, p. 504
Prochlorperazine, p. 514
Procyclidine, p. 514
Promazine, p. 517
Promethazine, p. 518
Solanidine, p. 541
Thenium, p. 566
Thiopropazate, p. 572
Tricyclamol, p. 583
Trimeprazine, p. 585

Blue

Embutramide, p. 325

BLUE-BLACK
Allylprodine, p. 180

BLUE-PURPLE
Methocarbamol, p. 414
Methotrimeprazine, p. 416
Neopine, p. 438
Noscapine, p. 451

BLUE-GREEN
Tolnaftate, p. 577

GREY-BLUE
Mebhydrolin, p. 397

PURPLE→BLUE
Dimethindene, p. 307

ORANGE→BLUE
Clidinium, p. 265

YELLOW→GREEN→BLUE
Pipethanate, p. 505

ORANGE→PURPLE→BLUE
Lucanthone, p. 394

ORANGE→GREEN→BLUE
Benactyzine, p. 209
Benzilonium, p. 214
Lachesine, p. 387
Pipenzolate, p. 502
Poldine, p. 506

PURPLE→BLUE-PURPLE
Nicocodine, p. 439

ORANGE→GREEN-BLUE
Dimenoxadole, p. 307

PURPLE-RED→BLUE-GREEN
Thioridazine, p. 573

BLUE-GREY→YELLOW-BROWN
Acetorphine, p. 172
Cyprenorphine, p. 278
Etorphine, p. 341

Green

Berberine, p. 219
Butoxamine, p. 231
Harman, p. 358
Norharman, p. 448
Norlevorphanol, p. 449
Oleandomycin, p. 455
Propranolol, p. 521
Protriptyline, p. 524
Pseudomorphine, p. 525
Tolonium, p. 577
Xenysalate, p. 596

BLUE-GREEN
Tolnaftate, p. 577

GREEN-YELLOW
Adrenolone, p. 176

GREEN-BROWN
Alcuronium, p. 177
Bufotenine, p. 227
Psilocin, p. 526

BROWN-GREEN
Harmaline, p. 358

GREY-GREEN
Cyproheptadine, p. 278
Deserpidine, p. 284
Naphazoline, p. 435
Oxypertine, p. 461
Phenindamine, p. 484
Protokylol, p. 523
Rescinnamine, p. 535

GREEN→BROWN
Octaverine, p. 452

YELLOW→GREEN
Chlorphenoxamine, p. 255
Chlortetracycline, p. 259
Demethylchlortetracycline, p. 281
Pramoxine, p. 508

RED→GREEN
Pentazocine, p. 473
Thiethylperazine, p. 570

BROWN→GREEN
Hordenine, p. 367
Narceine, p. 436
Tyramine, p. 592

GREY→GREEN
Pholedrine, p. 497

Yellow

Orange

Aletamine, p. 178
Anileridine, p. 197
Benzethidine, p. 212
Benzethonium, p. 213
Benzphetamine, p. 215
Carbetapentane, p. 238
Dehydroemetine, p. 280
Diampromide, p. 292
Dimethyltryptamine, p. 311
Dipyridamole, p. 318
Embramine, p. 324
Ethacridine, p. 331
Ethoheptazine, p. 336
Etoxeridine, p. 341
Fencamfamin, p. 343
Fenethylline, p. 343
Fentanyl, p. 345
Furethidine, p. 351
Harmine, p. 359
Hydroxypethidine, p. 375
Isothipendyl, p. 385
Ketobemidone, p. 387
Lymecycline, p. 394
Mepenzolate, p. 401
Mescaline, p. 404
Methacycline, p. 408
Methanthelinium, p. 409
Methylamphetamine, p. 420
Morpheridine, p. 430
Norbutrine, p. 447
Oxeladin, p. 459
Oxytetracycline, p. 463
Pamaquin, p. 464
Pentaquin, p. 472
Pethidine, p. 476
Phenethylamine, p. 482
Phentermine, p. 491
Piminodine, p. 501
Piperidolate, p. 503
Plasmocide, p. 506
Primaquine, p. 510
Proheptazine, p. 516
Propantheline, p. 519
Properidine, p. 520
Prothipendyl, p. 522
Psilocybin, p. 526
Rolitetracycline, p. 537
Spiramycin, p. 542
Tetracycline, p. 562
Trimethoprim, p. 586
Trimethoxyamphetamine, p. 587
Tryptamine, p. 590
Veratrine, p. 594
Xylometazoline, p. 597

YELLOW-ORANGE
Orphenadrine, p. 456
Pipradrol, p. 505

ORANGE-RED
Alverine, p. 182
Bethanidine, p. 222
Diphemanil, p. 314

ORANGE-BROWN
Nortriptyline, p. 450

RED-ORANGE
Chlorprothixene, p. 258

BROWN-ORANGE
Amitriptyline, p. 189
Azacosterol, p. 204

YELLOW→ORANGE
Isoetharine, p. 382
Proflavine, p. 515

ORANGE→PURPLE
Adrenaline, p. 175

ORANGE→BLUE
Clidinium, p. 265

ORANGE→RED
Cycrimine, p. 277

ORANGE→BROWN
Amphetamine, p. 192
Dexamphetamine, p. 287
Ethylnoradrenaline, p. 340
Mephentermine, p. 401
Phenformin, p. 483
Phenylpropylmethylamine, p. 495
Prolintane, p. 517

RED→ORANGE
Thebaine, p. 565

ORANGE→PURPLE→BLUE
Lucanthone, p. 394

ORANGE→GREEN→BLUE
Benactyzine, p. 209
Benzilonium, p. 214
Lachesine, p. 387
Pipenzolate, p. 502
Poldine, p. 506

ORANGE→PURPLE-BROWN
Metanephrine, p. 406
Normetanephrine, p. 449

ORANGE→GREEN-BLUE
Dimenoxadole, p. 307

ORANGE→RED-PURPLE
Carphenazine, p. 242

Red

Buphenine, p. 227
Dibutoline, p. 296
Dimethothiazine, p. 309
Fenpiprane, p. 345
Fluphenazine, p. 348
Mephenesin, p. 401
Methoxyphenamine, p. 418
Pericyazine, p. 475
Phenazopyridine, p. 480
Phenoperidine, p. 488
Phenoxypropazine, p. 490
Phenylephrine, p. 493
Prenylamine, p. 509
Thioproperazine, p. 572
Thiothixene, p. 574
Tolpropamine, p. 577
Tymazoline, p. 592
Vinblastine, p. 595

Brown

GREY-BROWN
Dihydroergotamine, p. 305 | Methylergometrine, p. 424

PURPLE→BROWN
Dimethylthiambutene, p. 310

GREEN→BROWN
Octaverine, p. 452

ORANGE→BROWN
Amphetamine, p. 192 | Dexamphetamine, p. 287 | Ethylnoradrenaline, p. 340 | Mephentermine, p. 401 | Phenformin, p. 483 | Phenylpropylmethylamine, p. 495 | Prolintane, p. 517

RED→BROWN
Tranylcypromine, p. 579

BROWN→PURPLE
Isoprenaline, p. 384

BROWN→GREEN
Hordenine, p. 367 | Narceine, p. 436 | Tyramine, p. 592

YELLOW→BROWN→PURPLE
Hydrocodone, p. 369 | Oxycodone, p. 460

BROWN→GREEN-GREY→GREY
Metazocine, p. 407

ORANGE→PURPLE-BROWN
Metanephrine, p. 406 | Normetanephrine, p. 449

GREY→PURPLE-BROWN
Diaveridine, p. 293

PURPLE-BROWN→GREEN
Methoxamine, p. 417

RED-PURPLE→BROWN
Chlophedianol, p. 244

GREY-GREEN→BROWN
Reserpine, p. 535

PURPLE-BROWN→GREY-GREEN
Alphacetylmethadol, p. 180 | Alphamethadol, p. 181

BLUE-GREY→YELLOW-BROWN
Acetorphine, p. 172 | Cyprenorphine, p. 278 | Etorphine, p. 341

Grey

Lysergide, p. 395 | Methoserpidine, p. 415 | Methysergide, p. 427

GREY-PURPLE
Benzhexol, p. 213 | Oxymorphone, p. 461 | Pyrrobutamine, p. 529 | Thenalidine, p. 565

GREY-BLUE
Mebhydrolin, p. 397

GREY-GREEN
Cyproheptadine, p. 278 | Deserpidine, p. 284 | Naphazoline, p. 435 | Oxypertine, p. 461 | Phenindamine, p. 484 | Protokylol, p. 523 | Rescinnamine, p. 535

GREY-BROWN
Dihydroergotamine, p. 305 | Methylergometrine, p. 424

PURPLE→GREY
Levophenacylmorphan, p. 391

GREY→GREEN
Pholedrine, p. 497

BROWN→GREEN-GREY→GREY
Metazocine, p. 407

GREY→PURPLE-BROWN
Diaveridine, p. 293

GREY-GREEN→BROWN
Reserpine, p. 535

PURPLE-BROWN→GREY-GREEN
Alphacetylmethadol, p. 180 | Alphamethadol, p. 181

BLUE-GREY→YELLOW-BROWN
Acetorphine, p. 172 | Cyprenorphine, p. 278 | Etorphine, p. 341

Ultraviolet Absorption Maxima

In the following tables no values below 220 mμ have been included, although several have been recorded in monographs in Part 2. Particulars of the solvents and the E(1%, 1 cm) values will be found in the monographs on the pages indicated. For the barbiturates, however, the E(1%, 1 cm) values in 0·05 M borax buffer are given on p. 99.

Table A gives the wavelengths of maximum absorption, together with the wavelengths of subsidiary peaks, for the compounds in acid solution. Table B gives these values in alkaline solution when values in acid solution are not recorded in the monographs in Part 2 or when the values in alkaline solution differ significantly from those in acid solution. Table C gives the values in neutral solution for compounds for which values in acid or alkaline solution are not recorded in the monographs in Part 2.

A. In Acid Solution—Wavelengths of Maximum Absorption (λ max)

λ *max* mμ	*Compound*	*Subsidiary Peaks* (mμ)
220	Clothiapine, p. 267	
	Cycloserine, p. 276	
	Ethylnoradrenaline, p. 340	278
	Methyldopa, p. 422	279
	Methyldopate, p. 423	280
	Thalidomide, p. 564	299·5
	Yohimbine, p. 598	272, 278, 287·5
220·5	Haloperidol, p. 357	248
221	Dibenzepin, p. 295	
	Hydroxychloroquine, p. 374	236, 250, 256·5, 329, 343
221·5	Chloroquine, p. 252	236, 257·5, 329·5, 343
222	Hydroxyamphetamine, p. 373	274
	Isoetharine, p. 382	278
	Isoprenaline, p. 384	278·5, 280
	Lysergic Acid, p. 395	281·5, 290
	Pentaquin, p. 472	265, 277, 331, 400
223	Aminohippuric Acid, p. 187	
	Primaquine, p. 510	261, 282, 334, 406
	Thenium Closylate, p. 566	268, 275
224	Amodiaquine, p. 190	238, 342
	Amopyroquine, p. 191	238, 342
	Cyproheptadine, p. 278	285
	Pholedrine, p. 497	275
	Procainamide, p. 512	
225	Cyclizine, p. 273	257, 262·5, 269
	Diamprodine, p. 292	257, 263
	Hexetidine, p. 361	
	Meclofenoxate, p. 398	277
	Oxypertine, p. 461	277, 302

λ max mμ	*Compound*	*Subsidiary Peaks* (mμ)
226	Cyclothiazide, p. 277	272
	Dimethoxanate, p. 309	254
	Embramine, p. 324	258
	Gallamine, p. 352	
	Levallorphan, p. 390	278
	Methylergometrine, p. 424	313
227	Benzocaine, p. 214	272, 278
	Decamethonium Iodide, p. 280	
	Dimethisoquin, p. 308	261, 269, 331, 343
	Normetanephrine, p. 449	277·5
	Protokylol, p. 523	281·5
	Pyrrobutamine, p. 529	
227, 268	Demethylchlortetracycline, p. 281	368
228	Amiphenazole, p. 188	261
	Berberine, p. 219	264, 345
	Butylated Hydroxyanisole, p. 232	292
	Mecamylamine, p. 397	
	Metabutethamine, p. 405	274
	Methohexitone, p. 415	
	Procaine, p. 513	272, 279
229	Aspirin, p. 201	276
	Benzoic Acid, p. 214	
229·5	Ethionamide, p. 335	276, 317
230	Bromodiphenhydramine, p. 224	
	Chloroprocaine, p. 251	288
	Etonitazene, p. 341	282
	Imolamine, p. 380	
	Meclozine, p. 398	261, 265·5, 272·5
	Phenazone, p. 480	
231	Clopenthixol, p. 266	269, 325
	Diperodon, p. 314	264, 270, 277
	Laudexium Methylsulphate, p. 388	280
	Pseudomorphine, p. 525	261
	Xenysalate, p. 596	319
232	Amicarbalide, p. 185	
	Chlorcyclizine, p. 247	258·5, 263·5, 270, 276
	Chlorpropamide, p. 257	
	Clonitazene, p. 266	285
	Diphemanil Methylsulphate, p. 314	
	Hexylcaine Hydrochloride, p. 363	275
	Hydroxyzine, p. 376	257, 263, 269
	Meprylcaine, p. 403	
	Piperocaine, p. 504	275
	Procarbazine, p. 513	
	Trimetazidine, p. 586	269
233	Benzamine, p. 210	274
	Clomiphene, p. 265	288
	Cocaine, p. 267	275
	Homochlorcyclizine, p. 366	258·5, 263·5, 270, 276
	Phenisonone, p. 485	284, 313

λ *max* mμ	*Compound*	*Subsidiary Peaks* (mμ)
234	Aconitine, p. 174	275
	Aminosalicylic Acid, p. 188	300
	Amylocaine, p. 196	275
	Benzoylecgonine, p. 215	275
	Heteronium Bromide, p. 360	
	Methaqualone, p. 411	269
	Prothionamide, p. 522	275
	Thenalidine, p. 565	
235	Cinchonine, p. 263	315
	Digitoxin, p. 302	340, 420, 485
	Propoxycaine, p. 521	298
	Thonzylamine, p. 574	273, 313
236	Cinchonidine, p. 262	316
236·5	Amydricaine, p. 194	277
	Phenyramidol, p. 495	308
237	Methapyrilene, p. 410	313
237·5	Chloropyrilene, p. 251	312
238	Penthienate Methobromide, p. 473	
238·5	Halopyramine, p. 357	221·5, 314
239	Mepyramine Maleate, p. 403	316
	Thenyldiamine, p. 566	315
	Tripelennamine, p. 588	314
240	Amitriptyline, p. 189	
	Dihydrallazine, p. 304	274, 308
	Ouabain, p. 457	325, 515
	Paraphenylenediamine, p. 467	244, 248, 255, 260
	Tacrine, p. 560	323·5, 336
241	Antazoline Hydrochloride, p. 198	291
	Diazepam, p. 294	284, 359
	Physostigmine *N*-Oxide, p. 499	300
242	Cetoxime, p. 243	290
	Oleandomycin, p. 455	
	Prothipendyl, p. 522	
243	Acepromazine, p. 169	278, 374
	Acetophenazine, p. 172	278, 374
	Carphenazine, p. 242	277
	Methacycline, p. 408	340
	Propantheline Bromide, p. 519	281
244·5	Isothipendyl, p. 385	315
245	Ajmaline, p. 177	290
	Ascorbic Acid, p. 201	
	Chlordiazepoxide, p. 248	306
246	Amprolium Hydrochloride, p. 193	263
	Phenoperidine, p. 488	250
	Physostigmine, p. 498	302
246·5	Harmine, p. 359	319, 366

λ *max* mμ	*Compound*	*Subsidiary Peaks* (mμ)
247	Cinchocaine, p. 262	318
	Norharman, p. 448	300
	Proguanil, p. 516	
	Thiamine, p. 570	
247·5	Fluanisone, p. 346	275, 305, 360
248	Azapetine, p. 205	
248·5	Pipamperone, p. 501	
249	Ethopropazine, p. 337	299, 362
	Framycetin, p. 350	305, 362
	Hydrastinine, p. 368	306, 363
	Lobeline, p. 393	
	Promethazine, p. 518	300
250	Allopurinol, p. 179	231
	Chlorproguanil, p. 256	
	Diethazine, p. 300	298
	Histapyrrodine, p. 365	295
	Hydroquinidine, p. 372	316, 345
	Hydroquinine, p. 372	316, 345
	Methoxypromazine, p. 418	278, 303
	Papaverine, p. 464	284, 310
	Quinine, p. 532	316, 346
	Trimipramine, p. 587	
250, 256	Pemoline, p. 470	261·5, 268
250, 256·5	Phenampromide, p. 479	
251	Desipramine, p. 285	275
	Imipramine, p. 379	
	Levophenacylmorphan, p. 391	
	Trimeprazine, p. 585	302
251, 257·5	Phenformin, p. 483	263·5, 267
251·5	Diphenidol, p. 316	248, 259
	Methimazole, p. 413	211
	Methotrimeprazine, p. 416	302
252	Hydroxyquinoline, p. 375	309, 319, 365
	Promazine, p. 517	300
253	Diethylpropion, p. 301	
	Orthocaine, p. 456	
	Pecazine, p. 470	300
	Pipazethate, p. 502	
253·5	Norbutrine, p. 447	285
254	Chlorhexidine, p. 249	
	Cinnarizine, p. 263	227·5, 291·5
	Tropicamide, p. 589	
254·5	Perphenazine, p. 475	306
255	Aniline, p. 197	249, 261
	Chlorpromazine, p. 256	307
	Opipramol, p. 455	280

λ *max* mμ	*Compound*	*Subsidiary Peaks* (mμ)
255	Pipamazine, p. 501	
	Strychnine, p. 545	
	Thiethylperazine, p. 570	307
256	Amidopyrine, p. 185	
	Fluopromazine, p. 347	304
	Methsuximide, p. 418	
	Phenmetrazine Hydrochloride, p. 486	250, 261, 267
	Thiopropazate, p. 572	305
	Trifluoperazine, p. 584	
256, 250	Pemoline, p. 470	261·5, 268
256·5	Cycrimine, p. 277	246·5, 251, 263
	Ephedrine, p. 327	251, 262·5
	Hydroxyphenamate, p. 375	246·5, 250·5, 262·5
	Norpseudoephedrine, p. 450	246·5, 250·5, 262·5, 266
	Phendimetrazine, p. 481	250·5, 260·5, 267
256·5, 250	Phenampromide, p. 479	
257	Alphameprodine, p. 181	247, 251·5, 263
	Amphetamine, p. 192	251·5, 263
	Atropine Methobromide, p. 203	251, 263
	Atropine Methonitrate, p. 203	251, 263
	Chlormethiazole, p. 250	
	Dextropropoxyphene, p. 290	251·5, 263
	Diphenhydramine, p. 315	252
	Etafedrine, p. 330	247, 251, 263
	Lucanthone, p. 394	223, 331
	Methyl Phenidate, p. 419	246·5, 251, 263
	Methylamphetamine, p. 420	251·5, 263
	Methylephedrine, p. 423	251, 263
	Phenglutarimide Hydrochloride, p. 483	251, 263
	Phenylpropanolamine, p. 494	251, 263
	Phenylpropylmethylamine, p. 495	251·5, 263
	Properidine, p. 520	251, 263
	Styramate, p. 546	247, 251, 263
	Trimeperidine, p. 584	242, 247, 251, 263
257·5	Adiphenine, p. 175	248, 253, 264
	Allylprodine, p. 180	251·5, 263·5
	Benzethidine, p. 212	252, 263·5
	Dexamphetamine, p. 287	252, 265
	Ethoheptazine, p. 336	246, 251·5, 263·5
	Fentanyl, p. 345	251, 263
	Glycopyrronium Bromide, p. 355	251, 263
	Hyoscine, p. 376	251, 263·5
	Hyoscine Methobromide, p. 377	251, 263·5
	Hyoscine Methonitrate, p. 378	251, 263·5
	Paraquat, p. 468	
	Phenelzine, p. 482	247·5, 252, 262·5
	Phenethylamine, p. 482	242, 247, 251·5, 263
257·5, 251	Phenformin, p. 483	263·5, 267
258	Aletamine, p. 178	247·5, 252·5, 264
	Anileridine, p. 197	
	Atropine, p. 202	252, 264

λ *max* mμ	*Compound*	*Subsidiary Peaks* (mμ)
258	Benactyzine, p. 209	252, 262, 264
	Benzhexol, p. 213	247, 252, 264
	Benzilonium Bromide, p. 214	252, 264
	Benzphetamine, p. 215	253, 263, 268
	Betaprodine, p. 221	248, 252·5, 264, 268
	Bibenzonium Bromide, p. 222	247·5, 252·5, 264, 268
	Butethamate, p. 230	247, 252·5, 264
	Caramiphen, p. 237	252, 264·5
	Clidinium Bromide, p. 265	252, 263, 268
	Diminazene, p. 312	
	Diphenylpyraline, p. 317	
	Etoxeridine, p. 341	252, 264
	Etymide, p. 342	263
	Eucatropine, p. 342	252, 264, 268
	Hexocyclium Methylsulphate, p. 363	248, 252, 264, 268
	Homatropine, p. 365	252, 264, 267
	Lachesine Chloride, p. 387	252, 262, 264, 268
	Mephentermine, p. 401	247·5, 252, 264
	Noracymethadol, p. 445	253, 264, 269
	Oxethazaine, p. 459	248, 252, 264, 267
	Oxyphenonium Bromide, p. 463	252, 264, 268
	Pipenzolate Bromide, p. 502	252, 262
	Piperidolate, p. 503	252, 264
	Pipethanate, p. 505	252, 262
	Pipradrol, p. 505	252·5
	Poldine Methylsulphate, p. 506	252, 262
	Procyclidine, p. 514	252, 264
	Prolintane, p. 517	248, 252, 264
258·5	Alverine, p. 182	252·5, 264, 268
	Carbetapentane, p. 238	252, 264·5
	Doxapram, p. 322	248, 252·5, 264, 268·5
	Fencamfamin, p. 343	248, 253, 264·5, 268
	Oxeladin, p. 459	252·5, 264·5
	Racemoramide, p. 534	253·5, 264
259	Alphamethadol, p. 181	253·5
	Ambutonium Bromide, p. 183	253, 265
	Aminopentamide, p. 187	253, 265
	Azacyclonol, p. 204	253·5
	Benztropine, p. 216	253
	Chlophedianol, p. 244	253·5, 265
	Chlorphenoxamine, p. 255	253, 265, 275
	Fenpipramide, p. 344	253, 265
	Fenpiprane, p. 345	254, 268·5
	Isopropamide Iodide, p. 384	265
	Levomoramide, p. 391	254, 265
	Methadone, p. 408	253, 265, 292
	Valethamate Bromide, p. 593	253, 265
259, 292	Normethadone Hydrochloride, p. 449	253, 265
259·5	Phenindamine, p. 484	
260	Aminacrine, p. 185	313, 326, 381, 400, 422
	Metyrapone, p. 429	

λ *max* mμ	*Compound*	*Sudsidiary Peaks* (mμ)
260	Neostigmine Methylsulphate, p. 438	266
	Nicotine, p. 440	
	Nicotinyl Alcohol, p. 442	
260, 264·5	Tolpropamine, p. 577	273
260·5	Nicotinic Acid, p. 441	266·5
261	Cyclomethycaine, p. 275	
	Dextromoramide, p. 290	256, 267
	Dibromopropamidine, p. 295	
	Dimethothiazine, p. 309	235, 306
	Doxylamine, p. 322	
	Nicocodine, p. 439	267
	Nicotinamide, p. 440	
	Nifenazone, p. 442	
	Pargyline, p. 469	251, 256, 268
261·5	Nicomorphine, p. 439	268
262	Acriflavine, p. 175	238, 450
	Debrisoquine, p. 279	270
262, 266	Pheniramine, p. 485	
262·5	Phencyclidine, p. 481	252·5, 257·5, 269
263	Mepivacaine, p. 402	271
	Thioridazine, p. 573	230, 313
	Veratrine, p. 594	293
263·5	Fenfluramine, p. 344	259, 270·5
	Nikethamide, p. 443	
264	Carbinoxamine, p. 239	
	Cetalkonium Chloride, p. 243	258, 270
	Orphenadrine, p. 456	
	Tranylcypromine, p. 579	258, 271
264·5	Bisacodyl, p. 223	
	Nialamide, p. 439	
264·5, 260	Tolpropamine, p. 577	273
265	Acetazolamide, p. 170	
	Brompheniramine, p. 225	
	Brucine, p. 225	300
	Captodiame, p. 236	
	Chlormezanone, p. 250	258
	Chlorpheniramine, p. 254	
	Chlortetracycline, p. 259	228, 319
	Dexbrompheniramine, p. 288	
	Dexchlorpheniramine, p. 289	
	Ethinamate, p. 334	
	Isoniazid, p. 383	
	Leptazol, p. 389	
	Pempidine, p. 471	
	Phenamidine, p. 478	
	Tetrahydrozoline, p. 563	260, 272
265, 272	Phanquone, p. 476	292

λ *max* mμ	*Compound*	*Subsidiary Peaks* (mμ)
266	Bialamicol, p. 222	
	Carbutamide, p. 241	272
	Xylometazoline, p. 597	
266, 262	Pheniramine, p. 485	
267	Ethomoxane, p. 337	
	Iproniazid, p. 381	
267·5	Butanilicaine, p. 229	274·5
268	Dinitro-orthocresol, p. 312	
	Ethylmethylthiambutene, p. 339	226, 285
	Mescaline, p. 404	
	Pericyazine, p. 475	233
	Phenoxybenzamine, p. 489	262, 274
	Phenoxypropazine, p. 490	263, 274·5
	Sulphafurazole, p. 549	
268, 227	Demethylchlortetracycline, p. 281	368
268·5	Amisometradine, p. 189	
	Lymecycline, p. 394	356
269	Amolanone Hydrochloride, p. 191	265, 276·5
	Bephenium Embonate, p. 219	263, 275
	Histamine, p. 364	
	Isoxsuprine, p. 386	274
	Ketamine, p. 387	264, 276
	Oxytetracycline Dihydrate, p. 463	320, 352
	Pyrazinamide, p. 527	312
	Pyridostigmine Bromide, p. 527	
	Trimethoxyamphetamine, p. 587	
	Viomycin Sulphate, p. 595	
269·5	Ethacridine, p. 331	364, 410
270	Aminophylline, p. 567	
	Distigmine Bromide, p. 319	
	Methyclothiazide, p. 419	315
	Phenylephrine, p. 493	
	Phenyltoloxamine, p. 495	276
	Polythiazide, p. 506	310
	Tetracycline, p. 562	356
	Theophylline, p. 567	
270·5	Bretylium Tosylate, p. 224	256, 264
270·5, 277	Benzethonium Chloride, p. 213	265
271	Bufylline, p. 227	
	Embutramide, p. 325	276·5
	Guanoclor, p. 356	277
	Trimethoprim, p. 586	
272	Caffeine, p. 234	
	Cyclopenthiazide, p. 276	315
	Pyrimethamine, p. 528	
272, 265	Phanquone, p. 476	292
273	Apomorphine, p. 199	

λ *max* mμ	*Compound*	*Subsidiary Peaks* (mμ)
273	Edrophonium Chloride, p. 324	
	Oxedrine, p. 458	
	Proxyphylline, p. 525	
274	Acepifylline, p. 169	
	Buphenine, p. 227	
	Clemizole, p. 264	
	Hordenine, p. 367	
	Piperoxan, p. 504	
274·5	Fenethylline, p. 343	
275	Guanoxan, p. 356	
	Thymoxamine, p. 575	
276	Diaveridine, p. 293	
	Hyoscine Butylbromide, p. 377	
	Isometheptene, p. 383	
	Orciprenaline, p. 455	280
	Phentolamine, p. 492	
	Triprolidine, p. 588	230, 290
277	Bufotenine, p. 227	296
	Desomorphine, p. 286	
	Metronidazole, p. 429	
	Narceine, p. 436	
	Racemethorphan, p. 534	
277, 270·5	Benzethonium Chloride, p. 213	265
277·5	Nitrazepam, p. 443	
	Phenazocine, p. 479	
278	Ambenonium Chloride, p. 183	271·5, 292
	Bamifylline, p. 206	
	Chloramphenicol, 246	
	Dextromethorphan, p. 289	
	Levomethorphan, p. 390	
	Tryptamine, p. 590	272·5, 287
278·5	Naepaine, p. 433	273, 290
	Racemorphan, p. 534	
279	Chloroxylenol, p. 254	
	Chlorzoxazone, p. 260	
	Dextrorphan, p. 291	
	Diamorphine, p. 292	
	Ketobemidone, p. 387	
	Leucinocaine, p. 389	
	Levorphanol, p. 391	
	Noradrenaline, p. 445	
	Phenomorphan, p. 488	
279·5	Dopamine, p. 321	
	Mepacrine, p. 400	222
280	Adrenaline, p. 175	
	Hydrocodone, p. 369	
	Metopon, p. 428	

λ *max* mμ	*Compound*	*Subsidiary Peaks* (mμ)
280	Oxycodone, p. 460	
	Streptomycin, p. 544	
280·5	Vancomycin Hydrochloride, p. 593	
281	Azathioprine, p. 205	
	Hydromorphone, p. 371	
	Naphazoline, p. 435	271, 288, 291
	Oxymorphone, p. 461	
	Phentermine, p. 491	252, 257·5, 264
	Thebacon, p. 565	
281·5	Emetine, p. 325	
282	Chlorisondamine Chloride, p. 249	274, 290
	Dyclonine, p. 323	221
282·5	Dihydrocodeine, p. 304	
283	Acetorphine, p. 172	
	Acetyldihydrocodeine, p. 174	
	Benzthiazide, p. 216	
	Carbamazepine, p. 238	
	Dihydromorphine, p. 305	
	Dipyridamole, p. 318	236, 398
	Homidium Bromide, p. 366	242
	Methyldesorphine, p. 422	
	Myrophine, p. 433	
	Nicoumalone, p. 442	304
	Pholcodine, p. 496	
	Thebaine, p. 565	
284	Benzylmorphine, p. 218	
	Hydromorphinol, p. 371	
	Morphine, p. 431	
	Neopine, p. 438	
284·5	Morphine *N*-Oxide, p. 432	
285	Ethylmorphine, p. 340	
	Nalorphine, p. 434	
	Normorphine, p. 450	
	Tolonium Chloride, p. 577	245
286	Dimethylthiambutene, p. 310	227, 267·5
287	Cyprenorphine, p. 278	
	Etorphine, p. 341	
287·5	Diethylthiambutene, p. 302	225, 268
288	Diphenadione, p. 315	238, 277, 306, 314
288·5	Propranolol, p. 521	305, 319·5
290	Thialbarbitone, p. 569	239
	Thiopentone, p. 571	239
291	Carbimazole, p. 238	227
	Pyridoxine Hydrochloride, p. 528	
292	Phenadoxone, p. 478	253, 259, 266
	Rotenone, p. 537	235

λ *max* mμ	*Compound*	*Subsidiary Peaks* (mμ)
292, 259	Normethadone Hydrochloride, p. 449	253, 265
293	Dipipanone, p. 317	252·5, 259, 265
296	Methylpentynol, p. 425	
296·5	Quinapyramine Sulphate, p. 531	248, 325, 348
298	Pentazocine, p. 473	
300	Buformin, p. 226	
	Norbormide, p. 446	283
302	Salicylic Acid, p. 539	
	Thiabendazole, p. 568	243
306	Guanethidine, p. 356	
307·5	Benzydamine, p. 217	
309	Dimefline, p. 306	245
	Dioxyline, p. 313	285, 335
310	Diquat, p. 319	
312	Ergometrine, p. 328	
313	Metabutoxycaine, p. 405	
	Pyrithidium Bromide, p. 529	255
315	Ergotamine, p. 328	
332	Cotarnine, p. 271	253
345	Acinitrazole, p. 174	237
351	Hydroxocobalamin, p. 373	274, 525
360	Triamterene, p. 581	
362	Furaltadone, p. 351	255
390	Deslanoside, p. 286	235, 325, 480
	Digoxin, p. 303	230, 320, 490
	Lanatoside C, p. 388	230, 480
398·5	Ambazone, p. 182	

B. In Alkaline Solution—Wavelengths of Maximum Absorption (λ max)

In this table wavelengths of maximum absorption in alkaline solution are given only for those compounds for which maxima in acid solution are not recorded in the monographs in Part 2 or for which the maxima in alkaline solution differ significantly from the maxima in acid solution.

λ *max* mμ	*Compound*	*Subsidiary Peaks* (mμ)
223	Chlortetracycline, p. 259	253, 346
224	Allantoin, p. 178	
227	Ethacrynic Acid, p. 331	280
228	Bromvaletone, p. 225	

λ *max* mμ	*Compound*	*Subsidiary Peaks* (mμ)
228	Chlorothiazide, p. 253	292
	Rescinnamine, p. 535	301
229	Frusemide, p. 350	272, 335
234·5	Saccharin, p. 538	268
237	Acetylcarbromal, p. 172	
237·5	Pamaquin, p. 464	287·5, 297·5, 362
238	Phenylephrine, p. 493	291
239	Cresol, p. 271	290
240	Allobarbitone (pH 10), p. 179	
	Allylbarbituric Acid (pH 10), p. 179	
	Amylobarbitone (pH 10), p. 195	
	Aprobarbitone (pH 10), p. 200	
	Barbitone (pH 10), p. 207	
	Butallylonal (pH 10), p. 229	
	Butobarbitone (pH 10), p. 231	
	Cyclobarbitone (pH 10), p. 274	
	Edrophonium Chloride, p. 324	294
	Heptabarbitone (pH 10), p. 359	
	Hexobarbitone (pH 10 and 13), p. 362	
	Ibomal (pH 10), p. 378	
	Levallorphan, p. 390	299
	Levorphanol, p. 391	299
	Metharbitone (pH 10 and 13), p. 412	
	Methylphenobarbitone (pH 10 and 13), p. 425	
	Narcobarbital (pH 10 and 13), p. 437	
	Nealbarbitone (pH 10), p. 437	
	Pentobarbitone (pH 10), p. 473	
	Phenobarbitone (pH 10), p. 486	
	Phenylmethylbarbituric Acid (pH 10), p. 494	
	Probarbital (pH 10), p. 511	
	Quinalbarbitone (pH 10), p. 530	
	Secbutobarbitone (pH 10), p. 540	
	Talbutal (pH 10), p. 560	
	Vinbarbitone (pH 10), p. 594	
241	Thonzylamine, p. 574	273, 279, 312
242	Hexoestrol, p. 363	295
	Salicylamide, p. 538	328
243	Chloropyrilene, p. 251	308
	Chlorzoxazone, p. 260	287·5
246	Dichlorophen, p. 297	305
	Diethylpropion, p. 301	
	Eugenol, p. 342	296
248	Bisacodyl, p. 223	
249	Cetoxime, p. 243	300
	Hexachlorophane, p. 360	320
	Prothipendyl, p. 522	

λ *max* mμ	*Compound*	*Subsidiary Peaks* (mμ)
250	Methohexitone (pH 10 and 13), p. 415	
250·5	Morphine, p. 431	296
252	Sulphaquinoxaline, p. 555	
253	Clemizole, p. 264	267, 274, 282
	Sulphafurazole, p. 549	
254	Oxyphenbutazone, p. 462	
	Sulphanilamide, p. 553	
255	Allobarbitone (pH 13), p. 179	
	Allylbarbituric Acid (pH 13), p. 179	
	Amylobarbitone (pH 13), p. 195	
	Aprobarbitone (pH 13), p. 200	
	Barbitone (pH 13), p. 207	
	Butallylonal (pH 13), p. 229	
	Butobarbitone (pH 13), p. 231	
	Carbutamide, p. 241	
	Cyclobarbitone (pH 13), p. 274	
	Heptabarbitone (pH 13), p. 359	
	Ibomal (pH 13), p. 378	
	Nealbarbitone (pH 13), p. 437	
	Pentobarbitone (pH 13), p. 473	
	Phenobarbitone (pH 13), p. 486	
	Phenylmethylbarbituric Acid (pH 13), p. 494	
	Probarbital (pH 13), p. 511	
	Quinalbarbitone (pH 13), p. 530	
	Secbutobarbitone (pH 13), p. 540	
	Talbutal (pH 13), p. 560	
	Vinbarbitone (pH 13), p. 594	
256	Folic Acid, p. 349	283, 365
259	Nalidixic Acid, p. 434	338
	Stilboestrol, p. 543	
260	Chlordiazepoxide, p. 248	243
	Sulphinpyrazone, p. 557	
264	Methyclothiazide, p. 419	318
	Phenylbutazone, p. 492	
	Polythiazide, p. 506	315
265	Aminosalicylic Acid, p. 188	298
269	Bephenium Embonate, p. 219	275, 288, 300, 365
	Sulphadimethoxine, p. 548	
270	Teclothiazide, p. 561	315
272	Isocarboxazid, p. 382	
273	Bendrofluazide, p. 210	329
	Theobromine, p. 567	
274	Hydroflumethiazide, p. 370	333
275	Procainamide, p. 512	
278	Pentazocine, p. 473	

λ *max* mμ	*Compound*	*Subsidiary Peaks* (mμ)
280	Idoxuridine, p. 379	
284	Diphenadione, p. 315	246, 275, 312, 323
285	Mefenamic Acid, p. 399	
286	Phenol, p. 487	
296	Chloroxylenol, p. 254	
297	Hexylresorcinol, p. 364	
298	Ethinyloestradiol, p. 335	
298·5	Parachlorophenol, p. 466	
301	Cyprenorphine, p. 278	
	Etorphine, p. 341	
305	Nialamide, p. 439	238
	Thialbarbitone (pH 10), p. 569	255
	Thialbarbitone (pH 13), p. 569	
	Thiopentone (pH 10), p. 571	255
	Thiopentone (pH 13), p. 571	
308	Warfarin, p. 596	
312	Amiphenazole, p. 188	
	Dicoumarol, p. 298	
319·5	Pentachlorophenol, p. 471	
370	Dinitro-orthocresol, p. 312	265, 409

C. In Neutral Solution—Wavelengths of Maximum Absorption (λ max)

The compounds listed below are those whose wavelengths of maximum absorption in acid or alkaline solution are not quoted in Part 2.

λ *max* mμ	*Compound*	*Subsidiary Peaks* (mμ)
220	Deserpidine, p. 284	272
	Naphthalene, p. 436	266, 275, 286
222	Riboflavine, p. 536	267, 371·5, 445
224	Endrin, p. 326	
225	Hydroquinone, p. 373	295
226	Betanaphthol, p. 221	274, 285, 322, 330
228	Dienoestrol, p. 300	276
	Methoxychlor, p. 417	
	Tolbutamide, p. 576	257, 262, 267, 274
230	Benzyl Benzoate, p. 217	
	Oxazepam, p. 458	315
	Tropacocaine, p. 589	273
232	Dehydroemetine, p. 280	284
236	Quinidine, p. 531	278, 332

λ *max* mμ	*Compound*	*Subsidiary Peaks* (mμ)
238	Methyl Salicylate, p. 420	306
	Spironolactone, p. 542	
	Triamcinolone, p. 580	
240	Betamethasone, p. 220	
	Cephaloridine, p. 243	
	Cortisone Acetate, p. 271	
	Deoxycortone Acetate, p. 283	
	Dequalinium, p. 284	326, 335
	Dimethisterone, p. 308	
	Ethisterone, p. 336	
	Fludrocortisone Acetate, p. 346	
	Fluocinolone Acetonide, p. 346	
	Hydrallazine Hydrochloride, p. 367	260, 303, 315
	Hydrocortisone, p. 370	
	Methyltestosterone, p. 426	
	Nandrolone, p. 435	
	Norethisterone, p. 447	
	Norethynodrel, p. 448	
	Nortriptyline Hydrochloride, p. 450	
	Prednisone, p. 509	
	Progesterone, p. 515	
	Testosterone, p. 561	
242	Acetanilide, p. 170	
	Salol, p. 539	310
243	Colchicine, p. 269	350
	Methaphenilene, p. 410	
245	Benzaldehyde, p. 210	279, 289
	Santonin, p. 540	
246	Methanthelinium Bromide, p. 409	282
247	Chlorotrianisene, p. 254	307
	Octaverine, p. 452	321, 358
248	Ethosuximide, p. 338	
	Probenecid, p. 512	225
249	Paracetamol, p. 465	
	Phytomenadione, p. 499	245, 263, 271, 327
250	Menaphthone, p. 399	245, 263, 333
	Phenacetin, p. 477	
251, 257	Benzathine Penicillin, p. 211	263, 266, 320
252	Gelsemine, p. 353	
252·5, 258·5	Fenimide, p. 344	248, 265
254	Methdilazine, p. 412	304
	Phenothiazine, p. 489	317
255	Benzene, p. 211	
	Hyoscyamine, p. 378	247·5, 252, 264
256	Methyridine, p. 427	262
256·5	Pseudoephedrine Hydrochloride, p. 525	250·5, 262·5

λ *max* mμ	*Compound*	*Subsidiary Peaks* (mμ)
257	Bethanidine, p. 222	251
	Phenacemide, p. 477	
	Phensuximide, p. 491	251, 263
	Tolazoline, p. 576	263
	Tolnaftate, p. 577	
	Tricyclamol Chloride, p. 583	252, 263
257, 251	Benzathine Penicillin, p. 211	263, 266, 320
257·5	Glutethimide, p. 353	251·5, 263·5
258	Di-iodohydroxyquinoline, p. 306	
	Homatropine Methobromide, p. 365	252, 264
	Pethidine, p. 476	252, 264
	Phenytoin, p. 496	
	Primidone, p. 511	251, 264
	Prochlorperazine, p. 514	
	Trimetaphan Camsylate, p. 586	252, 264
258·5	Nitrobenzene, p. 444	
258·5, 252·5	Fenimide, p. 344	248, 265
259	Alphacetylmethadol, p. 180	
	Cetylpyridinium Chloride, p. 244	
	Ethotoin, p. 338	265
	Pheneturide, p. 483	265
259, 261·5	Phenprobamate, p. 491	248·5, 253·5, 265, 268·5
261	Buclizine, p. 226	254, 266
	Proflavine Hemisulphate, p. 515	458
261·5, 259	Phenprobamate, p. 491	248·5, 253·5, 265, 268·5
261·6	Toluene, p. 578	249, 253·5, 255·3, 259·7, 264·5, 268·2
263	Dexamethasone, p. 287	240
	Lignocaine, p. 392	278
	Prednisolone, p. 508	240
263·5	Denatonium Benzoate, p. 282	269
264	Sulphaguanidine, p. 550	
265	Calciferol, p. 234	
267	Aminometradine, p. 187	
	Pentamidine, p. 472	
	Propamidine, p. 519	
	Reserpine, p. 535	294
	Sulphamethoxypyridazine, p. 553	
	Sulphaphenazole, p. 554	
268	Domiphen Bromide, p. 321	274
	Phenoxymethylpenicillin, p. 490	263, 275
269	Phenindione, p. 484	320

λ *max* mμ	*Compound*	*Subsidiary Peaks* (mμ)
291	Griseofulvin, p. 355	
	Phthalylsulphathiazole, p. 498	260
293	Alcuronium Chloride, p. 177	
294	Butyl Aminobenzoate, p. 232	
	Isobutyl Aminobenzoate, p. 381	223
295	Hydrastine, p. 368	
308	Cytisine, p. 279	235
310	Noscapine, p. 451	291
320	Ergotoxine Esylate, p. 329	
327	Dithiazanine Iodide, p. 320	276
329	Dieldrin, p. 299	
344	Harmaline, p. 358	260, 376
351	Aloin, p. 180	268, 295·5
361	Cyanocobalamin, p. 272	278, 550
375	Nitrofurazone, p. 445	260
405	Phenazopyridine, p. 480	238, 267, 277
508	Viprynium Embonate, p. 595	239, 358

Infra-red Peaks

Method of using the infra-red data

On each of the infra-red spectra reproduced on pp. 727–93, the major peaks have been labelled 'A', 'B', or 'C' in decreasing order of intensity. With some spectra (e.g. that of amphetamine) selection of these peaks presents no difficulty; with others (e.g. that of brucine) there are a number of peaks of almost equal intensity and therefore several peaks have to carry the same designation. The choice of whether two absorbing bands carry the same letter or different ones has been somewhat arbitrary, but this is of no practical importance as the relative intensity of such bands is not reproducible owing to variations between different instruments.

The table is used as follows. Assume that the spectrum reproduced below is that of the unknown compound.

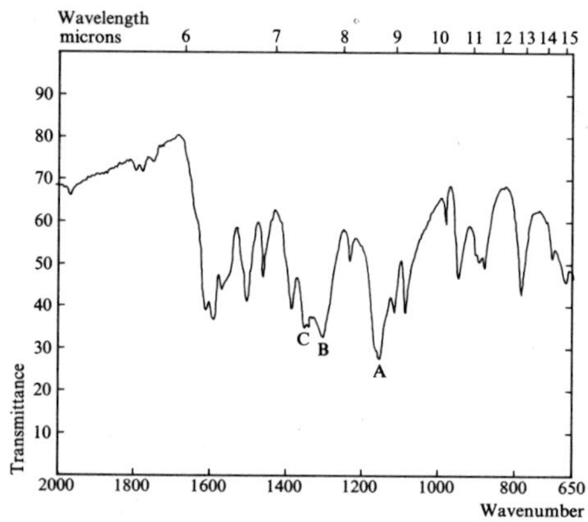

It will be seen that the three major peaks are at 1157 cm^{-1} (A), 1305 cm^{-1} (B), and 1342 cm^{-1} (C). Turn to the table and list all the peaks (a) between 1156 and 1158 cm^{-1}, (b) between 1304 and 1306 cm^{-1}, and (c) between 1341 and 1343 cm^{-1}, thus:

1156 Methylpentynol (B)
Pyridostigmine Bromide (B)
1157 Chlorothiazide (A)
Tolbutamide (A)
1158 Butethamate (B)
Carbetapentane (C)
Cyclopenthiazide (A)
Methyclothiazide (A)

1304 Metaraminol (A)
Nalorphine Hydrobromide (C)
Phenindamine (A)
1305 Aspirin (C)
Chlorothiazide (B)
Nicotinyl Alcohol (A)

1341 Hydroflumethiazide (B)
1342 Chlorothiazide (C)
Tybamate (B)
1343 Cyclopenthiazide (B)
Methysergide Maleate (C)

Chlorothiazide is the only compound occurring on all three lists so its spectrum (p. 734) is now compared with that of the unknown. It will be seen to be identical. Had there been no resemblance, comparison should have been made with the spectrum of cyclopenthiazide which occurs on two of the lists. If it is still impossible to obtain agreement a wider coverage must be used. Lists should be drawn up of all the compounds with peaks (a) between 1154 and 1160 cm^{-1}, (b) between 1302 and 1308 cm^{-1}, and (c) between 1339 and 1345 cm^{-1}.

Should the unknown have several peaks of almost equal intensity, a corresponding number of lists must be made.

Principal Peaks in Ascending Order of Wavenumber

cm^{-1}	*Compound*	*Spectrum on page*
650	Chlormethiazole (B), p. 250	779
660	Pilocarpine (C), p. 500	756
667	Diamthazole (B), p. 293	783
675	Nicotinyl Alcohol (A), p. 442	792
688	Amiphenazole (C), p. 188	729
689	Diethylpropion (C), p. 301	784
690	Bamipine (B), p. 206	775
	Edrophonium Chloride (B), p. 324	785
	Tranylcypromine Sulphate (C), p. 579	767
691	Cinnarizine (B), p. 263	736
693	Oxazepam (C), p. 458	749
694	Caramiphen (C), p. 237	778
695	Alverine (A), p. 182	771
	Aminopentamide (A), p. 187	772
	Amphetamine (A), p. 192	729
	Captodiame (B), p. 236	777
	Pemoline (C), p. 470	751
	Phenmetrazine Hydrochloride (B), p. 486	754
696	Benzhexol (A), p. 213	775
	Bromodiphenhydramine (C), p. 224	776
	Cycrimine (A), p. 277	782
	Doxapram (C), p. 322	785
	Mephentermine (C), p. 401	790
	Procyclidine Hydrochloride (A), p. 514	759
697	Biperiden (A), p. 223	776
	Diphenidol (A), p. 316	785
	Etafedrine (A), p. 330	786
	Pargyline (A), p. 469	793
698	Cetalkonium Chloride (C), p. 243	778
	Fencamfamin (A), p. 343	786
	Fenpiprane (B), p. 345	786
	Methylamphetamine Hydrochloride (B), p. 420	746
	Phenadoxone Hydrochloride (B), p. 478	752
	Pipenzolate Bromide (B), p. 502	757
699	Diphenhydramine Theoclate (A), p. 315	785
	Embramine (C), p. 324	785
700	Adiphenine (C), p. 175	771
	Azacyclonol (A), p. 204	774
	Benztropine (B), p. 216	775
	Chlophedianol (A), p. 244	733
	Doxylamine (A), p. 322	785
	Ethotoin (C), p. 338	740
	Lobeline (B), p. 393	789
	Phencyclidine Hydrochloride (B), p. 481	753
	Phenindione (B), p. 484	754

cm^{-1}	*Compound*	*Spectrum on page*
700	Phenylpropanolamine Hydrochloride (A), p. 494	755
	Pseudoephedrine Hydrochloride (A), p. 525	760
	Tolpropamine Hydrochloride (A), p. 577	767
701	Diphenidol (A), p. 316	785
	Norbormide (B), p. 446	792
	Pipradrol Hydrochloride (A), p. 505	757
702	Cinnarizine (A), p. 263	736
	Methylephedrine (A), p. 423	791
	Nitrazepam (B), p. 443	748
703	Ephedrine (A), p. 327	740
704	Phenadoxone Hydrochloride (B), p. 478	752
705	Bibenzonium Bromide (A), p. 222	776
	Isopropamide Iodide (C), p. 384	744
708	Benzoic Acid (A), p. 214	731
	Cyclizine (A), p. 273	782
710	Amydricaine (C), p. 194	773
	Amylocaine (C), p. 196	773
	Isocarboxazid (B), p. 382	743
	Tridihexethyl Chloride (B), p. 583	767
711	Benzamine (C), p. 210	775
	Mephentermine (B), p. 401	790
	Piperocaine Hydrochloride (B), p. 504	757
712	Nicotine (A), p. 440	748
716	Phenacemide (C), p. 477	752
717	Tridihexethyl Chloride (A), p. 583	767
721	Tolazoline (C), p. 576	767
722	Cetalkonium Chloride (B), p. 243	778
725	Bamipine (A), p. 206	775
727	Tolpropamine Hydrochloride (A), p. 577	767
729	Oxyphenonium Bromide (C), p. 463	750
731	Norharman (C), p. 448	792
733	Biperiden (B), p. 223	776
735	Phenothiazine (A), p. 489	754
736	Pericyazine (B), p. 475	752
737	Amphetamine (B), p. 192	729
	Methyl Nicotinate (B), p. 419	745
740	Benzyl Nicotinate (C), p. 218	775
	Pipradrol Hydrochloride (A), p. 505	757
	Thiabendazole (B), p. 568	766
741	Yohimbine Hydrochloride (B), p. 598	770
742	Alverine (B), p. 182	771
	Benztropine (C), p. 216	775
	Methylephedrine (A), p. 423	791
	Nortriptyline Hydrochloride (B), p. 451	792
	Tetrahydrozoline Hydrochloride (B), p. 563	765

cm⁻¹	*Compound*	*Spectrum on page*
744	Nicotinamide (B), p. 440	748
	Nicotinic Acid (B), p. 441	748
745	Azacyclonol (B), p. 204	774
	Bamipine (A), p. 206	775
	Caffeine (B), p. 234	733
	Cyclizine (C), p. 273	782
	Ephedrine (C), p. 327	740
	Imipramine (C), p. 379	789
	Mephenesin (C), p. 401	744
746	Pargyline (B), p. 469	793
	Phenylpropanolamine Hydrochloride (B), p. 494	755
747	Chlorpromazine (B), p. 256	780
	Desipramine (B), p. 285	783
	Diprophylline (C), p. 317	785
	Methylamphetamine Hydrochloride (A), p. 420	746
	Norharman (C), p. 448	792
	Pipamazine (C), p. 501	757
748	Azapetine (A), p. 205	774
	Clemizole (A), p. 264	781
	Diethazine (B), p. 300	784
	Hexocyclium Methylsulphate (C), p. 363	742
	Methoxypromazine Maleate (C), p. 418	745
	Phenytoin (C), p. 496	756
	Promazine Hydrochloride (B), p. 517	759
	Trimeprazine Tartrate (B), p. 585	768
749	Bibenzonium Bromide (C), p. 222	776
	Cyproheptadine (A), p. 278	782
	Diphenidol (C), p. 316	785
	Prothipendyl Hydrochloride (B), p. 523	760
750	Aminacrine (B), p. 185	772
	Aminopentamide (B), p. 187	772
	Amolanone (C), p. 191	773
	Hydrallazine (A), p. 367	788
	Methixene (A), p. 414	791
	Pecazine Hydrochloride (B), p. 470	751
	Phenothiazine (C), p. 489	754
	Proxyphylline (C), p. 525	760
751	Norbormide (C), p. 446	792
752	Acetanilide (A), p. 170	727
	Amitriptyline (A), p. 189	772
	Apomorphine (C), p. 199	773
	Chlorcyclizine (C), p. 247	779
	Domiphen Bromide (B), p. 321	739
753	Protriptyline Hydrochloride (A), p. 524	760
754	Buclizine (B), p. 226	776
	Cinchonidine (A), p. 262	780
755	Bephenium Hydroxynaphthoate (A), p. 219	775
	Cycrimine (C), p. 277	782
	Phenylbutazone (C), p. 492	755
	Procyclidine Hydrochloride (C), p. 514	759
	Thioridazine Hydrochloride (C), p. 573	793
756	Chlophedianol (A), p. 244	733
	Isocarboxazid (A), p. 382	743
	Nortriptyline Hydrochloride (A), p. 451	792

cm^{-1}	*Compound*	*Spectrum on page*
757	Butriptyline (A), p. 231	777
	Clopenthixol (C), p. 266	781
	Desipramine (C), p. 285	783
	Phenmetrazine Hydrochloride (B), p. 486	754
	Promethazine Hydrochloride (A), p. 518	759
758	Salicylic Acid (A), p. 539	762
759	Bibenzonium Bromide (C), p. 222	776
	Cyclizine (C), p. 273	782
760	Aminacrine (A), p. 185	772
	Benzhexol (C), p. 213	775
	Chlordiazepoxide (C), p. 248	779
	Cinchonine (A), p. 263	780
	Mepivacaine (C), p. 402	790
	Phencyclidine Hydrochloride (C), p. 481	753
	Phenoxypropazine Maleate (B), p. 490	755
761	Pseudoephedrine Hydrochloride (B), p. 525	760
762	Lignocaine (B), p. 392	789
764	Dequalinium Chloride (C), p. 284	737
	Prilocaine Hydrochloride (B), p. 510	758
	Strychnine (B), p. 545	763
765	Amitriptyline (B), p. 189	772
	Clemizole (B), p. 264	781
	Cyproheptadine (B), p. 278	782
766	Phenindione (C), p. 484	754
767	Ambenonium Chloride (C), p. 183	772
	Chloropyrilene (C), p. 251	779
	Dichloralphenazone (B), p. 296	738
768	Nortriptyline Hydrochloride (C), p. 451	792
	Pecazine Hydrochloride (C), p. 470	751
770	Butanilicaine (C), p. 229	777
	Phenazone (B), p. 480	753
	Tripelennamine Hydrochloride (C), p. 588	768
772	Protriptyline Hydrochloride (B), p. 524	760
773	Diphenidol (C), p. 316	785
775	Amitriptyline (C), p. 189	772
	Triprolidine Hydrochloride (A), p. 588	768
776	Chlorprothixene (A), p. 258	735
	Cyproheptadine (C), p. 278	782
	Tolpropamine Hydrochloride (A), p. 577	767
779	Hydroxyquinoline (B), p. 375	788
780	Naphazoline (A), p. 435	792
788	Nicotinyl Alcohol (C), p. 442	792
790	Apomorphine (C), p. 199	773
791	Naphazoline (B), p. 435	792
795	Benactyzine (A), p. 209	775
797	Cyproheptadine (A), p. 278	782
799	Meclozine (C), p. 398	790
	Protriptyline Hydrochloride (A), p. 524	760

cm^{-1}	*Compound*	*Spectrum on page*
800	Cinchonidine (C), p. 262	780
801	Chlorzoxazone (B), p. 260	735
802	Chlorbutol (A), p. 246	734
	Tolpropamine Hydrochloride (B), p. 577	767
805	Morphine (A), p. 431	747
808	Ethionamide (B), p. 335	740
810	Chlorphentermine (B), p. 255	780
	Nicotine (C), p. 440	748
811	Pericyazine (C), p. 475	752
815	Amodiaquine (C), p. 190	772
	Primaquine Phosphate (B), p. 510	758
817	Dichlorophen (B), p. 297	738
820	Hordenine (B), p. 367	787
828	Dienoestrol (C), p. 300	738
830	Butylchloral Hydrate (A), p. 233	733
	Ethchlorvynol (C), p. 333	740
	Oxazepam (C), p. 458	749
832	Bamethan (A), p. 206	774
	Chlorprothixene (C), p. 258	735
	Haloperidol (A), p. 357	741
833	Prothionamide (B), p. 522	760
838	Chloral Hydrate (A), p. 245	733
845	Chlorbutol (B), p. 246	734
865	Ethionamide (B), p. 335	740
872	Testosterone (C), p. 561	765
892	Dexamethasone (C), p. 287	737
899	Cinchonidine (B), p. 262	780
906	Thiabendazole (C), p. 568	766
910	Decamethonium Iodide (A), p. 280	782
912	Prednisone (C), p. 509	758
913	Hexamethonium Bromide (A), p. 361	787
917	Methylpentynol (A), p. 425	746
918	Azapetine (B), p. 205	774
925	Hydrastinine (B), p. 368	788
935	Ethchlorvynol (A), p. 333	740
945	Hexamethonium Bromide (C), p. 361	787
	Morphine (C), p. 431	747
946	Paraldehyde (B), p. 466	751
950	Acetylcholine Chloride (A), p. 173	771
	Ethchlorvynol (B), p. 333	740
953	Choline Chloride (C), p. 261	735

cm^{-1}	*Compound*	*Spectrum on page*
1032	Hydrastinine (A), p. 368	788
	Hyoscyamine (C), p. 378	743
1033	Butriptyline (C), p. 231	777
	Oxycodone (C), p. 460	750
1035	Atropine (B), p. 202	730
	Chlophedianol (B), p. 244	733
	Cotarnine (C), p. 271	781
	Strophanthin-K (B), p. 544	763
1036	Chlorthalidone (B), p. 259	780
1037	Embutramide (C), p. 325	785
	Hydrastine (A), p. 368	788
	Normetanephrine Hydrochloride (B), p. 449	749
1038	Noscapine (C), p. 451	749
1039	Diprophylline (B), p. 317	785
	Methylephedrine (A), p. 423	791
1040	Quinidine (C), p. 531	761
1041	Ethinamate (B), p. 334	740
	Hyoscine (B), p. 376	789
	Mephenesin (B), p. 401	744
1042	Hydrocortisone (C), p. 370	743
1043	Pholcodine (C), p. 496	756
1044	Methoxamine (C), p. 417	791
1050	Dimercaprol (B), p. 307	739
	Lincomycin (B), p. 393	789
	Phenelzine (C), p. 482	753
1051	Butylchloral Hydrate (C), p. 233	733
	Testosterone (B), p. 561	765
1052	Codeine (A), p. 268	736
1054	Benactyzine (C), p. 209	775
	Benztropine (A), p. 216	775
1055	Digoxin (C), p. 303	738
1057	Etafedrine (C), p. 330	786
1059	Styramate (B), p. 546	763
1060	Amprotropine (C), p. 194	773
	Hyoscine (C), p. 376	789
1061	Chloramphenicol (B), p. 246	734
	Testosterone (B), p. 561	765
1064	Paraquat (C), p. 468	792
1065	Azacosterol (A), p. 204	774
	Tybamate (C), p. 591	769
1066	Bamethan (B), p. 206	774
	Pericyazine (C), p. 475	752
1067	Bromodiphenhydramine (A), p. 224	776
1068	Papaverine (B), p. 464	751

cm⁻¹	*Compound*	*Spectrum on page*
1069	Fenfluramine (C), p. 344	786
	Meprobamate (B), p. 403	744
1070	Metronidazole (C), p. 429	791
1071	Strophanthin-K (A), p. 544	763
1075	Digoxin (A), p. 303	738
	Lincomycin (B), p. 393	789
	Urethane (C), p. 593	769
1078	Chloral Hydrate (B), p. 245	733
1080	Pyrrobutamine (B), p. 529	761
1081	Dimefline (C), p. 306	784
	Iproniazid (B), p. 381	743
	Meclozine (C), p. 398	790
1082	Hydroxyzine (A), p. 376	788
1083	Phenmetrazine Hydrochloride (A), p. 486	754
1084	Carbinoxamine (A), p. 239	778
	Chlorphentermine (C), p. 255	780
	Serotonin (A), p. 540	762
1085	Heteronium Bromide (C), p. 360	787
	Veratrine (B), p. 594	769
1086	Hydromorphinol (A), p. 371	743
1088	Acetylcholine Chloride (C), p. 173	771
	Chlorphenoxamine Hydrochloride (A), p. 255	735
1089	Carbutamide (C), p. 241	778
	Cotarnine (A), p. 271	781
1090	Ambazone (A), p. 182	772
	Butylchloral Hydrate (B), p. 233	733
	Cinchonidine (B), p. 262	780
	Clopenthixol (B), p. 266	781
	Demecolcine (C), p. 281	737
	Phenacemide (B), p. 477	752
	Phenadoxone Hydrochloride (B), p. 478	752
1092	Aconitine (A), p. 174	771
	Apronal (C), p. 200	730
	Fenpiprane (B), p. 345	786
1093	Hexetidine (B), p. 361	787
	Pheneturide (C), p. 483	753
1094	Bromodiphenhydramine (B), p. 224	776
1095	Bibenzonium Bromide (B), p. 222	776
	Embramine (B), p. 324	785
	Paraldehyde (A), p. 466	751
1098	Troxidone (C), p. 590	769
1100	Diphenhydramine Theoclate (B), p. 315	785
1102	Fencamfamin (C), p. 343	786
	Hydroxyamphetamine (C), p. 373	788
1104	Atropine Methobromide (C), p. 203	774
	Chlorprothixene (B), p. 258	735
	Pilocarpine (C), p. 500	756

cm^{-1}	*Compound*	*Spectrum on page*
1106	Cocaine (C), p. 267	736
	Trifluoperazine Hydrochloride (A), p. 584	768
1108	Bamethan (C), p. 206	774
	Benzamine (C), p. 210	775
	Benzyl Nicotinate (B), p. 218	775
	Orphenadrine Citrate (C), p. 456	749
	Phenelzine (B), p. 482	753
1109	Isobutyl Aminobenzoate (C), p. 381	789
1110	Amylocaine (C), p. 196	773
	Carbinoxamine (B), p. 239	778
	Cinchonine (B), p. 263	780
	Methyl Nicotinate (B), p. 419	745
	Pholedrine Sulphate (A), p. 497	756
1111	Clomiphene (B), p. 265	781
	Dichlorophen (C), p. 297	738
	Hydromorphinol (A), p. 371	743
	Mephentermine (A), p. 401	790
	Veratrine (C), p. 594	769
1112	Benzhexol (B), p. 213	775
1114	Doxapram (B), p. 322	785
	Phenoxybenzamine (B), p. 489	793
1115	Fluphenazine (A), p. 348	787
	Leptazol (B), p. 389	744
	Lobeline (C), p. 393	789
1117	Cycrimine (B), p. 277	782
	Fluopromazine (A), p. 347	787
1118	Dexamphetamine Sulphate (A), p. 287	737
	Morphine (C), p. 431	747
	Pholcodine (A), p. 496	756
	Sparteine Sulphate (A), p. 542	763
1119	Fenfluramine (A), p. 344	786
	Methocarbamol (B), p. 414	745
1120	Ambazone (A), p. 182	772
	Anileridine (B), p. 197	729
	Benzethonium Chloride (C), p. 213	793
	Carbetapentane (B), p. 238	778
	Reserpine (A), p. 535	762
	Tranylcypromine Sulphate (A), p. 579	767
	Tubocurarine Chloride (C), p. 591	769
1121	Deserpidine (A), p. 284	737
	Nalorphine Hydrobromide (C), p. 434	747
1122	Dicyclomine (A), p. 299	784
1123	Picrotoxin (B), p. 500	756
1125	Sulphasomidine (A), p. 556	765
1126	Amidopyrine (C), p. 185	728
	Methylpentynol (B), p. 425	746
1128	Chlormezanone (B), p. 250	734
	Dicyclomine (A), p. 299	784
1129	Sulphaguanidine (A), p. 550	764

cm⁻¹	*Compound*	*Spectrum on page*
1130	Fencamfamin (C), p. 343	786
	Hydroxyzine (A), p. 376	788
	Meclozine (C), p. 398	790
1131	Buclizine (B), p. 226	776
1135	Arecoline (C), p. 201	774
	Chlorcyclizine (B), p. 247	779
1138	Cinnarizine (B), p. 263	736
	Sulphasomidine (B), p. 556	765
1140	Methyl Phenidate (C), p. 419	746
1142	Fluphenazine (C), p. 348	787
	Hydrallazine (C), p. 367	788
1143	Frusemide (A), p. 350	741
	Sulphamerazine (A), p. 550	764
1144	Sulphanilamide (A), p. 553	764
	Thebaine Hydrochloride (B), p. 565	793
1145	Adiphenine (B), p. 175	771
	Chlormezanone (B), p. 250	734
	Dioxyline (C), p. 313	784
	Hydrochlorothiazide (B), p. 368	742
	Sulphacetamide Sodium (A), p. 547	763
1147	Carbutamide (B), p. 241	778
1148	Pethidine Hydrochloride (C), p. 476	752
	Sulphaphenazole (A), p. 554	764
	Suxamethonium Chloride (B), p. 559	765
1149	Methyltestosterone (B), p. 426	746
1150	Atropine Methobromide (C), p. 203	774
	Chlorbutol (C), p. 246	734
	Clopenthixol (B), p. 266	781
	Cyclizine (B), p. 273	782
	Hexylresorcinol (C), p. 364	742
	Sulphadiazine (A), p. 547	764
1151	Acetomenaphthone (B), p. 171	727
	Haloperidol (B), p. 357	741
	Hydroflumethiazide (A), p. 370	743
1152	Methoxypromazine Maleate (C), p. 418	745
	Sulphamethoxypyridazine (A), p. 553	764
1153	Atropine (C), p. 202	730
	Cyclothiazide (B), p. 277	782
1154	Caramiphen (B), p. 237	778
	Dicyclomine (C), p. 299	784
	Hyoscyamine (B), p. 378	743
	Neostigmine Bromide (C), p. 438	748
1155	Benzthiazide (B), p. 216	731
	Nalorphine Hydrobromide (C), p. 434	747
1156	Methylpentynol (B), p. 425	746
	Pyridostigmine Bromide (B), p. 527	760
1157	Chlorothiazide (A), p. 253	734
	Tolbutamide (A), p. 576	767

cm⁻¹	*Compound*	*Spectrum on page*
1158	Butethamate (B), p. 230	777
	Carbetapentane (C), p. 238	778
	Cyclopenthiazide (A), p. 276	737
	Methyclothiazide (A), p. 419	745
1159	Chlorpropamide (B), p. 257	735
	Fluopromazine (C), p. 347	787
1160	Ambazone (A), p. 182	772
	Fenfluramine (B), p. 344	786
	Hydrochlorothiazide (B), p. 368	742
	Yohimbine Hydrochloride (C), p. 598	770
1161	Fluphenazine (C), p. 348	787
1162	Amprotropine (B), p. 194	773
	Bendrofluazide (A), p. 210	731
	Normetanephrine Hydrochloride (A), p. 449	749
1163	Chlorthalidone (C), p. 259	780
1164	Butyl Aminobenzoate (B), p. 232	732
1165	Butacaine (A), p. 228	777
	Chlorotrianisene (C), p. 254	734
	Hyoscine (B), p. 376	789
	Methyl Phenidate (B), p. 419	746
	Stilboestrol (C), p. 543	763
1166	Amethocaine (C), p. 184	772
	Pethidine Hydrochloride (C), p. 476	752
1167	Acetazolamide (A), p. 170	727
1168	Aminobenzoic Acid (B), p. 186	728
	Cyclothiazide (B), p. 277	782
	Pilocarpine (B), p. 500	756
1170	Benzocaine (C), p. 214	731
	Naepaine (C), p. 433	792
	Paraldehyde (A), p. 466	751
	Saccharin (B), p. 538	762
1172	Disulphamide (A), p. 320	739
	Homatropine (A), p. 365	742
	Isobutyl Aminobenzoate (B), p. 381	789
1173	Caramiphen (C), p. 237	778
1174	Paraquat (A), p. 468	792
1175	Benzthiazide (A), p. 216	731
	Hydrochlorothiazide (A), p. 368	742
1177	Chlorisondamine Chloride (C), p. 249	734
1179	Anileridine (C), p. 197	729
1180	Hydroflumethiazide (A), p. 370	743
1181	Phenglutarimide Hydrochloride (C), p. 483	753
1182	Hexachlorophane (B), p. 360	742
1183	Aspirin (A), p. 201	730
1184	Trimetaphan Camsylate (B), p. 586	768

cm^{-1}	*Compound*	*Spectrum on page*
1185	Hexylresorcinol (B), p. 364	742
	Pholedrine Sulphate (C), p. 497	756
1187	Metronidazole (A), p. 429	791
1188	Alverine (B), p. 182	771
	Bretylium Tosylate (A), p. 224	732
	Dicyclomine (C), p. 299	784
1190	Apoatropine (A), p. 198	773
	Benzilonium Bromide (C), p. 214	731
	Brucine (B), p. 225	732
1191	Benztropine (C), p. 216	775
1192	Norbutrine (C), p. 447	792
1194	Butethamate (C), p. 230	777
	Phenglutarimide Hydrochloride (B), p. 483	753
1195	Amicarbalide (A), p. 185	772
	Amprotropine (C), p. 194	773
	Desferrioxamine (B), p. 285	783
1197	Yohimbine Hydrochloride (C), p. 598	770
1198	Bisacodyl (B), p. 223	776
	Stilboestrol (A), p. 543	763
1199	Dienoestrol (A), p. 300	738
	Oxymetazoline Hydrochloride (B), p. 460	750
1200	Acetomenaphthone (A), p. 171	727
	Glutethimide (C), p. 353	741
	Methyl Phenidate (C), p. 419	746
	Nitrofurantoin (C), p. 444	749
	Physostigmine (A), p. 498	756
1204	Benzquinamide (C), p. 216	775
1206	Butoxamine (B), p. 231	777
1207	Pyridoxine Hydrochloride (C), p. 528	761
1208	Dioxyline (C), p. 313	784
1210	Acinitrazole (B), p. 174	771
	Diperodon (A), p. 314	784
	Noradrenaline Acid Tartrate (B), p. 445	749
	Quinuronium Sulphate (A), p. 533	762
1211	Lobeline (C), p. 393	789
	Naphazoline (C), p. 435	792
1212	Bisacodyl (A), p. 223	776
1215	Methocarbamol (B), p. 414	745
	Methoxamine (B), p. 417	791
	Neostigmine Bromide (B), p. 438	748
	Nicotinyl Alcohol (A), p. 442	792
	Oxybuprocaine Hydrochloride (A), p. 460	750
1216	Metaraminol (B), p. 406	790
	Orphenadrine Citrate (B), p. 456	749
1217	Dimethoxanate (C), p. 309	784
	Edrophonium Chloride (B), p. 324	785
	Haloperidol (C), p. 357	741

cm^{-1}	*Compound*	*Spectrum on page*
1218	Pemoline (A), p. 470	751
	Pethidine Hydrochloride (B), p. 476	752
1219	Heteronium Bromide (B), p. 360	787
	Phenindione (C), p. 484	754
1220	Acepromazine (C), p. 169	771
	Acetophenazine (C), p. 172	771
	Benzilonium Bromide (B), p. 214	731
	Deserpidine (A), p. 284	737
	Diethylpropion (B), p. 301	784
	Pipenzolate Bromide (C), p. 502	757
	Reserpine (A), p. 535	762
	Trimetaphan Camsylate (A), p. 586	768
1221	Theobromine (B), p. 567	765
1222	Promethazine Hydrochloride (B), p. 518	759
	Thiopropazate Hydrochloride (A), p. 572	766
1224	Hexocyclium Methylsulphate (A), p. 363	742
	Lucanthone (B), p. 394	789
1225	Bephenium Hydroxynaphthoate (B), p. 219	775
	Imipramine (C), p. 379	789
	Mepacrine (A), p. 400	790
	Oxyphenonium Bromide (A), p. 463	750
	Pipazethate (B), p. 502	757
	Testosterone (C), p. 561	765
1226	Dichlorophen (A), p. 297	738
	Furaltadone (C), p. 351	741
	Furazolidone (A), p. 351	741
1227	Droperidol (C), p. 323	739
1228	Bamethan (A), p. 206	774
	Desipramine (C), p. 285	783
	Domiphen Bromide (A), p. 321	739
	Emetine (C), p. 325	786
	Tubocurarine Chloride (B), p. 591	769
1229	Paraquat (C), p. 468	792
1230	Primaquine Phosphate (C), p. 510	758
	Sulphaguanidine (B), p. 550	764
1231	Benactyzine (B), p. 209	775
1232	Hydrocortisone (C), p. 370	743
1234	Thebaine Hydrochloride (A), p. 565	793
1235	Hydrastinine (A), p. 368	788
	Phenyltoloxamine Citrate (C), p. 495	755
	Quinine (A), p. 532	761
1237	Fluopromazine (C), p. 347	787
1238	Bamipine (B), p. 206	775
	Fluanisone (A), p. 346	786
1239	Nitrofurantoin (B), p. 444	749
1240	Benzethonium Chloride (A), p. 213	793
	Chloroprocaine (B), p. 251	779
	Chlorpromazine (C), p. 256	780

cm^{-1}	*Compound*	*Spectrum on page*
1263	Butoxamine (C), p. 231	777
	Metaraminol (A), p. 406	790
1264	Bamethan (C), p. 206	774
	Sulphacetamide Sodium (B), p. 547	763
1265	Apomorphine (A), p. 199	773
1268	Codeine (B), p. 268	736
	Phenylephrine Hydrochloride (C), p. 493	755
1269	Dimethisterone (B), p. 308	739
	Methotrimeprazine (C), p. 416	791
1270	Amethocaine (B), p. 184	772
	Veratrine (A), p. 594	769
1271	Berberine (B), p. 219	776
	Methimazole (C), p. 413	745
1272	Bemegride (B), p. 209	731
	Butethamine (A), p. 230	777
	Butyl Aminobenzoate (A), p. 232	732
1273	Aconitine (A), p. 174	771
	Papaverine (C), p. 464	751
	Pyridoxine Hydrochloride (B), p. 528	761
1274	Adrenaline (A), p. 175	727
	Procaine Hydrochloride (A), p. 513	758
1275	Amylocaine (A), p. 196	773
	Bamipine (B), p. 206	775
	Butacaine (A), p. 228	777
	Cocaine (A), p. 267	736
	Oxyphenbutazone (C), p. 462	750
	Phensuximide (B), p. 491	755
1276	Benzamine (B), p. 210	775
	Hexachlorophane (B), p. 360	742
	Noscapine (B), p. 451	749
	Quinuronium Sulphate (C), p. 533	762
1277	Naepaine (B), p. 433	792
1278	Benzyl Nicotinate (A), p. 218	775
	Carbimazole (B), p. 238	733
	Dimefline (B), p. 306	784
	Isobutyl Aminobenzoate (A), p. 381	789
	Piperocaine Hydrochloride (A), p. 504	757
1279	Tymazoline (C), p. 592	793
1280	Benzocaine (A), p. 214	731
	Ethylnoradrenaline (A), p. 340	786
	Tubocurarine Chloride (C), p. 591	769
1282	Amydricaine (A), p. 194	773
	Methsuximide (C), p. 418	791
1283	Alcuronium Chloride (C), p. 177	727
	Chlorcyclizine (C), p. 247	779
1284	Methyl Nicotinate (A), p. 419	745
	Paraquat (C), p. 468	792
1285	Brucine (B), p. 225	732
	Cyclizine (C), p. 273	782

cm^{-1}	*Compound*	*Spectrum on page*
1324	Hydroflumethiazide (B), p. 370	743
	Nicotinamide (A), p. 440	748
	Nicotinic Acid (A), p. 441	748
1325	Fluphenazine (B), p. 348	787
1326	Metharbitone (B), p. 412	745
1327	Hydromorphinol (A), p. 371	743
1330	Benzoic Acid (C), p. 214	731
	Deserpidine (B), p. 284	737
	Dienoestrol (C), p. 300	738
	Di-iodohydroxyquinoline (A), p. 306	738
	Fenfluramine (C), p. 344	786
	Reserpine (B), p. 535	762
1331	Ethylnoradrenaline (B), p. 340	786
1334	Saccharin (A), p. 538	762
1335	Isoniazid (C), p. 383	744
	Methaqualone (C), p. 411	790
1336	Chlormezanone (C), p. 250	734
	Hydrochlorothiazide (A), p. 368	742
	Tolbutamide (B), p. 576	767
1337	Cinchocaine (C), p. 262	780
	Cyclothiazide (C), p. 277	782
1340	Bendrofluazide (B), p. 210	731
	Bethanechol Chloride (B), p. 221	776
	Urethane (B), p. 593	769
1341	Hydroflumethiazide (B), p. 370	743
1342	Chlorothiazide (C), p. 253	734
	Tybamate (B), p. 591	769
1343	Cyclopenthiazide (B), p. 276	737
	Methysergide Maleate (C), p. 427	747
1345	Acinitrazole (A), p. 174	771
	Azacosterol (C), p. 204	774
	Chlorthalidone (C), p. 259	780
	Furazolidone (A), p. 351	741
	Nitrofurantoin (A), p. 444	749
1346	Amiphenazole (C), p. 188	729
1347	Bamipine (B), p. 206	775
	Clamoxyquin (B), p. 264	781
1348	Bephenium Hydroxynaphthoate (B), p. 219	775
1350	Barbituric Acid (C), p. 208	730
1351	Chloramphenicol (C), p. 246	734
	Trimipramine Maleate (B), p. 587	768
1352	Furaltadone (B), p. 351	741
	Lysergic Acid (B), p. 395	789
	Nitrazepam (A), p. 443	748
1353	Phenoxypropazine Maleate (B), p. 490	755
1355	Pamaquin (C), p. 464	750

cm^{-1}	*Compound*	*Spectrum on page*
1393	Cycloguanil (A), p. 274	782
	Pamaquin (B), p. 464	750
	Piperazine Citrate (B), p. 503	757
1394	Mephentermine (C), p. 401	790
1395	Dexbrompheniramine Maleate (C), p. 288	783
	Pheneturide (B), p. 483	753
1396	Ethionamide (B), p. 335	740
1397	Cinchocaine (C), p. 262	780
1398	Prothionamide (A), p. 522	760
1399	Cycloserine (B), p. 276	782
1400	Brucine (B), p. 225	732
	Clemizole (B), p. 264	781
	Pempidine Tartrate (A), p. 471	751
	Tridihexethyl Chloride (C), p. 583	767
1402	Chlorpromazine (C), p. 256	780
	Methyldopa (C), p. 422	791
	Thioridazine Hydrochloride (B), p. 573	793
1406	Phenobarbitone (B), p. 486	754
1407	Denatonium Benzoate (C), p. 282	783
1408	Acetophenazine (A), p. 172	771
	Carphenazine (B), p. 242	778
	Meprobamate (C), p. 403	744
	Thiabendazole (A), p. 568	766
	Thialbarbitone Sodium (C), p. 569	766
1409	Chlormethiazole (A), p. 250	779
	Hydroxyquinoline (C), p. 375	788
	Thiopentone Sodium (B), p. 571	766
1410	Acepromazine (B), p. 169	771
	Phenacemide (C), p. 477	752
1412	Barbituric Acid (C), p. 208	730
	Nikethamide (C), p. 443	748
	Noradrenaline Acid Tartrate (C), p. 445	749
	Phenindamine (B), p. 484	754
1413	Cropropamide (C), p. 272	781
	Prothipendyl Hydrochloride (A), p. 523	760
1414	Iproniazid (C), p. 381	743
1416	Apronal (B), p. 200	730
	Bamifylline (C), p. 206	774
	Pipazethate (C), p. 502	757
1417	Crotethamide (C), p. 272	781
	Fluopromazine (B), p. 347	787
	Metyrapone (C), p. 429	747
1418	Dimercaprol (C), p. 307	739
	Ethionamide (A), p. 335	740
1420	Prothionamide (A), p. 522	760
1421	Sparteine Sulphate (B), p. 542	763
	Triprolidine Hydrochloride (C), p. 588	768

cm^{-1}	*Compound*	*Spectrum on page*
1447	Diphenidol (B), p. 316	785
	Hydroxychloroquine (B), p. 374	788
	Methylephedrine (B), p. 423	791
	Procyclidine Hydrochloride (B), p. 514	759
	Prothipendyl Hydrochloride (B), p. 523	760
	Sparteine Sulphate (B), p. 542	763
1448	Alverine (B), p. 182	771
	Chloroquine (C), p. 252	779
	Chlorphenoxamine Hydrochloride (C), p. 255	735
	Diphenhydramine Theoclate (C), p. 315	785
	Etafedrine (B), p. 330	786
	Morphine (B), p. 431	747
	Oxycodone (C), p. 460	750
	Pholcodine (C), p. 496	756
	Pipradrol Hydrochloride (A), p. 505	757
1449	Fencamfamin (B), p. 343	786
1450	Brucine (B), p. 225	732
	Captodiame (A), p. 236	777
	Cetalkonium Chloride (A), p. 243	778
	Norharman (B), p. 448	792
	Pemoline (C), p. 470	751
	Tolpropamine Hydrochloride (B), p. 577	767
	Tridihexethyl Chloride (C), p. 583	767
1451	Clopenthixol (A), p. 266	781
	Debrisoquine (C), p. 279	782
1452	Amphetamine (C), p. 192	729
	Cinnarizine (C), p. 263	736
	Cycloguanil (A), p. 274	782
	Imipramine (B), p. 379	789
1453	Clothiapine (B), p. 267	781
	Hexylresorcinol (C), p. 364	742
1455	Acepromazine (A), p. 169	771
	Acetophenazine (A), p. 172	771
	Amolanone (C), p. 191	773
	Azacosterol (B), p. 204	774
	Butriptyline (B), p. 231	777
	Carphenazine (A), p. 242	778
	Chlorpromazine (A), p. 256	780
	Desferrioxamine (C), p. 285	783
	Ephedrine (B), p. 327	740
	Ethotoin (B), p. 338	740
	Hexetidine (A), p. 361	787
	Pipamazine (B), p. 501	757
1456	Diethazine (A), p. 300	784
	Ethylnoradrenaline (B), p. 340	786
1458	Chlordiazepoxide (B), p. 248	779
	Dihydrallazine (C), p. 304	784
	Pamaquin (A), p. 464	750
	Pargyline (C), p. 469	793
	Pecazine Hydrochloride (A), p. 470	751
1459	Fluopromazine (C), p. 347	787
	Promethazine Hydrochloride (A), p. 518	759
	Pseudoephedrine Hydrochloride (C), p. 525	760

cm⁻¹	*Compound*	*Spectrum on page*
1460	Apomorphine (B), p. 199	773
	Butanilicaine (B), p. 229	777
	Clemizole (B), p. 264	781
	Diamthazole (C), p. 293	783
	Diaveridine (A), p. 293	783
	Dimethoxanate (C), p. 309	784
	Methotrimeprazine (A), p. 416	791
	Nikethamide (C), p. 443	748
	Thioridazine Hydrochloride (A), p. 573	793
1461	Trimeprazine Tartrate (A), p. 585	768
	Triprolidine Hydrochloride (B), p. 588	768
1462	Alcuronium Chloride (C), p. 177	727
	Carbinoxamine (C), p. 239	778
	Cetrimide (B), p. 244	778
	Mepacrine (B), p. 400	790
	Methixene (B), p. 414	791
	Promazine Hydrochloride (A), p. 517	759
	Thiethylperazine Maleate (A), p. 571	766
	Thiopropazate Hydrochloride (A), p. 572	766
1463	Chlophedianol (B), p. 244	733
	Emetine (C), p. 325	786
	Methyprylone (C), p. 426	747
1464	Pericyazine (A), p. 475	752
	Phenylephrine Hydrochloride (B), p. 493	755
	Prilocaine Hydrochloride (C), p. 510	758
1465	Ambenonium Chloride (C), p. 183	772
	Chlorpheniramine (B), p. 254	779
	Methaqualone (C), p. 411	790
	Phenoxypropazine Maleate (A), p. 490	755
1466	Methimazole (A), p. 413	745
	Methysergide Maleate (B), p. 427	747
	Nalorphine Hydrobromide (B), p. 434	747
1467	Metronidazole (C), p. 429	791
1468	Chlorproguanil (C), p. 256	780
	Chlorprothixene (C), p. 258	735
	Cycrimine (C), p. 277	782
	Hexetidine (A), p. 361	787
1469	Hordenine (B), p. 367	787
1470	Dexbrompheniramine Maleate (B), p. 288	783
	Dibromopropamidine (C), p. 295	783
	Doxylamine (B), p. 322	785
	Methoxypromazine Maleate (A), p. 418	745
	Protriptyline Hydrochloride (B), p. 524	760
1474	Metformin (C), p. 407	790
1475	Acetylcholine Chloride (C), p. 173	771
	Leptazol (A), p. 389	744
	Methylamphetamine Hydrochloride (C), p. 421	746
	Morphine (C), p. 431	747
	Sulphamethoxypyridazine (A), p. 553	764
1476	Phenothiazine (B), p. 489	754
1477	Azamethonium Bromide (A), p. 204	774
	Choline Chloride (B), p. 261	735

cm⁻¹	*Compound*	*Spectrum on page*
1478	Chlorcyclizine (C), p. 247	779
	Cotarnine (B), p. 271	781
1479	Decamethonium Iodide (A), p. 280	782
	Edrophonium Chloride (A), p. 324	785
1480	Amodiaquine (B), p. 190	772
	Cetrimide (A), p. 244	778
	Chlorisondamine Chloride (B), p. 249	734
	Chlorzoxazone (C), p. 260	735
	Hydrastinine (A), p. 368	788
	Strychnine (C), p. 545	763
	Sulphasomidine (A), p. 556	765
	Tolpropamine Hydrochloride (B), p. 577	767
1481	Hexamethonium Bromide (B), p. 361	787
	Pheniramine Maleate (B), p. 485	754
1482	Buclizine (B), p. 226	776
	Desipramine (A), p. 285	783
	Thialbarbitone Sodium (A), p. 569	766
1483	Bromodiphenhydramine (B), p. 224	776
1484	Acetylcarbromal (A), p. 172	727
	Carbinoxamine (C), p. 239	778
	Diazepam (B), p. 294	738
	Dichloralphenazone (C), p. 296	738
	Di-iodohydroxyquinoline (B), p. 306	738
	Folic Acid (C), p. 349	741
	Propantheline Bromide (B), p. 519	759
	Thiopentone Sodium (A), p. 571	766
1485	Acinitrazole (C), p. 174	771
	Butoxamine (A), p. 231	777
	Captodiame (C), p. 236	777
	Dexbrompheniramine Maleate (B), p. 288	783
	Dibromopropamidine (B), p. 295	783
	Imipramine (A), p. 379	789
	Metronidazole (B), p. 429	791
	Sulphamethoxypyridazine (A), p. 553	764
1486	Chlorhexidine (C), p. 249	779
	Chlorpheniramine (B), p. 254	779
	Phenazone (C), p. 480	753
1487	Chlorphentermine (A), p. 255	780
	Dichlorophen (C), p. 297	738
	Metformin (C), p. 407	790
1488	Amprolium Hydrochloride (B), p. 193	773
	Chloropyrilene (A), p. 251	779
	Nortriptyline Hydrochloride (C), p. 451	792
	Prothipendyl Hydrochloride (C), p. 523	760
	Trimipramine Maleate (A), p. 587	768
1489	Meclozine (A), p. 398	790
	Pyrithidium Bromide (B), p. 529	793
1490	Amopyroquine (B), p. 191	773
	Chlorphenoxamine Hydrochloride (B), p. 255	735
	Lignocaine (A), p. 392	789
	Mepyramine (A), p. 403	790
1492	Amisometradine (B), p. 189	729
	Fenpiprane (A), p. 345	786

cm⁻¹	*Compound*	*Spectrum on page*
1515	Cycloguanil (A), p. 274	782
	Pyrithidium Bromide (C), p. 529	793
	Stilboestrol (B), p. 543	763
1516	Methyldopate (C), p. 423	791
	Tubocurarine Chloride (A), p. 591	769
1517	Hydroxyamphetamine (B), p. 373	788
	Warfarin Sodium (A), p. 596	770
1518	Oxyphenbutazone (C), p. 462	750
1519	Pholedrine Sulphate (B), p. 497	756
	Procainamide Hydrochloride (A), p. 512	758
1522	Amprolium Hydrochloride (B), p. 193	773
1523	Lincomycin (B), p. 393	789
	Mepivacaine (B), p. 402	790
1525	Chlorproguanil (A), p. 256	780
1526	Chloramphenicol (C), p. 246	734
	Cycloserine (B), p. 276	782
1527	Chlorhexidine (A), p. 249	779
	Methyldopate (A), p. 423	791
1529	Ethylnoradrenaline (A), p. 340	786
	Hydrallazine (A), p. 367	788
	Normetanephrine Hydrochloride (A), p. 449	749
1530	Allantoin (C), p. 178	728
	Buformin (B), p. 226	776
	Diperodon (B), p. 314	784
1534	Proguanil Hydrochloride (A), p. 516	759
1535	Amodiaquine (C), p. 190	772
	Leptazol (B), p. 389	744
	Metronidazole (A), p. 429	791
1536	Choline Theophyllinate (C), p. 568	735
	Pyridoxine Hydrochloride (A), p. 528	761
1537	Dihydrallazine (C), p. 304	784
	Phenformin Hydrochloride (B), p. 483	753
	Sulphaguanidine (B), p. 550	764
1538	Bamifylline (C), p. 206	774
	Chloroquine (B), p. 252	779
1540	Prilocaine Hydrochloride (B), p. 510	758
1543	Cinchocaine (B), p. 262	780
1544	Riboflavine (A), p. 536	762
1546	Fenethylline (C), p. 343	786
1548	Acetazolamide (C), p. 170	727
	Clothiapine (C), p. 267	781
	Diamthazole (C), p. 293	783
	Serotonin (B), p. 540	762
1550	Cycloserine (B), p. 276	782
	Denatonium Benzoate (A), p. 282	783
	Theobromine (C), p. 567	765

cm⁻¹	*Compound*	*Spectrum on page*
1552	Disulphamide (B), p. 320	739
	Isoniazid (B), p. 383	744
	Sulphacetamide Sodium (C), p. 547	763
	Tolbutamide (B), p. 576	767
1553	Chlorpropamide (C), p. 257	735
1555	Phenacetin (C), p. 477	752
1556	Aminacrine (A), p. 185	772
	Nicotinyl Alcohol (B), p. 442	792
1557	Carphenazine (C), p. 242	778
	Mepacrine (B), p. 400	790
1559	Quinalbarbitone Sodium (A), p. 530	761
	Sulphamerazine (C), p. 550	764
1560	Theophylline (C), p. 567	766
1561	Chlorpromazine (C), p. 256	780
1562	Demecolcine (A), p. 281	737
	Desferrioxamine (C), p. 285	783
1563	Amopyroquine (A), p. 191	773
	Paracetamol (B), p. 465	751
1565	Amodiaquine (A), p. 190	772
	Frusemide (C), p. 350	741
	Methaqualone (C), p. 411	790
1566	Colchicine (B), p. 269	736
	Methysergide Maleate (A), p. 427	747
1568	Phenformin Hydrochloride (A), p. 483	753
	Thiethylperazine Maleate (B), p. 571	766
1569	Dibromopropamidine (C), p. 295	783
1570	Clothiapine (A), p. 267	781
	Methimazole (B), p. 413	745
1572	Primaquine Phosphate (C), p. 510	758
	Quinuronium Sulphate (C), p. 533	762
	Triamterene (A), p. 581	767
1573	Chloroquine (A), p. 252	779
	Chlortetracycline (B), p. 259	780
	Demethylchlortetracycline (B), p. 281	783
	Methylergometrine Maleate (A), p. 424	746
1575	Chlorhexidine (C), p. 249	779
	Dihydrallazine (B), p. 304	784
	Mefenamic Acid (C), p. 399	744
	Proguanil Hydrochloride (C), p. 516	759
	Pyrimethamine (A), p. 528	761
	Riboflavine (B), p. 536	762
1576	Isopropamide Iodide (B), p. 384	744
1577	Cycloserine (A), p. 276	782
	Sulphadiazine (B), p. 547	764
1578	Metyrapone (B), p. 429	747
1579	Hydroxychloroquine (A), p. 374	788

cm^{-1}	*Compound*	*Spectrum on page*
1580	Metformin (A), p. 407	790
	Tetracycline Hydrochloride (B), p. 562	765
	Trimipramine Maleate (C), p. 587	768
1581	Bromvaletone (B), p. 225	732
1582	Demecolcine (B), p. 281	737
	Dexamphetamine Sulphate (C), p. 287	737
	Methoxypromazine Maleate (C), p. 418	745
	Phenoxypropazine Maleate (A), p. 490	755
1584	Carbinoxamine (C), p. 239	778
	Pheniramine Maleate (A), p. 485	754
1585	Carphenazine (B), p. 242	778
	Chlorpheniramine (A), p. 254	779
	Hydrallazine (C), p. 367	788
1587	Methotrimeprazine (B), p. 416	791
1588	Ethionamide (B), p. 335	740
	Phenyltoloxamine Citrate (B), p. 495	755
1589	Colchicine (C), p. 269	736
	Dibromopropamidine (A), p. 295	783
1590	Amicarbalide (B), p. 185	772
	Cinchonine (C), p. 263	780
	Clomiphene (A), p. 265	781
	Dexbrompheniramine Maleate (A), p. 288	783
	Doxylamine (B), p. 322	785
	Phenformin Hydrochloride (C), p. 483	753
1591	Droperidol (B), p. 323	739
	Lucanthone (B), p. 394	789
	Metaraminol (B), p. 406	790
1592	Alcuronium Chloride (B), p. 177	727
	Lysergic Acid (A), p. 395	789
	Phenylephrine Hydrochloride (A), p. 493	755
	Piperazine Citrate (A), p. 503	757
	Prothionamide (C), p. 522	760
	Sulphamerazine (B), p. 550	764
	Sulphaphenazole (C), p. 554	764
	Tripelennamine Hydrochloride (B), p. 588	768
1593	Amprolium Hydrochloride (B), p. 193	773
	Bamipine (A), p. 206	775
	Sulphanilamide (B), p. 553	764
1594	Carbamazepine (C), p. 238	778
1595	Chloroprocaine (A), p. 251	779
	Chloropyrilene (A), p. 251	779
	Methyclothiazide (B), p. 419	745
	Oxymetazoline Hydrochloride (A), p. 460	750
	Primaquine Phosphate (B), p. 510	758
1596	Cinchocaine (A), p. 262	780
	Clothiapine (A), p. 267	781
	Cyclothiazide (A), p. 277	782
	Denatonium Benzoate (B), p. 282	783
1597	Aminobenzoic Acid (A), p. 186	728
1598	Acetanilide (A), p. 170	727
	Amethocaine (A), p. 184	772

cm^{-1}	*Compound*	*Spectrum on page*
1598	Benzocaine (B), p. 214	731
	Butacaine (A), p. 228	777
	Cyclopenthiazide (A), p. 276	737
	Diaveridine (C), p. 293	783
	Halopyramine (B), p. 357	787
	Mepyramine (A), p. 403	790
1599	Carbutamide (B), p. 241	778
	Fluanisone (C), p. 346	786
	Hydroxyamphetamine (C), p. 373	788
	Methaqualone (B), p. 411	790
	Procainamide Hydrochloride (A), p. 512	758
	Warfarin Sodium (B), p. 596	770
1600	Butethamine (B), p. 230	777
	Butyl Aminobenzoate (C), p. 232	732
	Carbromal (C), p. 240	733
	Chlorotrianisene (C), p. 254	734
	Cyclomethycaine (C), p. 275	736
	Dimethisterone (C), p. 308	739
	Diperodon (C), p. 314	784
	Fenethylline (C), p. 343	786
	Hydrochlorothiazide (B), p. 368	742
	Methyldopa (A), p. 422	791
	Phenoxybenzamine (C), p. 489	793
	Tetrahydrozoline Hydrochloride (A), p. 563	765
1601	Folic Acid (B), p. 349	741
1602	Chlorproguanil (B), p. 256	780
	Diamthazole (C), p. 293	783
	Dimefline (C), p. 306	784
	Noradrenaline Acid Tartrate (C), p. 445	749
	Xylometazoline Hydrochloride (A), p. 597	770
1604	Amisometradine (B), p. 189	729
1605	Clomiphene (C), p. 265	781
	Dequalinium Chloride (A), p. 284	737
	Naepaine (A), p. 433	792
	Procaine Hydrochloride (B), p. 513	758
	Thebaine Hydrochloride (B), p. 565	793
1607	Isobutyl Aminobenzoate (A), p. 381	789
1608	Aminometradine (A), p. 187	728
	Betamethasone (B), p. 220	732
	Dihydrallazine (A), p. 304	784
	Hydroxychloroquine (C), p. 374	788
	Tolazoline (A), p. 576	767
1609	Edrophonium Chloride (A), p. 324	785
1610	Emylcamate (C), p. 326	739
	Prednisolone (B), p. 508	758
1611	Primaquine Phosphate (A), p. 510	758
1612	Tetracycline Hydrochloride (A), p. 562	765
	Triamterene (A), p. 581	767
1614	Chlorproguanil (B), p. 256	780
	Norbutrine (B), p. 447	792
1615	Debrisoquine (A), p. 279	782
	Naphazoline (A), p. 435	792
	Nitrazepam (B), p. 443	748

cm⁻¹	*Compound*	*Spectrum on page*
1615	Progesterone (C), p. 515	759
	Pyrithidium Bromide (A), p. 529	793
1616	Demethylchlortetracycline (A), p. 281	783
	Dexamethasone (B), p. 287	737
	Hexylresorcinol (C), p. 364	742
	Lucanthone (A), p. 394	789
1617	Chlortetracycline (A), p. 259	780
	Cropropamide (B), p. 272	781
	Crotethamide (B), p. 272	781
	Tymazoline (A), p. 592	793
1618	Phenacemide (C), p. 477	752
1619	Quinidine (C), p. 531	761
	Quinine (C), p. 532	761
1620	Azamethonium Bromide (C), p. 204	774
	Hydroquinidine (C), p. 372	788
	Metformin (B), p. 407	790
	Sulphaguanidine (A), p. 550	764
1624	Sulphanilamide (C), p. 553	764
1625	Chlordiazepoxide (A), p. 248	779
	Chloroprocaine (C), p. 251	779
	Hydrallazine (C), p. 367	788
	Mepacrine (C), p. 400	790
	Phenformin Hydrochloride (C), p. 483	753
1627	Choline Theophyllinate (A), p. 568	735
	Decamethonium Iodide (A), p. 280	782
	Nikethamide (A), p. 443	748
1628	Chlorhexidine (B), p. 249	779
	Desferrioxamine (A), p. 285	783
	Isoniazid (C), p. 383	744
	Pyrimethamine (A), p. 528	761
1629	Homidium Bromide (A), p. 366	787
1630	Diaveridine (B), p. 293	783
	Hexamethonium Bromide (C), p. 361	787
1631	Fenpiprane (B), p. 345	786
1632	Procainamide Hydrochloride (B), p. 512	758
1633	Benzquinamide (B), p. 216	775
	Dihydrallazine (B), p. 304	784
1634	Buformin (C), p. 226	776
1635	Carbutamide (C), p. 241	778
	Proguanil Hydrochloride (B), p. 516	759
1636	Bufylline (C), p. 227	777
	Choline Chloride (A), p. 261	735
1637	Amiphenazole (B), p. 188	729
	Dimefline (A), p. 306	784
	Phensuximide (C), p. 491	755
1638	Aminosalicylic Acid (C), p. 188	729
	Amprolium Hydrochloride (A), p. 193	773
	Paraquat (B), p. 468	792

cm⁻¹	*Compound*	*Spectrum on page*
1639	Amisometradine (A), p. 189	729
	Cinchocaine (B), p. 262	780
1640	Folic Acid (C), p. 349	741
	Hydrocortisone (A), p. 370	743
	Warfarin Sodium (C), p. 596	770
1641	Riboflavine (C), p. 536	762
1642	Aminometradine (B), p. 187	728
	Pyrithidium Bromide (A), p. 529	793
1643	Methylergometrine Maleate (B), p. 424	746
1644	Mefenamic Acid (B), p. 399	744
	Pipamazine (A), p. 501	757
1645	Aminacrine (A), p. 185	772
	Chlormezanone (A), p. 250	734
	Diaveridine (C), p. 293	783
	Lincomycin (A), p. 393	789
1647	Debrisoquine (B), p. 279	782
1648	Betamethasone (A), p. 220	732
	Quinalbarbitone Sodium (B), p. 530	761
1649	Brucine (A), p. 225	732
1650	Alcuronium Chloride (C), p. 177	727
	Bamifylline (A), p. 206	774
	Dimethisterone (A), p. 308	739
	Isopropamide Iodide (A), p. 384	744
	Mepivacaine (A), p. 402	790
	Methysergide Maleate (C), p. 427	747
	Paracetamol (A), p. 465	751
	Prednisolone (A), p. 508	758
	Testosterone (A), p. 561	765
1652	Allantoin (B), p. 178	728
	Dequalinium Chloride (B), p. 284	737
	Embutramide (A), p. 325	785
1653	Pemoline (B), p. 470	751
1654	Cropropamide (A), p. 272	781
1655	Aminacrine (A), p. 185	772
	Crotethamide (A), p. 272	781
	Dexamethasone (A), p. 287	737
	Metharbitone (A), p. 412	745
	Methyprylone (A), p. 426	747
	Phenacetin (A), p. 477	752
1656	Dichloralphenazone (A), p. 296	738
	Proxyphylline (A), p. 525	760
1657	Methyltestosterone (A), p. 426	746
	Salicylic Acid (C), p. 539	762
1658	Caffeine (A), p. 234	733
	Tolbutamide (A), p. 576	767
1659	Isoniazid (A), p. 383	744
	Progesterone (A), p. 515	759
1660	Acepifylline (A), p. 169	771
	Acetanilide (A), p. 170	727

cm^{-1}	*Compound*	*Spectrum on page*
1660	Amidopyrine (A), p. 185	728
	Demethylchlortetracycline (C), p. 281	783
	Diprophylline (A), p. 317	785
	Hexobarbitone (A), p. 362	742
	Phenacemide (A), p. 477	752
	Phenazone (A), p. 480	753
	Styramate (A), p. 546	763
	Theophylline (A), p. 567	766
1661	Carbutamide (A), p. 241	778
	Chlorpropamide (A), p. 257	735
1662	Lignocaine (A), p. 392	789
1663	Chlortetracycline (C), p. 259	780
1664	Fenethylline (A), p. 343	786
	Strychnine (A), p. 545	763
1665	Bufylline (A), p. 227	777
	Iproniazid (C), p. 381	743
1666	Tetracycline Hydrochloride (C), p. 562	765
1667	Methocarbamol (A), p. 414	745
1668	Bemegride (A), p. 209	731
	Frusemide (B), p. 350	741
	Prednisone (A), p. 509	758
1670	Acetophenazine (B), p. 172	771
	Isocarboxazid (A), p. 382	743
1672	Amicarbalide (B), p. 185	772
	Metyrapone (A), p. 429	747
	Pheneturide (A), p. 483	753
1673	Cycloguanil (A), p. 274	782
	Haloperidol (C), p. 357	741
1674	Barbitone (A), p. 207	730
1675	Acepromazine (B), p. 169	771
	Ambenonium Chloride (A), p. 183	772
	Vinbarbitone (A), p. 594	769
1676	Apronal (A), p. 200	730
	Choline Theophyllinate (B), p. 568	735
1678	Carbamazepine (A), p. 238	778
1680	Amisometradine (C), p. 189	729
	Benzocaine (B), p. 214	731
	Denatonium Benzoate (C), p. 282	783
1681	Diazepam (A), p. 294	738
1682	Chloramphenicol (A), p. 246	734
	Diethylpropion (A), p. 301	784
	Methaqualone (A), p. 411	790
1683	Butobarbitone (A), p. 231	732
	Isobutyl Aminobenzoate (B), p. 381	789
	Oxyphenbutazone (A), p. 462	750
1684	Methylphenobarbitone (A), p. 425	746
1685	Butacaine (B), p. 228	777
	Chlorthalidone (A), p. 259	780

cm^{-1}	*Compound*	*Spectrum on page*
1685	Doxapram (A), p. 322	785
	Naepaine (C), p. 433	792
	Pentobarbitone (A), p. 473	752
	Thialbarbitone Sodium (B), p. 569	766
1686	Benzoic Acid (A), p. 214	731
	Glutethimide (A), p. 353	741
	Phensuximide (A), p. 491	755
1687	Allobarbitone (A), p. 179	728
	Lobeline (A), p. 393	789
	Oxazepam (A), p. 458	749
1688	Allylbarbituric Acid (A), p. 179	728
	Aspirin (B), p. 201	730
	Droperidol (A), p. 323	739
	Folic Acid (A), p. 349	741
	Meprobamate (A), p. 403	744
	Methyprylone (B), p. 426	747
	Thiopentone Sodium (C), p. 571	766
1689	Amylobarbitone (B), p. 195	729
	Aprobarbitone (A), p. 200	730
1690	Emylcamate (A), p. 326	739
	Fluanisone (A), p. 346	786
	Procaine Hydrochloride (A), p. 513	758
	Proxyphylline (B), p. 525	760
	Quinalbarbitone Sodium (C), p. 530	761
	Theobromine (A), p. 567	765
1691	Progesterone (B), p. 515	759
1692	Carbromal (A), p. 240	733
	Nitrazepam (A), p. 443	748
1693	Cyclobarbitone (A), p. 274	736
1694	Butanilicaine (A), p. 229	777
1695	Caffeine (A), p. 234	733
	Nealbarbitone (A), p. 437	747
	Tybamate (A), p. 591	769
1696	Acetylcarbromal (C), p. 172	727
	Cyclomethycaine (B), p. 275	736
1697	Betamethasone (C), p. 220	732
1698	Bamifylline (B), p. 206	774
	Chloroprocaine (B), p. 251	779
	Oxybuprocaine Hydrochloride (A), p. 460	750
	Phenglutarimide Hydrochloride (A), p. 483	753
1699	Metharbitone (A), p. 412	745
	Phenadoxone Hydrochloride (A), p. 478	752
1700	Acepifylline (A), p. 169	771
	Anileridine (A), p. 197	729
	Bromvaletone (A), p. 225	732
	Cocaine (B), p. 267	736
	Diprophylline (A), p. 317	785
	Phenindione (A), p. 484	754
	Prilocaine Hydrochloride (A), p. 510	758
	Theophylline (B), p. 567	766
1701	Prednisolone (C), p. 508	758
	Trimetaphan Camsylate (A), p. 586	768

cm^{-1}	*Compound*	*Spectrum on page*
1702	Butacaine (B), p. 228	777
	Butethamine (C), p. 230	777
	Hydrocortisone (B), p. 370	743
1703	Phenobarbitone (A), p. 486	754
	Piperocaine Hydrochloride (A), p. 504	757
1704	Apronal (B), p. 200	730
1705	Diperodon (A), p. 314	784
	Fenethylline (B), p. 343	786
	Methsuximide (A), p. 418	791
	Saccharin (A), p. 538	762
	Yohimbine Hydrochloride (A), p. 598	770
1706	Oxazepam (B), p. 458	749
1707	Barbitone (C), p. 207	730
	Methylphenobarbitone (A), p. 425	746
	Prednisone (B), p. 509	758
1708	Norbormide (A), p. 446	792
	Pethidine Hydrochloride (A), p. 476	752
	Phenylbutazone (A), p. 492	755
1709	Digoxin (B), p. 303	738
1710	Allantoin (A), p. 178	728
	Amylocaine (B), p. 196	773
	Apoatropine (A), p. 198	773
	Barbituric Acid (A), p. 208	730
	Glutethimide (B), p. 353	741
1711	Neostigmine Bromide (A), p. 438	748
1712	Arecoline (A), p. 201	774
	Bethanechol Chloride (A), p. 221	776
	Bufylline (B), p. 227	777
	Butobarbitone (A), p. 231	732
	Hexobarbitone (A), p. 362	742
	Hyoscyamine (A), p. 378	743
1713	Aconitine (B), p. 174	771
	Ethinamate (A), p. 334	740
	Phenytoin (A), p. 496	756
	Urethane (A), p. 593	769
1714	Benzamine (A), p. 210	775
1715	Amydricaine (B), p. 194	773
	Aprobarbitone (A), p. 200	730
1716	Allylbarbituric Acid (A), p. 179	728
	Amylobarbitone (A), p. 195	729
	Ethotoin (A), p. 338	740
	Nitrofurantoin (A), p. 444	749
1717	Pipazethate (A), p. 502	757
1718	Atropine Methobromide (B), p. 203	774
	Bemegride (C), p. 209	731
	Caramiphen (A), p. 237	778
	Dimethoxanate (A), p. 309	784
	Orphenadrine Citrate (A), p. 456	749
1719	Nealbarbitone (A), p. 437	747
	Oxycodone (A), p. 460	750
	Oxyphenonium Bromide (B), p. 463	750

cm^{-1}	*Compound*	*Spectrum on page*
1754	Barbitone (B), p. 207	730
	Bisacodyl (C), p. 223	776
1755	Acetylcarbromal (B), p. 172	727
	Furaltadone (A), p. 351	741
1756	Phenobarbitone (A), p. 486	754
1760	Hydrastine (A), p. 368	788
	Vinbarbitone (A), p. 594	769
1762	Chlorzoxazone (A), p. 260	735
1768	Phenytoin (B), p. 496	756
1780	Picrotoxin (A), p. 500	756
1795	Amolanone (A), p. 191	773
1802	Troxidone (B), p. 590	769

Infra-red Spectra

The infra-red spectra reproduced on the following pages were obtained from two different instruments which produce spectra of different sizes. For ease of comparison, the reproductions have been reduced so that the horizontal wavenumber–wavelength axes of the two types of spectra are of the same width. The two types of spectra are arranged separately (pp. 727–70 and 771–93), each in alphabetical order, and a combined alphabetical index to them is given below.
For details of the method of using these spectra see under Infra-red Peaks, p. 688.

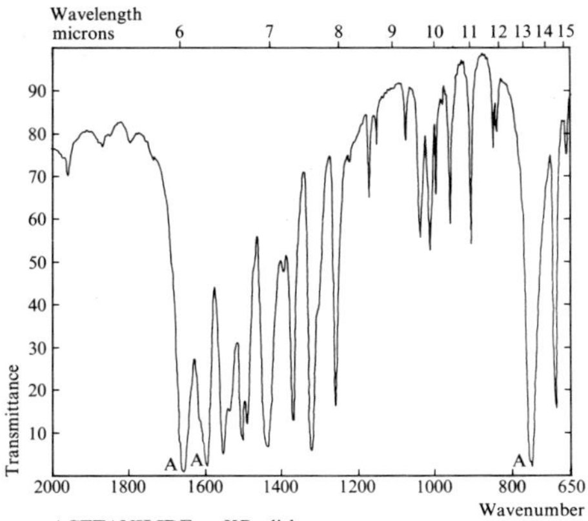

ACETANILIDE — KBr disk
A 752 or 1598 or 1660

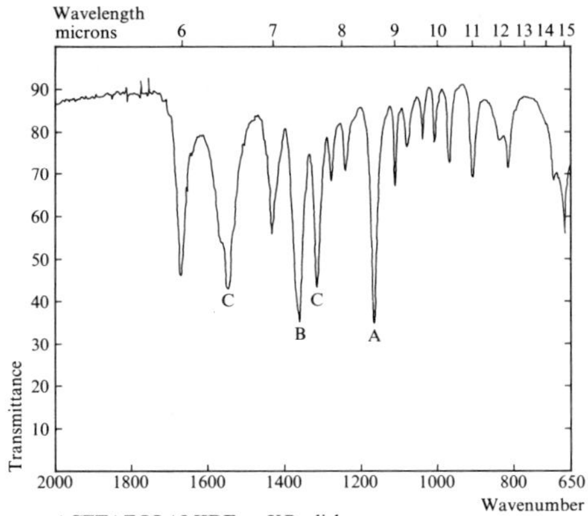

ACETAZOLAMIDE — KBr disk
A 1167, B 1363, C 1316 or 1548

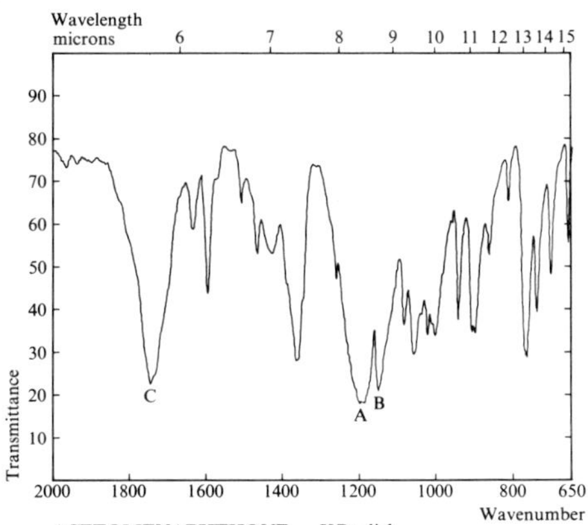

ACETOMENAPHTHONE — KBr disk
A 1200, B 1151, C 1740

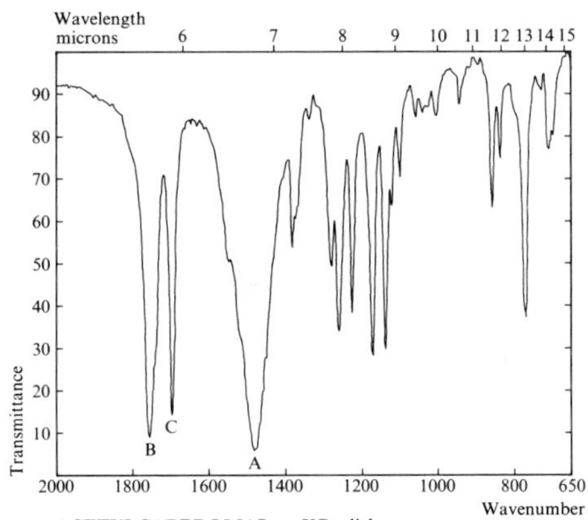

ACETYLCARBROMAL — KBr disk
A 1484, B 1755, C 1696

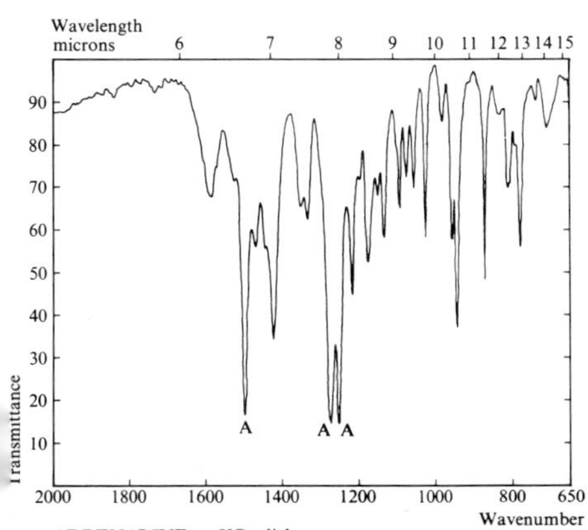

ADRENALINE — KBr disk
A 1253 or 1274 or 1500

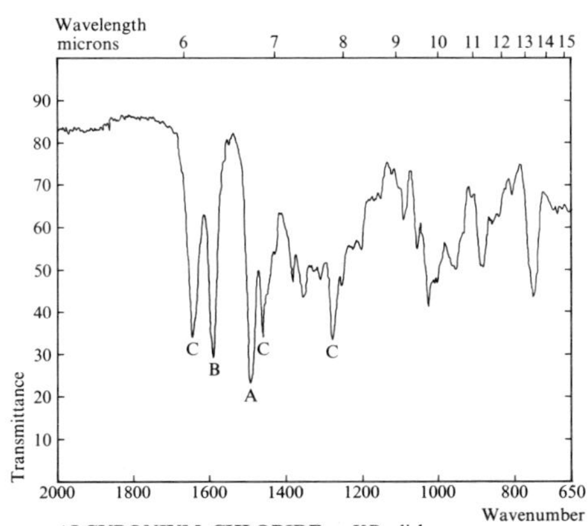

ALCURONIUM CHLORIDE — KBr disk
A 1495, B 1592, C 1283 or 1462 or 1650

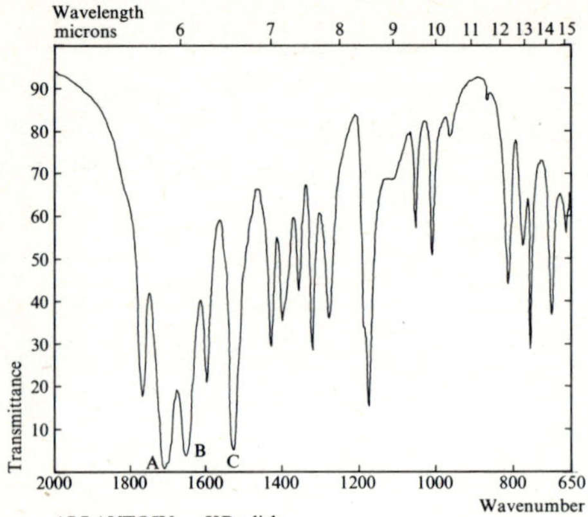

ALLANTOIN — KBr disk
A 1710, B 1652, C 1530

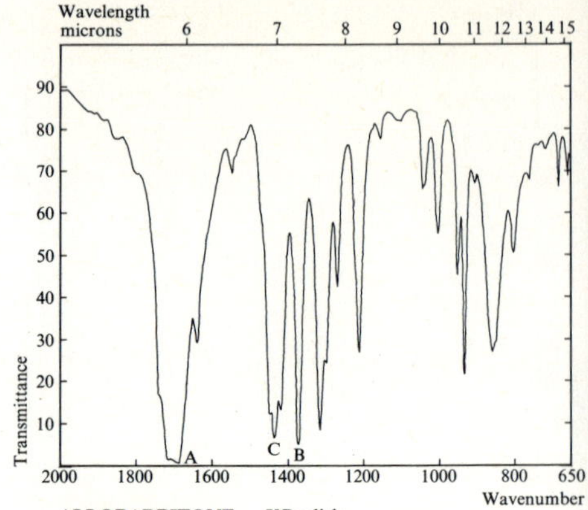

ALLOBARBITONE — KBr disk
A 1687, B 1375, C 1437

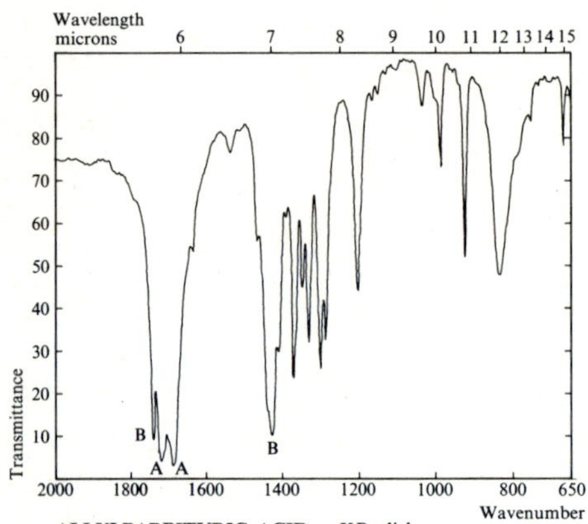

ALLYLBARBITURIC ACID — KBr disk
A 1688 or 1716, B 1428 or 1740

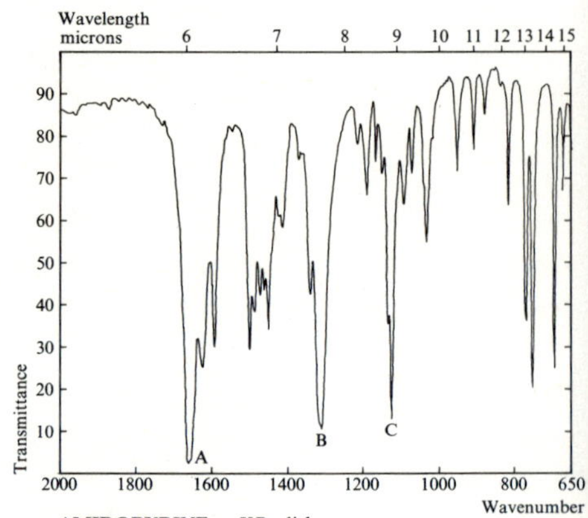

AMIDOPYRINE — KBr disk
A 1660, B 1315, C 1126

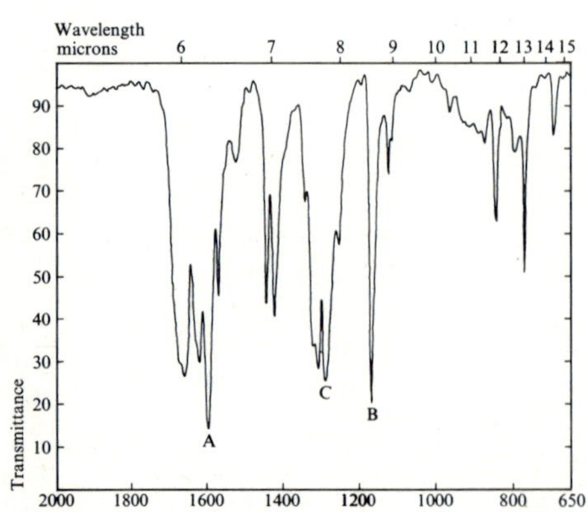

AMINOBENZOIC ACID — KBr disk
A 1597, B 1168, C 1290

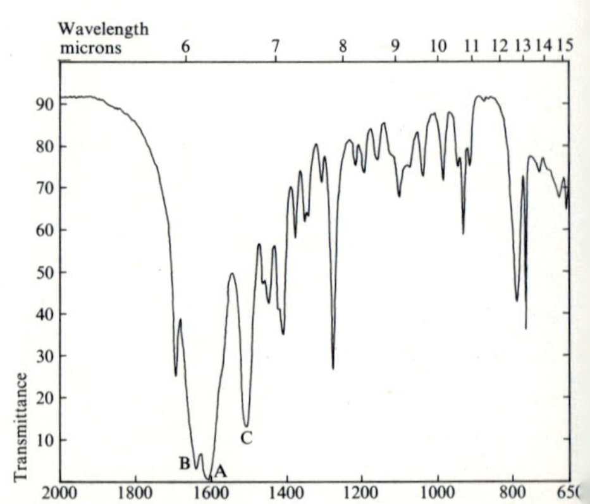

AMINOMETRADINE — KBr disk
A 1608, B 1642, C 1508

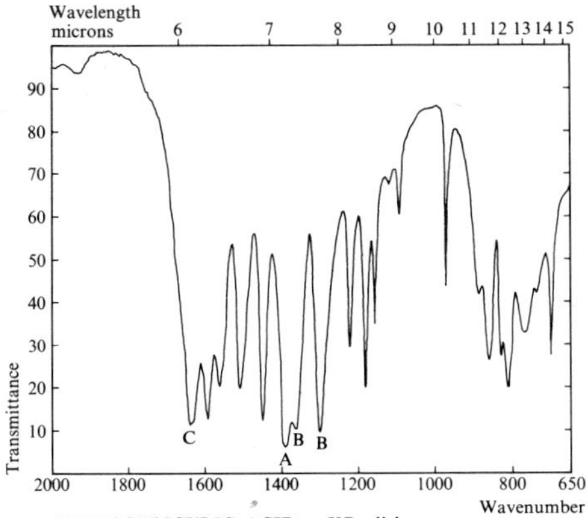

AMINOSALICYLIC ACID — KBr disk
A 1392, B 1301 or 1363, C 1638

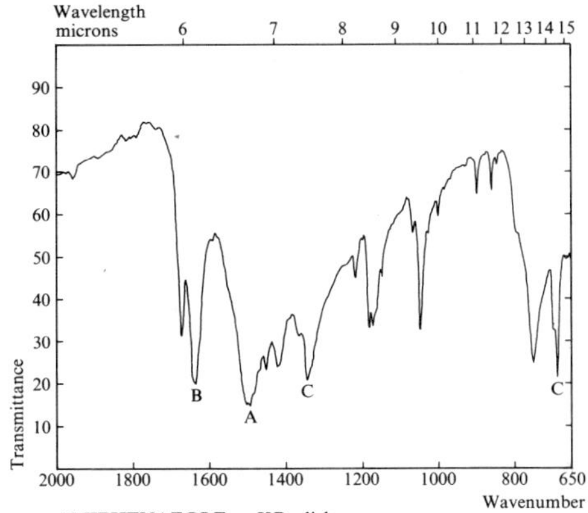

AMIPHENAZOLE — KBr disk
A 1495, B 1637, C 688 or 1346

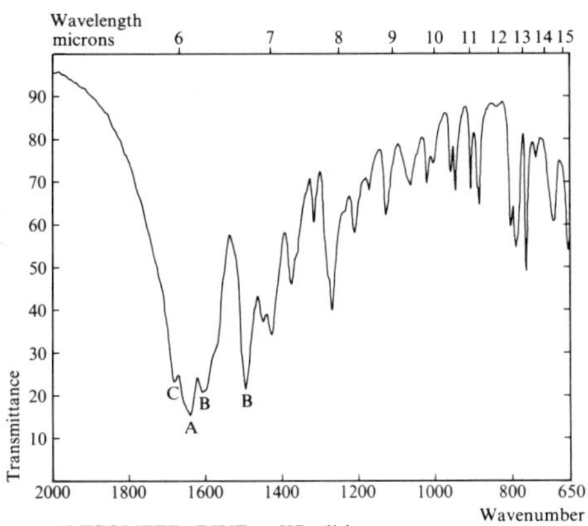

AMISOMETRADINE — KBr disk
A 1639, B 1492 or 1604, C 1680

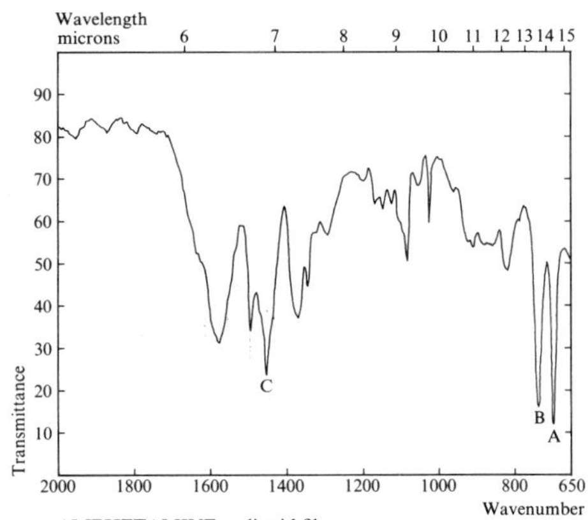

AMPHETAMINE — liquid film
A 695, B 737, C 1452

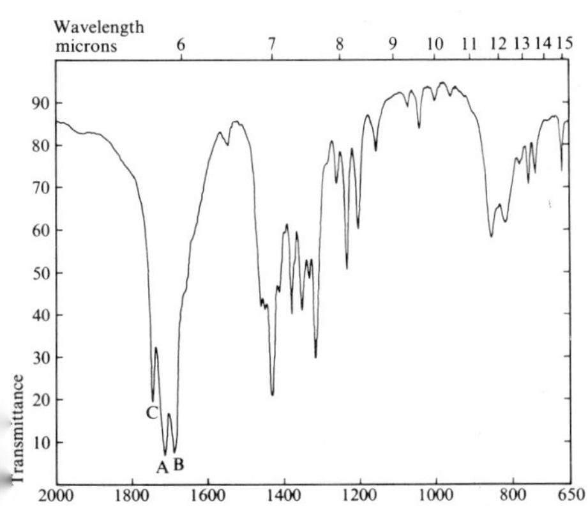

AMYLOBARBITONE — KBr disk
A 1716, B 1689, C 1745

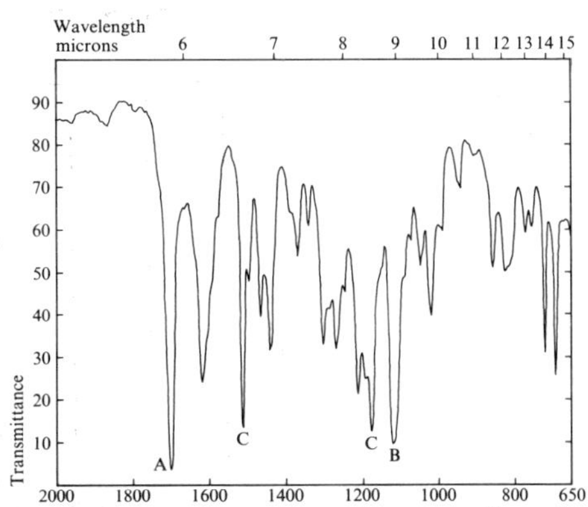

ANILERIDINE — KCl disk
A 1700, B 1120, C 1179 or 1512

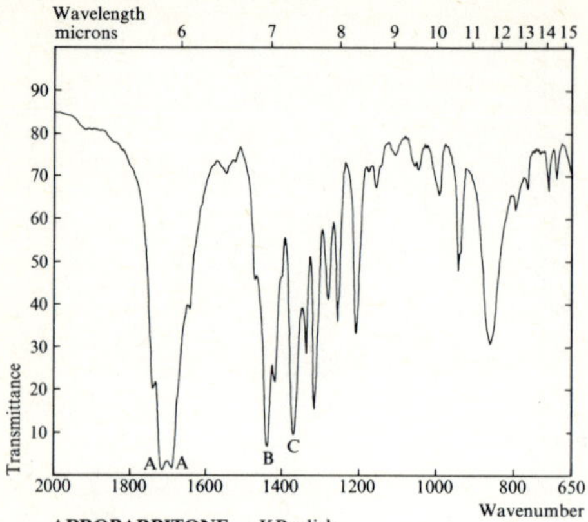

APROBARBITONE — KBr disk
A 1689 or 1715, B 1439, C 1376

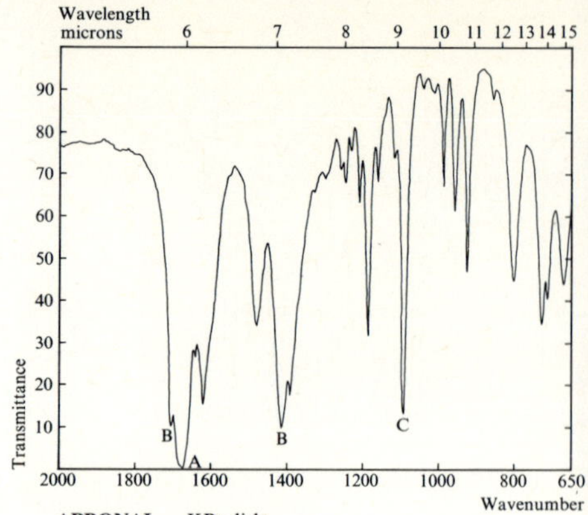

APRONAL — KBr disk
A 1676, B 1416 or 1704, C 1092

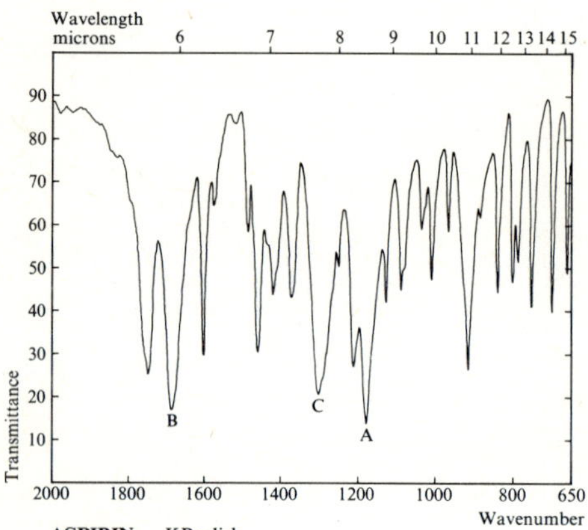

ASPIRIN — KBr disk
A 1183, B 1688, C 1305

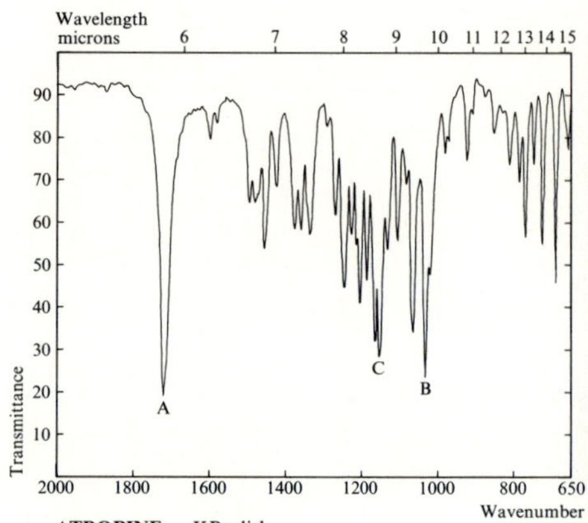

ATROPINE — KBr disk
A 1720, B 1035, C 1153

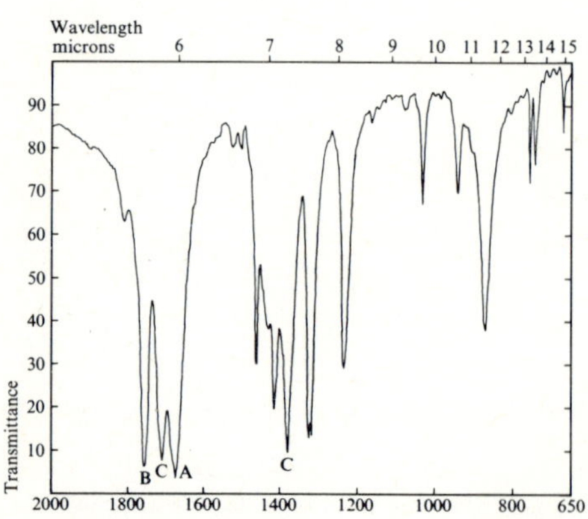

BARBITONE — KBr disk
A 1674, B 1754, C 1380 or 1707

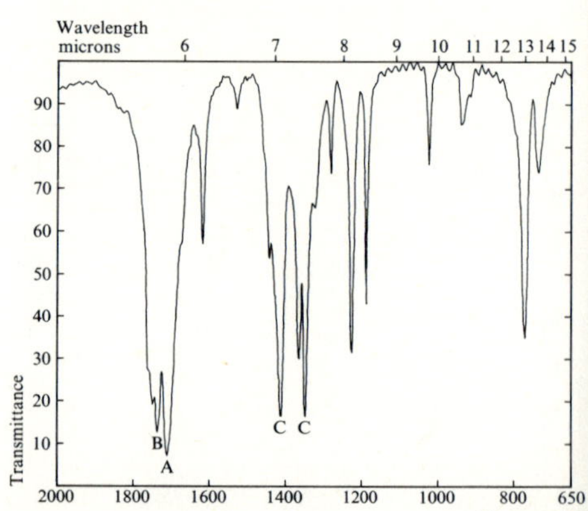

BARBITURIC ACID — KBr disk
A 1710, B 1734, C 1350 or 1412

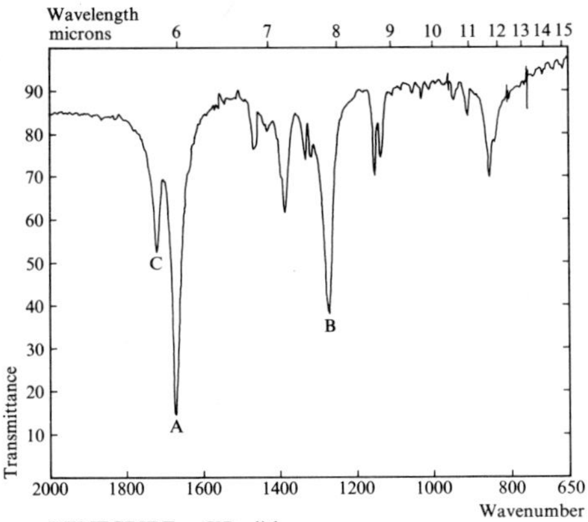

BEMEGRIDE — KBr disk
A 1668, B 1272, C 1718

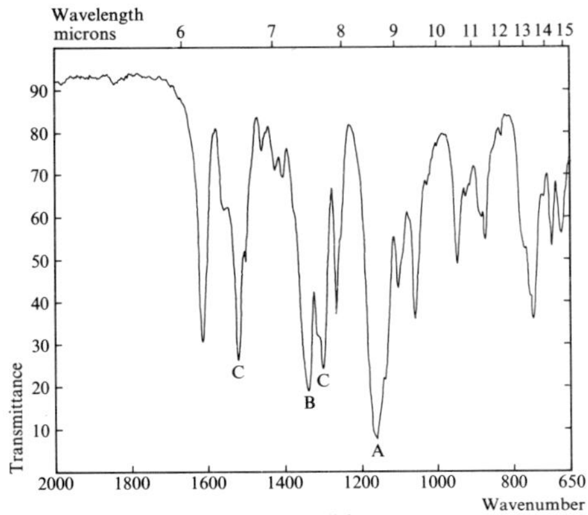

BENDROFLUAZIDE — KBr disk
A 1162, B 1340, C 1302 or 1512

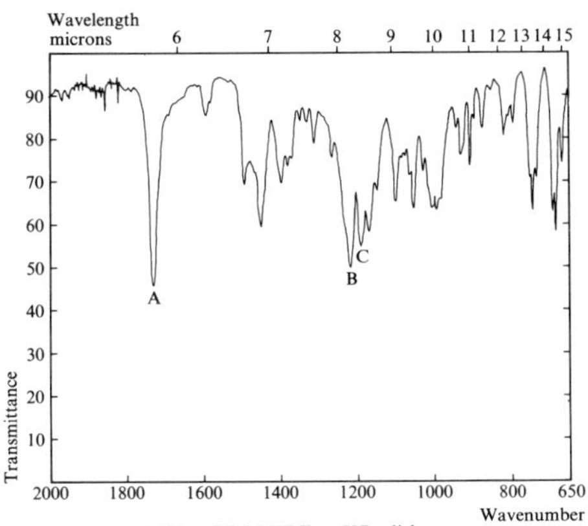

BENZILONIUM BROMIDE — KBr disk
A 1728, B 1220, C 1190

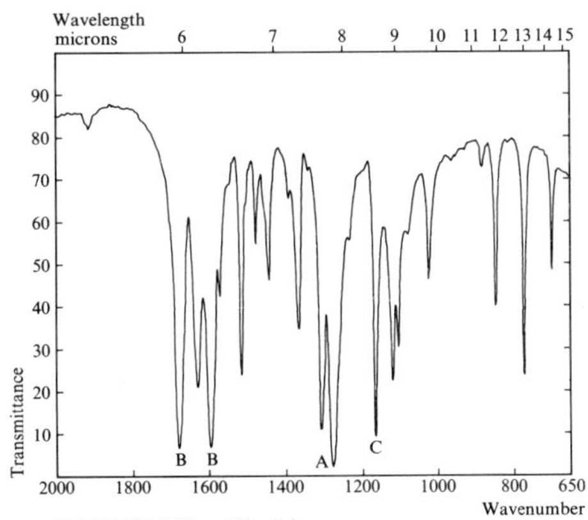

BENZOCAINE — KBr disk
A 1280, B 1598 or 1680, C 1170

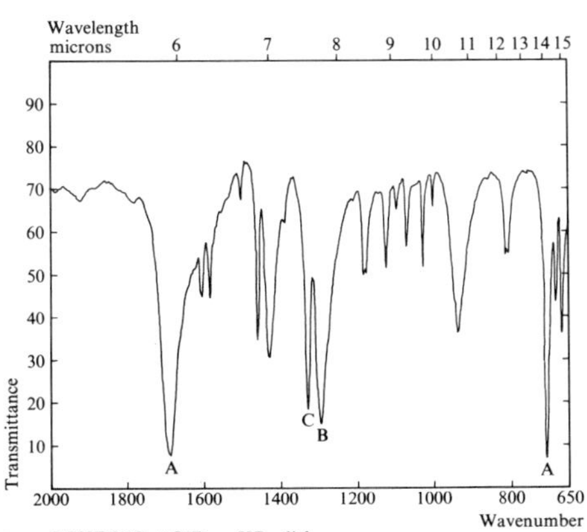

BENZOIC ACID — KBr disk
A 708 or 1686, B 1294, C 1330

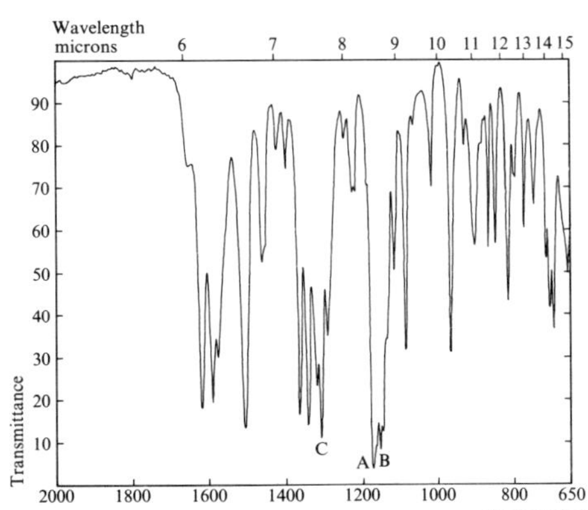

BENZTHIAZIDE — KBr disk
A 1175, B 1155, C 1311

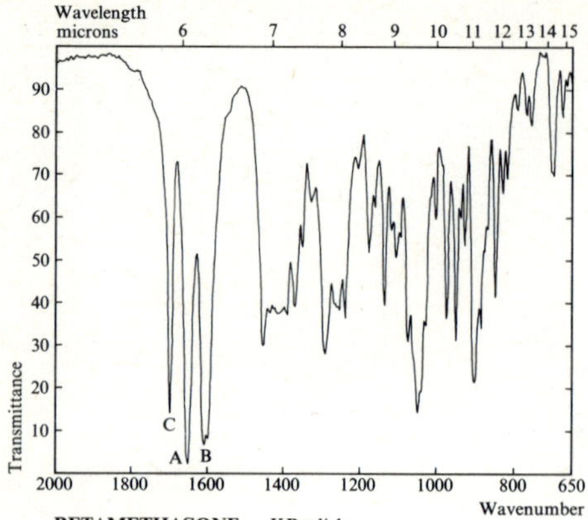

BETAMETHASONE — KBr disk
A 1648, B 1608, C 1697

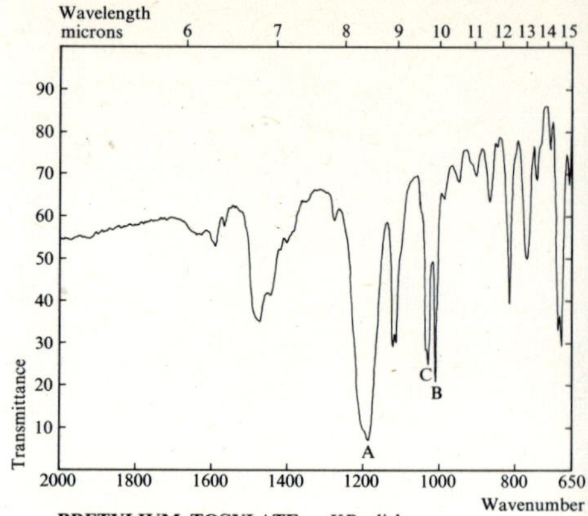

BRETYLIUM TOSYLATE — KBr disk
A 1188, B 1012, C 1032

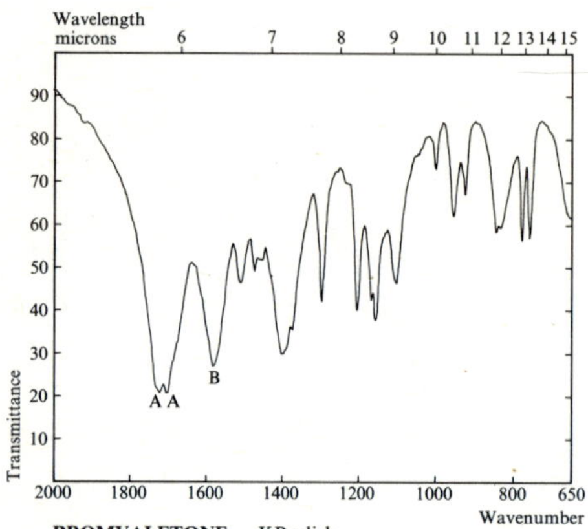

BROMVALETONE — KBr disk
A 1700 or 1721, B 1581

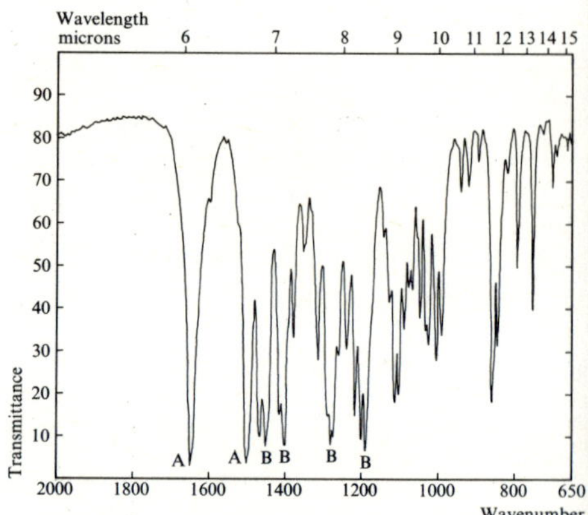

BRUCINE — KBr disk
A 1500 or 1649, B 1190 or 1285 or 1400 or 1450

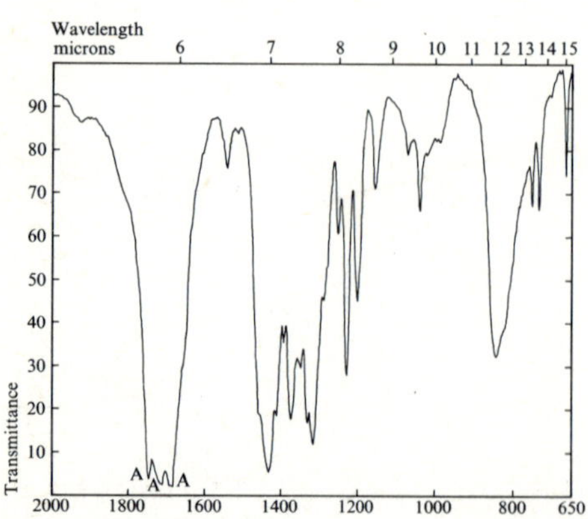

BUTOBARBITONE — KBr disk
A 1683 or 1712 or 1745

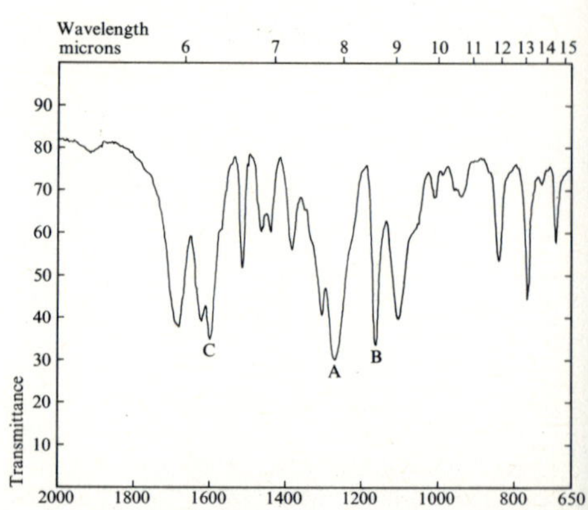

BUTYL AMINOBENZOATE — KBr disk
A 1272, B 1164, C 1600

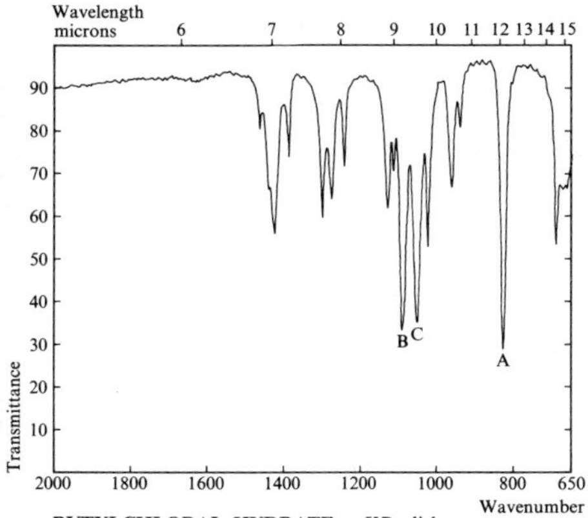

BUTYLCHLORAL HYDRATE — KBr disk
A 830, B 1090, C 1051

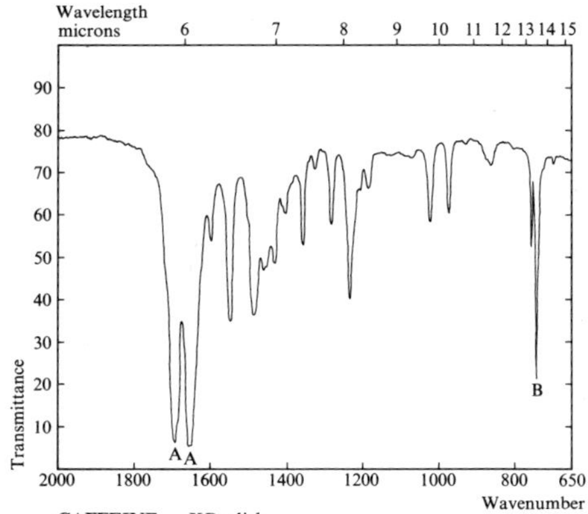

CAFFEINE — KBr disk
A 1658 or 1695, B 745

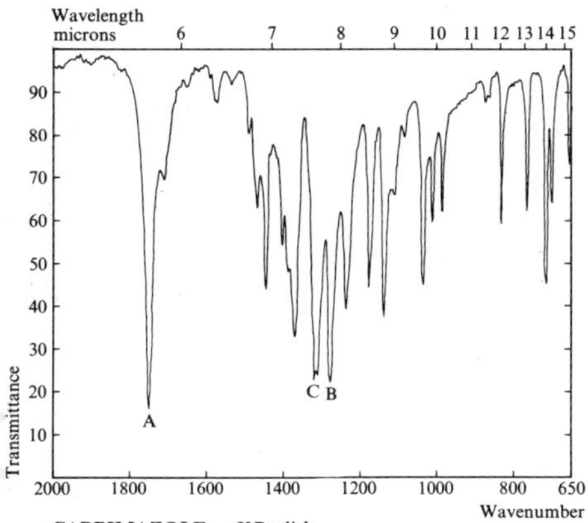

CARBIMAZOLE — KBr disk
A 1748, B 1278, C 1320

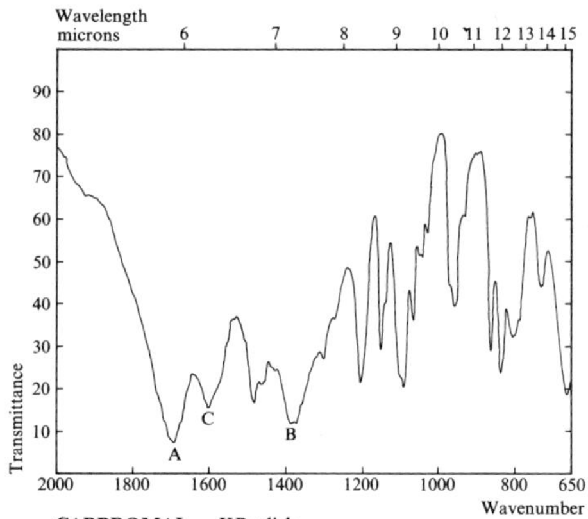

CARBROMAL — KBr disk
A 1692, B 1388, C 1600

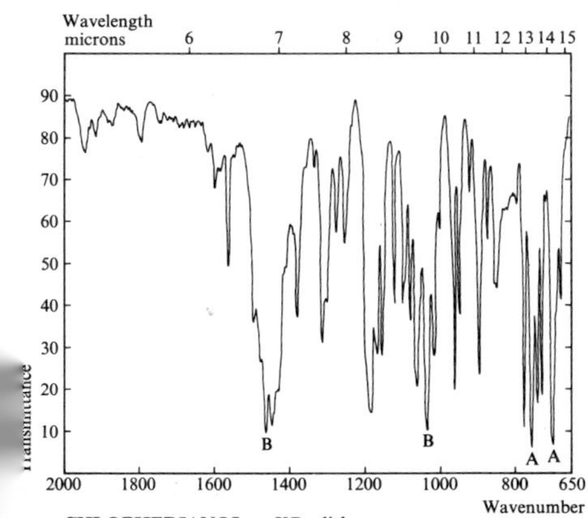

CHLOPHEDIANOL — KBr disk
A 700 or 756, B 1035 or 1463

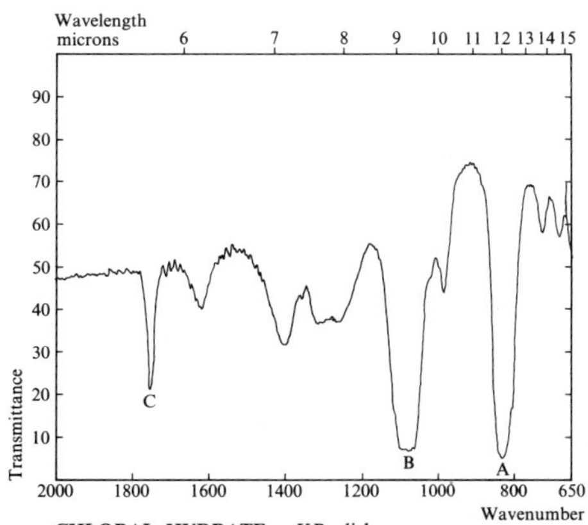

CHLORAL HYDRATE — KBr disk
A 838, B 1078, C 1750

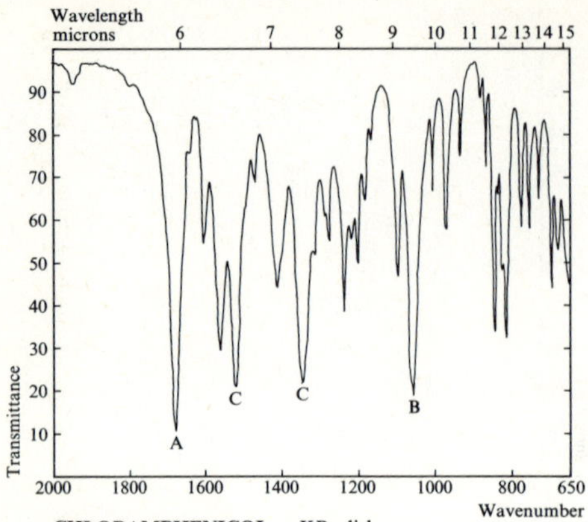

CHLORAMPHENICOL — KBr disk
A 1682, B 1061, C 1351 or 1526

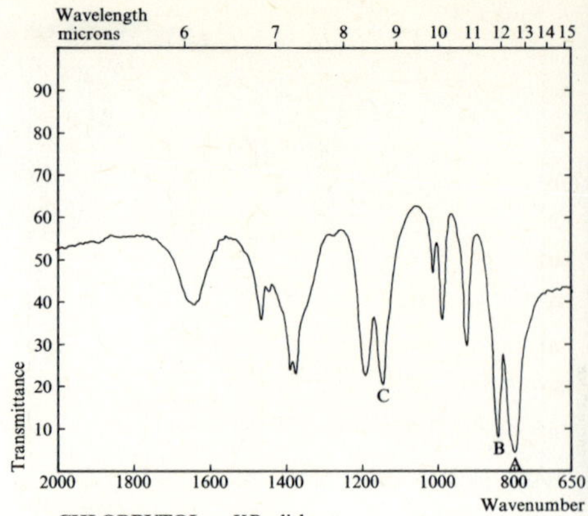

CHLORBUTOL — KBr disk
A 802, B 845, C 1150

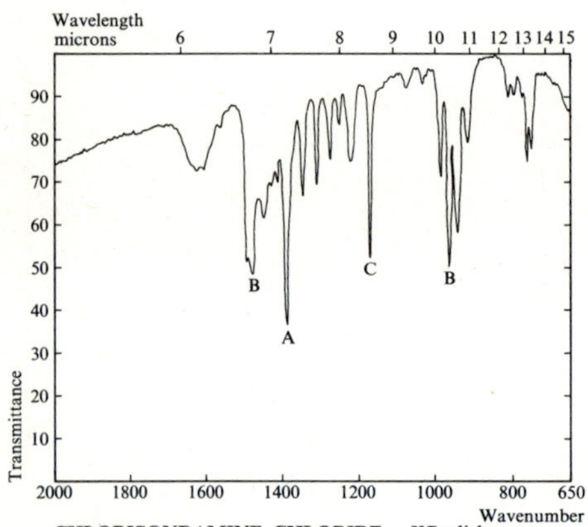

CHLORISONDAMINE CHLORIDE — KBr disk
A 1392, B 964 or 1480, C 1177

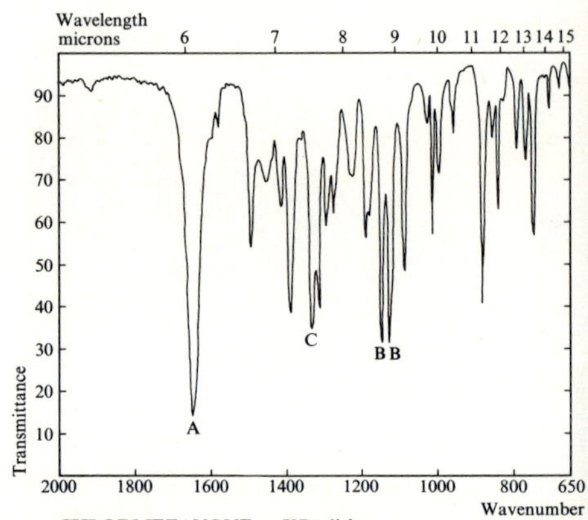

CHLORMEZANONE — KBr disk
A 1645, B 1128 or 1145, C 1336

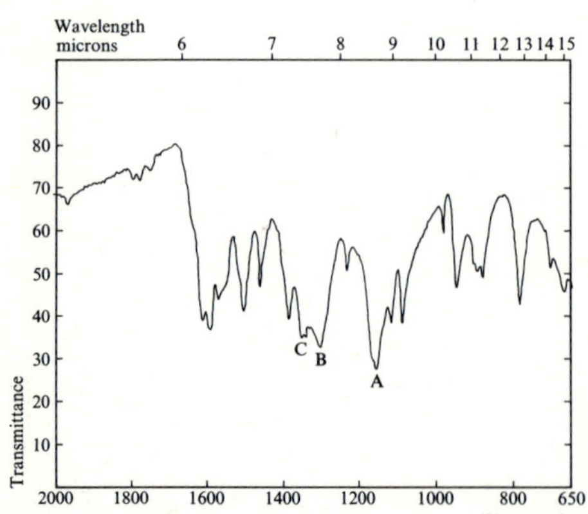

CHLOROTHIAZIDE — KBr disk
A 1157, B 1305, C 1342

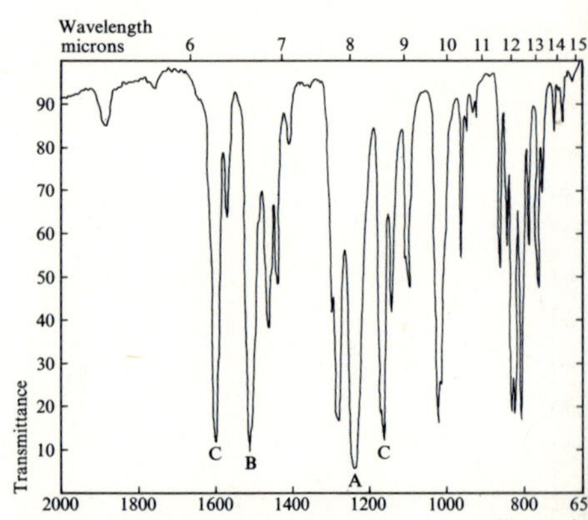

CHLOROTRIANISENE — KBr disk
A 1246, B 1514, C 1165 or 1600

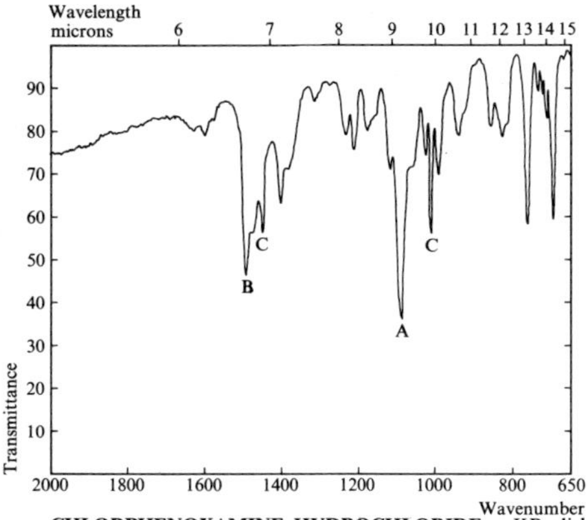

CHLORPHENOXAMINE HYDROCHLORIDE — KBr disk
A 1088, B 1490, C 1010 or 1448

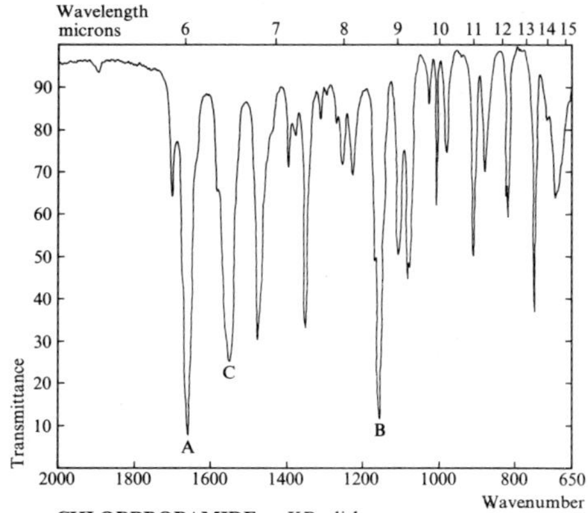

CHLORPROPAMIDE — KBr disk
A 1661, B 1159, C 1553

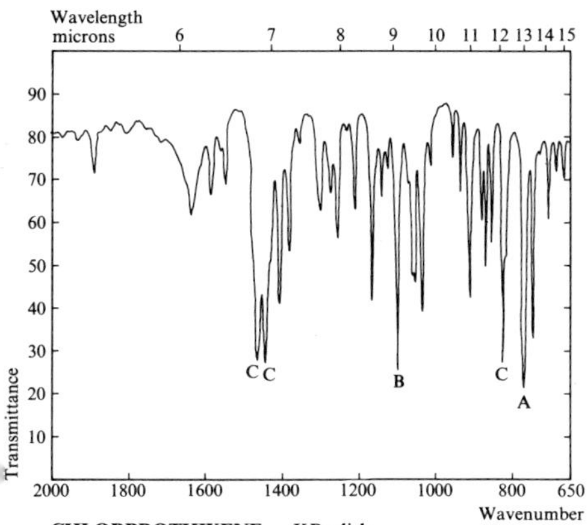

CHLORPROTHIXENE — KBr disk
A 776, B 1104, C 832 or 1446 or 1468

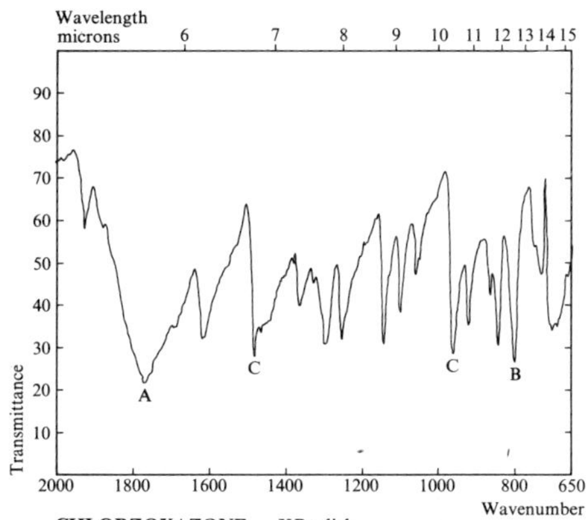

CHLORZOXAZONE — KBr disk
A 1762, B 801, C 962 or 1480

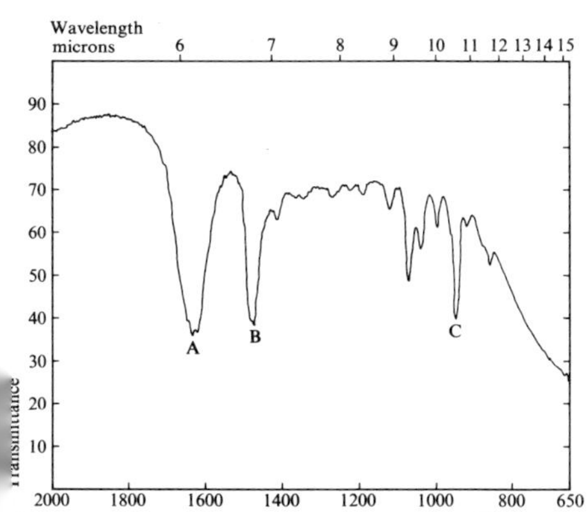

CHOLINE CHLORIDE — capillary film between KBr windows
A 1636, B 1477, C 953

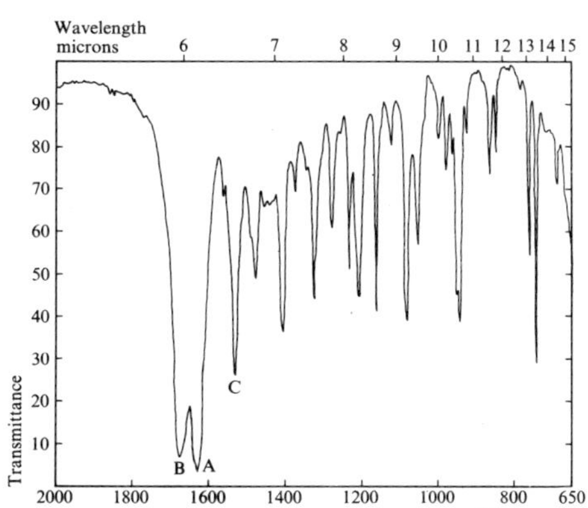

CHOLINE THEOPHYLLINATE — KBr disk
A 1627, B 1676, C 1536

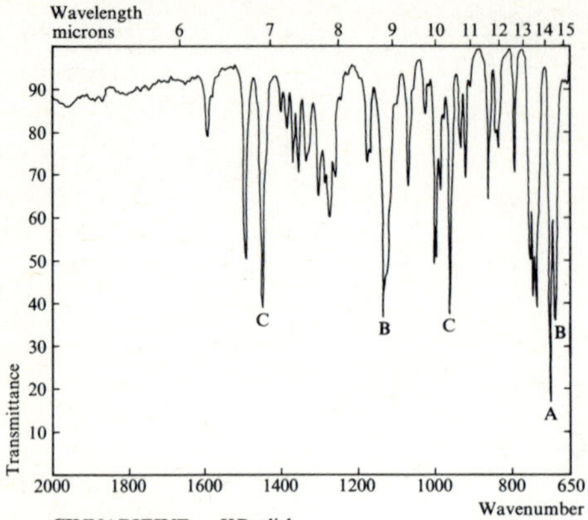

CINNARIZINE — KBr disk
A 702, B 691 or 1138, C 964 or 1452

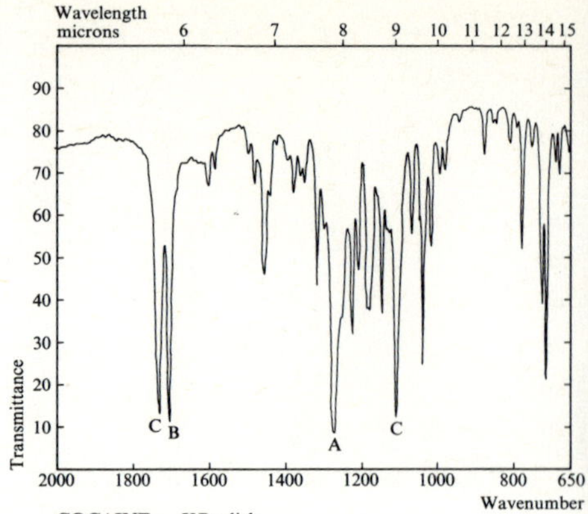

COCAINE — KBr disk
A 1275, B 1700, C 1106 or 1728

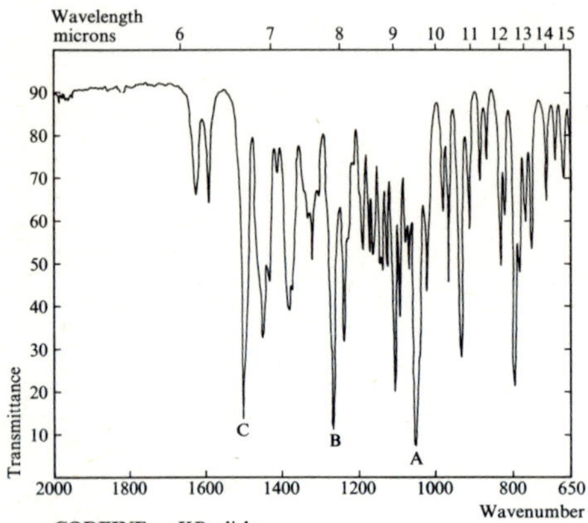

CODEINE — KBr disk
A 1052, B 1268, C 1500

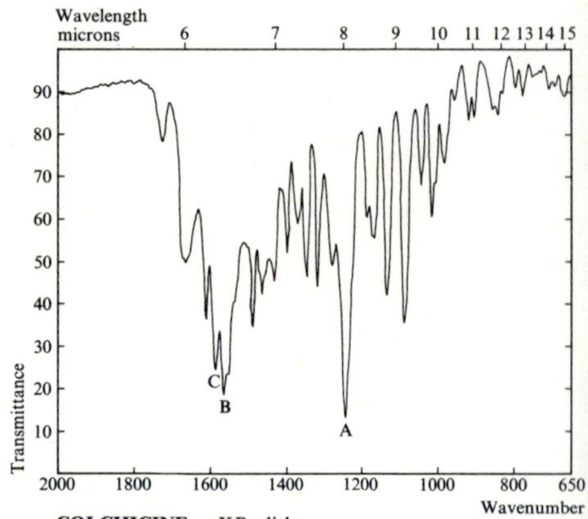

COLCHICINE — KBr disk
A 1248, B 1566, C 1589

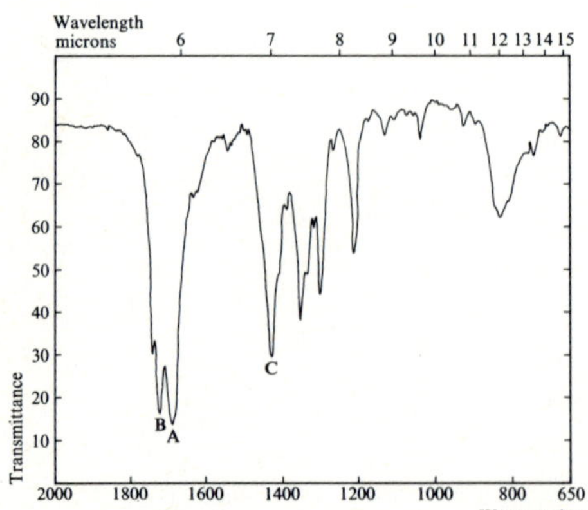

CYCLOBARBITONE — KBr disk
A 1693, B 1725, C 1430

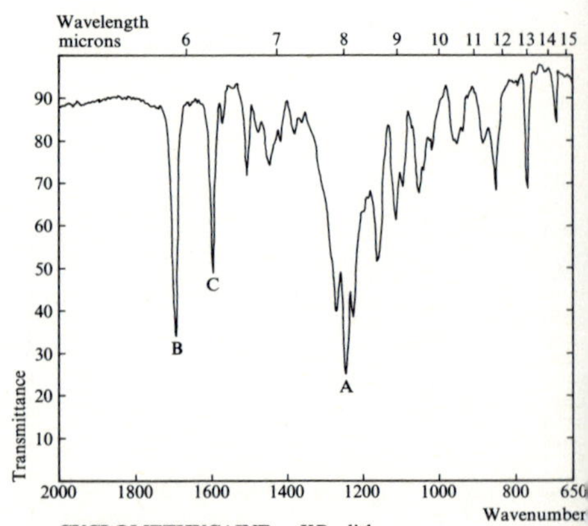

CYCLOMETHYCAINE — KBr disk
A 1247, B 1696, C 1600

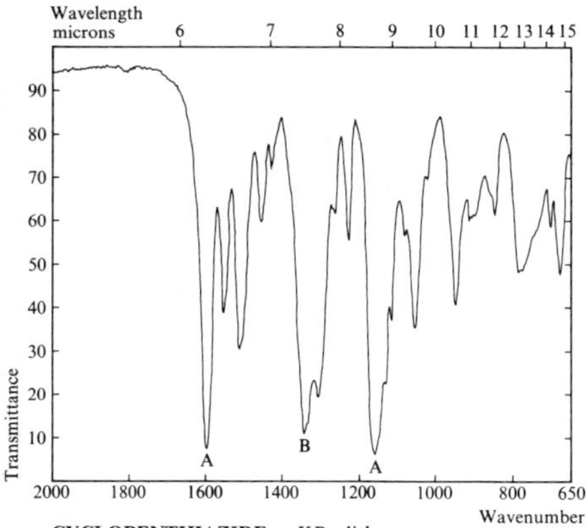

CYCLOPENTHIAZIDE — KBr disk
A 1158 or 1598, B 1343

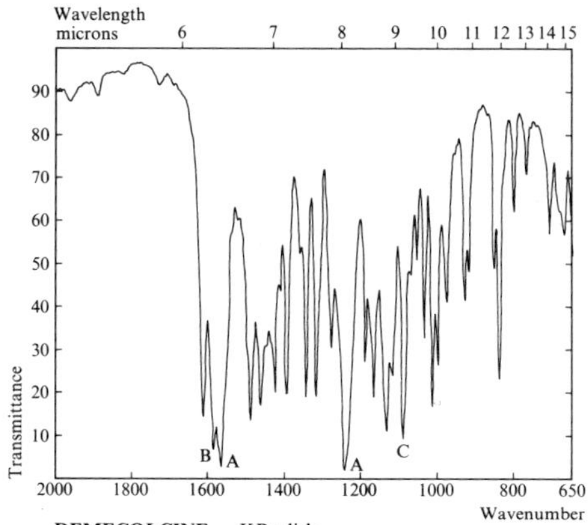

DEMECOLCINE — KBr disk
A 1241 or 1562, B 1582, C 1090

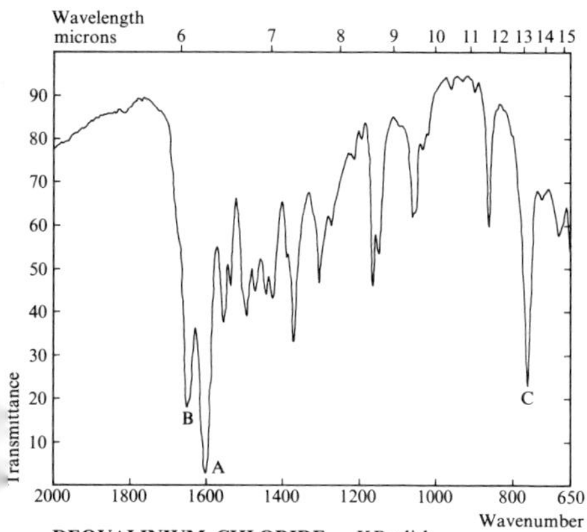

DEQUALINIUM CHLORIDE — KBr disk
A 1605, B 1652, C 764

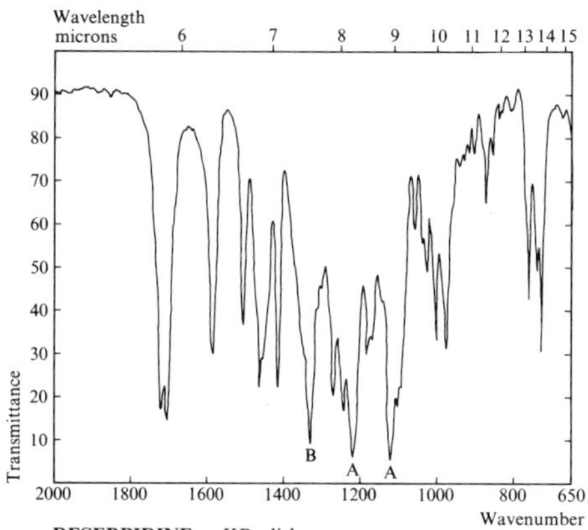

DESERPIDINE — KBr disk
A 1121 or 1220, B 1330

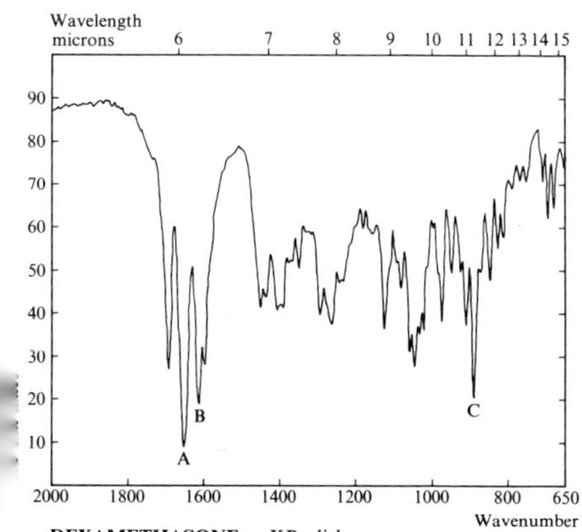

DEXAMETHASONE — KBr disk
A 1655, B 1616, C 892

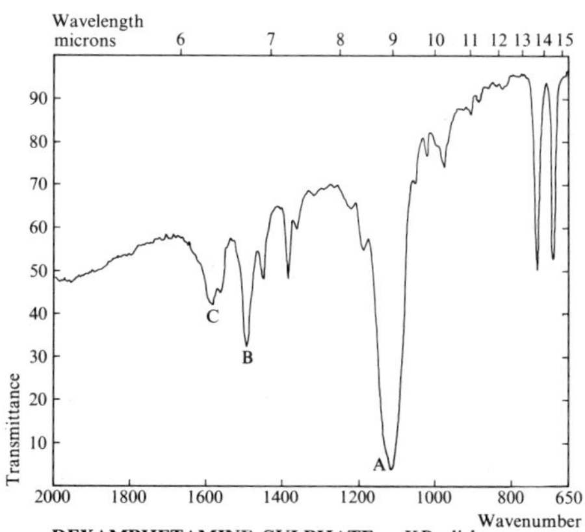

DEXAMPHETAMINE SULPHATE — KBr disk
A 1118, B 1495, C 1582

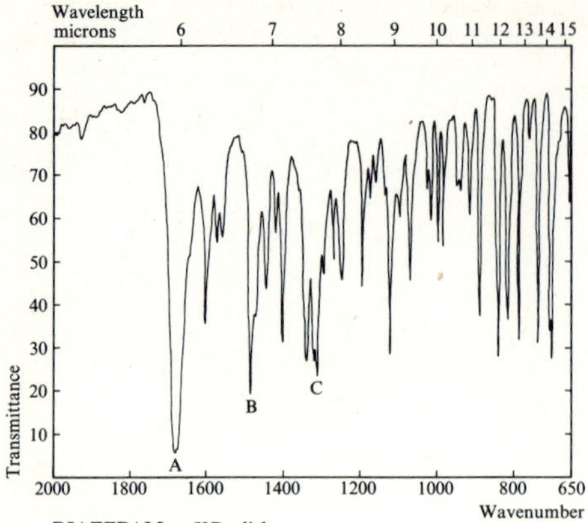

DIAZEPAM — KBr disk
A 1681, B 1484, C 1313

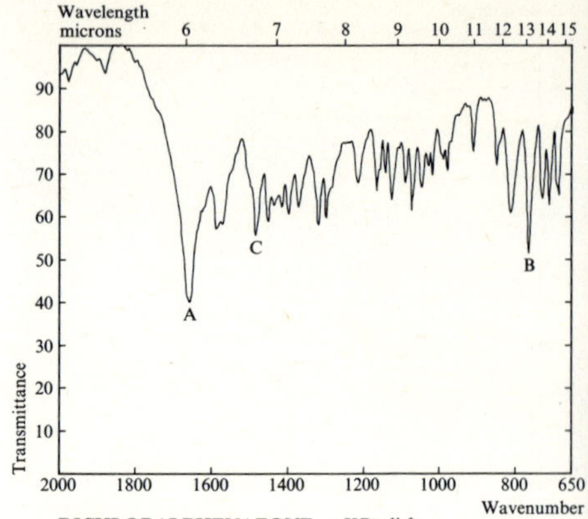

DICHLORALPHENAZONE — KBr disk
A 1656, B 767, C 1484

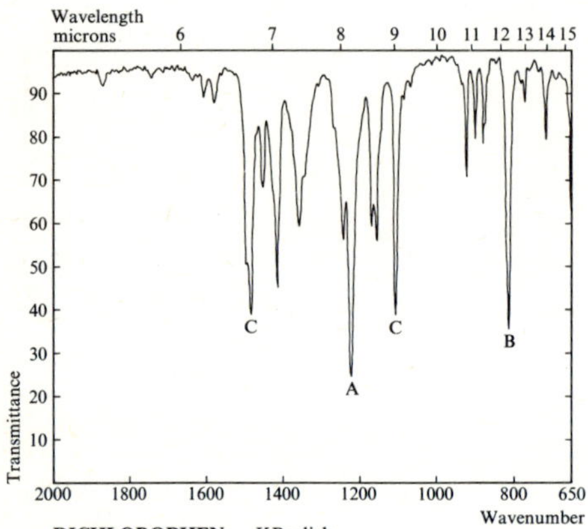

DICHLOROPHEN — KBr disk
A 1226, B 817, C 1111 or 1487

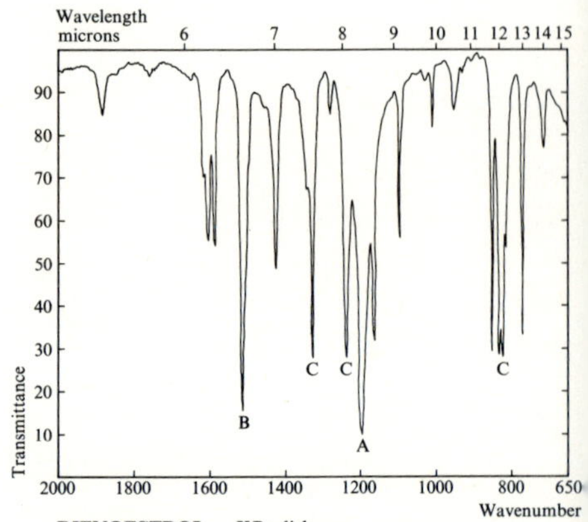

DIENOESTROL — KBr disk
A 1199, B 1513, C 828 or 1241 or 1330

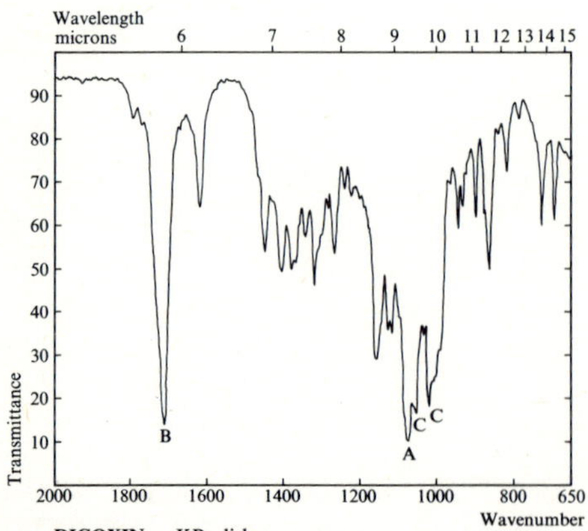

DIGOXIN — KBr disk
A 1075, B 1709, C 1020 or 1055

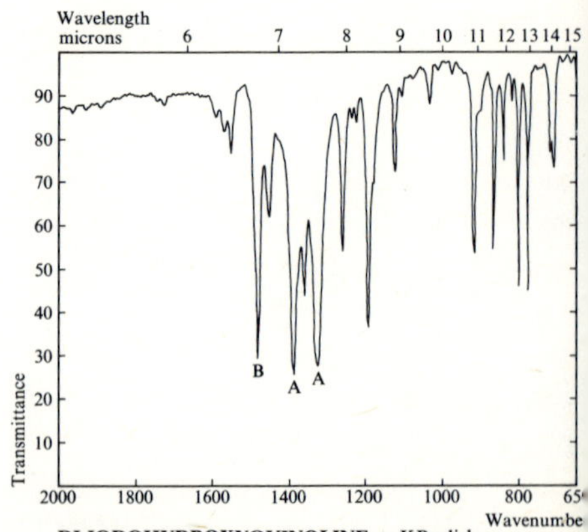

DI-IODOHYDROXYQUINOLINE — KBr disk
A 1330 or 1390, B 1484

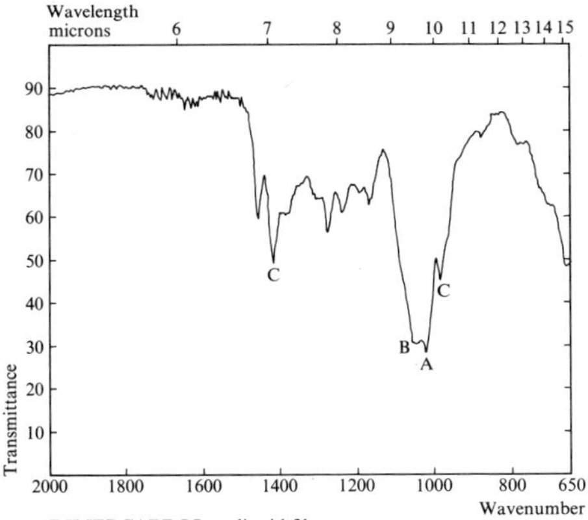

DIMERCAPROL — liquid film
A 1022, B 1050, C 990 or 1418

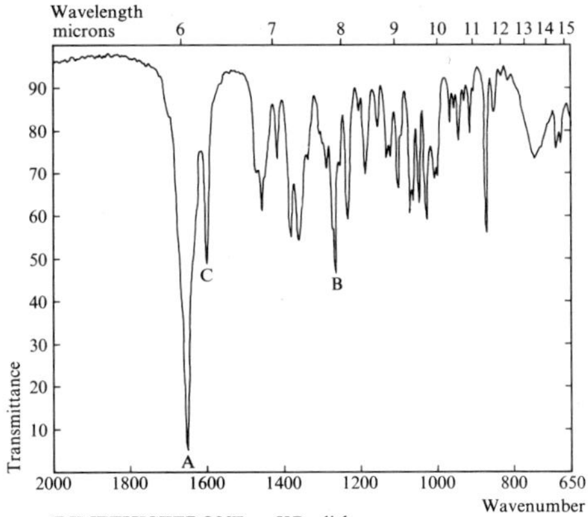

DIMETHISTERONE — KBr disk
A 1650, B 1269, C 1600

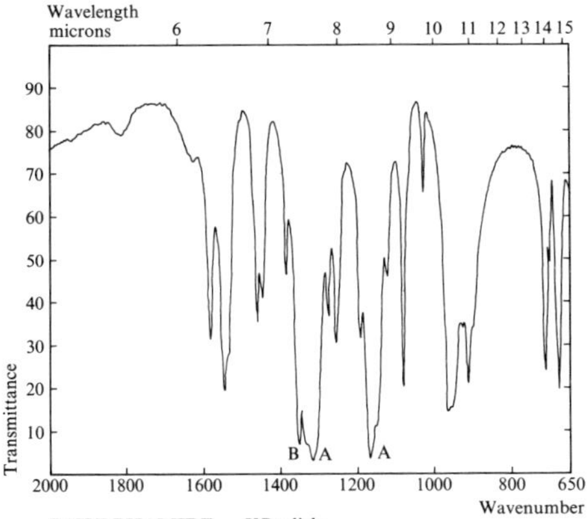

DISULPHAMIDE — KBr disk
A 1172 or 1320, B 1552

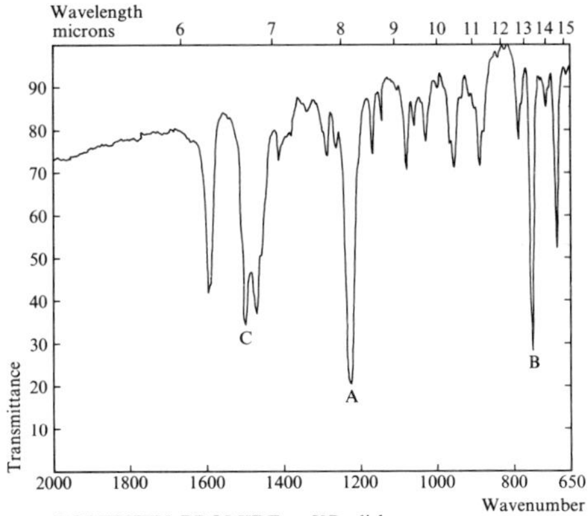

DOMIPHEN BROMIDE — KBr disk
A 1228, B 752, C 1500

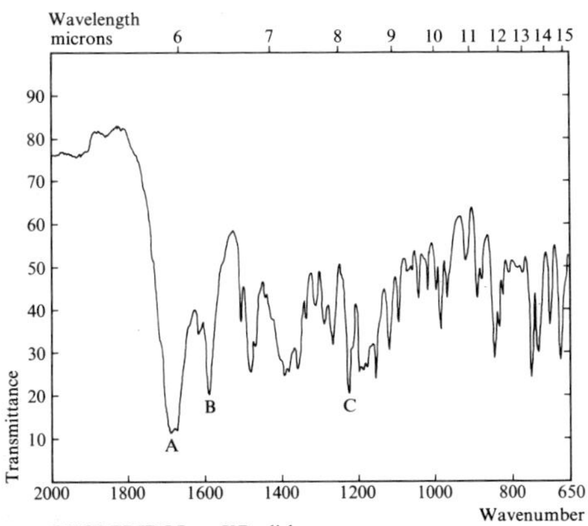

DROPERIDOL — KBr disk
A 1688, B 1591, C 1227

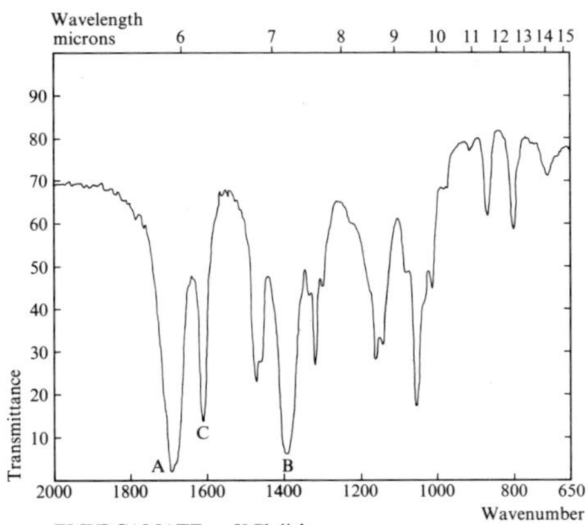

EMYLCAMATE — KCl disk
A 1690, B 1392, C 1610

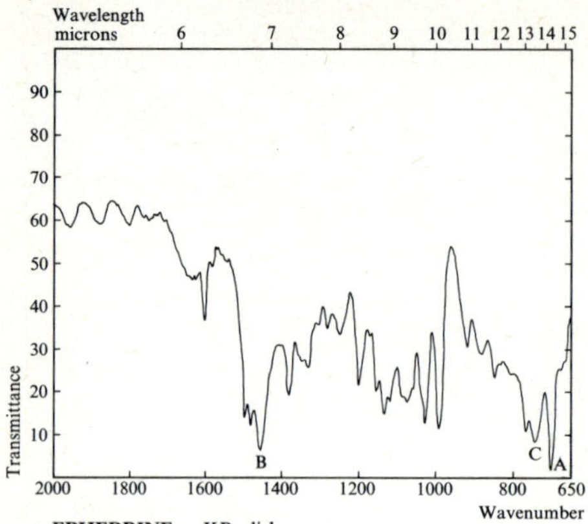

EPHEDRINE — KBr disk
A 703, B 1455, C 745

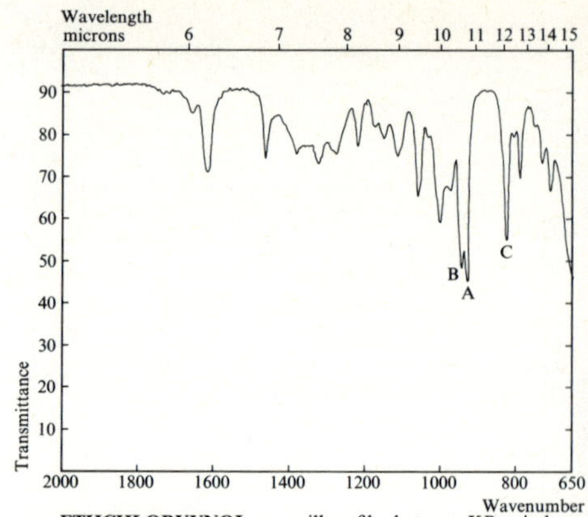

ETHCHLORVYNOL — capillary film between KBr windows
A 935, B 950, C 830

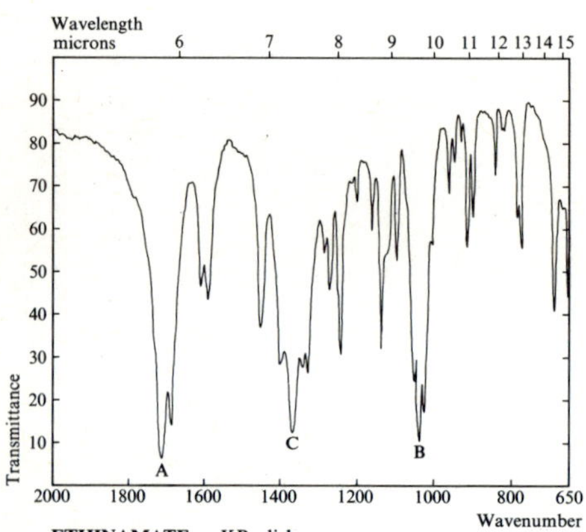

ETHINAMATE — KBr disk
A 1713, B 1041, C 1370

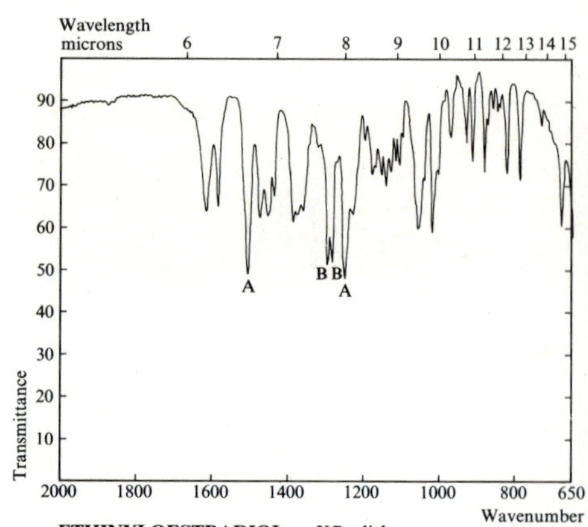

ETHINYLOESTRADIOL — KBr disk
A 1252 or 1505, B 1285 or 1298

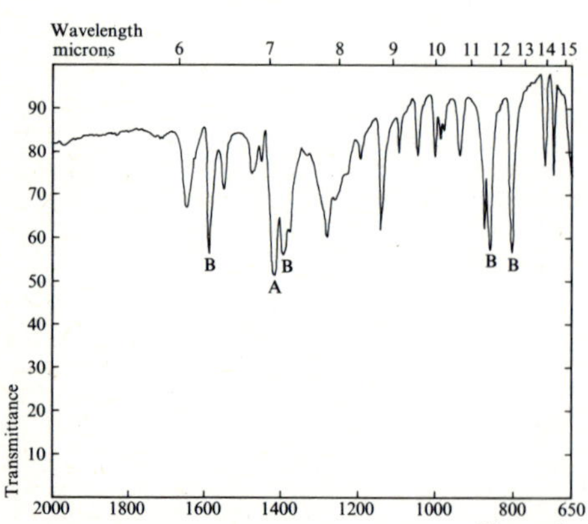

ETHIONAMIDE — KBr disk
A 1418, B 808 or 865 or 1396 or 1588

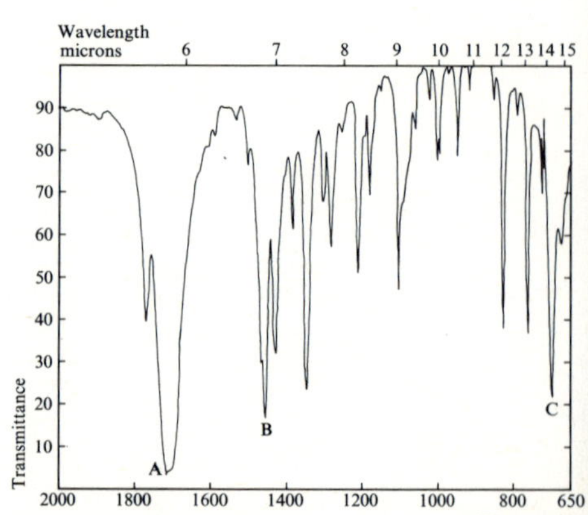

ETHOTOIN — KBr disk
A 1716, B 1455, C 700

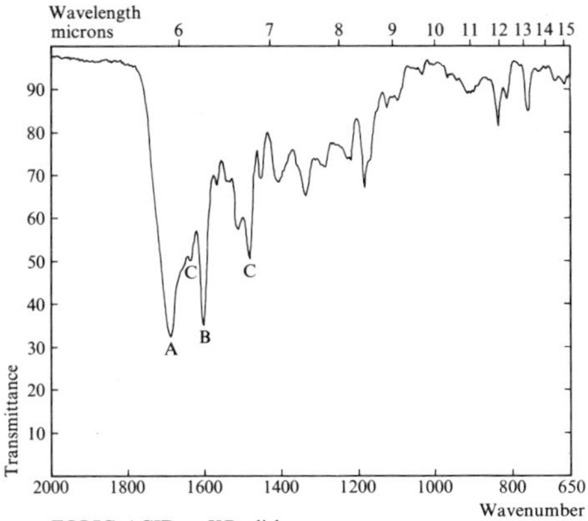

FOLIC ACID — KBr disk
A 1688, B 1601, C 1484 or 1640

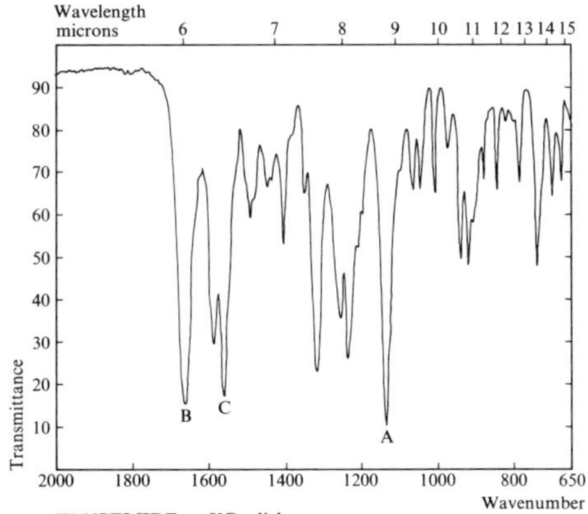

FRUSEMIDE — KBr disk
A 1143, B 1668, C 1565

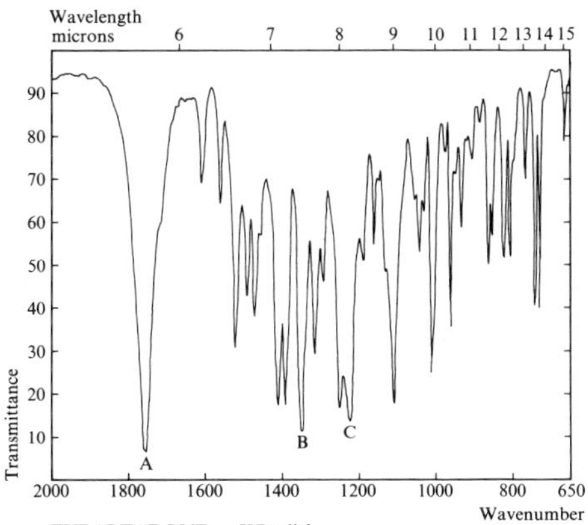

FURALTADONE — KBr disk
A 1755, B 1352, C 1226

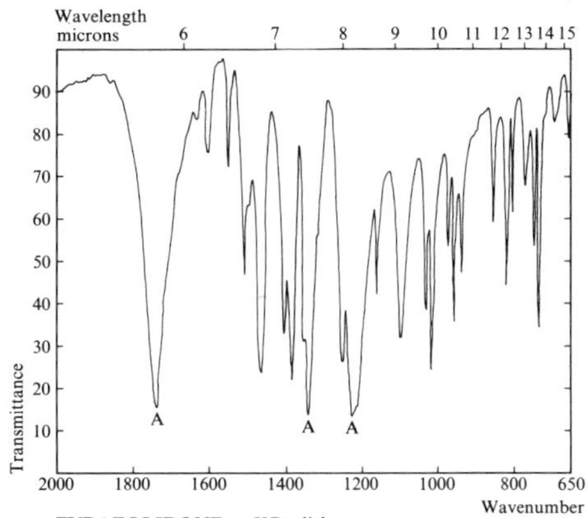

FURAZOLIDONE — KBr disk
A 1226 or 1345 or 1738

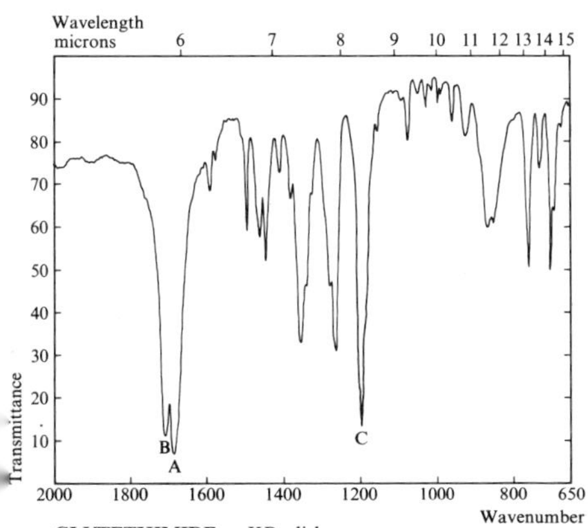

GLUTETHIMIDE — KBr disk
A 1686, B 1710, C 1200

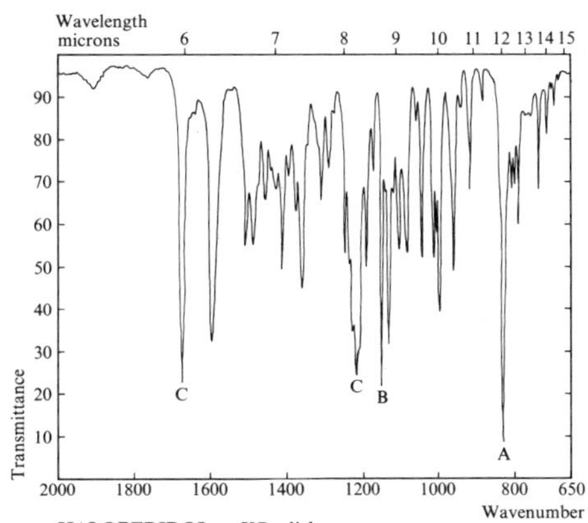

HALOPERIDOL — KBr disk
A 832, B 1151, C 1217 or 1673

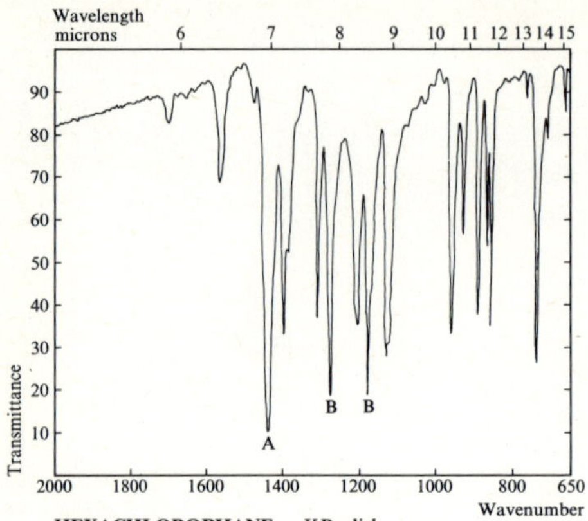

HEXACHLOROPHANE — KBr disk
A 1442, B 1182 or 1276

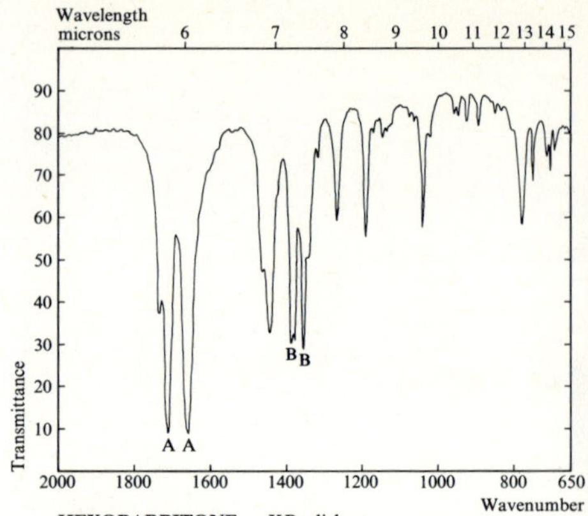

HEXOBARBITONE — KBr disk
A 1660 or 1712, B 1358 or 1390

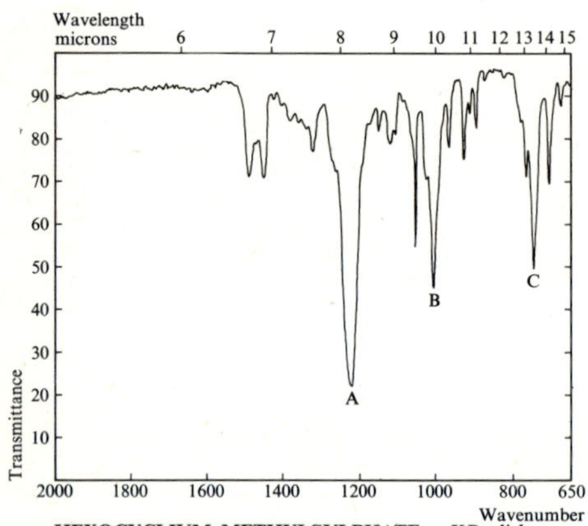

HEXOCYCLIUM METHYLSULPHATE — KBr disk
A 1224, B 1005, C 748

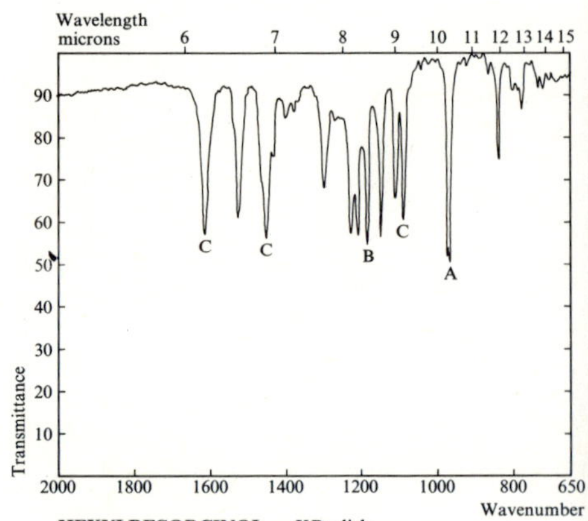

HEXYLRESORCINOL — KBr disk
A 970, B 1185, C 1150 or 1453 or 1616

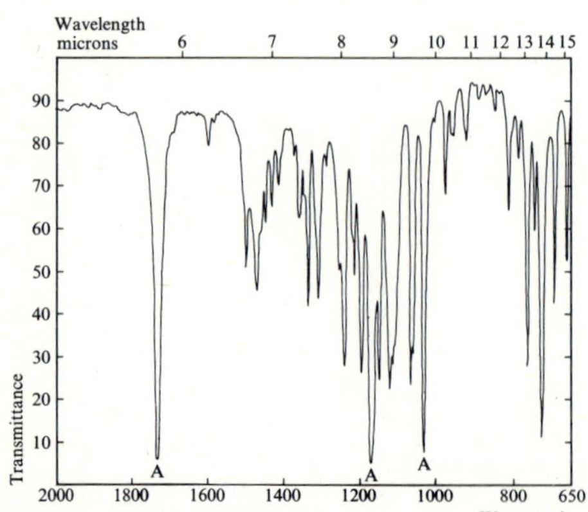

HOMATROPINE — KBr disk
A 1172 or 1730 or 1032

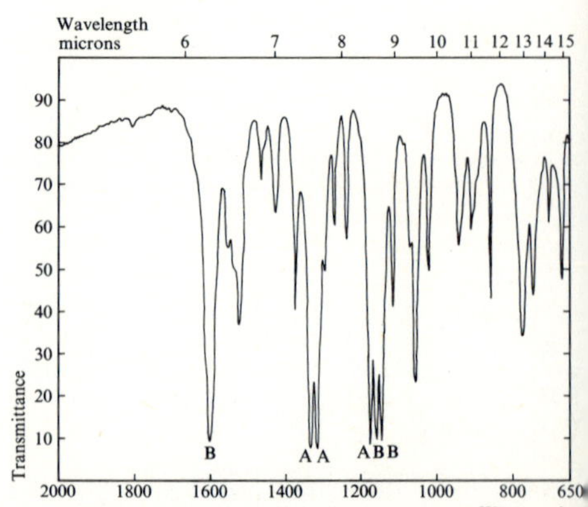

HYDROCHLOROTHIAZIDE — KBr disk
A 1175 or 1318 or 1336, B 1145 or 1160 or 1600

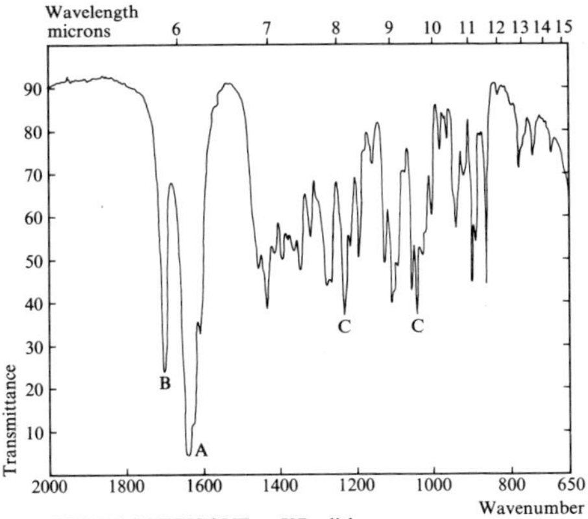

HYDROCORTISONE — KBr disk
A 1640, B 1702, C 1042 or 1232

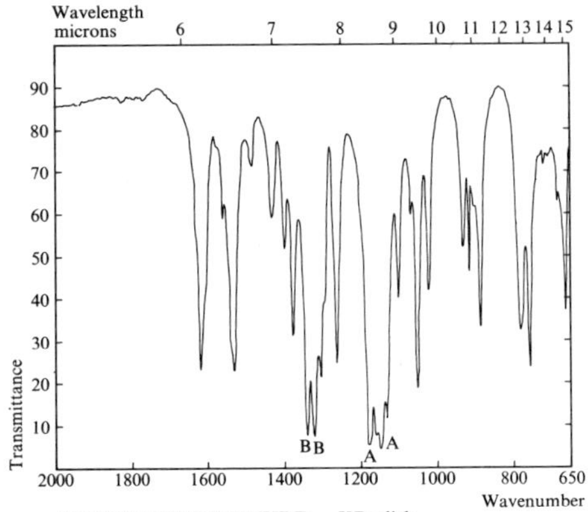

HYDROFLUMETHIAZIDE — KBr disk
A 1151 or 1180, B 1324 or 1341

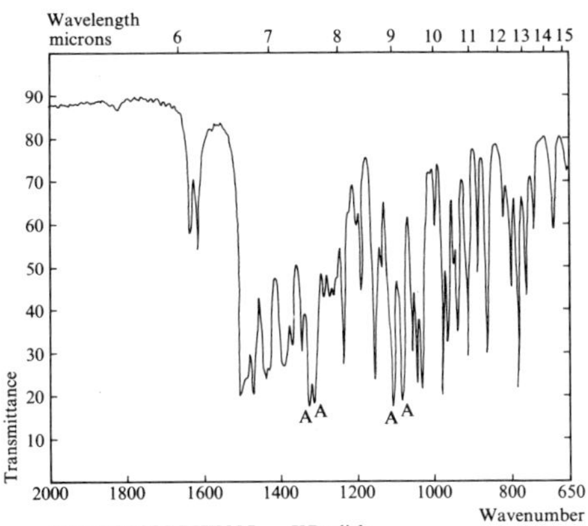

HYDROMORPHINOL — KBr disk
A 1086 or 1111 or 1318 or 1327

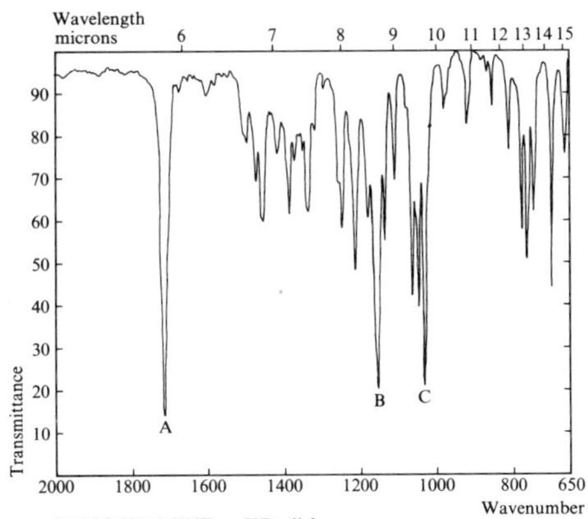

HYOSCYAMINE — KBr disk
A 1712, B 1154, C 1032

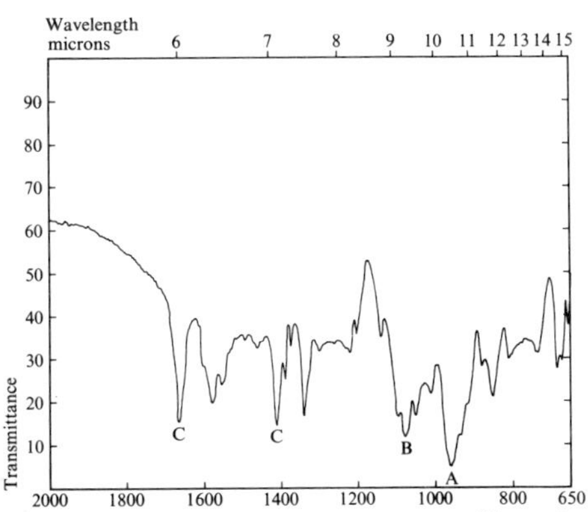

IPRONIAZID — KBr disk
A 961, B 1081, C 1414 or 1665

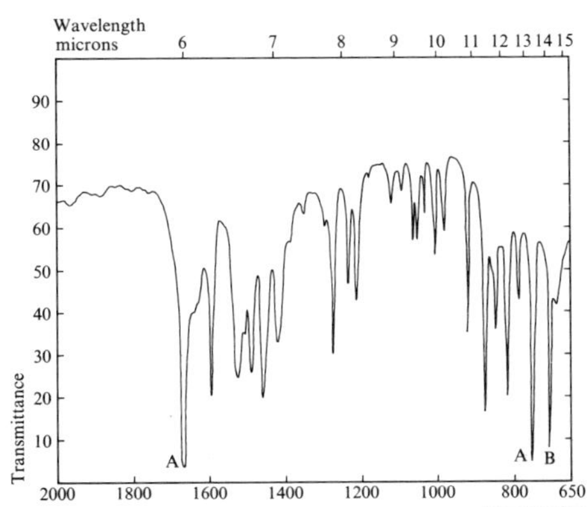

ISOCARBOXAZID — KBr disk
A 756 or 1670, B 710

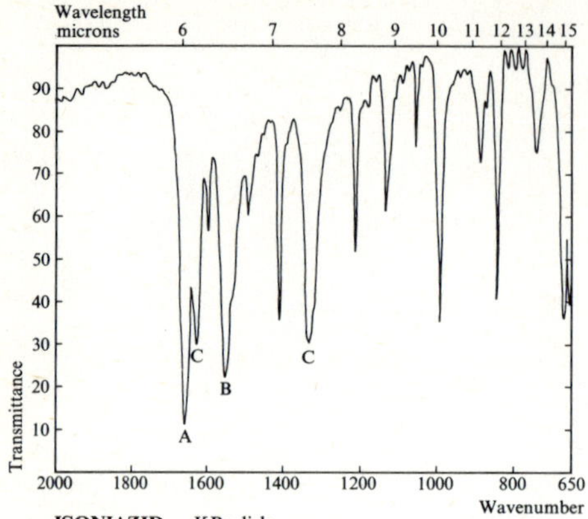

ISONIAZID — KBr disk
A 1659, B 1552, C 1335 or 1628

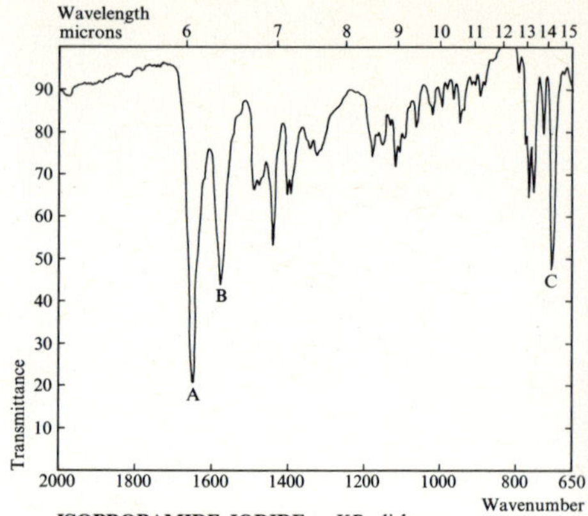

ISOPROPAMIDE IODIDE — KBr disk
A 1650, B 1576, C 705

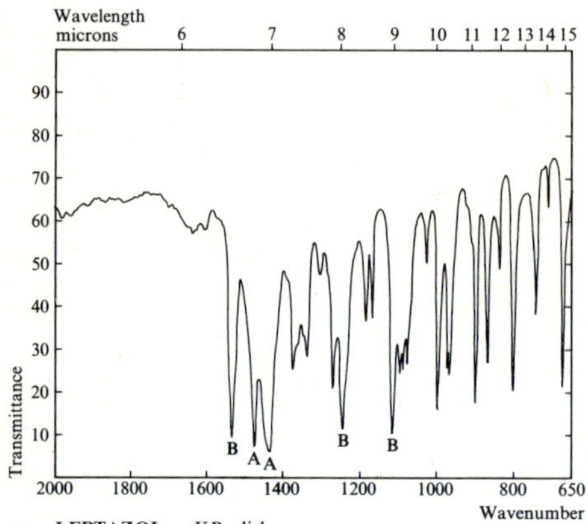

LEPTAZOL — KBr disk
A 1435 or 1475, B 1115 or 1250 or 1535

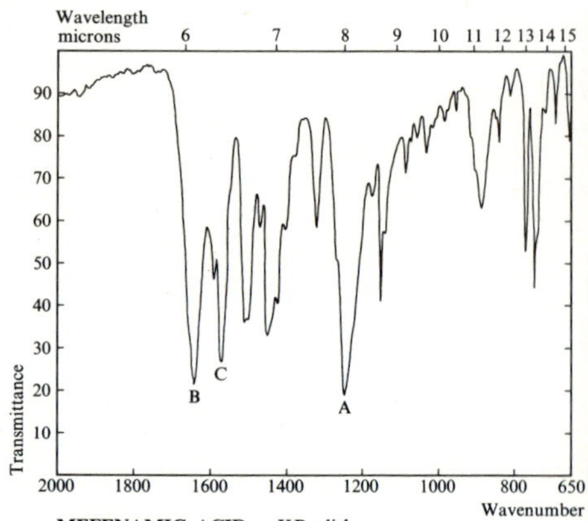

MEFENAMIC ACID — KBr disk
A 1253, B 1644, C 1575

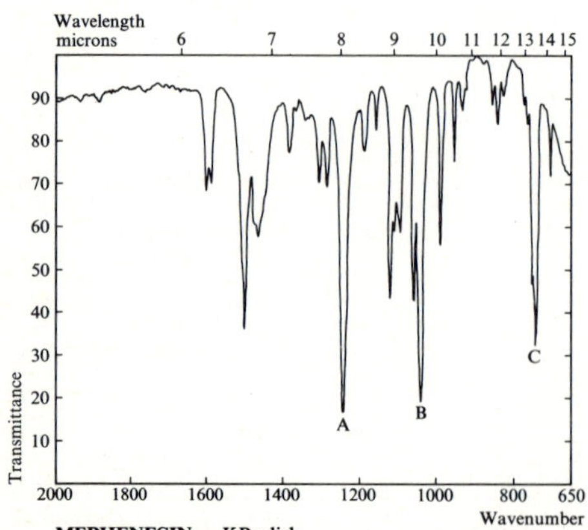

MEPHENESIN — KBr disk
A 1245, B 1041, C 745

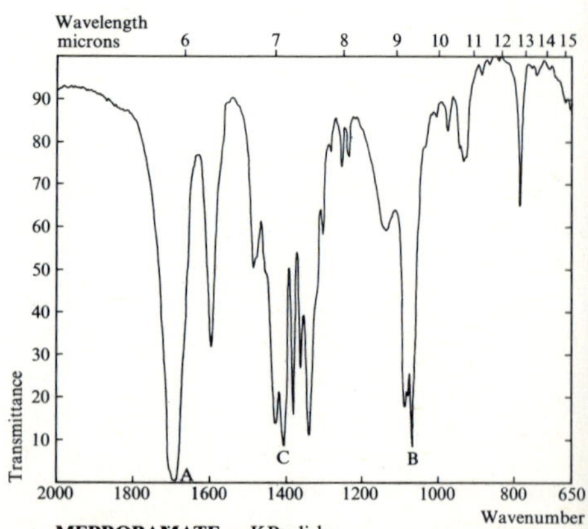

MEPROBAMATE — KBr disk
A 1688, B 1069, C 1408

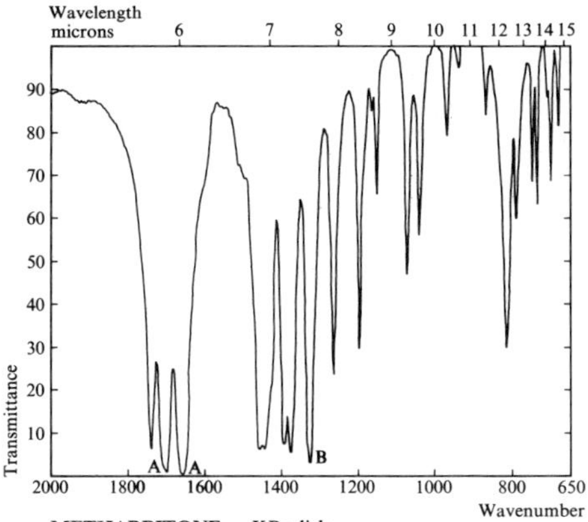

METHARBITONE — KBr disk
A 1655 or 1699, B 1326

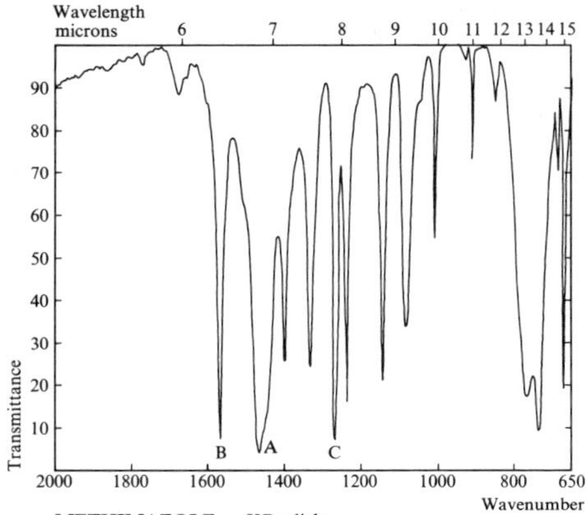

METHIMAZOLE — KBr disk
A 1466, B 1570, C 1271

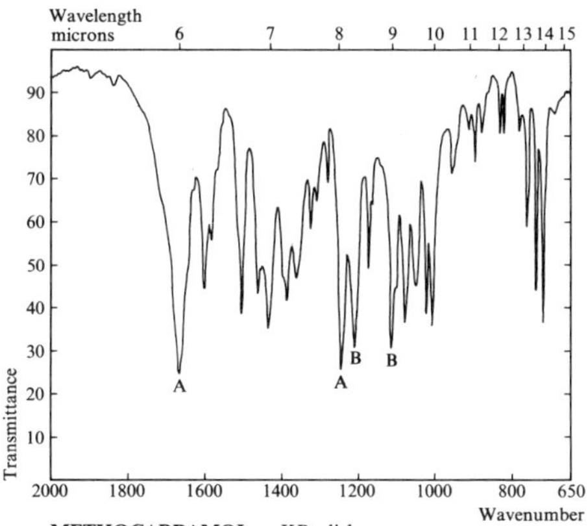

METHOCARBAMOL — KBr disk
A 1248 or 1667, B 1119 or 1215

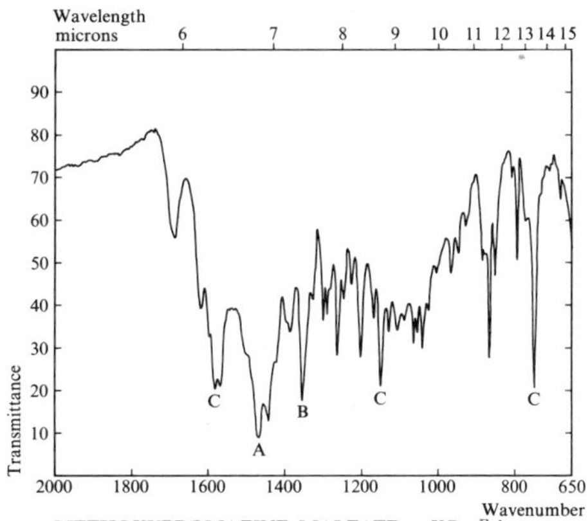

METHOXYPROMAZINE MALEATE — KBr disk
A 1470, B 1356, C 748 or 1152 or 1582

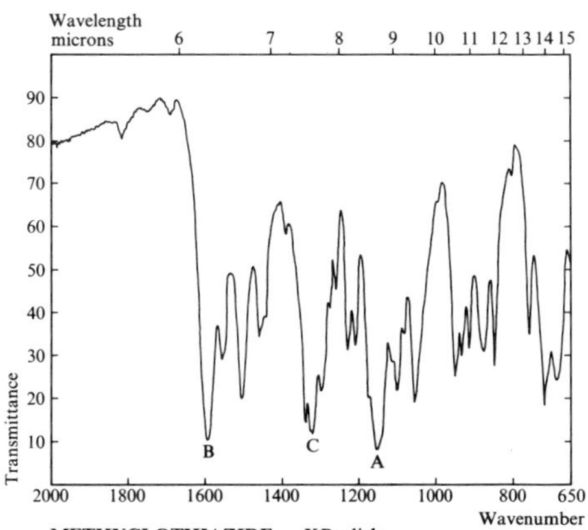

METHYCLOTHIAZIDE — KBr disk
A 1158, B 1595, C 1320

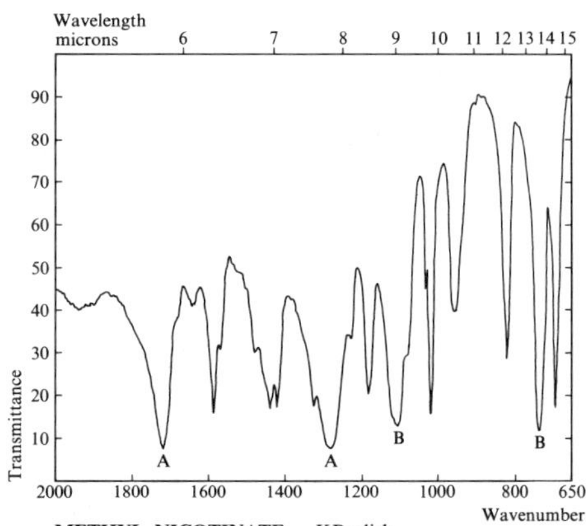

METHYL NICOTINATE — KBr disk
A 1284 or 1720, B 737 or 1110

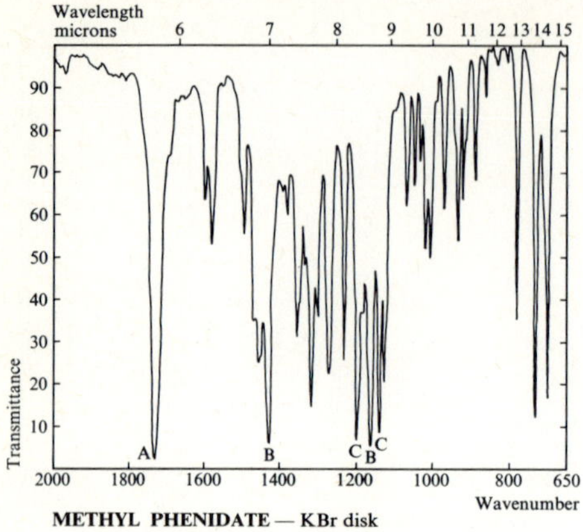

METHYL PHENIDATE — KBr disk
A 1728, B 1165 or 1431, C 1140 or 1200

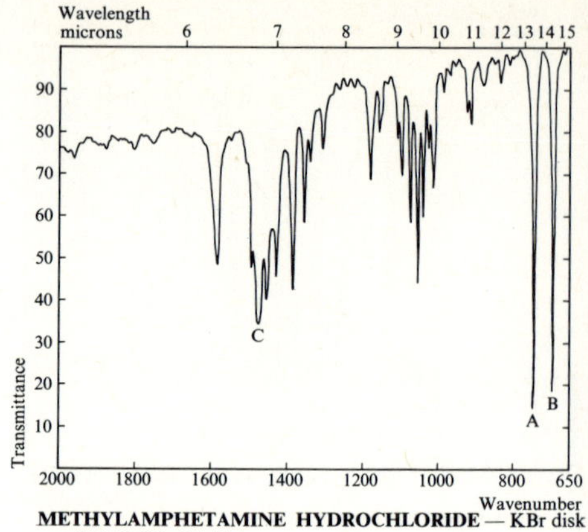

METHYLAMPHETAMINE HYDROCHLORIDE — KBr disk
A 747, B 698, C 1475

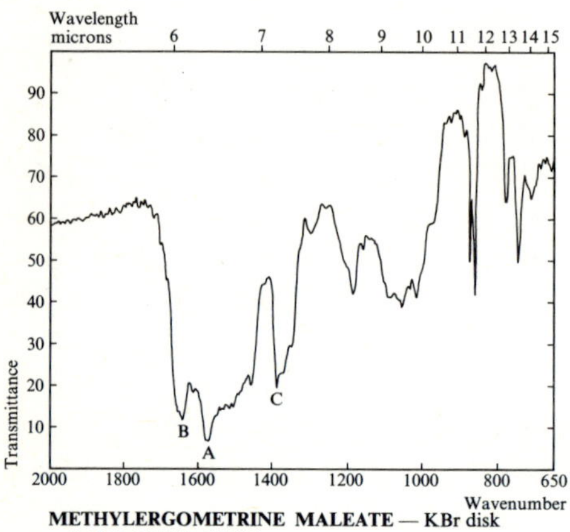

METHYLERGOMETRINE MALEATE — KBr disk
A 1573, B 1643, C 1383

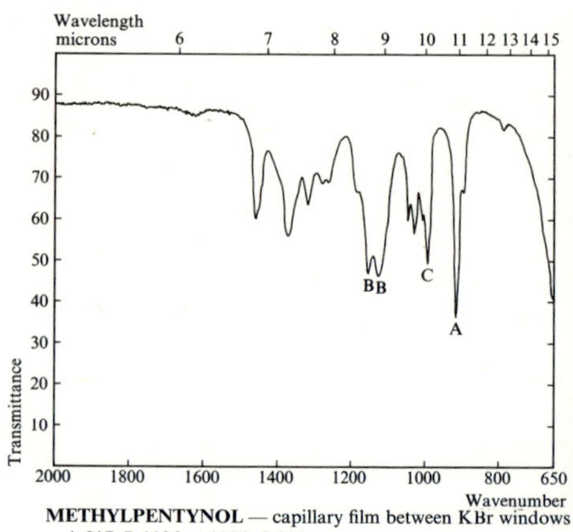

METHYLPENTYNOL — capillary film between KBr windows
A 917, B 1126 or 1156, C 995

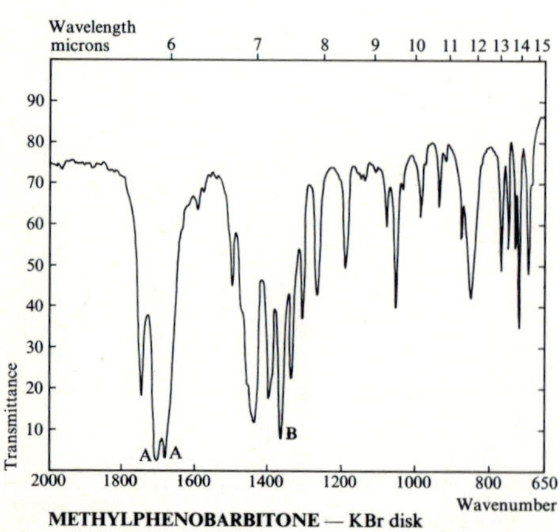

METHYLPHENOBARBITONE — KBr disk
A 1684 or 1707, B 1365

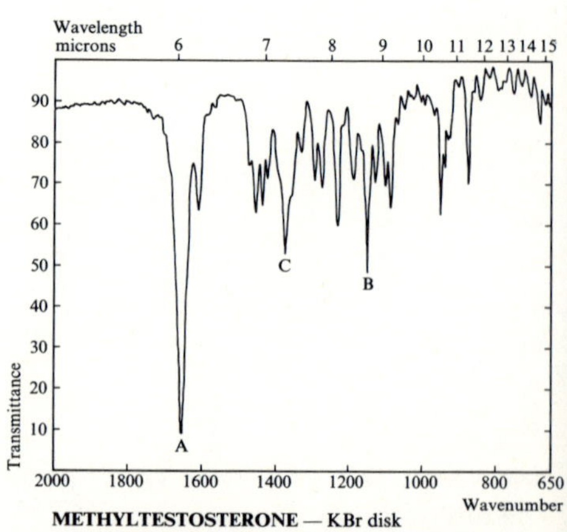

METHYLTESTOSTERONE — KBr disk
A 1657, B 1149, C 1375

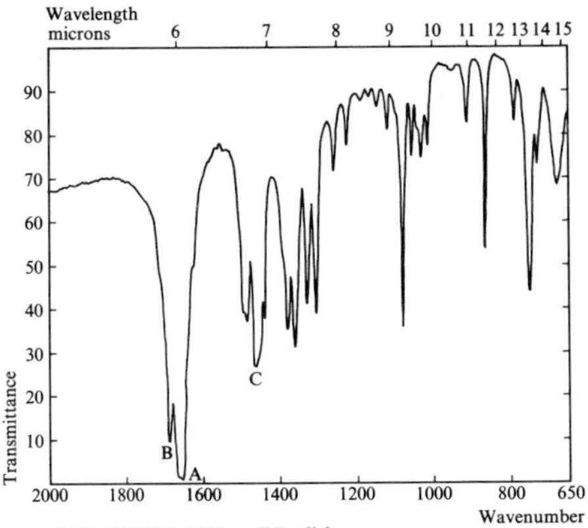

METHYPRYLONE — KBr disk
A 1655, B 1688, C 1463

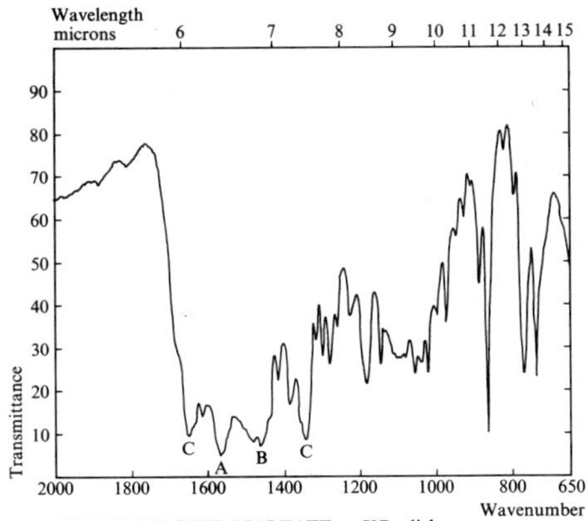

METHYSERGIDE MALEATE — KBr disk
A 1566, B 1466, C 1343 or 1650

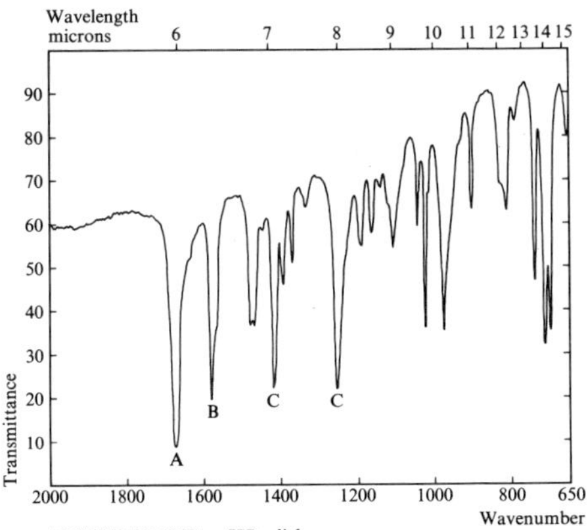

METYRAPONE — KBr disk
A 1672, B 1578, C 1255 or 1417

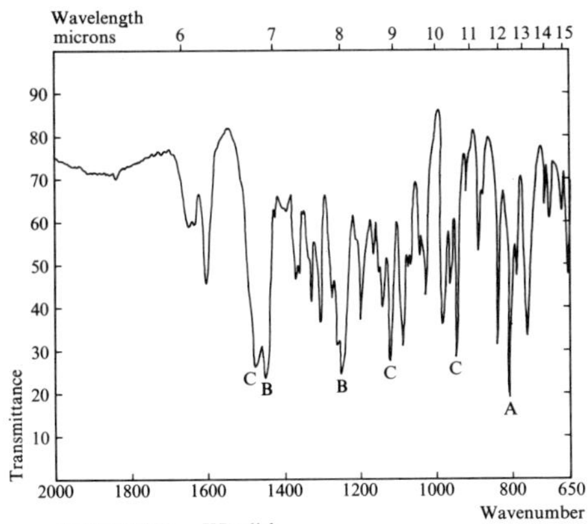

MORPHINE — KBr disk
A 805, B 1243 or 1448, C 945 or 1118 or 1475

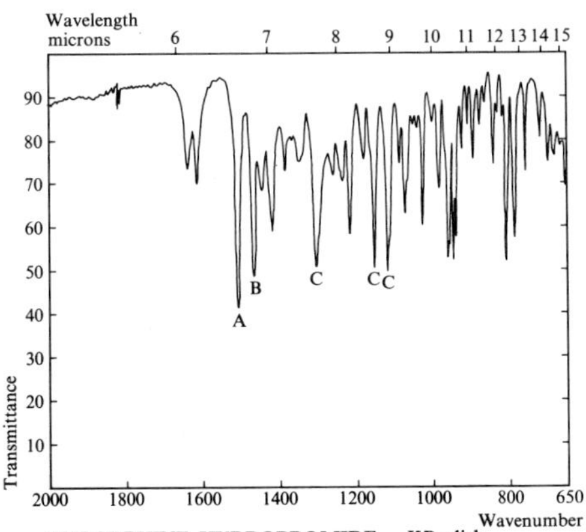

NALORPHINE HYDROBROMIDE — KBr disk
A 1505, B 1466, C 1121 or 1155 or 1304

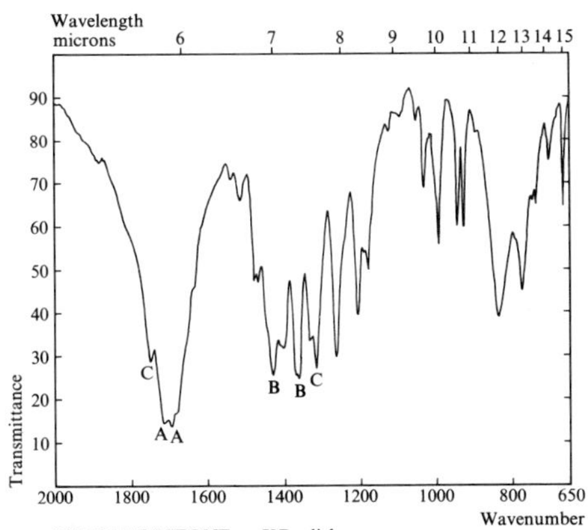

NEALBARBITONE — KBr disk
A 1695 or 1719, B 1364 or 1430, C 1320 or 1752

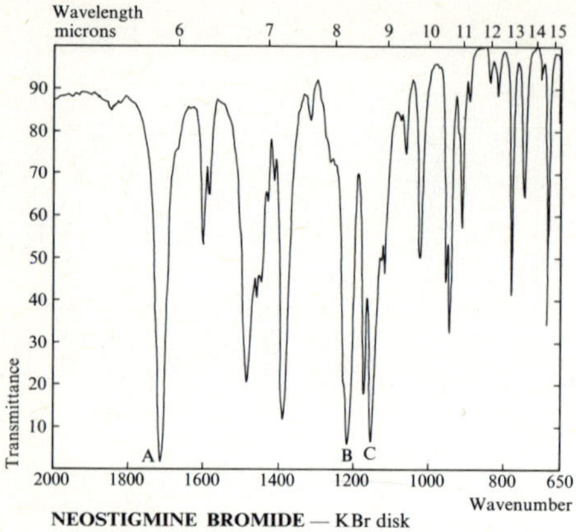

NEOSTIGMINE BROMIDE — KBr disk
A 1711, B 1215, C 1154

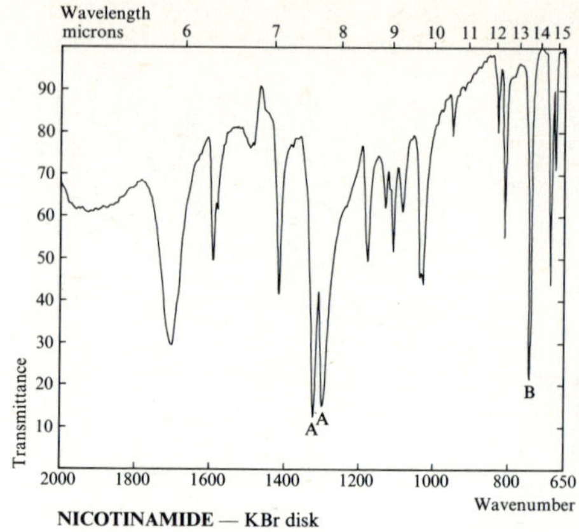

NICOTINAMIDE — KBr disk
A 1300 or 1324, B 744

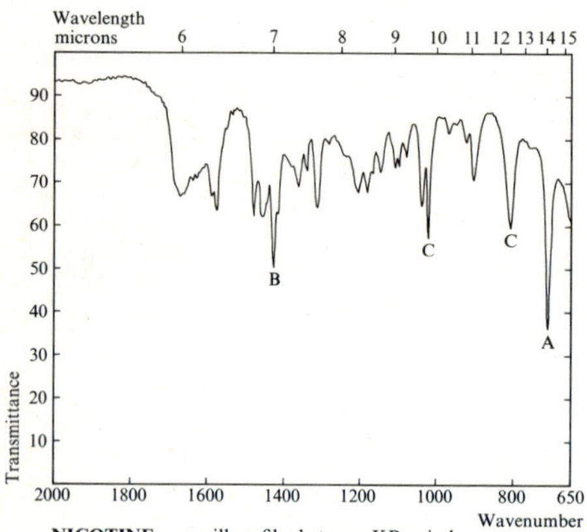

NICOTINE — capillary film between KBr windows
A 712, B 1429, C 810 or 1022

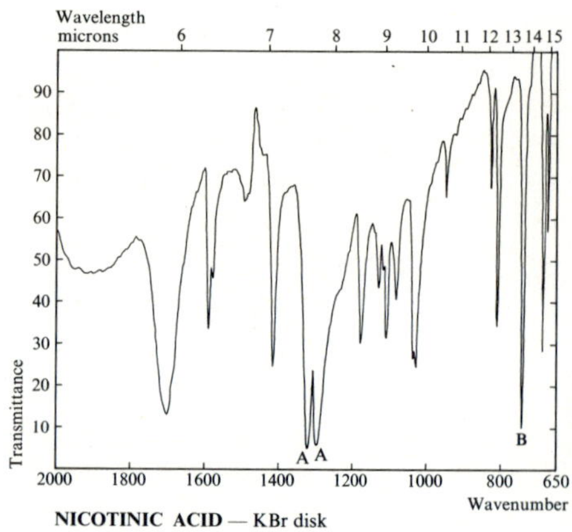

NICOTINIC ACID — KBr disk
A 1300 or 1324, B 744

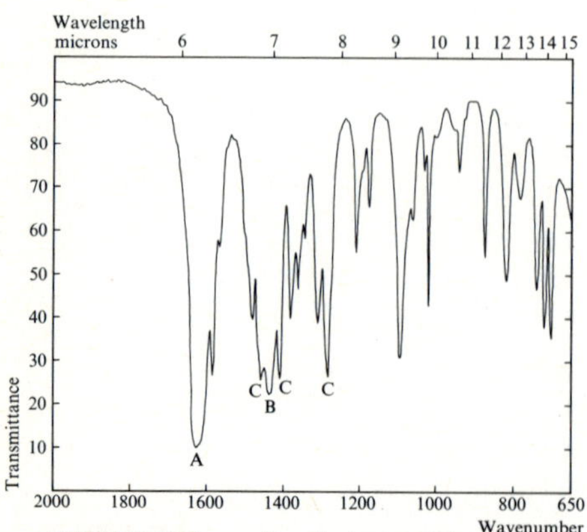

NIKETHAMIDE — capillary film between KBr windows
A 1627, B 1437, C 1285 or 1412 or 1460

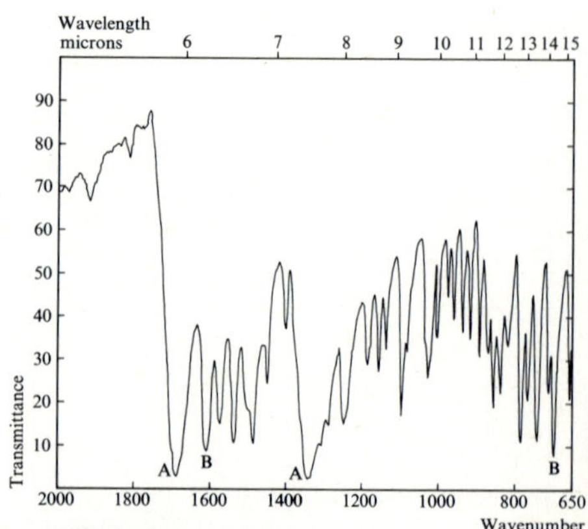

NITRAZEPAM — KBr disk
A 1352 or 1692, B 702 or 1615

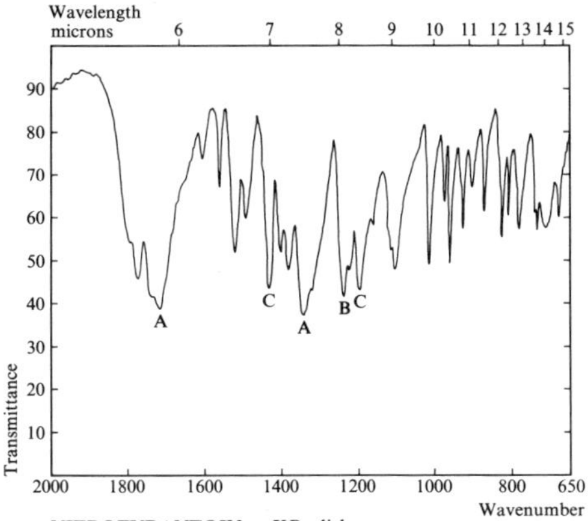

NITROFURANTOIN — KBr disk
A 1345 or 1716, B 1239, C 1200 or 1435

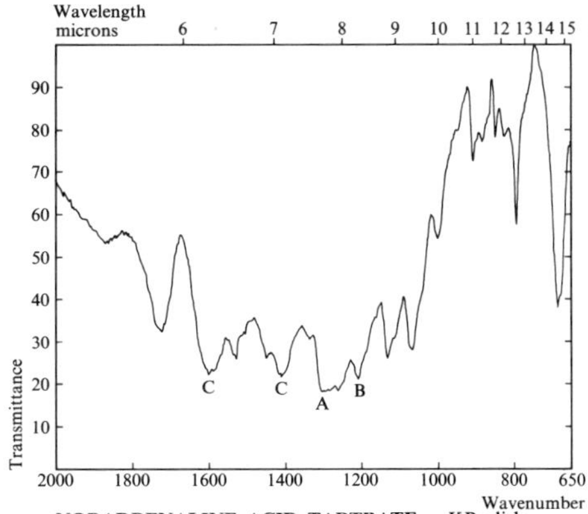

NORADRENALINE ACID TARTRATE — KBr disk
A 1300, B 1210, C 1412 or 1602

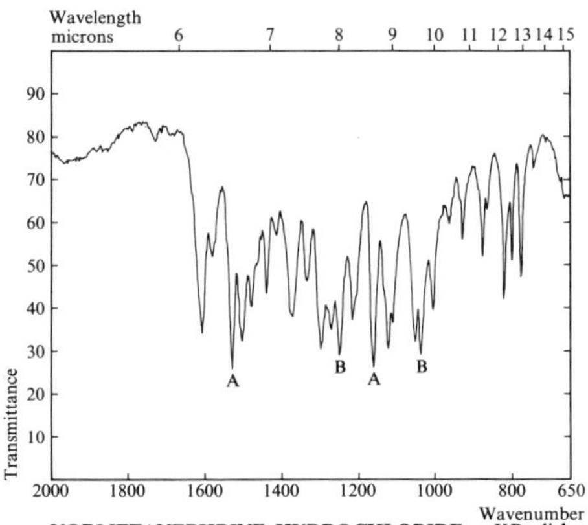

NORMETANEPHRINE HYDROCHLORIDE — KBr disk
A 1162 or 1529, B 1037 or 1250

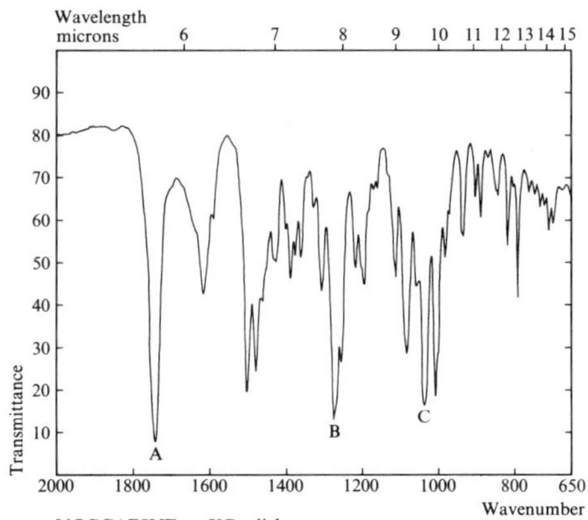

NOSCAPINE — KBr disk
A 1745, B 1276, C 1038

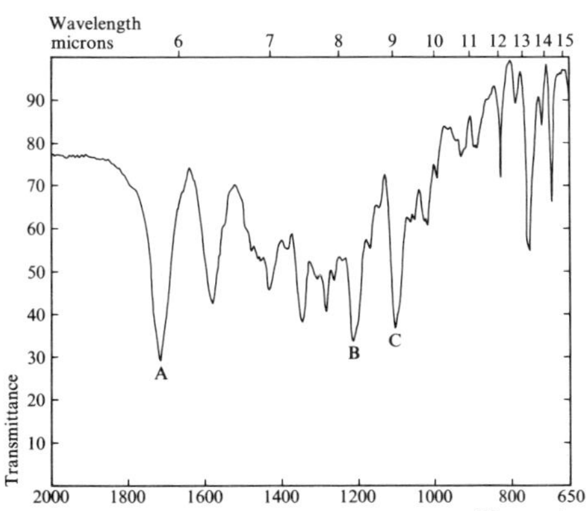

ORPHENADRINE CITRATE — KBr disk
A 1718, B 1216, C 1108

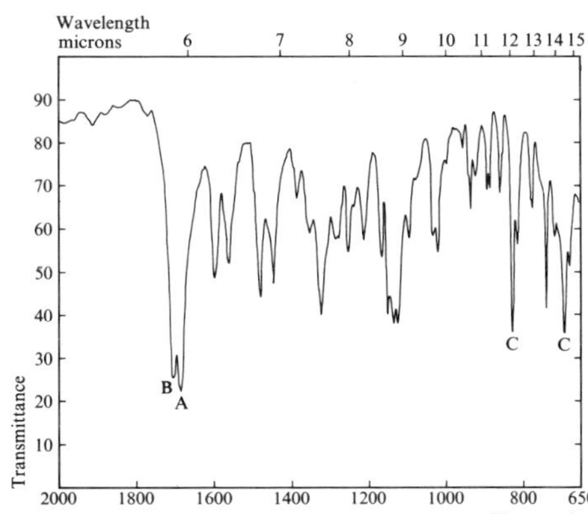

OXAZEPAM — KBr disk
A 1687, B 1706, C 693 or 830

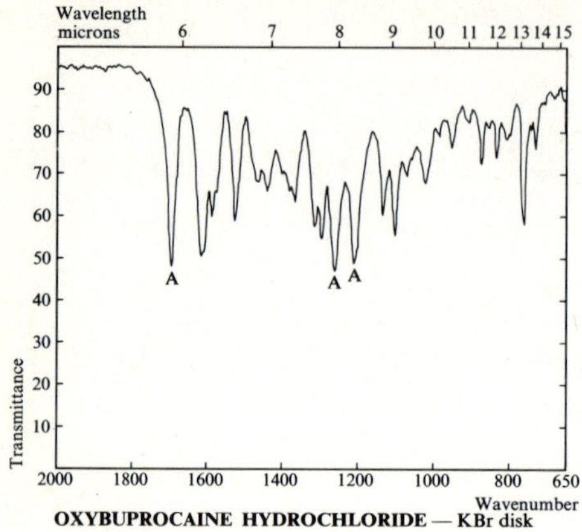

OXYBUPROCAINE HYDROCHLORIDE — KBr disk
A 1215 or 1262 or 1698

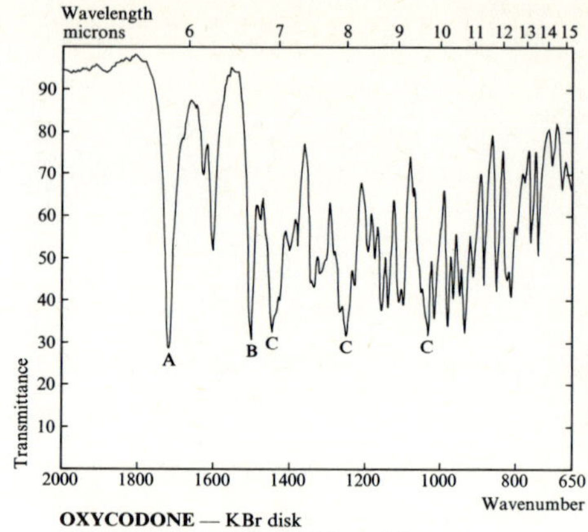

OXYCODONE — KBr disk
A 1719, B 1501, C 1033 or 1255 or 1448

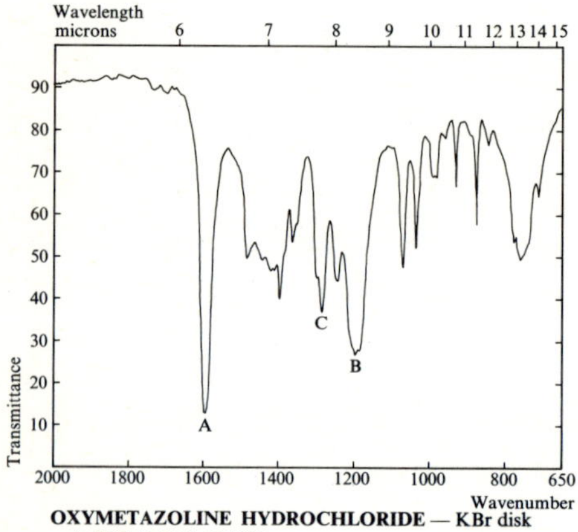

OXYMETAZOLINE HYDROCHLORIDE — KBr disk
A 1595, B 1199, C 1285

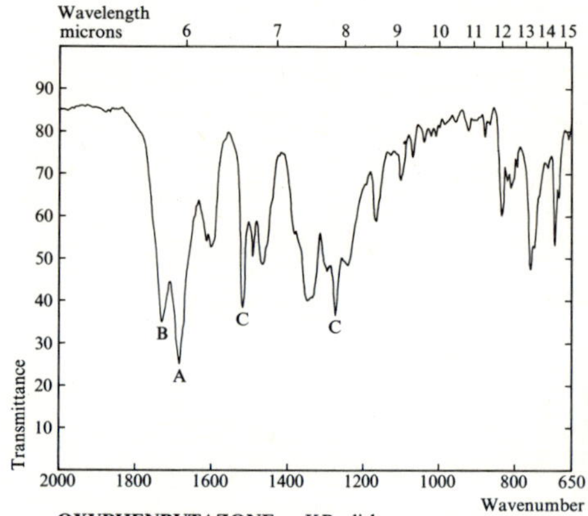

OXYPHENBUTAZONE — KBr disk
A 1683, B 1725, C 1275 or 1518

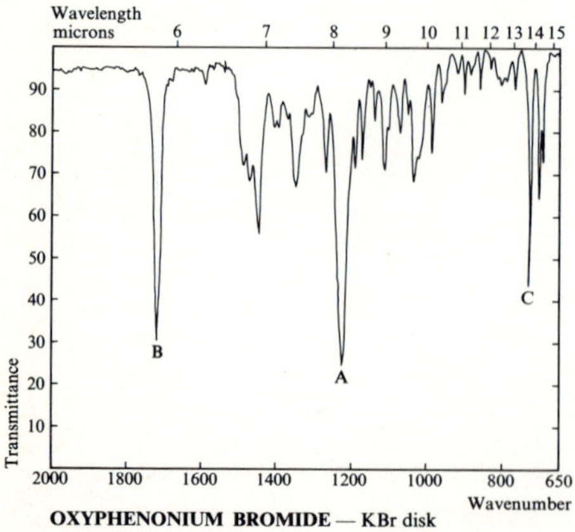

OXYPHENONIUM BROMIDE — KBr disk
A 1225, B 1719, C 729

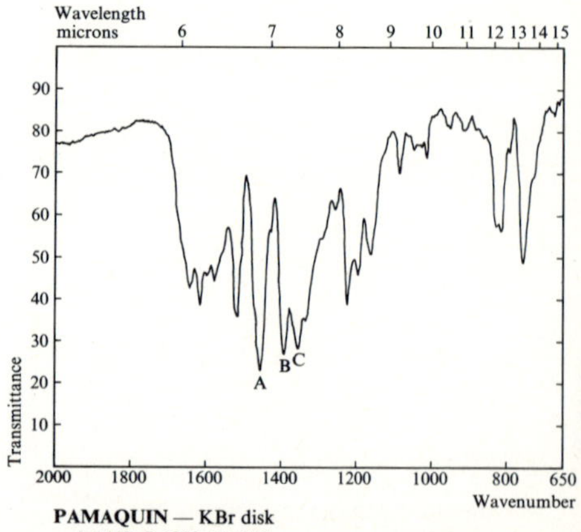

PAMAQUIN — KBr disk
A 1458, B 1393, C 1355

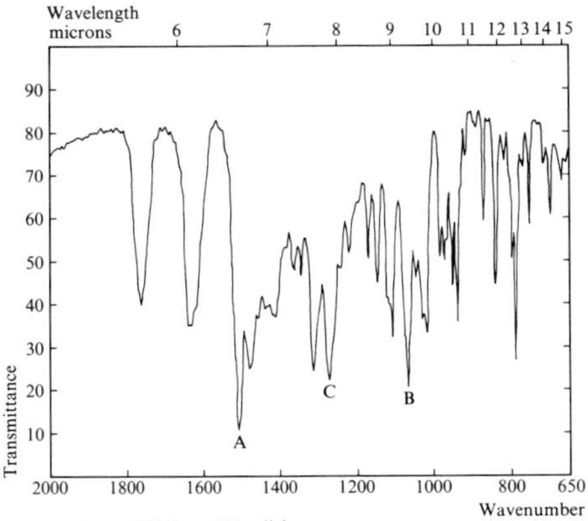

PAPAVERINE — KBr disk
A 1507, B 1068, C 1273

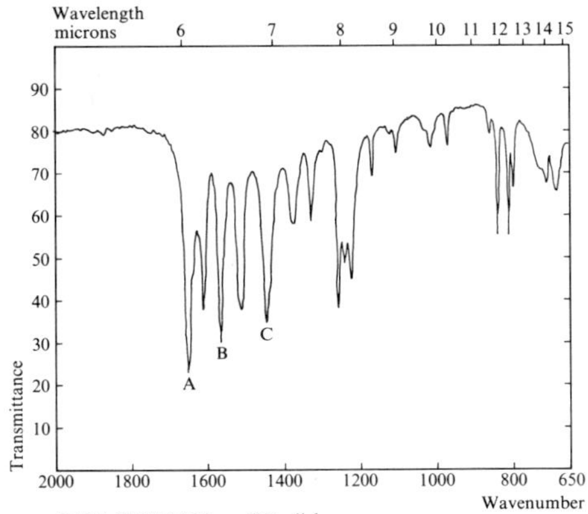

PARACETAMOL — KBr disk
A 1650, B 1563, C 1443

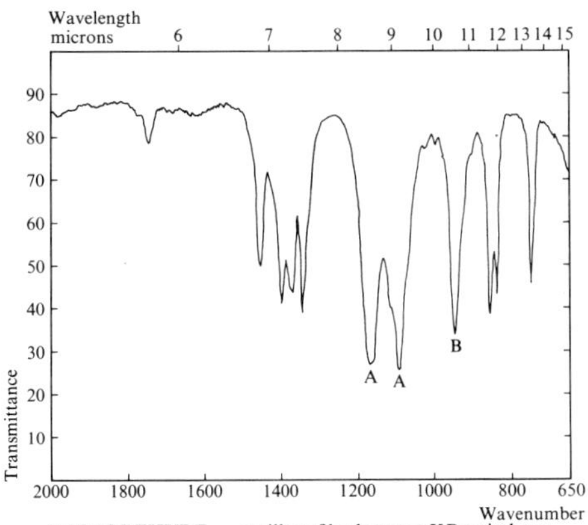

PARALDEHYDE — capillary film between KBr windows
A 1095 or 1170, B 946

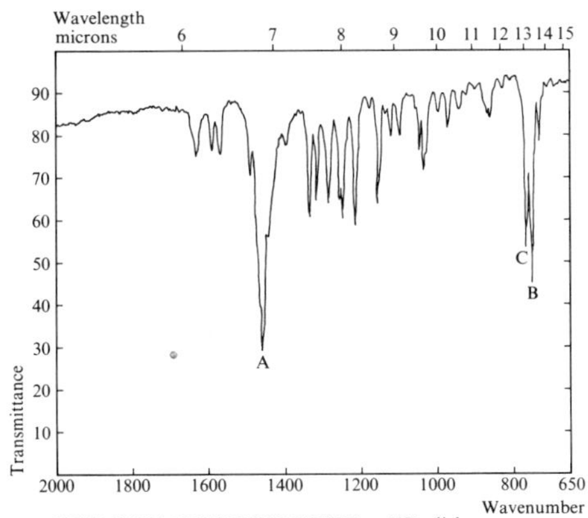

PECAZINE HYDROCHLORIDE — KBr disk
A 1458, B 750, C 768

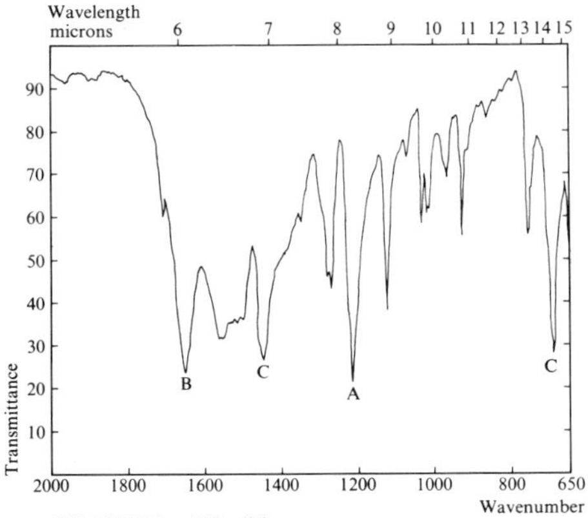

PEMOLINE — KBr disk
A 1218, B 1653, C 695 or 1450

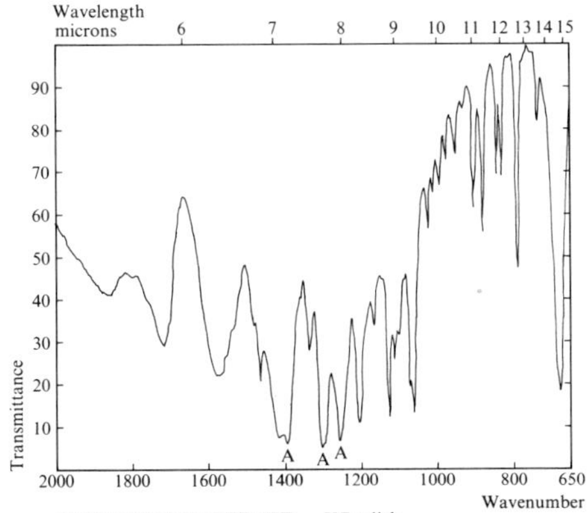

PEMPIDINE TARTRATE — KBr disk
A 1261 or 1308 or 1400

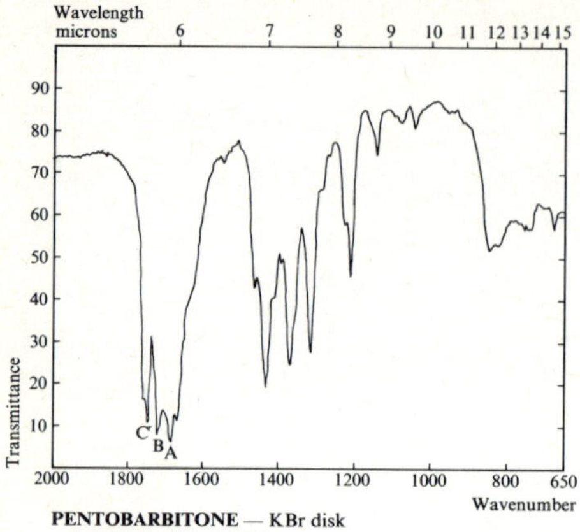

PENTOBARBITONE — KBr disk
A 1685, B 1719, C 1744

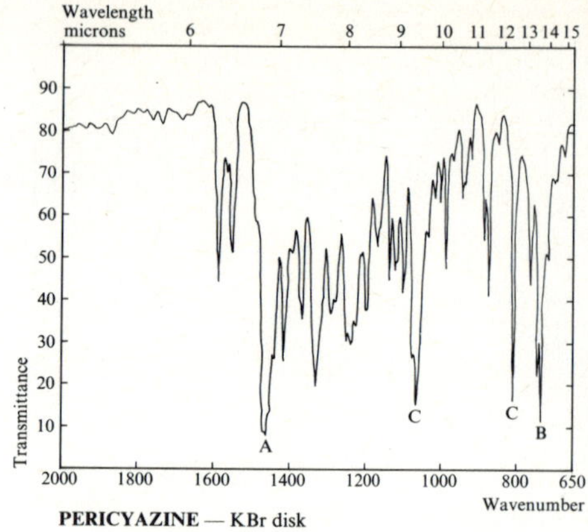

PERICYAZINE — KBr disk
A 1464, B 736, C 811 or 1066

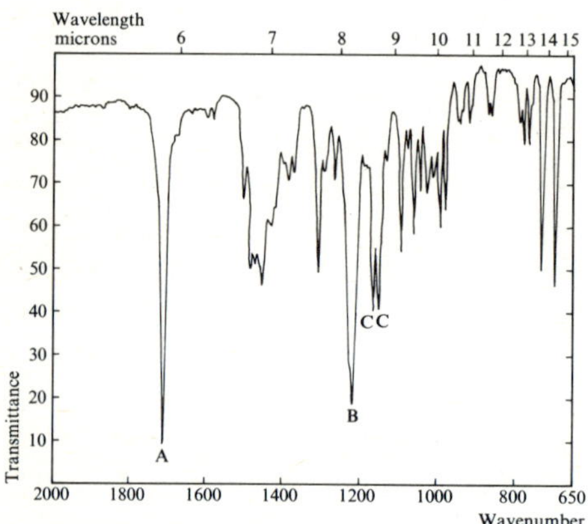

PETHIDINE HYDROCHLORIDE — KBr disk
A 1708, B 1218, C 1148 or 1166

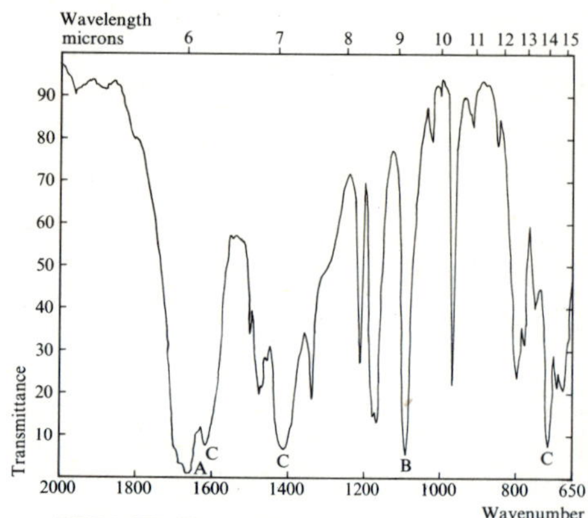

PHENACEMIDE — KBr disk
A 1660, B 1090, C 716 or 1410 or 1618

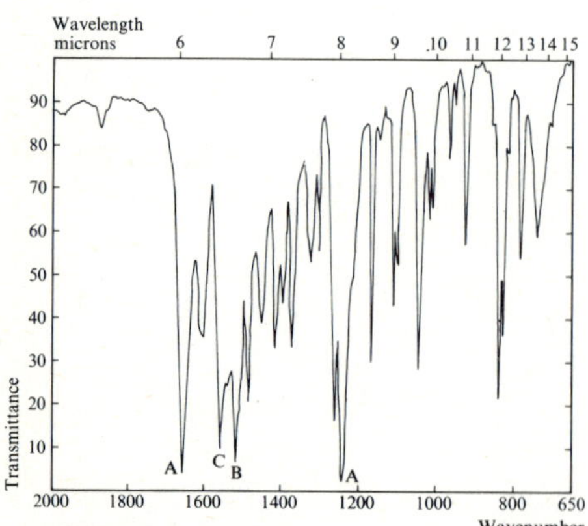

PHENACETIN — KBr disk
A 1243 or 1655, B 1513, C 1555

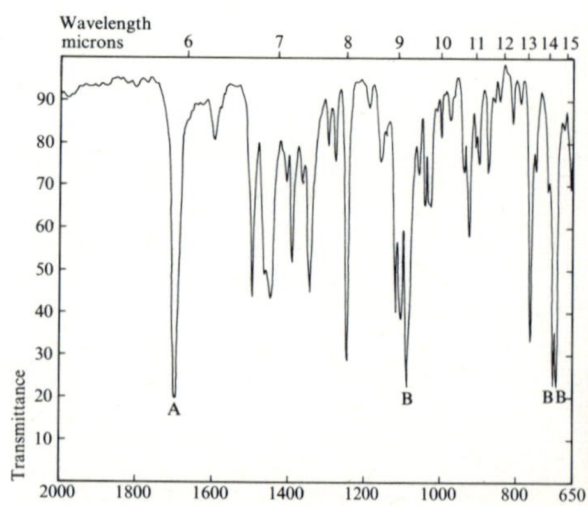

PHENADOXONE HYDROCHLORIDE — KBr disk
A 1699, B 698 or 704 or 1090

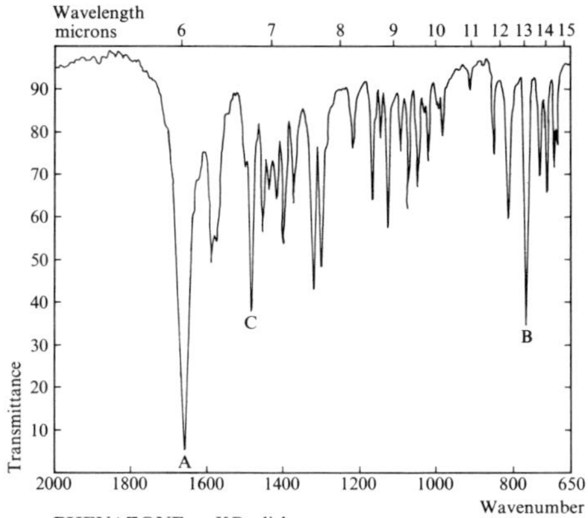

PHENAZONE — KBr disk
A 1660, B 770, C 1486

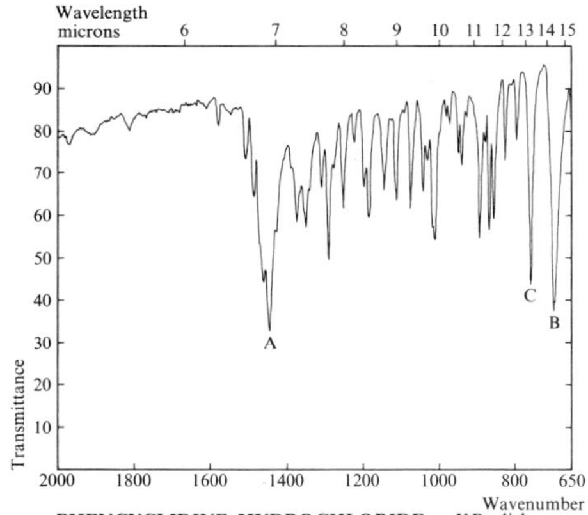

PHENCYCLIDINE HYDROCHLORIDE — KBr disk
A 1446, B 700, C 760

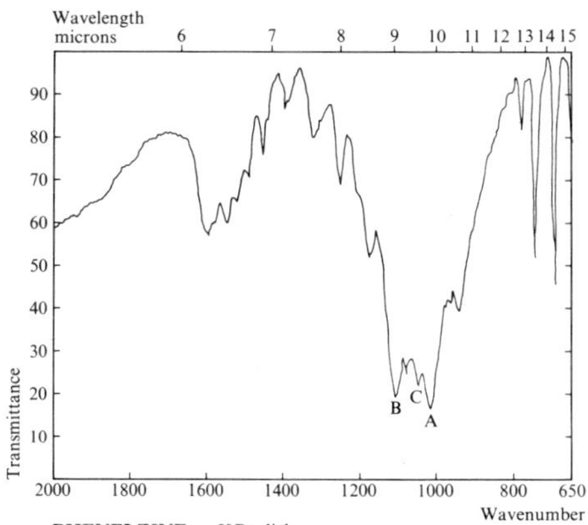

PHENELZINE — KBr disk
A 1016, B 1108, C 1050

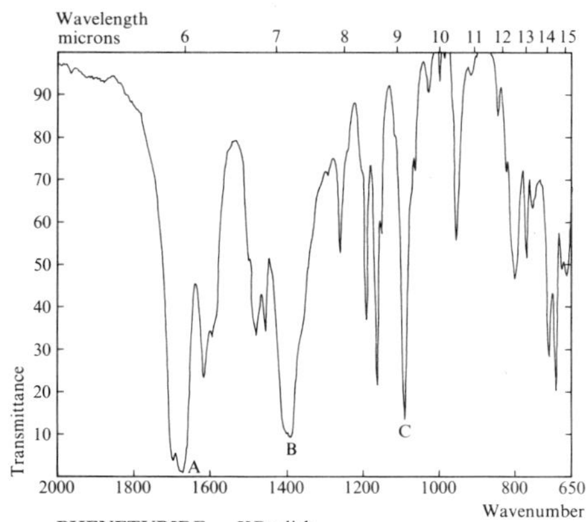

PHENETURIDE — KBr disk
A 1672, B 1395, C 1093

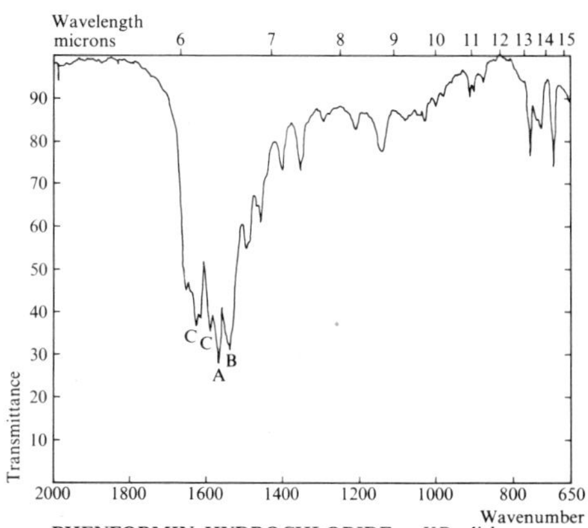

PHENFORMIN HYDROCHLORIDE — KBr disk
A 1568, B 1537, C 1590 or 1625

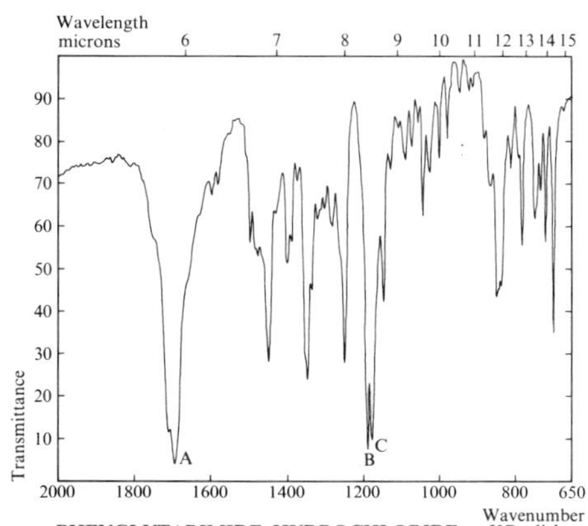

PHENGLUTARIMIDE HYDROCHLORIDE — KBr disk
A 1698, B 1194, C 1181

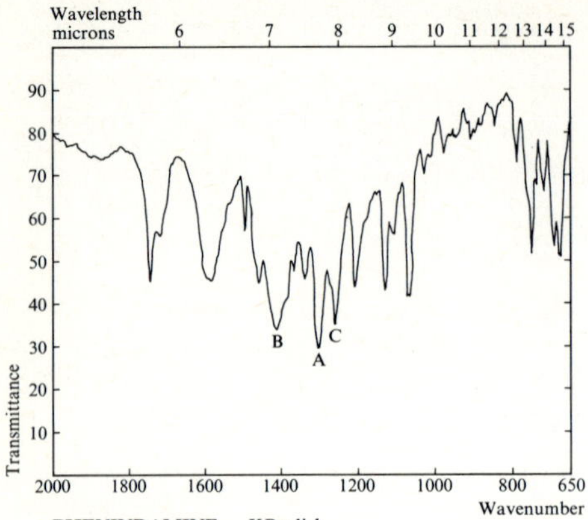

PHENINDAMINE — KBr disk
A 1304, B 1412, C 1261

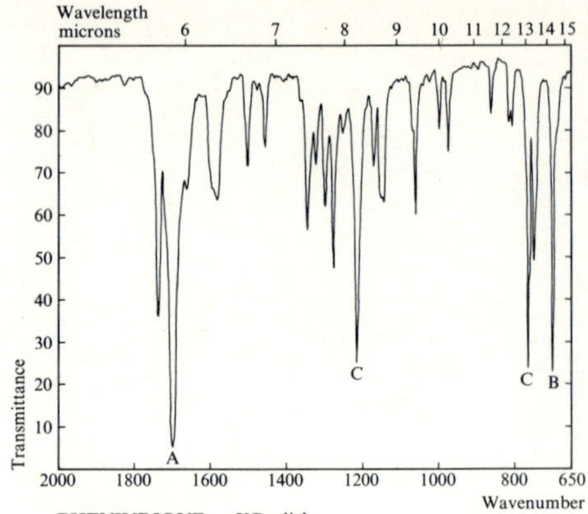

PHENINDIONE — KBr disk
A 1700, B 700, C 766 or 1219

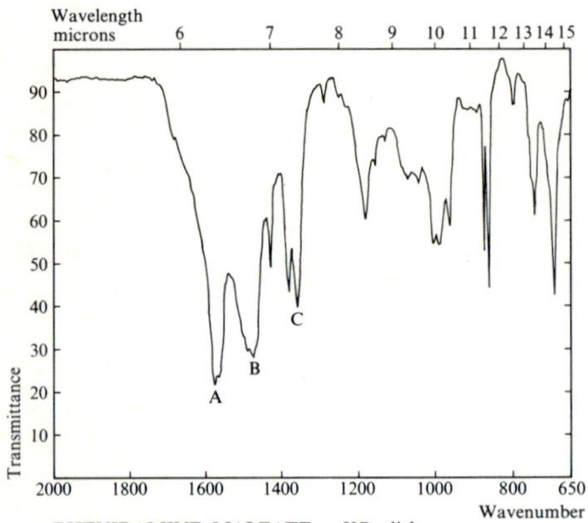

PHENIRAMINE MALEATE — KBr disk
A 1584, B 1481, C 1366

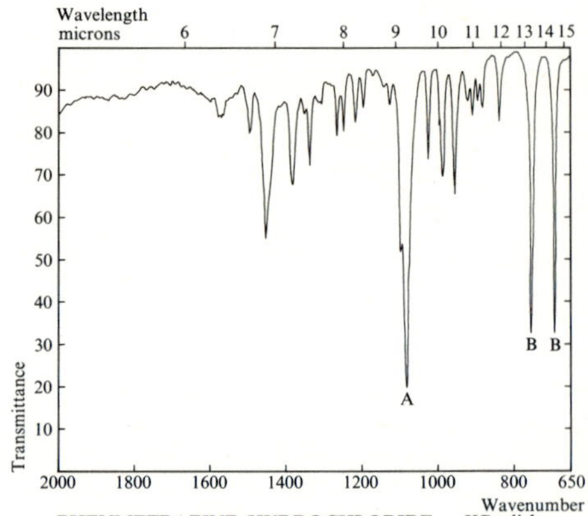

PHENMETRAZINE HYDROCHLORIDE — KBr disk
A 1083, B 695 or 757

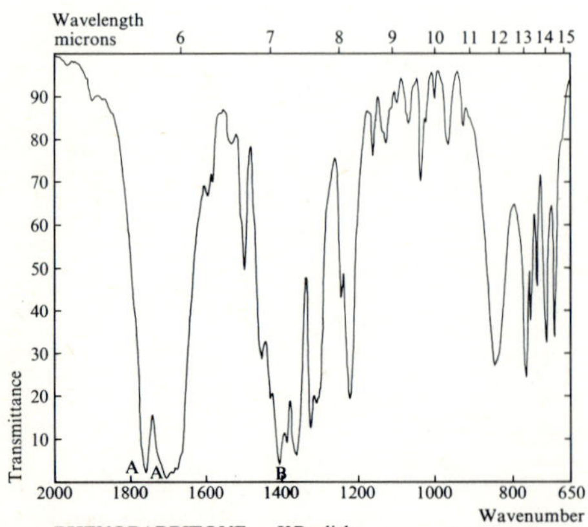

PHENOBARBITONE — KBr disk
A 1703 or 1756, B 1406

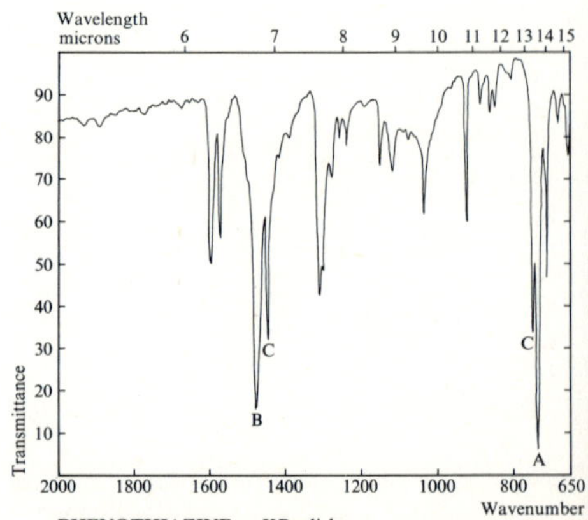

PHENOTHIAZINE — KBr disk
A 735, B 1476, C 750 or 1445

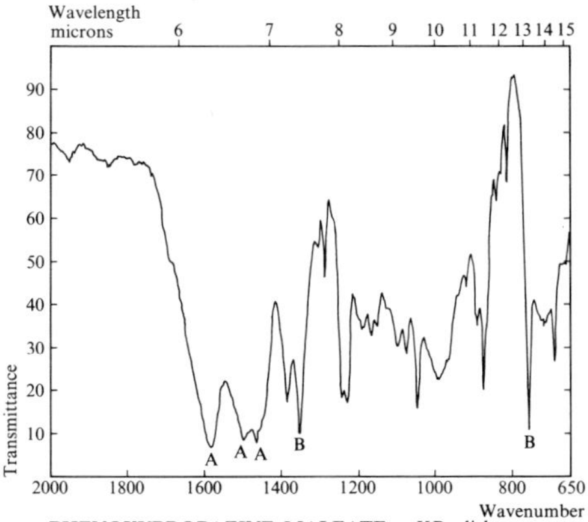

PHENOXYPROPAZINE MALEATE — KBr disk
A 1465 or 1500 or 1582, B 760 or 1353

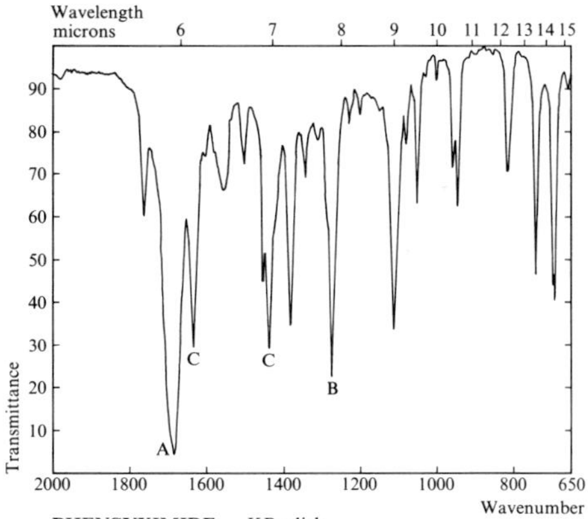

PHENSUXIMIDE — KBr disk
A 1686, B 1275, C 1439 or 1637

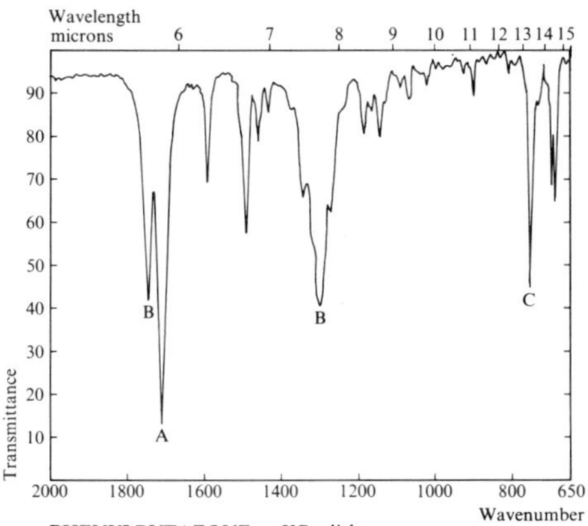

PHENYLBUTAZONE — KBr disk
A 1708, B 1300 or 1743, C 755

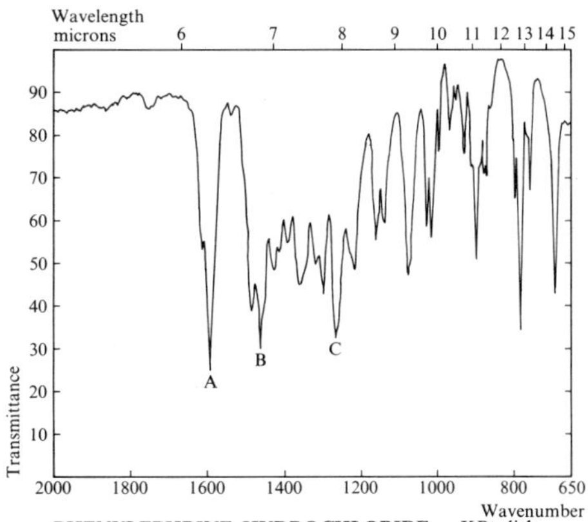

PHENYLEPHRINE HYDROCHLORIDE — KBr disk
A 1592, B 1464, C 1268

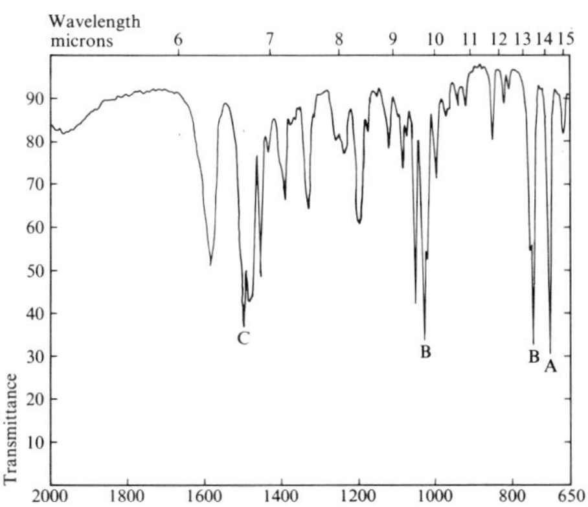

PHENYLPROPANOLAMINE HYDROCHLORIDE — KBr disk
A 700, B 746 or 1030, C 1500

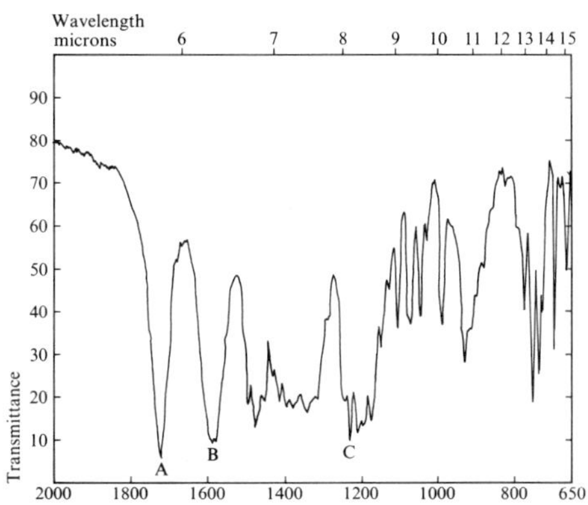

PHENYLTOLOXAMINE CITRATE — KBr disk
A 1722, B 1588, C 1235

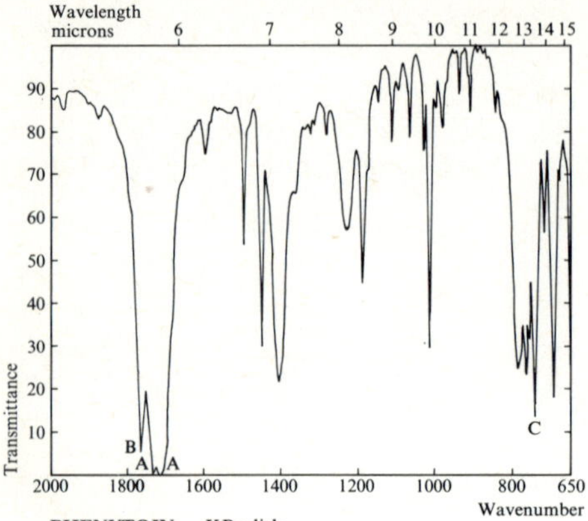

PHENYTOIN — KBr disk
A 1713 or 1747, B 1768, C 748

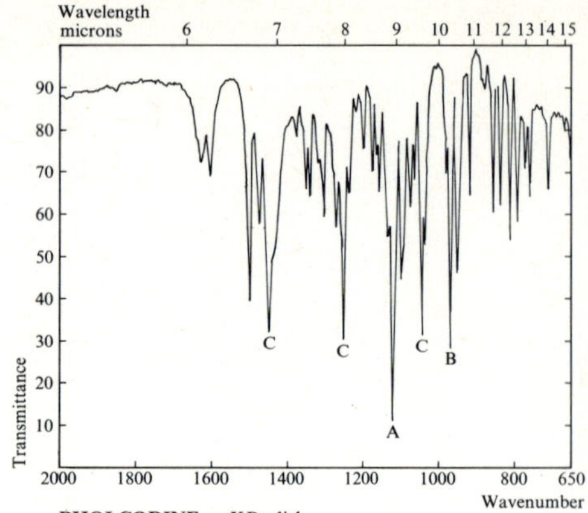

PHOLCODINE — KBr disk
A 1118, B 969, C 1043 or 1250 or 1448

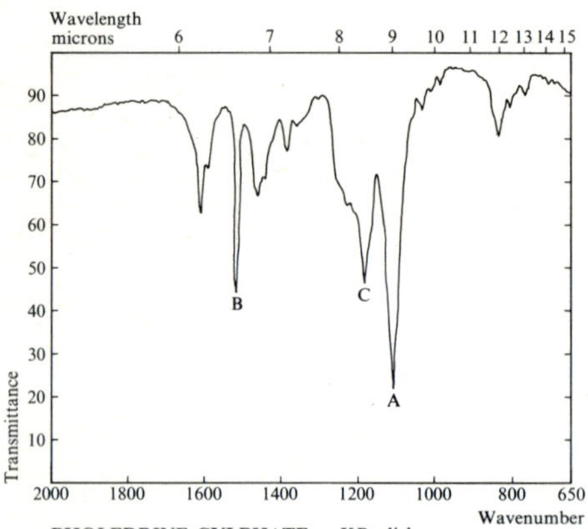

PHOLEDRINE SULPHATE — KBr disk
A 1110, B 1519, C 1185

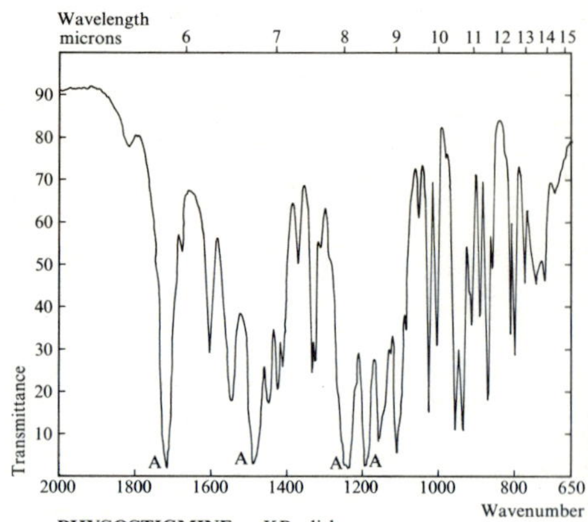

PHYSOSTIGMINE — KBr disk
A 1200 or 1243 or 1495 or 1724

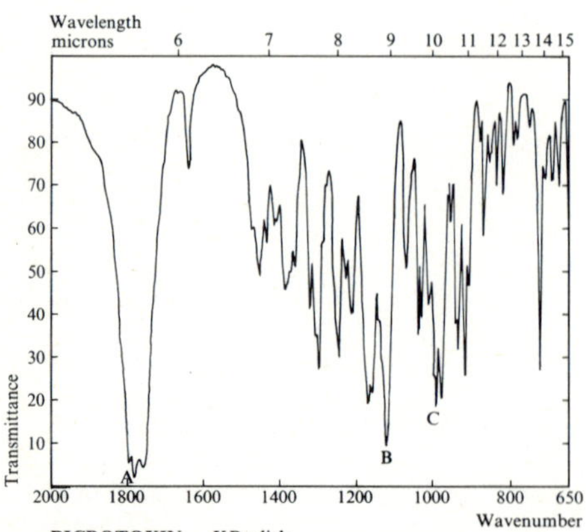

PICROTOXIN — KBr disk
A 1780, B 1123, C 990

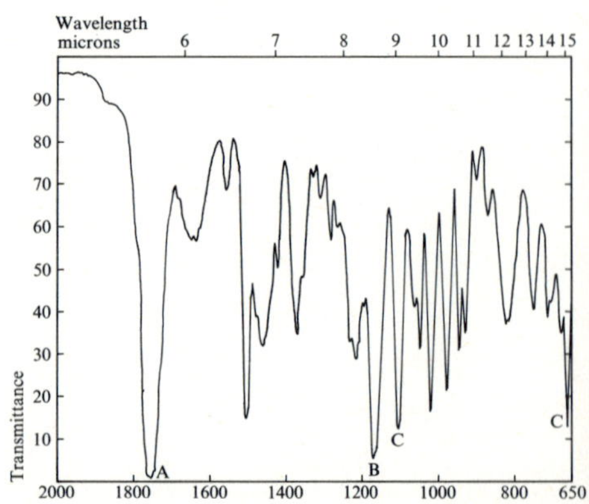

PILOCARPINE — capillary film between KBr windows
A 1752, B 1168, C 660 or 1104

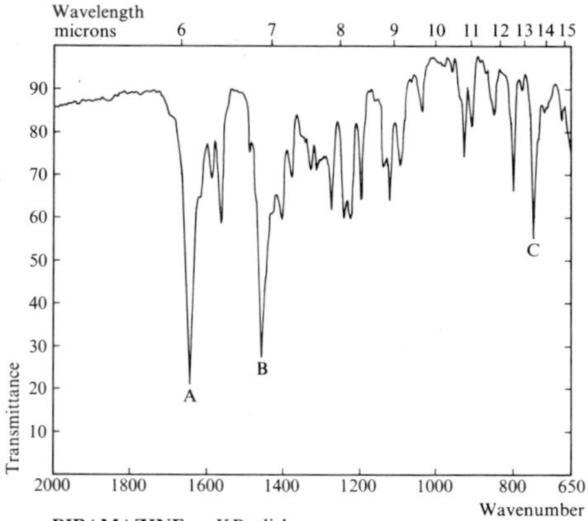

PIPAMAZINE — KBr disk
A 1644, B 1455, C 747

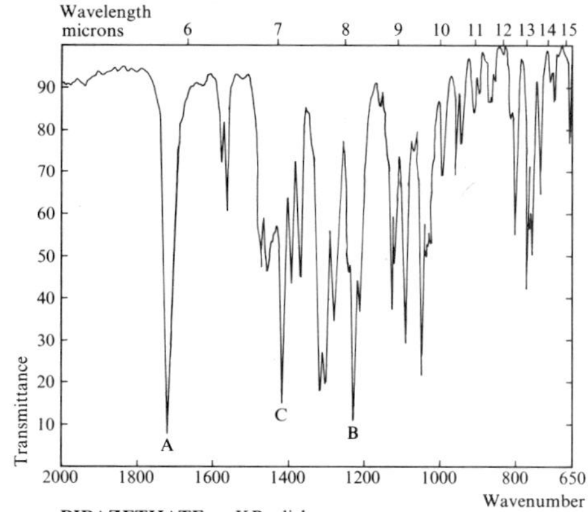

PIPAZETHATE — KBr disk
A 1717, B 1225, C 1416

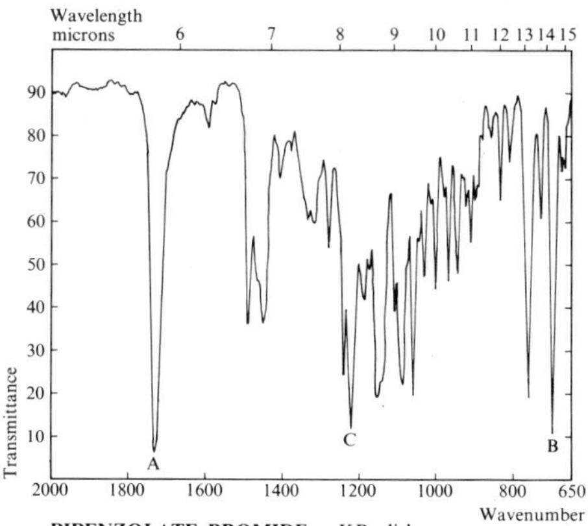

PIPENZOLATE BROMIDE — KBr disk
A 1726, B 698, C 1220

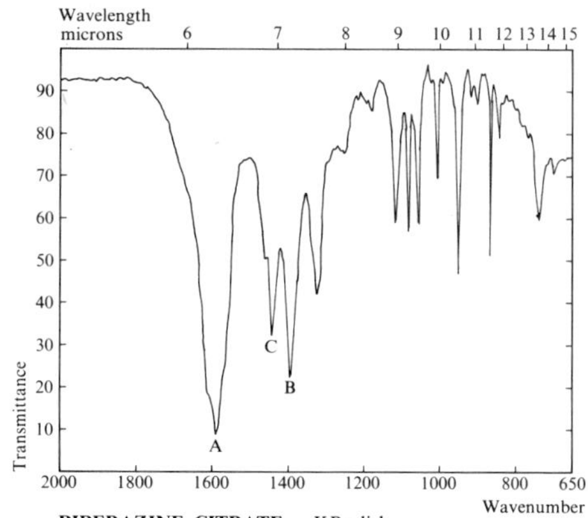

PIPERAZINE CITRATE — KBr disk
A 1592, B 1393, C 1442

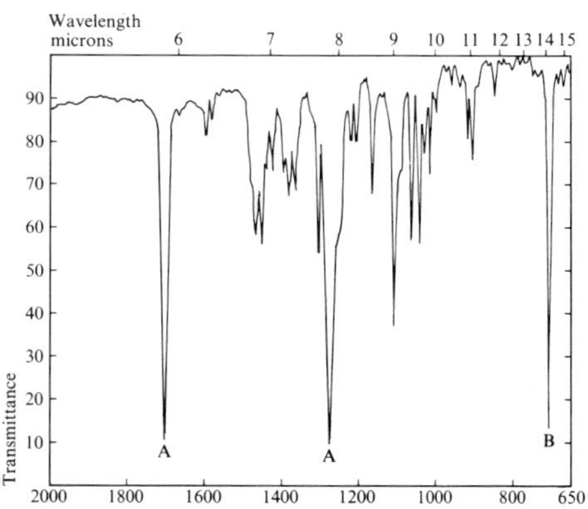

PIPEROCAINE HYDROCHLORIDE — KBr disk
A 1278 or 1703, B 711

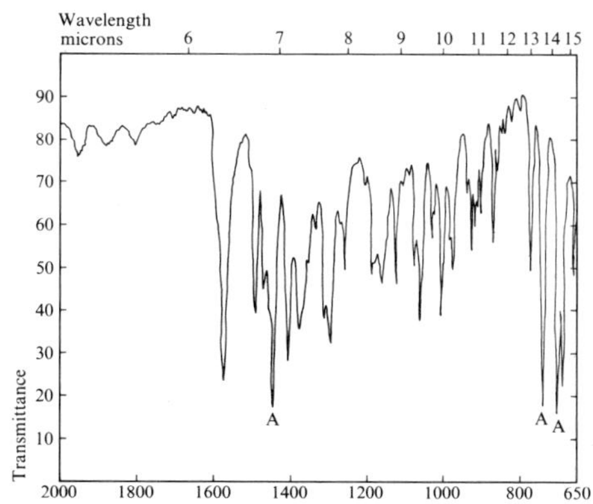

PIPRADROL HYDROCHLORIDE — KBr disk
A 701 or 740 or 1448

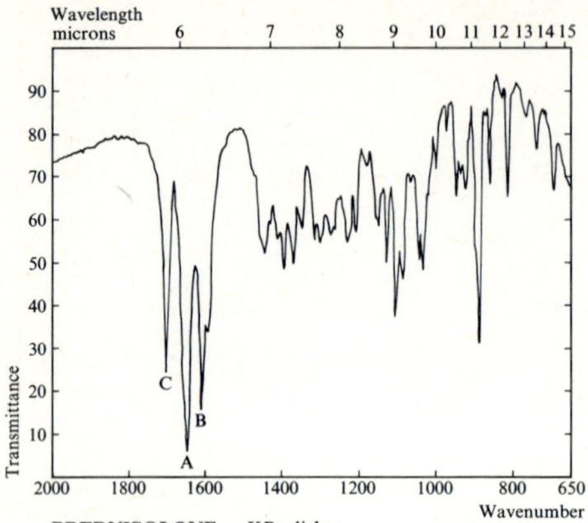

PREDNISOLONE — KBr disk
A 1650, B 1610, C 1701

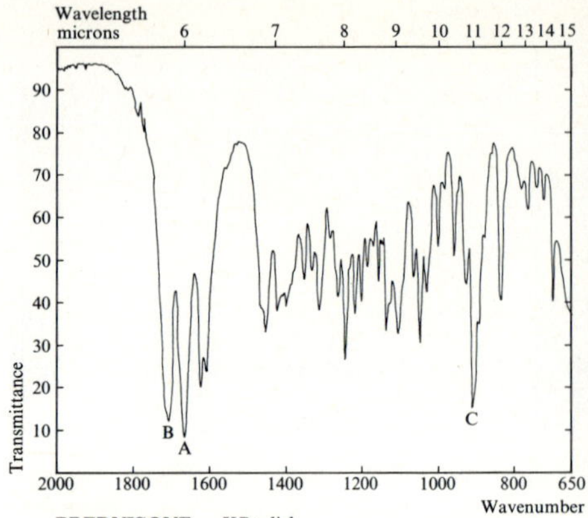

PREDNISONE — KBr disk
A 1668, B 1707, C 912

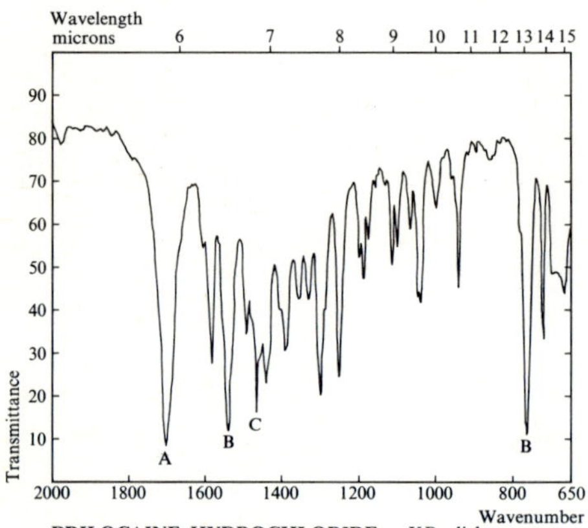

PRILOCAINE HYDROCHLORIDE — KBr disk
A 1700, B 764 or 1540, C 1464

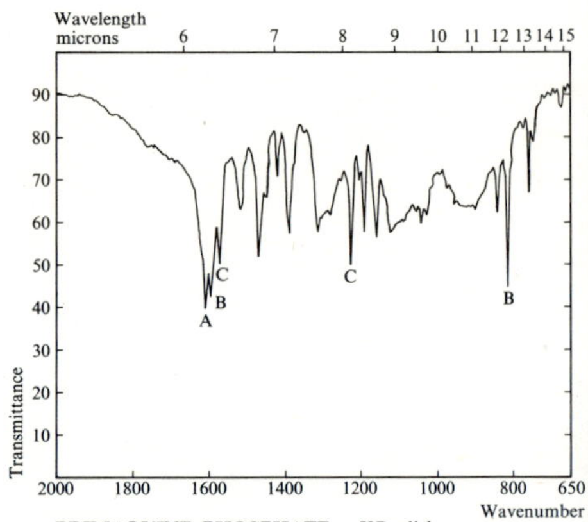

PRIMAQUINE PHOSPHATE — KBr disk
A 1611, B 815 or 1595, C 1230 or 1572

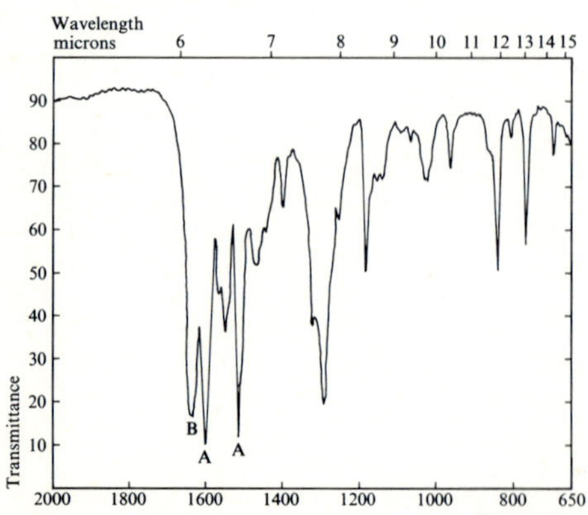

PROCAINAMIDE HYDROCHLORIDE — KBr disk
A 1519 or 1599, B 1632

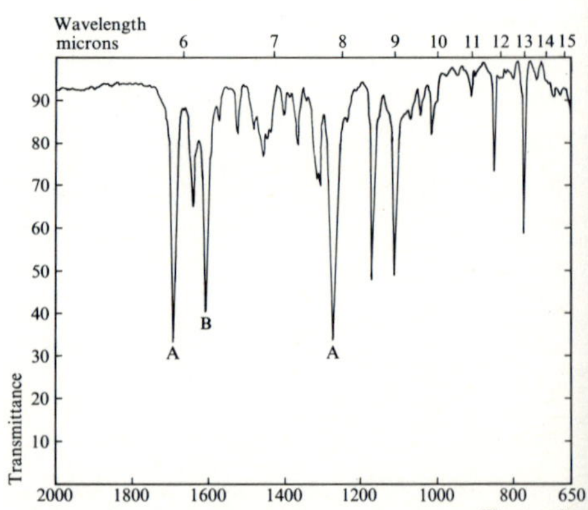

PROCAINE HYDROCHLORIDE — KBr disk
A 1274 or 1690, B 1605

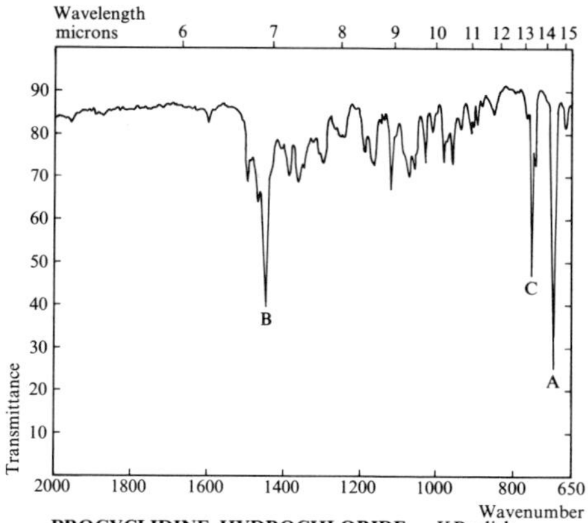

PROCYCLIDINE HYDROCHLORIDE — KBr disk
A 696, B 1447, C 755

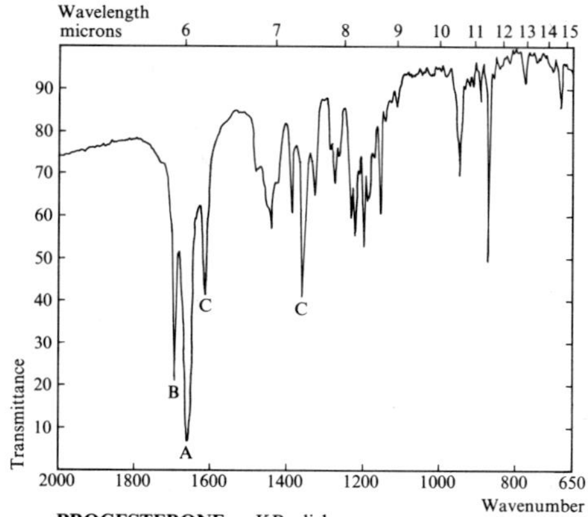

PROGESTERONE — KBr disk
A 1659, B 1691, C 1358 or 1615

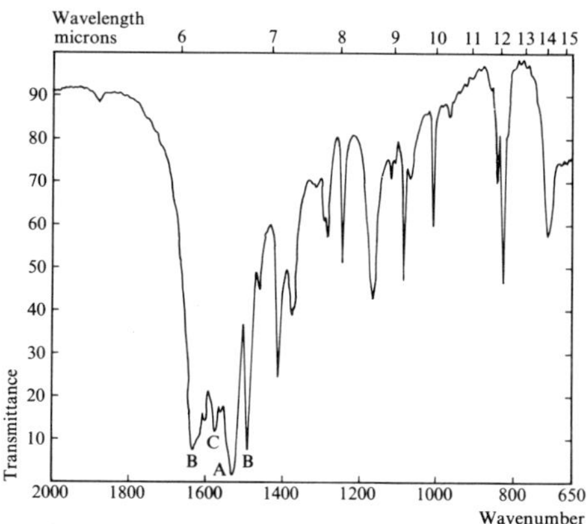

PROGUANIL HYDROCHLORIDE — KBr disk
A 1534, B 1492 or 1635, C 1575

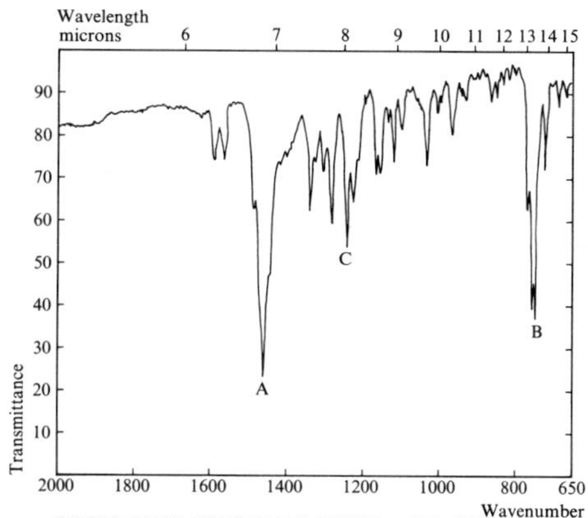

PROMAZINE HYDROCHLORIDE — KBr disk
A 1462, B 748, C 1245

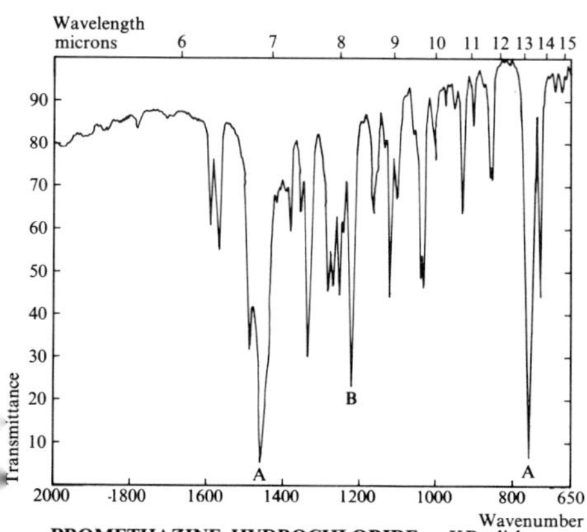

PROMETHAZINE HYDROCHLORIDE — KBr disk
A 757 or 1459, B 1222

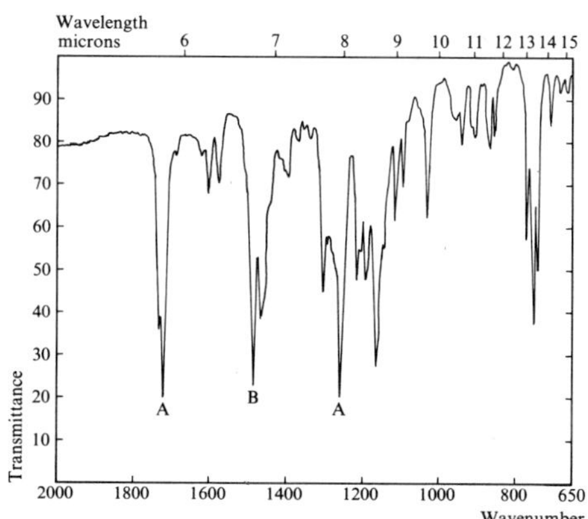

PROPANTHELINE BROMIDE — KBr disk
A 1260 or 1719, B 1484

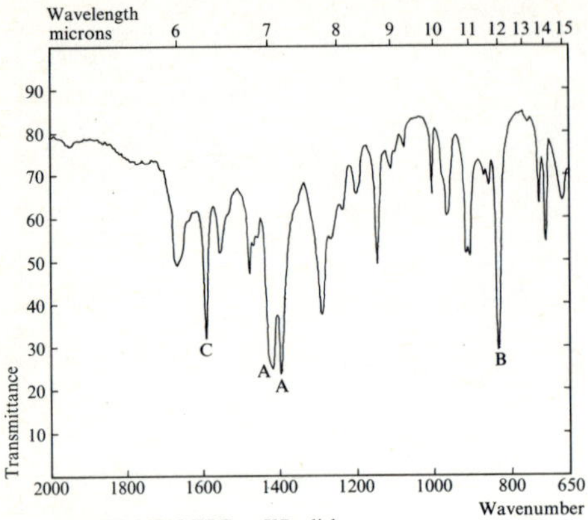

PROTHIONAMIDE — KBr disk
A 1398 or 1420, B 833, C 1592

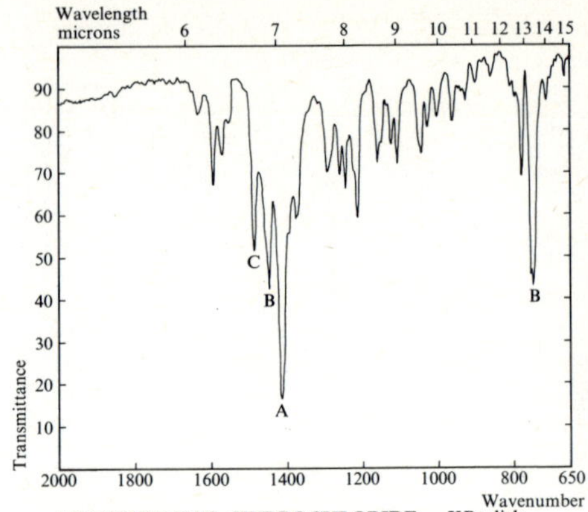

PROTHIPENDYL HYDROCHLORIDE — KBr disk
A 1413, B 749 or 1447, C 1488

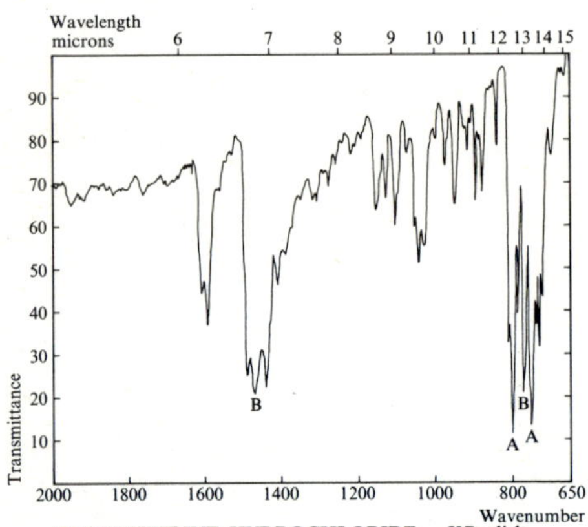

PROTRIPTYLINE HYDROCHLORIDE — KBr disk
A 753 or 799, B 772 or 1470

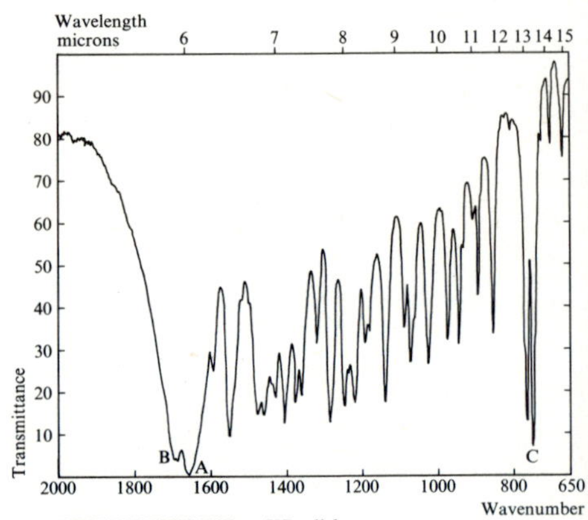

PROXYPHYLLINE — KBr disk
A 1656, B 1690, C 750

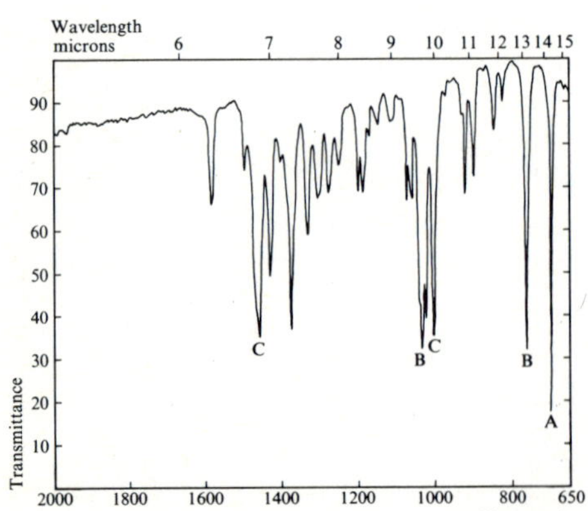

PSEUDOEPHEDRINE HYDROCHLORIDE — KBr disk
A 700, B 761 or 1031, C 1000 or 1459

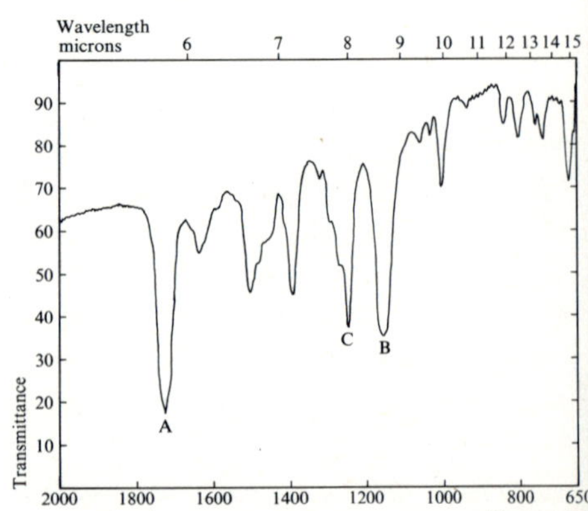

PYRIDOSTIGMINE BROMIDE — KBr disk
A 1728, B 1156, C 1249

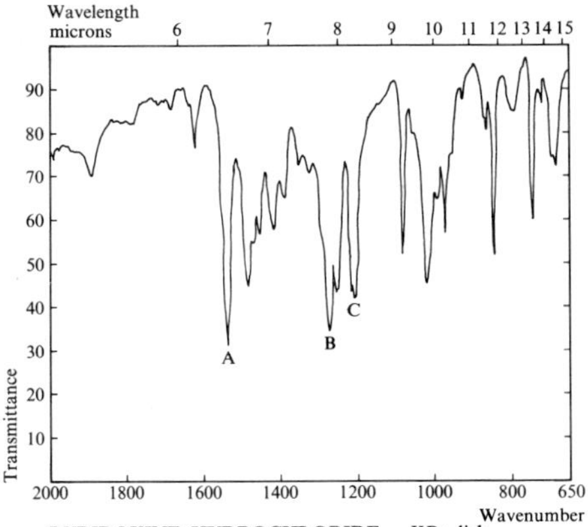

PYRIDOXINE HYDROCHLORIDE — KBr disk
A 1536, B 1273, C 1207

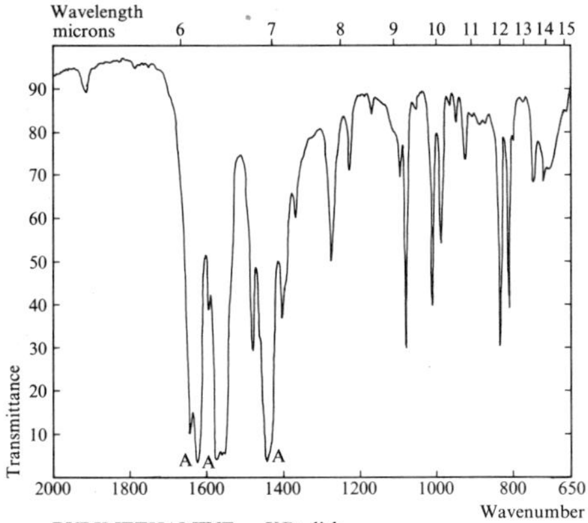

PYRIMETHAMINE — KBr disk
A 1445 or 1575 or 1628

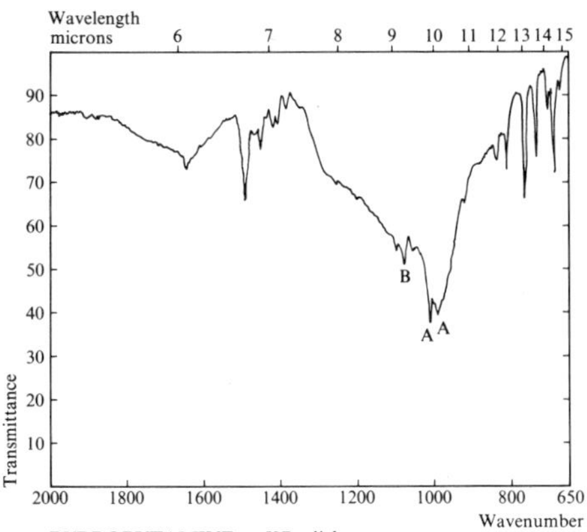

PYRROBUTAMINE — KBr disk
A 989 or 1009, B 1080

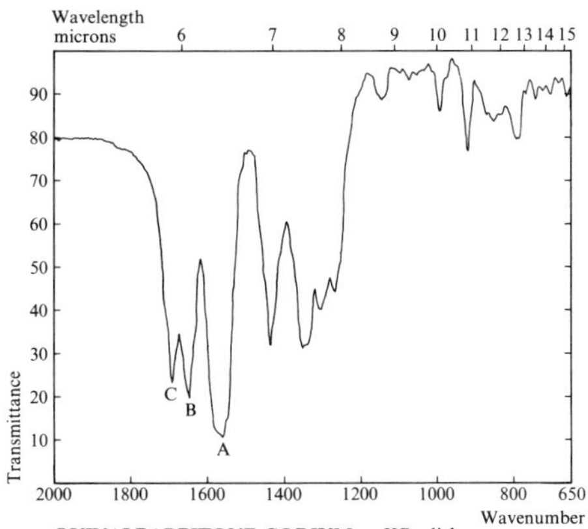

QUINALBARBITONE SODIUM — KBr disk
A 1559, B 1648, C 1690

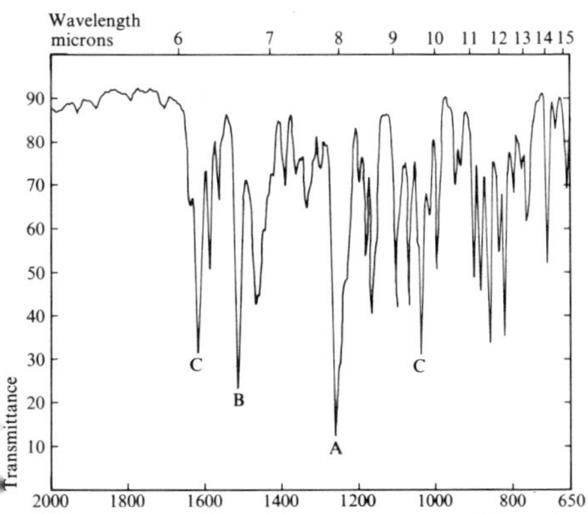

QUINIDINE — KBr disk
A 1258, B 1514, C 1040 or 1619

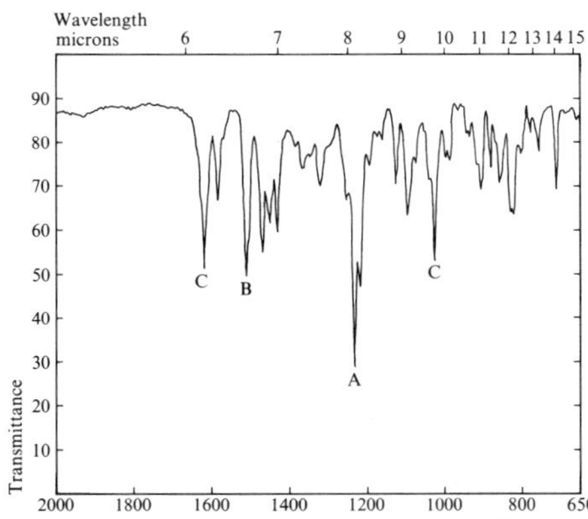

QUININE — KBr disk
A 1235, B 1510, C 1030 or 1619

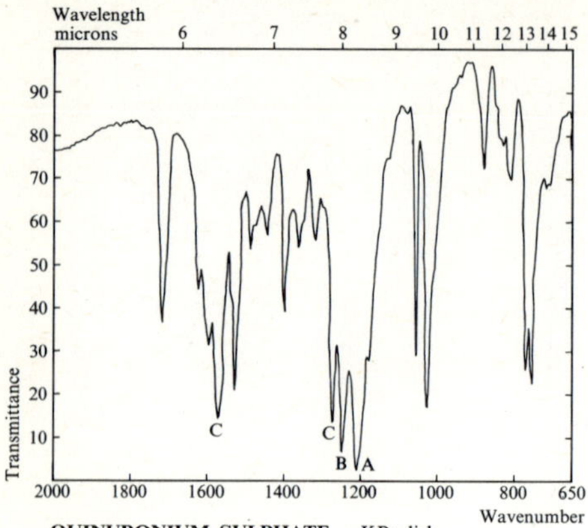

QUINURONIUM SULPHATE — KBr disk
A 1210, B 1248, C 1276 or 1572

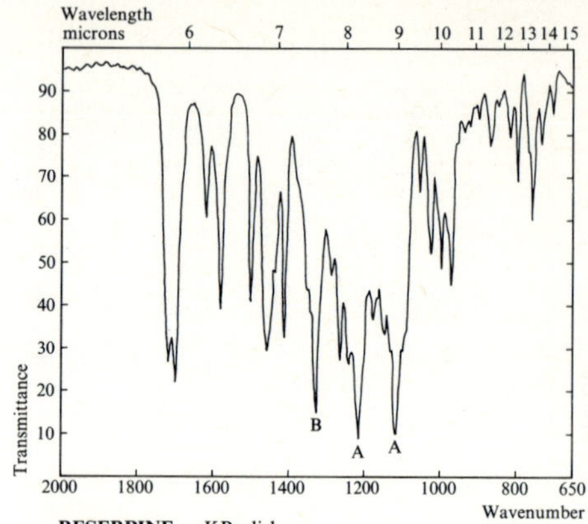

RESERPINE — KBr disk
A 1120 or 1220, B 1330

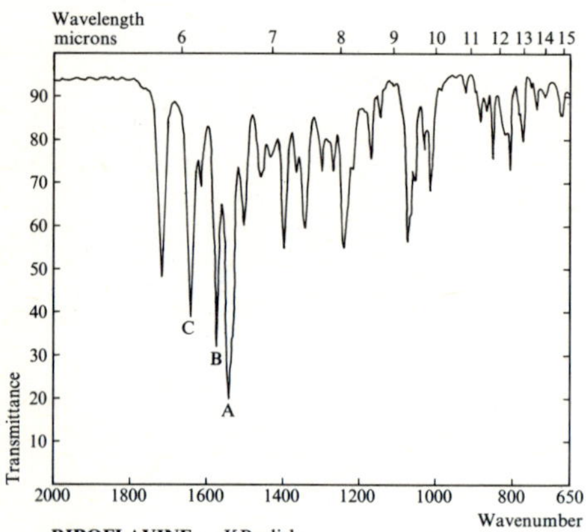

RIBOFLAVINE — KBr disk
A 1544, B 1575, C 1641

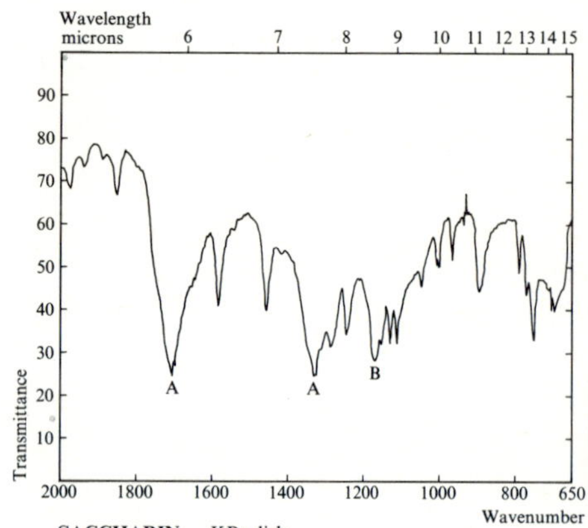

SACCHARIN — KBr disk
A 1334 or 1705, B 1170

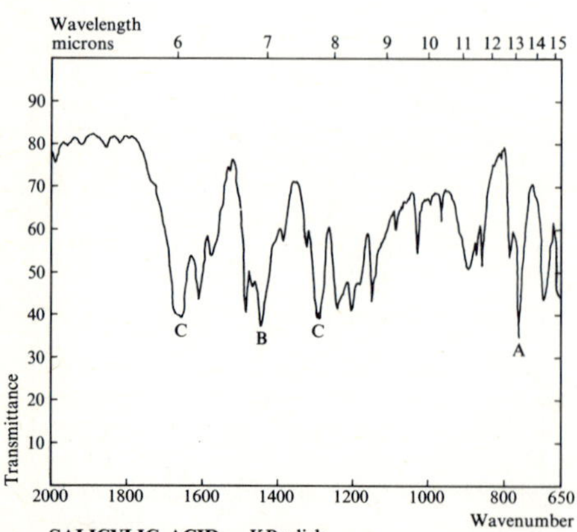

SALICYLIC ACID — KBr disk
A 758, B 1446, C 1288 or 1657

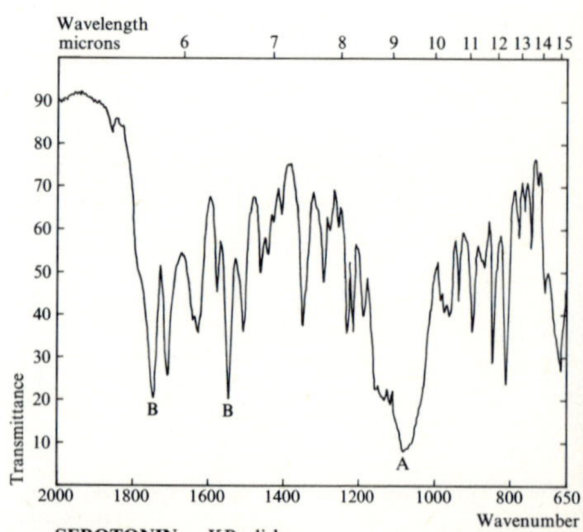

SEROTONIN — KBr disk
A 1084, B 1548 or 1747

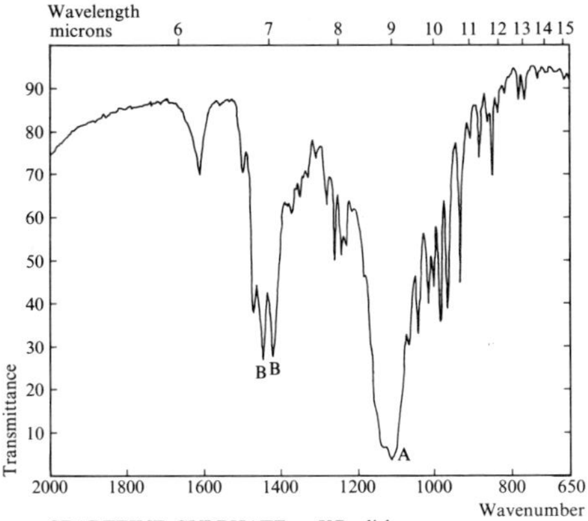

SPARTEINE SULPHATE — KBr disk
A 1118, B 1421 or 1447

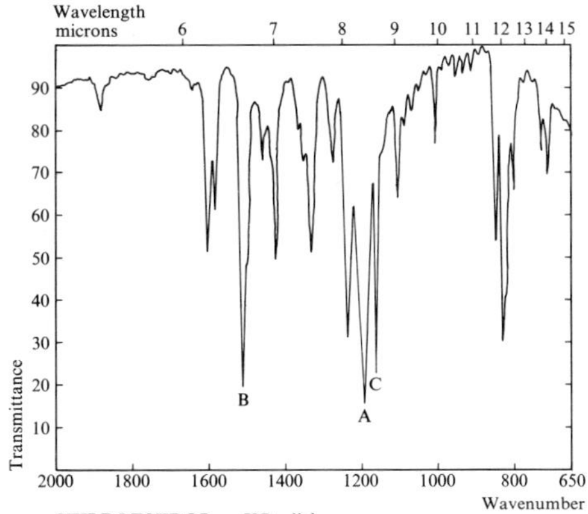

STILBOESTROL — KBr disk
A 1198, B 1515, C 1165

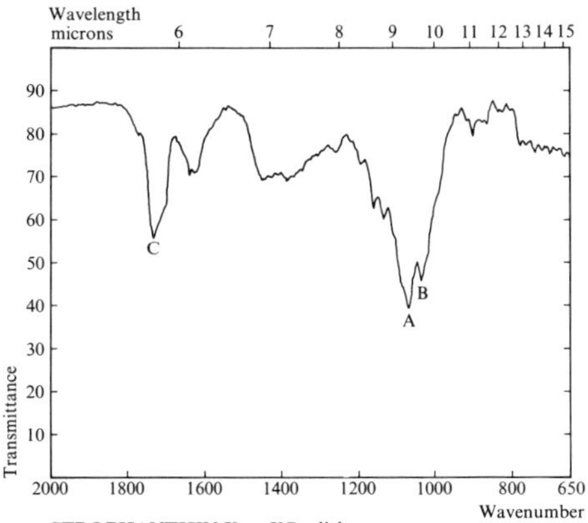

STROPHANTHIN-K — KBr disk
A 1071, B 1035, C 1733

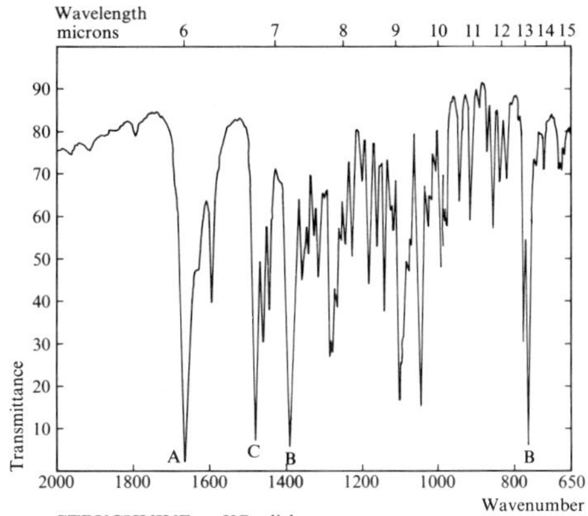

STRYCHNINE — KBr disk
A 1664, B 764 or 1392, C 1480

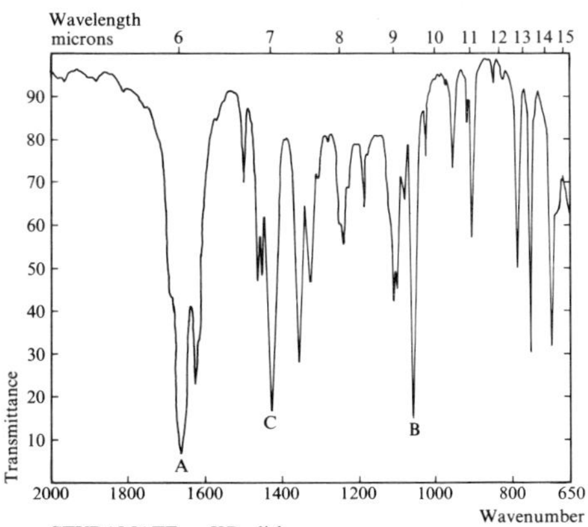

STYRAMATE — KBr disk
A 1660, B 1059, C 1425

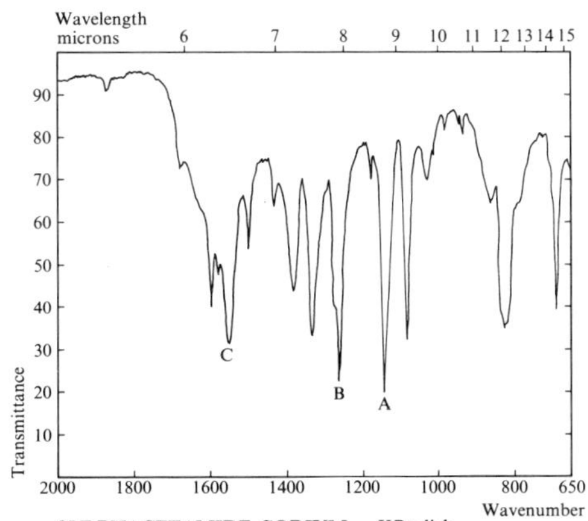

SULPHACETAMIDE SODIUM — KBr disk
A 1145, B 1264, C 1552

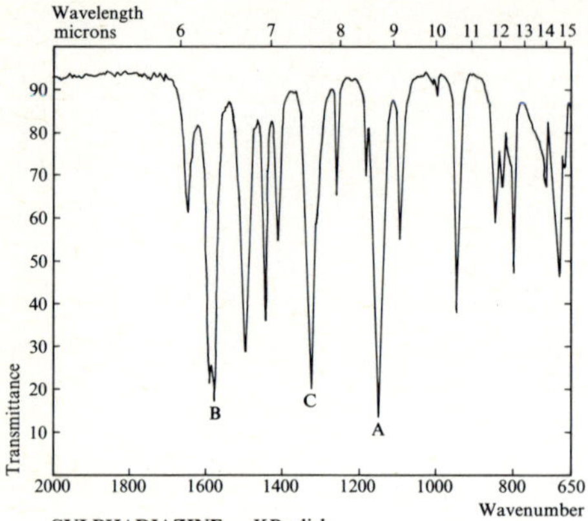

SULPHADIAZINE — KBr disk
A 1150, B 1577, C 1323

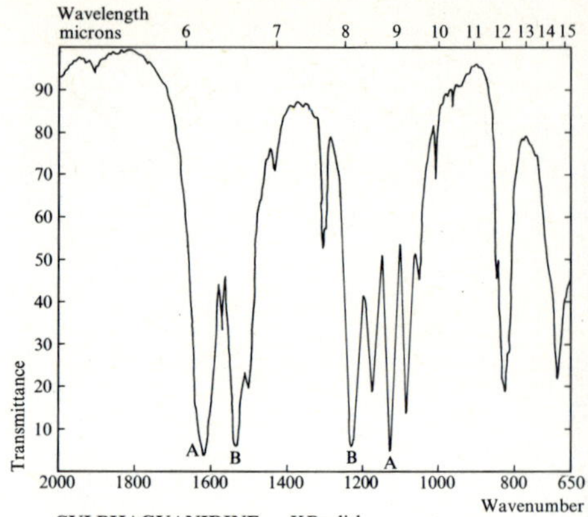

SULPHAGUANIDINE — KBr disk
A 1129 or 1620, B 1230 or 1537

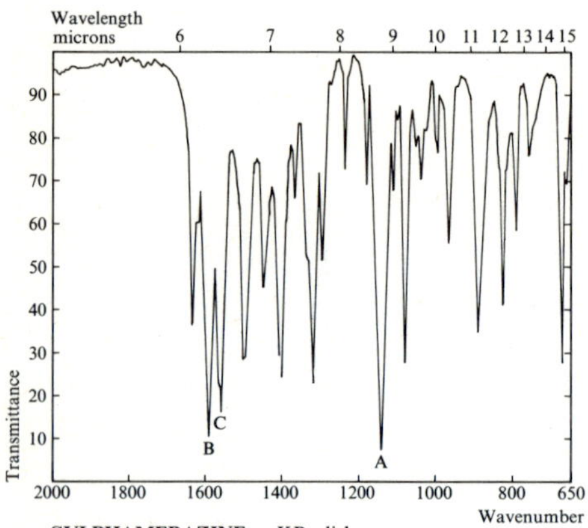

SULPHAMERAZINE — KBr disk
A 1143, B 1592, C 1559

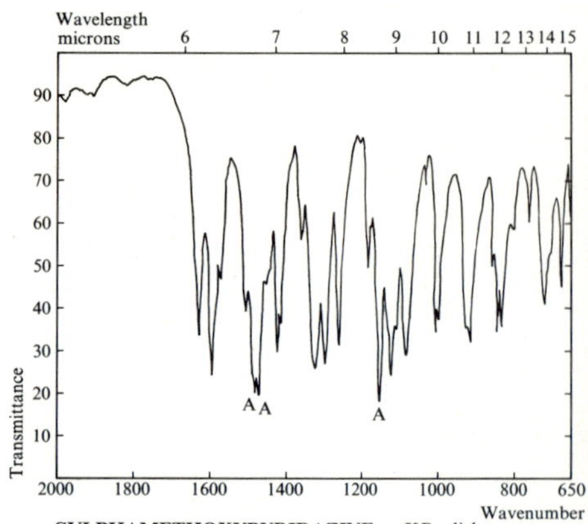

SULPHAMETHOXYPYRIDAZINE — KBr disk
A 1152 or 1475 or 1485

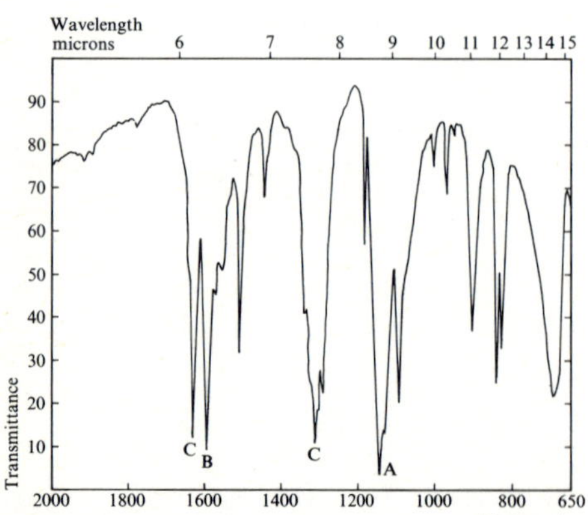

SULPHANILAMIDE — KBr disk
A 1144, B 1593, C 1312 or 1624

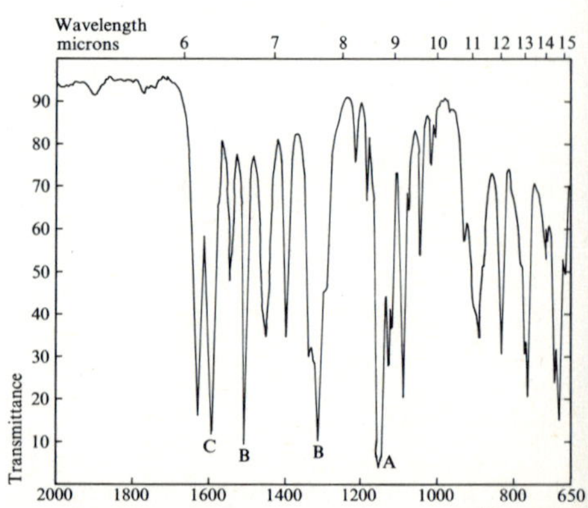

SULPHAPHENAZOLE — KBr disk
A 1148, B 1507 or 1313, C 1592

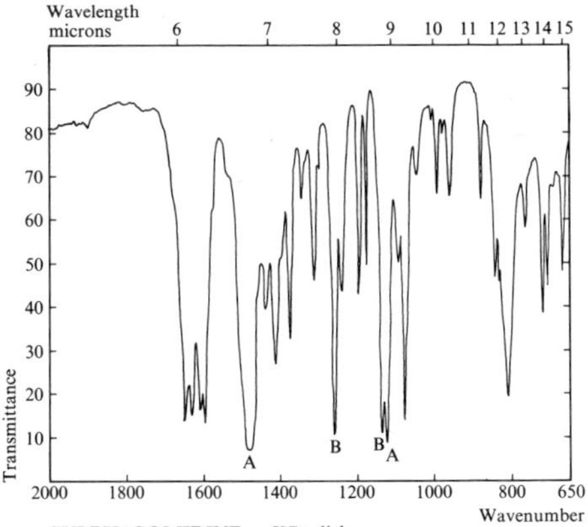

SULPHASOMIDINE — KBr disk
A 1125 or 1480, B 1138 or 1260

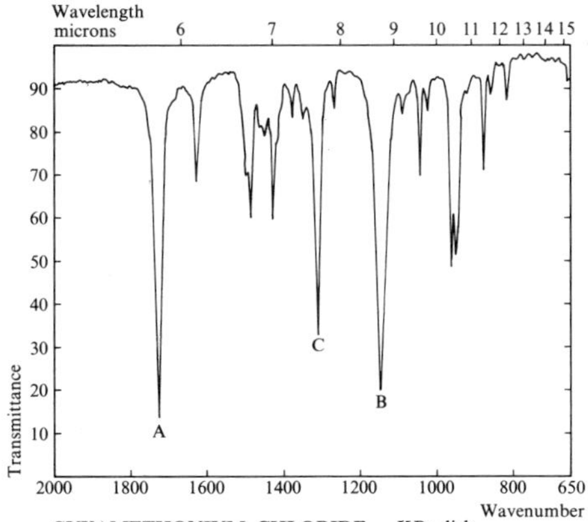

SUXAMETHONIUM CHLORIDE — KBr disk
A 1724, B 1148, C 1308

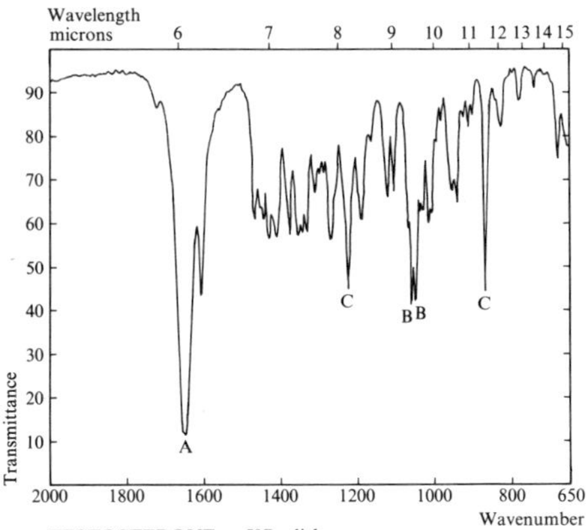

TESTOSTERONE — KBr disk
A 1650, B 1051 or 1061, C 872 or 1225

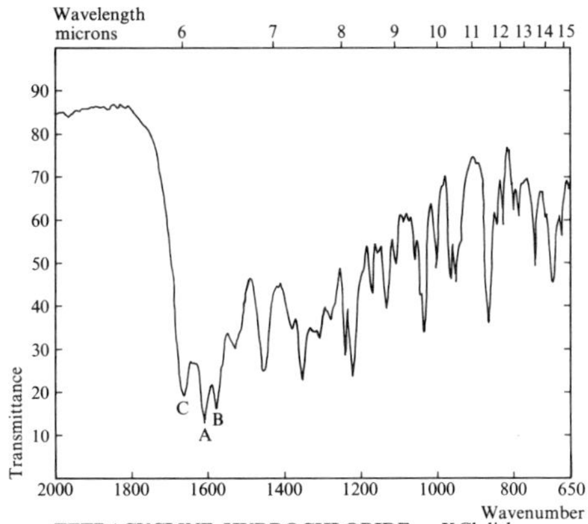

TETRACYCLINE HYDROCHLORIDE — KCl disk
A 1612, B 1580, C 1666

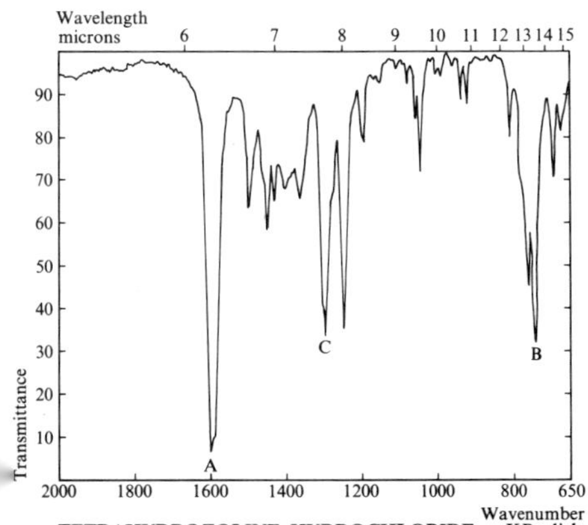

TETRAHYDROZOLINE HYDROCHLORIDE — KBr disk
A 1600, B 742, C 1293

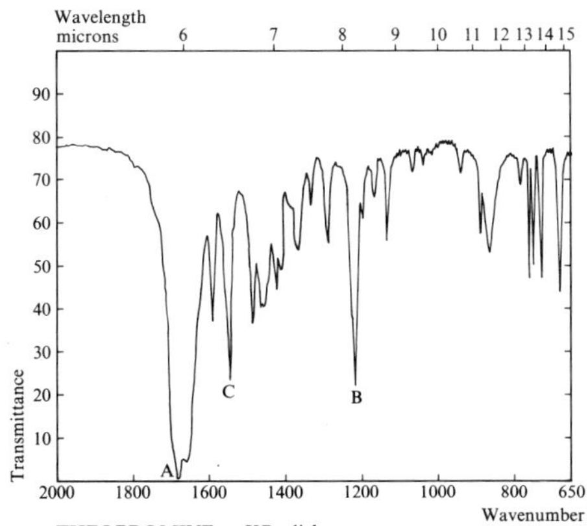

THEOBROMINE — KBr disk
A 1690, B 1221, C 1550

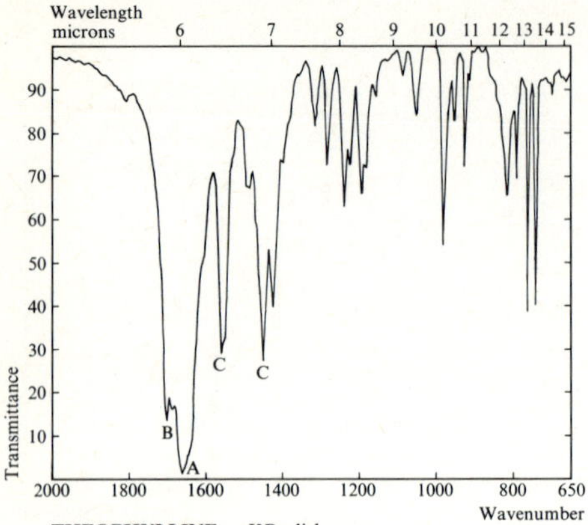

THEOPHYLLINE — KBr disk
A 1660, B 1700, C 1445 or 1560

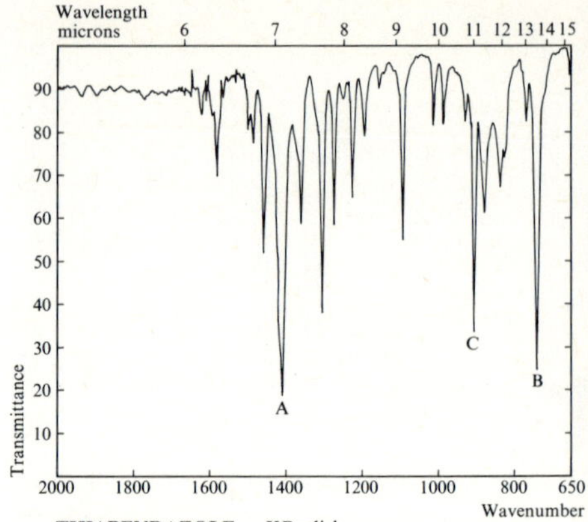

THIABENDAZOLE — KBr disk
A 1408, B 740, C 906

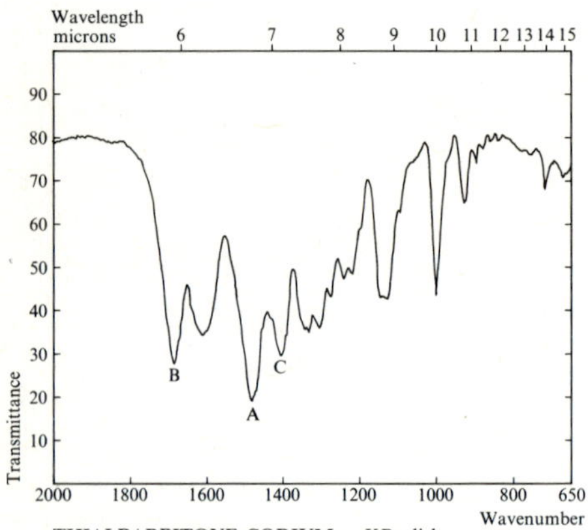

THIALBARBITONE SODIUM — KBr disk
A 1482, B 1685, C 1408

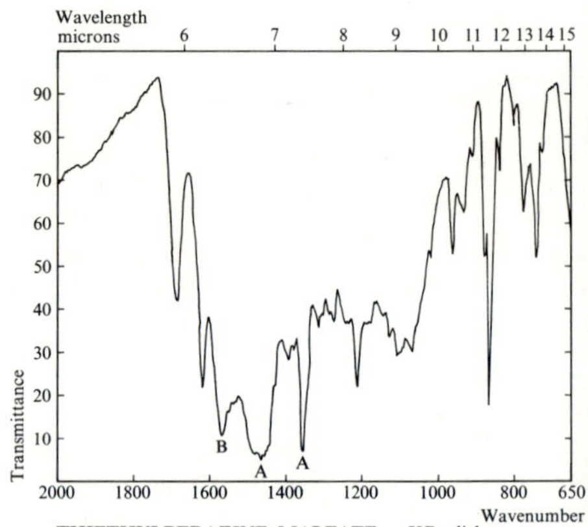

THIETHYLPERAZINE MALEATE — KBr disk
A 1356 or 1462, B 1568

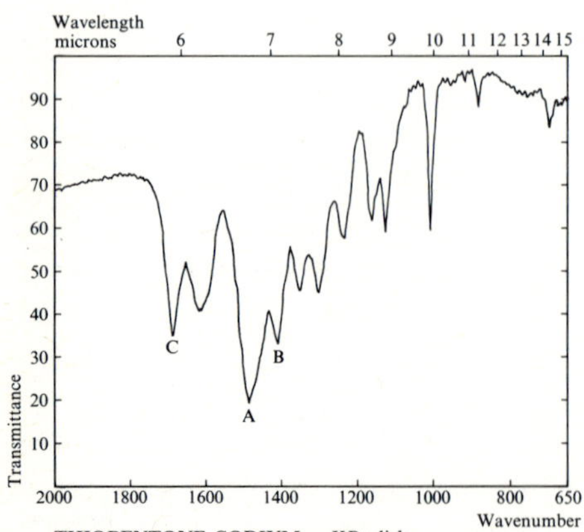

THIOPENTONE SODIUM — KBr disk
A 1484, B 1409, C 1688

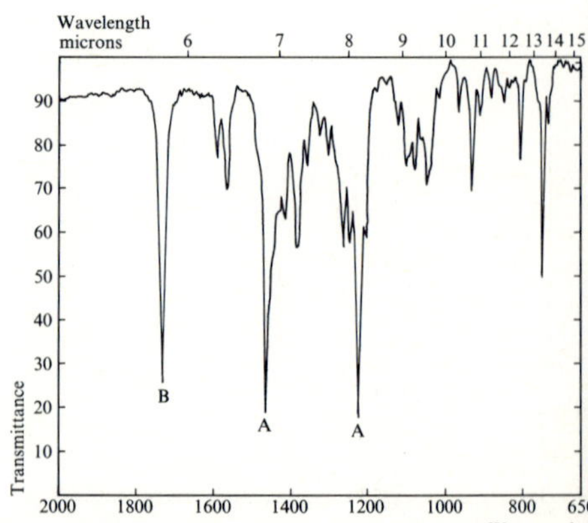

THIOPROPAZATE HYDROCHLORIDE — KBr disk
A 1222 or 1462, B 1728

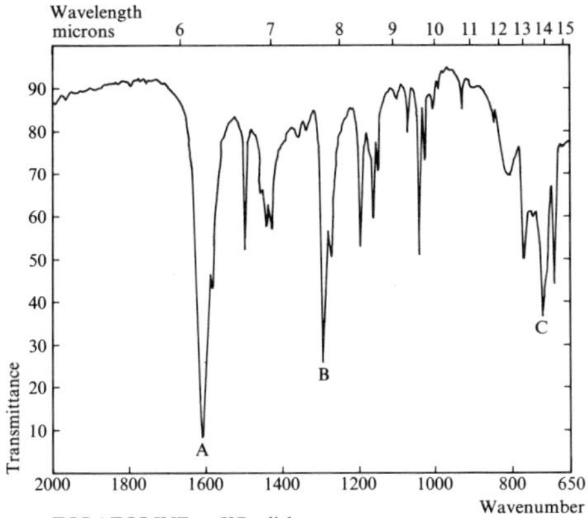

TOLAZOLINE — KBr disk
A 1608, B 1296, C 721

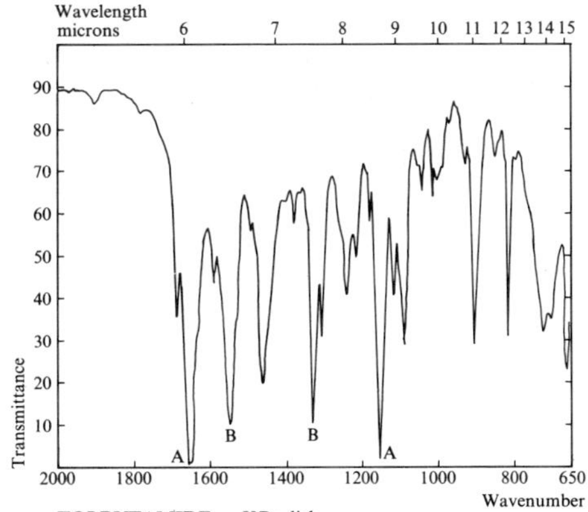

TOLBUTAMIDE — KBr disk
A 1157 or 1658, B 1336 or 1552

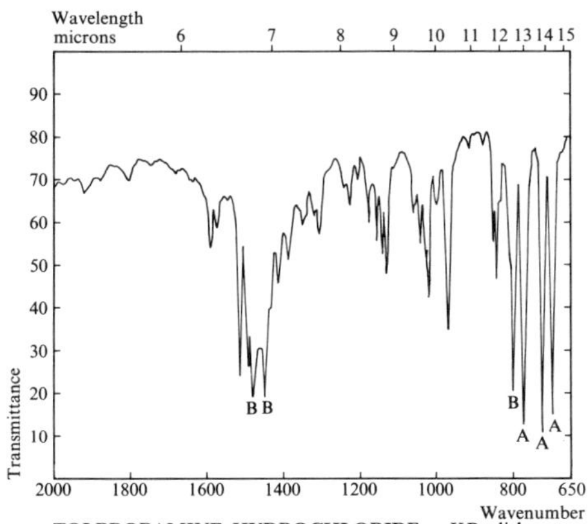

TOLPROPAMINE HYDROCHLORIDE — KBr disk
A 700 or 727 or 776, B 802 or 1450 or 1480

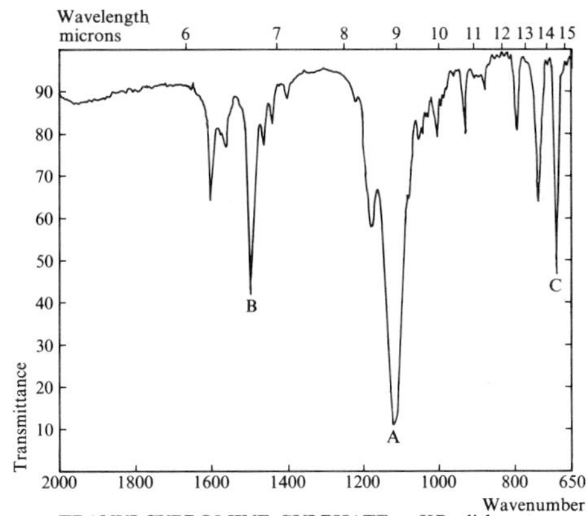

TRANYLCYPROMINE SULPHATE — KBr disk
A 1120, B 1497, C 690

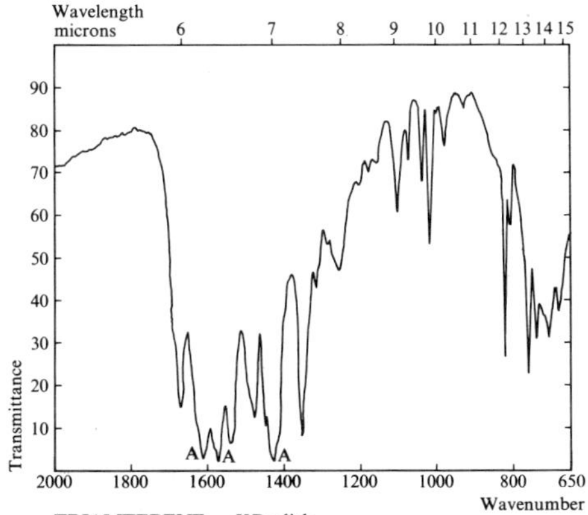

TRIAMTERENE — KBr disk
A 1428 or 1572 or 1612

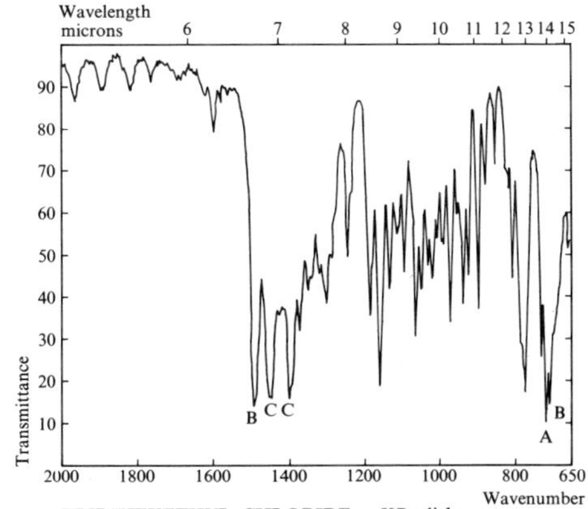

TRIDIHEXETHYL CHLORIDE — KBr disk
A 717, B 710 or 1492, C 1400 or 1450

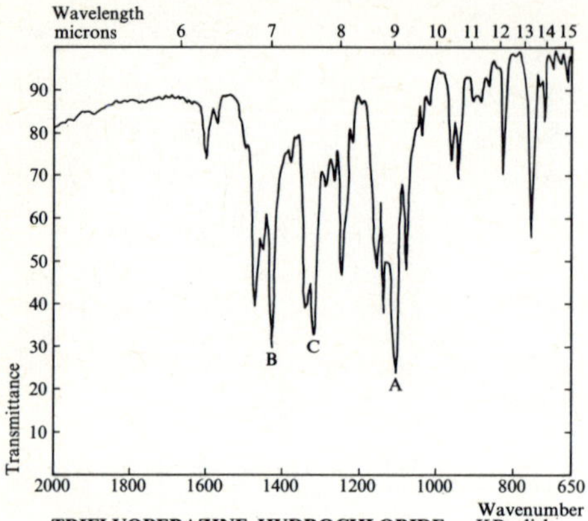

TRIFLUOPERAZINE HYDROCHLORIDE — KBr disk
A 1106, B 1426, C 1316

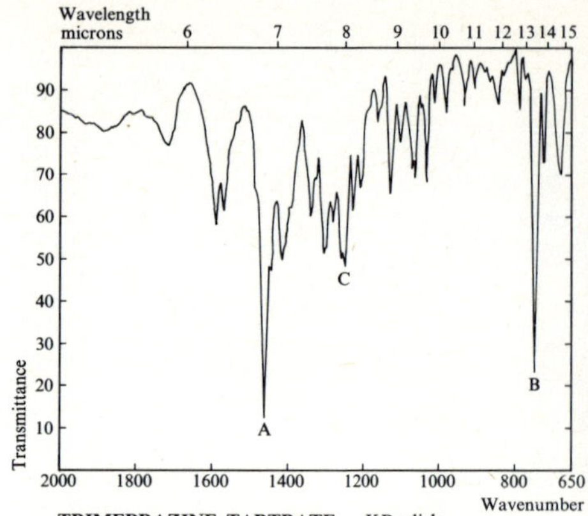

TRIMEPRAZINE TARTRATE — KBr disk
A 1461, B 748, C 1248

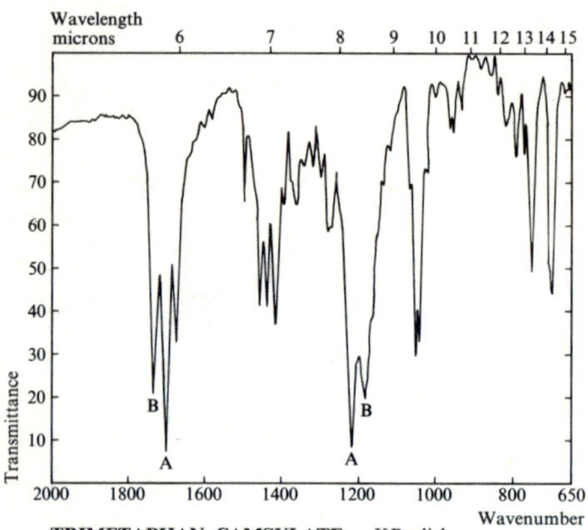

TRIMETAPHAN CAMSYLATE — KBr disk
A 1220 or 1701, B 1184 or 1735

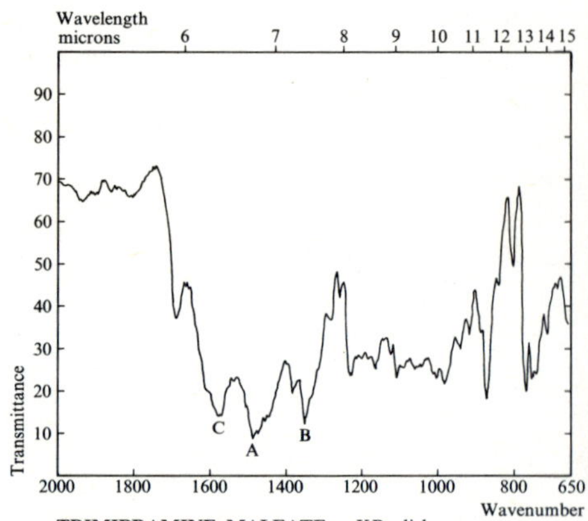

TRIMIPRAMINE MALEATE — KBr disk
A 1488, B 1351, C 1580

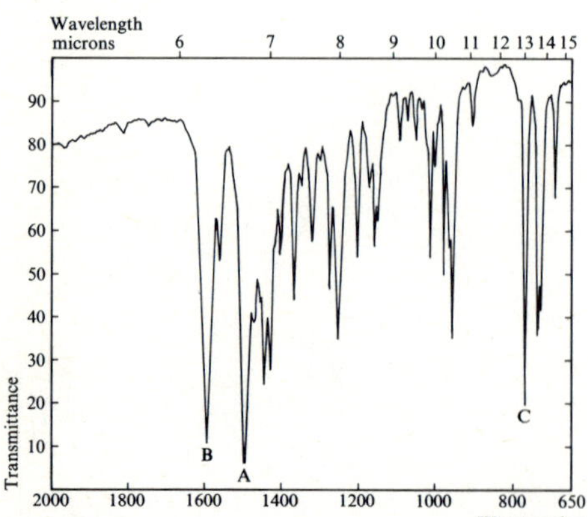

TRIPELENNAMINE HYDROCHLORIDE — KBr disk
A 1496, B 1592, C 770

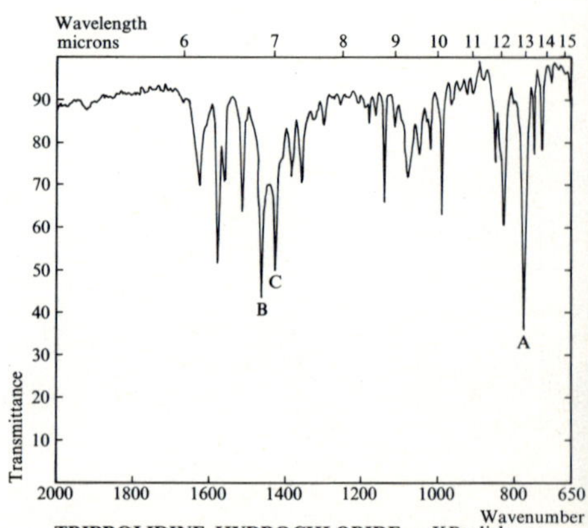

TRIPROLIDINE HYDROCHLORIDE — KBr disk
A 775, B 1461, C 1421

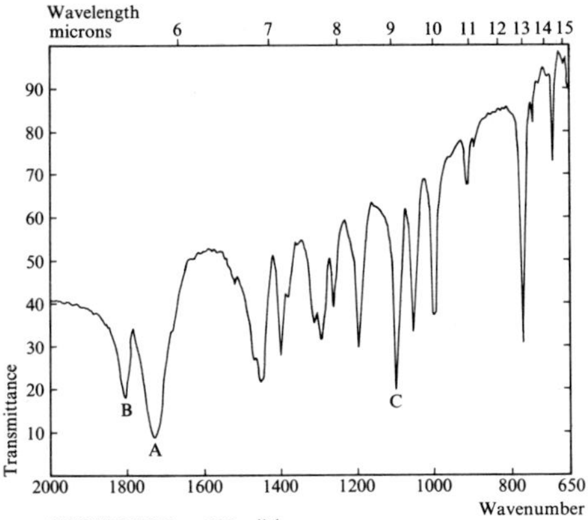

TROXIDONE — KBr disk
A 1730, B 1802, C 1098

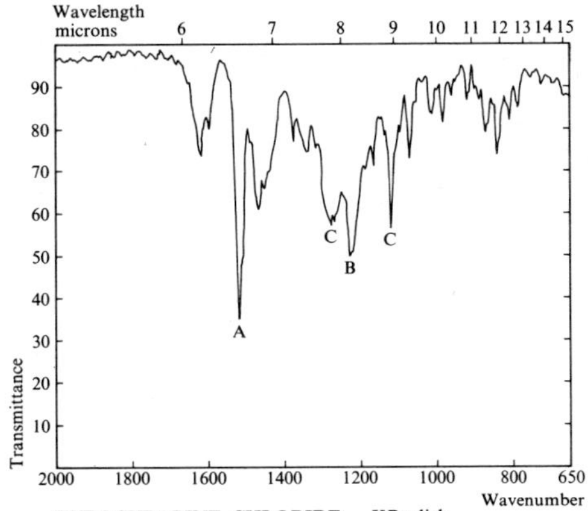

TUBOCURARINE CHLORIDE — KBr disk
A 1516, B 1228, C 1120 or 1280

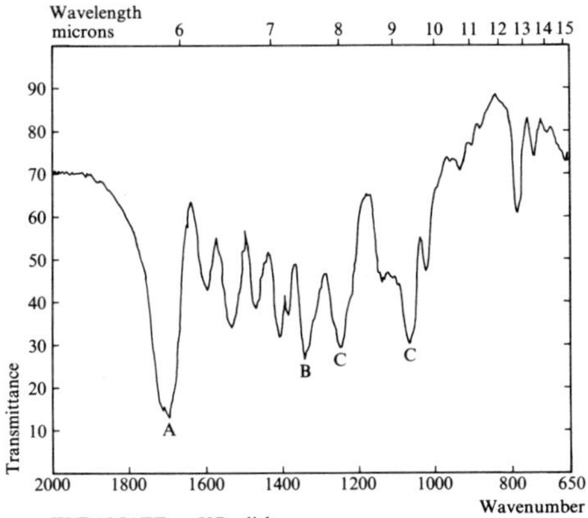

TYBAMATE — KBr disk
A 1695, B 1342, C 1065 or 1250

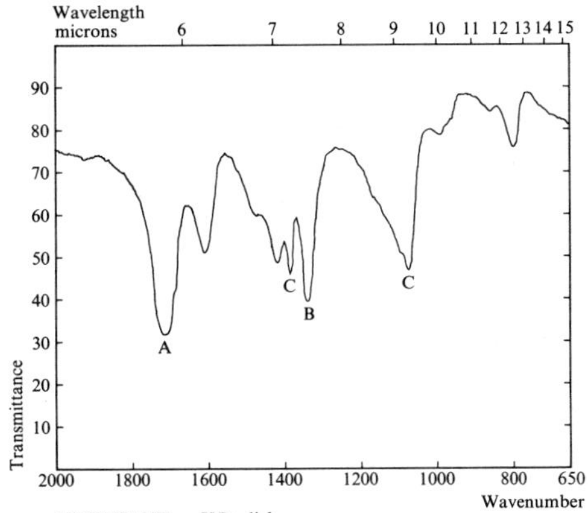

URETHANE — KBr disk
A 1713, B 1340, C 1075 or 1385

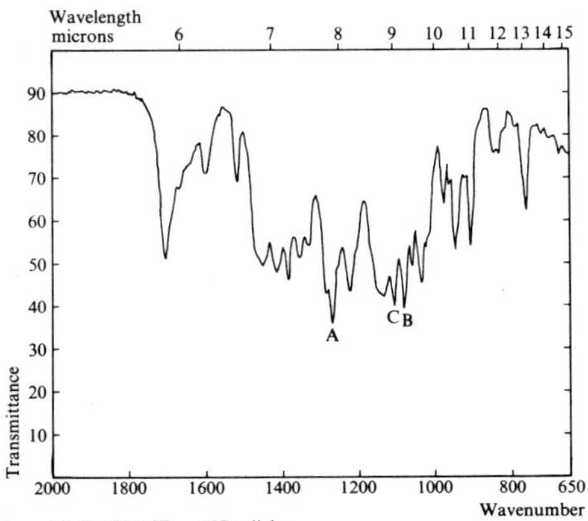

VERATRINE — KBr disk
A 1270, B 1085, C 1111

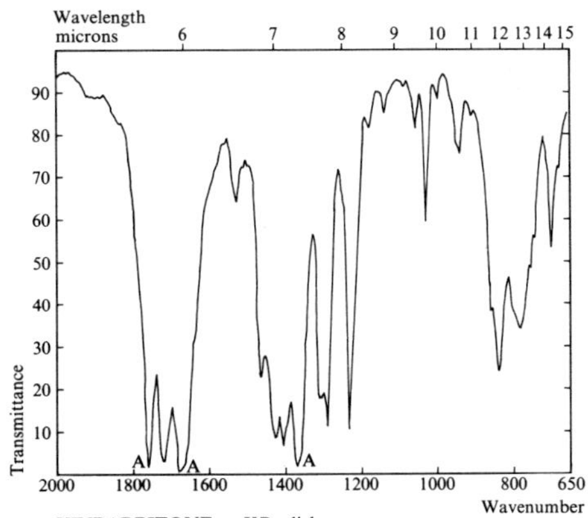

VINBARBITONE — KBr disk
A 1370 or 1675 or 1760

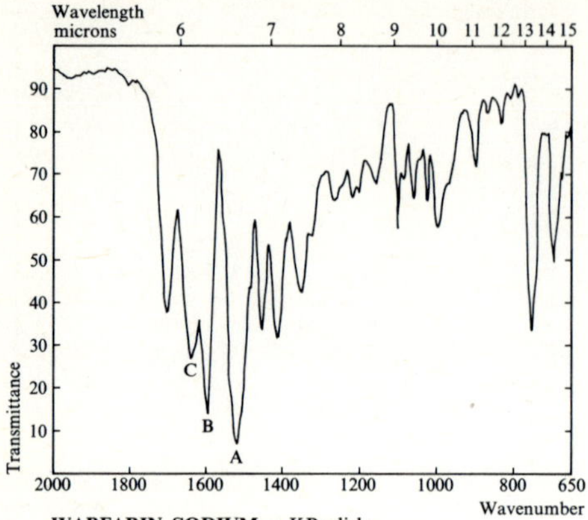

WARFARIN SODIUM — KBr disk
A 1517, B 1599, C 1640

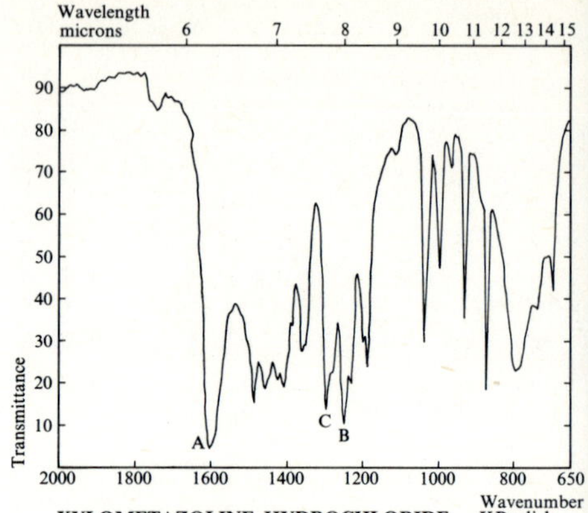

XYLOMETAZOLINE HYDROCHLORIDE — KBr disk
A 1602, B 1253, C 1298

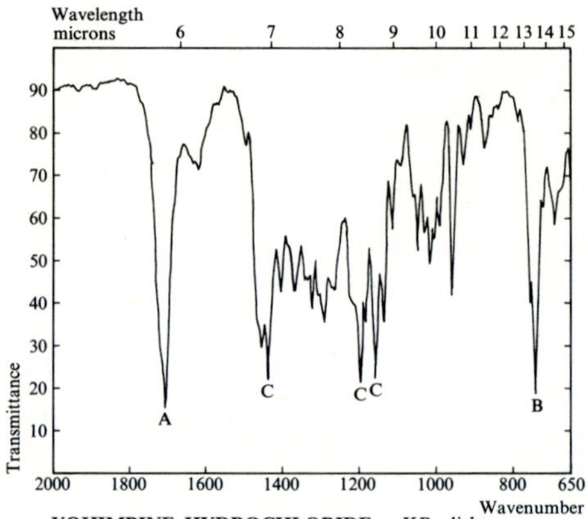

YOHIMBINE HYDROCHLORIDE — KBr disk
A 1705, B 741, C 1160 or 1197 or 1436

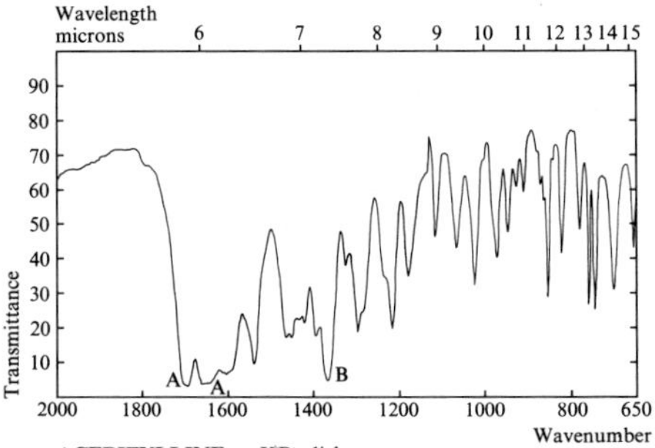

ACEPIFYLLINE — KBr disk
A 1660 or 1700, B 1370

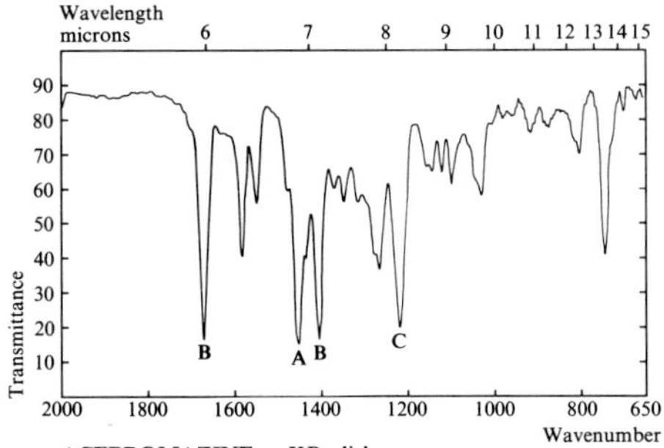

ACEPROMAZINE — KBr disk
A 1455, B 1410 or 1675, C 1220

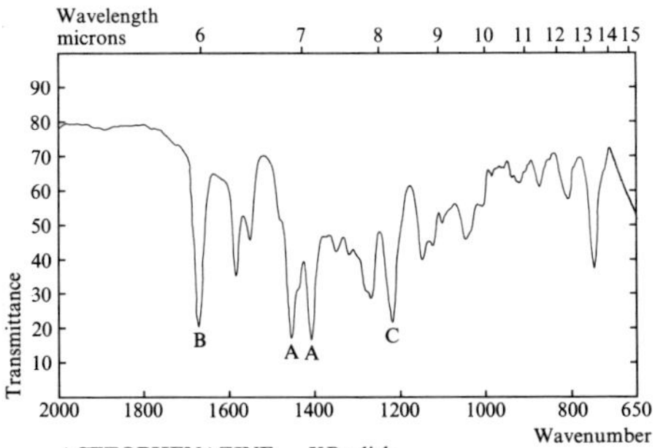

ACETOPHENAZINE — KBr disk
A 1408 or 1455, B 1670, C 1220

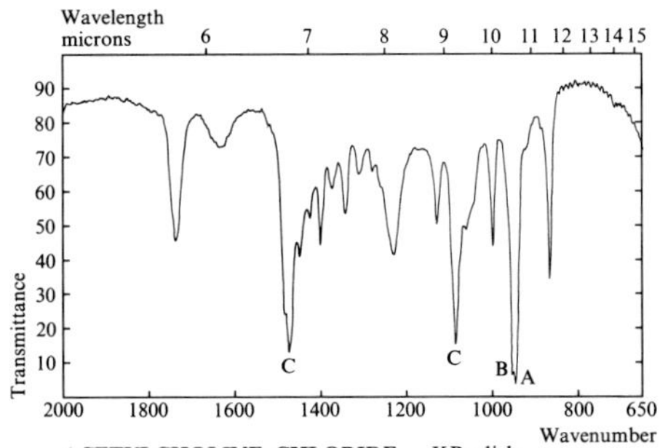

ACETYLCHOLINE CHLORIDE — KBr disk
A 950, B 955, C 1088 or 1475

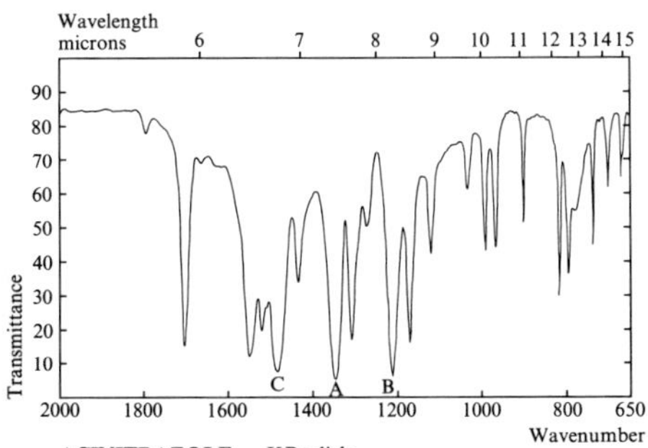

ACINITRAZOLE — KBr disk
A 1345, B 1210, C 1485

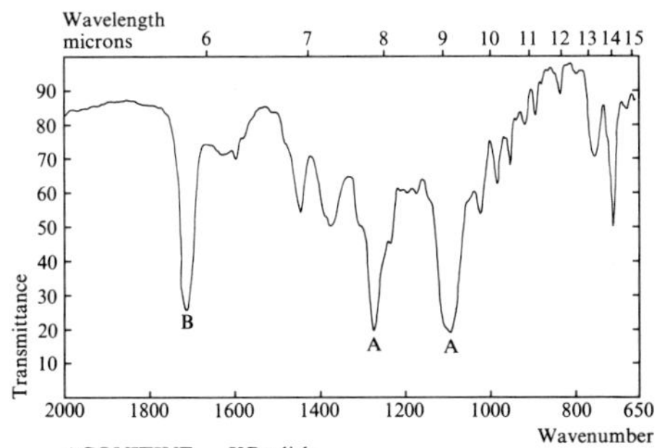

ACONITINE — KBr disk
A 1092 or 1273, B 1713

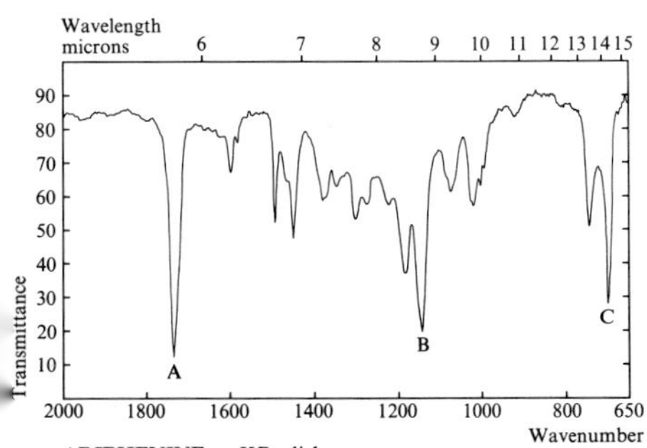

ADIPHENINE — KBr disk
A 1736, B 1145, C 700

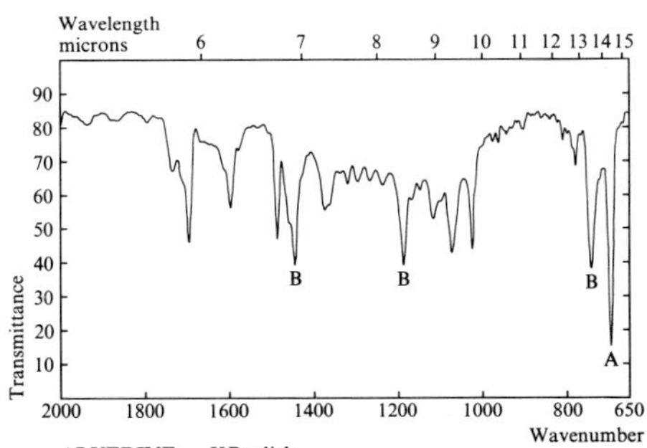

ALVERINE — KBr disk
A 695, B 742 or 1188 or 1448

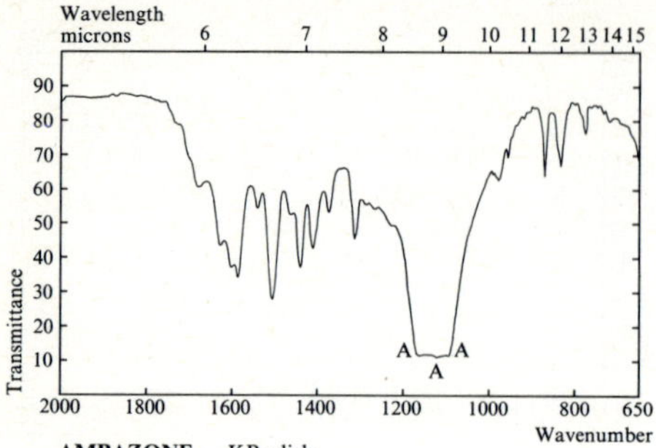

AMBAZONE — KBr disk
A 1090 or 1120 or 1160

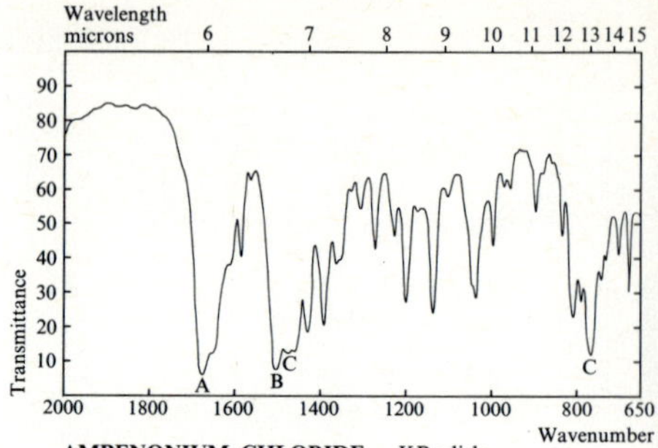

AMBENONIUM CHLORIDE — KBr disk
A 1675, B 1505, C 767 or 1465

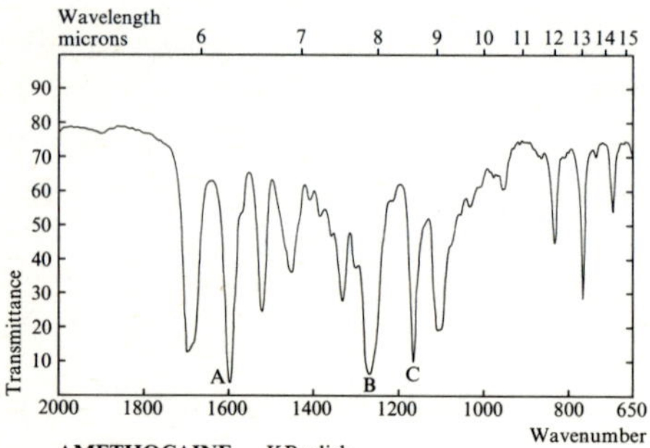

AMETHOCAINE — KBr disk
A 1598, B 1270, C 1166

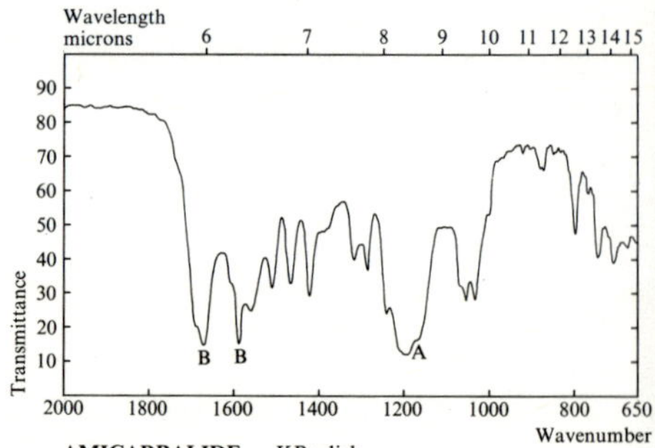

AMICARBALIDE — KBr disk
A 1195, B 1590 or 1672

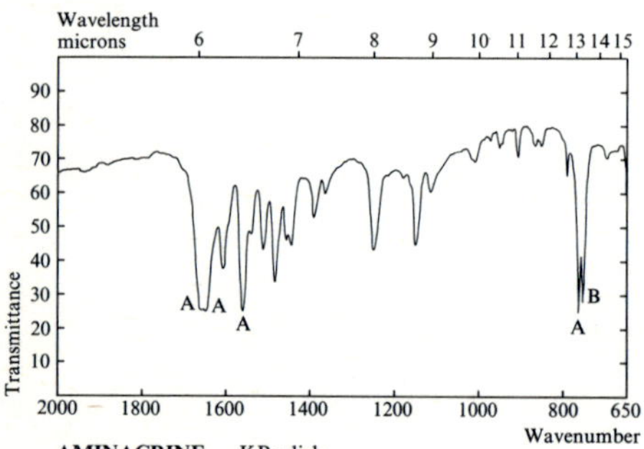

AMINACRINE — KBr disk
A 760 or 1556 or 1645 or 1655, B 750

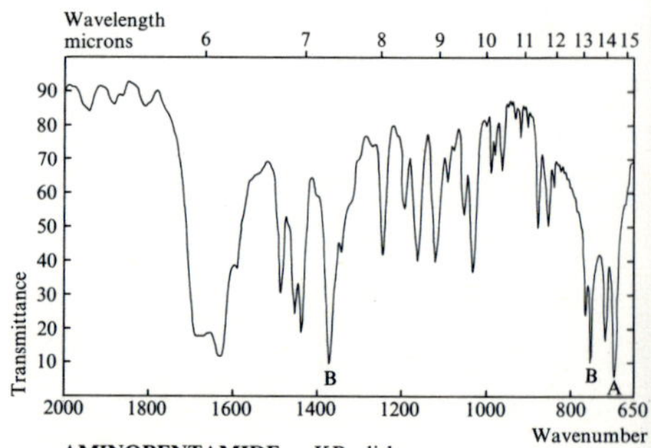

AMINOPENTAMIDE — KBr disk
A 695, B 750 or 1370

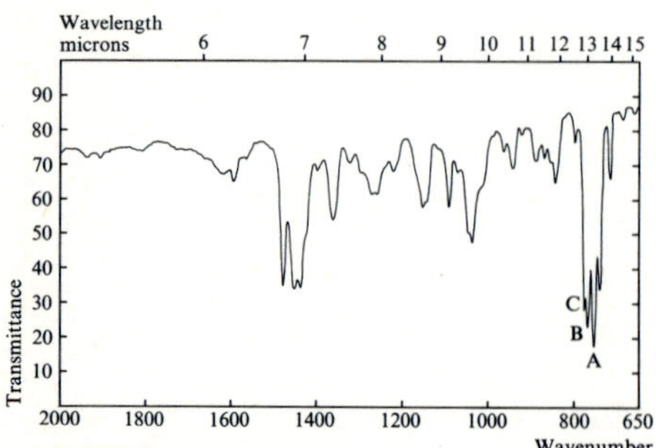

AMITRIPTYLINE — KBr disk
A 752, B 765, C 775

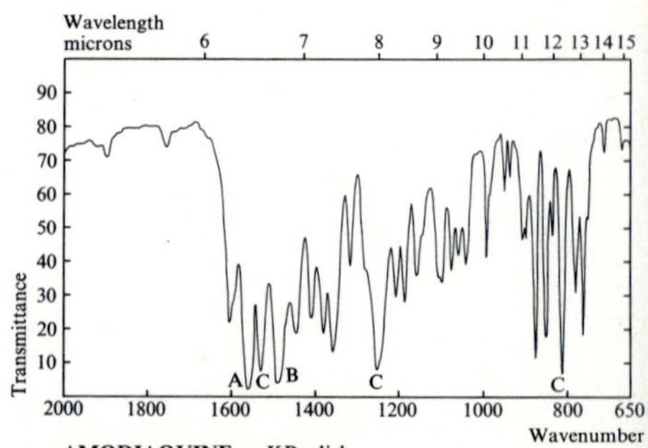

AMODIAQUINE — KBr disk
A 1565, B 1480, C 815 or 1255 or 1535

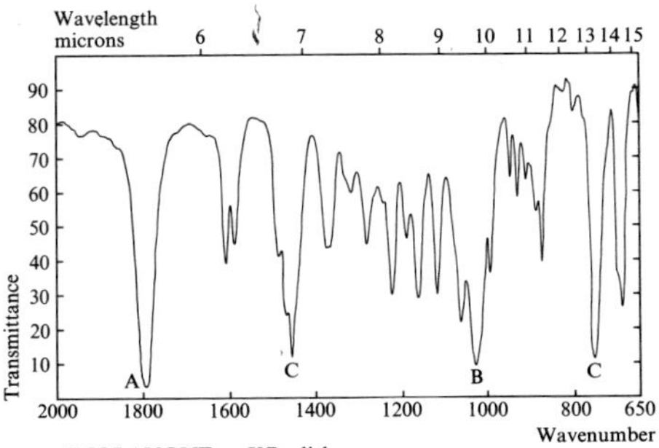

AMOLANONE — KBr disk
A 1795, B 1025, C 750 or 1455

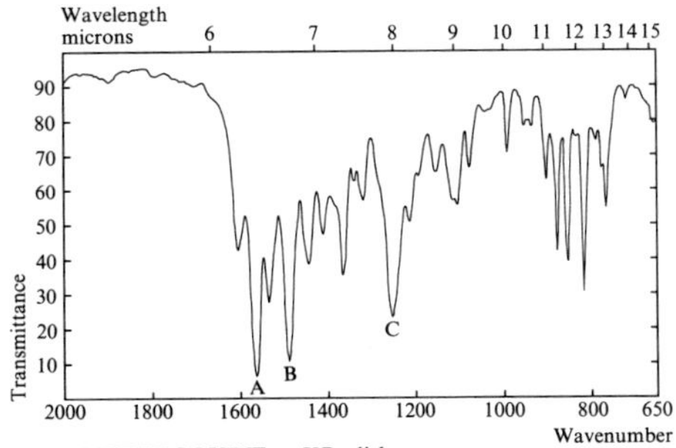

AMOPYROQUINE — KBr disk
A 1563, B 1490, C 1252

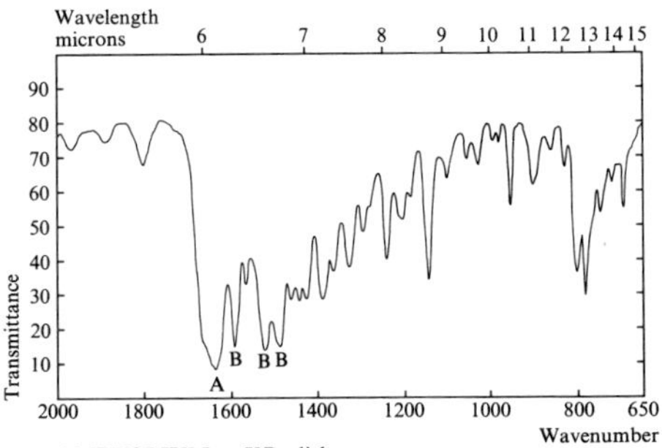

AMPROLIUM — KBr disk
A 1638, B 1488 or 1522 or 1593

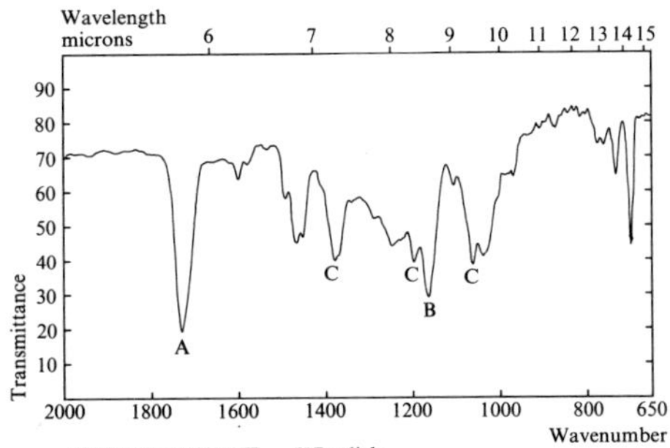

AMPROTROPINE — KBr disk
A 1730, B 1162, C 1060 or 1195 or 1378

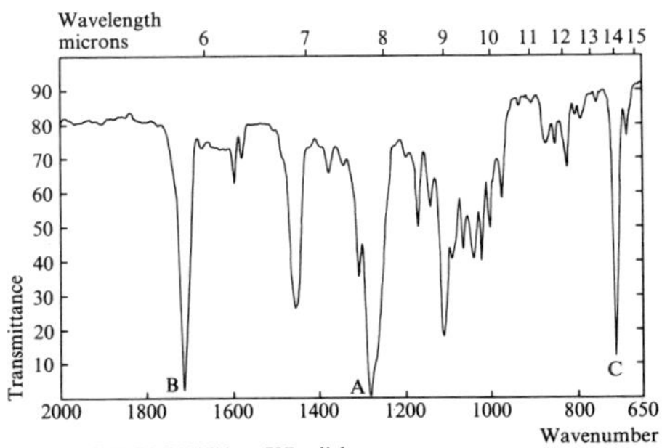

AMYDRICAINE — KBr disk
A 1282, B 1715, C 710

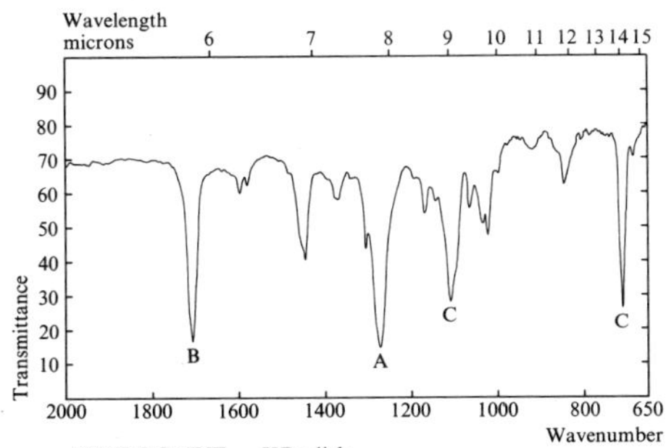

AMYLOCAINE — KBr disk
A 1275, B 1710, C 710 or 1110

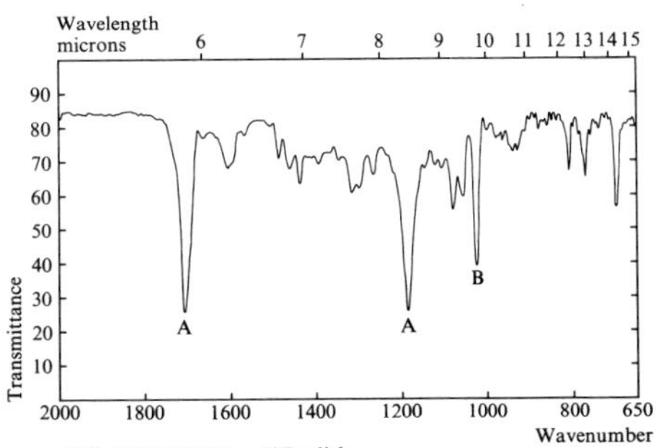

APOATROPINE — KBr disk
A 1190 or 1710, B 1025

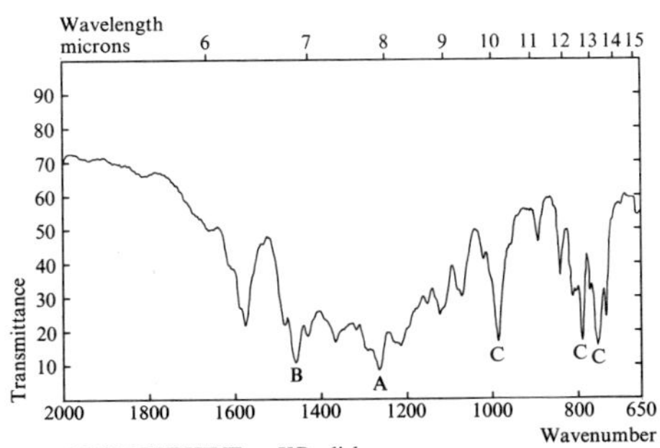

APOMORPHINE — KBr disk
A 1265, B 1460, C 752 or 790 or 985

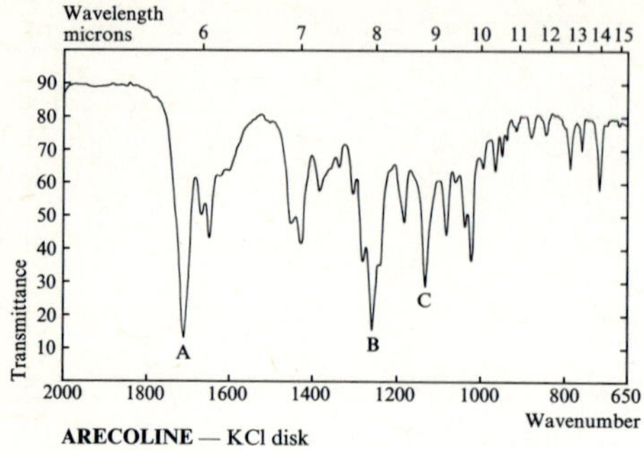

ARECOLINE — KCl disk
A 1712, B 1262, C 1135

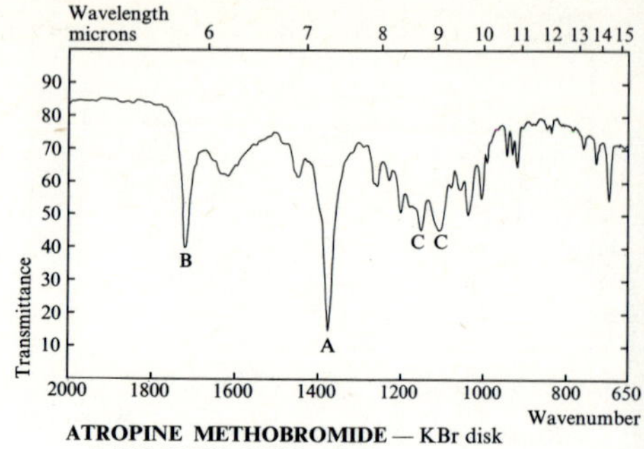

ATROPINE METHOBROMIDE — KBr disk
A 1377, B 1718, C 1104 or 1150

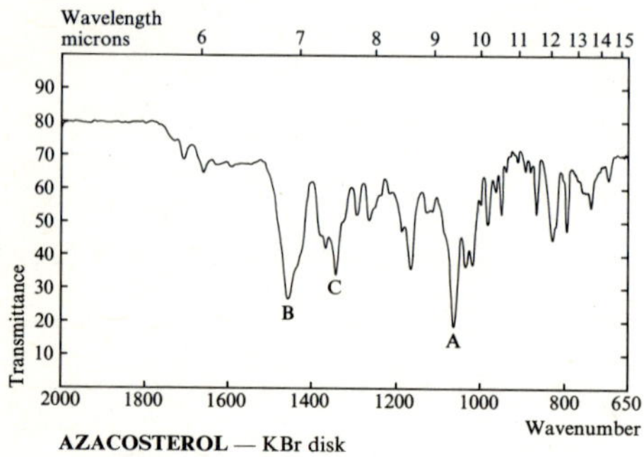

AZACOSTEROL — KBr disk
A 1065, B 1455, C 1345

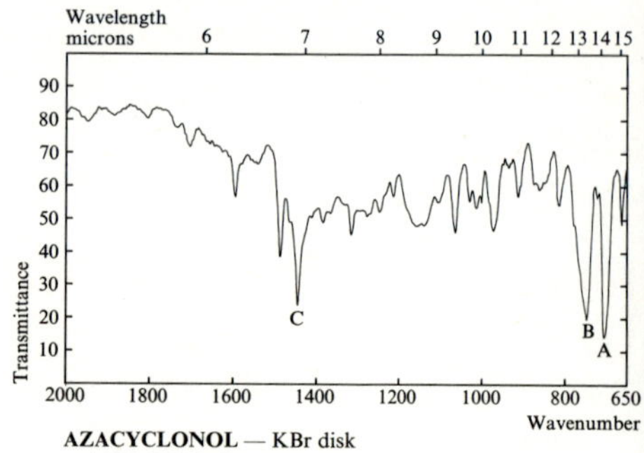

AZACYCLONOL — KBr disk
A 700, B 745, C 1445

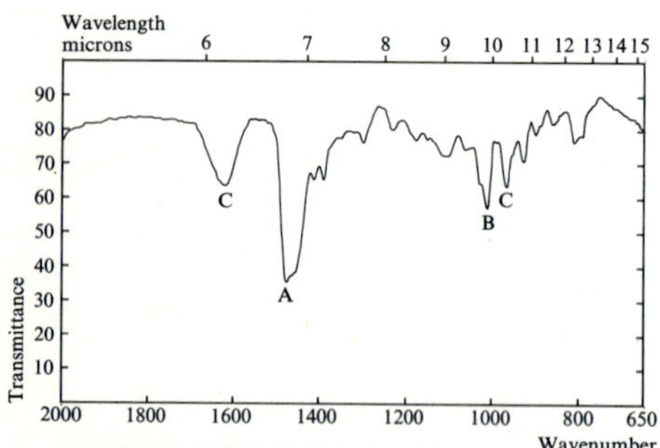

AZAMETHONIUM BROMIDE — KBr disk
A 1477, B 1014, C 968 or 1620

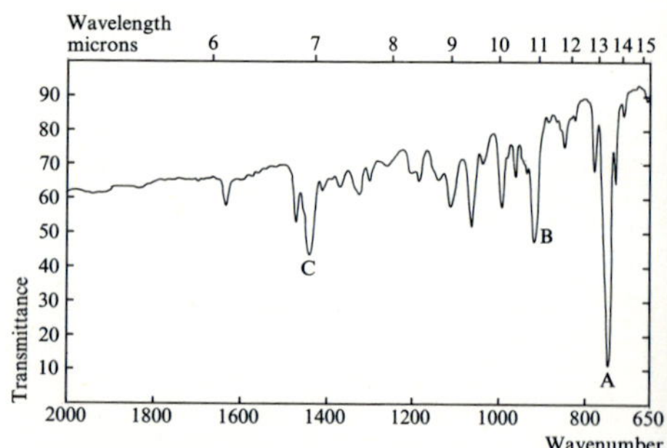

AZAPETINE — KBr disk
A 748, B 918, C 1440

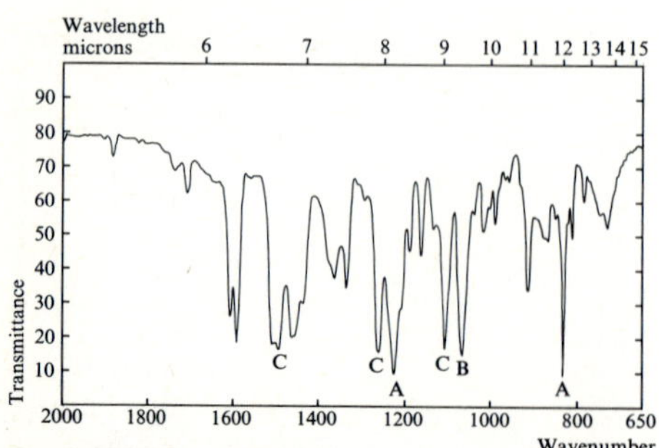

BAMETHAN — KBr disk
A 832 or 1228, B 1066, C 1108 or 1264 or 1494

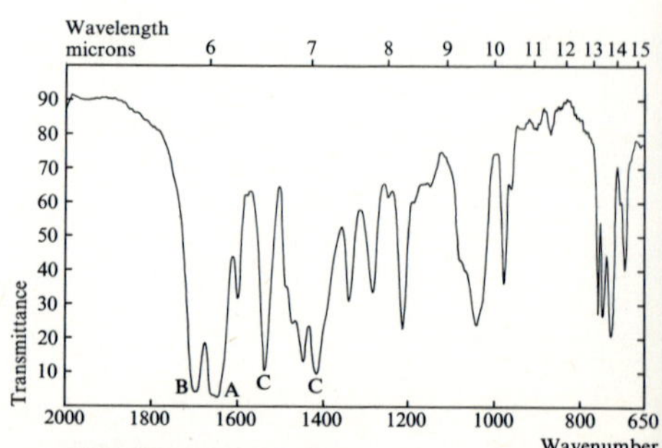

BAMIFYLLINE — KBr disk
A 1650, B 1698, C 1416 or 1538

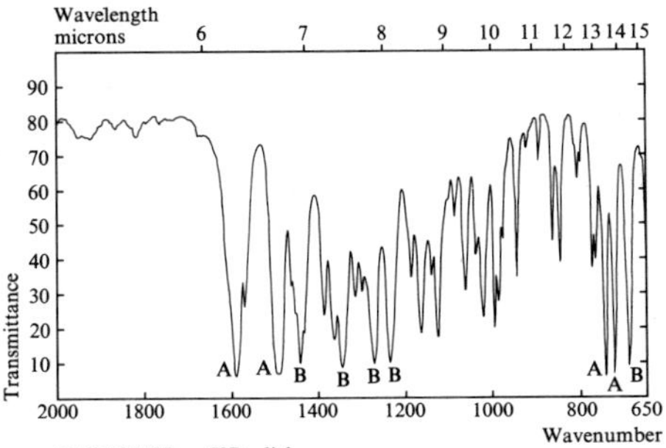

BAMIPINE — KBr disk
A 725 or 745 or 1495 or 1593,
B 690 or 1238 or 1275 or 1347 or 1445

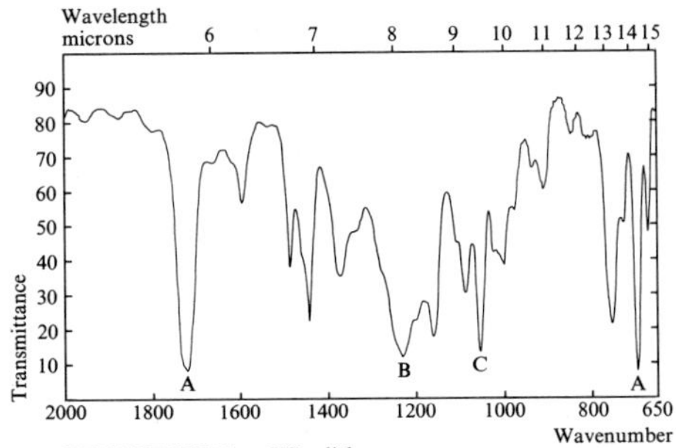

BENACTYZINE — KBr disk
A 795 or 1723, B 1231, C 1054

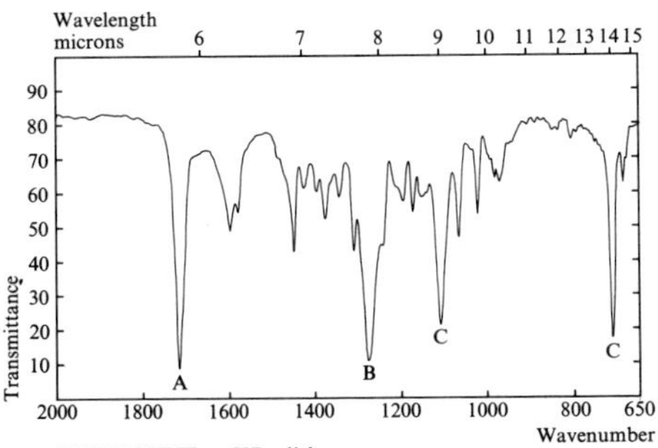

BENZAMINE — KBr disk
A 1714, B 1276, C 711 or 1108

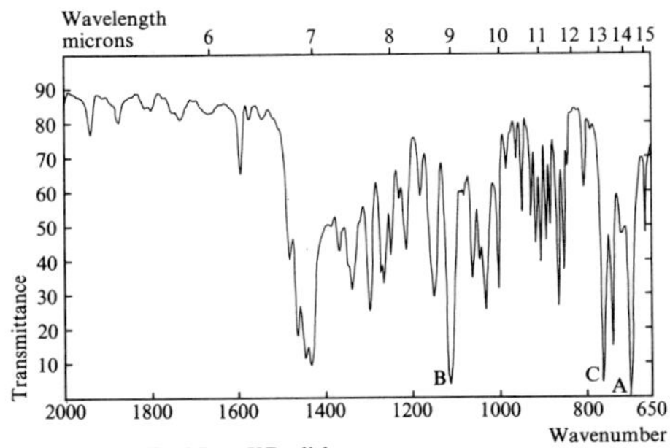

BENZHEXOL — KBr disk
A 696, B 1112, C 760

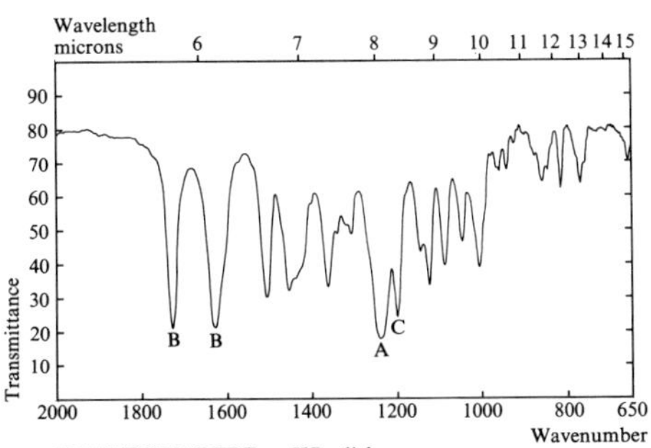

BENZQUINAMIDE — KBr disk
A 1244, B 1633 or 1733, C 1204

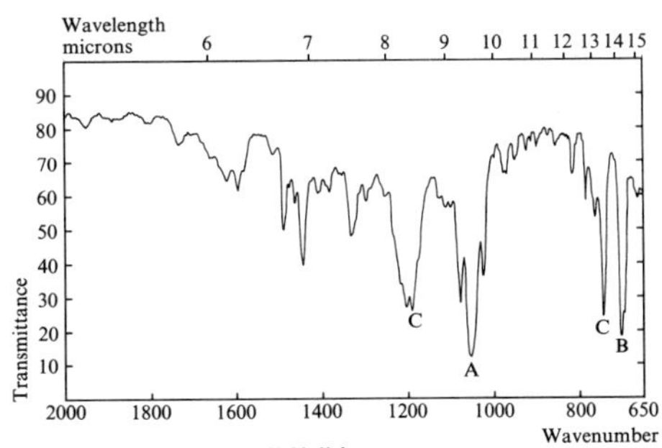

BENZTROPINE — KCl disk
A 1054, B 700, C 742 or 1191

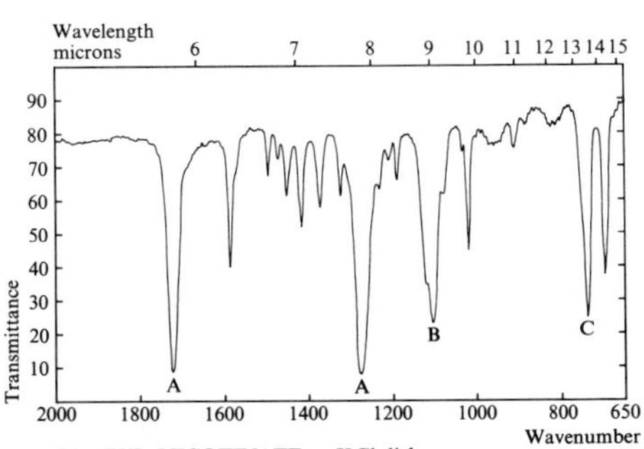

BENZYL NICOTINATE — KCl disk
A 1278 or 1724, B 1108, C 740

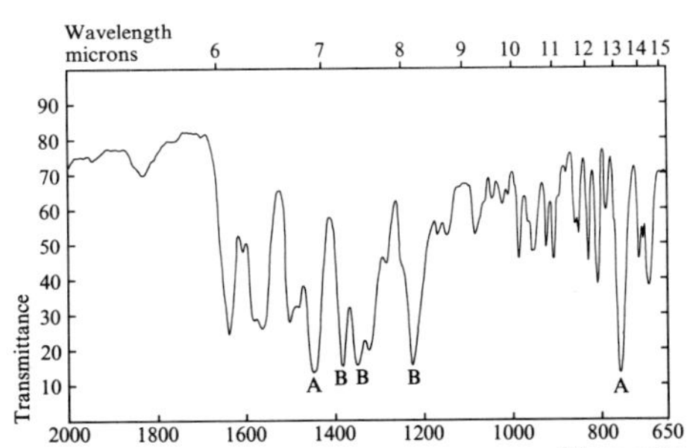

BEPHENIUM HYDROXYNAPHTHOATE — KBr disk
A 755 or 1445, B 1225 or 1348 or 1382

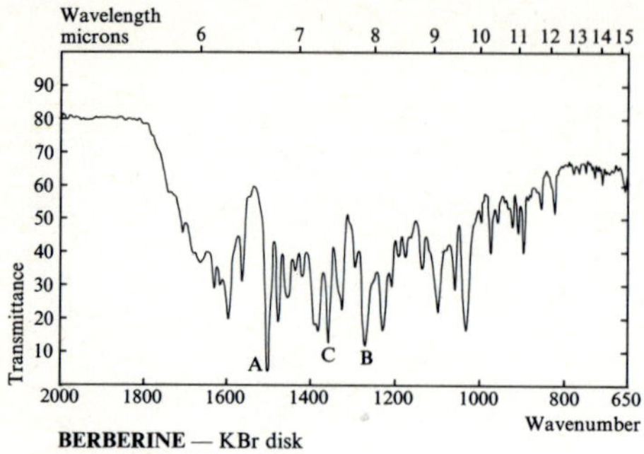

BERBERINE — KBr disk
A 1505, B 1271, C 1360

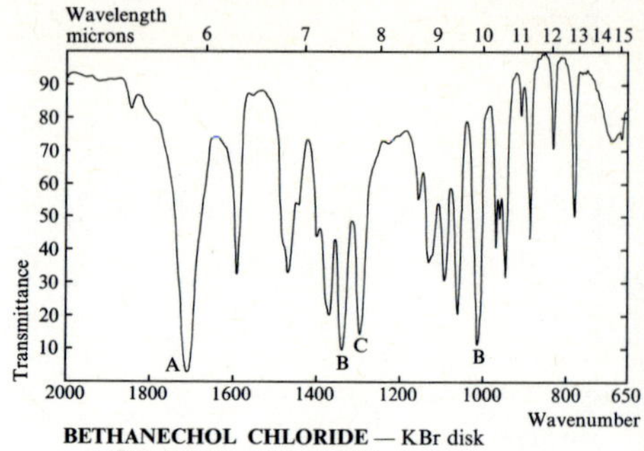

BETHANECHOL CHLORIDE — KBr disk
A 1712, B 1014 or 1340, C 1300

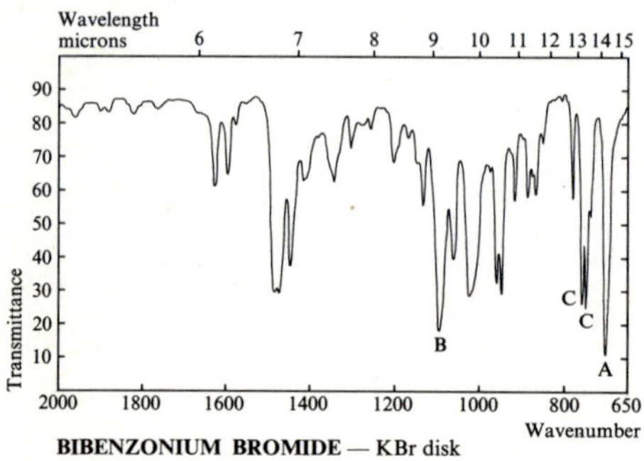

BIBENZONIUM BROMIDE — KBr disk
A 705, B 1095, C 749 or 759

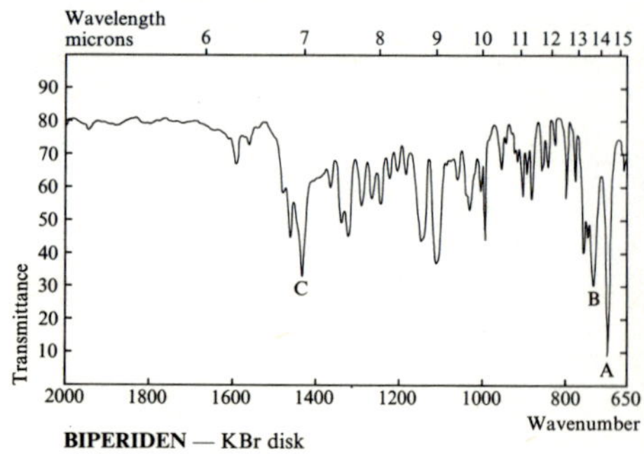

BIPERIDEN — KBr disk
A 697, B 733, C 1436

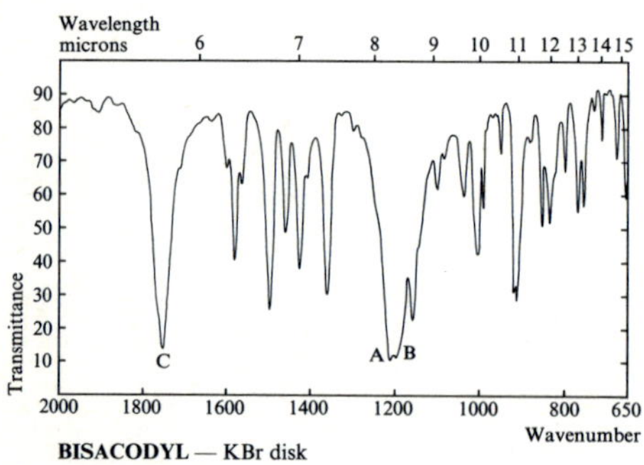

BISACODYL — KBr disk
A 1212, B 1198, C 1754

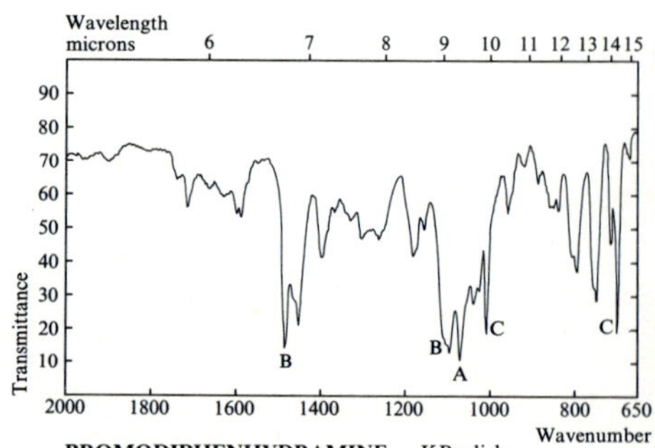

BROMODIPHENHYDRAMINE — KBr disk
A 1067, B 1094 or 1483, C 696 or 1007

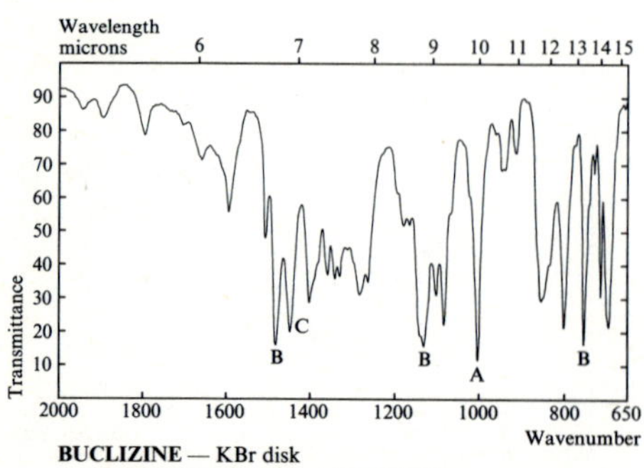

BUCLIZINE — KBr disk
A 1002, B 754 or 1131 or 1482, C 1447

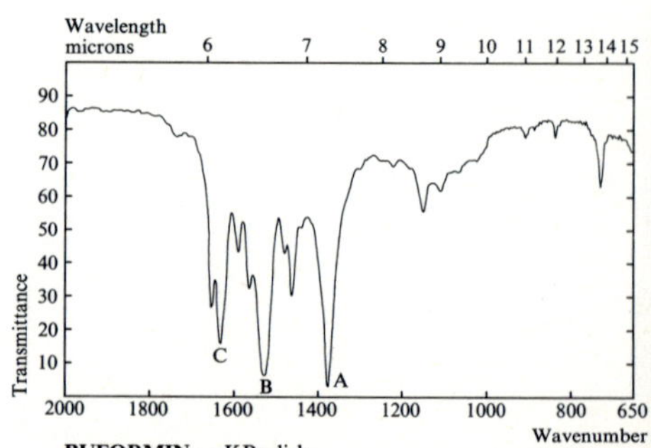

BUFORMIN — KBr disk
A 1378, B 1530, C 1634

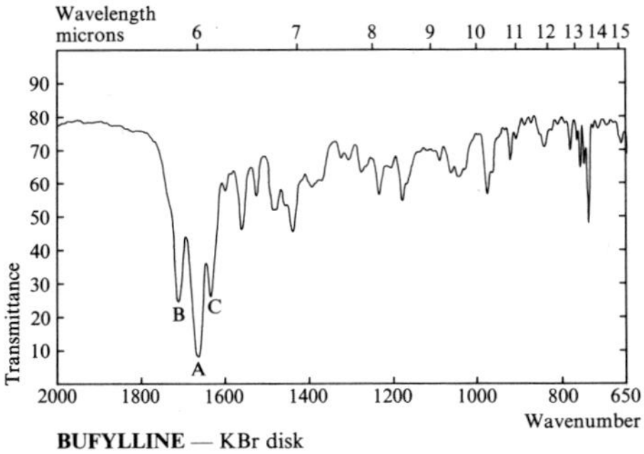

BUFYLLINE — KBr disk
A 1665, B 1712, C 1636

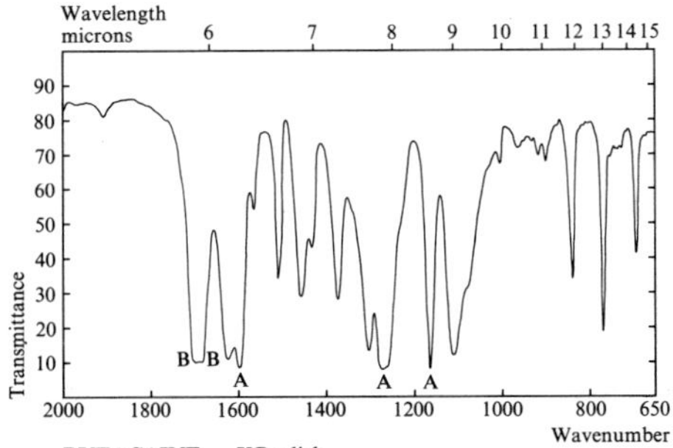

BUTACAINE — KBr disk
A 1165 or 1275 or 1598, B 1685 or 1702

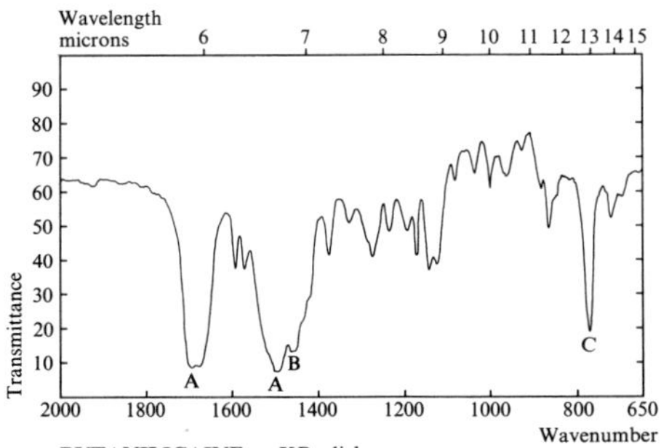

BUTANILICAINE — KBr disk
A 1495 or 1694, B 1460, C 770

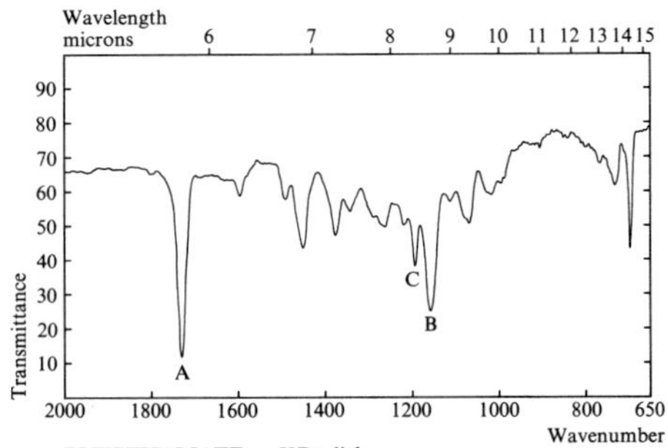

BUTETHAMATE — KBr disk
A 1730, B 1158, C 1194

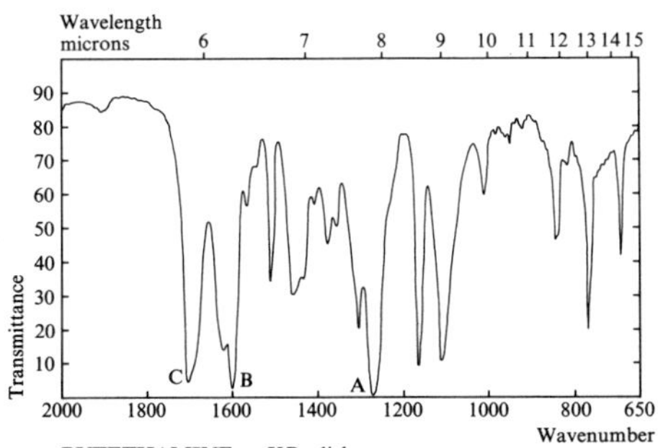

BUTETHAMINE — KBr disk
A 1272, B 1600, C 1702

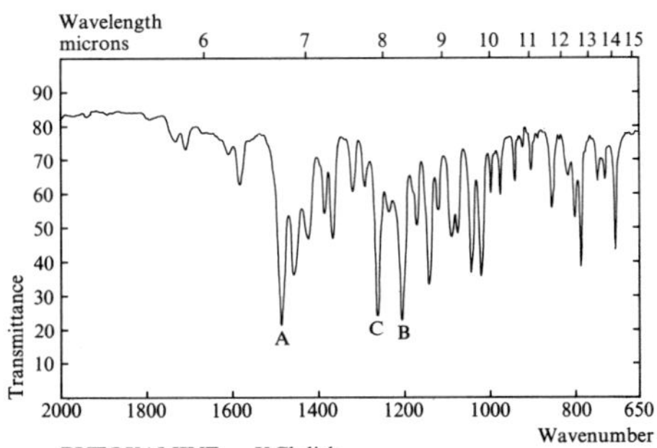

BUTOXAMINE — KCl disk
A 1485, B 1206, C 1263

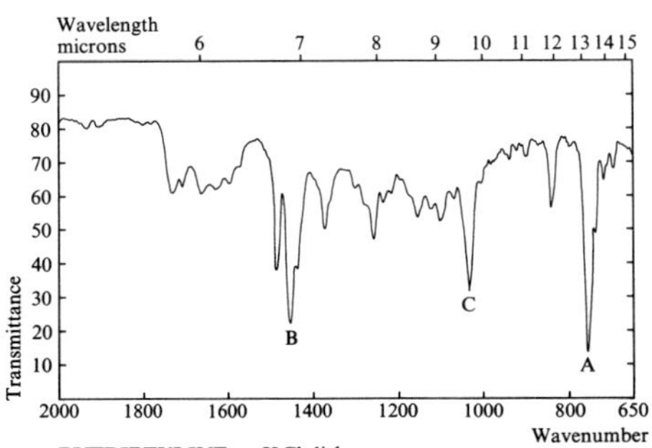

BUTRIPTYLINE — KCl disk
A 757, B 1455, C 1033

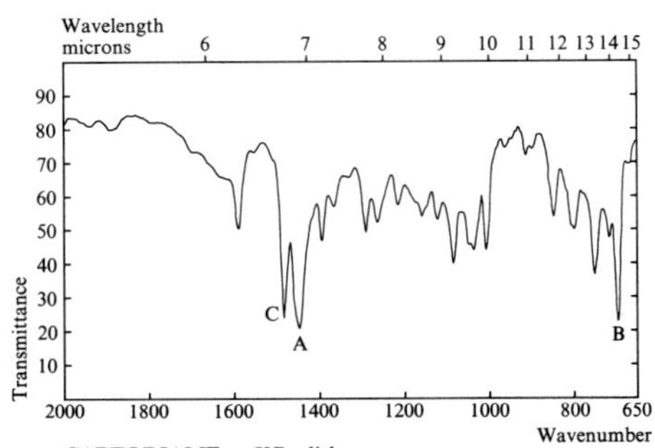

CAPTODIAME — KBr disk
A 1450, B 695, C 1485

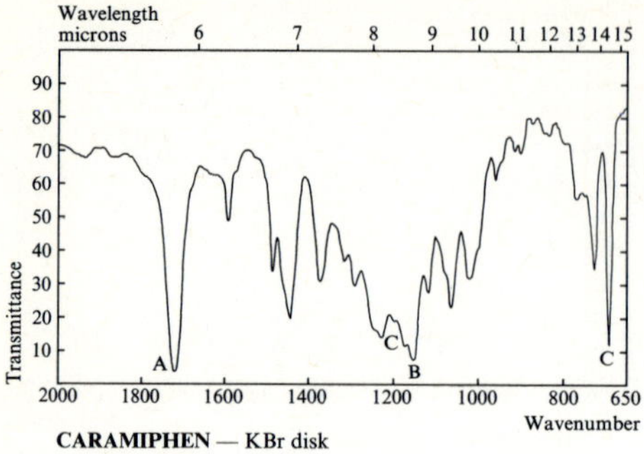

CARAMIPHEN — KBr disk
A 1718, B 1154, C 694 or 1173

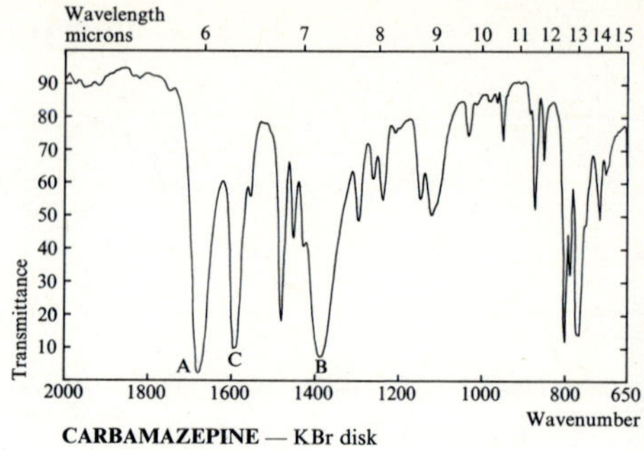

CARBAMAZEPINE — KBr disk
A 1678, B 1388, C 1594

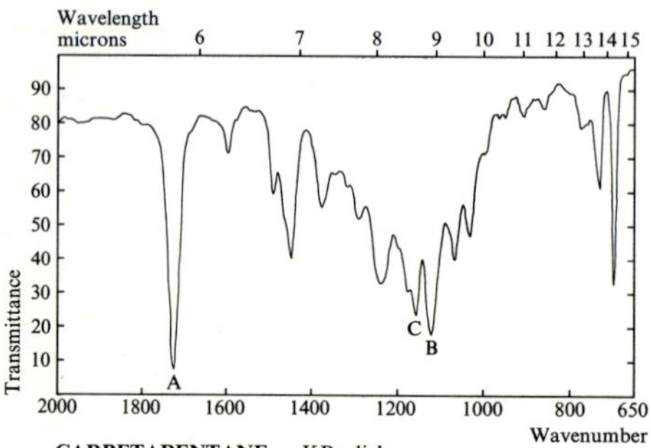

CARBETAPENTANE — KBr disk
A 1725, B 1120, C 1158

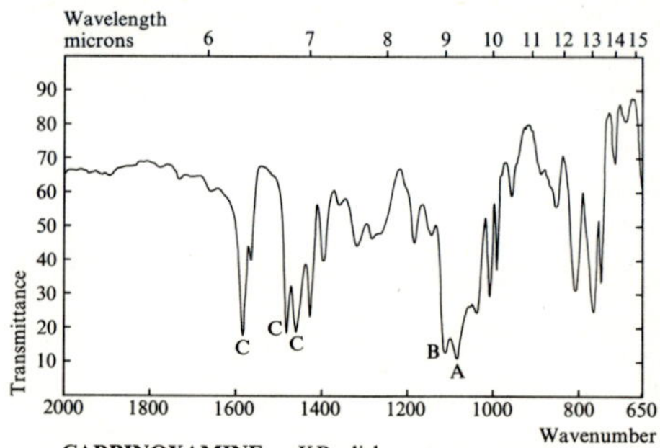

CARBINOXAMINE — KBr disk
A 1084, B 1110, C 1462 or 1484 or 1584

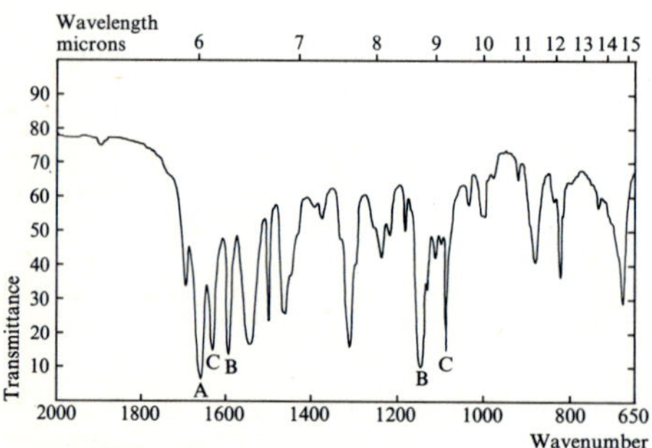

CARBUTAMIDE — KBr disk
A 1661, B 1147 or 1599, C 1089 or 1635

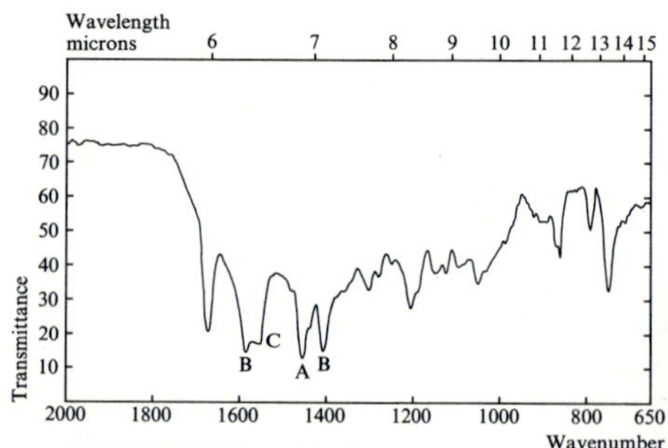

CARPHENAZINE — KBr disk
A 1455, B 1408 or 1585, C 1557

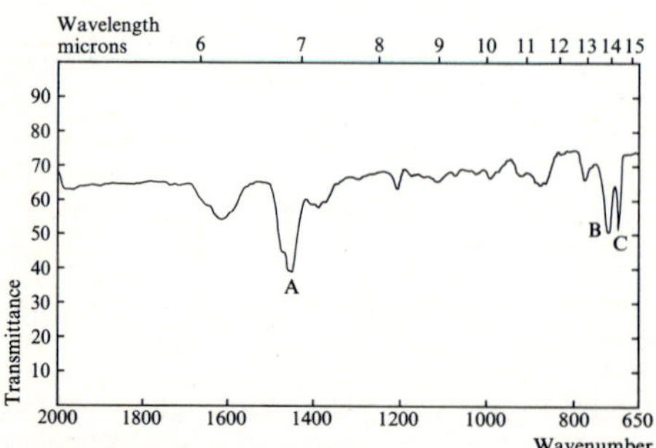

CETALKONIUM CHLORIDE — KBr disk
A 1450, B 722, C 698

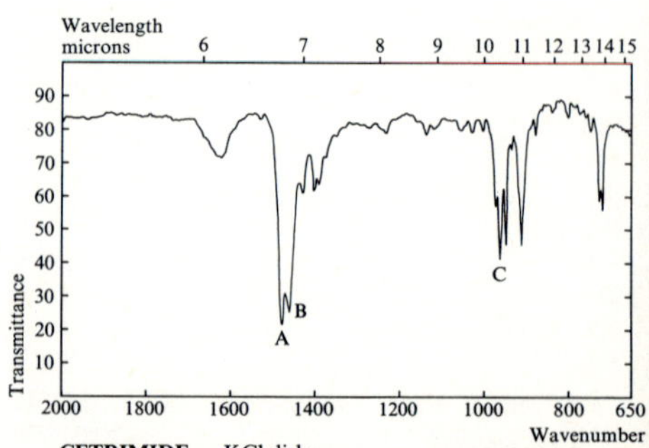

CETRIMIDE — KCl disk
A 1480, B 1462, C 961

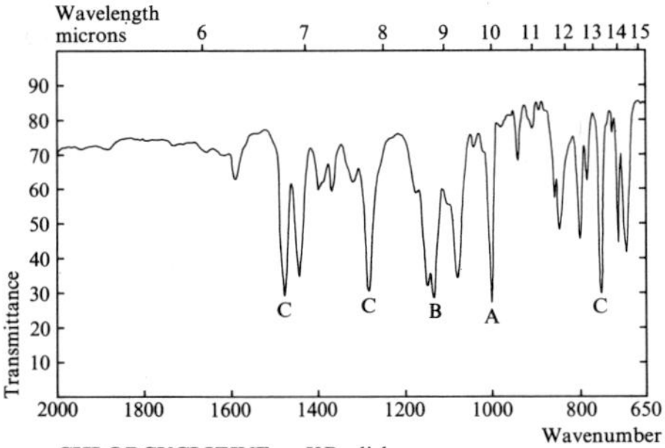

CHLORCYCLIZINE — KBr disk
A 1000, B 1135, C 752 or 1283 or 1478

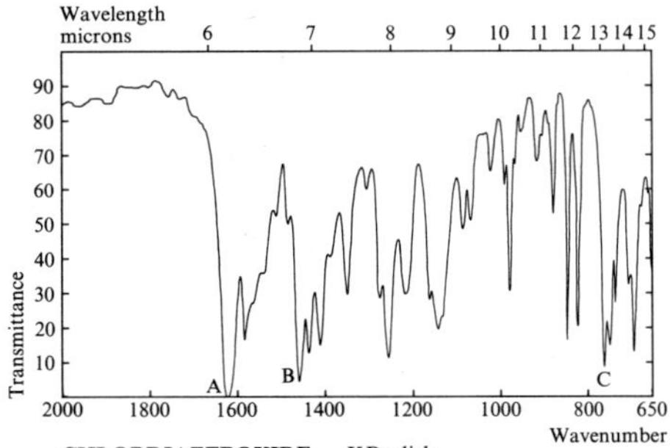

CHLORDIAZEPOXIDE — KBr disk
A 1625, B 1458, C 760

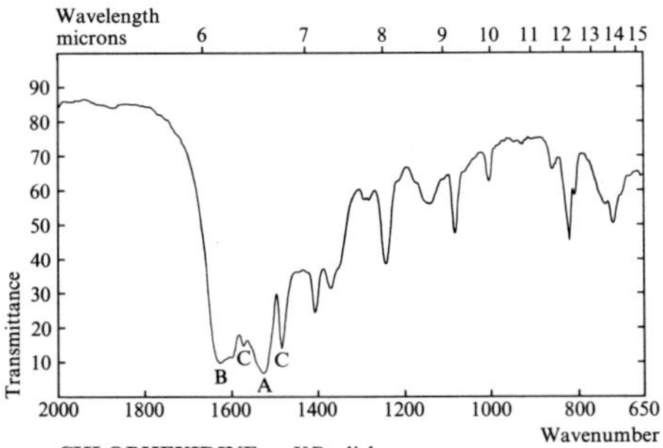

CHLORHEXIDINE — KBr disk
A 1527, B 1628, C 1486 or 1575

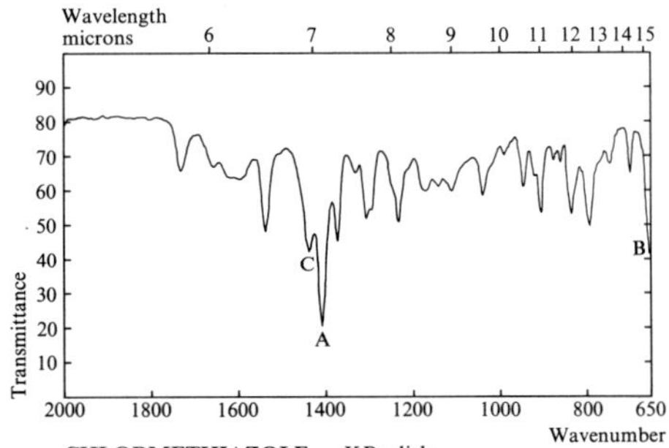

CHLORMETHIAZOLE — KBr disk
A 1409, B 650, C 1438

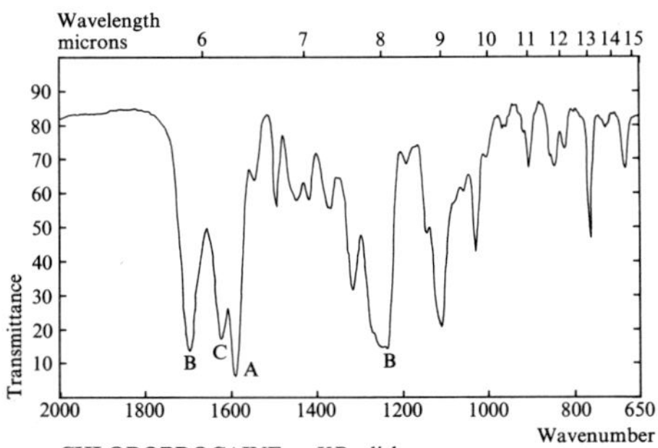

CHLOROPROCAINE — KBr disk
A 1595, B 1240 or 1698, C 1625

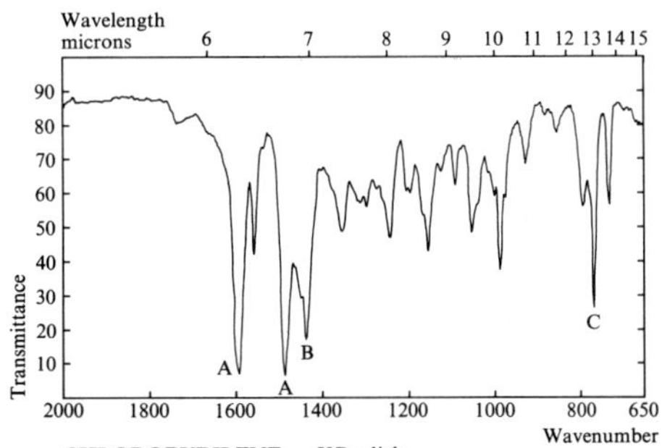

CHLOROPYRILENE — KBr disk
A 1488 or 1595, B 1437, C 767

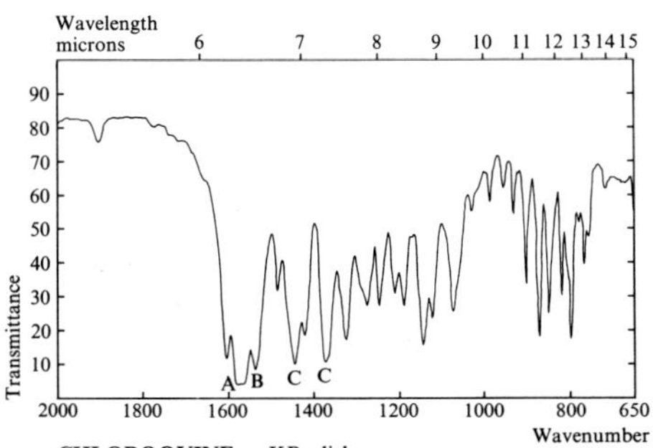

CHLOROQUINE — KBr disk
A 1573, B 1538, C 1372 or 1448

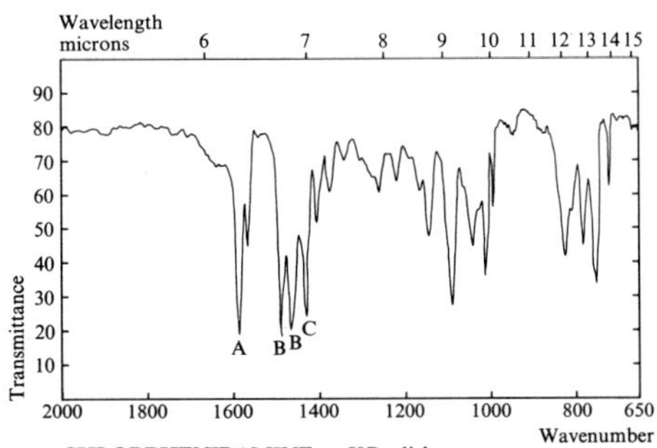

CHLORPHENIRAMINE — KBr disk
A 1585, B 1465 or 1486, C 1430

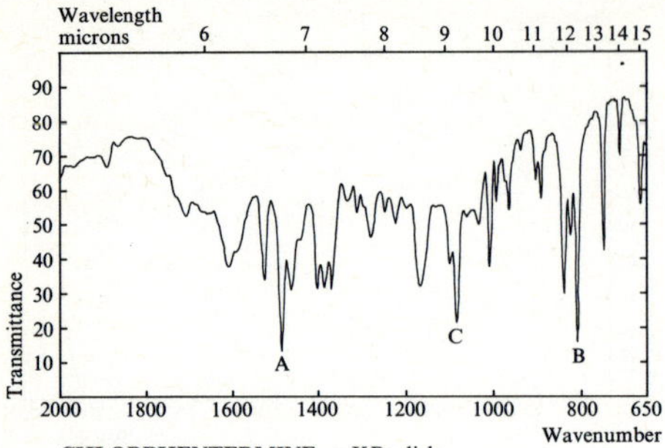

CHLORPHENTERMINE — KBr disk
A 1487, B 810, C 1084

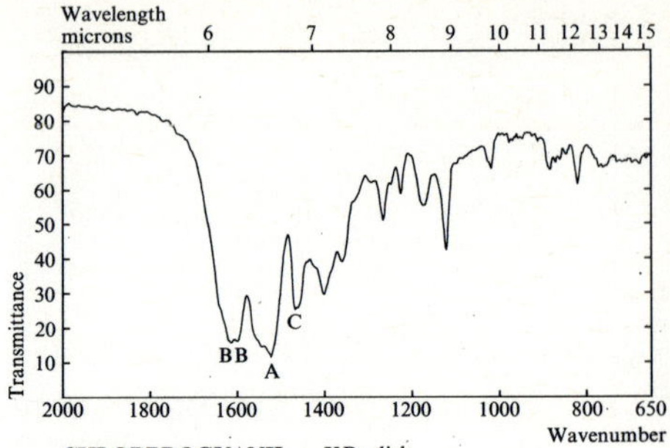

CHLORPROGUANIL — KBr disk
A 1525, B 1602 or 1614, C 1468

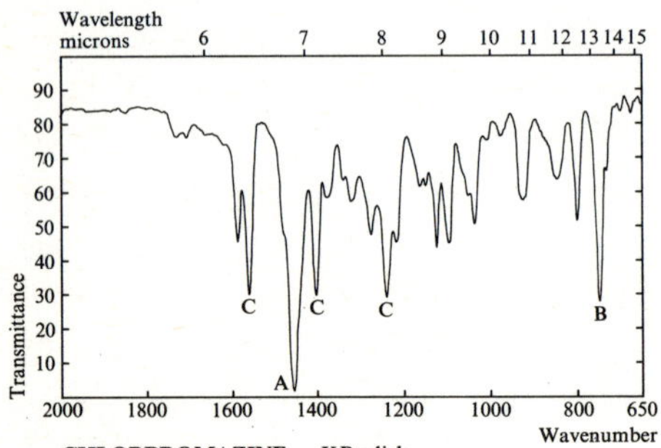

CHLORPROMAZINE — KBr disk
A 1455, B 747, C 1240 or 1402 or 1561

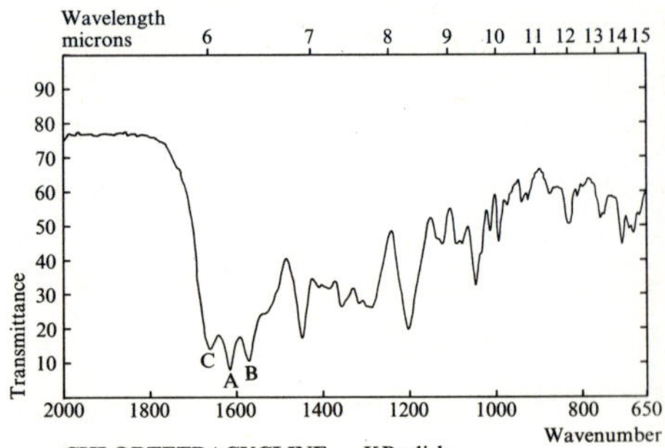

CHLORTETRACYCLINE — KBr disk
A 1617, B 1573, C 1663

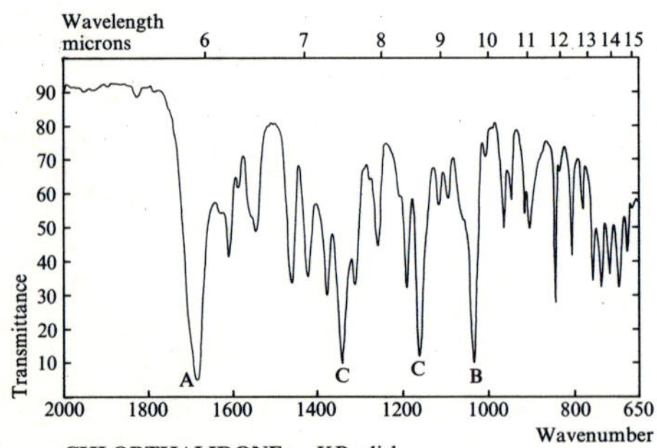

CHLORTHALIDONE — KBr disk
A 1685, B 1036, C 1163 or 1345

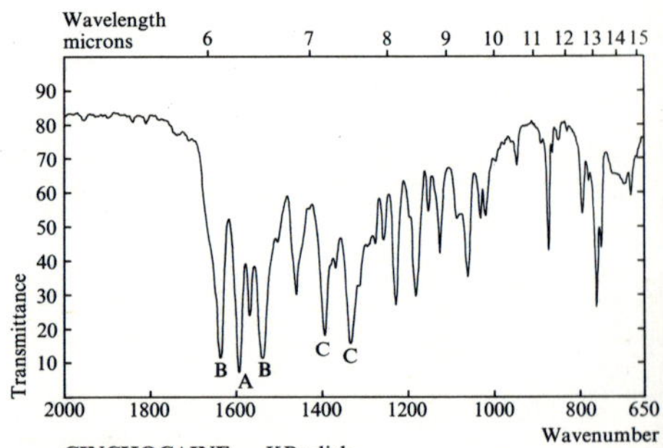

CINCHOCAINE — KBr disk
A 1596, B 1543 or 1639, C 1337 or 1397

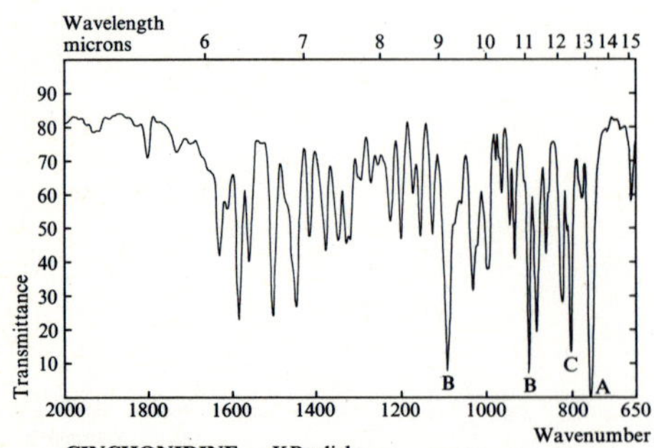

CINCHONIDINE — KBr disk
A 754, B 899 or 1090, C 800

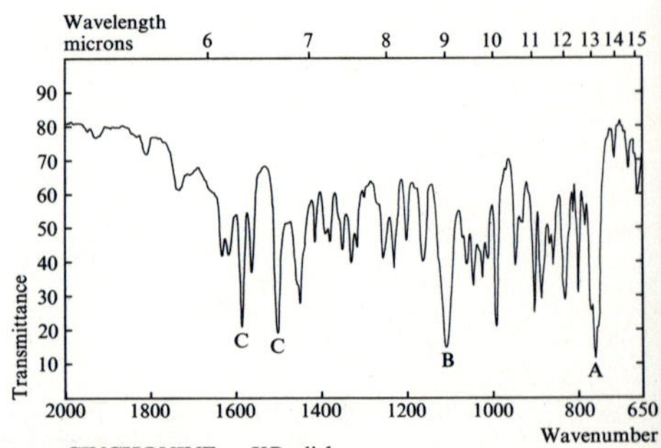

CINCHONINE — KBr disk
A 760, B 1110, C 1505 or 1590

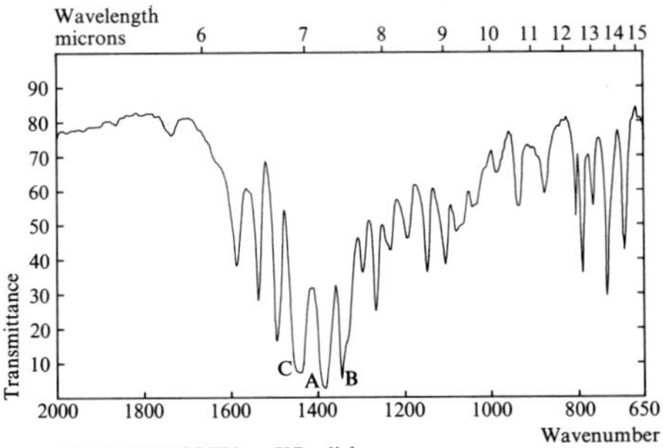

CLAMOXYQUIN — KBr disk
A 1387, B 1347, C 1444

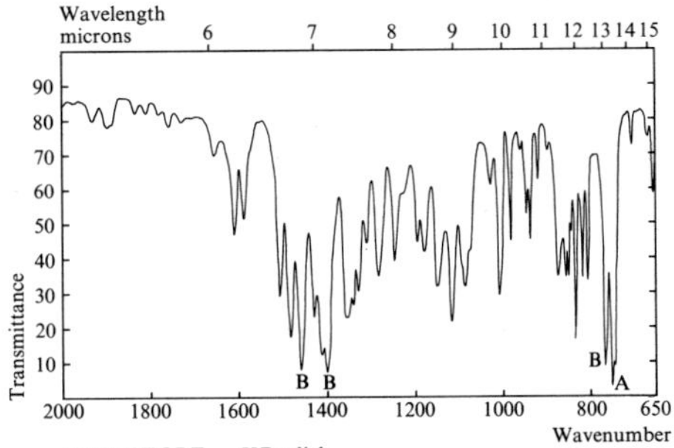

CLEMIZOLE — KBr disk
A 748, B 765 or 1400 or 1460

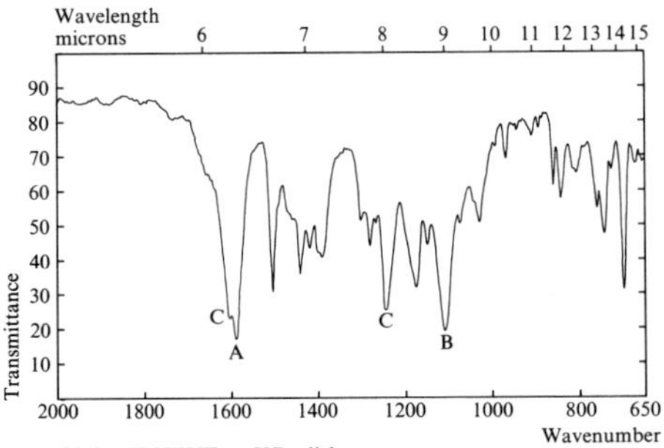

CLOMIPHENE — KBr disk
A 1590, B 1111, C 1245 or 1605

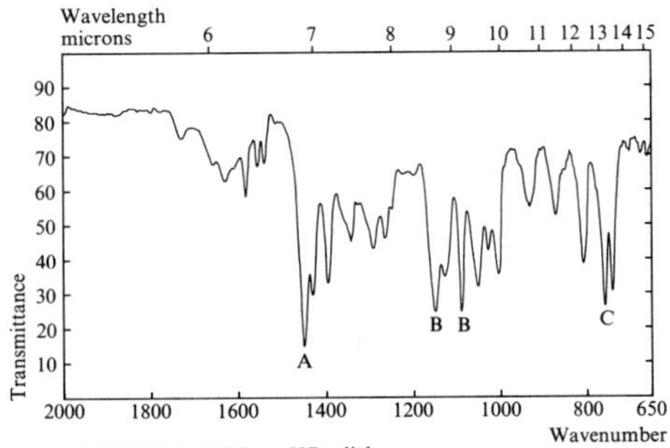

CLOPENTHIXOL — KBr disk
A 1451, B 1090 or 1150, C 757

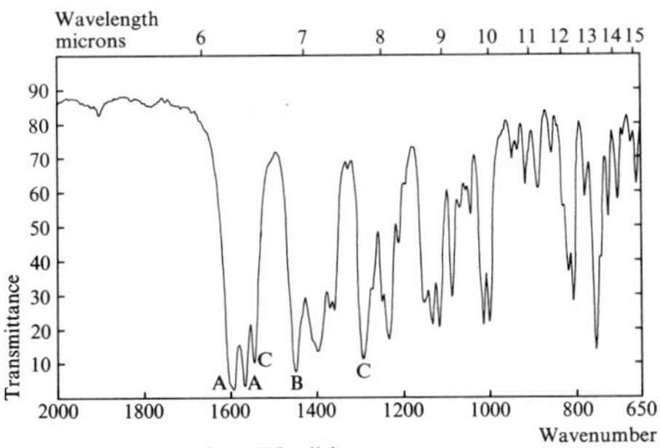

CLOTHIAPINE — KBr disk
A 1570 or 1596, B 1453, C 1295 or 1548

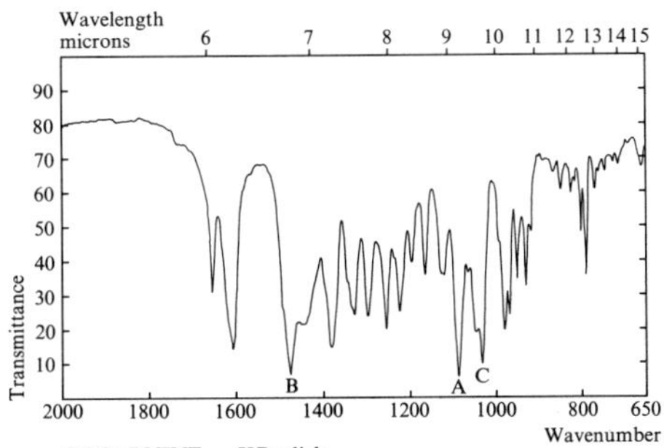

COTARNINE — KBr disk
A 1089, B 1478, C 1035

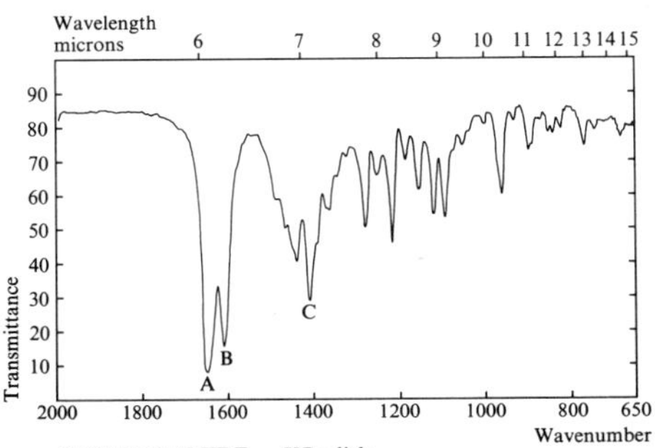

CROPROPAMIDE — KBr disk
A 1654, B 1617, C 1413

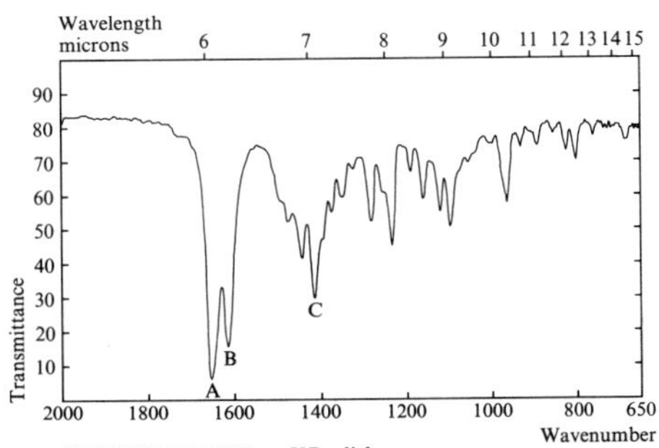

CROTETHAMIDE — KBr disk
A 1655, B 1617, C 1417

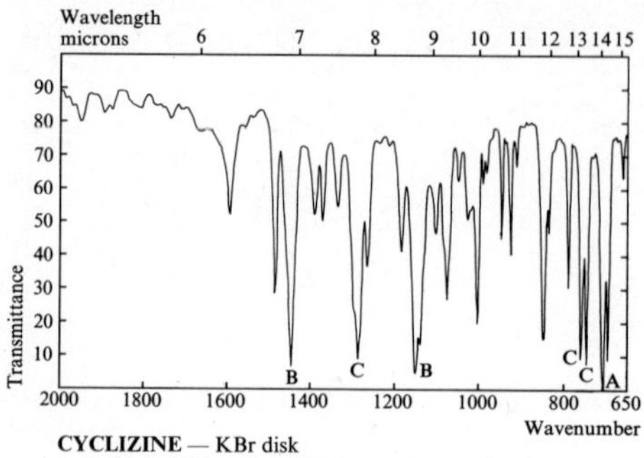

CYCLIZINE — KBr disk
A 708, B 1150 or 1447, C 745 or 759 or 1285

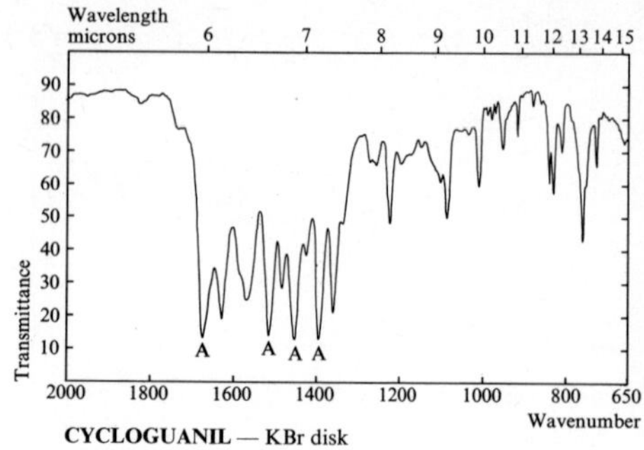

CYCLOGUANIL — KBr disk
A 1393 or 1452 or 1515 or 1673

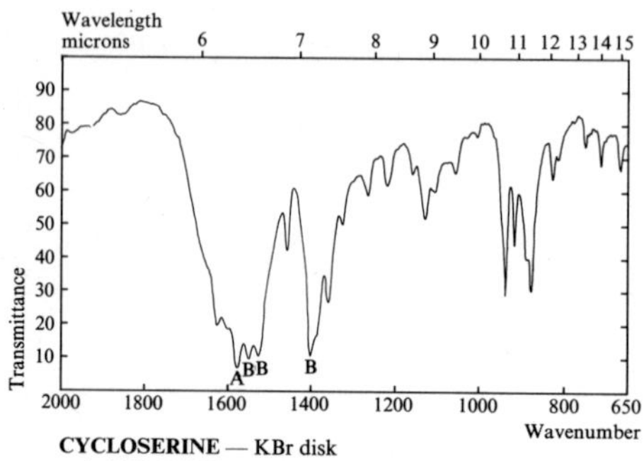

CYCLOSERINE — KBr disk
A 1577, B 1399 or 1526 or 1550

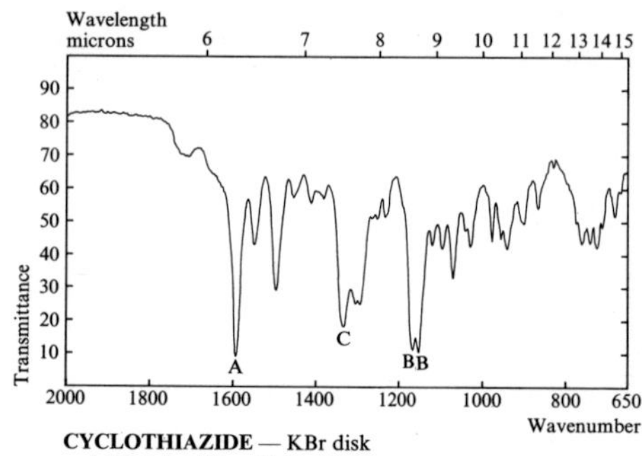

CYCLOTHIAZIDE — KBr disk
A 1596, B 1153 or 1168, C 1337

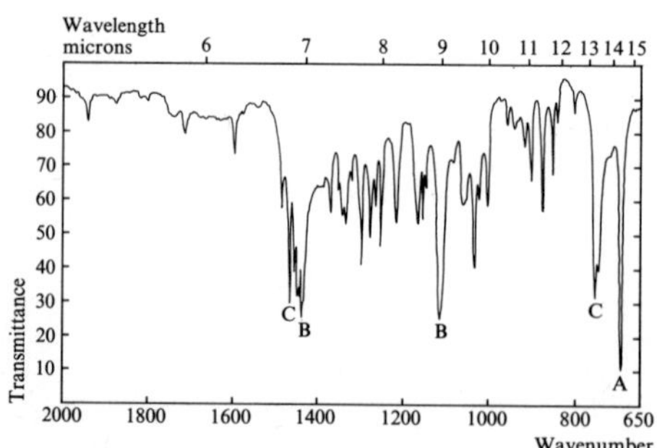

CYCRIMINE — KBr disk
A 696, B 1117 or 1438, C 755 or 1468

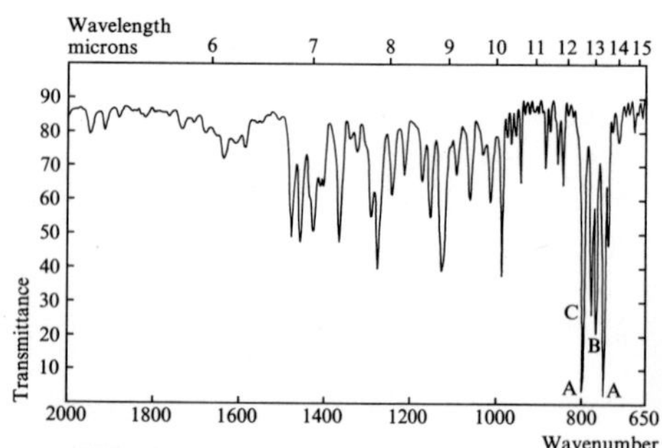

CYPROHEPTADINE — KBr disk
A 749 or 797, B 765, C 776

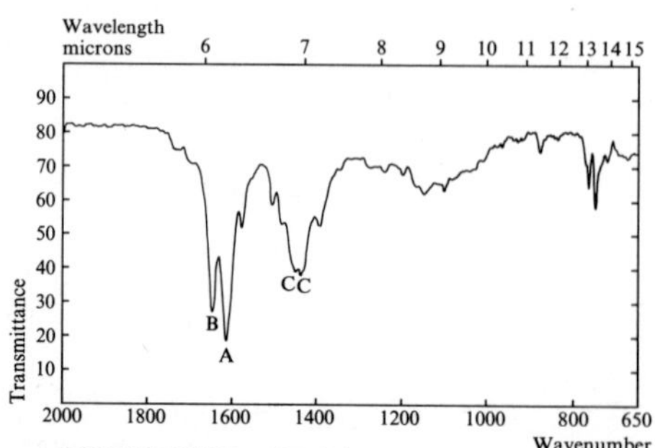

DEBRISOQUINE — KBr disk
A 1615, B 1647, C 1439 or 1451

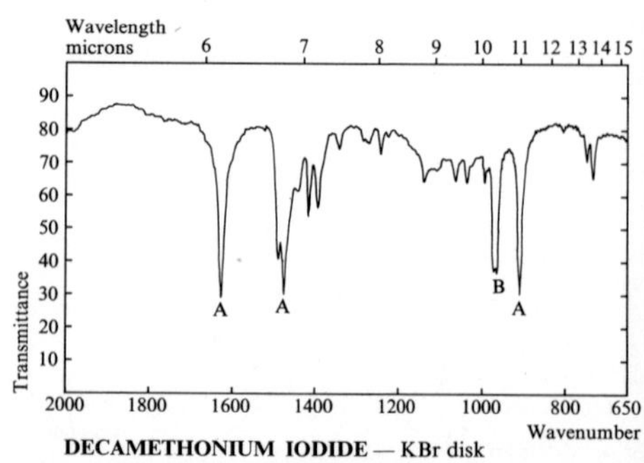

DECAMETHONIUM IODIDE — KBr disk
A 910 or 1479 or 1627, B 965

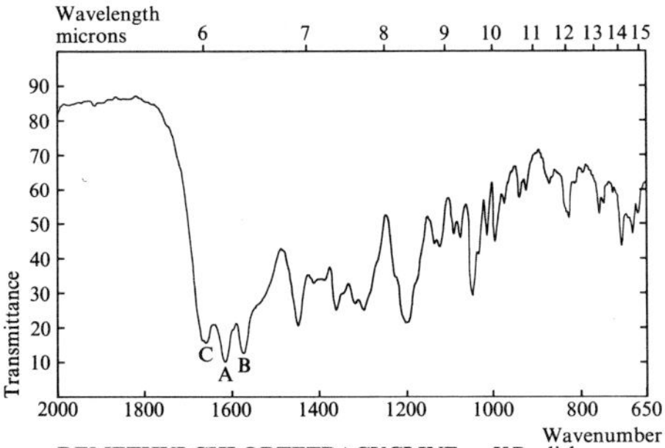

DEMETHYLCHLORTETRACYCLINE — KBr disk
A 1616, B 1573, C 1660

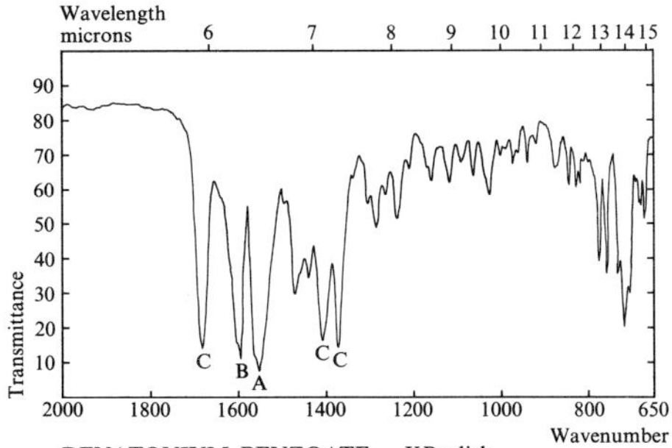

DENATONIUM BENZOATE — KBr disk
A 1550, B 1596, C 1370 or 1407 or 1680

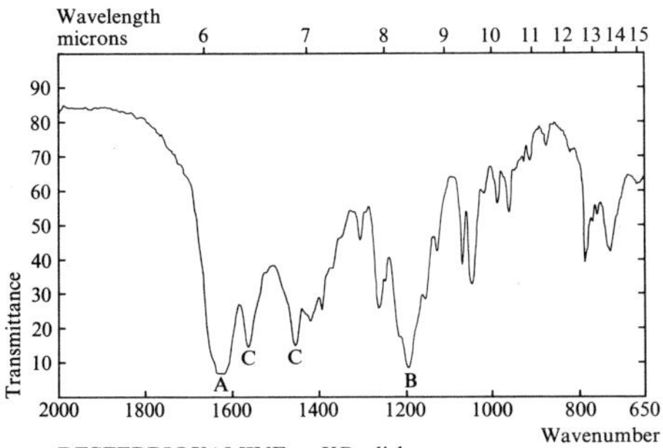

DESFERRIOXAMINE — KBr disk
A 1628, B 1195, C 1455 or 1562

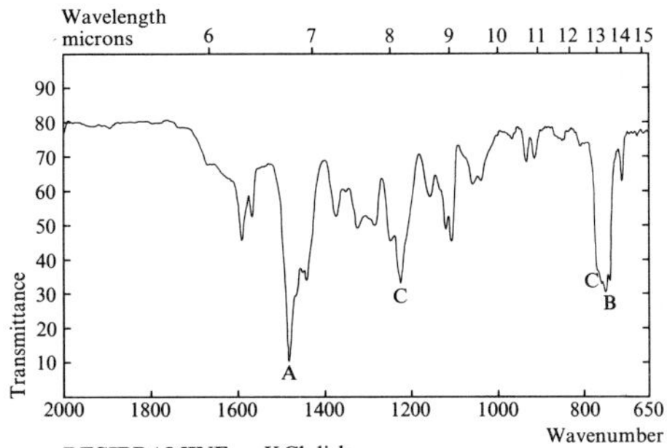

DESIPRAMINE — KCl disk
A 1482, B 747, C 757 or 1228

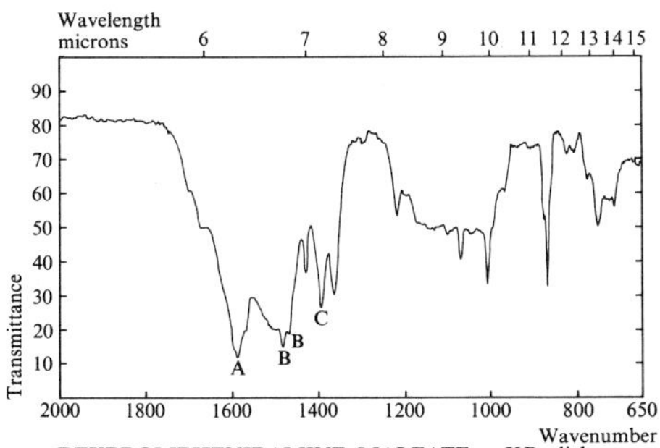

DEXBROMPHENIRAMINE MALEATE — KBr disk
A 1590, B 1470 or 1485, C 1395

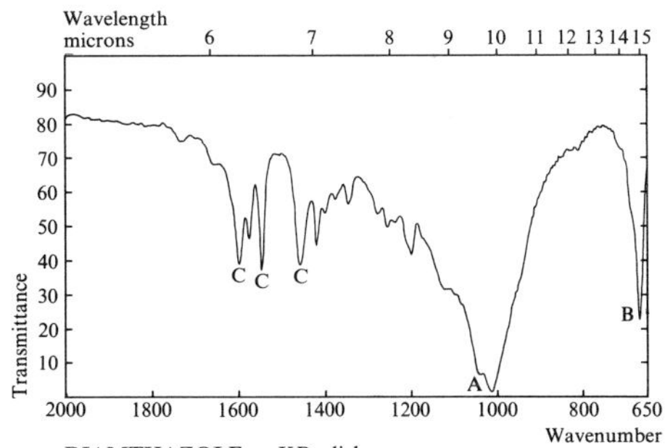

DIAMTHAZOLE — KBr disk
A 1015, B 667, C 1460 or 1548 or 1602

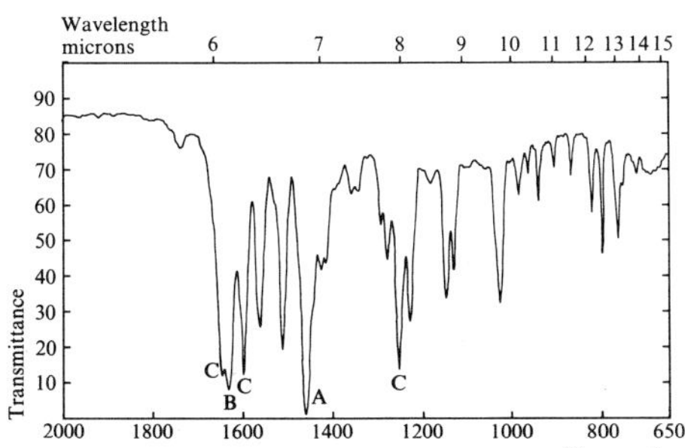

DIAVERIDINE — KBr disk
A 1460, B 1630, C 1252 or 1598 or 1645

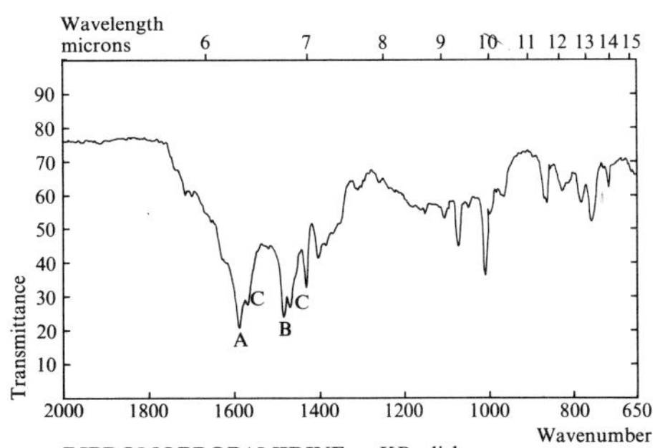

DIBROMOPROPAMIDINE — KBr disk
A 1589, B 1485, C 1470 or 1569

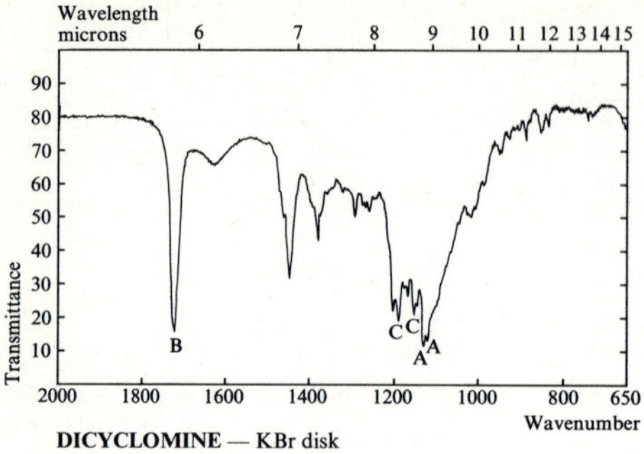

DICYCLOMINE — KBr disk
A 1122 or 1128, B 1724, C 1154 or 1188

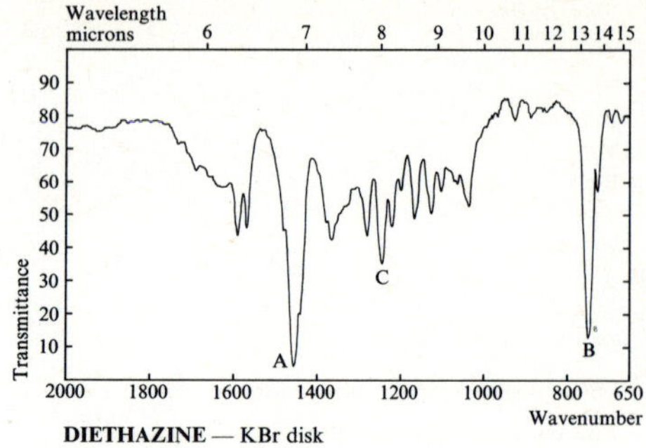

DIETHAZINE — KBr disk
A 1456, B 748, C 1245

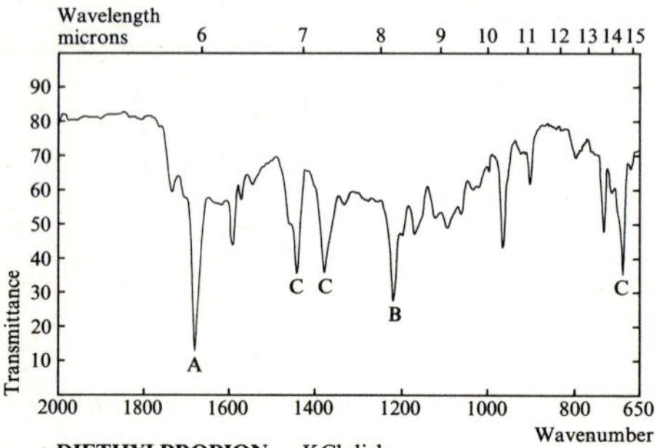

DIETHYLPROPION — KCl disk
A 1682, B 1220, C 689 or 1378 or 1445

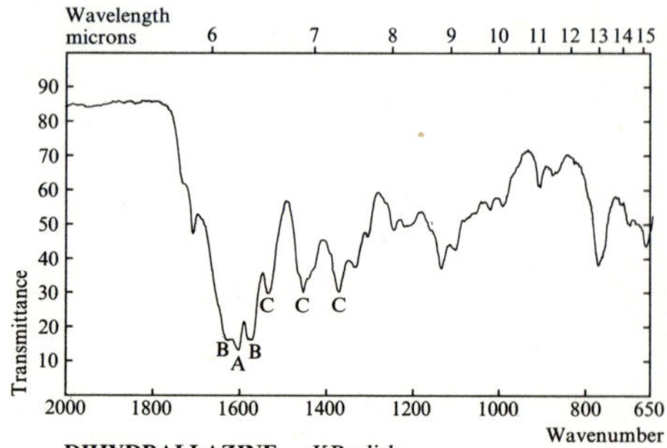

DIHYDRALLAZINE — KBr disk
A 1608, B 1575 or 1633, C 1375 or 1458 or 1537

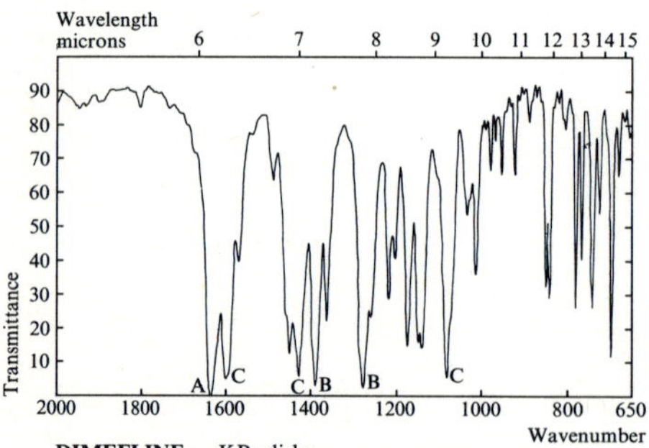

DIMEFLINE — KBr disk
A 1637, B 1278 or 1389, C 1081 or 1428 or 1602

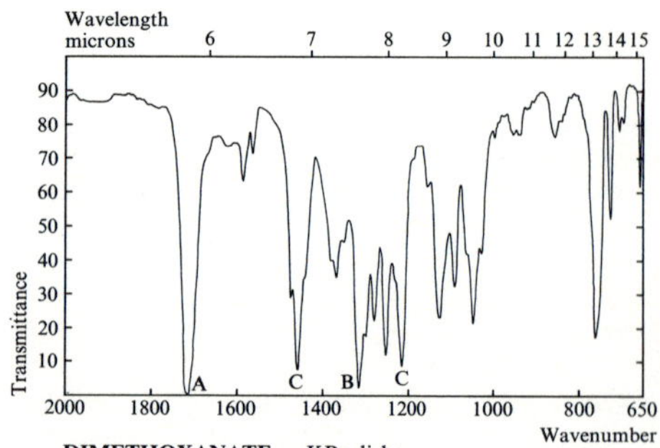

DIMETHOXANATE — KBr disk
A 1718, B 1317, C 1217 or 1460

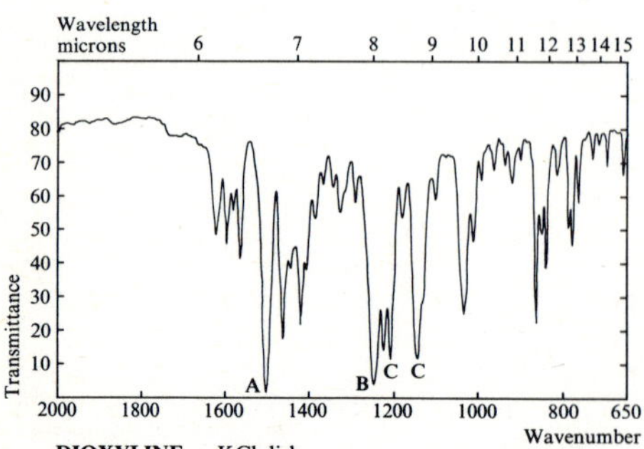

DIOXYLINE — KCl disk
A 1504, B 1247, C 1145 or 1208

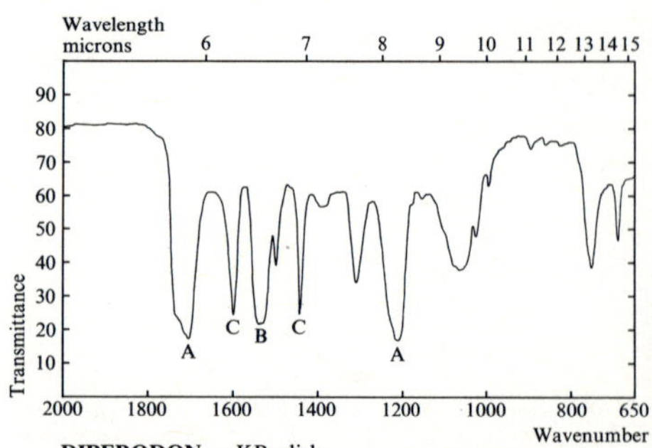

DIPERODON — KBr disk
A 1210 or 1705, B 1530, C 1442 or 1600

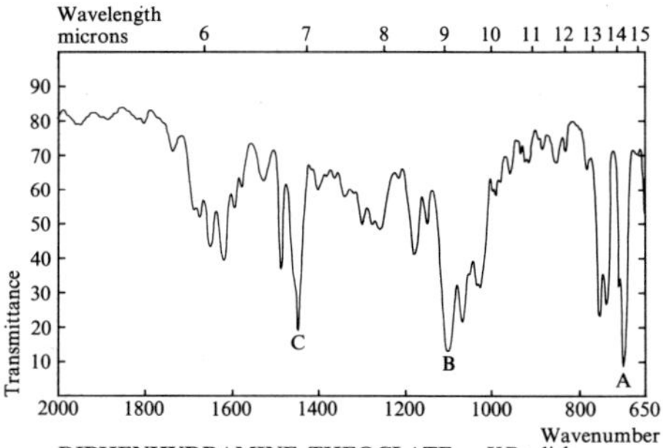

DIPHENHYDRAMINE THEOCLATE — KBr disk
A 699, B 1100, C 1448

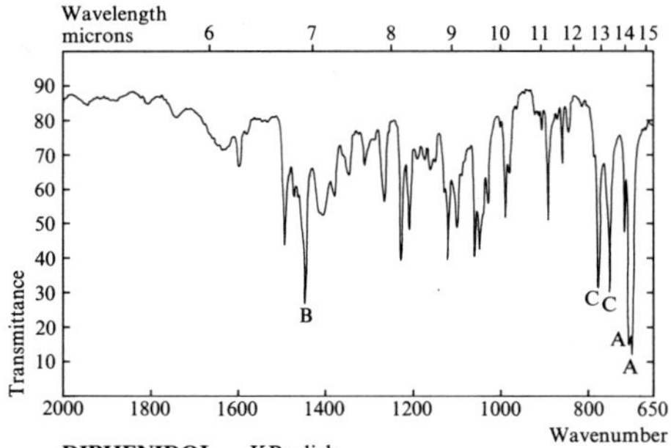

DIPHENIDOL — KBr disk
A 697 or 701, B 1447, C 749 or 773

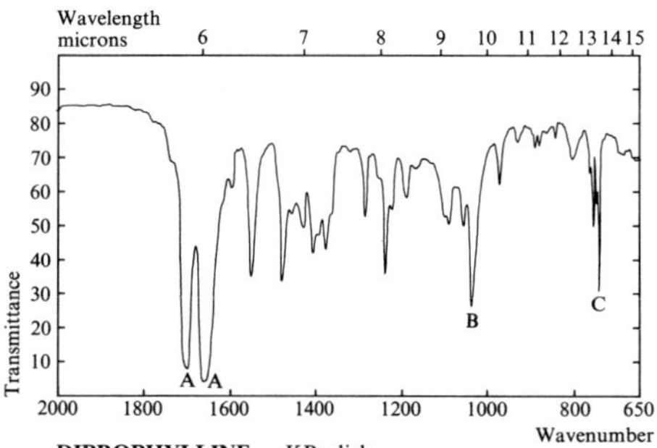

DIPROPHYLLINE — KBr disk
A 1660 or 1700, B 1039, C 747

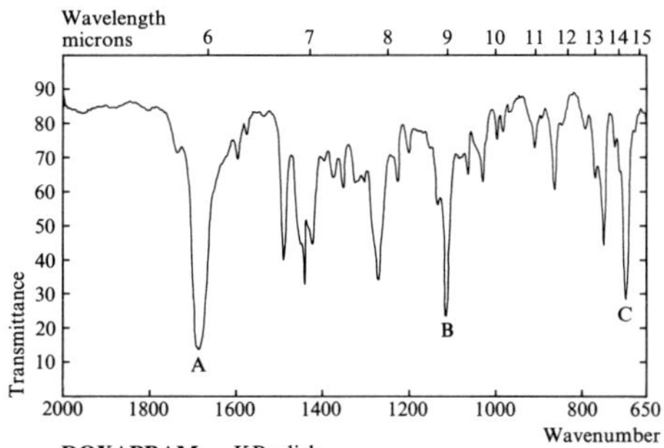

DOXAPRAM — KBr disk
A 1685, B 1114, C 696

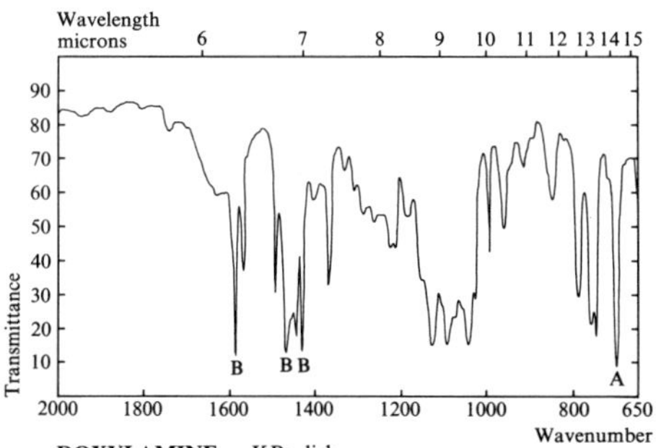

DOXYLAMINE — KBr disk
A 700, B 1431 or 1470 or 1590

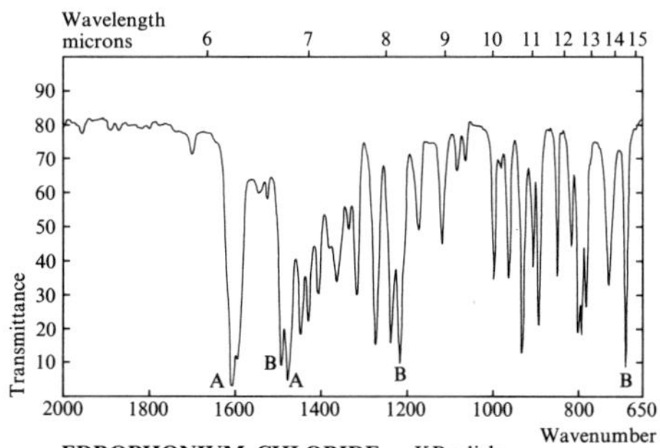

EDROPHONIUM CHLORIDE — KBr disk
A 1479 or 1609, B 690 or 1217 or 1495

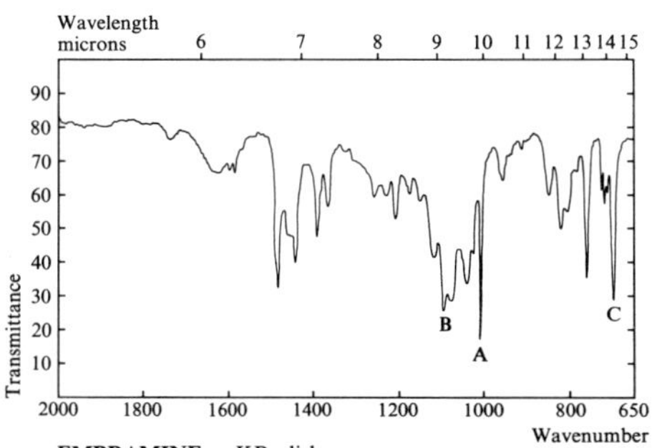

EMBRAMINE — KBr disk
A 1009, B 1095, C 699

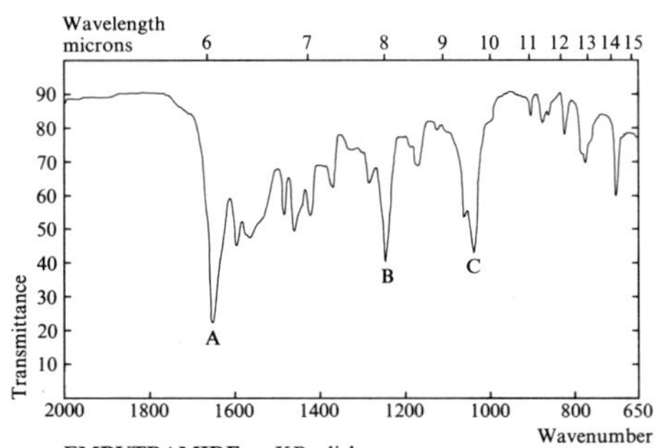

EMBUTRAMIDE — KBr disk
A 1652, B 1248, C 1037

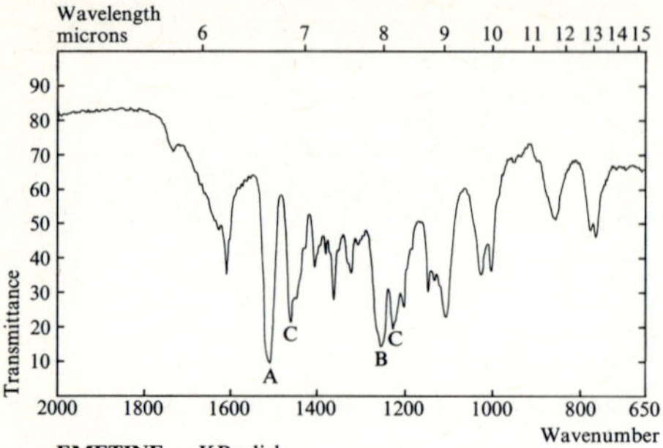

EMETINE — KBr disk
A 1514, B 1256, C 1228 or 1463

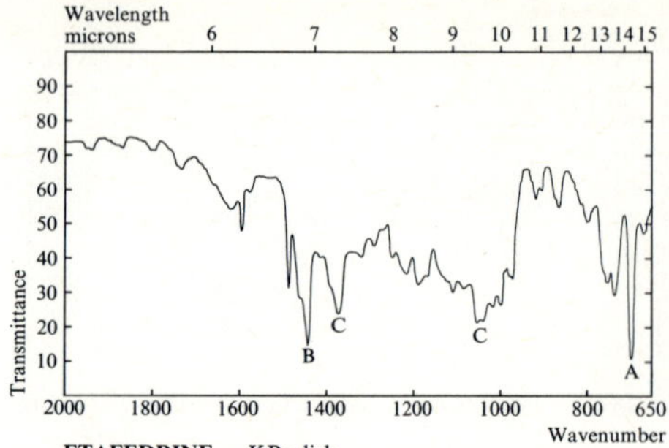

ETAFEDRINE — KBr disk
A 697, B 1448, C 1057 or 1375

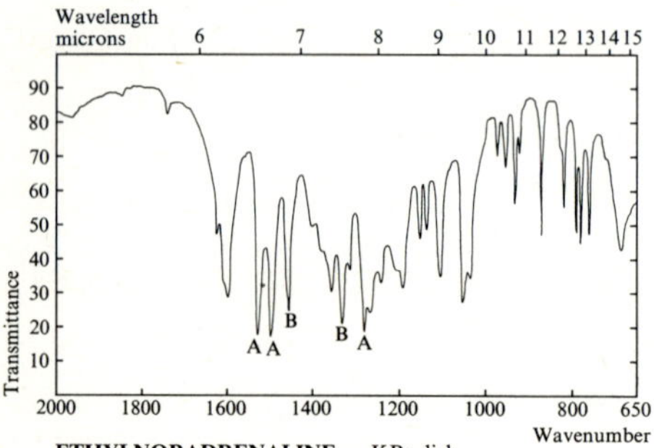

ETHYLNORADRENALINE — KBr disk
A 1280 or 1500 or 1529, B 1331 or 1456

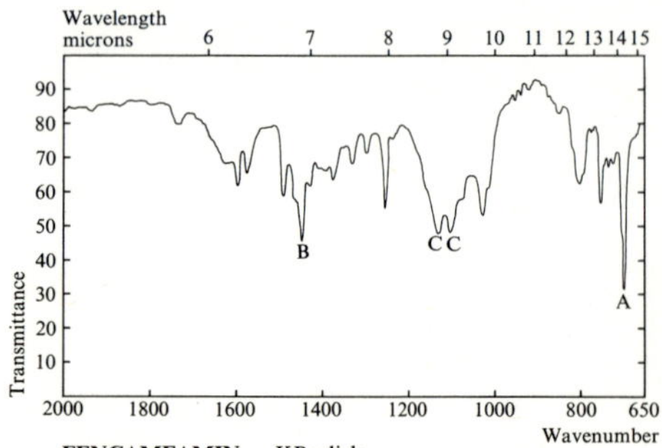

FENCAMFAMIN — KBr disk
A 698, B 1449, C 1102 or 1130

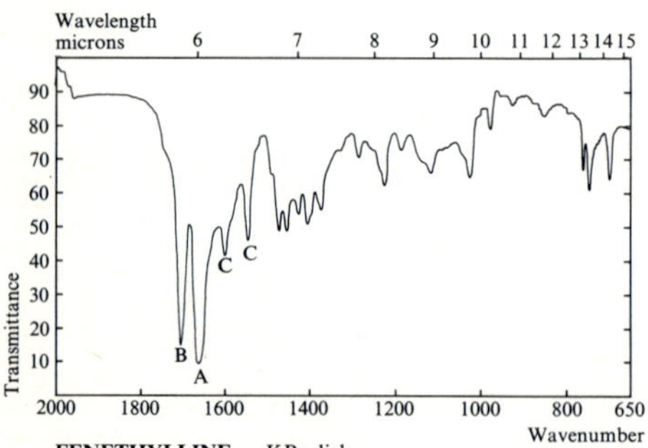

FENETHYLLINE — KBr disk
A 1664, B 1705, C 1546 or 1600

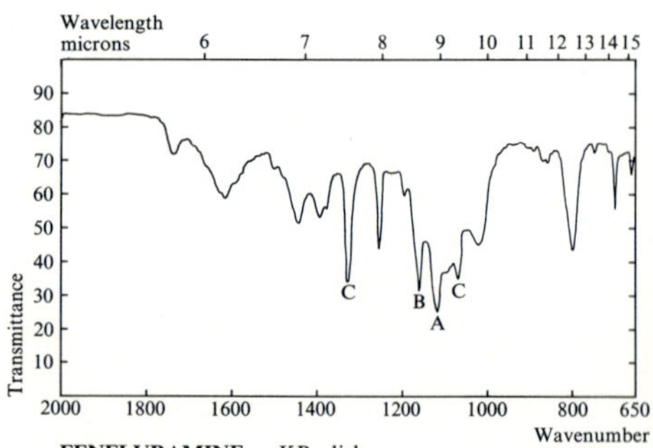

FENFLURAMINE — KBr disk
A 1119, B 1160, C 1069 or 1330

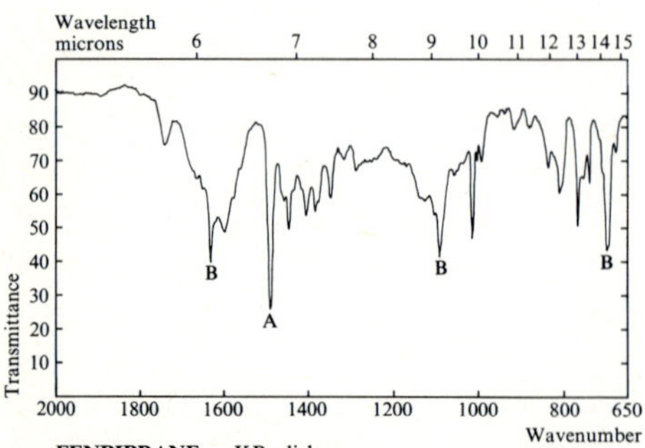

FENPIPRANE — KBr disk
A 1492, B 698 or 1092 or 1631

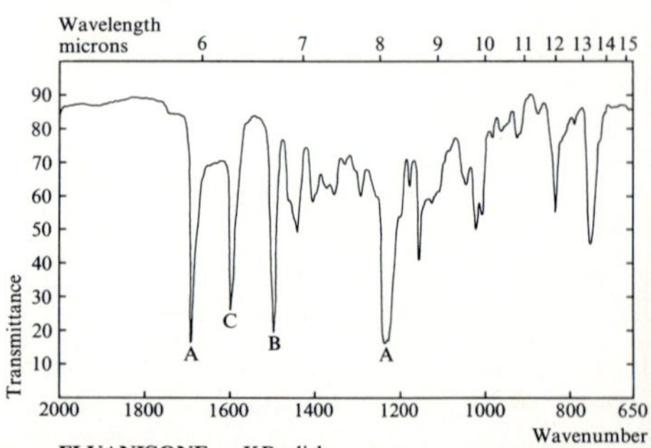

FLUANISONE — KBr disk
A 1238 or 1690, B 1499, C 1599

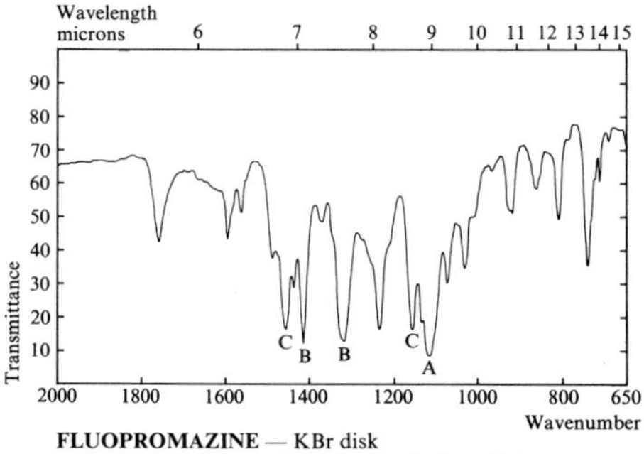

FLUOPROMAZINE — KBr disk
A 1117, B 1319 or 1417, C 1159 or 1237 or 1459

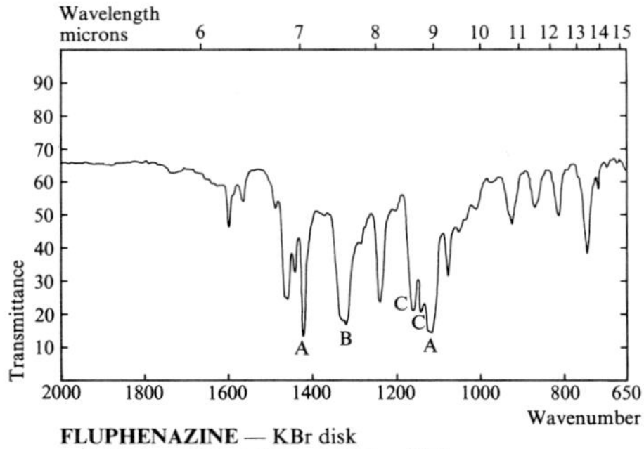

FLUPHENAZINE — KBr disk
A 1115 or 1425, B 1325, C 1142 or 1161

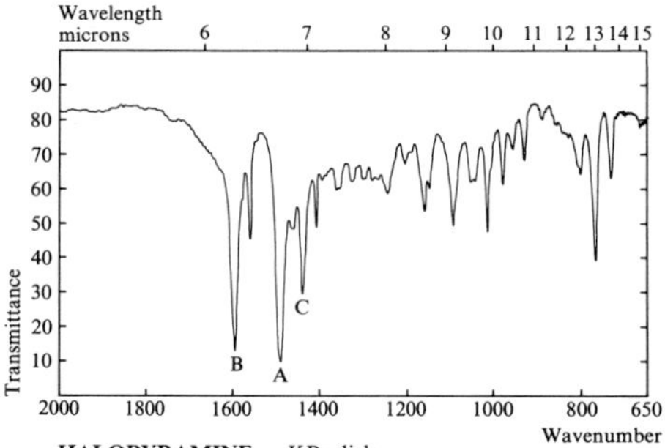

HALOPYRAMINE — KBr disk
A 1494, B 1598, C 1442

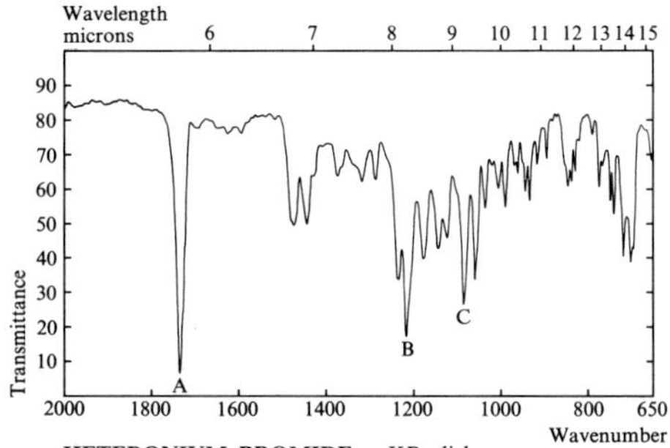

HETERONIUM BROMIDE — KBr disk
A 1735, B 1219, C 1085

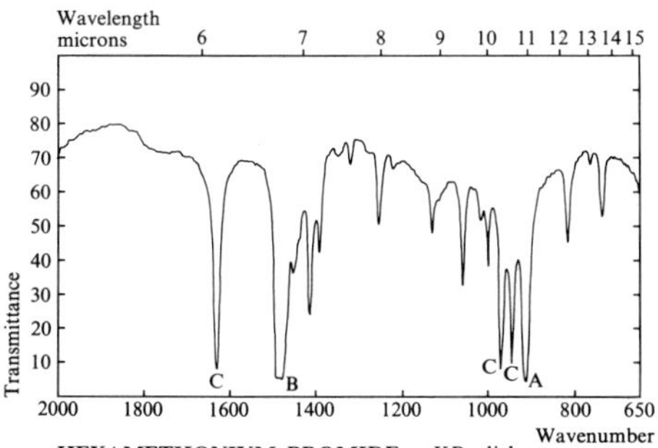

HEXAMETHONIUM BROMIDE — KBr disk
A 913, B 1481, C 945 or 970 or 1630

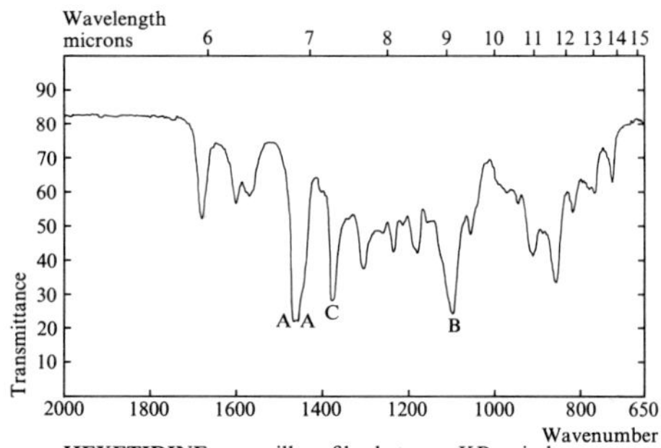

HEXETIDINE — capillary film between KBr windows
A 1455 or 1468, B 1093, C 1375

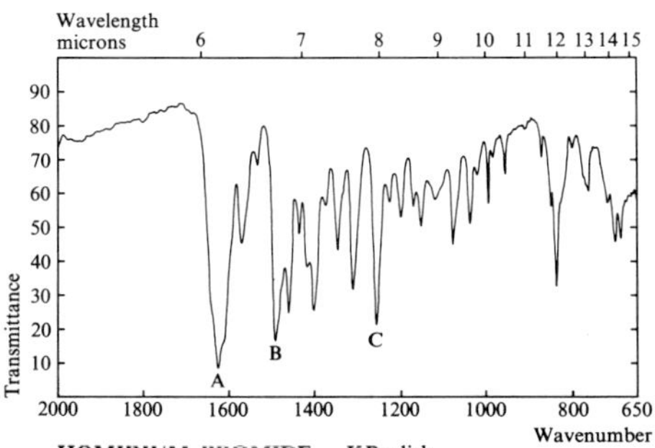

HOMIDIUM BROMIDE — KBr disk
A 1629, B 1492, C 1259

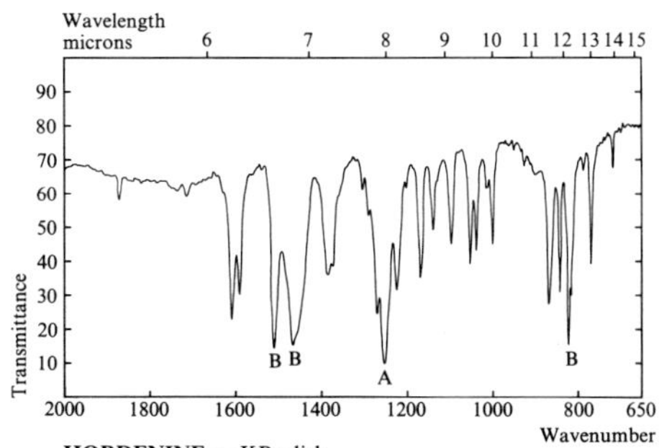

HORDENINE — KBr disk
A 1252, B 820 or 1469 or 1512

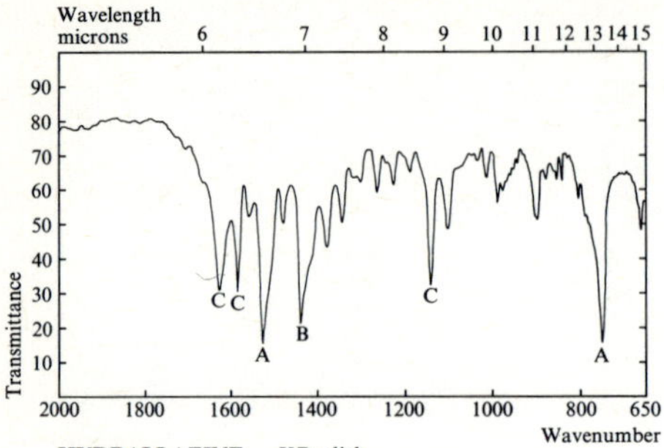

HYDRALLAZINE — KBr disk
A 750 or 1529, B 1439, C 1142 or 1585 or 1625

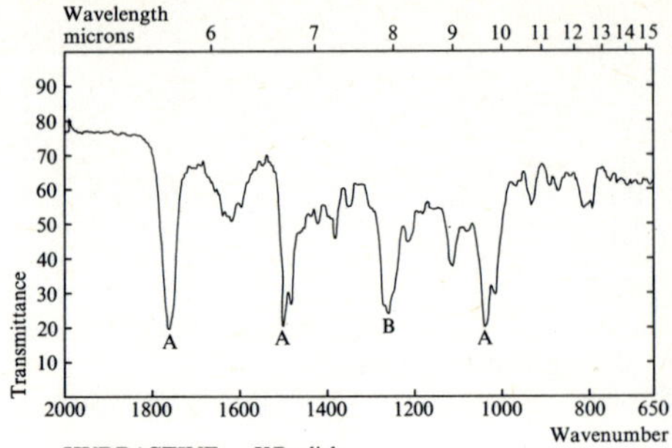

HYDRASTINE — KBr disk
A 1037 or 1501 or 1760, B 1260

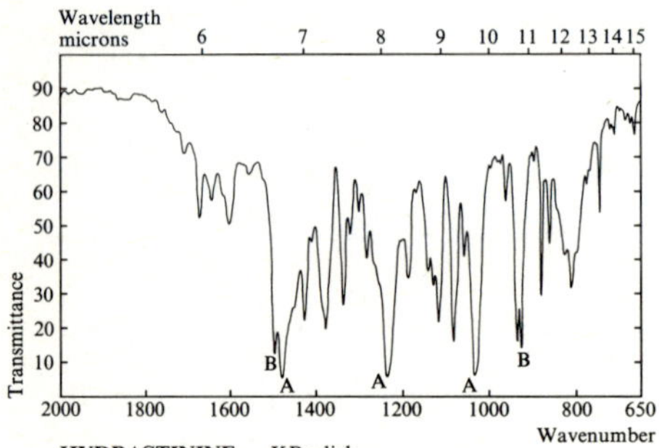

HYDRASTININE — KBr disk
A 1032 or 1235 or 1480, B 925 or 1499

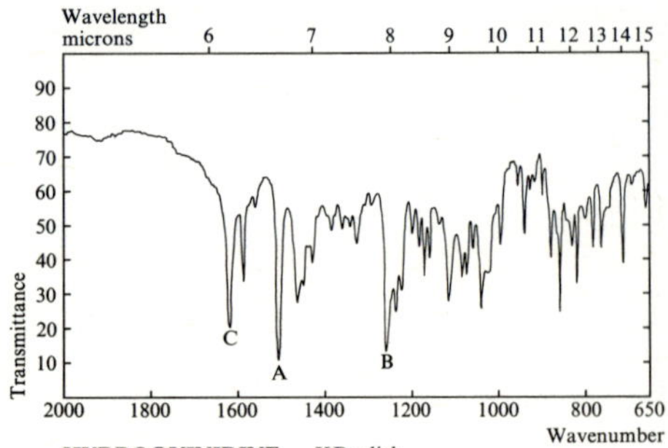

HYDROQUINIDINE — KBr disk
A 1509, B 1261, C 1620

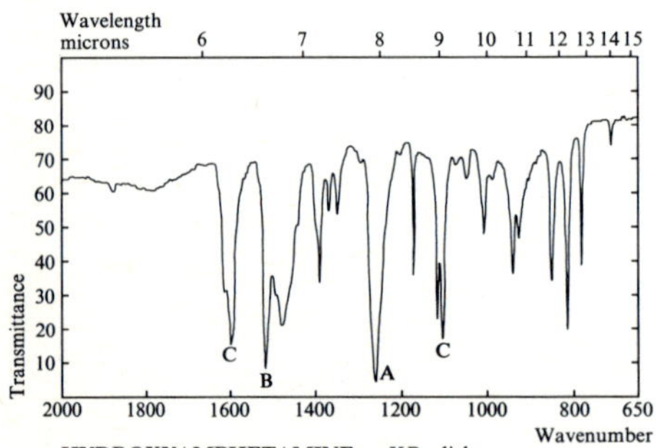

HYDROXYAMPHETAMINE — KBr disk
A 1259, B 1517, C 1102 or 1599

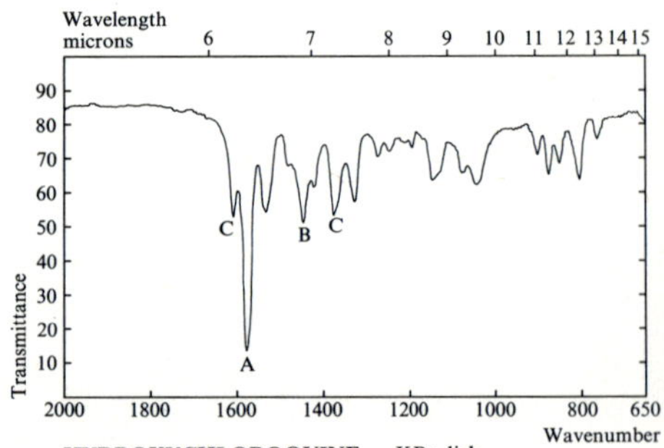

HYDROXYCHLOROQUINE — KBr disk
A 1579, B 1447, C 1372 or 1608

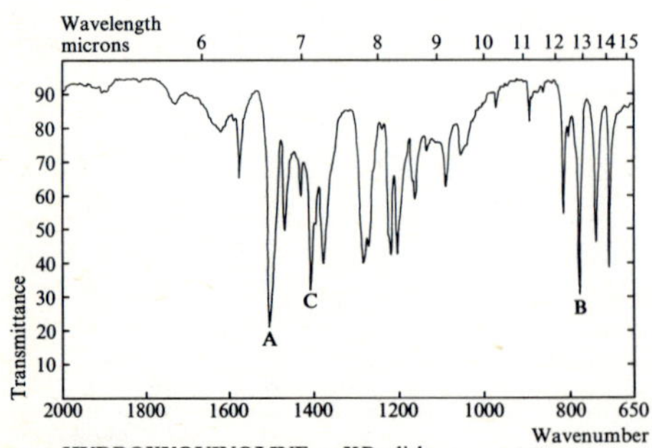

HYDROXYQUINOLINE — KBr disk
A 1509, B 779, C 1409

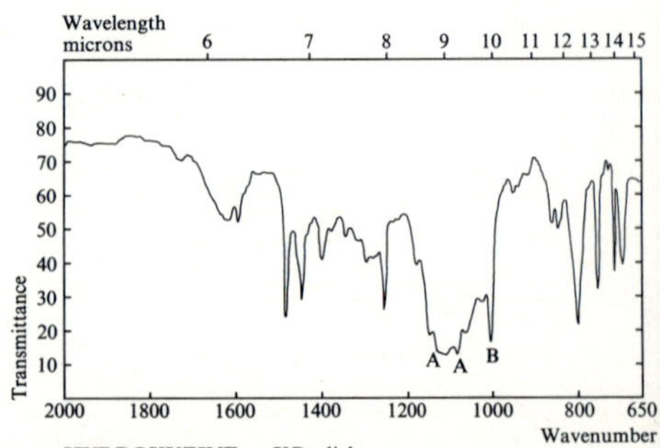

HYDROXYZINE — KBr disk
A 1082 or 1130, B 1005

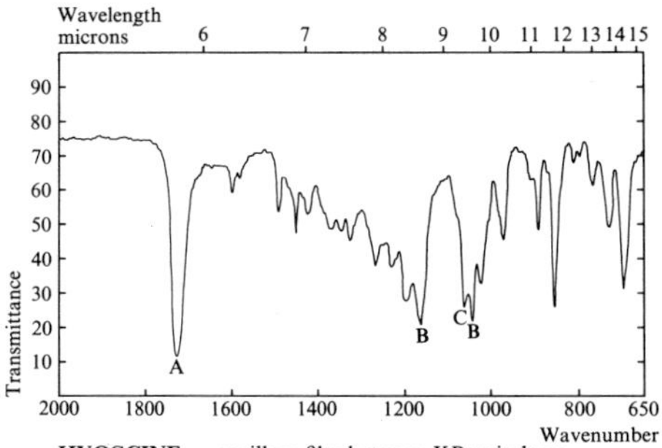

HYOSCINE — capillary film between KBr windows
A 1725, B 1041 or 1165, C 1060

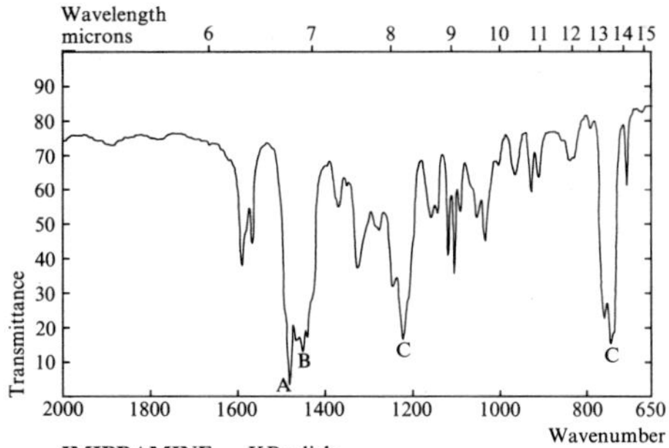

IMIPRAMINE — KBr disk
A 1485, B 1452, C 745 or 1225

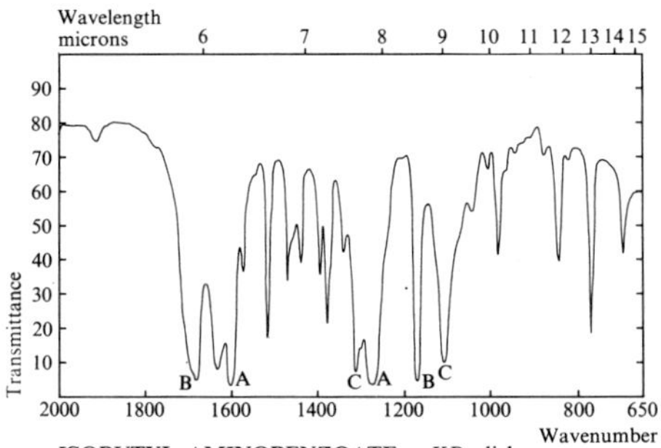

ISOBUTYL AMINOBENZOATE — KBr disk
A 1278 or 1607, B 1172 or 1683, C 1313 or 1109

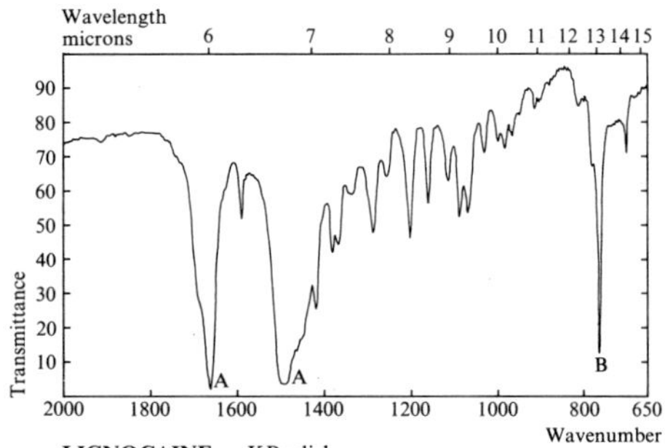

LIGNOCAINE — KBr disk
A 1490 or 1662, B 762

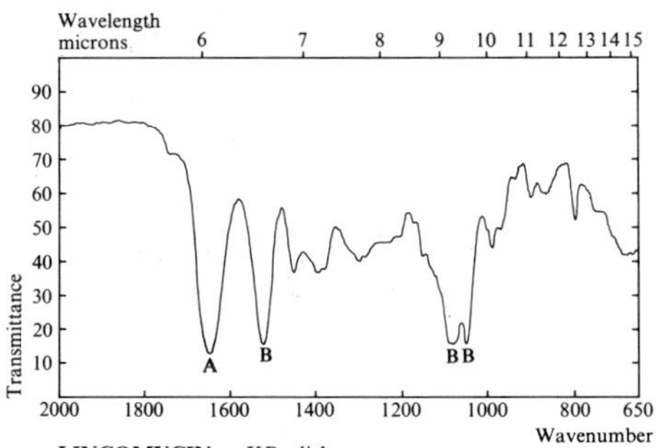

LINCOMYCIN — KBr disk
A 1645, B 1050 or 1075 or 1523

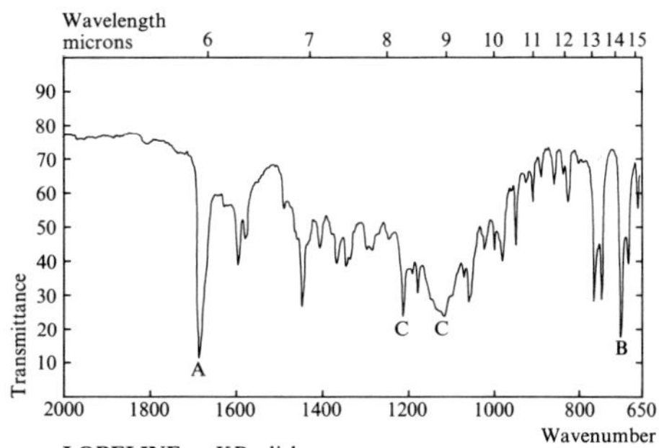

LOBELINE — KBr disk
A 1687, B 700, C 1115 or 1211

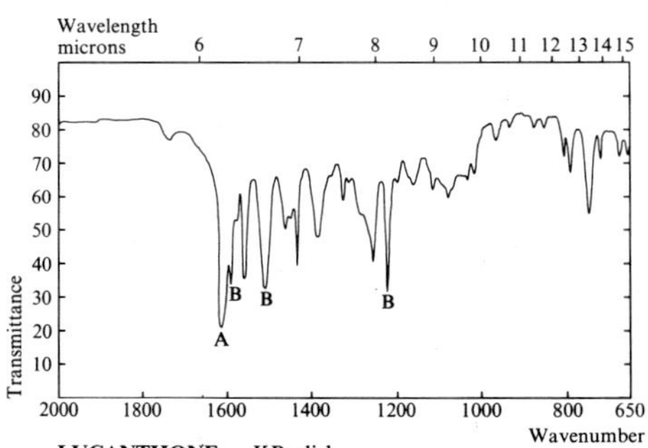

LUCANTHONE — KBr disk
A 1616, B 1224 or 1512 or 1591

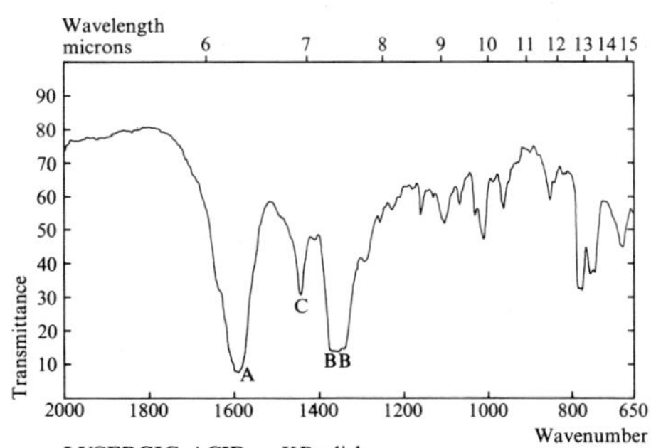

LYSERGIC ACID — KBr disk
A 1592, B 1352 or 1372, C 1445

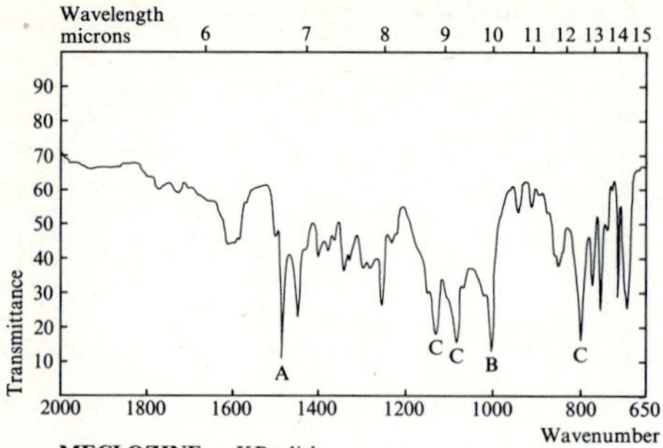

MECLOZINE — KBr disk
A 1489, B 1001, C 799 or 1081 or 1130

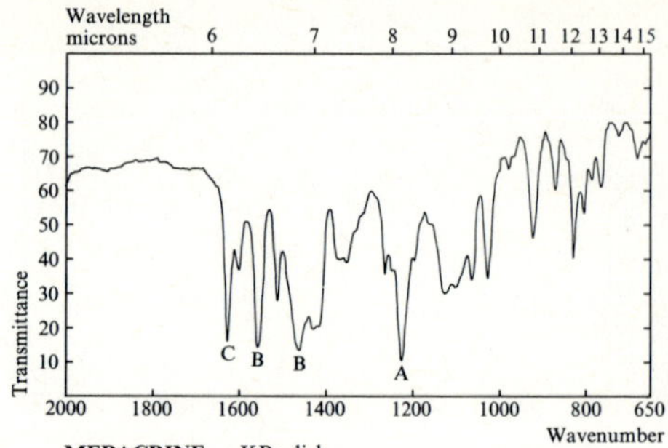

MEPACRINE — KBr disk
A 1225, B 1462 or 1557, C 1625

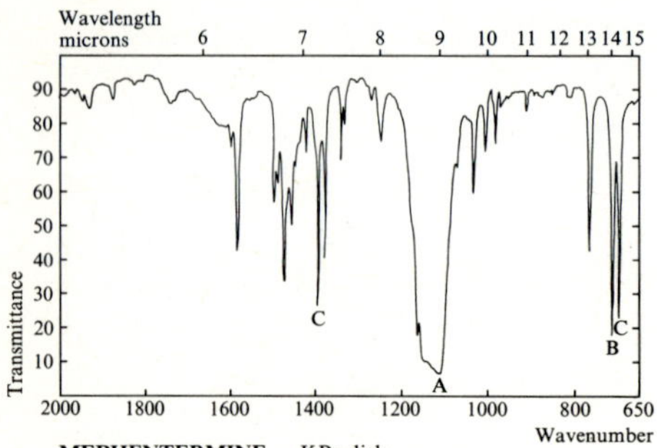

MEPHENTERMINE — KBr disk
A 1111, B 711, C 696 or 1394

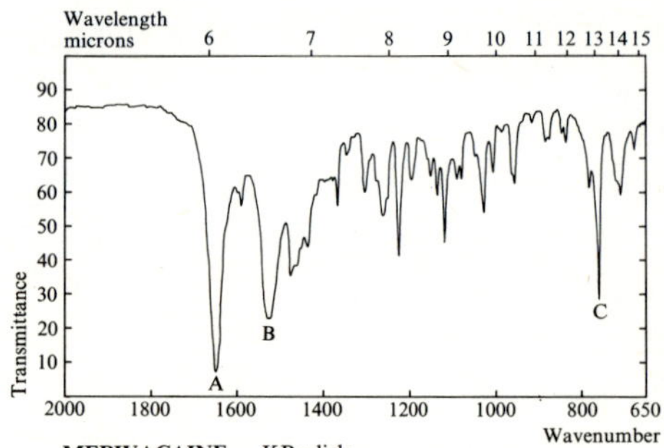

MEPIVACAINE — KBr disk
A 1650, B 1523, C 760

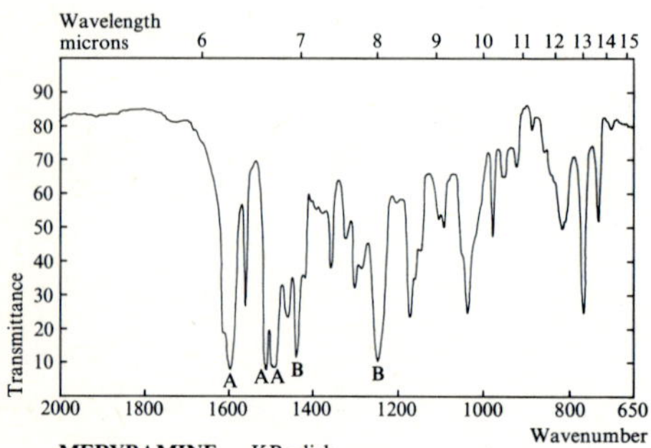

MEPYRAMINE — KBr disk
A 1490 or 1512 or 1598, B 1247 or 1441

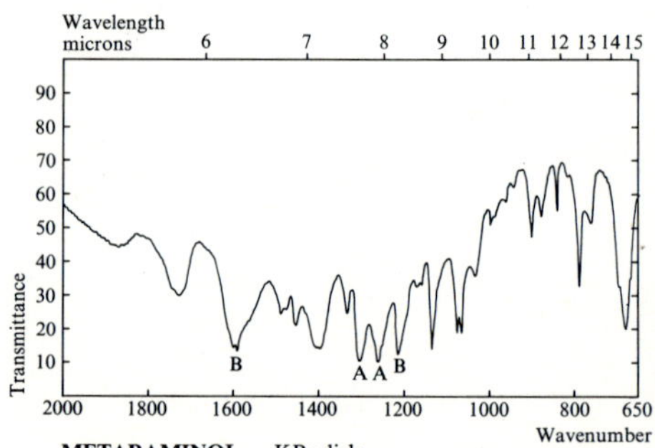

METARAMINOL — KBr disk
A 1263 or 1304, B 1216 or 1591

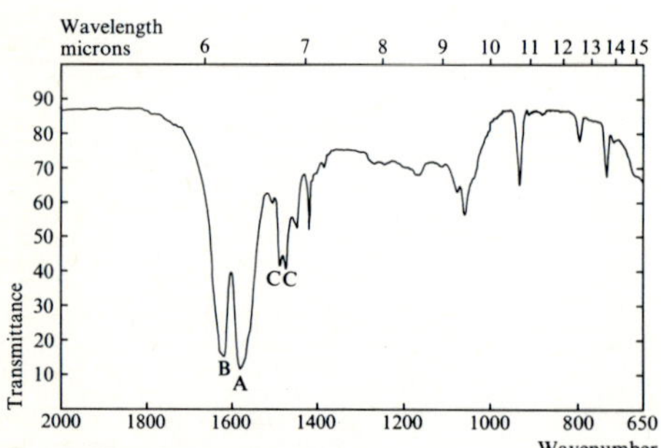

METFORMIN — KBr disk
A 1580, B 1620, C 1474 or 1487

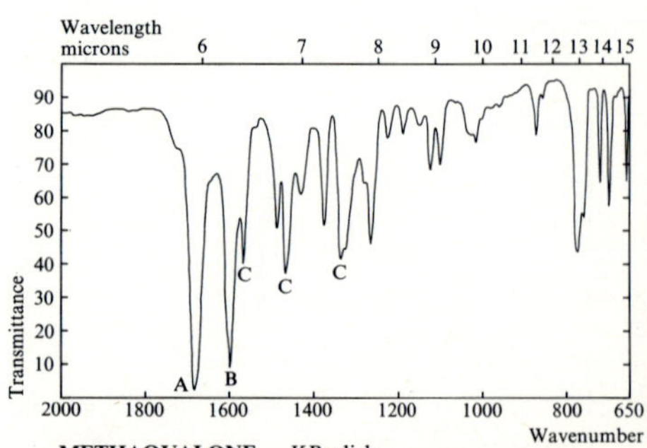

METHAQUALONE — KBr disk
A 1682, B 1599, C 1335 or 1465 or 1565

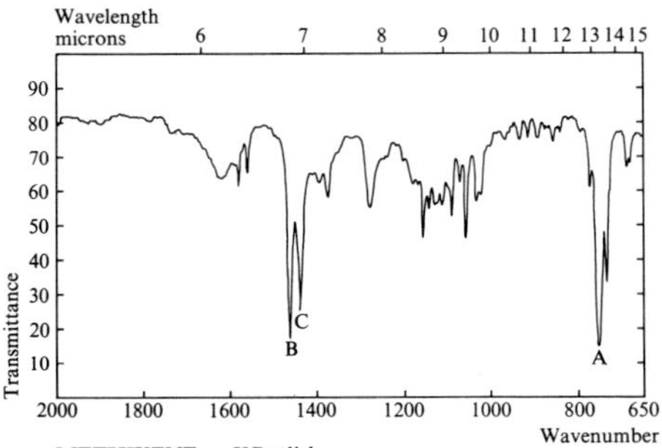

METHIXENE — KBr disk
A 750, B 1462, C 1439

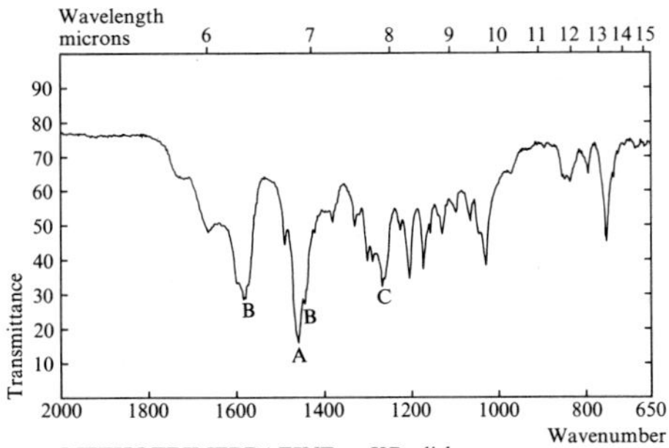

METHOTRIMEPRAZINE — KBr disk
A 1460, B 1446 or 1587, C 1269

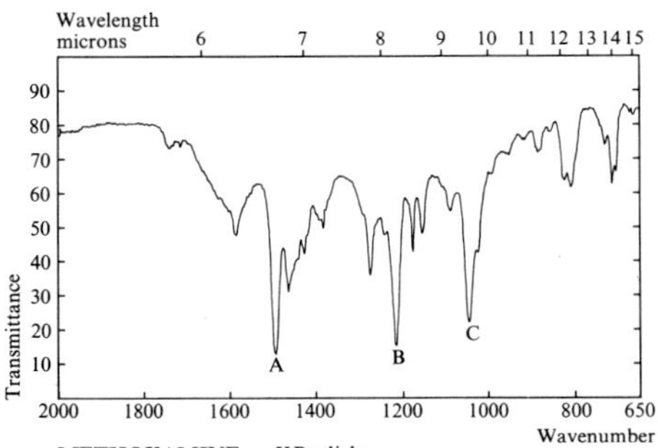

METHOXAMINE — KBr disk
A 1496, B 1215, C 1044

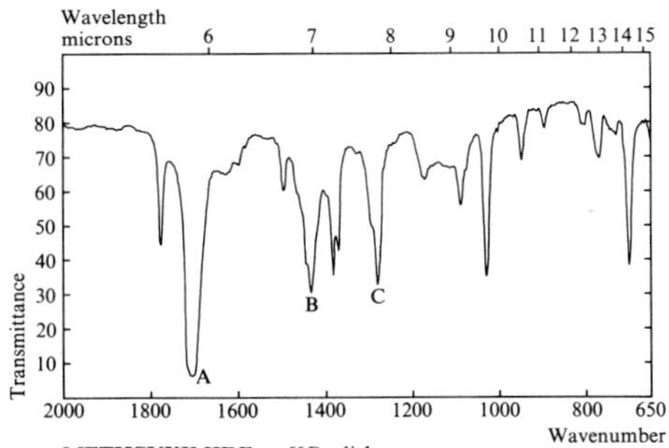

METHSUXIMIDE — KBr disk
A 1705, B 1435, C 1282

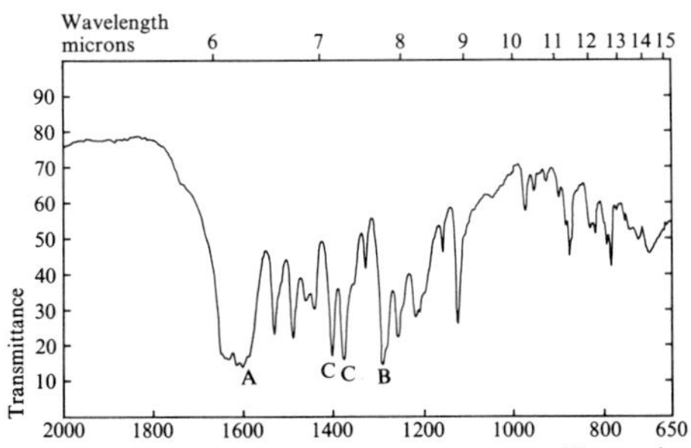

METHYLDOPA — KBr disk
A 1600, B 1288, C 1374 or 1402

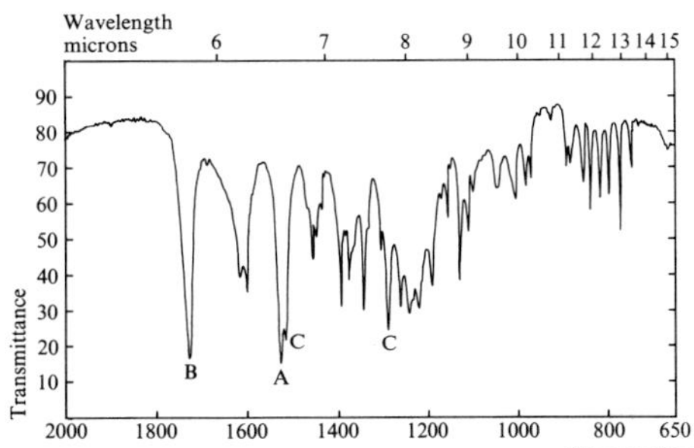

METHYLDOPATE — KBr disk
A 1527, B 1726, C 1290 or 1516

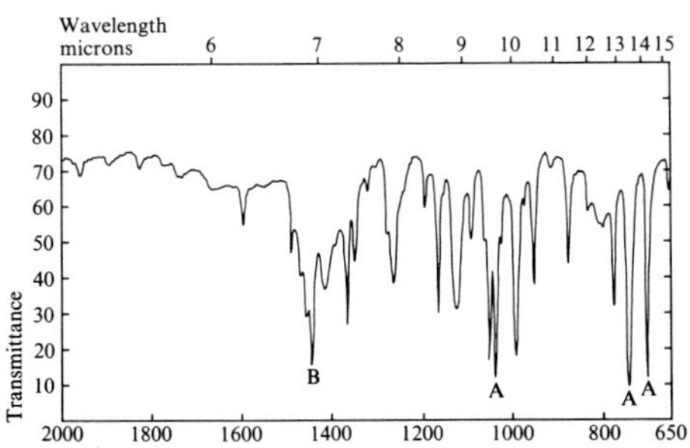

METHYLEPHEDRINE — KBr disk
A 702 or 742 or 1039, B 1447

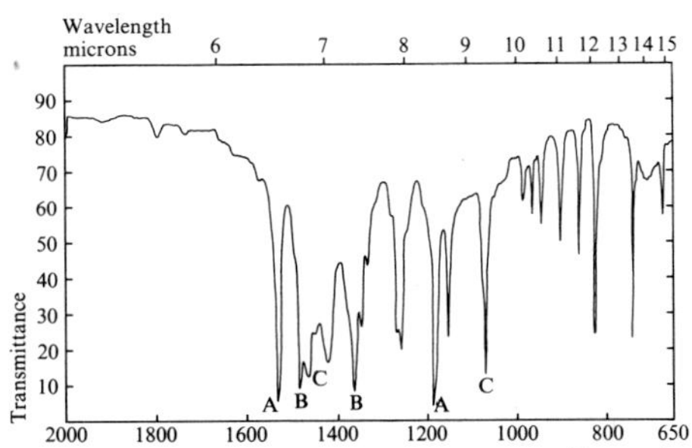

METRONIDAZOLE — KBr disk
A 1187 or 1535, B 1365 or 1485, C 1070 or 1467

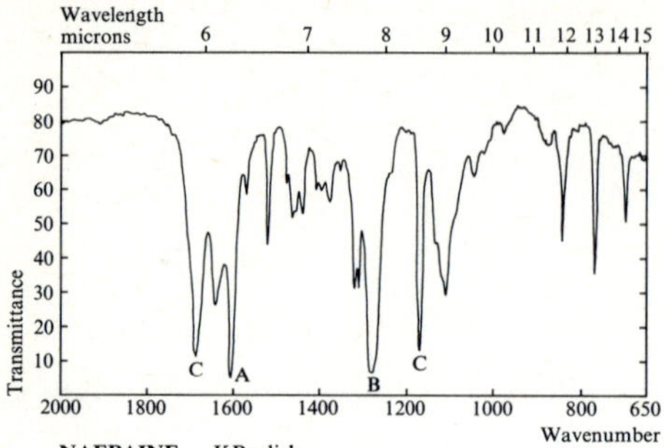

NAEPAINE — KBr disk
A 1605, B 1277, C 1170 or 1685

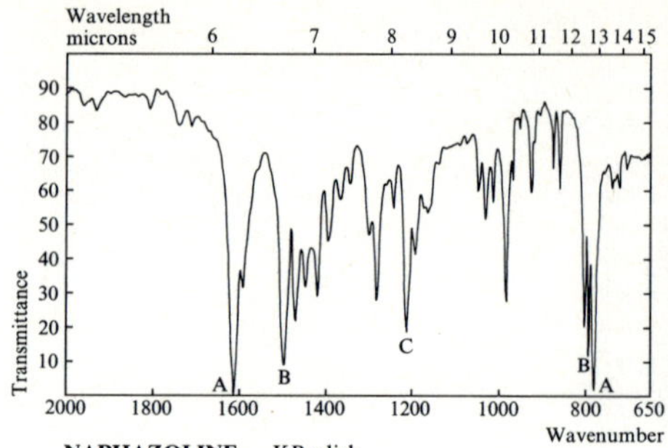

NAPHAZOLINE — KBr disk
A 780 or 1615, B 791 or 1499, C 1211

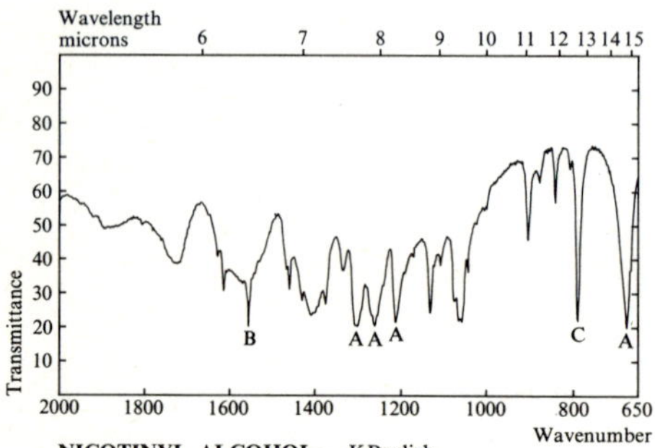

NICOTINYL ALCOHOL — KBr disk
A 675 or 1215 or 1262 or 1305, B 1556, C 788

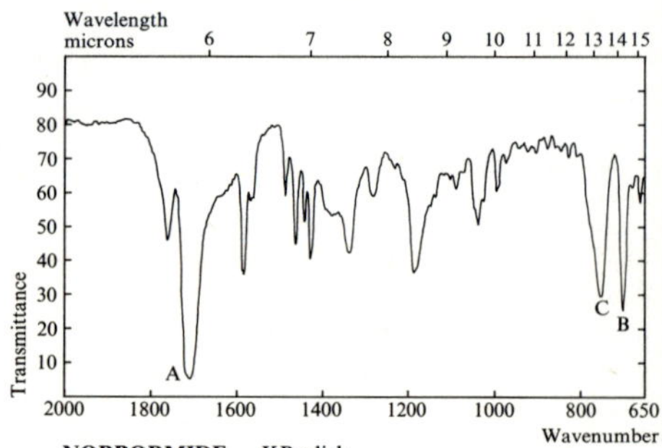

NORBORMIDE — KBr disk
A 1708, B 701, C 751

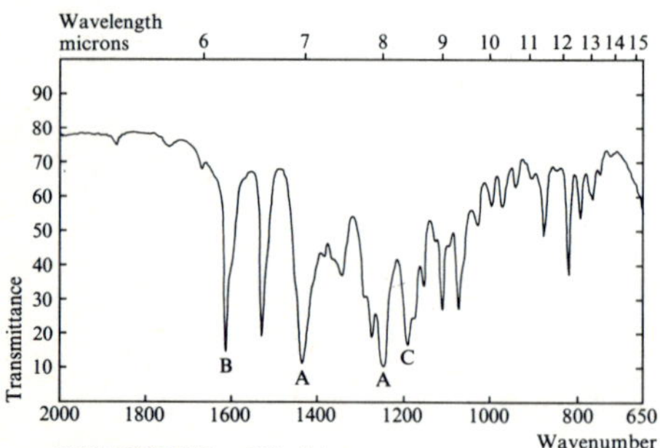

NORBUTRINE — KBr disk
A 1247 or 1437, B 1614, C 1192

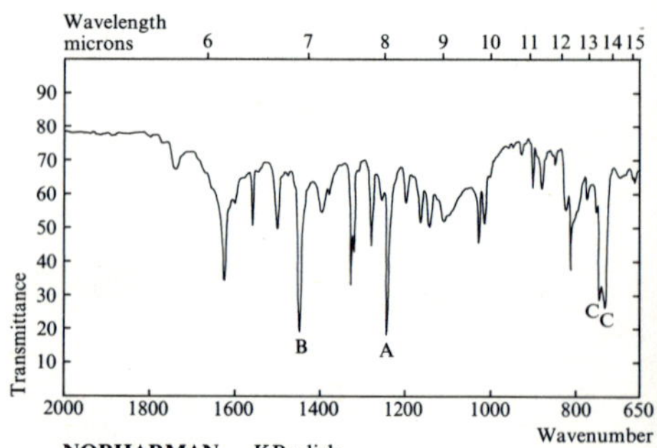

NORHARMAN — KBr disk
A 1247, B 1450, C 731 or 747

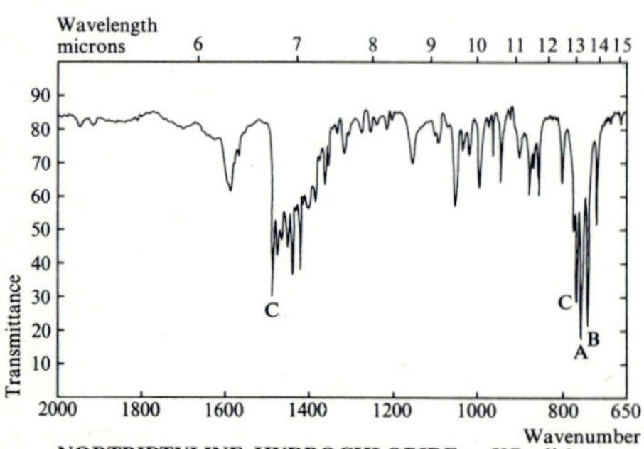

NORTRIPTYLINE HYDROCHLORIDE — KBr disk
A 756, B 742, C 768 or 1488

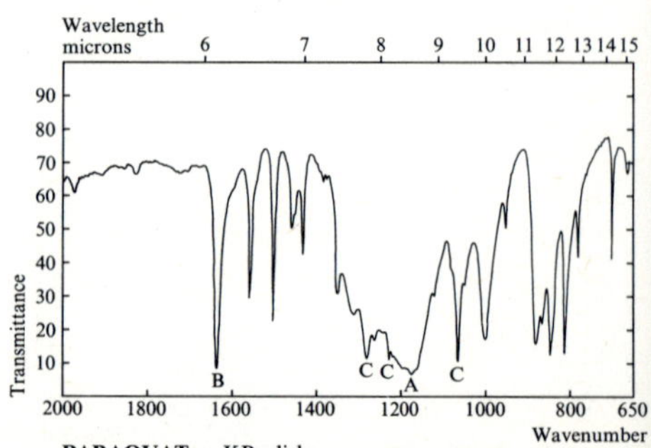

PARAQUAT — KBr disk
A 1174, B 1638, C 1064 or 1229 or 1284

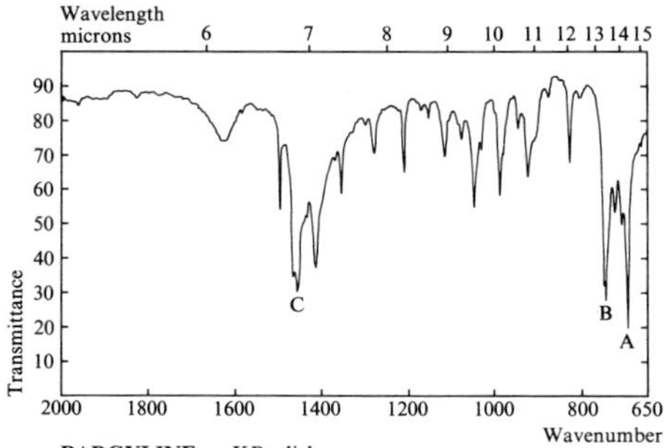

PARGYLINE — KBr disk
A 697, B 746, C 1458

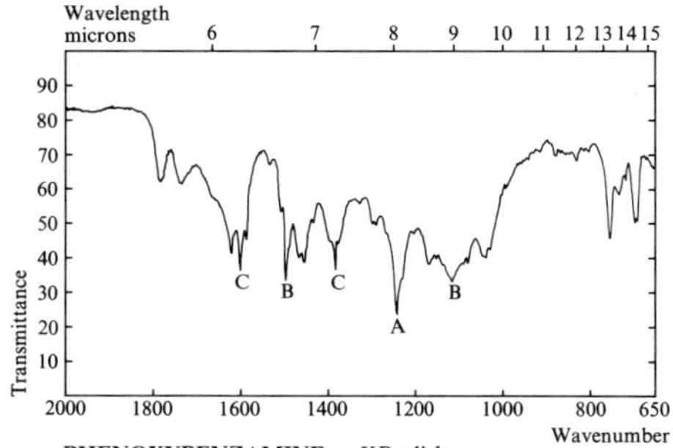

PHENOXYBENZAMINE — KBr disk
A 1242, B 1114 or 1497, C 1384 or 1600

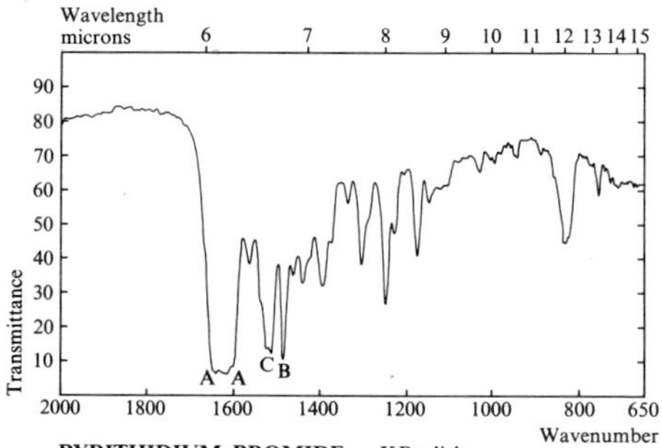

PYRITHIDIUM BROMIDE — KBr disk
A 1615 or 1642, B 1489, C 1515

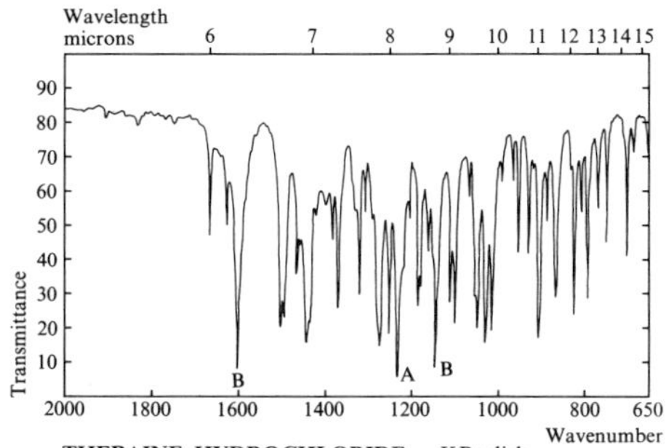

THEBAINE HYDROCHLORIDE — KBr disk
A 1234, B 1144 or 1605

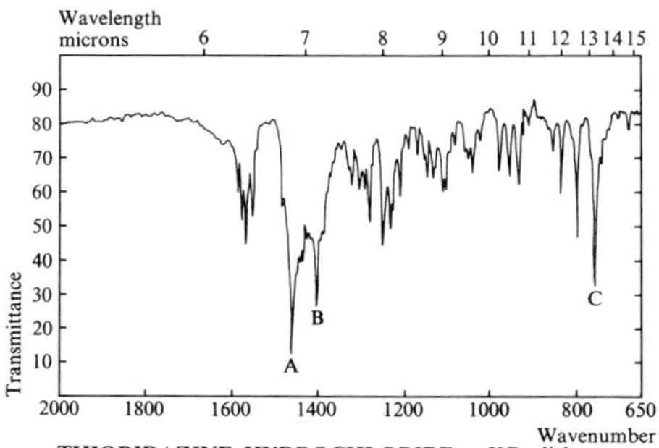

THIORIDAZINE HYDROCHLORIDE — KBr disk
A 1460, B 1402, C 755

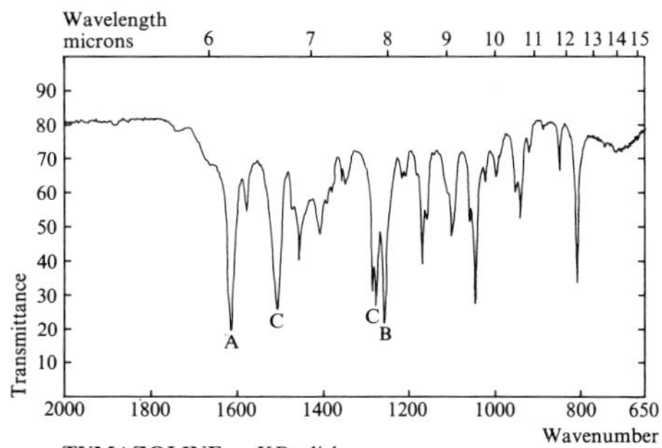

TYMAZOLINE — KBr disk
A 1617, B 1258, C 1279 or 1508

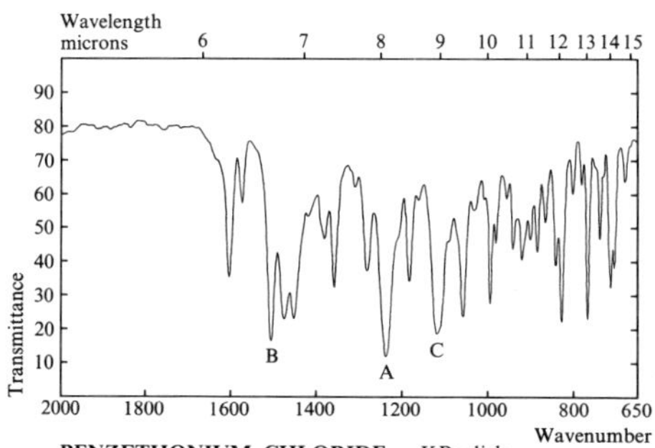

BENZETHONIUM CHLORIDE — KBr disk
A 1240, B 1505, C 1120

PART 4: Appendixes

Appendix 1: Reagents

The names of all the reagents listed and defined below are printed in *italic type* wherever they occur in descriptions of tests in the text of Part 2.

Acetate Buffer (pH 4·58): mix 25 ml of 1N hydrochloric acid with 50 ml of 1M sodium acetate and dilute to 250 ml with water.

Acetic Acid: Glacial Acetic Acid: contains not less than 99·0% w/w of $CH_3 \cdot CO_2H$.

Acetic Acid, Dilute: contains approximately 6% w/w of $CH_3 \cdot CO_2H$.

Acetic Acid Spray, 5% Aqueous: 5 volumes of *acetic acid* diluted to 100 volumes with water.

This spray is used as a location reagent in thin-layer chromatography—see System T16, p. 55.

Aluminium Chloride Solution: dissolve 35·9 g of anhydrous aluminium chloride in sufficient water to produce 100 ml, add 0·5 g of decolorising charcoal, stir for 10 minutes, filter, and add to the filtrate, with continuous stirring, sufficient of a 10% w/v solution of sodium hydroxide to adjust the pH to about 1·5.

Care should be exercised in dissolving the anhydrous aluminium chloride in the water.

Ammonia Solution, Dilute: dilute 37·5 ml of *strong ammonia solution* to 100 ml with water: contains about 10% w/w of NH_3.

Ammonia Solution, Strong: contains 27 to 35% of NH_3: weight per ml about 0·88 g.

Ammonium Thiocyanate Solution: dissolve 5 g of ammonium thiocyanate in sufficient water to produce 100 ml.

***p*-Anisaldehyde Spray:** dissolve 0·5 ml of *p*-anisaldehyde in 50 ml of *acetic acid* and 1 ml of *hydrochloric acid.*

This spray is used as a location reagent in thin-layer chromatography—see System T14, p. 54.

Antimony Pentachloride in Chloroform: pass dry chlorine gas into molten antimony trichloride: dissolve the resultant yellow fuming liquid in chloroform.

Beam's Reagent: dissolve 5 g of potassium hydroxide in sufficient ethanol to produce 100 ml. After spraying, heat locally.

This reagent is used as a location reagent in the thin-layer chromatographic detection of cannabidiol—see under Cannabis, p. 236.

Benzalkonium Chloride Solution: an aqueous solution containing 49 to 51% w/v of alkylbenzyldimethylammonium chlorides (see also p. 210).

Betanaphthol Spray, Alkaline: contains 4% w/v of betanaphthol in 2N sodium hydroxide.

This spray is used as a location reagent in paper and thin-layer chromatography, following *diazotisation* (p. 807) of the chromatographic paper or thin-layer plate.

Bicarbonate Buffer (pH 11): dissolve 8·401 g of sodium bicarbonate and 3·6 g of sodium hydroxide in sufficient water to produce 1000 ml.

Borate Buffer Solution: suspend 4 g of boric acid in 70 ml of water, add 27 ml of 1N sodium hydroxide, and dilute to 100 ml with water. pH about 9·5.

Borax Buffer (0·05M): dissolve 19·05 g of borax in sufficient water to produce 1000 ml. pH about 9·2 at 25°.

Bromine Solution: Bromine Water: a saturated solution of bromine in water.

Bromine–Starch–Potassium Iodide: as a location reagent in paper chromatography, expose the chromatographic paper to bromine vapour, allow the paper to hang in the air until almost all the bromine has evaporated (test a corner of the paper), then spray with a solution of starch (2% w/v of starch in water containing 1% of potassium iodide).

Bromocresol Green Spray: dissolve 0·5 g of bromocresol green in sufficient ethanol to produce 100 ml.

This spray is used as a location reagent in paper chromatography.

Bromocresol Purple Spray: dissolve 0·05 g of bromocresol purple in sufficient ethanol to produce 100 ml.

This spray is used as a location reagent in thin-layer chromatography—see System T23, p. 58.

Bromophenol Blue Spray: dissolve 0·05 g of bromophenol blue in 10 ml of acetone and dilute the solution to 100 ml with a 1% w/v solution of silver nitrate in acetone:water (1:3).

This spray is used as a location reagent in thin-layer chromatography—see System T16, p. 55.

Chloramine Solution: dissolve 4 g of chloramine-T in sufficient water to produce 100 ml.

Cobalt Thiocyanate Solution: dissolve 6·8 g of cobalt chloride and 4·3 g of ammonium thiocyanate in sufficient water to produce 100 ml.

Congo Red Spray: dissolve 0·4 g of congo red in sufficient of a solution of ethanol:water (1:1) to produce 100 ml.

This spray is used as a location reagent in paper chromatography—see System P11, p. 39.

Cyanogen Bromide Solution: add, drop by drop, a 10% w/v solution of potassium cyanide in water to *bromine solution* until the colour disappears.

This solution must be freshly prepared.

***o*-Dianisidine Spray, Diazotised:** dissolve 2 g of *o*-dianisidine in 1000 ml of 1N hydrochloric acid, leave overnight, filter, and mix 25 ml of this solution with

1·5 ml of a 5% solution of sodium nitrite in water. After 5 minutes, add 25 ml of 2M potassium phosphate solution.

This spray is used as a location reagent in paper chromatography—see System P8, p. 38.

2,6-Dichlorophenolindophenol Solution: warm 0·1 g of 2,6-dichlorophenolindophenol sodium salt with 100 ml of water and filter.

This solution must not be used later than 3 days after preparation.

***p*-Dimethylaminobenzaldehyde Spray:** dissolve 1 g of *p*-dimethylaminobenzaldehyde in 100 ml of ethanol and add 10 ml of *hydrochloric acid.*

This spray is used as a location reagent in paper and thin-layer chromatography.

Dimethylformamide–Sodium Acetate Trihydrate Solution: mix 50 ml of dimethylformamide with sufficient water to produce 500 ml and dilute 10 ml of this solution to 100 ml with a solution containing 1·8% w/v of sodium acetate and 0·14% v/v of *acetic acid* (this amount of solution is sufficient for dissolving up to 50 mg of nitrofurantoin).

Disodium Methyl Arsonate Solution: dissolve 5 g of disodium methyl arsonate in sufficient water to produce 100 ml.

Dithizone Solution: dissolve 3·75 mg of 1,5-diphenylthiocarbazone in sufficient chloroform to produce 100 ml.

DPST Solution: mix 1 volume of a 0·1% w/v solution of 2,5-diphenyl-3-(4-styrylphenyl)tetrazolium chloride in ethanol with 9 volumes of 2N sodium hydroxide immediately before use.

This solution is used as a location reagent in paper chromatography—see System P13, p. 40.

DPST Spray: dilute 5 ml of a 0·5% w/v solution of 2,5-diphenyl-3-(4-styrylphenyl)tetrazolium chloride in ethanol to 50 ml with 2N sodium hydroxide immediately before use.

This spray is used as a location reagent in thin-layer chromatography—see System T18, p. 56.

Dragendorff Spray: (a) mix together 2 g of bismuth subnitrate, 25 ml of *acetic acid*, and 100 ml of water; (b) dissolve 40 g of potassium iodide in 100 ml of water. Mix together 10 ml of (a), 10 ml of (b), 20 ml of *acetic acid*, and 100 ml of water.

This spray is used as a general location reagent for nitrogenous bases in paper and thin-layer chromatography.

Duquenois Spray: (a) dissolve 0·8 g of vanillin and 1 ml of acetaldehyde in 40 ml of ethanol (this solution is unstable and should be prepared immediately before use); (b) *hydrochloric acid.* Spray with (a) and then with (b).

This spray may be used as a location reagent in the thin-layer chromatographic detection of cannabidiol.

Ferric Chloride Solution: a 5% w/v solution of ferric chloride in water.

Ferric Chloride Spray: as for *ferric chloride solution*, p. 799.

This spray is used as a location reagent in paper chromatography—see System P12, p. 39.

Ferrous Sulphate Solution: a 2% w/v solution of ferrous sulphate in freshly boiled and cooled water.

This solution must be freshly prepared.

Fluorescein Spray: mix 10 ml of a saturated solution of fluorescein in *acetic acid* with 15 ml of *acetic acid* and 25 ml of *strong hydrogen peroxide solution.*

This spray must be freshly prepared.

It is used as a location reagent in thin-layer chromatography—see System T10, p. 52.

Folin–Ciocalteu Reagent: *Stock Solution*: dissolve 100 g of sodium tungstate and 25 g of sodium molybdate in 800 ml of water in a 1500-ml flask, add 50 ml of *phosphoric acid* and 100 ml of *hydrochloric acid* and reflux for 10 hours. Cool, add 150 g of lithium sulphate, 50 ml of water, and 4 to 6 drops of bromine, and allow to stand for 2 hours. Boil for 15 minutes to remove the excess of bromine, cool, filter, and dilute to 1000 ml with water.

This stock solution should be stored at a temperature not exceeding 4° and used within 4 months of its preparation; it has a golden-yellow colour and must not be used if any trace of green colour is present.

For use, dilute 1 volume of this stock solution with 2 volumes of water.

Formaldehyde Solution: Formalin: an aqueous solution containing 34 to 38% w/w of formaldehyde.

Forrest Reagent: mix together 25 ml of a 0·2% w/v solution of potassium dichromate in water, 25 ml of 30% w/w sulphuric acid, 25 ml of 20% w/w perchloric acid, and 25 ml of 50% w/w nitric acid.

FPN Reagent: mix together 5 ml of a 5% w/v solution of ferric chloride in water, 45 ml of 20% w/w perchloric acid, and 50 ml of 50% w/w nitric acid.

FPN Spray: as for *FPN reagent* (above).

This spray is used as a location reagent in paper chromatography.

Furfural–Hydrochloric Acid Spray: as a location reagent in paper chromatography, spray furfural very lightly on the paper, then spray more heavily with *hydrochloric acid.*

Gold Bromide Solution: dissolve 5 g of gold chloride and 5 g of sodium bromide in sufficient water to produce 100 ml.

Gold Bromide–Hydrochloric Acid Solution: dissolve 5 g of gold chloride and 5 g of sodium bromide in sufficient *hydrochloric acid* to produce 100 ml.

Gold Chloride Solution: dissolve 5 g of gold chloride in sufficient water to produce 100 ml.

Gold Cyanide Solution: dissolve 5 g of gold chloride in 100 ml of water and add solid sodium cyanide until the precipitate first formed redissolves.

Hydrochloric Acid: Concentrated: contains 35 to 38% w/w of HCl.

Hydrogen Peroxide Solution, Strong: 100 volume: contains 26 to 28% w/w of H_2O_2 in water.

Iodine Vapour: warm iodine crystals in a large beaker on a water-bath. As a location reagent in paper chromatography, hang the paper in the vapour.

Iodine–Carbon Tetrachloride Spray: dissolve 1 g of iodine in sufficient carbon tetrachloride to produce 100 ml.

This spray is used as a location reagent in thin-layer chromatography.

Iodobismuthous Acid Solution: mix 40 mg of bismuth carbonate with 0·5 ml of 1N sulphuric acid and add 5 ml of a 10% w/v solution of potassium iodide, 1 ml of 1N sulphuric acid, and 25 ml of water.

Iodoplatinate Spray: dissolve 0·25 g of platinic chloride and 5 g of potassium iodide in sufficient water to produce 100 ml.

This spray is used as a general location reagent for nitrogenous bases in paper and thin-layer chromatography.

NOTE. With thin-layer systems employing alkaline buffered plates or alkaline solvents, *acidified iodoplatinate spray* (see below) must be used.

Iodoplatinate Spray, Acidified: add 2 ml of *hydrochloric acid* to 100 ml of *iodoplatinate spray* (above).

Iodoplatinate Spray, Strongly Acid: mix together 1 ml of a 5% w/v platinic chloride solution, 9 ml of a 10% sodium iodide solution, 2 ml of water, and 3 ml of *hydrochloric acid.*

This spray is used as a location reagent for certain weak bases in thin-layer chromatography.

Lead Acetate Solution: dissolve 10 g of lead acetate in sufficient water to produce 100 ml.

Lead Iodide Solution: adjust a 30% w/v solution of potassium acetate in water to pH 6 with 2N acetic acid and saturate with lead iodide.

Liebermann's Reagent: dissolve 10 g of potassium nitrite in sufficient *sulphuric acid* to produce 100 ml.

Marquis Reagent (for chromatography): mix 1 ml of *formaldehyde solution* with 10 ml of *sulphuric acid.*

This location reagent is not sprayed; it must be poured over the chromatographic paper or thin-layer plate.

Marquis Reagent (for colour tests): mix 2 drops of *formaldehyde solution* with 1 ml of *sulphuric acid.*

Mercuric Bicarbonate Solution (400 μg of mercuric ions per ml): dissolve 0·5 g of mercuric chloride in 50 ml of water with 3 drops of *nitric acid.* Dilute 1 ml of this solution to 25 ml with water and add 0·42 g of sodium bicarbonate.

Mercuric Chloride Solution: dissolve 5 g of mercuric chloride in sufficient water to produce 100 ml.

Mercuric Nitrate Solution: dissolve 40 g of mercuric oxide (red or yellow) in a mixture of 32 ml of *nitric acid* and 15 ml of water.

Store in glass containers protected from light.

Mercurous Nitrate Spray: a saturated solution of mercurous nitrate in water.

This spray is used as a location reagent in thin-layer chromatography—see Systems T10 and T11, p. 52.

Millon's Reagent: dissolve 3 ml of mercury in 27 ml of cold *fuming nitric acid* and dilute the solution with an equal volume of water.

As a location reagent in paper chromatography, it is not sprayed but must be poured over the paper.

***N*-1-Naphthylethylenediamine Spray:** dissolve 100 mg of *N*-1-naphthylethylenediamine dihydrochloride in sufficient ethanol to produce 100 ml.

This spray is used as a location reagent in paper and thin-layer chromatography following *diazotisation* (p. 807).

Nessler's Reagent: dissolve 3·5 g of potassium iodide and 1·25 g of mercuric chloride in 80 ml of water and add a cold saturated solution of mercuric chloride in water, with constant stirring, until a slight red precipitate remains; dissolve 12 g of sodium hydroxide in this solution and add a little more of the saturated solution of mercuric chloride and sufficient water to produce 100 ml; allow to stand, and decant the clear liquid.

Ninhydrin Spray: dissolve 0·5 g of ninhydrin in sufficient acetone to produce 100 ml.

This spray is used as a location reagent in paper chromatography. The paper is lightly sprayed, then heated in an oven at 100° for 5 minutes.

Nitric Acid: Concentrated: contains 69 to 71% w/w of HNO_3.

Nitric Acid, Fuming: contains not less than 95% w/w of HNO_3.

***p*-Nitroaniline Solution, Diazotised:** dissolve 0·4 g of *p*-nitroaniline in 60 ml of 1N hydrochloric acid, cool to 15°, and add a 10% w/v solution of sodium nitrite in water until one drop of the mixture turns *starch-iodide paper* blue.

This solution must be freshly prepared.

***p*-Nitroaniline Spray, Diazotised:** (a) mix, immediately before spraying, 25 ml of a 0·3% w/v solution of *p*-nitroaniline in 8% w/v hydrochloric acid with 1·5 ml of a 5% w/v solution of sodium nitrite in water; (b) a 20% solution of sodium carbonate in water. Spray successively with (a) and (b).

This spray is used as a location reagent in paper chromatography—see System P15, p. 41.

***p*-Nitroaniline–Sodium Hydroxide Spray, Diazotised:** (i) solution as for (a) in *diazotised* p-*nitroaniline spray* (above); (ii) a 20% w/v solution of sodium hydroxide in ethanol:water (1:1). Spray successively with (i) and (ii).

This spray is used as a location reagent in paper and thin-layer chromatography.

Nitrogen Dioxide Vapour: produced by the action of nitric acid on copper turnings. For location in paper or thin-layer chromatography the paper or thin-layer plate is exposed to the nitrous fumes given off.

Palladium Chloride Spray: dissolve 0·5 g of palladium chloride in 100 ml of water, acidified to pH 3 with 2 or 3 drops of *hydrochloric acid.*

This spray is used as a location reagent in thin-layer chromatography—see System T15, p. 54.

Pauly's Reagent: used as a location reagent on paper chromatograms: mix 10 ml of a 1% w/v solution of sulphanilamide in 1N hydrochloric acid with 10 ml of a 5% w/v solution of sodium nitrite in water; allow to stand 1 minute, add 80 ml of n-butanol, and shake; separate the layers and spray the paper with the aqueous phase; allow to dry, and spray with a 10% w/v solution of sodium carbonate in water.

Perchloric Acid Spray: add 15 ml of 72% w/w perchloric acid to sufficient water to produce 100 ml.

This spray is used as a location reagent in thin-layer chromatography—see System T14, p. 54.

Phosphate Buffer (pH 4·5): dissolve 1·361 g of potassium dihydrogen phosphate in about 75 ml of water, adjust the pH to 4·5 ± 0·1 by the addition of 0·1N potassium hydroxide, and dilute to 100 ml with water.

Phosphate Buffer (pH 6·95): dissolve 0·624 g of disodium hydrogen phosphate dihydrate and 0·363 g of potassium dihydrogen phosphate in sufficient water to produce 100 ml.

Phosphate Buffer (pH 7·0): mix 50 ml of 0·2M potassium dihydrogen phosphate with 29·63 ml of 0·2N sodium hydroxide and dilute with water to 200 ml.

Phosphate Buffer (pH 7·4): (a) dissolve 9·465 g of anhydrous disodium hydrogen phosphate in water and dilute to 1000 ml; (b) dissolve 9·073 g of potassium dihydrogen phosphate in water and dilute to 1000 ml. Mix 80 ml of (a) with 20 ml of (b) to obtain a solution of pH 7·4.

Phosphoric Acid: contains 88 to 90% w/w of H_3PO_4.

Picric Acid: Trinitrophenol Solution: a saturated solution of picric acid in water.

Picrolonic Acid: a saturated solution of picrolonic acid in water.

Platinic Bromide Solution: dissolve 5 g of platinic chloride and 10 g of sodium bromide in sufficient water to produce 100 ml.

Platinic Chloride Solution: dissolve 5 g of platinic chloride in sufficient water to produce 100 ml.

Platinic Iodide Solution: dissolve 5 g of platinic chloride and 25 g of sodium iodide in sufficient water to produce 100 ml.

Potassium Bismuth Iodide Solution: dissolve 5 g of bismuth subnitrate and 25 g of potassium iodide in sufficient 2% w/w sulphuric acid to produce 100 ml.

Potassium Cadmium Iodide Solution: dissolve 1 g of cadmium iodide and 2 g of potassium iodide in sufficient water to produce 100 ml.

Potassium Chromate Solution: dissolve 5 g of potassium chromate in sufficient water to produce 100 ml.

Potassium Cupri-tartrate Solution: Fehling's Solution: (a) dissolve 34·64 g of copper sulphate in a mixture of 0·5 ml of *sulphuric acid* and sufficient water to produce 500 ml; (b) dissolve 176 g of sodium potassium tartrate and 77 g of sodium hydroxide in sufficient water to produce 500 ml. Mix equal volumes of solutions (a) and (b) immediately before use.

Potassium Cyanide Solution: dissolve 5 g of potassium cyanide in sufficient water to produce 100 ml.

Potassium Dichromate Solution, Acidified: dissolve 10 g of potassium dichromate in sufficient *dilute sulphuric acid* to produce 100 ml.

Potassium Ferrocyanide–Hydrochloric Acid Solution: mix equal volumes of 0·5N hydrochloric acid and a 1% solution of potassium ferrocyanide in water.

Potassium Iodide Solution: dissolve 5 g of potassium iodide in sufficient water to produce 100 ml.

Potassium Mercuric Iodide Solution: dissolve 1·5 g of mercuric chloride and 5 g of potassium iodide in sufficient water to produce 100 ml.

Potassium Permanganate Reagent, Acidified: dissolve 15 g of potassium permanganate and 75 ml of *phosphoric acid* in water and add sufficient water to produce 500 ml.

Potassium Permanganate Solution: mix 2 g of potassium permanganate with 5 drops of *phosphoric acid* and add sufficient water to produce 100 ml.

Potassium Permanganate Spray: dissolve 1 g of potassium permanganate in sufficient water to produce 100 ml.

This spray is used as a location reagent in paper and thin-layer chromatography.

It should be protected from light.

Potassium Tri-iodide Solution (1): dissolve 2 g of iodine and 4 g of potassium iodide in sufficient water to produce 100 ml.

Potassium Tri-iodide Solution (2): dissolve 0·1 g of iodine and 0·2 g of potassium iodide in sufficient water to produce 100 ml.

Potassium Tri-iodide Solution (3): dissolve 1 g of iodine and 50 g of potassium iodide in sufficient water to produce 100 ml.

Schiff's Reagent: dissolve 0·2 g of basic fuchsin in 120 ml of hot water, cool, and add 20 ml of a 10% w/v solution of sodium hydrogen sulphite and 2 ml of *hydrochloric acid*; dilute to 200 ml.

Store in the cold, protected from light.

Silver Ammonio-nitrate Solution: dissolve 2·5 g of silver nitrate in 80 ml of water and cautiously add *dilute ammonia solution* until the precipitate first formed is nearly dissolved; allow to stand, decant the clear liquid, and to it add sufficient water to produce 100 ml.

This solution should be freshly prepared.

Silver Nitrate Spray: (a) a 0·5% w/v solution of silver nitrate in methanol; (b) methanol:*strong ammonia solution* (9:1); (c) a 5% w/v solution of sodium hydroxide in methanol. Mix (a), (b), and (c) in the ratio 5:1:2.

This spray must be freshly prepared.

It is used as a location reagent in paper chromatography—see System P3, p. 35.

Sodium Carbonate Solution: dissolve 5 g of sodium carbonate in sufficient water to produce 100 ml.

Sodium Dithionite Solution, Alkaline: dissolve 1 g of sodium dithionite in sufficient 2N sodium hydroxide to produce 100 ml.

Sodium Naphthaquinone Spray: spray lightly with 0·1N sodium hydroxide then with a saturated solution of sodium 1,2-naphthaquinone-4-sulphonate in ethanol:water (1:1).

This spray is used as a location reagent in paper chromatography—see System P16, p. 41.

Sodium Nitroprusside Solution: dissolve 1 g of sodium nitroprusside in sufficient water to produce 100 ml.

Sodium Phosphate Solution: dissolve 5 g of disodium hydrogen phosphate in sufficient water to produce 100 ml.

Solution of Standard pH 2·0: mix 50 ml of 0·2M potassium chloride with 10·6 ml of 0·2N hydrochloric acid and dilute with freshly boiled and cooled water to 200 ml.

Starch Mucilage: triturate 0·5 g of starch, or 0·5 g of soluble starch, with 5 ml of water and add this, with constant stirring, to sufficient water to produce about 100 ml. Boil for a few minutes, cool, and filter.

Starch Mucilage must be freshly prepared.

Starch-iodide Paper: impregnate unglazed white paper with *starch mucilage* diluted with an equal volume of a 0·4% w/v solution of potassium iodide in water.

Styphnic Acid: dissolve 5 g of styphnic acid in sufficient water to produce 100 ml.

Sulphanilic Acid Spray, Diazotised: mix 25 ml of a 0·45% w/v solution of sulphanilic acid in 1N hydrochloric acid with 1·5 ml of a 5% w/v solution of sodium nitrite in water, allow to stand for 5 minutes, add 25 ml of 2M sodium carbonate solution, and shake. For location in paper chromatography (System P8, p. 38), spray the paper immediately with this solution and, 15 to 30 minutes later, spray with 3N hydrochloric acid; the spots may change colour or disappear.

Sulphuric Acid: Concentrated: contains 97 to 98% w/w of H_2SO_4.

Sulphuric Acid, Dilute: 2N: mix 104 g of *sulphuric acid* with 896 g of water and cool. The acid should be added gradually to the water.

Sulphuric Acid Spray, 50%: mix equal volumes of *sulphuric acid* and water, and cool. The acid should be added gradually to the water.

This spray is used as a location reagent in thin-layer chromatography—see System T20, p. 56.

Sulphuric Acid Spray, 0·2M: add gradually 1·98 g of *sulphuric acid* to 80 ml of water, cool, and adjust to 100 ml with water.

This spray is used as a location reagent in thin-layer chromatography—see Systems T21a, 21b, and 21c, p. 57.

Sulphuric Acid–Ethanol Spray: add gradually 2 volumes of *sulphuric acid* to 2 volumes of water; cool, then add 1 volume of ethanol.

This spray is used as a location reagent in thin-layer chromatography—see System T3, p. 47.

Titanous Chloride Solution: a 15% w/v solution of titanous chloride, $TiCl_3$, in 10% w/w hydrochloric acid.

Trinder's Reagent: dissolve 4 g of mercuric chloride in 85 ml of water with the aid of heat, cool, and add 12 ml of 1N hydrochloric acid and 4 g of ferric nitrate. When the ferric nitrate has dissolved, adjust the volume to 100 ml with water.

Trinitrobenzoic Acid Solution: a saturated solution of trinitrobenzoic acid in water.

Vanillin in Sulphuric Acid Solution: a 1% w/v solution of vanillin in *sulphuric acid.*

Zinc Chloride Solution: dissolve 5 g of zinc chloride in sufficient water to produce 100 ml.

Zwikker's Reagent Spray: mix 40 ml of a 10% w/v solution of copper sulphate in water with 10 ml of pyridine and add sufficient water to produce 100 ml.

This spray is used as a location reagent for barbiturates in thin-layer chromatography—see System T10, p. 52.

Appendix 2: Tests

The tests listed below are those mentioned in Parts 1 and 2. Details will be found on the pages indicated.

Alkaline Cobalt Test: Zwikker's Test (q.v.).

Alphanaphthol–Sodium Nitrite Test (Diazotisation: as a screening test for paracetamol and phenacetin), pp. 5 and 14.

Amalic Acid Test (for xanthine derivatives), p. 127.

Ammonium Molybdate Test: Fröhde's Test (for alkaloids and other nitrogenous bases), p. 133.

Ammonium Vanadate Test: Mandelin's Test (for alkaloids and other nitrogenous bases), p. 133.

Chen's Test (for adrenaline–ephedrine type drugs), p. 131.

Chromotropic Acid Test (for formaldehyde and methanol), p. 6.

Clarke–Kalayci Test. A location test for xanthine derivatives on paper chromatograms. Locate the spot on the paper chromatogram by examination under ultraviolet light and then expose to *bromine vapour* for 2 minutes; hold the paper in the steam over a boiling water-bath for 1 minute and heat the paper for five minutes in an oven at about 110° to 120°. Finally, expose the paper to ammonia vapour—a purple spot is formed. To avoid the use of large quantities of bromine it is advisable to cut out the section of paper containing the spot (Clarke and Kalayci, 1963).

Cobalt Acetate–Lithium Hydroxide Test: Zwikker's Test (q.v.).

Copper Sulphate Test (for sulphonamides), p. 131.

Diazotisation Test (for compounds containing a primary aromatic amino-group), p. 133.

In chromatography **diazotisation** is carried out as follows. Expose the chromatographic paper or thin-layer plate to *nitrogen dioxide vapour* (p. 803) and then spray with either *alkaline betanaphthol spray* (p. 797) or N-*1-naphthylethylenediamine spray* (p. 802).

Dichromate Test (screening test for alcohols etc.), pp. 4 and 6.

***p*-Dimethylaminobenzaldehyde Test,** p. 130.

Ethanol–Furfural Test (screening test for carbamates), p. 13.

Ethanolic Phloroglucinol–Hydrochloric Acid Test (screening test for ethchlorvynol), p. 12.

Ferric Chloride Test (for phenols and related compounds), pp. 4, 8, and 129.

Fluorescein–Hydrogen Peroxide Test (screening test for carbromal), p. 10.

Forrest Test (screening test for imipramine, trimipramine, etc.), pp. 4 and 13.

FPN Test (screening test for phenothiazines), pp. 4 and 10.

Fröhde's Test: Ammonium Molybdate Test (q.v.).

Fujiwara's Test (for certain trichloro-substituted hydrocarbons), pp. 4, 15, and 128.

Iodoform Test (for ethanol, acetaldehyde, etc.), pp. 6 and 132.

Mandelin's Test: Ammonium Vanadate Test (q.v.).

Marquis Test: Sulphuric Acid–Formaldehyde Test (q.v.).

McNally's Test (for salicylates), p. 131.

Paraformaldehyde–Phosphoric Acid Test (for solanine and solanidine), p. 132. This test may also be used to detect solanine and solanidine on paper chromatograms (Clarke, 1958): dissolve 1 g of paraformaldehyde in 100 ml of phosphoric acid.

Rothera's Test (screening test for ketones), p. 4.

Sulphuric Acid–Formaldehyde Test: Marquis Test (for alkaloids and other nitrogenous bases), p. 133.

Sulphuric Acid Tests—see pp. 123 to 125.

Thalleioquin Test (for quinine alkaloids), p. 131.

Vitali's Test (for alkaloids and other nitrogenous bases), p. 133.

Wintergreen Test (for alcohols or salicylates), p. 6.

Zwikker's Test: Alkaline Cobalt Test; Cobalt Acetate–Lithium Hydroxide Test (for barbiturates), pp. 9, 132, and 208.

Proprietary Test Materials

Clinistix: reagent strips impregnated with a buffered mixture of glucose oxidase, peroxidase, and *o*-tolidine; for the detection of glucose in urine.

Marketed by Ames Co. Division of Miles Laboratories Ltd, Stoke Poges, Bucks.

Dextrostix: reagent strips impregnated with a buffered mixture of glucose oxidase, peroxidase, and a chromogen system, and coated with a semi-permeable membrane; for the approximate estimation of glucose in blood.

Marketed by Ames Co. Division of Miles Laboratories Ltd, Stoke Poges, Bucks.

Ketostix: reagent strips impregnated with a buffered mixture of sodium nitroprusside and glycine; for the detection of ketones in urine, serum, plasma, and milk (but not in whole blood).

Marketed by Ames Co. Division of Miles Laboratories Ltd, Stoke Poges, Bucks.

Phenistix: reagent strips impregnated with ferric ammonium sulphate, magnesium sulphate, and cyclamic acid; for the detection in urine of phenylketones (e.g. salicylates) and some phenothiazine tranquillisers and their metabolites.
Marketed by Ames Co. Division of Miles Laboratories Ltd, Stoke Poges, Bucks.

Urastrat: test strips for the rapid quantitative estimation of urea nitrogen in serum and plasma.
Marketed by William R. Warner & Co. Ltd, Eastleigh, Hants.

Appendix 3: Bibliography

Titles of journals are abbreviated according to the style of the *World List of Scientific Periodicals*, Fourth Edn, London, Butterworths, 1963.

A.M.A. Council on Drugs (1962) *J. Am. med. Ass.* **179** 799

Abadie, S. H. and Samuels, M. (1965) *J. Am. med. Ass.* **192** 326

Abrahamsen, A. M. (1960) *Acta pharmac. tox.* **17** 288

Adams, J. T., Bigler, J. A., and Green, O. C. (1957) *J. Am. med. Ass.* **165** 1563

Adamski, S. (1965) *Acta Pol. pharm.* **22** 311

Addison, E. and Clark, R. G. (1963) *J. Pharm. Pharmac.* **15** 268

Adler, T. K., Fujimoto, J. M., Way, E. L., and Baker, E. M. (1955) *J. Pharmac. exp. Ther.* **114** 251

Adriani, J. (1960) *Clin. Pharmac. Ther.* **1** 645

Aebi, H., Lauber, E., Lehner, H., and Michaelis, W. (1964) *Arzneimittel-Forsch.* **14** 92

Afifi, A. M. and Way, E. L. (1967) *J. Pharm. Sci.* **56** 720

Akagi, M., Oketani, Y., and Takada, M. (1963) *Chem. pharm. Bull., Tokyo* **11** 62

Åkerman, B., Åström, A., Ross, S., and Telč, A. (1966) *Acta pharmac. tox.* **24** 389

Åkesson, H. O. and Wålinder, J. (1965) *Lancet* **1** 1271

Alexander, R. F., Forbes, G. B., and Hawkins, E. S. (1948) *Br. med. J.* **2** 518

Algeri, E. J. and Katsas, G. (1960) *J. forens. Sci.* **5** 217

Algeri, E. J. and McBay, A. J. (1953) *New Engl. J. Med.* **248** 423

Alha, A. and Tamminen, V. (1965) 'Infra-red Absorption Spectroscopy in Forensic Toxicological Practice', *Methods of Forensic Science*, ed. A. S. Curry, London and New York, Interscience Publishers Inc., Vol. 4, p. 265

Alha, A. R. (1966)—personal communication

Alha, A. R. and Ohela, K. (1955) *Acta pharmac. tox.* **11** 156

Alles, G. A. and Wisegarver, B. A. (1961) *Toxic. appl. Pharmac.* **3** 678

Allgén, L. G., Hellström, L., and Sant'Orp, C. J. (1963) *Acta psychiat. scand. Supp. 169* **39** 366

Almog, C. and Tal, E. (1967) *Br. med. J.* **3** 721

American Society for Testing Materials (1962) 'Molecular Formula List of Compounds, Names, and References to Published Infrared Spectra', *Special Technical Publication No. 331*

American Society for Testing Materials (1963) 'First Supplement to Molecular Formula List of Compounds, Names, and References to Published Infrared Spectra', *Special Technical Publication No. 331A*

Amundson, M. E. and Manthey, J. A. (1966) *J. pharm. Sci.* **55** 277

Amundson, M. E., Johnson, M. L., and Manthey, J. A. (1965) *J. pharm. Sci.* **54** 684

Analytical Methods Committee (1960) Report by the Metallic Impurities in Organic Matter Sub-committee: 'Methods for the Destruction of Organic Matter', *Analyst, Lond.* **85** 643

Annesley, P. T. and Mant, A. K. (1962) *Br. med. J.* **1** 233

Archer, A. W. and Haugas, E. A. (1960) *J. Pharm. Pharmac.* **12** 754

Arterberry, J. D., Durham, W. F., Elliott, J. W., and Wolfe, H. R. (1961) *Arch. envir. Hlth* **3** 476

Asatoor, A. M., London, D. R., Milne, M. D., and Simenhoff, M. L. (1963) *Br. J. Pharmac. Chemother.* **20** 285

Ascione, P. P., Zagar, J. B., and Chrekian, G. P. (1967) *J. pharm. Sci.* **56** 1393

Ashton, F. C. (1960) *Analyst, Lond.* **85** 685

Atkins, R., Cutting, C. J., and Mackintosh, T. F. (1965) *Br. med. J.* **1** 907

Axelrod, J. (1953a) *J. Pharmac. exp. Ther.* **109** 62

Axelrod, J. (1954) *J. Pharmac. exp. Ther.* **110** 315

Axelrod, L. R. (1953b) *J. biol. Chem.* **201** 59

Aycrigg, J. B. (1964) *Am. J. Psychiat.* **120** 1201

Baker, E. A. and Skerrett, E. J. (1960) *Analyst, Lond.* **85** 184

Bălintffy, I. and Kovács, J. (1955) *Acta vet. hung.* **5** 143

Ballard, C. W., Isaacs, J., and Scott, P. G. W. (1954) *J. Pharm. Pharmac.* **6** 971

Barbour, R. F., Pilkington, F., and Sargant, W. (1936) *Br. med. J.* **2** 957

Barker, S. A., Bourne, E. J., and Whiffen, D. H. (1956) 'Use of Infrared Analysis in the Determination of Carbohydrate Structure', *Methods of Biochemical Analysis*, ed. D. Glick, New York, Interscience Publishers Inc., Vol. 3, p. 213

Barron, D. W. and Milliken, T. G. (1960) *Lancet* **1** 262

Barry, J. A., Vasishth, R. C., and Shelton, F. J. (1962) *Analyt. Chem.* **34** 67

Barua, R. K. and Rao, M. V. K. (1964) *Analyst, Lond.* **89** 534

Bastow, R. A. (1967) *J. Pharm. Pharmac.* **19** 41

Beach, G. O., Fitzgerald, R. P., Holmes, R., Phibbs, B., and Stuckenhoff, H. (1964) *New Engl. J. Med.* **270** 1354

Becker, M. C. and Sugarman, G. (1952) *J. Am. med. Ass.* **149** 568

Beckett, A. H. and Brookes, L. G. (1967) *J. Pharm. Pharmac.* **19** *Supp.* 42S
Beckett, A. H. and Rowland, M. (1965) *J. Pharm. Pharmac.* **17** *Supp.* 109S
Beckett, A. H. and Triggs, E. J. (1966) *Nature, Lond.* **211** 1415
Beckett, A. H. and Wilkinson, G. R. (1965) *J. Pharm. Pharmac.* **17** *Supp.* 104S and 107S
Beckett, A. H., Boyes, R. N., and Appleton, P. J. (1966) *J. Pharm. Pharmac.* **18** *Supp.* 76S
Beckett, A. H., Boyes, R. N., and Parker, J. B. (1965a) *Anaesthesia* **20** 294
Beckett, A. H., Rowland, M., and Turner, P. (1965b) *Lancet* **1** 303
Beckett, A. H., Tucker, G. T., and Moffat, A. C. (1967) *J. Pharm. Pharmac.* **19** 273
Bedford, C., Child, K. J., and Tomich, E. G. (1959) *Nature, Lond.* **184** 364
Bell, D. B. and Scaff, J. (1963) *Hawaii med. J. inter-Isl. Nurs. Bull.* **22** 440
Bellamy, L. J. (1962a) *The Infrared Spectra of Complex Molecules*, London, Methuen & Co. Ltd
Bellamy, L. J. (1962b) 'Infrared Spectra of Compounds of Biological Interest', *Comprehensive Biochemistry*, ed. M. Florkin and E. H. Stotz, Amsterdam & New York, Elsevier Publishing Company, Vol. 3, p. 133
Belles, Q. C. and Littleman, M. L. (1960) *Analyt. Chem.* **32** 720
Bendersky, G. and Ramirez, C. (1960) *J. Am. med. Ass.* **173** 1789
Bennett, I. L. (1953) *Medicine (Baltimore)* **32** 531 and *Lancet* 1954 **1** 356
Berger, K. G., Sylvester, N. D., and Haines, D. M. (1960) *Analyst, Lond.* **85** 341
Bernstein, S. and Leff, R. (1967) *New Engl. J. Med.* **277** 638.
Best, W. R. (1963) *J. Am. med. Ass.* **185** 286
Betts, T. J. and Holloway, P. J. (1967) *J. Pharm. Pharmac.* **19** *Supp.* 97S
Bian Ru-rie, Fang Juei-ying, Wang Pei-chun, Jung Ting-kuo, and Li Cheng-koa (1964) *Acta pharm. sin.* **11** 531
Bidstrup, P. L. and Payne, D. J. H. (1951) *Br. med. J.* **2** 16
Bidstrup, P. L., Bonnell, J. A. L., and Harvey, D. G. (1952) *Lancet* **1** 794
Birner, J. (1961) *Analyt. Chem.* **33** 1955
Blanchard, A. J. and Mertens, G. A. (1958) *Can. med. Ass. J.* **79** 627
Blanke, R. V. (1960) *J. forens. Sci.* **5** 539
Blumenthal, M. D. and Reinhart, M. J. (1964) *J. Am. med. Ass.* **190** 154
Bogan, J. (1967)—personal communication
Bogan, J. and Smith, H. (1967) *J. forens. Sci. Soc.* **7** 37
Bogan, J. and Smith, H. (1968) *J. Pharm. Pharmac.* **20** 64
Bogan, J., Rentoul, E., and Smith, H. (1965) *J. forens. Sci. Soc.* **5** 97
Bogan, J., Rentoul, E., Smith, H., and Weir, W. P. (1966) *J. forens. Sci. Soc.* **6** 166
Boggiano, B. G., Condon, S., Davies, M. T., Jackman, G. B., Overell, B. G., Petrow, V., Stephenson, O., and Wild, A. M. (1960) *J. Pharm. Pharmac.* **12** 419
Böhme, H. and Kreutzig, L. (1964) *Arch. Pharm.* **297** 681
Bolt, A. G., Forrest, I. S., and Serra, M. T. (1966) *J. pharm. Sci.* **55** 1205
Bond, P. A. (1967) *Nature, Lond.* **213** 721
Bonnichsen, R. and Maehly, A. C. (1965) *J. forens. Sci. Soc.* **5** 201
Bonnichsen, R. and Maehly, A. C. (1966) *J. forens. Sci.* **11** 414
Bonnichsen, R., Maehly, A. C., and Moeller, M. (1966) *J. forens. Sci.* **11** 186
Bonnichsen, R., Maehly, A. C., and Nordlander, S. (1960) *J. Chromat.* **3** 190
Bösche, J. and Schmidt, G. (1966) *Arzneimittel-Forsch.* **16** 548
Bose, B. C. and Vijayvargiya, R. (1962) *J. Pharm. Pharmac.* **14** 58
Bose, B. C. and Vijayvargiya, R. (1964) *J. Pharm. Pharmac.* **16** 561
Boughton, O. D., Bryant, R., Ludwig, W. J., and Timma, D. L. (1966) *J. pharm. Sci.* **55** 951
Bowden, R. S. T., Baxter, M. K., Hodgman, S. F. J., and Wilkinson, E. (1960) *Vet. Rec.* **72** 102
Bowen, D. A. (1963) *Medicine Sci. Law* **3** 216
Bowman, E. R. and McKennis, H. (1962) *J. Pharmac. exp. Ther.* **135** 306
Boyland, E. and Nery, R. (1964) *Analyst, Lond.* **89** 520
Brancaccia, A., Fermariello, U., and Castellino, N. (1966) *Folia med., Napoli* **49** 729 and *Abstr. Wld Med.* 1967 **41** 567
Bratton, A. C. and Marshall, E. K. (1939) *J. biol. Chem.* **128** 537
Braun, G. A., Poos, G. I., and Soudijn, W. (1967) *Eur. J. Pharmac.* **1** 58
Breton, J., Caroff, J., Dérobert, L. (1964) *Annls Méd. lég. Crimin. Police scient.* **44** 265
Bridges, J. W. and Williams, R. T. (1963) *J. Pharm. Pharmac.* **15** 565
Bridges, R. G., Harrison, A., and Winteringham, F. P. W. (1956) *Nature, Lond.* **177** 86
Brink, N. G., Bonnichsen, R., and Theorell, H. (1954) *Acta pharmac. tox.* **10** 223
Brodie, B. B. (1956) *J. Pharm. Pharmac.* **8** 11
Brodie, B. B. and Axelrod, J. (1948) *J. Pharmac. exp. Ther.* **94** 29
Brodie, B. B. and Axelrod, J. (1949) *J. Pharmac. exp. Ther.* **97** 58
Brodie, B. B., Burns, J. J., Mark, L. C., Lief, P. A., Bernstein, E., and Papper, E. M. (1953) *J. Pharmac. exp. Ther.* **109** 26
Brodie, B. B., Lief, P. A., and Poet, R. (1948) *J. Pharmac. exp. Ther.* **94** 359
Brown, H. W. (1960) *Clin. Pharmac. Ther.* **1** 87
Brown, J. B. and Matthew, G. D. (1962) *Recent Progress in Hormone Research*, ed. G. Pincus, New York and London, Academic Press Inc., Vol. 18, p. 337
Brownie, A. C., Molen, H. J. van der, Nishizawa, E. E., and Eik-Nes, K. B. (1964) *J. clin. Endocr. Metab.* **24** 1091

Brownlee, G. and Spriggs, T. L. B. (1965) *J. Pharm. Pharmac.* **17** 429
Bruce, R. B., Pitts, J. E., Pinchbeck, F., and Newman, J. (1965) *J. mednl Chem.* **8** 157
Bulger, R. J., Sidell, S., and Kirby, W. M. (1963) *Ann. intern. Med.* **59** 593
Bullivant, C. M. (1966) *Br. med. J.* **1** 1272
Burn, J. I. and Coleman, S. J. (1961) *Antibiotic Med. clin. Ther.* **8** 37
Burns, J. and Snow, G. A. (1961) *Br. J. Anaesth.* **33** 102
Burns, J. J., Berger, B. L., Lief, P. A., Wollack, A., Papper, E. M., and Brodie, B. B. (1955) *J. Pharmac. exp. Ther.* **114** 289
Burnstein, N. and Stauss, H. K. (1965) *J. Am. med. Ass.* **194** 1139
Butler, R. A. and Freeman, J. (1962) *Br. J. Anaesth.* **34** 440
Butler, R. A. and Hill, D. W. (1961) *Nature, Lond.* **189** 488
Butler, T. C. (1964) *J. Pharm. exp. Ther.* **143** 23

Caccia, P. A. (1957) *Am. Rev. Tuberc. pulm. Dis.* **76** 1071
Caddy, B. and Fish, F. (1967) *J. Chromat.* **31** 584
Caddy, B., Fish, F., and Wilson, W. D. C. (1967) *J. Pharm. Pharmac.* **19** 851
Cahn, B., Brahen, L. S., Wiseman, E. H., and Pinson, R. (1963) *Curr. ther. Res.* **5** 301
Calesnick, B., Christensen, J. A., and Richter, M. (1966) *Proc. Soc. exp. Biol. Med.* **123** 17
Cameron, A. J. (1964) *Br. med. J.* **1** 594
Campbell, A. D., Coles, F. K., Eubank, L. L., and Huf, E. G. (1961) *J. Pharmac. exp. Ther.* **131** 18
Campbell, G. D. (1963) *Br. med. J.* **1** 59
Campbell, J. E. (1960) *J. forens. Sci.* **5** 501
Campbell, S. (1968) *Lancet* **1** 144
Caridis, D. T., McAndrew, G. N., and Matheson, N. A. (1967) *Lancet* **1** 51
Carr, A. A. (1965) *Archs intern. Med.* **115** 29
Catanese, B., Grasso, A., and Silvestrini, B. (1966) *Arzneimittel-Forsch.* **16** 1354
Cavett, J. W. (1938) *J. Lab. clin. Med.* **3** 543
Chapman, I. and Cheung, W. H. (1963) *J. Am. med. Ass.* **186** 595
Chapman, J. B. and Robson, P. (1965) *Lancet* **1** 1266
Charalampous, K. D., Orengo, A., Walker, K. E., and Kinross-Wright, J. (1964) *J. Pharmac. exp. Ther.* **145** 242
Charro Arias, A., Simal Lozano, J., and Creus, J. M. (1966) *An. R. Acad. Farm. Madr.* **32** 131
Chatten, L. G. and Levi, L. (1957) *Appl. Spectrosc.* **11** 177
Chissell, J. F. (1964) *J. Pharm. Pharmac.* **16** 490
Choulis, N. H. (1967) *J. pharm. Sci.* **56** 196
Christensen, C. B. (1966a) *Acta pharmac. tox.* **24** 139
Christensen, C. B. (1967) *Acta pharmac. tox.* **25** 465
Christensen, F. (1964) *Acta pharmac. tox.* **21** 23 and 299
Christensen, F. (1966b) *Acta pharmac. tox.* **24** 232
Clancy, D. J. and Kramm, D. E. (1963) *Analyt. Chem.* **35** 1987
Clark, C. and Chianta, M. (1957) *Ann. N.Y. Acad. Sci.* **69** 205
Clarke, E. G. C. (1958) *Nature, Lond.* **181** 1152
Clarke, E. G. C. (1960a) *Nature, Lond.* **188** 411
Clarke, E. G. C. (1960b) 'The Identification of Quaternary Ammonium Compounds', *Proceedings of the Fourth International Congress on Clinical Chemistry*, Edinburgh, Livingstone (E. & S.) Ltd, p. 161
Clarke, E. G. C. and Hawkins, A. E. (1960) *J. Pharm. Pharmac.* **12** 509
Clarke, E. G. C. and Hawkins, A. E. (1963) *J. Pharm. Pharmac.* **15** 390
Clarke, E. G. C. and Kalayci, S. (1963) *Lab. Pract.* **12** 1095 (refers to the citation on p. 24)
Clarke, E. G. C. and Kalayci, S. (1963) *Nature, Lond.* **198** 783 (refers to the citation on p. 807)
Clarke, E. G. C. and Sowter, S. (1964) *Nature, Lond.* **202** 795
Clarke, E. G. C. and Williams, M. (1955) *J. Pharm. Pharmac.* **7** 255
Clements, J. A., Forbes, St. J., Olliff, C. J., and Rogers, A. R. (1967) *J. Pharm. Pharmac.* **19** *Supp.* 103S
Cleverley, B. and Williams, P. P. (1959) *Chemy Ind.* **78** 49
Clow, W. M. and Smith, A. C. A. (1967) *Scott. med. J.* **12** 307
Coble, Y., Hildebrandt, P., Davis, J., Raasch, F., and Curley, A. (1967) *J. Am. med. Ass.* **202** 153
Cochin, J. and Daly, J. W. (1963a) *J. Pharmac. exp. Ther.* **139** 154
Cochin, J. and Daly, J. W. (1963b) *J. Pharmac. exp. Ther.* **139** 160
Cohen, E. N. (1963) *J. Lab. clin. Med.* **61** 338 and **62** 979
Cohen, E. N., Brewer, H. W., Bellville, J. W., and Sher, R. (1965) *Anesthesiology* **26** 140
Cohen, S. (1957) *J. Ass. off. agric. Chem.* **40** 224
Cole, A. R. H. (1956) *Fortschr. Chem. org. NatStoffe* **13** 1
Coleman, T. J. and Parke, D. V. (1963) *J. Pharm. Pharmac.* **15** 841
Combes, B., Damon, A., and Gottfried, E. (1956) *New Engl. J. Med.* **254** 223
Committee on Safety of Drugs (1965) *Adverse Reactions Series No. 3*
Committee on Toxicology (1960) *J. Am. med. Ass.* **172** 2077
Conacher, H. B. S. and Rees, D. I. (1966) *Analyst, Lond.* **91** 55
Conklin, J. D. and Hollifield, R. D. (1965) *Clin. Chem.* **11** 925
Conney, A. H. and Burns, J. J. (1960) *J. Pharmac. exp. Ther.* **128** 340
Consden, R. (1967)—personal communication
Corby, C. and Camps, F. E. (1960) *J. forens. Med.* **7** 206
Corby, C., Dunnett, N., Kimber, K. J., and Walls, H. J. (1963) 'Acute Fatal Quinine

Poisoning', *Forensic Immunology, Medicine, Pathology and Toxicology* (*International Congress Series No. 80*), Report of the Third International Meeting, Abridged Proceedings, Amsterdam/New York/London, Excerpta Medica Foundation, 1964, p. 118

Cotty, V., Zurzola, F., Beezley, T., and Rodgers, A. (1965) *J. pharm. Sci.* **54** 868

Cotty, V. F. and Ederma, H. M. (1966) *J. pharm. Sci.* **55** 837

Cox, E., Roxburgh, G., and Wright, S. E. (1959) *J. Pharm. Pharmac.* **11** 535

Crew, M. C., Coutinho, C. B., and DiCarlo, F. J. (1966) *J. pharm. Sci.* **55** 1137

Cromp, C. C. and Turney, F. G. (1967) *J. forens. Sci.* **12** 538

Cross, A. D. (1960) *Introduction to Practical Infra-red Spectroscopy*, London, Butterworths Scientific Publications

Cross, A. J. H., Hendey, R. A., and Stevens, S. G. E. (1960) *Analyst, Lond.* **85** 355

Crummett, W. B., Simek, J., and Stenger, V. A. (1964) *Analyt. Chem.* **36** 1834

Curry, A. S. (1955) *J. Pharm. Pharmac.* **7** 1072

Curry, A. S. (1957) *J. Pharm. Pharmac.* **9** 102

Curry, A. S. (1959) *J. Pharm. Pharmac.* **11** 411

Curry, A. S. (1960) *Nature, Lond.* **188** 58

Curry, A. S. (1962) *Br. med. J.* **1** 687

Curry, A. S. (1963a) 'The Coding of Analytical Data', *Forensic Immunology, Medicine, Pathology and Toxicology* (*International Congress Series No. 80*), Report of the Third International Meeting, Abridged Proceedings, Amsterdam/New York/London, Excerpta Medica Foundation, 1964, p. 145

Curry, A. S. (1963b) *Poison Detection in Human Organs*, Springfield, Ill., Charles C. Thomas, p. 41

Curry, A. S. (1963c) *Poison Detection in Human Organs*, Springfield, Ill., Charles C. Thomas, p. 68

Curry, A. S. (1963d) *Poison Detection in Human Organs*, Springfield, Ill., Charles C. Thomas, p. 95

Curry, A. S. (1964a) *Br. med. J.* **1** 354

Curry, A. S. (1964b) *J. Pharm. Pharmac.* **16** 265

Curry, A. S. (1967)—personal communication

Curry, A. S. and Phang, S. E. (1960) *J. Pharm. Pharmac.* **12** 437

Curzon, G. (1955) *Lancet* **2** 1361

Cuthill, J. M., Griffiths, A. B., and Powell, D. E. B. (1964) *Lancet* **1** 1076

Daglish, C. (1950) *Biochem. J.* **47** 452

Dal Cortivo, L. A. and Broich, J. R. (1966) *Analyt. Chem.* **38** 1959

Dalley, R. A. and Hainsworth, D. (1965) *J. forens. Sci. Soc.* **5** 99

Daniel, J. W. and Gage, J. C. (1966) *Br. J. ind. Med.* **23** 126

Datey, K. K., Deshmukh, S. N., Dalvi, C. P., and Purandare, N. M. (1967) *Br. med. J.* **3** 152

Daubney, C. G. and Nickolls, L. C. (1938) *Analyst, Lond.* **63** 560

Dauterman, W. C., Casida, J. E., Knaak, J. B., and Kowalczyk, T. (1959) *J. agric. Fd Chem.* **7** 188

Davidson, D. G. D. and Eastham, W. N. (1966) *Br. med. J.* **2** 497

Davis, B., Dodds, M. G., and Tomich, E. G. (1962) *J. Pharm. Pharmac.* **14** 249

Davis, T. W. M., Farmilo, C. G., and Osadchuk, M. (1963) *Analyt. Chem.* **35** 751

Davison, C., Zimmerman, E. F., and Smith, P. K. (1961) *J. Pharmac. exp. Ther.* **132** 207

Dawson, J. A., Donegan, L., and Thain, E. M. (1964) *Analyst, Lond.* **89** 495

De Fina, V. and Setnikar, I. (1966) *Boll. chim.-farm.* **105** 756

de Silva, J. A. F., Koechlin, B. A., and Bader, G. (1966) *J. pharm. Sci.* **55** 692

de Silva, J. A. F., Schwartz, M. A., Stefanovic, V., Kaplan, J., and D'Arconte, L. (1964) *Analyt. Chem.* **36** 2099

Defalque, R. J. (1961) *Clin. Pharmac. Ther.* **2** 665

Denton, S. (1962) *Analyst, Lond.* **87** 234

Dobriner, K., Jones, R. N., and Katzenellenbogen, E. R. (1953) *Infrared Absorption Spectra of Steroids—An Atlas*, London and New York, Interscience Publishers Inc., Vol. 1

Dollery, C. T., Emslie-Smith, D., and Muggleton, D. F. (1960) *Br. med. J.* **1** 521

Domino, E. F. (1962) *Clin. Pharmac. Ther.* **3** 599

Douglas, J. F., Ludwig, B. J., and Schlosser, A. (1962) *J. Pharmac. exp. Ther.* **138** 21

Douglas, J. S. and Nicholls, P. J. (1965) *J. Pharm. Pharmac.* **17** *Supp.* 115S

Doyle, A. E. and Morley, A. (1965) *Br. J. Pharmac. Chemother.* **24** 701

Dring, L. G., Smith, R. L., and Williams, R. T. (1966) *J. Pharm. Pharmac.* **18** 402

Driscoll, J. L., Martin, H. F., and Gudzinowicz, B. J. (1964) *J. Gas Chromat.* **2** 109

Duff, I. F. and Shull, W. H. (1949) *J. Am. med. Ass.* **139** 762

Duncan, W. A. M. (1959) *Br. J. Anaesth.* **31** 316

Duncan, W. A. M., Macdonald, G., and Thornton, M. J. (1962) *J. Pharm. Pharmac.* **14** 217

Durel, P., Couture, J., and Bassoullet, M. T. (1967) *Br. J. vener. Dis.* **43** 111

Dutta, S., Marks, B. H., and Smith, C. R. (1963) *J. Pharmac. exp. Ther.* **142** 223

Duyckaerts, G. (1959) *Analyst, Lond.* **84** 201

Dyfverman, A. (1963) 'Clinical Methods for the Determination of Metals in Forensic Toxicology', *Methods of Forensic Science*, ed. F. Lundquist, London and New York, Interscience Publishers Inc., Vol. 2, p. 171

Ebert, A. G. and Hess, S. M. (1965) *J. Pharmac. exp. Ther.* **148** 412

Edson, E. F. (1954) *Lancet* **1** 981

Edson, E. F. (1955) *Br. med. J.* **1** 841

Edson, E. F., Jones, K. F., and Watson, W. A. (1967) *Br. med. J.* **4** 554

Egyed, M. and Brisk, Y. (1965) *Refuah vet.* **22** 278

Eisner, H. J. and Wulf, R. J. (1963) *J. Pharmac. exp. Ther.* **142** 122

Ellard, G. A. and Naylor, R. F. (1961) *Lepr. Rev.* **32** 249

Ellinwood, E. H., Ewing, J. A., and Hoaken, P. C. S. (1962) *New Engl. J. Med.* **266** 185

Ellis, G. G., Comish, K. A., and Hewer, R. L. (1966) *Practitioner* **196** 557

Elmendorf, D. F., Cawthon, W. U., Muschenheim, C., and McDermott, W. (1952) *Am. Rev. Tuberc. pulm. Dis.* **65** 429

Elson, A. and Domino, E. F. (1963) *J. Am. med. Ass.* **183** 482

Emanuel, D. A., Rowe, G. G., Musser, M. J., and Philpot, Van B. (1956) *J. Am. med. Ass.* **161** 436

England, N. J. and McEachern, D. (1949) *Can. med. Ass. J.* **60** 173

Erben, J. (1967) *Arch. Tox.* **22** 410

Erne, K. (1958) *Acta pharmac. tox.* **14** 158

Esplin, D. W. and Woodbury, D. M. (1956) *J. Pharmac. exp. Ther.* **118** 129

FAO/WHO Expert Committee on Food Additives, Sixth Report (1962): 'Evaluation of the Toxicity of a Number of Antimicrobials and Antioxidants', *Tech. Rep. Ser. Wld Hlth Org., No. 228*

FAO/WHO Expert Committee on Pesticide Residues (1967): 'Pesticide Residues in Food', *Tech. Rep. Ser. Wld Hlth Org., No. 370*

Fairbairn, J. W. and El-Masry, S. (1967) *J. Pharm. Pharmac.* **19** *Supp.* 93S

Fales, H. M. and Pisano, J. J. (1962) *Anal. Biochem.* **3** 337

Farah, A. (1946) *J. Pharmac. exp. Ther.* **86** 248

Farmilo, C. G. and Davis, T. W. M. (1961) *J. Pharm. Pharmac.* **13** 767

Farmilo, C. G. and Genest, K. (1963) 'Narcotics and Related Bases', *Progress in Chemical Toxicology*, ed. A. Stolman, New York and London, Academic Press Inc., Vol. 1, p. 199

Fatteh, A. (1964) *J. forens. Med.* **11** 120

Feinblatt, B. I., Aceto, T., Beckhorn, G., and Bruck, E. (1966) *Am. J. Dis. Child.* **112** 218

Feldmann, R. J. and Maibach, H. I. (1965) *Archs Derm.* **91** 661

Feldstein, M. (1965) *J. forens. Sci.* **10** 207

Feldstein, M. and Klendshoj, N. C. (1954) *Analyt. Chem.* **26** 932

Fenwick, M. L. and Parker, V. H. (1955) *Analyst, Lond.* **80** 774

Fiddes, F. S. (1958) *Br. med. J.* **2** 779

Finkle, B. (1967a and b)—personal communication

Fishwick, F. B. and Taylor, A. (1967) *Analyst, Lond.* **92** 192

Fisk, A. J., Czerwinski, G. R., and Kenhart, J. H. (1965) *J. forens. Sci.* **10** 473

Flanagan, J. F. (1955) *Archs intern. Med.* **96** 277

Fluker, J. L. (1961) *Br. J. vener. Dis.* **36** 280

Foldes, F. F. (1960) *Clin. Pharmac. Ther.* **1** 345

Food Standards Committee Report on Antioxidants in Food (1963): Ministry of Agriculture, Fisheries and Food, London, H.M. Stationery Office, 1963

Foppiano, R. and Brown, B. B. (1965) *J. pharm. Sci.* **54** 206

Forbes, G., Weir, W. P., Smith, H., and Bogan, J. (1965) *J. forens. Sci. Soc.* **5** 183

Forist, A. A. (1967)—personal communication

Forrest, I. S. and Forrest, F. M. (1964) *Mind* **2** 38 and 62

Forrest, I. S., Forrest, F. M., and Mason, A. S. (1960) *Am. J. Psychiat.* **116** 1021

Forrest, I. S., Kanter, S. L., Sperco, J. E., and Wechsler, M. B. (1965) *Am. J. Psychiat.* **121** 1049

Fraser, H. F., Martin, W. R., Wolbach, A. B., and Isbell, H. (1961) *Clin. Pharmac. Ther.* **2** 287

Freedman, B. J. (1955) *Lancet* **2** 575

Freedman, L., Blitz, M., Gunsberg, E., and Zak, S. (1961) *J. Lab. clin. Med.* **58** 662

Freireich, A. W., Cinque, T. J., Xanthaky, G., and Landau, D. (1967) *New Engl. J. Med.* **277** 699

Fretwurst, F., Halberkann, J., and Reiche, F. (1930) *Münch. med. Wschr.* **77** 1573

Frey, H.-H., Sudendey, F., and Krause, D. (1959) *Arzneimittel-Forsch.* **9** 294

Friebel, H. and Sommer, S. (1960) *Dt. med. Wschr.* **85** 2192

Friedman, E. A., Greenberg, J. B., Merrill, J. P., and Dammin, G. J. (1962) *Am. J. Med.* **32** 891

Friestad, H. O. (1963) *Analyt. Chem.* **35** 1012

Frýdl, V. (1967) *Prakt. Lék.* **47** 596 per *Int. pharm. Abstr.* 1967 **4** 1413

Fulton, C. C. (1969) *Modern Microcrystal Tests for Drugs*, New York and London, Interscience Publishers Inc., in press

Funckes, A. J. (1960) *Archs envir. Hlth* **1** 404

Gadsden, R. H., Mellette, R. R., and Miller, W. C. (1958) *J. Am. med. Ass.* **168** 1220

Garhart, M. D., Witmer, F. J., and Tajima, Y. A. (1952) *Analyt. Chem.* **24** 851

Garratt, D. C. and Marshall, P. G. (1954) *J. Pharm. Pharmac.* **6** 950

Genest, K. and Farmilo, C. G. (1964) *J. Pharm. Pharmac.* **16** 250

Gettler, A. O. and Sunshine, I. (1951) *Analyt. Chem.* **23** 779

Ginn, E. H., Anderson, K. E., Mercier, R. K., Stevens, T. W., and Matter, B. J. (1968) *J. Am. med. Ass.* **203** 164

Ginther, G. B. and Finch, R. C. (1960) *Analyt. Chem.* **32** 1894

Gitelson, S., Aladjemoff, L., Ben-Hador, S., and Katznelson, R. (1966) *J. Am. med. Ass.* **197** 819

Glick, D., Fell, B. F., and Sjølin, K.-E. (1964) *Analyt. Chem.* **36** 1119

Gochman, N. and Gantt, C. L. (1962) *J. Pharmac. exp. Ther.* **135** 312
Golab, T. and Layne, D. S. (1962) *J. Chromat.* **9** 321
Goldbaum, L. R. (1952) *Analyt. Chem.* **24** 1604
Goldbaum, L. R. and Domanski, T. J. (1966) *J. forens. Sci.* **11** 233
Goldbaum, L. R., Williams, M., and Johnston, M. D. (1962) *J. forens. Sci.* **7** 499
Goldbaum, L. R., Williams, M. A., and Koppanyi, T. (1960) *Analyt. Chem.* **32** 81
Goldin, A. R., Rubenstein, A. H., Bradlow, B. A., and Elliott, G. A. (1964) *New Engl. J. Med.* **271** 1289
Goldstein, N. P., Jones, P. H., and Brown, J. R. (1959) *J. Am. med. Ass.* **171** 1306
Gomersall, R., Wilson, A. E., Mehra, S. K., and Davies, D. M. (1966) *Lancet* **2** 1416
Gonzales, T. A., Vance, M., Helpern, M., and Umberger, C. J. (1954) *Legal Medicine, Pathology and Toxicology*, 2nd Edn, New York, Appleton-Century-Crofts Inc., p. 1045
Gosselin, R. E., Gabourel, J. D., and Wills, J. H. (1960) *Clin. Pharmac. Ther.* **1** 597
Gothelf, B. and Karczmar, A. G. (1963) *Int. J. Neuro-pharmac.* **2** 95
Graham, J. D. P. (1960) *Br. med. J.* **1** 1256
Gray, L. S., Metcalfe, L. D., and Leslie, S. W. (1963) 'A Convenient Method for Collecting Gas Chromatography Fractions for Infrared Analysis', *Gas Chromatography, Intern. Symp.*, ed. L. Fowler, New York, Academic Press Inc., Vol. 4, p. 203
Greaves, J. H. and Ayres, P. (1967) *Nature, Lond.* **215** 877
Green, J. N. and Benson, B. C. (1961) *J. Pharm. Pharmac.* **13** 117T
Green, R. C. (1959) *J. Am. med. Ass.* **171** 1342
Greenwood, R. and Peachey, R. S. (1957) *Br. med. J.* **1** 742
Greer, H. D., Ward, H. P., and Corbin, K. B. (1965) *J. Am. med. Ass.* **193** 555
Gripe, R. P. (1951) *New Engl. J. Med.* **245** 803
Gunther, F. A., Blinn, R. C., and Barkley, J. H. (1963) *Analyst, Lond.* **88** 36
Gutch, C. F., Tomhave, W. G., and Stevens, S. C. (1965) *Ann. intern. Med.* **63** 128
Gwilt, J. R., Robertson, A., and McChesney, E. W. (1963) *J. Pharm. Pharmac.* **15** 440

Hadnagy, C., Huszár, I., and Tusa, A. (1964) *Ther. Umsch. med. Biblphie* **21** 103
Hall, C. A. and Allen, C. S. (1964) *J. Lab. clin. Med.* **63** 517
Hall, F. B. and Hine, C. H. (1966) *J. forens. Sci.* **11** 404
Halmos, P. B. (1965) *Br. med. J.* **2** 704
Hamence, J. H., Hall, P. S., and Caverly, D. J. (1965) *Analyst, Lond.* **90** 649
Hansen, J. M., Kristensen, M., Skovsted, L., and Christensen, L. K. (1966) *Lancet* **2** 265
Hansen, S. E. (1963) *Acta pharmac. tox.* **20** 286
Hansson, E. and Schmiterlöw, C. G. (1962) *J. Pharmac. exp. Ther.* **137** 91
Hansson, E., Hoffman, P., and Kristerson, L. (1965) *Acta pharmac. tox.* **22** 213
Harger, R. N. and Forney, R. B. (1959) *J. forens. Sci.* **4** 136
Harington, M. (1953) *Clin. Sci.* **12** 185
Harper, P. and Oakley, D. P. (1960) *Lancet* **2** 764
Harthorne, J. W., Marcus, A. M., and Kaye, M. (1963) *New Engl. J. Med.* **268** 33
Hartmann, C. H. and Oaks, D. M. (1965) *Aerograph Research Notes* Winter Issue, 1
Harvey, D. G., Bidstrup, P. L., and Bonnell, J. A. (1951) *Br. med. J.* **2** 13
Harvey, D. R. (1968) *Practitioner* **200** 180
Haskins, W. T. (1958) *Am. J. trop. Med. Hyg.* **7** 199
Häussler, A. and Hajdú, P. (1964) *Arzneimittel-Forsch.* **14** 710
Häussler, A. and Wicha, H. (1965) *Arzneimittel-Forsch.* **15** 81
Hawkins, A. E. (1959) *Br. J. appl. Phys.* **10** 99
Heaysman, L. T., Walker, E. A., and Lewis, D. T. (1967) *Analyst, Lond.* **92** 450
Henwood, C. R. (1967) *Nature, Lond.* **216** 1039
Herrett, R. J. and Buzard, J. A. (1960) *Analyt. Chem.* **32** 1676
Herrmann, B. (1964) *Arzneimittel-Forsch.* **14** 219
Hershenson, H. M. (1959) *Infrared Absorption Spectra: Index for 1945–1957*, London and New York, Academic Press Inc.
Hershenson, H. M. (1964) *Infrared Absorption Spectra: Index for 1958–1962*, London and New York, Academic Press Inc.
Herxheimer, A. and Haefeli, L. (1966) *Lancet* **2** 418
Hespe, W., Roos, A. M. de, and Nauta, W. T. (1965) *Archs int. Pharmacodyn. Thér.* **156** 180
Heyndrickx, A., De Leenheer, A., and Massart-Leen, A. M. (1965) *J. Pharm. Belg.* **20** 359
Heyndrickx, A., Maes, R., and De Leenheer, A. (1964) *J. Pharm. Belg.* **19** 161
Heyndrickx, A., Vercruysse, A., and Noë M. (1967) *J. Pharm. Belg.* **22** 127
Hindle, W. and Negus, D. (1960) *Br. med. J.* **1** 1507
Hobbs, D. C. (1968) *J. pharm. Sci.* **57** 105
Hodgkinson, A. and Zarembski, P. M. (1961) *Analyst, Lond.* **86** 16
Hoffman, H. and Roller, K. (1964) *Arzneimittel-Forsch.* **14** 1001
Holeček, V., Šafanda, J., and Doupník, L. (1965) *Rozhl. Tuberk.* **25** 475
Hollis, O. L. (1966) *Analyt. Chem.* **38** 309
Hollister, L. E. and Kosek, J. C. (1965) *J. Am. med. Ass.* **192** 1035
Holmes, R. W. and Love, J. (1952) *J. Am. med. Ass.* **148** 935
Holsinger, D. R., Hanlon, D. G., and Welch, J. S. (1958) *Proc. Staff Meet. Mayo Clin.* **33** 679
Holt, L. P. J. and Hawkins, C. F. (1965) *Br. med. J.* **1** 1354
Holubek, J. and Strouf, O. (1967) *Spectral Data and Physical Constants of Alkaloids*, London, Heyden & Son Ltd

Hood, J. W. and Toth, W. N. (1966) *J. Am. med. Ass.* **198** 1366 and *Pharm. J.* 1967 **2** 189
Hoole, A. (1966)—personal communication
Huang, T. C., Wefler, V., and Raftery, A. (1963) *Analyt. Chem.* **35** 1757
Hubley, C. E. and Levi, L. (1960a) 'Spectrum Analysis: B, Absorption Spectra Part 3: The Infrared Spectroscopic Method', *Toxicology: Mechanisms and Analytical Methods*, ed. C. P. Stewart and A. Stolman, New York, Academic Press Inc., Vol. 1, p. 513
Hubley, C. E. and Levi, L. (1960b) *National Bureau of Standards Compound Cards*, Washington D.C., National Research Council
Hubley, C. E., Levi, L., and Eagleson, A. D. (1960) 'Spectrum Analysis: B, Absorption Spectra Part 4: Atlas of Infrared Spectra; KBr Pellet Method', *Toxicology: Mechanisms and Analytical Methods*, ed. C. P. Stewart and A. Stolman, New York, Academic Press Inc., Vol. 1, p. 562
Hucker, H. B., Ahmad, P. M., Miller, E. A., and Brobyn, R. (1966) *Nature, Lond.* **209** 619
Hucker, H. B., Miller, J. K., Hochberg, A., Brobyn, R. D., Riordan, F. H., and Calesnick, B. (1967) *J. Pharmac. exp. Ther.* **155** 309
Hudanick, J. (1964) *J. pharm. Sci.* **53** 332
Hug, C. C. and Mellett, L. B. (1965) *J. Pharmac. exp. Ther.* **149** 446
Hug, C. C. and Woods, L. A. (1963) *J. Pharmac. exp. Ther.* **142** 248
Hughes, D. W. O'G. and Diamond, L. K. (1964) *Science, Wash.* **144** 296 and *Analyt. Abstr.* 1965 **12** 4061
Hughes, R. E. (1964) *Analyst, Lond.* **89** 618
Hummel, D. (1962) *Identification and Analysis for Surface-active Agents by Infrared and Chemical Methods*, trans. E. A. Wilkow, London and New York, Interscience Publishers Inc., Vols 1 and 2
Hunter, C. G., Robinson, J., and Richardson, A. (1963) *Br. med. J.* **1** 221
Hunter, D. (1950) *Br. med. J.* **1** 509

Idler, D. R., Kimball, N. R., and Truscott, B. (1966) *Steroids* **8** 865
Ilich, V., Delich, V., and Djurich, D. (1964) *Arkh. Farm.* **14** 299
Ings, R. M. J., Law, G. L., and Parnell, E. W. (1966) *Biochem. Pharmac.* **15** 515
Irudayasamy, A. and Natarajan, A. R. (1961) *Analyt. Chem.* **33** 630

Jackson, J. V. (1967)—personal communication
Jackson, J. V. and Moss, M. S. (1961) *Nature, Lond.* **192** 553
Jacobs, A. (1967a)—personal communication
Jacobs, J. C. (1967b) *J. Am. med. Ass.* **199** 932
Jacobsen, E. (1963) *Clin. Pharmac. Ther.* **4** 480
Jacoby, J. and Boyle, K. (1956) *J. Lab. clin. Med.* **48** 270
Jain, N. C. and Forney, R. B. (1967)—personal communication
Jain, N. C., Crim, D., Kaplan, H. L., Forney, R. B., and Hughes, F. W. (1967a) *J. forens. Sci.* **12** 497
Jain, N. C., Fontan, C. R., and Kirk, P. L. (1965) *J. Pharm. Pharmac.* **17** 362
Jain, N. C., Kaplan, H., and Forney, R. B. (1967b)—personal communication
Jakovljevic, I. M. (1962) *J. pharm. Sci.* **51** 187
Jakovljevic, I. M. (1963) *Analyt. Chem.* **35** 1513
Jakovljevic, I. M., Fose, J. M., and Kuzel, N. R. (1962) *Analyt. Chem.* **34** 411
James, A. T. and Martin, A. J. P. (1952) *Biochem. J.* **50** 679
James, V. H. T. (1967)—personal communication
Janicki, C. A., Brenner, R. J., and Schwartz, B. E. (1966) *J. pharm. Sci.* **55** 1077
Janovsky, R. C. (1960) *J. Am. med. Ass.* **172** 155
Jeannerod, M., Motin, J., and Saury, A. (1965) *Lyon méd.* **214** 13
Jóhannesson, T. and Lausen, H. H. (1961) *Acta pharmac. tox.* **18** 398
Johnson, C. D. and Revill, J. P. (1965) *Acta pharmac. tox.* **22** 112
Johnson, D. E., Millar, J. D., and Burchfield, H. P. (1963) *Life Sciences, Oxford* **12** 959
Johnson, D. P. (1956) *J. Ass. off. agric. Chem.* **39** 490
Johnson, H. R. M. (1960) *J. forens. Med.* **7** 198
Johnson, H. R. M. and Koumides, O. (1965) *Br. med. J.* **2** 629
Johnson, P. C. and Masters, Y. F. (1962) *J. Lab. clin. Med.* **59** 993
Johnson, R. E., Sargent, F., Robinson, P. F., and Consolazio, F. C. (1945) *Ind. Engng Chem. analyt. Edn* **17** 384
Johnston, J. P., Kane, P. O., and Kibby, M. R. (1967) *J. Pharm. Pharmac.* **19** 1
Johnston, V. D. and Porcaro, P. J. (1964) *Analyt. Chem.* **36** 124
Joint Committee of the Pharmaceutical Society and the Society for Analytical Chemistry on Methods of Assay of Crude Drugs (1961) *Analyst, Lond.* **86** 748
Jones, B. M., Ratcliffe, R. J. M., and Stevens, S. G. E. (1965) *J. Pharm. Pharmac.* **17** 52S
Jones, E. M. and Williams, B. (1966) *Br. med. J.* **1** 466
Jones, L. R. (1956) *Analyt. Chem.* **28** 39
Jones, R. and Page, B. C. (1964) *Analyt. Chem.* **36** 35
Jones, R. O. (1949) *Can. med. Ass. J.* **60** 609

Kaempe, B. (1965) *Acta pharmac. tox.* **23** 15
Kaempe, B. (1967) *Acta pharmac. tox.* **25** 155
Kamm, J. J. and Van Loon, E. J. (1966) *Clin. Chem.* **12** 789
Kanagaratnam, K., Wong Hock·Boon, and Tan Kwang Hoh (1960) *Lancet* **1** 538
Karawya, M. S., Wahba, S. K., and Kozman, A. R. (1967) *J. Pharm. Pharmac.* **19** 332
Karlin, H. (1960) *New Engl. J. Med.* **262** 1076
Karliner, J. S. (1967) *J. Am. med. Ass.* **199** 1006
Karlog, O. (1957) *Acta pharmac. tox.* **14** 92
Kaul, P. N. (1962) *J. Pharm. Pharmac.* **14** 237

Kaul, P. N., Brochmann-Hanssen, E., and Way, E. L. (1961a) *J. pharm. Sci.* **50** 244

Kaul, P. N., Brochmann-Hanssen, E., and Way, E. L. (1961b) *J. pharm. Sci.* **50** 840

Kaye, S. (1961) *Handbook of Emergency Toxicology*, 2nd Edn, Springfield, Ill., Charles C. Thomas

Kaye, S. and Haag, H. B. (1964) *Toxic. appl. Pharmac.* **6** 316

Kazantzis, G., McLaughlin, A. I., and Prior, P. F. (1964) *Br. J. ind. Med.* **21** 46

Kazyak, L. and Knoblock, E. C. (1963) *Analyt. Chem.* **35** 1448

Keay, G. R. (1968) *Analyst, Lond.* **93** 28

Keeney, A. H. and Mellinkoff, S. M. (1951) *Ann. intern. med.* **34** 331 and *J. Am. med. Ass.* **146** 401

Keller, R. E. and Ellenbogen, W. C. (1952) *J. Pharmac. exp. Ther.* **106** 77

Kelly, C. A. and Auerbach, M. E. (1961) *J. pharm. Sci.* **50** 490

Kelso, T., Toll, H. W., Pinkerton, D. C., and Kier, L. C. (1965) *J. forens. Sci.* **10** 313

Kemal, H. (1927) *Biochem. Z.* **187** 461

Kendall, A. C. (1954) *Br. med. J.* **2** 1461

Kennedy, W. P. U., Murdoch, J. McC., and Wallace, A. T. (1963) *Br. med. J.* **2** 962

Kern, W. (1963) *Analyt. Chem.* **35** 50

Kerr, F., Patel, A. R., Scott, P. D. R., and Tompsett, S. L. (1968) *Br. med. J.* **3** 290

Kessler, R. H. (1962) *Clin. Pharmac. Ther.* **3** 109

Khoury, A. J. and Cali, L. J. (1967) *J. pharm. Sci.* **56** 1485

Kiel, F. W. (1964) *J. Am. med. Ass.* **190** 398

Kiese, M. (1965) *Ann. N.Y. Acad. Sci.* **123** 141

Kimber, K. J. (1965)—personal communication

Kimber, K. J. (1966)—personal communication

Kimmel, H. B. and Walkenstein, S. S. (1967) *J. pharm. Sci.* **56** 538

King, J. S. (1951) *J. Am. pharm. Ass.* (*Sci. Edn*) **40** 424

Kirk, P. L., Gibor, A., and Parker, K. P. (1958) *Analyt. Chem.* **30** 1418

Klendshoj, N. C. and Feldstein, M. (1955) *Can. J. med. Technol.* **17** 74

Klendshoj, N. C. and Rejent, T. A. (1966) *J. forens. Sci.* **11** 75

Kliment, J. (1965) *Chslká Pediat.* **20** 900

Knudsen, E. T., Robinson, G. N., and Stevens, S. (1961) *Br. med. J.* **2** 198

Koe, B. K. and Pinson, R. (1964) *J. mednl Chem.* **7** 635

Koechlin, B. A. and d'Arconte, L. (1963) *Analyt. Biochem.* **5** 195

Koechlin, B. A., Schwartz, M. A., Krol, G., and Oberhausli, W. (1965) *J. Pharmac. exp. Ther.* **148** 399

Kofler, M. (1945) *Helv. chim. Acta* **28** 702

Kohn, K. W. (1961) *Analyt. Chem.* **33** 862

Korzun, B. P., Brody, S. M., and Tishler, F. (1964) *J. pharm. Sci.*, **53** 976

Koshy, K. T. and Mitchner, H. (1963) *J. pharm. Sci.* **52** 802

Koshy, K. T., Conwell, R. C., and Duvall, R. N. (1967) *J. pharm. Sci.* **56** 269

Koumides, O. (1967)—personal communication

Kozelka, F. L. and Hine, C. H. (1941) *Ind. Engng Chem. analyt. Edn* **13** 905 and *Analyst, Lond.* 1942 **67** 174

Kraml, M., Dubuc, J., and Dvornik, D. (1965) *J. pharm. Sci.* **54** 655

Kuhn, L. P. (1950) *Analyt. Chem.* **22** 276

Kum-Tatt, L. (1961) *J. Pharm. Pharmac.* **13** 759

Kum-Tatt, L. and Leong, P. C. (1964) *Analyst, Lond.* **89** 674

Kunin, C. M. and Finland, M. (1961) *Clin. Pharmac. Ther.* **2** 51

Kunin, C. M., Chalmers, T. C., Leevy, C. M., Sebastyen, S. C., Lieber, C. S., and Finland, M. (1960) *New Engl. J. Med.* **262** 380

Kunin, C. M., Glazko, A. J., and Finland, M. (1959) *J. clin. Invest.* **38** 1498

Kuntzman, R., Klutch, A., Tsai, I., and Burns, J. J. (1965) *J. Pharmac. exp. Ther.* **149** 29

Ladomery, L. G., Ryan, A. J., and Wright, S. E. (1967) *J. Pharm. Pharmac.* **19** 383 and 388

Lander, H. and Bonnin, J. M. (1962) *Med. J. Aust.* **2** 297

Langley, P. F., Lewis, J. D., Mansford, K. R. L., and Smith, D. (1963) *J. Pharm. Pharmac.* **15** 100

Langley, P. F., Lewis, J. D., Mansford, K. R. L., and Smith, D. (1966) *Biochem. Pharmac.* **15** 1821

Laubscher, F. A. (1966) *J. Am. med. Ass.* **198** 1120

Laurie, N. M. (1950) *Can. med. Ass. J.* **63** 298

Laves, W. (1960) *J. forens. Med.* **7** 186

Laws, E. Q. and Webley, D. J. (1959) *Analyst, Lond.* **84** 28

Lawson, A. A. H. and Brown, S. S. (1966) *Br. med. J.* **2** 1455

Leggan, H. W. (1961) *Analyt. Chem.* **33** 1295

Lehner, H., Lauener, H., and Schmutz, J. (1964) *Arzneimittel-Forsch.* **14** 89

Leibman, K. C. and Hindman, J. D. (1964) *Analyt. Chem.* **36** 348

Lester, D. (1964) *Analyt. Chem.* **36** 1810

Lester, D. and Greenberg, L. A. (1947) *J. Pharmac. exp. Ther.* **90** 68

Levi, L. and Hubley, C. E. (1956) *Analyt. Chem.* **28** 1591

Levi, L., Hubley, C. E., and Hinge, R. A. (1955) *Bull. Narcot.* **7** 42

Levine, R. and Berger, S. (1960) *Clin. Pharmac. Ther.* **1** 227

Lewis, M. A. (1967) *Br. med. J.* **4** 38

Lindfors, R. (1963) *Annls Med. exp. Biol. Fenn.* **41** 355

Lipkin, D. and Kushnick, T. (1967) *J. Am. med. Ass.* **201** 57

Lloyd, J. B. F. (1967) *J. forens. Sci. Soc.* **7** 198

Lockett, M. F. and Patel, U. G. (1961) *J. Pharm. Pharmac.* **13** 536

Lodi, E. (1964) *Farmaco, Edn prat.* **19** 560

Loge, J. P. (1965) *J. Am. med. Ass.* **193** 110

London, I. and Poet, R. B. (1957) *Proc. Soc. exp. Biol. Med.* **94** 191
Longuet-Higgins, H. C. and Murrell, J. N. (1955) *Proc. phys. Soc.* **68A** 601
Lorenzetti, O. J., Tye, A., and Nelson, J. W. (1966) *J. pharm. Sci.* **55** 105
Loubeyre, M. J. and Farkas (1951) *Algér. méd.* **55** 857
Loughridge, L. W. (1962) *Lancet* **2** 1133
Lous, P. (1954) *Acta pharmac. tox.* **10** 147 and 261
Lovelock, J. E. (1958a) *J. Chromat.* **1** 35
Lovelock, J. E. (1958b) *Nature, Lond.* **182** 1663
Lovelock, J. E. (1961) *Analyt. Chem.* **33** 162
Lovelock, J. E. and Lipsky, S. R. (1960) *J. Am. chem. Soc.* **82** 431
Lowry, O. H., Graham, H. T., Harris, F. B., Priebat, M. K., Marks, A. R., and Bregman, R. U. (1954) *J. Pharmac. exp. Ther.* **112** 116
Lubash, G. D., Phillips, R. E., and Shields, J. D. (1964) *Archs intern. Med.* **114** 530
Lucas, G. H. W. and Korczak-Fabierkiewicz, C. (1964) *J. forens. Sci.* **9** 353
Luckens, M. M. (1966) *J. forens. Sci.* **11** 64
Lukas, D. S. and Peterson, R. E. (1966) *J. clin. Invest.* **45** 782
Lund, A. (1964) *Medicine, Sci. Law* **4** 194
Lundquist, F. and Wolthers, J. (1958) *Acta pharmac. tox.* **14** 265
Lurie, A. O., Villee, C. A., and Reid, D. E. (1966) *J. clin. Endocr. Metab.* **26** 742
Lynch, P. G. (1967) *J. forens. Med.* **14** 118
Lyness, W. I. and Quackenbush, F. W. (1955) *Analyt. Chem.* **27** 1978

McBay, A. J. (1966) *New Engl. J. Med.* **274** 1257
McBay, A. J. (1967)—personal communication
McBay, A. J. and Katsas, G. G. (1957) *New Engl. J. Med.* **257** 97
MacCaig, J. N. and Edmondson, J. S. (1965) *Br. med. J.* **1** 923
McCallum, N. E. W. (1955) *J. Pharm. Pharmac.* **7** 276
McChesney, E. W. and McAuliff, J. P. (1961) *Antibiotics Chemother.* **11** 800
McChesney, E. W., Banks, W. F., McAuliff, J. P. (1962) *Antibiotics Chemother.* **12** 583
McChesney, E. W., Conway, W. D., Banks, W. F., Rogers, J. E., and Shekosky, J. M. (1966) *J. Pharmac. exp. Ther.* **151** 482
McChesney, E. W., Froelich, E. J., Lesher, G. Y., Crain, A. V. R., and Rosi, D. (1964) *Toxic. appl. Pharmac.* **6** 292
McCoubrey, A. (1962) *J. Pharm. Pharmac.* **14** 798
Machata, G. (1961) *Dt. Z. ges. gericht. Med.* **51** 447
McIsaac, W. M. and Kanda, M. (1964) *J. Pharm. exp. Ther.* **143** 7
McLaughlin, J. L., Goyan, J. E., and Paul, A. G. (1964) *J. pharm. Sci.* **53** 306
McNamara, D. G., Brewer, E. J., and Ferry, G. D. (1964) *New Engl. J. Med.* **271** 1106
McWilliam, I. G. and Dewar, R. A. (1958) *Gas Chromatography*, ed. D. H. Desty, London, Butterworths Scientific Publications, p. 142
Maehly, A. C. and Bonnichsen, R. (1966) *Dt. Z. ges. gericht. Med.* **57** 446
Maggs, R. J. and Swan, D. F. K. (1966) *Column* (W. G. Pye Gas Chromatography Bulletin) **1** (3) 2
Magnussen, G. (1947) *Ugeskr. Laeg.* **109** 359 and *Abstr. Wld Med.* 1948 **3** 132
Majumdar, M. K. and Majumdar, S. K. (1967) *Analyt. Chem.* **39** 215
Manning, J. J. (1955) *Bull. Narcot.* **7** 85
Mant, A. K. (1961) *Medicine, Sci. Law* **1** 170
Marcus, F. I., Kapadia, G. J., and Kapadia, G. G. (1964) *J. Pharmac. exp. Ther.* **145** 203
Maren, T. H., Mayer, E., and Wadsworth, B. C. (1954) and Maren, T. H., Ash, V. I., and Bailey, E. M. (1954) *Johns Hopkins Hosp. Bull.* **95** 199 and 244
Marion, L., Ramsay, D. A., and Jones, R. N. (1951) *J. Am. chem. Soc.* **73** (1) 305
Mark, L. C. (1963) *Clin. Pharmac. Ther.* **4** 504
Markham, T. N., Dodson, V. N., and Eckberg, D. L. (1967) *J. Am. med. Ass.* **202** 1102
Markowitz, H. A. and McGinley, J. M. (1964) *J. Am. med. Ass.* **189** 950
Marks, B. H., Dutta, S., Gauthier, J., and Elliott, D. (1964) *J. Pharmac. exp. Ther.* **145** 351
Martin, J. F. and Wright, S. E. (1960) *J. Pharmac. exp. Ther.* **128** 329
Martin, J. L. and Shaw, W. H. C. (1963) *Analyst, Lond.* **88** 292
Martin, R. J. and Alexander, T. G. (1967) *J. Ass. off. analyt. Chem.* **50** 1362
Martin, R. J. and Alexander, T. G. (1968) *J. Ass. off. analyt. Chem.* **51** 159
Mason, M. F., Foerster, E., Patterson, W., and Drummond, W. (1966) *J. forens. Sci.* **11** 243
Mason, M. F., Wallace, S. M., Foerster, E., and Drummond, W. (1965) *J. forens. Sci.* **10** 136
Masuoka, D., Appelgren, L.-E., and Hansson, E. (1967) *Acta pharmac. tox.* **25** 113
Matter, B. J., Donat, P. E., Brill, M. L., and Ginn, H. E. (1965) *Archs intern. Med.* **116** 18
Maunder, M. J. de F., Egan, H., and Roburn, J. (1964a) *Analyst, Lond.* **89** 157
Maunder, M. J. de F., Egan, H., Godly, E. W., Hammond, E. W., Roburn, J., and Thomson, J. (1964b) *Analyst, Lond.* **89** 168
Maynert, E. W. (1952) *J. biol. Chem.* **195** 397
Maynert, E. W. (1965) *J. Pharmac. exp. Ther.* **150** 118
Mellinger, T. J., Mellinger, E. M., and Smith, W. T. (1964) *Am. J. Psychiat.* **120** 1111
Merchant, H. C., Choksi, N. D., and Ramamoorthy, K. (1963) *Indian J. med. Sci.* **17** 857
Mesley, R. J. and Johnson, C. A. (1965) *J. Pharm. Pharmac.* **17** 329
Middleton, G. and Stuckey, R. E. (1953) *Analyst, Lond.* **78** 532

Miller, A. H. and Pedley, E. (1950) *Br. med. J.* **1** 1115
Miller, R. G. J. (1965) *Laboratory Methods in Infrared Spectroscopy*, London, Heyden & Son Ltd
Millhouse, J., Davies, D. M., and Wraith, S. R. (1966) *Lancet* **2** 1251
Milthers, K. (1961) *Acta pharmac. tox.* **18** 199
Milthers, K. (1962) *Acta pharmac. tox.* **19** 235
Mindlin, R. L. (1966) *New Engl. J. Med.* **275** 112
Ministry of Aviation Technical Information and Library Services (1960) *An Index of Published Infrared Spectra*, London, H.M. Stationery Office, Vols 1 and 2
Misra, A. L., Jacoby, H. I., and Woods, L. A. (1961b) *J. Pharmac. exp. Ther.* **132** 311
Misra, A. L., Mule, S. J., and Woods, L. A. (1961a) *Nature, Lond.* **190** 82
Mitchell, L. C. (1956) *J. Ass. off. agric. Chem.* **39** 484 and 985
Mitchell, R. G. (1951) *Lancet* **2** 57
Møller, K. O. (1953) *Bull. Narcot.* **5** (No. 4) 11
Momose, T., Ueda, Y., Yamamoto, K., Masumura, T., and Ohta, K. (1963) *Analyt. Chem.* **35** 1751
Moore, P. A. (1957) *Vet. Rec.* **69** 1079
Morton, R. A. and Stubbs, A. L. (1946) *Analyst, Lond.* **71** 348
Moss, D. G. (1954) *J. clin. Path.* **7** 344
Moss, M. S. (1964)—personal communication
Moss, M. S. (1965) *Symposium on Identification of Drugs and Poisons*, The Pharmaceutical Society of Great Britain, 1965, p. 27
Moss, M. S. and Jackson, J. V. (1961) *J. Pharm. Pharmac.* **13** 361
Moss, M. S. and Kenyon, M. W. (1964) *Analyst, Lond.* **89** 802
Moss, M. S. and Rylance, H. J. (1966) *J. Pharm. Pharmac.* **18** 13
Moss, M. S. and Rylance, H. J. (1967) *J. Endocr.* **37** 129
Moy, T. W. and Wetherell, H. R. (1967) *J. forens. Sci.* **12** 241
Murgu, N. (1964) *Pharmazie* **19** 724

Nagashima, R., Levy, G., and Nelson, E. (1968) *J. pharm. Sci.* **57** 58
Nakamura, G. R. and Ukita, T. (1967) *J. pharm. Sci.* **56** 294
Narrod, S. A., Wilk, A. L., and King, C. T. G. (1965) *J. Pharmac. exp. Ther.* **147** 380
Needleman, P. and Krantz, J. C. (1965) *Biochem. Pharmac.* **14** 1225
Nelson, E., O'Reilly, I., and Chulski, T. (1960) *Clinica. chim. Acta* **5** 774
Neudert, W. and Roepke, H. (1965) *Atlas of Steroid Spectra*, Berlin, Heidelberg, New York, Springer-Verlag
Neve, H. K. (1961) *Acta pharmac. tox.* **17** 404
Nickolls, L. C. (1956) *The Scientific Investigation of Crime*, London, Butterworths, p. 382
Nickolls, L. C. (1960) *Analyst, Lond.* **85** 840
Nickolls, L. C. and Teare, D. (1954) *Br. med. J.* **2** 1384
Nielsen, K., Kaempe, B., and Jensen-Holm, J. (1965) *Acta pharmac. tox.* **22** 224
Nigro, S. A. (1968) *J. Am. med. Ass.* **203** 301
Niyogi, S. K., Cordova, V. F., and Rieders, F. (1965) *Nature, Lond.* **206** 716
Norn, S. (1965) *Acta pharmac. tox.* **22** 115

O'Dea, A. E. and Liss, M. (1953) *New Engl. J. Med.* **249** 566
Oelschlaeger, H., Volke, J., and Kurek, E. (1964) *Arch. Pharm. Chemi* **297** 431
Ogilvie, R. I., Douglas, D. E., Lochead, J. R., Moscovich, M. D., and Kaye, M. (1966) *Can. med. Ass. J.* **95** 954
Olesen, O. V. (1966) *Acta pharmac. tox.* **24** 183
Olesen, O. V. (1967) *Acta pharmac. tox.* **25** 123
Oliver, A. P. (1951) *Analyst, Lond.* **76** 730
Oroszlan, S. I. and Maengwyn-Davies, G. D. (1960) *J. Am. pharm. Ass.* (*Sci. Edn*) **49** 507
Ovechkin, G. V. (1963) *Zh. obshch. Khim.* **33** (6) 1923
Owen, L. N. (1955) *Vet. Rec.* **67** 561

Palframan, J. F. and Walker, E. A. (1967) *Analyst, Lond.* **92** 71
Papworth, D. S. (1965) *J. forens. Sci. Soc.* **5** 66
Parke, D. V., Pollock, S., and Williams, R. T. (1963) *J. Pharm. Pharmac.* **15** 500
Parker, K. D. and Kirk, P. L. (1961) *Analyt. Chem.* **33** 1378
Parker, K. D., Fontan, C. R., and Kirk, P. C. (1963) *Analyt. Chem.* **35** 356
Parker, K. D., Hine, C. H., Nomof, N., and Elliott, H. W. (1966) *J. forens. Sci.* **11** 152
Pechtold, F. (1964) *Arzneimittel-Forsch.* **14** 972
Peets, E. A., Sweeney, W. M., Place, V. A., *et al.* (1965) *Am. Rev. resp. Dis.* **91** 51
Pekkarinen, A. and Pitkänen, M.-E. (1955) *Scand. J. clin. Lab. Invest.* **7** 1
Perlman, P. L., Johnson, C. B., and Kosinski, R. E. (1953a) *J. Am. pharm. Ass.* (*Sci. Edn*) **42** 483
Perlman, P. L., Sutter, D., and Johnson, C. B. (1953b) *J. Am. pharm. Ass.* (*Sci. Edn*) **42** 750
Perry, H. M., Comens, P., and Yunice, A. (1962) *J. Lab. clin. Med.* **59** 456
Pfaff, J. and Forbeck, D. L. (1961) *J. forens. Sci.* **6** 134
Pfeffer, M., Schor, J. M., Gluck, N., Semmel, M. G., and Griboff, S. (1968) *J. pharm. Sci.* **57** 36
Phang, S., Dutt, M. C., Tee, T. S. (1961) *J. Pharm. Pharmac.* **13** 319
Phillips, B. M. and Miya, T. S. (1964) *J. pharm. Sci.* **53** 1098
Picchioni, A. L. (1960) *Am. J. Hosp. Pharm.* **17** 303
Picchioni, A. L. (1965) *Am. J. Hosp. Pharm.* **22** 486
Pleat, G. B., Harley, J. H., and Wiberley, S. E. (1951) *J. Am. pharm. Ass.* (*Sci. Edn*) **40** 107
Pollack, B. (1964) *Am. J. Psychiat.* **121** 189
Pollard, G. E., Saltman, W. M., and Yin, P. (1955) *J. Ass. off. agric. Chem.* **38** 478

Polster, H. (1965) *Arch. Tox.* **20** 271
Pontius, D. J. (1962) *Analyt. Chem.* **34** 168
Poole, J. W. and Gardocki, J. F. (1963) *J. pharm. Sci.* **52** 486
Popham, R. D. and Davies, D. M. (1964) *Br. med. J.* **1** 677
Porter, G. S. and Beresford, J. (1966) *J. Pharm. Pharmac.* **18** 223
Portmann, G. A., McChesney, E. W., Stander, H., and Moore, W. E. (1966) *J. pharm. Sci.* **55** 59
Porush, I., Shimamura, A., and Takahashi, L. T. (1965) *J. pharm. Sci.* **54** 1809
Powell, L. W., Mann, G. T., and Kaye, S. (1958) *New Engl. J. Med.* **259** 716
Prain, J. H. (1950) *Br. med. J.* **1** 1375
Prelog, V. and Jeger, O. (1960) 'Steroid Alkaloids: The Solanum Group', *The Alkaloids*, ed. R. H. F. Manske, New York, London, Academic Press Inc., Vol. VII, p. 343
Price, W. C., Bradley, J. E. S., Fraser, R. D. B., and Quilliam, J. P. (1954) *J. Pharm. Pharmac.* **6** 522
Pulver, R. (1943) *Schweiz. med. Wschr.* **73** 124
Pütter, J. (1964) *Arzneimittel-Forsch.* **14** 1198

Quinby, G. E. (1964) *J. Am. med. Ass.* **187** 202
Quinby, G. E., Hayes, W. J., Armstrong, J. F., and Durham, W. F. (1965) *J. Am. med. Ass.* **191** 175
Qureshi, E. H. (1964) *J. Am. med. Ass.* **188** 470

Radecka, C. and Nigam, I. C. (1966) *J. pharm. Sci.* **55** 861
Raekallio, J., Jääskeläiner, A. J., and Mäkinen, P.-L. (1967) *J. forens. Sci.* **12** 238
Rainsford, S. G. and Davies, T. A. L. (1965) *Br. J. ind. Med.* **22** 21
Rajzman, A. (1960) *Analyst, Lond.* **85** 116
Rajzman, A. (1963) *Analyst, Lond.* **88** 117
Ramsey, L. L. and Clifford, P. A. (1949) *J. Ass. off. agric. Chem.* **32** 788
Randall, L. O., Iliev, V., and Brandman, O. (1956) *Archs int. Pharmacodyn. Thér.* **106** 388
Randall, L. O., Scheckel, C. L., and Banziger, R. F. (1965) *Curr. ther. Res.* **7** 590
Rasmussen, J. (1965) *Lancet* **2** 850
Reid, I. S. (1960) *Papua New Guin. med. J.* **4** 65 and *Trop. Dis. Bull.* 1961 **58** 658
Reizenstein, P. (1967) *Blood* **29** 494
Renault, J., Cartron, J.-C., and Généras, G. (1966) *Annls Biol. clin.* **24** 939
Report by the Malathion Panel (1960), set up jointly by the Scientific Subcommittee of the Interdepartmental Advisory Committee on Poisonous Substances used in Agriculture and Food Storage, the Analytical Methods Committee of the Society for Analytical Chemistry, and the Association of British Manufacturers of Agricultural Chemicals, *Analyst, Lond.* **85** 915
Report by the Prophylactics in Animal Feeds Subcommittee of the Analytical Methods Committee (1964) of the Society for Analytical Chemistry, *Analyst, Lond.* **89** 505
Report by the Prophylactics in Animal Feeds Subcommittee of the Analytical Methods Committee (1966) of the Society for Analytical Chemistry, *Analyst, Lond.* **91** 672
Richardson, M. L. (1967) *Talanta* **14** 385
Rieders, F. and Frere, F. J. (1963) *J. forens. Sci.* **8** 46
Ringrose, C. A. D. (1962) *Can. med. Ass. J.* **87** 712
Rives, H. F., Ward, B. B., and Hicks, M. L. (1949) *J. Am. med. Ass.* **140** 1022
Roberts, G., Jones, R. N., and Gallagher, B. S. (1958) *Infrared Absorption Spectra of Steroids—An Atlas*, London and New York, Interscience Publishers Inc., Vol. 2
Roberts, J. B., Thomas, B. H., Hossain, M. A., and Wilson, A. (1967) *J. Pharm. Pharmac.* **19** 133
Rockley, G. J. (1965) *Br. med. J.* **2** 632
Rogers, A. R. (1966) *J. Soc. cosmet. Chem. Br. Edn* **17** 641
Rogers, E. W. (1958) *Br. med. J.* **2** 1576
Roland, C. B. (1959) *J. Am. med. Ass.* **171** 1806
Root, M. A. and Comer, J. P. (1953) *Fedn Proc. Fedn Am. Socs exp. Biol.* **12** 362
Rosenkrantz, H. (1955) 'Analysis of Steroids by Infrared Spectrometry', *Methods of Biochemical Analysis*, ed. D. Glick, New York, Interscience Publishers Inc., Vol. 2, p. 1
Rosenkrantz, H. (1957) 'The Infrared Analysis of Vitamins, Hormones, and Coenzymes', *Methods of Biochemical Analysis*, ed. D. Glick, New York, Interscience Publishers Inc., Vol. 5, p. 407
Rosenwald, R. J. and Russell, D. H. (1961) *New Engl. J. Med.* **264** 927
Rosin, R. D. (1967) *Br. med. J.* **4** 33
Ross, Hugh M. and Gordon, A. (1964) *Can. med. Ass. J.* **91** 1124
Rowland, M. and Riegelman, S. (1967) *J. pharm. Sci.* **56** 717
Rubenstein, C. J. (1964) *J. Am. med. Ass.* **187** 647
Ruskin, D. B. (1948) *J. Am. med. Ass.* **137** 1031
Ruzicka, J., Thomson, J., and Wheals, B. B. (1967) *J. Chromat.* **30** 92
Rylander, G. (1966) *Läkartidningen* **63** 4973 and *Int. pharm. Abstr.* 1967 **4** 341

Sadtler Standard Infrared Spectra, *Sadtler Infrared Spectra of Commercial Products*, Philadelphia, Sadtler Research Laboratories, Inc.
Sakaguchi, T. and Taguchi, K. (1955) *Pharm. Bull., Tokyo* **3** 303
Sakurai, Y. and Ito, K. (1960) *Chem. pharm. Bull., Tokyo* **8** 655
Saltzman, A. (1950) *J. Lab. clin. Med* **35** 123
Sammul, O. R., Brannon, W. L., and Hayden, A. L. (1964) *J. Ass. off. agric. Chem.* **47** 918
Sandberg, A. A. and Slaunwhite, W. R. (1965) *J. clin. Invest.* **44** 694

Sanderson, J. H., Cowdell, R. H., and Higgins, G. (1966) *Lancet* **2** 803

Sandler, S. and Strom, R. (1960) *Analyt. Chem.* **32** 1890

Sawyer, R., Cox, B. G., Dixon, E. J., and Thomson, J. (1967) *J. Sci. Fd Agric.* **18** 287

Scapini, G. and Gardini, G. P. (1964) *Ateneo parmense* **35** 328

Schach von Wittenau, M. and Delahunt, C. S. (1966) *J. Pharmac. exp. Ther.* **152** 164

Schatz, F. and Jahn, U. (1966) *Arzneimittel-Forsch.* **16** 866

Schoenheimer, R. and Sperry, W. M. (1934) *J. biol. Chem.* **106** 745

Schreiber, E. C., Min, B. H., Zeiger, A. V., and Lang, J. F. (1968) *J. Pharmac. exp. Ther.* **159** 372

Schuldiner, J. A. (1949) *Analyt. Chem.* **21** 298

Schultz, J. C., Adamson, J. S., Workman, W. W., and Norman, T. D. (1963) *New Engl. J. Med.* **269** 999

Schulz, E. P. and Szalkowski, C. R. (1961) *Analyt. Chem.* **33** 795

Schumacher, H., Smith, R. L., Stagg, R. B. L., and Williams, R. T. (1964) *Pharm. Acta Helv.* **39** 394

Schüppel, R. and Soehring, K. (1965) *Pharm. Acta Helv.* **40** 105

Schwär, T. G. (1965) *J. forens. Med.* **12** 142

Schwartz, M. A. and Postma, E. (1966) *J. pharm. Sci.*, **55** 1358

Schwartz, M. A., Koechlin, B. A., Postma, E., Palmer, S., and Krol, G. (1965) *J. Pharmac. exp. Ther.* **149** 423

Scott, C. A., Nowell, P. T., and Wilson, A. (1962) *J. Pharm. Pharmac.* **14** 31T

Scott, J. L., Finegold, S. M., Belkin, G. A., and Lawrence, J. S. (1965) *New Engl. J. Med.* **272** 1137

Sekules, G. and Guadagnini, G. (1964) *Boll. chim.-farm.* **103** 432 and *Int. pharm. Abstr.* 1965 **2** 288

Shaffer, A. (1953) *Bull. Narcot.* **5** 35

Shanahan, R. (1967)—personal communication

Sheppard, H., D'Asaro, B. S., and Plummer, A. J. (1956) *J. Am. pharm. Ass.* (*Sci. Edn*) **45** 681

Sheppard, H., Mowles, T. F., and Plummer, A. J. (1960) *J. Am. pharm. Ass.* (*Sci. Edn*) **49** 722

Shimanouchi, T., Tsuboi, M., and Kyogoku, Y. (1964) 'Infrared Spectra of Nucleic Acids and Related Compounds', *Advances in Chemical Physics*, ed. J. Duchesne, London, Interscience Publishers Inc., Vol. 7, p. 435

Shimkin, P. M. and Shaivitz, S. A. (1966) *J. Am. med. Ass.* **196** 662

Shin, Y. S. and Lee, J. C. (1961) *Analyt. Chem.* **33** 1220

Shulgin, A. T., Bunnell, S., and Sargent, T. (1961) *Nature, Lond.* **189** 1011

Siang, S. C. (1960) *Br. med. J.* **1** 1412

Silvestrov, V. P., Malor, Y. S., and Feofilova, V. G. (1963) *Lab. Delo.* No. 5, 16

Siminoff, R. and Saunders, P. R. (1958) *J. Pharmac. exp. Ther.* **124** 252

Simmons, J. H. and Tattan, J. O'G. (1966) *Clin. Chem.* **12** 697

Skerrett, E. J. and Baker, E. A. (1960) *Analyst, Lond.* **85** 606

Skinner, R. F. (1967) *J. forens. Sci.* **12** 230

Smith, E. L., Martin, J. L., Gregory, R. J., and Shaw, W. H. C. (1962) *Analyst, Lond.* **87** 183

Smith, G. M., Parson, M. E., and Whitehouse, M. W. (1964) *J. Pharm. Pharmac.* **16** 830

Smith, L. L. and Foell, T. (1962) *J. Chromat.* **9** 339

Smith, J. N., Smithies, R. H., and Williams, R. T. (1953) *Biochem. J.* **54** 225

Smythies, J. R., Johnston, V. S., Bradley, R. J., Benington, F., Morin, R. D., and Clark, L. C. (1967) *Nature, Lond.* **216** 128

Snavely, M. K. and Grasselli, J. G. (1964) 'The Use of Thin-Layer Chromatography with Infrared Spectroscopy', *Developments in Applied Spectroscopy*, ed. J. E. Forette and E. Lauterman, New York, Plenum Press, Vol. 3, p. 119

Snyder, F. H., Klahm, G. R., and Werner, H. W. (1948) *J. Am. pharm. Ass.* (*Sci. Edn*) **37** 420

Snyder, S. H., Faillace, L., and Hollister, L. (1967) *Science, Wash.* **158** 669

Solursh, L. P. and Clement, W. R. (1968) *Can. med. Ass. J.* **98** 407

Soudijn, W., Van Wijngaarden, I., and Allewijn, F. (1967) *Eur. J. Pharmac.* **1** 47

Sparagana, M., Mason, W. B., and Keutmann, E. H. (1962) *Analyt. Chem.* **34** 1157

Spedding, H. (1964) 'Infrared Spectroscopy and Carbohydrate Chemistry', *Advances in Carbohydrate Chemistry*, ed. M. L. Wolfrom, London and New York, Academic Press Inc., Vol. 19, p. 23

Spencer, R. D. and Beggs, B. H. (1966) *J. Chromat.* **21** 52

Spinelli, P. and Ciuffi, M. (1966) *Boll. chim.-farm.* **105** 849

Stainier, C., Bosly, J., Dutrieux, Fr., and Stainier, R. (1963) *Pharm. Acta Helv.* **38** 587

Staub, H. (1950) *Archs Neurol. Psychiat.* **65** 330

Steel, M. and Johnstone, J. M. (1959) *Br. med. J.* **2** 118

Steentoft, A. (1967)—personal communication

Steer, C. (1951) *Lancet* **1** 1419

Stevens, H. M. (1965) *Medicine, Sci. Law* **5** 157

Stevens, H. M. (1967) *J. forens. Sci. Soc.* **7** 184

Stevenson, G. W. (1960) *Analyt. Chem.* **32** 1522

Stevenson, G. W. (1961) *Analyt. Chem.* **33** 1374

Stewart, G. T., Coles, H. M. T., Nixon, H. H., and Holt, R. J. (1961a) *Br. med. J.* **2** 200

Stewart, R. D. and Andrews, J. T. (1966) *J. Am. med. Ass.* **195** 904

Stewart, R. D. and Dodd, H. C. (1964) *Am. ind. Hyg. Ass. J.* **25** 439

Stewart, R. D. and Erley, D. S. (1965) 'Detection of Volatile Organic Compounds and Toxic Gases in Humans by Rapid Infrared Techniques', *Progress in Chemical Toxicology*, ed. A. Stolman, London and New York, Academic Press Inc., Vol. 2, p. 183

Stewart, R. D., Boettner, E. A., and Stubbs, B. T. (1961b) *Nature, Lond.* **191** 1008
Stewart, R. D., Dodd, H. C., Erley, D. S., and Holder, B. B. (1965) *J. Am. med. Ass.* **193** 1097
Stewart, R. D., Gay, H. H., Erley, D. S., Hake, C. L., and Peterson, J. E. (1961c) *J. occup. Med.* **3** 586
Stewart, R. D., Torkelson, T. R., Hake, C. L., and Erley, D. S. (1960) *J. Lab. clin. Med.* **56** 148
Stinnett, J. L., Valentine, J., and Abrutyn, E. (1968) *J. Am. med. Ass.* **204** 69
Street, H. V. (1960) *Clinica chim. Acta* **5** 938
Street, H. V. (1962) *J. forens. Sci.* **7** 222
Stubbs, B. J., Stewart, R. D., and Boettner, E. A. (1962) *J. Lab. clin. Med.* **59** 667
Stur, O. and Zweymüller, E. (1961) *Dt. med. Wschr.* **86** 1474
Sunshine, I. and Bäumler, J. (1963) *Nature, Lond.* **199** 1103
Sunshine, I. and Fike, W. W. (1964) *New Engl. J. Med.* **271** 487
Sunshine, I. and Gerber, S. R. (1963) *Spectrophotometric Analysis of Drugs including Atlas of Spectra*, Springfield, Ill., Charles C. Thomas
Svendsen, A. B. and Brochmann-Hanssen, E. (1962) *J. pharm. Sci.* **51** 494
Swissman, N. and Jacoby, J. (1964) *Clin. Pharmac. Ther.* **5** 136
Szász, G., Szászné-Zacskó, M., and Polánkay, V. (1965) *Acta pharm. hung.* **35** 207
Szymanski, H. A. (1963) *Infrared Band Handbook*, New York, Plenum Press

Tabor, C. W., Freeman, M. V., Baily, J., and Smith, P. K. (1951) *J. Pharmac. exp. Ther.* **102** 98
Takemori, A. E. and Mannering, G. J. (1958) *J. Pharmac. exp. Ther.* **123** 171
Taniguchi, K., Kakimoto, Y., and Armstrong, M. D. (1964) *J. Lab. clin. Med.* **64** 469
Taylor, A., Rea, R. E., and Kirby, D. R. (1964) *Analyst, Lond.* **89** 497
Taylor, J. D. and Krause, R. A. (1962) *Fedn Proc. Fedn Am. Socs exp. Biol.* **21** 181
Taylor, J. J. (1965) *J. forens. Sci. Soc.* **5** 188
Terplan, M. and Unger, A. M. (1966) *J. Am. med. Ass.* **198** 322
Thomas, R. (1960) *Analyst, Lond.* **85** 551
Thompson, G. W. (1964) *Jl R. Army med. Cps* **110** 113
Thomson, G. W. (1956) *Circulation* **14** 757 and *J. Am. med. Ass.* (1957) **163** 324
Tichner, J. B. and Enselberg, C. D. (1951) *New Engl. J. Med.* **245** 723
Tiess, D. (1966a and b)—personal communication
Tobias, M. (1949) *Br. med. J.* **1** 1098
Tocco, D. J., Egerton, J. R., Bowers, W., Christensen, V. W., and Rosenblum, C. (1965) *J. Pharmac. exp. Ther.* **149** 263
Tompsett, S. L. (1958) *Clinica. Chim. Acta* **3** 149
Tompsett, S. L. (1962) *Acta pharmac. tox.* **19** 365
Tompsett, S. L. (1964) *Acta pharmac. tox.* **21** 20
Tompsett, S. L. (1966)—personal communication
Tompsett, S. L. (1967a) *Analyst, Lond.* **92** 534
Tompsett, S. L. (1967b)—personal communication
Tompsett, S. L. (1967c)—personal communication
Tompsett, S. L., Forshall, W., and Smith, D. C. (1961) *Acta pharmac. tox.* **18** 75
Trinder, P. (1954) *Biochem. J.* **57** 301
Turner, L. K. (1963) *J. forens. Sci. Soc.* **4** 39
Turner, L. K. (1964a)—personal communication
Turner, L. K. (1964b) *J. forens. Med.* **11** 24
Turner, L. K. (1965) 'Searching for Drug Metabolites in Viscera', *Methods of Forensic Science*, ed. A. S. Curry, London and New York, Interscience Publishers Inc., Vol. 4, p. 177
Turner, L. K. (1966)—personal communication
Turner, P., Young, J. H., and Scowen, E. F. (1966) *J. Pharm. Pharmac.* **18** 550

Umberger, C. J. (1954) 'Inorganic and Organic Poisons Volatile with Steam', *Legal Medicine, Pathology and Toxicology*, 2nd Edn, New York, Appleton-Century-Crofts Inc., p. 1064
Umberger, C. J. and Adams, G. (1952) *Analyt. Chem.* **24** 1309
Urbanyi, T., Sloniewsky, D., and Tishler, S. (1966) *J. pharm. Sci.* **55** 730

Vadodaria, D. J., Desai, B. R., and Mukherji, S. P. (1965) *Indian J. Pharm.* **27** 257
Valaes, T., Doxiadis, S. A., and Fessas, P. (1963) *J. Pediat.* **63** 904
Vallance, W. B. (1955) *Lancet* **2** 850
Valôv, P. (1946) *Ind. Engng Chem. analyt. Edn* **18** 456
Van Der Molen, H. J. and Groen, D. (1965) *J. clin. Endocr. Metab.* **25** 1625
Večerková, J., Kakáč, B., Večerek, B., and Ledvina, M. (1967) *Die Pharmazie* **22** 30
Vedsø, S. (1961) *Acta pharmac. tox.* **18** 119 and 157
Venkataraman, P., Eidus, L., and Tripathy, S. P. (1968) *Tubercle, Lond.* **49** 210
Vercruysse, A. and Deslypere, P. (1964) *J. forens. Med.* **11** 107
Vest, M. (1966) *Schweiz. med. Wschr.* **96** 920
Vickers, C. (1966) *J. Pharm. Pharmac.* **18** *Supp.* 17S
Vidic, E. (1957) *Arzneimittel-Forsch.* **7** 314
Villandy, J. (1967)—personal communication
Vlahakis, E. (1964) *Med. J. Aust.* **2** 506
Von Wittenau, M. S. and Delahunt, C. S. (1966) *J. Pharmac. exp. Ther.* **152** 164

Waarst, V. (1964) *Arch. Pharm. Chemi* **71** 116

Wacker, W. E. C., Haynes, H., Druyan, R., Fisher, W., and Coleman, J. E. (1965) *J. Am. med. Ass.* **194** 1231
Waddell, W. J. (1963) *Fedn Proc. Fedn Am. Socs exp. Biol.* **22** 480
Wagner, J., Kraus, P., and Večerek, B. (1955) *Čslká Farm.* **4** 389
Walaszek, E. J., Kocsis, J. J., Leroy, G. V., and Geiling, E. M. (1960) *Arch. int. Pharmacodyn.* **125** 371
Walkenstein, S. S., MacMullen, J. A., Knebel, C., and Seifter, J. (1958) *J. Am. pharm. Ass.* (*Sci. Edn*) **47** 20
Walkenstein, S. S., Wiser, R., Gudmundson, C. H., Kimmel, H. B., and Corradino, R. A. (1964) *J. pharm. Sci.* **53** 1181
Walker, G. W. (1964)—personal communication
Walkley, J. E., Pagnotto, L. D., and Elkins, H. B. (1961) *Am. ind. Hyg. Ass. J.* **22** 362
Wallace, H. E., Neumayer, F., and Gutch, C. F. (1964a) *Am. J. Dis. Child.* **108** 657
Wallace, J. E. (1966) *J. forens. Sci.* **11** 552
Wallace, J. E. (1967) *J. pharm. Sci.* **56** 1437
Wallace, J. E. and Dahl, E. V. (1967) *J. forens. Sci.* **12** 484
Wallace, J. E., Biggs, J. D., and Dahl, E. V. (1965) *J. forens. Sci.* **10** 179
Wallace, J. E., Wilson, W. J., and Dahl, E. V. (1964b) *J. forens. Sci.* **9** 342
Walls, H. J. (1958) *J. forens. Med.* **5** 27
Wanntorp, H. (1960) *Acta pharmac. tox.* **16** *Supp.* 2
Warembourg, H., Voisin, C., Le Dantec, G., Corsin, L., and Cauvin, P. (1964) *Lille méd.* **9** 192
Warren, R. J., Thompson, W. E., Zarembo, J. E., and Eisdorfer, I. B. (1967) *J. pharm. Sci.* **56** 1496
Way, E. L. and Adler, T. K. (1962) '*The Biological Disposition of Morphine and its Surrogates*', Geneva, World Health Organisation, p. 66
Way, E. L., Kemp, J. W., Young, J. M., and Grassetti, D. R. (1960) *J. Pharmac. exp. Ther.* **129** 144
Way, E. L., Peng, C.-T., Allawala, N., and Daniels, T. C. (1955) *J. Am. pharm. Ass.* (*Sci. Edn*) **44** 65
Wear, J. B., Shanahan, R., and Ratliff, R. K. (1962) *J. Am. med. Ass.* **181** 587
Welch, R. M. and Connery, A. H. (1965) *Clin. Chem.* **11** 1064
Weller, R. W. and Metcalfe, J. (1949) *New Engl. J. Med.* **241** 17
Welles, J. S., McMahon, R. E., and Doran, W. J. (1963) *J. Pharmac. exp. Ther.* **139** 166
Westervelt, F. B. (1966) *Ann. intern. Med.* **64** 1229
White, A. G., Beckett, A. H., and Brookes, L. G. (1967) *Br. med. J.* **1** 740
White, L. L. R. (1962) *Br. med. J.* **1** 691
Wick, A. N., Stewart, C. J., and Serif, G. S. (1960) *Diabetes*, **9** 163
Williams, A. F., Murray, W. J., and Gibbs, B. H. (1966) *Nature, Lond.* **210** 816
Williams, L. A., Linn, M. S., and Zak, B. (1961) *J. forens. Sci.* **6** 119
Willimott, S. G. (1933) *Analyst, Lond.* **58** 431
Willner, K. (1963) *Arzneimittel-Forsch.* **13** 26
Wilson, D. (1965)—personal communication
Wilson, G. S. (1959) *Mon. Bull. Minist. Hlth* **18** 207
Wilson, T. and Edeson, J. F. B. (1954) *Med. J. Malaya* **9** 115
Wilson, W. J. (1966)—personal communication
Winek, C. L., Wellon, D. C., and Wecht, C. H. (1967) *Lancet* **1** 683
Wood, R. (1960) *Analyst, Lond.* **85** 21
Woods, L. A. (1956) *Fedn Proc. Fedn Am. Socs exp. Biol.* **15** 502
Woods, L. A., Cochin, J., Fornefeld, E. J., McMahon, F. G., and Seevers, M. H. (1951) *J. Pharmac. exp. Ther.* **101** 188
Woods, L. A., Muehlenbeck, H. E., and Mellett, L. B. (1956) *J. Pharmac. exp. Ther.* **117** 117
Woodward, D. J. and Solomon, J. D. (1956) *J. Am. med. Ass.* **162** 1308
Wright, J. T. and Johns, R. G. S. (1953) *J. clin. Path.* **6** 78
Wright, L. T. and Rothman, M. (1951) *J. Am. med. Ass.* **145** 844
Wright, S. E. (1962) *J. Pharm. Pharmac.* **14** 613
Wullen, H. and Stainier, E. (1967) *J. Pharm. Belg.* **22** 291

Xanthaky, G., Freireich, A. W., Matusiak, W., and Lukash, L. (1966) *J. Am. med. Ass.* **198** 1212

Yates, C. M., Todrick, A., and Tait, A. C. (1963) *J. Pharm. Pharmac.* **15** 432
Yatzidis, H., Oreopoulos, D., Triantaphyllidis, D., Voudiclari, S., Tsaparas, N., Gavras, C., and Stavroulaki, A. (1965) *Lancet* **2** 216
Youberg, D. R. (1960) *New Engl. J. Med.* **263** 1130
Young, J. P. W. (1967) *Br. med. J.* **1** 301

Zaar, B. and Grönwall, A. (1961) *Scand. J. clin. Lab. Invest.* **13** 588
Zalis, E. and Parmley, L. F. (1963) *Archs intern. Med.* **112** 822
Zeigler, D. W. and McGuire, J. M. (1953) *Antibiotics Chemother.* **3** 67
Zicha, V. L., Weist, F., Schmid, E., and Schmid, S. (1964) *Arzneimittel-Forsch.* **14** 699
Zuckerman, A. J. and Chazan, A. A. (1958) *Br. med. J.* **2** 1338
Zwikker, J. J. L. and Steenhauer, A. J. (1942) *Pharm. Weekbl. Ned.* **79** 241

General Index

General Index

C

D

F

G

M

O

P

S

T

U

V

W

X

Y

Z